SEDATION

A GUIDE TO PATIENT MANAGEMENT

SIXTH EDITION

Stanley F. Malamed, DDS

Emeritus Professor of Anesthesia and Medicine
School of Dentistry
University of Southern California
Los Angeles, California

ELSEVIER

ELSEVIER

3251 Riverport Lane
St. Louis, Missouri 63043

Notices

Knowledge and best practice in this field are constantly changing. As new research and experience broaden our understanding, changes in research methods, professional practices, or medical treatment may become necessary.

Practitioners and researchers must always rely on their own experience and knowledge in evaluating and using any information, methods, compounds, or experiments described herein. In using such information or methods they should be mindful of their own safety and the safety of others, including parties for whom they have a professional responsibility.

With respect to any drug or pharmaceutical products identified, readers are advised to check the most current information provided (i) on procedures featured or (ii) by the manufacturer of each product to be administered, to verify the recommended dose or formula, the method and duration of administration, and contraindications. It is the responsibility of practitioners, relying on their own experience and knowledge of their patients, to make diagnoses, to determine dosages and the best treatment for each individual patient, and to take all appropriate safety precautions.

To the fullest extent of the law, neither the Publisher nor the authors, contributors, or editors, assume any liability for any injury and/or damage to persons or property as a matter of products liability, negligence or otherwise, or from any use or operation of any methods, products, instructions, or ideas contained in the material herein.

Library of Congress Cataloging-in-Publication Data

Names: Malamed, Stanley F., 1944- author.
Title: Sedation : a guide to patient management / Stanley F. Malamed.
Description: Sixth edition. | St. Louis, Missouri : Elsevier, [2018] | Includes bibliographical references and index.
Identifiers: LCCN 2017008725 | ISBN 9780323400534 (pbk. : alk. paper)
Subjects: | MESH: Anesthesia, Dental–methods | Conscious Sedation–methods | Pain–prevention & control | Dental Anxiety–prevention & control
Classification: LCC RK512.S44 | NLM WO 460 | DDC 615/.782–dc23 LC record available at https://lccn.loc.gov/2017008725

Previous editions copyrighted 2010, 2003, 1995, 1989, 1985

Senior Content Strategist: Jennifer Flynn-Briggs
Senior Content Development Manager: Laurie Gower
Publishing Services Manager: Jeff Patterson
Book Production Specialist: Carol O'Connell
Design Direction: Ryan Cook

Printed in India

Last digit is the print number: 9 8 7 6 5 4

Dedication

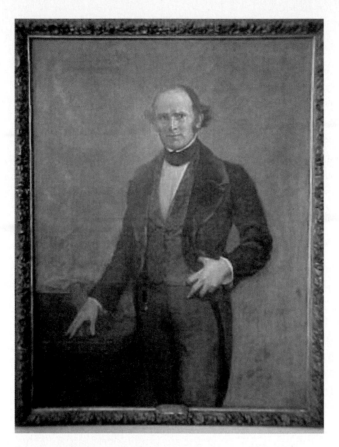

Horace Wells (1815–1848) (Courtesy the Horace Wells Museum, Hartford, Conn.)

To Francis Foldes, MD, for having instilled in me an everlasting fascination in the art and science of anesthesiology; to Norman Trieger, DMD, MD, and Thomas Pallasch, DDS, MS, for having made possible a career that has provided me with continued challenge, interest, and enjoyment, one that I would change for no other; and to Horace Wells, DDS, who 173 years ago discovered anesthesia.

And . . . to my wife Beverly; children Heather, Jennifer, and Jeremy; and our wonderful grandchildren Matthew, Rachel, Gabriella, Ashley, Rebecca, Elijah, and Ethan . . . who make it all worthwhile.

Contributors

DANIEL L. ORR II, BS, DDS, MS (ANESTHESIOLOGY), PHD, JD, MD

Professor and Director
Oral and Maxillofacial Surgery and Anesthesiology
School of Dental Medicine
University of Nevada Las Vegas
Las Vegas, Nevada;
Clinical Professor
Oral and Maxillofacial Surgery and Anesthesiology for Dentistry
School of Medicine
University of Nevada Las Vegas
Las Vegas, Nevada

JASON W. BRADY, DMD*

Attending Dentist Anesthesiologist
Dental Anesthesiology
NYU Lutheran Medical Center
New York, New York;
Adjunct Faculty
Department of Endodontics, Oral and Maxillofacial Surgery, and Orthodontics
Ostrow School of Dentistry
University of Southern California
Los Angeles, California

*Dr. Jason Brady, DMD, a dentist anesthesiologist, updated the chapters on monitoring during sedation and anesthesia (Chapter 5) and Chapters 30 and 31 in Section VI on general anesthesia. Dr. Brady represents, to me, the future of anesthesiology in dentistry and is a welcome addition to this textbook.

Preface

Hartford, Connecticut, December 10, 1844 . . . More than 170 years ago Samuel Cooley, a clerk in a retail store, ran around a stage in an intoxicated state, little realizing the major role he was playing in forever altering the degree of pain and suffering that patients throughout the world would experience during surgery. Cooley had come to attend a popular science lecture in which advances in science were demonstrated. One demonstration was of the intoxicating effects of "laughing gas," which Cooley volunteered to inhale. Also in attendance that fateful evening was Horace Wells, a local dentist who, on seeing Cooley injure his leg but continue to run about as though nothing had happened, considered there might be a clinical application for this "laughing gas." On the following day, December 11, 1844, nitrous oxide ("laughing gas") was administered to Dr. Horace Wells, rendering him unconscious and able to have a wisdom tooth extracted without any awareness of pain.

The world had forever been changed. But had it?

"In 1845 the New York Daily Tribune published a detailed account of an amputation. The operation took place at New York Hospital, a five-acre nest of low brick buildings, located on what is now Lower Broadway. The patient was a young man, cradled tenderly the whole time by his father and at the same time held firmly—and brusquely—in place by the attendants. As the surgeons—there were two—made their cuts, the boy's screams were so full of misery that everyone who could left the room. The first part of the operation complete, the young man watched 'with glazed agony' as the chief surgeon pushed a saw past the sliced muscles, still twitching, and listened as the blade cut through the bone in three heavy passes, back and forth. That was the only noise in the room, for the boy had stopped screaming."[1]

One hundred and seventy years after the discovery of anesthesia so much is taken for granted. Local anesthetics are administered to patients when a surgical procedure might be ever so slightly painful. Yet in 1844 these drugs did not exist. When patients require treatment, a variety of techniques are available to help manage their fears—intravenous sedation; intramuscular sedation; oral, rectal, transmucosal, and intranasal sedation; and general anesthesia. These routes and techniques of drug administration were not available in 1844.

No longer does a patient about to undergo dental or surgical procedures face that prospect with utter hopelessness and despair. Dentistry has long recognized that many persons are frightened of the dental experience and, to its credit, has taken steps to prepare the dental profession to recognize and manage these patients. In its approach to the management of pain and anxiety, the dental profession has remained in the forefront of all the health care professions.

Publication of the Guidelines for the Teaching of Pain and Anxiety Control and the Management of Related Complications (ADA, 1979) put forth a cohesive document aimed at providing well-constructed standards for teaching the future generations of dental students and dentists safe and effective techniques of managing pain and anxiety. A dentist graduating from a dental school in the United States in the past 40 years has received training (albeit to varying degrees of clinical proficiency) in these important areas. For phobic patients seeking dentists able to manage their dental fears, the search is usually short. More and more dentists promote their ability and desire to "cater to cowards." The public has been the ultimate beneficiary of that chance encounter between Mr. Samuel Cooley and Dr. Horace Wells in December 1844.

This sixth edition of *Sedation: A Guide to Patient Management* is, as were its predecessors, designed for the student of medicine or dentistry on a doctoral, postdoctoral, or continuing dental education level. It is meant to be comprehensive, providing basic concepts needed to fully understand the drugs and techniques and how they work, step-by-step descriptions of the various techniques, and a look at the potential complications and emergencies that might arise. More than anything else, this edition of *Sedation* is designed to be used in conjunction with a course in sedation that provides for the clinical management of patients in a controlled (supervised) environment. Only through this type of program can the techniques described in this book be used safely and effectively in a dental or medical practice.

Changes have occurred in several areas in this edition. In addition to general text and photographic updates of all chapters, Chapter 5, Monitoring During Sedation, and Section VI, General Anesthesia (Chapters 30 and 31), have been extensively rewritten so as to address the realities of contemporary drug use in the dental profession. I have invited Jason W. Brady, DMD, a dentist anesthesiologist, to reorganize these three chapters.

As with previous editions of *Sedation,* the ultimate aim of this book remains the same: to help dental patients, to enable them to receive the quality of care they truly deserve, and to enable them to receive this care in an atmosphere of relaxation, mental ease, and safety.

How times have changed in 173 years!

—*Stanley F. Malamed*

REFERENCE

1. Fenster JM: *Ether day: the strange tale of America's greatest medical discovery and the haunted men who made it*, New York, 2001, HarperCollins.

About This Book

This book is divided into eight sections. Section I is introductory, presenting an outline of the "problem" that all members of the dental profession face: the problem of fear and anxiety that confronts dentists throughout the world on a daily basis.

Section II introduces the concept of sedation and the spectrum of pain and anxiety control. The dental and medical professions have at their disposal an array of techniques that may be used in patient management. The availability of these to the dentist will increase the likelihood of a successful treatment outcome. Also included in Section II are chapters on preoperative physical evaluation of the patient and monitoring of the patient during the various sedative procedures. I have invited Dr. Jason Brady, a dentist anesthesiologist, to update the chapter on monitoring. Section II ends with an introduction to two nondrug techniques of sedation: iatrosedation and hypnosis. These techniques are extremely valuable in the management of virtually all patients.

Sections III, IV, and V present an in-depth look at the subject of pharmacosedation. Section III presents discussions of several techniques of sedation, including oral, rectal, and intramuscular. Considerable attention is devoted to the clinical pharmacology of the drugs discussed in an attempt to discourage the use of drugs that might be deemed inappropriate for certain procedures and to encourage the use of others that have proved to be safe and effective. Several drug categories (including barbiturates) have been deemphasized in this sixth edition, reflecting changes in drug utilization in the area of sedation. At the same time, other categories, such as benzodiazepines, have become more prominent, reflecting their increasing usage in sedation in both medicine and dentistry.

Sections IV and V are each devoted to one technique: Section IV to inhalation sedation and Section V to intravenous sedation. Because I believe that these are the two most effective and, when used properly, the safest of all sedative procedures, I have presented a complete and up-to-date discussion of these valuable techniques. It cannot be overemphasized that in the absence of considerable supervised clinical experience, the reading of these sections does *not* constitute preparation adequate to permit anyone to safely use these techniques of drug administration.

Section VI provides an introduction to general anesthesia, another important method of pain and anxiety control. Training in this area requires a considerably greater length of time: a minimum of 3 years of full-time training. Dr. Brady has extensively updated these chapters.

Section VII addresses the subject of emergencies in the dental office. Preparation for and management of emergencies are reviewed in this section. The most important aspect of training for emergencies—prevention—has been the subject of all of the chapters that precede this section. Although it may appear to some that the subject of emergencies and complications takes up an inappropriately large part of this book, it is my belief that this subject can never be discussed too often or too thoroughly. When the techniques discussed in this book are used properly, the number of emergencies and complications that occur are minimal. Although the absence of complications is our goal, success at achieving this goal does have inherent risks: the doctor may become complacent with a technique that works "all the time" and therefore become a little less vigilant. It is at times like this that problems do occur. If the doctor is aware of the possible complications associated with a procedure, then these may be recognized and managed more effectively if and when they do develop.

Finally, Section VIII discusses four groups of "special" patients. Management of the pediatric, geriatric, medically compromised, and disabled patient requires a degree of knowledge and training on the part of the doctor and dental staff beyond that needed for the typical patient. These four groups of patients are not uncommon in the dental office and, unfortunately, present all too many doctors with significant problems during management. It is paramount that the doctor be aware of the subtle changes in treatment protocol that may be required during treatment of these patients. A doctor knowledgeable in the management of these groups will have available a greatly expanded pool of potential patients.

Dan Orr II, BS, DDS, MS (Anesthesiology), PhD, JD, MD, has updated the chapter on legal considerations in sedation and general anesthesia. Dr. Orr is a practicing oral and maxillofacial surgeon who also has an extensive background in dentistry, medicine, and anesthesia (in all aspects of its definition) as well as the legal system. This chapter should be required reading, and the sage advice therein heeded by all who practice the art and science of sedation and general anesthesia.

Acknowledgments

Many people have been involved in the development of this sixth edition of *Sedation: A Guide to Patient Management.*

Through the first five editions of *Sedation* (which was initially published in 1985), the figures were in black and white. The fifth edition replaced them with color photographs, greatly enhancing the visual aspects of the textbook.

Many of the visuals for the product shots were provided by Rose Dodson of Sedation Resource to whom I am deeply indebted.

I wish to thank Drs. Jason W. Brady and Dan Orr II for continuing to make valuable contributions to this textbook.

As always, thanks must be proffered to those friendly folks at Elsevier: Brian Loehr, Senior Content Developmental Specialist; Jolynn Gower, Content Development Manager; Laurie Gower, Senior Content Development Manager; and Carol O'Connell, Book Production Specialist, for doggedly keeping after me to keep those printed pages coming!

—*Stanley F. Malamed*
West Hills, California
February 2017

Note: The treatment modalities and the indications and dosages of all drugs in Sedation: A Guide to Patient Management *have been recommended in the medical literature. Unless specifically indicated, drug dosages are those recommended for adult patients. The package insert for each drug should be consulted for use and dosages as approved by the U.S. Food and Drug Administration. Because standards of usage change, it is advisable to keep abreast of revised recommendations, particularly those concerning new drugs.*

Sedation in Dentistry

A Historic Perspective

The words *fear, anxiety,* and *pain* have long been associated with dentistry. Throughout the years the general public has thought, and been taught, that dentistry hurts. The public's image of the dentist has borne this out. Surveys have consistently shown that although dentistry as a profession is highly respected by the public,[1] the image of the dentist as one who enjoys hurting people is still retained by a majority of persons. In a survey of the most common fears of adults, fear of going to the dentist ranked second only to the fear of public speaking (Table 1).[2]

Is this image of the dentist justified? Of course not; indeed, it never truly was. Unfortunately, however, our predecessors in dentistry did not have at their disposal the vast array of equipment and drugs for the management of pain and anxiety that are available today. History has recorded that members of the dental profession have consistently been in the forefront in the research and development of new techniques and medications for the management of pain and anxiety. Horace Wells (a dentist) and William T. G. Morton (dentist and physician), in the 1840s, were the founders of anesthesia and the first to use nitrous oxide (N_2O) (Wells) and ether (Morton) for the management of pain during surgical procedures.[3] Before this time, dental care consisted to a great degree of the removal of root tips without any form of anesthetic, except for alcohol, which was frequently used preoperatively (and perhaps still is).[4] Surgery before the introduction of anesthesia consisted almost exclusively of the amputation of limbs that had become infected and gangrenous.[3] As in dentistry, these procedures were of necessity performed without the aid of any form of anesthesia except for laudanum, a drink of opium and alcohol.

In the area of intravenous (IV) medications and outpatient general anesthesia, the dental profession again led the way. With the introduction of IV barbiturates in the late 1930s, Victor Goldman and Stanley Drummond-Jackson in England and Adrian Hubbell in the United States pioneered techniques of IV general anesthesia for ambulatory oral surgery patients.[5,6] It was not until the 1970s that the medical profession, realizing the merits of short-stay surgery, began to use these same techniques.[7]

Dentistry has indeed been at the forefront in the fight against pain. Today virtually all dental procedures may be successfully completed in the absence of any patient discomfort through the administration of local anesthetics and/or the use of other techniques (e.g., hypnosis, acupuncture). However, the dental

consumers, our patients, may not be aware of this, or they may consider that the injection of a local anesthetic is the most traumatic part of the entire dental procedure.[8,9] How then are we to manage these patients?

As dentistry developed, dentists gained the reputation of being "tooth doctors." Dental education was for many years predicated on the fact that the dentist was responsible for the oral cavity of the patient, and dental school curricula illustrated this. Previously, dentists were trained to manage their patients' dental requirements only. The possible interaction between dental treatment and the overall health of the patient was either unknown or ignored.

As medicine became increasingly sophisticated, it became apparent that dental care could and indeed did have a significant effect on the overall health of patients. Dental schools amended their curricula, adding courses in medicine and physical evaluation.[10] The dentist became even more alert to the fact that treatment in the oral cavity could profoundly influence a patient's well-being and conversely that the patient's health could significantly affect the type of dental treatment offered. The use of the patient-completed medical history questionnaire became a standard in the 1950s, followed by the routine recording of vital signs (1970s). The direction in the late 1990s and still today is toward more in-depth training in physical evaluation, including heart and lung auscultation.

Unfortunately, until the late 1960s and early 1970s, few dental schools in the United States (the University of Pittsburgh, The Ohio State University, and Loma Linda University being notable exceptions) provided the graduating dentist with a thorough background in the recognition and management of fear and anxiety. Until recently, the dentist could only treat the teeth of a patient who was known to be healthy enough (physically) to withstand the stresses of dental therapy. The "mind" of the patient (the patient's psychological attitude toward dentistry) was almost entirely ignored. The absence, at all levels of education, of training programs in the recognition and management of anxiety implied that anxiety did not exist or that it was of little or no importance. The doctor would treat the patient as well as he or she could given the clinical circumstances, and quite often the quality of the dentistry demonstrated the difficulty in patient management. General anesthesia was always available for those few patients who were absolutely unable to tolerate treatment; however, the most common type of dentistry performed under general

Table 1	Our Most Common Fears
FEAR	PERCENTAGE
Public speaking	27
Going to dentist	21
Heights	20
Mice	12
Flying	9
Other/no fears	11

From *Dental Health Advisor*, Spring 1987 (survey of 1000 adults).

anesthesia was exodontia. For conservative dental care, little or no thought was given to the patient's state of mind during treatment.

Under the sponsorship of three organizations—the American Dental Association (ADA), the American Dental Society of Anesthesiology (ADSA), and the American Dental Education Association (ADEA)—five "Workshops on Pain Control" were held (1964, 1965, 1971, 1977, and 1989). From these workshops came the Guidelines for Teaching the Comprehensive Control of Pain and Anxiety in Dentistry, which established an outline for three levels of training in various techniques of pain and anxiety control: the predoctoral dental program, the postdoctoral (residency) program, and continuing dental education.[11]

The 1970s saw the establishment by dental schools of viable programs in the area of sedation. Although the level of training still varies considerably from school to school, the dental student today receives at a minimum a background in the subject of anxiety and fear of dentistry and the techniques available in their management. Dentists today are aware that many patients are fearful of receiving dental treatment. This awareness is the first step required for the effective treatment of the patient's fears and anxieties. Add to this the almost universal availability of one or more techniques of sedation (usually iatrosedation, oral sedation, and inhalation sedation), and it becomes possible for the dentist to effectively and safely manage virtually all patients seeking care.

In the past few years, however, it has also become quite obvious that some dentists (and physicians) who had not received training in the use of these techniques while in school have begun to use them in their private practices without the benefit of appropriate postgraduate training programs. In all too many cases the result has been death or serious injury to patients.[12,13] Lawmakers in many states have taken action to halt this trend, either by prohibiting dentists from using certain techniques of sedation or anesthesia[14,15] or by requiring a special permit or license if the doctor is to use the techniques.[16] The Dentists Insurance Company (TDIC) in California published a retrospective study of deaths related to drug administration in dental practice.[17] Three major areas of fault were found to be present in almost all instances of negative outcome:
1. Inadequate preoperative evaluation of the patient
2. Inadequate monitoring during the procedure

3. Lack of knowledge of the pharmacology of the drugs being administered

Though written in 1983, these factors are, sadly, still commonly seen when problems do arise.

Whenever drugs are administered to a patient, it is essential that the doctor be fully cognizant of these three areas, as well as of any others that are involved in the ultimate safety of a drug technique. Failure to adequately prepare ourselves to administer drugs safely to patients can only result in these techniques being taken forcibly away from us.

One of my goals in preparing this book was to provide the doctor with appropriate background information concerning the various techniques of sedation that are most frequently used in the typical outpatient setting. As was stated in the preface, this book is not intended to be used as a sole source of knowledge concerning these techniques. Only when used in conjunction with a course of study that involves use of these procedures in the actual management of patients can a doctor become truly capable of safely administering the drugs discussed in this book. Of greater importance perhaps is the level of training required for each of these techniques. At the end of the chapter or section on each technique, recommendations are presented that outline the level of training deemed appropriate for the doctor to be able to use the technique in a safe and effective manner.

As is mentioned throughout this textbook, no single technique of sedation can ever be considered a panacea. Failures are to be expected on occasion with every technique of sedation. Although failures are frustrating for the doctor, they must be considered an unavoidable aspect of any sedation procedure, for as long as some patients retain even the slightest degree of consciousness, they will respond inappropriately to stimulation. It is only with the loss of consciousness (general anesthesia) that a significantly greater success rate can be expected; however, most doctors (both dentists and physicians) do not have the training necessary to use techniques in which unconsciousness is purposefully induced. As the doctor becomes more experienced with the techniques of sedation, failure rates decrease. Patients will sense a doctor's unease and unfamiliarity with a "new" technique, and this uncertainty is transferred to the patient, thereby decreasing the chance of a successful result. With increased experience, the doctor will become increasingly comfortable with the procedure and so, too, will the patient, thereby increasing the likelihood of success.

The greater the number of routes of sedation that a doctor has available for patient management, the greater the probability of a successful result. The only way to become successful with these techniques is to receive appropriate supervised training.

REFERENCES

1. Professions with prestige (National Opinion Research Center report on job status), Washington Post 115, p WH5, March 31, 1991.

2. Dental Health Advisor, Spring, 1987.
3. Bankoff G: *The conquest of pain: the story of anesthesia*, London, 1946, MacDonald.
4. Sykes WS: *Essays on the first hundred years of anaesthesia*, Edinburgh, 1960, E & S Livingstone.
5. Drummond-Jackson SL: Evipal anesthesia in dentistry. *Dental Cosmos* 77:130, 1935.
6. Hubbell AO, Adams RC: Intravenous anesthesia for dental surgery with sodium ethyl (1-methylbutyl) thiobarbituric acid. *J Am Dent Assoc* 27:1186, 1940.
7. White PF: Outpatient anesthesia: an overview. In White PF, editor: *Outpatient anesthesia*, New York, 1990, Churchill Livingstone.
8. Fiset L, Milgrom P, Weinstein P, et al: Psychophysiological responses to dental injections. *J Am Dent Assoc* 111:578, 1985.
9. Matsuura H: Analysis of systemic complications and deaths during dental treatment in Japan. *Anesth Prog* 36:219, 1990.
10. Curricular guide for physical evaluation. *J Dent Educ* 48:219, 1984.
11. Guidelines for teaching the Comprehensive Control of Pain and Anxiety in Dentistry. Council on Dental Education, American Dental Association. *J Dent Educ* 53:305, 1989.
12. Newcomer K: Dentist waited outside while patient died, Rocky Mountain News, August 4, 1992.
13. Child dies in dentist's chair. News2Houston.com, September 8, 2001.
14. Alaska State Board of Dental Examiners, Juneau, AK.
15. Christie B: Scotland to ban general anaesthesia in dental surgeries. *BMJ* 320:598, 2000.
16. American Dental Association: *Department of state and government affairs*, Chicago, 2008, The Association.
17. de Julien LF: Causes of severe morbidity/mortality cases. *J Calif Dent Assoc* 11:45, 1983.

Contents

Section I

Chapter 1: Pain and Anxiety in Dentistry

chapter 1

Pain and Anxiety in Dentistry

CHAPTER OUTLINE

BASIC FEARS
DENTAL FEARS

August 14, 1984

Dear Dr. Malamed,

I am writing to you in hope that you can give me some information on dentists who use conscious sedation in their practice. In reading the Los Angeles Times article June 4, 1984 … I finally found the right course I could take to get my teeth worked on.

For the last 5 years I have been trying to find a solution to my problem. I have an overwhelming fear of dentists and a very sensitive mouth. When I read the article and found out about various types of anesthesia that are available to dentists, I found light at the end of the tunnel. I do not, however, know how to find these dentists who are trained in the field … I would appreciate any help you can give me.

Thank you

The writer of the preceding letter is unusual, not because of her fear of dentistry, but because she was able to write this letter in an effort to seek help for herself.

Another, more recent letter:

June 23, 2007

Dear Dr. Malamed,

Thank you for recommending XXXX, DDS, when I explained to you I was in need of dental work, probably for a root-canal as described by my current dentist who was not proficient in the use of nitrous-oxide, and that I am a very apprehensive and squeamish patient.

I would never have been able to even make the appointment without assurances from all that the procedure would be painless and that this dentist had the skills to curb my anxieties. Your recommendation and assurances are much appreciated.

Fear of dentistry has been recognized for many years. A 1987 survey of 1000 adult Americans rated "going to the dentist" second only to "fear of public speaking" as the most common fear[1] (Fig. 1.1). In a 2009 survey of 1969 Dutch adults ages 18 to 93 years, 24.3% acknowledged having dental fear (behind only snakes [34.8%], heights [30.8%] and injuries [27.2%])[2] (Fig. 1.2). Sixteen percent of 1000 "'affluent Americans'" in a 2014 survey listed dentistry as a common fear.[3] Hollywood movies, such as *Marathon Man* (1976), *Little Shop of Horrors* (1986), and *The Dentist* (1996), exaggerate the evil and sadistic qualities of our profession.

Fear of dentistry (also known as odontophobia) is real, it is palpable, and it is a problem.

Many adults in North America still avoid visits to the dentist out of fear.

In the United States it is estimated that somewhere between 6% and 14% of the population (14 million to 34 million persons) voluntarily avoid seeking dental care because of their fear of dentistry.[4] These individuals delay treatment until they are in such pain that home remedies are no longer effective. They are categorized as severely anxious patients and represent a dual problem in management because the dentist will have to treat both the patients' acute dental problem (usually pain and infection) and their psychological emergency. I once gave a speech titled "The Pain of Fear."[5] This title aptly describes the dilemma faced by both the acutely fearful dental patient and the dentist asked to treat them. Fear of pain keeps the patient from seeking needed dental care until the pain, which is exacerbated by this fear, ultimately compels the patient to visit the dental office, urgent care, or a hospital emergency room. Such patients present the dentist with a significant problem. Attempts to treat these patients without addressing their fear usually lead to great frustration and increased stress for the dentist and an increased level of fear for the patient.[6]

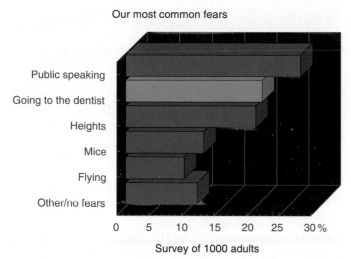

Figure 1.1 Most common fears. (From Dental Health Advisor, Spring 1987.)

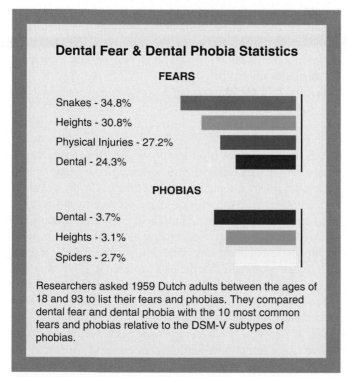

Figure 1.2 Dental fear and dental phobia statistics relative to other common fears from the DSM-V. (Data from Oosterink FM, Floor MD, de Jongh A, Hoogstraten J: Prevalence of dental fear and phobia relative to other fear and phobia subtypes. *Eur J Oral Sci* 117(2):135–143, 2009.)

Kahn, Cooper, and Mallenger surveyed a group of dentists and reported that 57% of those responding stated that the most stressful factor in their dental practices was the "difficult patient."[7]

Much more typically seen than the person with severe anxiety—the vast majority of those seen in the dental office—is the patient who does not harbor any irrational fears of dental treatment (Box 1.1). However, this patient does experience a

---

Box 1.1   Fear and Anxiety in Dental Patients

The terms *fear* and *anxiety* are often used interchangeably, as is the case in this text. However, there is a distinction to be made between them.

Fear tends to be a short-lived phenomenon, disappearing when the external danger or threat passes. It includes a feeling that something terrible is going to happen; physiologic changes, including tachycardia, profuse perspiration, and hyperventilation; and overt behavioral movements, such as becoming jittery or shaking. These clinical manifestations comprise what is called the *"fight or flight"* response.[4,8]

Anxiety, in contrast, is not likely to be dispelled as quickly. The emotional response is usually an internal one and is not readily recognized. Weiss and English[9] defined anxiety as "a specific unpleasurable state of tension which indicates the presence of some danger to the organism." Anxiety tends to be a learned response, acquired from personal experience or secondarily through the experiences of others. Anxiety arises from anticipation of an event, the outcome of which is unknown.[10]

Milgrom and Weinstein[4] state that a major difference between fear and anxiety is the immediacy of the threat to the person. A response to an immediate threat is fear. Properly used in the dental situation, the term *anxiety* describes reactions that develop in anticipation of or at the thought of dentistry, whereas *fear* refers to the reaction occurring at the dental office.

---

degree of heightened anxiety as the scheduled dental appointment nears. This apprehension over the forthcoming dental treatment does not prevent the patient from appearing in the office because this patient is genuinely concerned about maintaining oral hygiene and does not want to experience the pain of a toothache. This patient is categorized as having low-to-moderate anxiety and will appear on a regular basis for scheduled care because such a patient knows that avoidance of needed dental treatment will only lead to more significant (and painful) problems later. However, while in the dental office, this patient has somewhat sweaty palms and a more rapid heartbeat and admittedly would much rather be somewhere else.

In 1972 the Ad Hoc Committee on Research and Faculty Training in Pain Control in Dentistry reported that "the threat and fear of pain constitutes one of the great obstacles to the acceptance of dental services in the United States, considered by some to be greater than the financial barrier."[11] With the arrival of prepaid dental care and health insurance coverage for many millions of Americans, it has become quite obvious that it is not only the financial aspect of dental care that prevents patients from seeking treatment.

If this is so, then we in the dental profession have been neglecting a very important aspect of the management of our patients. With the great technical advances that have been achieved in dentistry in recent years, all areas of dental treatment can be undertaken with greater skill, a greater degree of accuracy, and less trauma and can be completed in less time. Yet despite these advances, the problems of fear and anxiety persist.

A large part of the problem can be assumed to be a carryover from the recent past when many dental patients were severely traumatized, both physically and psychologically, in the process of receiving routine dental care. Because of the lesser degree of scientific knowledge available at the time, a certain level of discomfort (pain) was to be expected. "Grin and bear it" was a commonly heard cliché.

The traumatized children of that era are the adults of today, and because they carry with them many psychological scars and bitter memories of "going to the dentist," today's dental professional is faced with a multiplicity of management problems when these patients appear for treatment.

Anxious patients present a problem to the dentist not only when they appear for treatment, but also when their children require treatment. Fear and anxiety are contagious, and even though apprehensive adults will usually make every attempt to mask their true feelings about "the dentist" (for it is "childish" to be afraid of the dentist), their feelings usually manage to make themselves evident to their children. Every dentist is familiar with the child who appears at his or her very first dental appointment already "knowing" that the drill is going to hurt. The problem of anxiety and its management in the pediatric patient are discussed more fully in Chapter 35.

This is our problem.

BASIC FEARS

What are the causes of our patients' fear of dentistry? Most persons harbor five universal fears:
1. Fear of pain
2. Fear of the unknown
3. Fear of helplessness and dependency
4. Fear of bodily change and mutilation
5. Fear of death

When the stress of the dental situation is superimposed onto these fears, many patients find themselves unable to successfully cope and they exhibit "dental phobia"—an irrational fear of dentistry and all that it represents.

Each of the aforementioned fears is easily transferred into the dental situation. As will be demonstrated, the *fear of pain* is easily the most significant fear harbored by the typical dental patient. How often does one hear the plaintive question "Is it going to hurt?" from a patient just before a procedure is to start? In fact, how do most patients select their dentist? Do they make their selection because of the superior quality of dental care or because the dentist has a reputation for being "painless" and caring? Each of us has heard a patient say, "It's nothing personal, doctor, but I don't like dentists." Milgrom

| 10. High standard of sterilization |
| 9. Prompt new-patient examination appointment |
| 8. Prompt emergency service |
| 7. Patients are happy with the results |
| 6. Dentists who listen, allow questions, treat dumb questions with dignity |
| 5. "Doctor, that was the most thorough dental examination I've ever had" |
| 4. Runs on time |
| 3. Staff who are:
    Kind, professional, caring, warm, helpful |
| 2. Does not hurt |
| 1. Painless injection |

Figure 1.3 Survey by patients reporting the most important factors of a dentist. (From de St Georges J: How dentists are judged by patients, *Dent Today* 23[8]:96–99, 2004.)

and Weinstein found that patients who were not experiencing dental pain when they appeared for routine treatment fully expected that at some time during their treatment they would experience pain, and the person most likely to inflict this pain on them was the dentist.[4]

A survey of the way patients evaluate their dentist (Fig. 1.3) demonstrated the two most important factors to be a dentist who (2) does not hurt and (1) gives a painless injection.[12]

Fear of the unknown is present in varying degrees whenever a person is confronted with a new situation, be it attempting to cross a furnished room for the first time in the dark of night or facing a new and threatening dental procedure. Fortunately, this fear can be effectively eliminated, or at least modulated, through an iatrosedative technique (see Chapter 6) called *preparatory communications*. The dentist need merely discuss the planned procedure with the patient, describing in nontechnical and nonthreatening terms the nature of the planned procedure. Description of the dental procedure is also a component of the informed consent process.

The fear of helplessness and dependency is unfortunately more difficult to eliminate in dentistry. Because of the nature of dental care, the patient is both unable to observe the treatment and is usually placed in a very vulnerable position—supine. Most persons experience a sense of unease at this time, especially when they are receiving treatment from a stranger—a dentist or hygienist with whom they are not well acquainted. As the patient becomes more familiar—and comfortable—with the dentist or hygienist, this feeling of helplessness should resolve.

In the area of pharmacosedation, the fear of helplessness and dependency also appears. Consider that we are asking already apprehensive patients to lie back in the dental chair (a vulnerable position) and to permit virtual strangers to administer drugs that alter their level of consciousness and decrease even further the degree of control that they maintain over their body. Examples of ways in which a patient's active participation may be enlisted during certain procedures are presented throughout this book. Such participation increases the patient's sense of control, thereby helping allay the feeling of helplessness.

One personality type—the authoritarian or "type A"—will prove very difficult to manage with the use of pharmacosedation. This individual, the "executive type," is a "take-charge" person who likes to be in complete control of his or her situation at all times. Where anxiety exists and pharmacosedation is indicated, this patient may prove somewhat more difficult to sedate successfully. The success of pharmacosedation is based in part on a patient's desire to simply "let go" and relax. Authoritarian patients often prove unwilling or unable to release control of their mind to the drug(s) used. The dentist will label this patient as "resistant" or say that the patient "fought the medication."

The fear of bodily change or mutilation is common in all aspects of medicine, but is especially evident in dentistry. The oral cavity is both richly innervated and a psychologically important region. All aspects of dental care have potentially great psychological overtones. Though at times these may seem illogical to the dentist, they must be dealt with for treatment to be successful. Changes in the size and shape or configuration of the body may have a profound effect on the patient's overall outlook and attitude toward life. The loss of teeth, for example, in today's society represents the process of growing old, a situation that might prove to be extremely disturbing psychologically to the patient.

The fear of death is also ever present. Placed in a vulnerable position in the dental chair, patients next have a multitude of hands and instruments placed into their mouth. Drugs are injected that remove the patient's ability to feel, and a high-speed handpiece is placed in the mouth, with a bur rotating several hundred thousand times per minute. Many sensations and thoughts race through the typical patient's mind at this time. Can I breathe with all this equipment and these hands in my mouth? Will I move my tongue too close to the drill and have it injured? Will the dentist slip and injure me? Add to this the feelings of a patient when the use of sedation is recommended in light of the many media reports of death and injury related to the use of drugs in dental offices.[13-16]

The fear of death in the dental office has probably been accentuated because of the seeming popularity of this subject in the mass media. Several nationwide television programs (e.g., *20/20*) have presented exposés on the dangers of anesthesia and sedation in dentistry.[17] Reaction from patients has been as expected: an increased reluctance to permit the dentist to administer any drugs, even local anesthetics and N_2O-O_2 sedation, for their treatment.

DENTAL FEARS

Table 1.1 presents the results of a survey of dental patients who were asked to list in order of fearfulness a number of situations that commonly occur in the dental office. As can be seen from this list, virtually any procedure that is performed in the dental office can be viewed as frightening by the patient.[18]

Most of these fear-producing situations are easily understood (e.g., extractions and drilling). However, several situations might easily be overlooked by the dentist. Being told that "you have bad teeth" (No. 3), "holding a syringe and needle in front of you" (No. 4), and "dentist laughs as he looks in your mouth" (No. 7) are almost entirely avoidable if the dentist is made aware of them. We all develop habits during our professional careers, most good, but a few of them bad. The manner in which we present ourselves to our patients may be the most important of all the habits that we develop. Through the use of proper treatment protocols combined with an appropriate professional attitude and demeanor, these three fear-producing situations may be eliminated or diminished.

Our profession has taken great strides toward the elimination of dental pain. With the many excellent local anesthetics available to us today, treatment-related pain need not be a problem. With the disposable equipment available today and the use of recommended injection technique, the injection of local anesthetic solution can become virtually 100% painless and atraumatic. Of interest, therefore, is the finding in Table 1.1 that the statement "dentist holds syringe in front of you" was considered to be more fear provoking than "dentist giving you a shot." The anticipation of the injection produces more fear than the actual injection.

Dental fear does exist. The first step in the management of a patient's fear of dentistry must be the recognition that it is present. All members of the dental and medical office staff must be ever alert to clues that signify the presence of heightened anxiety in a patient. The methods of recognizing the presence of anxiety and fear are discussed in Chapters 4 and 6.

Ignoring the presence of dental fears provokes many negative responses from the patient. One of the most common is the response of the pain-reaction threshold to heightened anxiety. Murray demonstrated that of the many variables that influence the pain reaction threshold of a patient, anticipation and anxiety appear to be the most important.[19,20] Apprehensive patients do in fact have a lowered pain-reaction threshold. The patient will respond adversely to stimulation (e.g., pressure) that in the more relaxed patient would not be interpreted as painful. When anxiety is reduced or eliminated through psychosedation, the patient's subjective experience of pain declines significantly.[21]

Pain and anxiety are related circularly. According to Schottstraedt, "Pain is a source of anxiety, anxiety is a factor that increases pain, and increased pain incites further anxiety."[22] Ignoring fear and anxiety increases the frustration and stress of the dentist and staff and increases the likelihood of stress-related emergency situations developing in the patient.

Ignoring a patient's fear of dentistry will not make the fear go away. Ignoring a patient's fear of dentistry may, however, make the patient go away. The following is a transcript of an

Table 1.1	Ranking of Dental Situations From the Most Fearful to the Least Fearful		
SITUATION	TOTAL GROUP	LOW-FEAR GROUP	HIGH-FEAR GROUP
Dentist is pulling your tooth	1	1	2
Dentist is drilling your tooth	2	2	1
Dentist tells you that you have bad teeth	3	3	3
Dentist holds syringe and needle in front of you	4	4	6
Dentist is giving you a shot	5	5	4
Having a probe placed in a cavity	6	6	5
Dentist laughs as he looks in your mouth	7	7	10
Dentist squirts air into a cavity	8	8	7
Sitting in the dentist's waiting room	9	9	8
Dentist laying out his instruments	10	10	13
Nurse tells you it's your turn	11	12	9
Getting in the dentist's chair	12	11	11
Dentist is putting in the filling	13	13	14
Thinking about going to the dentist	14	15	12
Dentist cleans your teeth with a steel probe	15	14	16
Getting in your car to go to the dentist	16	16	15
Dentist looks at your chart	17	17	17
Dentist places cotton in your mouth	18	18	18
Calling dentist to make an appointment	19	19	19
Dental assistant places bib on you	20	20	20
Dentist squirts water in your mouth	21	21	21
Making another appointment with the nurse	22	22	22
Dentist is cleaning your teeth	23	23	23
Dentist asks you to rinse your mouth	24	24	24
Dentist tells you he is through	25	25	25

From Gale E: Fears of the dental situation. *J Dent Res* 51:964, 1972.

interview with an apprehensive dental patient that illustrates this point:

I remember when I was in high school, I had a bad experience with a guy who I had to go to like every week for a couple of months and I hated going to this guy because he wasn't very ... he didn't have very much empathy for ... at least me ... I don't know about the rest of his patients. And he kept saying, "Oh, that doesn't hurt ... Come on, you're just a sissy," which wasn't cool ... He wasn't just hurting my mouth, but he was hurting my ego ... and when I was in high school, I just couldn't handle both.

But what he was doing was like he'd give me a prescription of a bunch of sedative pills to take before I went. So I'd take about a double dose, and I'd have to have somebody drive me to the dentist and there I was ... I don't know if they were like reds (secobarbital) or whatever, but I remember I felt out of it, but I felt uncomfortable. It wasn't a good experience. Going to him really, really, really touched off my fear of going back again because I didn't go back to the dentist for a long time after that.[23]

The remainder of this book is devoted to the various methods involved in the recognition of anxiety and its management. Today's dental and medical practitioners have at their disposal a plethora of techniques that are quite safe and effective in the management of a patient's fears and anxieties. Many of the techniques discussed involve the administration of drugs to the patient to achieve the desired goal, whereas other techniques may prove effective in the absence of drug administration. It is one of the goals of this book to help the dentist be able to select the appropriate psychosedative technique for a given patient so that fear of the dental situation may be managed in the least traumatic but still clinically effective manner.

Chanpong et al., in a telephone survey in Canada, sought to determine: *"Is there a need or demand for sedation and general anesthesia for dentistry among the adult Canadian population?"*[24] Of 1101 usable responses received, 7.6% stated that they had "missed, cancelled or avoided a dental appointment because of fear or anxiety." In response to the question *"How would you assess your feelings toward having dental treatment done?"* 5.5% assessed themselves as either "very afraid" (2.0%) or "terrified" (3.5%). In this "high-fear" group, 49.2% had missed, cancelled, or avoided a dental appointment because of fear or anxiety compared with only 5.2% of the "low-fear" or "no-fear" group. When asked about their interest in *sedation or general anesthesia which would allow you to undergo dental treatment while partially or completely asleep, in a safe, controlled environment,* 31.1% of the high-fear group was "definitely interested" with 54.1% of the same group "interested depending on the cost."

In the United States, Dionne et al. determined that 18.1% of responders would visit a dentist more often if given a drug to make them less nervous.[25]

The need is there …

The answer is there …

REFERENCES

1. Our most common fears, *Dent Health Advisor Spring*, 1987.
2. Oosterink FM, Floor MD, de Jongh A, Hoogstraten J: Prevalence of dental fear and phobia relative to other fear and phobia subtypes. *Eur J Oral Sci* 117(2):135–143, 2009.
3. Merrill Edge Report: Spring 2014 (June 1, 2014). Retirement fears don't inspire sacrifices. Page 2. www.merrilledge.com/Publish/Content/application/pdf/GWMOL/Merrill_Edge_Report_Spring_2014.pdf (Accessed 16 July 2015).
4. Milgrom P, Weinstein P: *Treating fearful dental patients*, Seattle, 1996, University of Washington in Seattle, Continuing Dental Education.
5. Malamed SF: The pain of fear. Lecture to the California Dental Society of Anesthesiology October 1975, San Francisco.
6. Friedman N: Iatrosedation. In McCarthy FM, editor: *Emergencies in dental practice*, ed 3, Philadelphia, 1979, WB Saunders.
7. Kahn RL, Cooper C, Mallenger M: Dentistry: what causes it to be a stressful profession? *Int Rev Appl Psych* 29:307, 1980.
8. Cannon WB: *Bodily changes in pain, hunger, fear and rage*, ed 2, New York, 1929, Appleton-Century-Crofts.
9. Weiss E, English OS: *Psychosomatic medicine*, Philadelphia, 1957, WB Saunders.
10. Pearson RE: Anxiety in the dental office. In Bennett CR, editor: *Conscious-sedation in dental practice*, ed 2, St Louis, 1978, Mosby.
11. National Institute of Health: Report of the Ad Hoc Committee II on research and faculty training in pain control in dentistry, Feb 9–10, 1972.
12. de St Georges J: How dentists are judged by patients. *Dent Today* 23(8):96–99, 2004.
13. Child dies in dentist's chair. Available at: www.News2Houston.com. 8 September 2001.
14. Not enough evidence to charge dentist, coroner says. Australian Broadcasting Company. Available at: www.abc.net.au/news. 22 September 2006.
15. Apodaca G: Girl, 2, dies after routine visit to the dentist. Available at: www.ABC13.com. 12 October 2006.
16. Owen M, Shelton DL, Gorner J: Patient dies during root canal. Principal's energy in life, work recalled. Available at: www.chicagotribune.com. 18 December 2007.
17. A visit to the dentist. 60 Minutes II. January 19, 1999, CBS Television.
18. Gale E: Fears of the dental situation. *J Dent Res* 51:964, 1972.
19. Murray JB: Psychology of the pain experience. In Weisenberg M, editor: *Pain: clinical and experimental perspectives*, St Louis, 1975, Mosby.
20. Murray JB: The puzzle of pain. *Percept Mot Skills* 28:887, 1969.
21. Jones A, Bentler PM, Petry G: The reaction of uncertainty concerning future pain. *J Abnorm Psychol* 71:87, 1966.
22. Schottstraedt WW: *Psychophysiologic approach in medical practice*, Chicago, 1960, Year Book Medical.
23. Interview, Department of Human Behavior, University of Southern California School of Dentistry, Los Angeles, 1975.
24. Chanpong B, Haas DA, Locker D: Need and demand for sedation or general anesthesia in dentistry: a national survey of the Canadian population. *Anesth Prog* 52(1):3–11, 2005.
25. Dionne RA, Gordon SM, McCullagh LM, et al: Assessing the need for anesthesia and sedation in the general population. *J Am Dent Assoc* 129(2):167–173, 1998.

Section II

SPECTRUM OF PAIN AND ANXIETY CONTROL

Sections II through VI present the answer to the problem presented in Section I—the problem of fear and anxiety in dentistry. The answer includes all of the techniques that can be termed *sedation* and those termed *general anesthesia*. This terminology is defined in this section (Section II).

In Chapter 2, the reader is introduced to the concept of sedation. The term is defined and then discussed in relation to general anesthesia, a state of unconsciousness that is often confused with sedation. The various stages of anesthesia, which include minimal, moderate, and deep sedation and general anesthesia, are described.

Chapter 3, The Spectrum of Pain and Anxiety Control, presents the wide range of patient management techniques available to the dentist and physician. Advantages and disadvantages of these techniques are discussed and the techniques compared.

Before the administration of any drug to a patient, or for that matter before treatment of any sort, it is imperative that the dentist fully evaluate the patient to determine his or her ability to withstand the stresses involved in the planned treatment. This evaluation must be even more comprehensive whenever a drug is to be administered to a patient during treatment. In addition, all patients receiving central nervous system (CNS) depressant drugs (sedation or general anesthesia) must be monitored to varying degrees throughout the procedure. Chapters 4 and 5 present extremely important guidelines that should be followed every time drug administration is considered. Failure to properly evaluate a patient before treatment (see Chapter 4) and failure to monitor the patient during treatment (see Chapter 5) have been implicated in many cases of morbidity and mortality.[1] The importance of these two chapters to the safety of the techniques that follow cannot be overstated.

In Chapter 6, the reader is introduced to the first of the two major categories of psychosedation—nondrug techniques (iatrosedative techniques). Although a number of nondrug techniques are available, two, iatrosedation and hypnosis, are used to a greater extent than others. Iatrosedation represents the building block upon which the success or failure of all pharmacosedative procedures (techniques involving the administration of drugs) will be based. Whether we are aware of it or not, all dentists employ iatrosedation in their office on every one of their patients. Hypnosis, on the other hand, is a technique that must be learned in a more formal setting. When used appropriately, its success rate in the management of both pain and fear is quite acceptable.

REFERENCE

1. de Julien LF: Causes of severe morbidity/mortality cases. *J Calif Dent Assoc* 11:45, 1983.

chapter 2

Introduction to Sedation

CHAPTER OUTLINE

DEFINITIONS
THE CONCEPT OF "RESCUE"

DEFINITIONS

The primary goal of this textbook is to aid the dentist in the management of pain and anxiety in the dental patient because it is these two items that, either singly or in combination, produce most of the difficulties associated with the delivery of patient care.

How can pain and anxiety be managed successfully and safely in the dental office? Pain associated with dental treatment is managed effectively through the administration of local anesthetics at the start of treatment. These chemicals block passage of the propagated nerve impulse beyond the site at which they are deposited. Although the tooth or soft tissues have received a noxious stimulus (e.g., drill, curette), the nerve impulse will travel only as far as the site at which the local anesthetic was deposited. The rapid influx of sodium ions into the interior of the nerve (the process responsible for continued propagation of the nerve impulse) is prevented, the impulse is terminated, and the patient experiences no discomfort.

As noted in Chapter 1, however, *fear* of pain is a major deterrent to the delivery of dental care. Patients who are not in pain fear the visit to the dental office because they believe that at some time during their dental treatment they will be hurt.[1] Fear of pain produces a heightened anxiety in these patients, a factor that may lead to the avoidance of dental care until they are in severe pain.

How can dentistry alter its image of being painful? It is a fact today that virtually all dental care can be completed without discomfort to the patient. With the availability of a variety of excellent local anesthetics, it is possible to achieve clinically adequate pain control in virtually all situations. The most difficult pain management problems usually occur in pulpally involved teeth (symptomatic irreversible pulpitis [SIP]) and, since the reintroduction of intraosseous anesthesia and the

introduction of articaine HCl, only rarely in this situation is effective pain control unattainable.[2-5]

The administration of a local anesthetic is also considered to be a traumatic procedure by most patients and indeed by many dentists (see Table 1.1).[6,7] Yet even this aspect of dental care need not be traumatic. Local anesthetic injections may be administered atraumatically anywhere in the oral cavity, including the palate. The technique of the atraumatic injection of local anesthetics is presented in various textbooks of local anesthesia.[8,9] The introduction of computer-controlled local anesthetic delivery (C-CLAD)[10,11] and buffered local anesthetics[12,13] have made painless anesthetic delivery more readily achievable.

Yet the possibility of pain and the "injection" of local anesthetics are not the only things about dentistry that induce fear in patients. Dentists with extensive clinical experience have probably heard patients express fear of almost every possible procedure that we are called upon to carry out.

How then can we manage these overtly fearful patients? The answer is to distract them, to take their attention away from what is being done for them (the patient would consider that we are doing things "to them") in their mouths. This can be accomplished through nondrug techniques, such as headsets with music, video, dark glasses, warm blankets, or through the administration of drugs that induce a state of consciousness (or, more precisely, an altered state of consciousness) in which a person is more relaxed and carefree. Over the years, many names have been given to this drug-induced state. Names such as chemamnesia,[14] sedamnesia,[15] twilight sleep,[16] relative analgesia,[17] and comedication[18] have been used to describe the state of altered consciousness that is now known as sedation.

Many definitions of sedation have been put forth over the years; however, in 1971, following the Third Pain Control Conference sponsored by the American Dental Association

(ADA), American Dental Society of Anesthesiology, and American Association of Dental Schools, the "Guidelines for Teaching the Comprehensive Control of Pain and Anxiety in Dentistry" were published.[19] These guidelines established a standard for the training of dental personnel in this area of patient management. The guidelines have undergone revision on several occasions over the ensuing years,[20,21] including 2007 when the House of Delegates of the ADA passed two documents representing significant revisions of the guidelines, including modification of the terms used to define the various levels of sedation.[22,23] The most recent update to the Guidelines was in 2016.[24,25]

In previous iterations, levels of sedation were defined as follows[20,21]:

Anxiolysis: a minimally depressed level of consciousness that retains the patient's ability to independently and continuously maintain an airway and respond appropriately to physical stimulation or verbal command and that is produced by a pharmacologic or nonpharmacologic method or a combination thereof. Although cognitive function and coordination may be modestly impaired, ventilatory and cardiovascular functions are unaffected.

Conscious sedation: a minimally depressed level of consciousness that retains the patient's ability to independently and continuously maintain an airway and respond appropriately to physical stimulation and verbal command and that is produced by a pharmacologic or nonpharmacologic method or combination thereof.

Deep sedation: a drug-induced depression of consciousness during which patients cannot be easily aroused, but respond purposefully following repeated or painful stimulation. The ability to independently maintain ventilatory function may be impaired. Patients may require assistance in maintaining a patent airway, and spontaneous ventilation may be inadequate. Cardiovascular function is usually maintained.

General anesthesia: a controlled state of unconsciousness accompanied by partial or complete loss of protective reflexes, including inability to independently maintain an airway and respond purposefully to physical stimulation or verbal command, and is produced by a pharmacologic or nonpharmacologic method or a combination thereof.

In 2002 the American Society of Anesthesiologists, the organization for medical specialists in anesthesia, in response to an increase in the use of sedation by physicians, many of whom had little background or training in anesthesiology, published "Practice Guidelines for Sedation and Analgesia by Nonanesthesiologists."[26]

In the introduction it is stated: "These Guidelines are designed to be applicable to procedures performed in a variety of settings (e.g., hospitals, freestanding clinics, physician, dental, and other offices) by practitioners who are not specialists in anesthesiology. Because minimal sedation (anxiolysis) entails minimal risk, the Guidelines specifically exclude it. Examples of minimal sedation include peripheral nerve blocks, local or topical anesthesia, and either (1) less than 50% nitrous oxide (N_2O) in oxygen with no other sedative or analgesic medications by any route; or (2) a single oral sedative or analgesic medication administered in doses appropriate for the unsupervised treatment of insomnia, anxiety, or pain."[26]

Another extremely important concept included in these guidelines is the principle of the need to be able to "rescue" a patient from unintended entry into a more profound level of central nervous system (CNS) depression than intended:

Because sedation is a continuum, it is not always possible to predict how an individual patient will respond. Hence, practitioners intending to produce a given level of sedation should be able to rescue patients whose level of sedation becomes deeper than initially intended. Individuals administering Moderate Sedation/Analgesia (Conscious Sedation) *should be able to rescue patients who enter a state of* Deep Sedation/Analgesia, *while those administering* Deep Sedation/Analgesia *should be able to rescue patients who enter a state of general anesthesia.*[24]

Rather than maintain a set of clinical standards slightly at variance with those of the anesthesiologists, and recognizing the expertise of the American Society of Anesthesiologists in this area, the House of Delegates of the ADA reviewed the ADA guidelines from 2002 and in October 2007 passed a revised document[22] and a new document providing guidelines for the teaching of sedation and anesthesia to dental students.[23]

The following definitions of levels of sedation are excerpted from these two ADA guidelines.[22,23]

Minimal sedation (this definition was previously associated with *anxiolysis*)—"a minimally depressed level of consciousness that retains the patient's ability to independently and continuously maintain an airway and respond appropriately to physical stimulation or verbal command and that is produced by a pharmacological or nonpharmacological method or a combination thereof. Although cognitive function and coordination may be modestly impaired, ventilatory and cardiovascular functions are unaffected."

"*Note:* In accord with this particular definition, the drug(s) and/or techniques used should carry a margin of safety wide enough never to render unintended loss of consciousness. Further, patients whose only response is reflex withdrawal from repeated painful stimuli would not be considered to be in a state of minimal sedation."

"When the intent is minimal sedation for adults, the appropriate initial dose of a single enteral drug is no more than the maximum recommended dose (MRD) of a drug that can be prescribed for unmonitored home use."

Moderate sedation (this definition was previously associated with *conscious sedation*)—"a drug-induced depression of consciousness during which patients respond *purposefully* to verbal commands, either alone or accompanied by light tactile stimulation. No interventions are required to maintain a patent airway, and spontaneous ventilation is adequate. Cardiovascular function is usually maintained."

Table 2.1	Continuum of Depth of Sedation: Definition of General Anesthesia and Levels of Sedation/Analgesia			
	MINIMAL SEDATION (ANXIOLYSIS)	MODERATE SEDATION/ ANALGESIA (CONSCIOUS SEDATION)	DEEP SEDATION/ ANALGESIA	GENERAL ANESTHESIA
Responsiveness	Normal response to verbal stimulation	Purposeful* response to verbal or tactile stimulation	Purposeful* response after repeated or painful stimulation	Unarousable, even with painful stimulation
Airway	Unaffected	No intervention required	Intervention may be required	Intervention often required
Spontaneous ventilation	Unaffected	Adequate	May be inadequate	Frequently inadequate

*Reflex withdrawal from painful stimulus is not considered a purposeful response.
From American Society of Anesthesiologists Task Force on Sedation and Analgesia by Non-Anesthesiologists: Practice guidelines for sedation and analgesia by non-anesthesiologists. *Anesthesiology* 96:1004–1017, 2002.

"*Note:* In accord with this particular definition, the drug(s) and/or techniques used should carry a margin of safety wide enough to render unintended loss of consciousness unlikely. Repeated dosing of an agent before the effects of previous dosing can be fully appreciated may result in a greater alteration of the state of consciousness than is the intent of the dentist. Further, patients whose only response is reflex withdrawal from repeated painful stimuli would not be considered to be in a state of moderate sedation."

Deep sedation "a drug-induced depression of consciousness during which patients cannot easily be aroused, but respond purposefully following repeated or painful stimulation. The ability to independently maintain ventilatory function may be impaired. Patients may require assistance in maintaining a patent airway, and spontaneous ventilation may be inadequate. Cardiovascular function is usually maintained."

General anesthesia "a drug-induced loss of consciousness during which patients are not arousable, even by painful stimulation. The ability to independently maintain ventilatory function is often impaired. Patients often require assistance in maintaining a patent airway, and positive pressure ventilation may be required because of depressed spontaneous ventilation or drug-induced depression of neuromuscular function. Cardiovascular function may be impaired."

Table 2.1 compares the different levels of CNS depression described in the American Society of Anesthesiologists' guidelines.

THE CONCEPT OF "RESCUE"

Recognizing that serious instances of morbidity and mortality have occurred associated with the administration of "sedation" by nonanesthesiologists, the guidelines from the American Society of Anesthesiologists included and stressed the important concept of "rescue":

Because sedation and general anesthesia are a continuum, it is not always possible to predict how an individual will

respond. Hence, practitioners intending to produce a given level of sedation should be able to diagnose and manage the physiologic consequences (rescue) for patients whose level of sedation becomes deeper than initially intended.

For all levels of sedation, the practitioner must have the training, skills, drugs and equipment to identify and manage such an occurrence until either assistance arrives (emergency medical service) or the patient returns to the intended level of sedation without airway or cardiovascular complications.

Preparation for and management of sedation- and general anesthesia–related urgencies and emergencies are thoroughly reviewed in Section VII, Chapters 32 to 34.

The principle governing a health care provider's responsibility to the victim during a medical emergency is quite similar to the definition of "rescue" previously presented. It has been stated by this author on literally hundreds of occasions as follows: "The obligation of the health-care provider to their patient during a medical emergency is simple: To try to keep the victim alive until one of two things occur: (1) they recover, or (2) help arrives on the scene to take over their management, provided that 'help' is better qualified in emergency management than you."[27]

SUMMARY

The reader must be aware and never forget that there are no distinct stages of anesthesia. One level of CNS depression (e.g., minimal sedation) seamlessly blends into the next level (moderate sedation) that then seamlessly becomes deep sedation and, eventually, when consciousness is lost, general anesthesia.

The next chapter introduces the many techniques of sedation and general anesthesia available for use by the dental and medical professions for the management of both pain and anxiety. In subsequent sections of this book, each of these techniques is reviewed in considerable depth so as to impart to the reader a degree of knowledge that will, when combined with adequate clinical and didactic training, permit these techniques to be employed safely and effectively.

REFERENCES

1. Milgrom P, Weinstein P: *Treating fearful dental patients*, Seattle, 1996, University of Washington in Seattle, Continuing Dental Education.
2. Jensen J, Nusstein J, Drum M, et al: Anesthetic efficacy of a repeated intraosseous injection following a primary intraosseous injection. *J Endod* 34(2):126–130, 2008.
3. Bigby J, Reader A, Nusstein J, et al: Articaine for supplemental intraosseous anesthesia in patients with irreversible pulpitis. *J Endod* 32(11):1044–1047, 2006.
4. Robertson D, Nusstein J, Reader A, et al: The anesthetic efficacy of articaine in buccal infiltration of mandibular posterior teeth. *J Am Dent Assoc* 138(8):1104–1112, 2007.
5. Kanaa MD, Whitworth JM, Corbett IP, et al: Articaine and lidocaine mandibular buccal infiltration anesthesia: a prospective randomized double-blind cross-over study. *J Endod* 32(4):296–298, 2006.
6. Gale E: Fears of the dental situation. *J Dent Res* 51:964, 1972.
7. Fiset L, Milgrom P, Weinstein P, et al: Psychophysiological responses to dental injections. *J Am Dent Assoc* 111:578, 1985.
8. Malamed SF: *Handbook of local anesthesia*, ed 5, St Louis, 2004, CV Mosby.
9. Jastak JT, Yagiela JA, Donaldson D: *Local anesthesia of the oral cavity*, Philadelphia, 1995, Saunders.
10. Hochman M, Chiarello D, Hochman CB, et al: Computerized local anesthetic delivery vs. traditional syringe technique. Subjective pain response. *N Y State Dent J* 63(7):24–29, 1997.
11. Ashkenazi M, Blumer S, Eli I: Effectiveness of computerized delivery of intrasulcular anesthetic in primary molars. *J Am Dent Assoc* 136(10):1418–1425, 2005.
12. Malamed SF, Hersh E, Poorsattar S, Falkel M: Faster onset and more comfortable injection with alkalinized 2% lidocaine with epinephrine 1:100,000. *Compendium* 34(spec issue#1):1–11, 2013.
13. Malamed SF, Tavana S, Falkel M: Faster onset and more comfortable injection with alkalinized 2% lidocaine with epinephrine 1:100,000. *Compend Contin Educ Dent* 34(Spec1):10–20, 2013.
14. Monheim LJ: *General anesthesia in dental practice*, ed 3, St Louis, 1968, Mosby.
15. Carnow R, Schaffer AB: Application of the concept of augmenter-moderator-reducer to dental patient management. In Spiro SR, editor: *Amnesia-analgesia techniques in dentistry*, Springfield, IL, 1972, Charles C. Thomas.
16. Berns J: Twilight sedation: a substitute for lengthy office intravenous anesthesia. *J Conn State Dent Assoc* 37:4, 1963.
17. Langa H: *Relative analgesia in dental practice: inhalation analgesia with nitrous oxide*, Philadelphia, 1968, WB Saunders.
18. Hamburg HL: *The joy of sedation: a beginner's manual to newer sedative techniques for the dentist and dental student*, Hamburg, NY, 1978, Hamburg.
19. American Dental Association, Council on Dental Education: Guidelines for teaching the comprehensive control of pain and anxiety in dentistry. *J Dent Educ* 36:62, 1972.
20. American Dental Association, Council on Dental Education: Guidelines for teaching the comprehensive control of pain and anxiety in dentistry. *J Dent Educ* 53:305, 1989.
21. American Dental Association: *Guidelines for the use of conscious sedation, deep sedation, and general anesthesia for dentists*, Oct. 2002, ADA House of Delegates, The Association.
22. American Dental Association: *Council on Dental Education: Guidelines for the use of sedation and general anesthesia by dentists*, as adopted by the Oct. 2007 ADA House of Delegates, Chicago, 2007, The Association.
23. American Dental Association: *Council on Dental Education: Guidelines for teaching pain control and sedation in dentists and dental students*, as adopted by the Oct. 2007 ADA House of Delegates, Chicago, 2007, The Association.
24. American Dental Association: *Council on Dental Education. Guidelines for the use of sedation and general anesthesia by dentists*. Adopted by the ADA House of Delegates, Chicago, 2016, The American Dental Association.
25. American Dental Association: *Council on Dental Education. Guidelines for teaching pain control and sedation to dentists and dental students*. Adopted by the ADA House of Delegates, Chicago, 2016, The American Dental Association.
26. American Society of Anesthesiologists Task Force on Sedation and Analgesia by Non-Anesthesiologists: Practice guidelines for sedation and analgesia by non-anesthesiologists. *Anesthesiology* 96:1004–1017, 2002.
27. Malamed SF: *Medical emergencies in the dental office*, St Louis, 2015, Elsevier.

chapter 3

The Spectrum of Pain and Anxiety Control

CHAPTER OUTLINE

NO ANESTHESIA
IATROSEDATION
OTHER NONDRUG PSYCHOSEDATIVE
TECHNIQUES
ROUTES OF DRUG ADMINISTRATION
  Oral
  Rectal
  Topical

Sublingual
Intranasal
Transdermal
Subcutaneous
Intramuscular
Inhalation (Pulmonary)
Intravenous
GENERAL ANESTHESIA

A variety of techniques are available to dental and medical professionals to aid their management of a patient's fears and anxieties regarding dental care and surgery. To some this statement may be self-evident; however, to others the availability of a variety of techniques may come as something of a surprise. The aim of this chapter is to introduce the concept of the *spectrum of pain and anxiety control*. This spectrum, which is presented graphically in Fig. 3.1, illustrates that there are indeed quite a number of techniques available to manage patients' fears and anxieties. This chapter introduces the various techniques included in this spectrum, and subsequent chapters and sections describe them in depth.

The vertical bar about three-quarters of the way across the spectrum in Fig. 3.1 denotes a very significant barrier: the point at which consciousness is lost. Techniques to the right of the bar fall under the heading of general anesthesia, whereas techniques to its left may be termed *psychosedation, sedation, conscious sedation,* or as recently redefined: *minimum, moderate,* or *deep sedation*.[1-3]

Techniques of sedation may further be divided into those requiring the administration of drugs to achieve a desirable clinical effect and those that do not. The former are termed *pharmacosedation* techniques, the latter *iatrosedation* techniques. These terms are further defined elsewhere in this text.

The bar representing the point at which unconsciousness occurs is significant in that it identifies a level of training that must be achieved by the dentist before various techniques can even be considered for use. Without elaborating at this point

(educational requirements for specific techniques are discussed in the appropriate sections of this book), it may be stated that the absolute minimum of training recommended for the use of general anesthesia is 3 years in an accredited residency program. These guidelines for general anesthesia and those for techniques of sedation have been accepted by the American Dental Association, the American Dental Society of Anesthesiology, and the American Dental Education Association.[2,3]

The duration of time required to adequately prepare the dentist to use the various techniques of sedation safely and effectively will vary from technique to technique and from dentist to dentist. Many dentists and dental hygienists are fully prepared upon graduating from dental school to enter into private practice, knowledgeable in the safe and effective use of some of these techniques (e.g., inhalation sedation with N_2O-O_2). Many others, however, will not have obtained this ability, and for these health care professionals, continuing education courses are available. In the United States, for inhalation sedation with nitrous oxide (N_2O) and oxygen (O_2), a minimum course of 14 hours, including patient management, is recommended; for intravenous (IV) moderate sedation, a minimum of 60 hours, including patient management, is required.[3]

In recent years, outpatient surgery in the practice of medicine has increased in popularity. Minor surgical procedures on the limbs, trunk, and face are easily completed with the administration of local anesthetics by general surgeons, dermatologists, cosmetic, and plastic and reconstructive surgeons.[4-7] Until

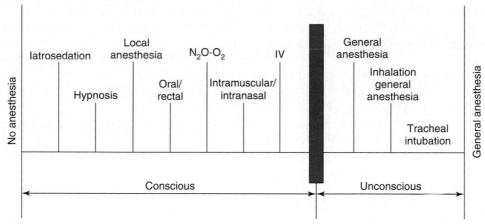

Figure 3.1 Spectrum of pain and anxiety control. Illustration of the range of techniques available in medicine and dentistry for patient management. Vertical bar represents the loss of consciousness.

recently, however, little consideration was given to the degree of patient anxiety toward this type of surgical procedure. The patient faces these nondental surgical procedures with the same dread as may be seen in dental patients. The techniques and concepts discussed in this book are as appropriate for nondental surgery as they are in dentistry.

Many techniques of pain and anxiety control are available to the health care professional. Which ones, if any, are used is a very personal choice. Some dentists are comfortable using a technique that others might be uncomfortable using. Having several techniques available at his or her disposal enables the dentist to tailor the appropriate sedation technique to a given patient. There is no panacea, nor is any one technique always indicated or always effective. To rely solely on one technique for moderate sedation is to invite the occasional failure.

NO ANESTHESIA

The extreme left-hand portion of the spectrum of pain and anxiety control (see Fig. 3.1) comprises a small group of patients who require absolutely no sedation or local anesthesia during their dental treatment. Although quite rare, it is probable that a dentist or hygienist will be called upon to treat one or more of these persons at some time. For whatever reason—anatomic, physiologic, psychological, cultural, or religious—these patients either do not feel pain or do not react to it, and they are able to tolerate any form of dental treatment without the need for any sort of drug intervention.

Although such patients may not feel any pain in the course of their treatment, such may not be the case with the dentist or hygienist asked to treat them. The following incident actually took place: The patient, a pleasant 26-year-old woman requiring periodontal surgery (soft tissue), requested that the dentist not use any drugs at all during her treatment because she did not require them. After a futile attempt to dissuade the patient from what was assumed to be a foolhardy course, the dentist agreed to begin the surgical procedure without local anesthesia only if the patient would consent to receive it if at any time

during the surgery pain was present. The surgical procedure required approximately 45 minutes to complete during which time the patient displayed absolutely no evidence of discomfort to the complete amazement of the (numerous) dental personnel who had gathered around to watch. Vital signs (blood pressure, heart rate, and rhythm) monitored during the procedure demonstrated essentially no deviation from baseline values. Not so with the dentist and assistant. Following the procedure, which proceeded uneventfully, they were bathed in perspiration. The dentist commented that he felt quite uncomfortable throughout the procedure because he knew that the patient *should* be in pain. Indeed, he stopped many times to ask the patient how she was feeling. He also said that he could almost feel the pain for the patient. "I was uncomfortable for the patient," he said. At the next surgical appointment, the dentist and assistant were quite pleased when the patient consented to their request to give her local anesthesia for the surgery. When asked why she had changed her mind, the patient stated that she did it for the sake of the dentist and the assistant. She had noticed *their* discomfort at the prior visit and, although she still did not require the pain-controlling drug, thought it prudent to receive it to allow the dentist to be more relaxed during her treatment.

It is important to separate this small group of patients who truly do not require anesthetics from those patients who similarly request that they not receive local anesthesia because they are quite fearful of injections. It is somewhat easier to recognize such a patient before starting the planned procedure. However, if the dentist is unable to recognize the patient's anxiety and proceeds to dental treatment, it usually becomes painfully obvious, to both the dentist and the patient, to which group the patient truly belongs.

IATROSEDATION

Iatrosedation, defined as the relief of anxiety through the dentist's behavior, is the building block for all other forms of psychosedation. The term and the technique of *iatrosedation* were created many years ago by Dr. Nathan Friedman, then chairman and founder of the Department of Human Behavior, University of Southern California School of Dentistry.[8] Discussed in depth in Chapter 6, iatrosedation may briefly be described as a process involving several steps: recognition by the dentist of the patient's anxieties toward dentistry, management of the information gathered by the dentist from the patient, and a commitment by the dentist to aid the patient during dental treatment.

Simply stated, iatrosedation is a technique of communication between the dentist and the patient that creates a bond of trust and confidence. Patients possessing trust and confidence in their health care provider (physician, dentist, or other health care professional) are well on their way to being more relaxed and cooperative, without the need for supplemental pharmacosedation.[9]

Another important benefit of the use of iatrosedation in the practice of medicine and dentistry is the prevention of possible medicolegal complications. Lack of effective communication between the health care professional and patient is a leading cause of suits brought against medical and dental professionals. In some estimates, up to 37% of all malpractice actions are a result of a lack of communication and trust between the doctor and patient.[10]

In some situations, iatrosedation alone may remove all of a patient's fears and anxieties concerning the treatment, permitting treatment to proceed in a "normal" manner, without the need for pharmacosedation. More often, however, iatrosedation will produce a decrease in the patient's level of anxiety to the point where the use of supplemental pharmacosedation will enable the patient to more readily accept and tolerate the planned treatment.

OTHER NONDRUG PSYCHOSEDATIVE TECHNIQUES

In addition to iatrosedation, other techniques are available to decrease a patient's fear and anxiety toward dentistry without the administration of drugs.

Hypnosis has been used for many years for the management of both pain and anxiety. When employed by a trained hypnotherapist, in the proper clinical environment, and on the appropriate patient, hypnosis has proved to be a highly effective means of achieving both a relaxed and a pain-free treatment environment.[11]

Other nondrug techniques for achieving pain and anxiety control are available. Some are not new, having been introduced to the medical and dental professions decades ago. Interest in these techniques has waxed and waned over the years. They may prove to be effective in the hands of some medical and dental practitioners. Textbooks that provide in-depth coverage of these potentially valuable procedures are available and recommended.

Nondrug techniques are mentioned here for the sake of completeness. Developments in this field are occurring so rapidly that it is virtually impossible to include all of them in our compendium of available techniques. Nondrug techniques for the management of either pain or anxiety, or both, include acupuncture,[12] acupressure, audioanalgesia (e.g., music),[13] biofeedback,[14] electroanesthesia (e.g., transcutaneous electrical nerve stimulation [TENS], electroanesthesia [EA], electronic dental anesthesia [EDA]),[15] and electrosedation.

ROUTES OF DRUG ADMINISTRATION

To this point in discussing the management of treatment-related anxiety, we have not yet employed any technique that requires administration of a drug. Sedation produced without administration of drugs is termed *iatrosedation*. The use of drugs to control anxiety is termed *pharmacosedation*. Iatrosedation by itself will allow us to manage but a small percentage of our fearful patients. One advantage possessed by iatrosedative techniques is their ability to increase the effectiveness of any drugs that might be needed for the definitive management of the patient's dental fears. Even though we may have to turn to pharmacosedation, the great majority of patients in whom iatrosedation has been used will require smaller doses of the drug(s) to bring about a comparable degree of moderate sedation.[16]

There are many routes through which drugs may be administered (Table 3.1). The first 13 of these routes are used within the practice of medicine, with the first 10 used in dentistry. The intraperitoneal route is used in veterinary medicine. These routes are as follows:

1. Oral
2. Rectal
3. Topical
4. Sublingual
5. Intranasal (IN)
6. Transdermal
7. Subcutaneous (SC)
8. Intramuscular (IM)
9. Inhalation (pulmonary)
10. Intravenous (IV)
11. Intraarterial (IA)
12. Intrathecal (within the spinal cord)
13. Intramedullary
14. Intraperitoneal

Oral

The oral route is the most commonly used route of drug administration. It possesses advantages over parenteral routes of administration that make it useful in various situations involving the management of pain and anxiety. This route, however, has a number of significant disadvantages that must also be considered. Advantages include an almost universal acceptance by patients, ease of administration, and relative safety. Patients today are accustomed to taking drugs by mouth. It is quite rare to come upon an adult patient who objects to the oral route of administration. The younger child, however, often proves to be an unwilling recipient of orally administered drugs. Unwanted drug effects, such as overdosage, idiosyncrasy,

Table 3.1	Comparison of Routes of Drug Administration					
Route	**Cooperation***	**First-Pass Effect**	**Used for Sedation†**	**Children/Adults**	**Titration**	**Maximal Sedation Level Recommended‡**
Topical	2	–	0	na	–	na
Sublingual	2	–	1	–/+	–	1
Intranasal	1	–	2	+/–	–	2
Oral	2	+	1	+/+	–	2
Rectal	1	+	1	+/+	–	2
Transdermal	1	–	1	–/+	–	1
Subcutaneous	1	–	0	na	–	1
IM/SM	0	–	2/1	+/+	–	2
Inhalation	2	–	2	+/+	+	2
Intravenous	2	–	2	+/+	+	3
Intraarterial	2	–	0	na	–	na
Intrathecal (spinal)	2	–	0	na	+	na
Intramedullary	1	–	0	na	+	na
Intraperitoneal	0	–	0	na	–	na

IM, Intramuscular; *na*, not applicable; *SM*, submucosal.
*Key: Cooperation required, 2; cooperation not critical, 1; cooperation not necessary, 0.
†Strongly recommended, 2; somewhat recommended, 1; not recommended, 0.
‡Deep sedation, 3; moderate sedation, 2; minimal sedation, 1.

allergy, and drug side effects, may occur whenever any drug is administered by any route, but such reactions are less likely to be noted when a drug is administered orally. When they do occur, they are normally less intense than those reactions that develop following parenteral administration. This is not meant to imply that life-threatening situations do not arise following oral drug administration. Indeed, cardiac arrest and anaphylaxis after oral drug administration have been reported.[17,18]

Disadvantages of oral drug administration include a long latent period, unreliable drug absorption, an inability to easily achieve a desired drug effect (titration is not possible), and a prolonged duration of action. These represent significant disadvantages that serve to limit the clinical use of the oral route in the management of pain and anxiety in the outpatient environment.

Orally administered drugs must reach the stomach and small intestine, where most absorption into the circulatory system occurs. For most drugs, the onset of clinical effectiveness is not noted for approximately 30 minutes, the latent period. Drug absorption continues, and a peak plasma concentration, equivalent to the greatest degree of clinical effectiveness (e.g., pain or anxiety relief), is reached. With most orally administered drugs, this maximal clinical effect develops approximately 60 minutes after administration. Because of this slow onset of action and the delay in reaching maximal effect, it is impossible to titrate via the oral route. *Titration is defined as the administration of small incremental doses of a drug until a desired clinical action is observed.* The ability to titrate endows the administrator with control over a drug's actions and its ultimate effect. Titration

eliminates the need to make an educated "guesstimate" of the appropriate dose of a drug for a patient. The lack of ability to titrate via the oral route of administration is a considerable handicap to the effective use of this technique when central nervous system (CNS)–depressant drugs are administered. The clinician must administer a predetermined dose to the patient. This dose will be determined after consideration of a number of factors (discussed fully in Chapter 7). However, once the drug is administered, it becomes impossible to quickly enhance its actions, should the initial dose prove inadequate, or to rapidly reverse its effects, should an undesirable reaction develop.

The duration of action of most orally administered pain- and anxiety-controlling drugs is prolonged, approximately 3 to 4 hours. This duration is unacceptable for most dental procedures (for sedative drugs especially) because the patient will remain under the influence of the drug well into the posttreatment period and therefore be unable to leave the dentist's office unescorted. Patients receiving CNS-depressant drugs via the oral route must be advised against operating potentially dangerous machinery or driving a car (see drug package insert for all oral CNS depressants).

Orally administered drugs may be safely and effectively used for the management of pain in the postoperative period and for the management of anxiety in the preoperative period. Because of the significant disadvantages associated with it, the oral route of drug administration is not highly recommended for routine use in the management of intraoperative pain and anxiety. The oral route of drug administration is fully discussed in Chapter 7.

Rectal

The rectal route of drug administration is only occasionally employed in dentistry. Its primary use is in pediatric dentistry, where it is more common to encounter patients who are either unwilling or unable to take drugs by mouth.[19,20]

Advantages and disadvantages of the rectal route are similar to those of the oral route of drug administration. Rectal drug administration is discussed more fully in Chapter 8.

The techniques of drug administration that follow are those in which the drug is absorbed directly from its site of administration into the systemic circulation, effectively bypassing the gastrointestinal (GI) tract. Such techniques are given the name *parenteral* in contradistinction to the oral and rectal routes of administration in which drugs are absorbed from the GI tract into the enterohepatic circulation before entering the systemic circulation. These routes are termed *enteral* routes of administration. Common usage of the term *parenteral* usually denotes drug administration by injection with a syringe (e.g., IM, SC, IV). Though injection is not required, both intranasal and sublingual administration are properly termed parenteral techniques because drug absorption occurs directly into the systemic circulation.

Topical

The absorption of drugs through intact skin is quite poor; however, topically applied local anesthetics can be used to produce anesthesia of tissues where a layer of keratinized skin is absent, such as the mucous membranes of the mouth, nose, throat, trachea, bronchi, esophagus, stomach, urethra, bladder, vagina, and rectum.[21,22] Topical anesthesia, as used in dentistry, is a highly effective method of relieving some of the fear and pain potentially involved in the administration of injectable local anesthetics.[23,24] Topical application of drugs other than local anesthetics is not common.

Sublingual

Certain drugs can be administered sublingually (i.e., they can be absorbed into the blood through the mucous membranes of the oral cavity). Examples of the clinical use of sublingual drug administration include nitroglycerin for management of anginal pain[25] and triazolam for moderate sedation.[26]

An advantage of sublingual drug administration is that the drug enters directly into the systemic circulation, bypassing the enterohepatic circulation. In this way, the drug does not undergo the hepatic first-pass effect in which a percentage of the drug is biotransformed before ever having the opportunity to enter the systemic circulation and to reach its target organ (e.g., brain).[27]

Intranasal

IN drug administration has become significantly more popular since publication of the fourth edition of this text in 2003. IN drugs have been used primarily in pediatrics as a means of circumventing the need for injection or oral drug administration in uncooperative or precooperative patients.[28–32] Additionally, IN drugs have been employed with increasing frequency in emergency medicine as a means of terminating status epilepticus in younger patients in whom venous cannulation is difficult to achieve.[33,34] Absorption of IN drugs occurs directly into the systemic circulation, bypassing the enterohepatic circulation. Clinical trials have demonstrated that the absorption and bioavailability of intranasally administered drugs were close to those of IV administration, with peak plasma levels occurring 10 minutes after administration.[35,36]

Midazolam, a water-soluble benzodiazepine,[28-37] and sufentanil,[37-39] an opioid analgesic, have received the most attention via the IN route.

Transdermal

The transdermal route is a means of administering a drug, bypassing the GI tract, without the need for injection.[40] The drugs most frequently administered transdermally are scopolamine (primarily for the prevention of motion sickness and postsurgical nausea and vomiting),[41,42] nitroglycerin (for angina pectoris),[43] nicotine (for smoking cessation),[44] and opioids, such as fentanyl (for postsurgical analgesia).[45,46]

Transdermal drug administration is considered when a long-term course of drug therapy is necessary. Although rarely necessary in dentistry, there are situations (e.g., after surgery) in which transdermally administered analgesics might prove advantageous. Potential drawbacks to transdermal drug administration include the development of decreased responsiveness to the drug[47] and adverse skin reactions at the site of application.[48]

Subcutaneous

The subcutaneous (SC or SQ) route involves the injection of a drug beneath the skin into the subcutaneous tissues. It is useful for the administration of nonvolatile, water- or fat-soluble hypnotic and opioid drugs.[49] Drugs capable of producing tissue irritation, such as diazepam, are not recommended for SC administration.

The rate of drug absorption into the cardiovascular system (CVS) varies with the blood supply to the tissue. Subcutaneous tissues have a relatively limited blood supply; therefore absorption of drugs following SC administration is usually prolonged.

This slow rate of absorption following SC injection limits the effectiveness of this route in dentistry. Other more rapidly effective and controllable techniques are preferred and available.

Intramuscular

IM administration is a parenteral technique that maintains several advantages over enteral techniques, making it potentially useful in the management of pain and anxiety. However, the IM route pales in comparison with other parenteral methods of administration, especially the inhalation and IV routes. Of the major techniques used in dentistry (oral, IN, IM, inhalation, and IV), IM is the least commonly used.

Submucosal (SM) drug administration is similar to IM administration and was most often employed in pediatric dentistry. Its advantages and disadvantages are similar to those discussed for IM administration, except that the absorption of the drug is somewhat more rapid than that with the IM route.[50,51] Clinical consequences of this are significant, including a somewhat more rapid onset of action of the drug. Because of this more rapid onset, it is also possible for undesirable drug actions to develop more rapidly and to be somewhat more intense than those following IM administration. Problems associated with the SM route are reviewed in Chapter 10.

Advantages of IM administration over enteral routes include a more rapid onset of action (shorter latent period, approximately 10 minutes) and a more rapid onset of maximal clinical effect (approximately 30 minutes). Another advantage is the usually more reliable absorption of a drug into the CVS following IM rather than oral administration. In other words, 50 mg of a drug administered intramuscularly produces a more pronounced clinical effect than the same dose of drug given by mouth or rectally. Patient cooperation is not as critical as it is with most other techniques. This advantage is of particular importance in younger pediatric patients who are unwilling or unable to cooperate during drug administration. The child needs to be restrained only momentarily while the IM drug is administered.

Disadvantages of IM administration include its 10-minute latent period, a time factor that makes titration impossible. In addition, it is impossible to rapidly reverse the effect of a drug should overdose or other complications develop; patients may not be willing to accept the injection necessary to administer the drug; the prolonged duration of action (about 2 to 4 hours or more) requires that the patient be accompanied from the dentist's office by a responsible companion; and there is a possibility of injury to the tissues at the site of the injection caused by either the drug or the needle.

Several sites are available for IM injections. Whichever site is selected, it is important to become familiar with the anatomy of that area before administering any drug via the IM route.

As with the oral route, the IM route has several significant disadvantages. The IM route is not commonly used in dental practice; however, there are situations in which this route is valuable (e.g., drug administration during a medical emergency [e.g., epinephrine in anaphylaxis]). The inability to titrate IM drugs makes it unwise to attempt to achieve deep sedation or to attempt to control pain with this route unless the drug administrator is well trained in general anesthesia and maintains continual contact with the patient (i.e., does not send the patient home). In adult patients, there are limited indications for the administration of pain- and anxiety-controlling drugs via the IM route because the IV route is more effective, reliable, and controllable. One indication is when a longer duration of drug action is desirable, as in postsurgical pain relief or when naloxone is employed following IV drug administration. In patients with disabilities and in uncooperative or precooperative children, however, techniques that require any degree of patient cooperation (oral, inhalation, IV) are likely to prove impossible to use effectively, and the IM route (or, more commonly today, IN route) may be the only means of sedation available. General anesthesia may prove to be the only alternative treatment available to this patient. IM and SM administration of drugs for pain and anxiety control are discussed further in Chapter 10.

Inhalation (Pulmonary)

A variety of gaseous agents may be administered by inhalation to produce either sedation or general anesthesia. In dental practice, however, the inhalation route is virtually synonymous with the use of N_2O and O_2. N_2O, the first general anesthetic, has been in clinical use since 1844 in both medicine and dentistry. It is estimated that more than 35% of dentists practicing in the United States use this agent as an aid in patient management,[52] though in pediatric dentistry inhalation sedation is the most used sedation technique.[53] In addition, 31 states (2014 data) have enacted legislation permitting dental hygienists to administer N_2O-O_2.[54]

The advantages and disadvantages discussed here relate to inhalation anesthetics in general and to the use of N_2O-O_2 in particular. The latent period observed in the inhalation route is quite short. Arguably the inhalation route provides the most rapid onset of clinical action. After rapid passage through the mouth or nose, the trachea, and the lungs, the drug enters into the CVS. With some inhalation agents, such as N_2O, clinical effects may become noticeable as quickly as 15 to 30 seconds after inhalation. This extremely short latent period is used to advantage to permit titration of the drug to the patient. The ability to titrate is a major reason why N_2O-O_2 inhalation sedation is considered by many (including this author) to be the most ideal sedative technique currently available. In addition, the administrator of the gases possesses the ability to reverse the actions of the drug rapidly, should this become necessary. Indeed, the inhalation route is the only one in which drug actions can be quickly adjusted to either increase or decrease the depth of sedation. With IV sedation, drug action may easily be enhanced; however, it is not possible to lessen the level of sedation unless a specific pharmacologic antagonist is available.

Recovery from inhalation moderate sedation is also quite rapid and complete. In an outpatient medical or dental practice, rapid recovery is important because it permits the doctor to discharge virtually all patients receiving N_2O-O_2 from the office unaccompanied by a responsible adult companion. Most patients may return to their work, drive a motor vehicle, or operate machinery without undue concern for their well-being. The latter is an advantage possessed only by inhalation sedation using N_2O-O_2.

A few disadvantages are associated with the use of the inhalation route. N_2O is not a very potent anesthetic, and when given with at least 20% O_2 (as it always should be), there will be a certain percentage of patients in whom this technique will fail to produce the desired results. Patient cooperation is required for the successful use of inhalation sedation; the lack of such cooperation is a significant disadvantage. This will most often be observed in the management of disruptive children and children and adults with disabilities. In the dental setting, patients must be capable of breathing through their nose. As used in the operating theater setting as a component of a general anesthetic, inhalation agents may be delivered through both the mouth and nose; this is, of course, not possible in dentistry. Dental patients unable to breathe through their nose will find the use of inhalation sedation quite uncomfortable. Physicians and other health care professionals employing N_2O-O_2 while treating patients at sites other than the oral cavity (e.g., arm, foot) will be able to use either the nose and/or mouth as a portal of entry for the gaseous agents, an advantage over their dental colleagues.

Two minor disadvantages of the inhalation route include the size and cost of the equipment and the additional training and expense required for the safe administration of N_2O-O_2. It is especially important that all health care personnel employing inhalation sedation be well trained in all aspects of its clinical application.

N_2O-O_2 inhalation sedation is the technique of choice for most dental procedures and many minor surgical procedures that require intraoperative anxiety control. Pain, however, is not consistently controlled when N_2O-O_2 is employed, and its use as an analgesic in lieu of local anesthesia cannot be recommended primarily because of the high degree of effectiveness and safety of local anesthetics and because of the increased incidence of unwanted side effects that may accompany the increased concentration of N_2O required to produce profound analgesia. Inhalation sedation is described in depth in Section IV, Chapters 11 through 19.

Intravenous

The IV route of drug administration represents the most effective method of ensuring predictable and adequate sedation in virtually all patients. Effective blood levels of drugs are achieved quite rapidly.

Advantages of IV drug administration include its short latent period of about 20 to 25 seconds (permitting drugs to be titrated) and the ability to rapidly enhance the action of a drug, if necessary. In clinical practice, a drug used intravenously for sedation will require approximately 2 to 5 minutes for titration to the desired effect to be achieved. An additional advantage possessed by many intravenously administered CNS-depressant drugs is that they provide amnesic periods of varying duration. Dental or surgical procedures (e.g., colonoscopy[55]) that are feared by the patient, such as the injection of local anesthetics, may be carried out during the amnesic period.

Disadvantages of drugs administered by IV include an inability to reverse the actions of all drugs after they have been injected. Although it is possible to reverse the actions of some drugs (e.g., opioids, anticholinergics, and benzodiazepines) through the use of specific drug antagonists, this is not always the case. The rapid onset of action of intravenously injected drugs and their accentuated clinical actions can lead to more exaggerated problems, such as overdosage, side effects, and allergic manifestations, than are seen with other, less effective, routes of drug administration. The entire office staff must therefore be well trained in the use of these drugs and in the recognition and management of associated adverse reactions and emergencies.

Patient cooperation is a requirement if venipuncture is to be successful. Many children will not permit venipuncture to be performed; therefore IV sedation is rarely indicated or attempted in these disruptive patients. Conversely a cooperative child, willing to sit still and permit venipuncture to proceed, probably does not require a technique such as IV sedation for his or her dental care. Intraoral injections of local anesthetics might possibly be carried out with a little more patience on the part of the dentist and perhaps with another technique of sedation, such as inhalation sedation. However, patients with disabilities (both physical and mental) are usually good candidates for IV sedation. These patients may be incapable of cooperation during dental therapy, but, once sedated, frequently become quite manageable.

IV sedation may not be suitable for all dentists and physicians. Most doctors are uncomfortable with the technique during their early exposure to it; however, as they gain clinical experience, they gradually become more comfortable and relaxed. A small percentage, however, remain uneasy with the technique and will be unable to provide a quality of dental or surgical care up to their usual standard. It is important to remember that regardless of the route of drug administration used, the quality of the dental or surgical care delivered should not be compromised.

IV sedation is not a panacea. Indeed, no technique of sedation is a panacea. Although the IV route provides the most effective technique of sedation available, the occasional patient will be encountered in whom IV drugs within recommended (e.g., reasonable) doses prove ineffective. A concern of many involved with the teaching of IV sedation is that intravenously administered drugs will always prove to be effective if a large enough dose is administered. In many cases, however, this course of action will result in the loss of consciousness (general anesthesia, not sedation), and unless the doctor and staff are well versed in recognizing and managing the unconscious patient, grave complications may develop (the concept of 'Rescue' is discussed in Chapter 2).

The IV route of administration is most often reserved for the management of the more fearful patient. Drugs and techniques are available that permit the effective management of fear for varying lengths of time. IV drug administration is occasionally used for patients in whom it is difficult to achieve adequate pain control following local anesthetic administration alone. Small doses of opioid analgesics administered intravenously in conjunction with intraoral local anesthesia may produce adequate pain control without increased risk to the patient. IV sedation is discussed in detail in Section V, Chapters 20 through 29.

To this point we have been able to manage successfully approximately 99% of our dental patients using one or more of the techniques discussed. In the remaining 1%, various factors, such as intense fear or biologic variability, act to produce management failures. General anesthesia is usually required for these patients.

We now approach a very important barrier in the spectrum of pain and anxiety control (see Fig. 3.1). As we cross this barrier, we are dealing with the unconscious patient and with general anesthesia. The patient can no longer respond to command, and his or her protective reflexes are no longer intact.

GENERAL ANESTHESIA

The importance of general anesthesia in dentistry is illustrated by the fact that in excess of 5 million persons annually receive general anesthesia on an ambulatory basis in the United States, the overwhelming majority of these in outpatient dental settings (private practice, surgicenters).[56] About 16% of all general anesthetics administered in the United States annually are administered in conjunction with dental care.[57]

General anesthesia was the first technique of pain and anxiety control introduced into the practice of medicine and dentistry. Though still used extensively in the practice of medicine (although the use of sedation is growing rapidly), its use in dentistry has declined since the introduction of the techniques of sedation, primarily IV sedation with midazolam. Several advantages to general anesthesia are a rapid onset of action, high effectiveness, and reliability. However, its disadvantages frequently outweigh the advantages. These include an increased risk to the patient and the requirement of an intensive training program (minimum 3 years) in anesthesiology to prepare the dentist to manage the unconscious patient safely.[2,3] The majority of general anesthetics employed in dentistry are for oral surgical procedures; however, there are many indications for their use in other procedures, such as restorations and hygiene, especially in the disruptive child or in the child or adult patient with a physical or mental disability.[58]

The step from management of the conscious patient (minimal, moderate sedation) to management of the unconscious patient (general anesthesia) is a significant one, requiring an absolute minimum of 3 years of training in the principles and techniques of general anesthesia.[2,3] General anesthesia is further discussed in Section VI, Chapters 30 and 31.

REFERENCES

1. American Society of Anesthesiologists Task Force on Sedation and Analgesia by Non-Anesthesiologists: Practice guidelines for sedation and analgesia by non-anesthesiologists. *Anesthesiology* 96(4):1004–1017, 2002.
2. House of Delegates American Dental Association: Guidelines for the use of sedation and general anesthesia by dentists, Adopted Oct 2016, ADA House of Delegates. www.ada.org.
3. House of Delegates American Dental Association: Guidelines for teaching pain control and sedation to dentists and dental students, adopted Oct. 2016, ADA House of Delegates. Available at www.ada.org.
4. Bing J, McAuliffe MS, Lupton JR: Regional anesthesia with monitored anesthesia care for dermatologic laser surgery. *Dermatol Clin* 20(1):123–134, 2002.
5. Olsha O, Feldman A, Odenheimer DB, Frankel D: Local anesthesia for inguinal hernia repair in adolescents. *Hernia* 11(6):497–500, 2007.
6. Bernal-Sprekelsen M, Schmelzer A: Local anesthesia of the head and neck. *Anesth Pain Control* 1.81, 1992.
7. Davis JE: Ambulatory surgery ... how far can we go? *Med Clin North Am* 77:365, 1993.
8. Friedman N: Iatrosedation. In McCarthy FM, editor: *Emergencies in dental practice*, ed 3, Philadelphia, 1979, WB Saunders.
9. Milgrom P: Treatment of the distrustful patient. In Weinstein P, Milgrom P, Getz T, editors: *Treating fearful dental patients: a patient management handbook*, ed 2, Seattle, 1995, University of Washington Press.
10. Shapiro RS, Simpson DE, Lawrence SL: A survey of sued and nonsued physicians and suing patients. *Arch Intern Med* 149:2190, 1989.
11. Roberts K: Hypnosis in dentistry. *Dent Update* 33(5):312–314, 2006.
12. Thayer ML: The use of acupuncture in dentistry. *Dent Update* 34(4):244–246, 249–250, 2007.
13. Wismeijer AA, Vingerhoets AJ: The use of virtual reality and audiovisual eyeglass systems as adjunct analgesic techniques: a review of the literature. *Ann Behav Med* 30(3):268–278, 2005.
14. Little JW: Complementary and alternative medicine: impact on dentistry. *Oral Surg Oral Med Oral Pathol Oral Radiol Endod* 98(2):137–145, 2004.
15. Meechan JG, Gowans AJ, Welbury RR: The use of patient-controlled transcutaneous electronic nerve stimulation (TENS) to decrease the discomfort of regional anaesthesia in dentistry: a randomised controlled clinical trial. *J Dent* 26(5-6):417–420, 1998.
16. Malamed SF: A most powerful drug. *J Calif Acad Gen Dent* 4:17, 1979.
17. Chugh SS, Socoteanu C, Reinier K, et al: A community-based evaluation of sudden death associated with therapeutic levels of methadone. *Am J Med* 121(1):66–71, 2008.
18. Gill CJ, Michaelides PL: Dental drugs and anaphylactic reactions: report of a case. *Oral Surg* 50:30, 1980.
19. Flaitz CM, Nowak AJ, Hicks MJ: Evaluation of anterograde amnesic effect of rectally administered diazepam in the sedated pedodontic patient. *J Dent Child* 53:17, 1986.
20. Jensen B, Matsson L: Benzodiazepines in child dental care: a survey of its use among general practitioners and paediatric dentists in Sweden. *Swed Dent J* 25(1):31–38, 2001.
21. Ernst AA, Marvez-Valls E, Nick TG, et al: TAC (lidocaine-adrenaline-tetracaine) versus TAC (tetracaine-adrenaline-cocaine) for topical anesthesia in face and scalp lacerations. *Am J Emerg Med* 13(2):151–154, 1995.
22. Erdurmus M, Aydin B, Usta B, et al: Patient comfort and surgeon satisfaction during cataract surgery using topical anesthesia with or without dexmedetomidine sedation. *Eur J Ophthalmol* 18(3):361–367, 2008.
23. Carr MP, Horton JE: Clinical evaluation and comparison of 2 topical anesthetics for pain caused by needle sticks and scaling and root planning. *J Periodontol* 72(4):479–484, 2001.

24. Deepika A, Rao CR, Vinay C, et al: Effectiveness of two flavored topical anesthetic agents in reducing injection pain in children: a comparative study. *J Clin Pediatr Dent* 37(1):15–18, 2012.

25. Diker E, Ertuerk A, Akguen G: Is sublingual nifedipine administration superior to oral administration in the active treatment of hypertension? *Angiology* 43:477, 1992.

26. Pickrell JE, Hosaka K, Jackson DL, et al: Expanded studies of the pharmacokinetics and clinical effects of multidose sublingual triazolam in healthy volunteers. *J Clin Psychopharmacol* 29(5):426–431, 2009.

27. Konttinen VK, Maunuksela EL, Sarvela J: Premedication with sublingual triazolam compared with oral diazepam. *Can J Anaesth* 40(9):829–834, 1993.

28. Wood M: The safety and efficacy of intranasal midazolam sedation combined with inhalation sedation with nitrous oxide and oxygen in paediatric dental patients as an alternative to general anaesthesia. *SAAD Dig* 26:12–22, 2010.

29. Johnson E, Briskie D, Majewski R, et al: The physiologic and behavioral effects of oral and intranasal midazolam in pediatric dental patients. *Pediatr Dent* 32(3):229–238, 2010.

30. Heard C, Smith J, Creighton P, et al: A comparison of four sedation techniques for pediatric dental surgery. *Paediatr Anaesth* 20(10):924–930, 2010.

31. Chopra R, Mittal M, Bansal K, Chaudhuri P: Buccal midazolam spray as an alternative to intranasal route for conscious sedation in pediatric dentistry. *J Clin Pediatr Dent* 38(2):171–173, 2013.

32. Lam C, Udin RD, Malamed SF, et al: Midazolam premedication in children: a pilot study comparing intramuscular and intranasal administration. *Anesth Prog* 52(2):56–61, 2005.

33. Sanchez Fernandez I, Loddenkemper T: Therapeutic choices in convulsive status epilepticus. *Expert Opin Pharmacother* 16(4):487–500, 2015.

34. Mula M: The safety and tolerability of intranasal midazolam in epilepsy. *Expert Rev Neurother* 14(7):735–740, 2014.

35. Rey E, Delaunay L, Pons G, et al: Pharmacokinetics of midazolam in children: comparative study of intranasal and intravenous administration. *Eur J Clin Pharmacol* 41:355–357, 1991.

36. Walbergh EJ, Wills RJ, Eckhert J: Plasma concentrations of midazolam in children following intranasal administration. *Anesthesiology* 74:233, 1991.

37. Lundeberg S, Roelofse JA: Aspects of pharmacokinetics and pharmacodynamics of sufentanil in pediatric practice. *Paediatr Anaesth* 21(3):274–279, 2011.

38. Roelofse JA, Shipton EA, de la Harpe CJ: Intranasal sufentanil/midazolam versus ketamine/midazolam for analgesia/sedation in the pediatric population prior to undergoing multiple dental extractions under general anesthesia: a prospective, double-blind, randomized comparison [see comment]. *Anesth Prog* 51(4):114–121, 2004.

39. Bayrak F, Gunday I, Memis D, et al: A comparison of oral midazolam, oral tramadol, and intranasal sufentanil premedication in pediatric patients. *J Opioid Manage* 3(2):74–78, 2007.

40. Asmussen B: Transdermal therapeutic systems: actual state and future developments. *Methods Find Exp Clin Pharmacol* 13:343, 1991.

41. Pergolizzi JV, Jr, Philip BK, Leslie JB, et al: Perspectives on transdermal scopolamine for the treatment of postoperative nausea and vomiting. *J Clin Anesth* 24(4):334–345, 2012.

42. Santamaria LB, Fodale V, Mandolfino T, et al: Transdermal scopolamine reduces nausea, vomiting and sialorrhea in the postoperative period in teeth and mouth surgery. *Minerva Anesthesiol* 57:686, 1991.

43. Cowan JC, Beatt KJ, Williams DO, Reid DS: Transdermal nitroglycerin. *Lancet* 2(8460):899, 1985.

44. Doggrell SA: Which is the best primary medication for long-term smoking cessation–nicotine replacement therapy, bupropion or varenicline? *Expert Opin Pharmacother* 8(17):2903–2915, 2007.

45. Abrisham SM, Ghahramani R, Heiranizadeh N, et al: Pahlavanhosseini H: Reduced morphine consumption and pain severity with transdermal fentanyl patches following total knee arthroplasty. *Knee Surg Sports Traumatol Arthrosc* 22(7):1580–1584, 2014.

46. Merivirta R, Aarimaa V, Aantaa R, et al: Postoperative fentanyl patch versus subacromial bupivacaine infusion in arthroscopic shoulder surgery. *Arthroscopy* 29(7):1129–1134, 2013.

47. Parker JO: Nitrate tolerance: a problem during continuous nitrate administration. *Eur J Clin Pharmacol* 38(Suppl 1):21, 1990.

48. Hogan DJ, Maibach HI: Adverse dermatologic reactions to transdermal drug delivery systems. *J Am Acad Dermatol* 22(Pt 1):811, 1990.

49. Dugas R: Subcutaneous drug administration. An alternative used in palliative care. *Can Fam Physician* 47:266–267, 2001.

50. Roberts SM, Wilson CF, Seale NS, et al: Evolution of morphine as compared to meperidine when administered to moderately anxious pediatric dental patients. *Pediatr Dent* 14:306, 1992.

51. Donaldson M, Goodchild JH: Maximum cumulative doses of sedation medications for in-office use. *Gen Dent* 55(2):143–148, 2007.

52. Jastak JT, Donaldson D: Nitrous oxide. *Anesth Prog* 38:172, 1991.

53. Haupt M: Project USAP 2000—Use of sedative agents by pediatric dentists: a 15-year follow-up survey. *Pediatr Dent* 24:289–294, 2002.

54. States where dental hygienists can administer nitrous oxide. American Dental Hygienists Association, Chicago, IL, November 2014. Available at www.adha.org. (Accessed 21 July 2015).

55. Triantafillidis JK, Merikas E, Nikolakis D, Papalois AE: Sedation in gastrointestinal endoscopy: current issues. *World J Gastroenterol* 19(4):463–481, 2013.

56. Flick WG, Katsnelson A, Alstrom H: Illinois dental anesthesia and sedation survey for. *Anesth Prog* 54(2):52–58, 2007, 2006.

57. Stapleton M, Sheller B, Williams BJ, et al: Combining procedures under general anesthesia. *Pediatr Dent* 29(5):397–402, 2007.

58. Savanheimo N, Sundberg SA, Virtanen JI, Vehkalahti MM: Dental care and treatments provided under general anaesthesia in the Helsinki Public Dental Service. *BMC Oral Health* 12:45, 2012.

chapter 4

Physical and Psychological Evaluation

*B*efore a new patient is treated, it is important that the dentist and staff become acquainted with the patient's medical history. This is true in all situations, regardless of whether or not the patient is to receive drugs for pain or anxiety control. Because dental care can have a profound effect on both the physical and psychological well-being of the patient, it is extremely important for the person treating the patient to know beforehand the most likely problems to be encountered. It has been stated that "when you prepare for an emergency, the emergency ceases to exist."[1] Prior knowledge of a patient's physical status enables the dentist to modify the proposed treatment plan to better meet the patient's limit of tolerance. This is of special importance whenever the administration of a drug for the management of pain (e.g., local anesthetic) or anxiety (e.g., central nervous system [CNS] depressant) is planned. The administration of certain drugs used in dentistry is specifically (relatively or absolutely) contraindicated in patients with some disease states. Knowledge of these contraindications is critical if potentially serious complications are to be prevented.

GOALS OF PHYSICAL AND PSYCHOLOGICAL EVALUATION

In the following discussion, a comprehensive but easy-to-use program of physical evaluation is described.[2,3] Used as recommended, it allows the dentist to accurately determine any potential risk presented by the patient before the start of treatment. The following are the goals that are sought in the use of this system:

1. To determine the patient's ability to tolerate **physically** the stresses involved in the planned dental treatment
2. To determine the patient's ability to tolerate **psychologically** the stresses involved in the planned dental treatment
3. To determine whether treatment modification is indicated to enable the patient to better tolerate the stresses of dental treatment
4. To determine whether the use of sedation is indicated
5. To determine which technique of sedation is most appropriate for the patient
6. To determine whether contraindications exist to (1) the planned dental treatment and (2) any of the drugs to be used.

The first two goals involve the patient's ability to tolerate the stress involved in the planned dental care. Stress may be of either a physiologic or psychological nature. Patients with underlying medical problems may be less able to tolerate the usual levels of stress associated with various types of dental care. These patients are more likely to experience an acute exacerbation of their underlying medical problem(s) during periods of increased stress. Such disease processes include angina pectoris, seizure disorders, asthma, and sickle cell disease. Although most of these patients will be able to tolerate the planned dental care in relative safety, it is the obligation of the dentist and staff to determine whether this problem does exist and the severity of the problem and how it might impact the proposed dental treatment plan.

Excessive stress can also prove detrimental to the nonmedically compromised (e.g., "healthy") patient. Fear, anxiety, and acute pain produce abrupt changes in the homeostasis of the body that may prove detrimental. Many "healthy" patients suffer from fear-related emergencies, including hyperventilation and vasodepressor syncope (vasovagal syncope, "fainting").

The third goal is to determine whether or not to modify the usual treatment regimen for a patient to enable the patient to better tolerate the stress of treatment. In some cases, a healthy patient will be psychologically unable to tolerate the planned treatment. Treatment may be modified to minimize the stress faced by this patient. The medically compromised patient will also benefit from treatment modification aimed at minimizing stress. The stress-reduction protocols (SRPs) discussed in this chapter are designed to aid the dentist in minimizing treatment-related stress in both the healthy and medically compromised patient.

When it is believed that the patient will require some assistance in coping with his or her dental treatment, the use of psychosedation should be considered. The last three goals involve the determination of the need for use of psychosedation, selection of the most appropriate technique, and selection of the most appropriate drug(s) for patient management.

PHYSICAL EVALUATION

The term *physical evaluation* is used to discuss the steps involved in fulfilling the aforementioned goals. Physical evaluation in dentistry consists of the following three components:
1. Medical history questionnaire
2. Physical examination
3. Dialog history

With the information (database) collected from these three steps, the dentist will be better able to (1) determine the physical and psychological status of the patient (establish a risk factor classification for the patient); (2) seek medical consultation, if indicated; and (3) appropriately modify the planned dental treatment, if indicated. Each of the three steps in the evaluation process is discussed in general terms, with specific emphasis placed on its importance in the evaluation of the patient for whom pharmacosedation is considered.

Medical History Questionnaire

The use of a written, patient-completed medical history questionnaire is a moral and legal necessity in the practice of both medicine and dentistry. These questionnaires provide the dentist with valuable information about the physical, and in some cases the psychological, condition of the prospective patient.

Many types of medical history questionnaires are available; however, most are simply modifications of two basic types: the "short" form and the "long" form. The *short-form* medical history questionnaire provides basic information concerning a patient's medical history and is best suited for use by a dentist with considerable clinical experience in physical evaluation. When using the short-form history, the dentist must have a firm grasp of the appropriate dialog history required to aid in a determination of the relative risk presented by the patient. The dentist should also be experienced in the use of the techniques of physical evaluation and their interpretation. Unfortunately, most dentists use the short form or a modification of it in their office primarily as a convenience to their patients and themselves. The *long form,* on the other hand, provides a more detailed database concerning the physical condition of the prospective patient. It is used most often in teaching situations and represents a more ideal instrument for teaching physical evaluation.

Computer-generated medical history questionnaires have been developed and are increasing in popularity.[4,5] These questionnaires permit patients to enter their responses to questions electronically on a computer. Whenever a positive response is given, the computer asks additional questions related to the positive response. In effect, the computer asks the questions called for in the dialog history.

Any medical history questionnaire can prove to be extremely valuable or entirely worthless. The ultimate value of the questionnaire resides in the ability of the dentist to interpret the significance of the answers and to elicit additional information through physical examination and dialog history.

In this sixth edition of *Sedation,* I have again included as the prototypical adult health history questionnaire one that has been developed by the University of the Pacific (UOP) School of Dentistry in conjunction with MetLife (Fig. 4.1). Fig. 4.2 is an example of a pediatric medical history questionnaire.

This health history has been translated into 36 different languages, comprising the languages spoken by 95% of the persons on this planet. The cost of the translation was supported by several organizations, including the California Dental Association, but most extensively by MetLife Dental. The health history (see Fig. 4.1), translations of the health history (Fig. 4.3), the interview sheet (Fig. 4.4), medical consultation form (Fig. 4.5), and protocols for the dental management of medically complex patients may be found on the UOP website at *www.dental.pacific.edu* under Dental Professionals and then under Health History Forms. Protocols for management of medically complex patients can be found at the same website under Dental Practice Documents. Translations of the medical history form can also be found at *www.metdental.com* under Multi-Language Medical Health History Forms Available.

The health history was translated, keeping the same question-numbering sequence. Thereby a dentist who speaks English and is caring for a patient who does not can ask the patient

MetLife	**HEALTH HISTORY**	University of the Pacific
	English	

Patient Name:_____   Patient Identification Number:_____

Birth Date:_____

I. CIRCLE APPROPRIATE ANSWER (leave blank if you do not understand question):

1.	Yes	No	Is your general health good?
2.	Yes	No	Has there been a change in your health within the last year?
3.	Yes	No	Have you been hospitalized or had a serious illness in the last three years?
			If YES, why?_____
4.	Yes	No	Are you being treated by a physician now? For what? _____
			Date of last medical exam?_____Date of last dental exam _____
5.	Yes	No	Have you had problems with prior dental treatment?
6.	Yes	No	Are you in pain now?

II. HAVE YOU EXPERIENCED:

7.	Yes	No	Chest pain (angina)?	18.	Yes	No	Dizziness?
8.	Yes	No	Swollen ankles?	19.	Yes	No	Ringing in ears?
9.	Yes	No	Shortness of breath?	20.	Yes	No	Headaches?
10.	Yes	No	Recent weight loss, fever, night sweats?	21.	Yes	No	Fainting spells?
11.	Yes	No	Persistent cough, coughing up blood?	22.	Yes	No	Blurred vision?
12.	Yes	No	Bleeding problems, bruising easily?	23.	Yes	No	Seizures?
13.	Yes	No	Sinus problems?	24.	Yes	No	Excessive thirst?
14.	Yes	No	Difficulty swallowing?	25.	Yes	No	Frequent urination?
15.	Yes	No	Diarrhea, constipation, blood in stools?	26.	Yes	No	Dry mouth?
16.	Yes	No	Frequent vomiting, nausea?	27.	Yes	No	Jaundice?
17.	Yes	No	Difficulty urinating, blood in urine?	28.	Yes	No	Joint pain, stiffness?

III. DO YOU HAVE OR HAVE YOU HAD:

29.	Yes	No	Heart disease?	40.	Yes	No	AIDS?
30.	Yes	No	Heart attack, heart defects?	41.	Yes	No	Tumors, cancer?
31.	Yes	No	Heart murmurs?	42.	Yes	No	Arthritis, rheumatism?
32.	Yes	No	Rheumatic fever?	43.	Yes	No	Eye diseases?
33.	Yes	No	Stroke, hardening of arteries?	44.	Yes	No	Skin diseases?
34.	Yes	No	High blood pressure?	45.	Yes	No	Anemia?
35.	Yes	No	Asthma, TB, emphysema, other lung diseases?	46.	Yes	No	VD (syphilis or gonorrhea)?
36.	Yes	No	Hepatitis, other liver disease?	47.	Yes	No	Herpes?
37.	Yes	No	Stomach problems, ulcers?	48.	Yes	No	Kidney, bladder disease?
38.	Yes	No	Allergies to: drugs, foods, medications, latex?	49.	Yes	No	Thyroid, adrenal disease?
39.	Yes	No	Family history of diabetes, heart problems, tumors?	50.	Yes	No	Diabetes?

IV. DO YOU HAVE OR HAVE YOU HAD:

51.	Yes	No	Psychiatric care?	56.	Yes	No	Hospitalization?
52.	Yes	No	Radiation treatments?	57.	Yes	No	Blood transfusions?
53.	Yes	No	Chemotherapy?	58.	Yes	No	Surgeries?
54.	Yes	No	Prosthetic heart valve?	59.	Yes	No	Pacemaker?
55.	Yes	No	Artificial joint?	60.	Yes	No	Contact lenses?

V. ARE YOU TAKING:

61.	Yes	No	Recreational drugs?	63.	Yes	No	Tobacco in any form?
62.	Yes	No	Drugs, medications, over-the-counter medicines (including aspirin), natural remedies?	64.	Yes	No	Alcohol?

Please list:_____

VI. WOMEN ONLY:

65.	Yes	No	Are you or could you be pregnant or nursing?	66.	Yes	No	Taking birth control pills?

VII. ALL PATIENTS:

67.	Yes	No	Do you have or have you had any other diseases or medical problems NOT listed on this form?

If so, please explain:_____

To the best of my knowledge, I have answered every question completely and accurately. I will inform my dentist of any change in my health and/or medication.

Patient's signature:_____   Date:_____

RECALL REVIEW:

1. Patient's signature_____   Date:_____

2. Patient's signature_____   Date:_____

3. Patient's signature_____   Date:_____

The Health History is created and maintained by the University of the Pacific School of Dentistry, San Francisco, California.
Support for the translation and dissemination of the Health Histories comes from MetLife Dental Care.

Figure 4.1 Adult health history questionnaire. (Reprinted with permission from University of the Pacific Arthur A. Dugoni School of Dentistry in San Francisco, CA.)

to complete the health history in his or her own language. The dentist then compares the English health history with the patient's translated health history, scanning the translated version for "yes" responses. When a "yes" is found, the dentist is able to look at the question number and match it to the question number on the English version. For example, the dentist would know that a "yes" response to question 34 on the non-English version is the same as question 34 on the English version and relates to high blood pressure (HBP). For that matter, a Chinese-speaking dentist could also use the multilanguage health history with an English-speaking patient and have the same cross-referenced information. A dentist who speaks Spanish could

Child's Name: _____ Date of Birth: _____ Age _____ Date: _____
Address: _____ Telephone: ( )
Physician's name (Medical Doctor): _____ Telephone: ( )

Please circle the appropriate answer

1. Does your child have a health problem? .... YES NO
2. Was your child a patient in a hospital? .... YES NO
3. Date of last physical exam: _____
4. Is your child now under medical care? .... YES NO
5. Is your child taking medication now? .... YES NO
   If so, for what? _____.
6. Has your child ever had a serious illness or operation? YES NO
7. If so, explain: _____
8. Does your child have (or ever had) any of the following diseases?
   a. Rheumatic fever or rheumatic heart disease ... YES NO
   b. Congenital heart disease .... YES NO
   c. Cardiovascular disease (heart trouble, heart attack, coronary insufficiency, coronary occlusion, high blood pressure, arteriosclerosis, stroke) .... YES NO
   d. Allergy? Food □, Medicine □, Other □ .. YES NO
   e. Asthma □ Hay Fever □ .... YES NO
   f. Hives or a skin rash .... YES NO
   g. Fainting spells or seizures .... YES NO
   h. Hepatitis, jaundice or liver disease .... YES NO
   i. Diabetes .... YES NO
   j. Inflammatory rheumatism (painful or swollen joints) .... YES NO
   k. Arthritis .... YES NO
   l. Stomach ulcers .... YES NO
   m. Kidney trouble .... YES NO
   n. Tuberculosis (TB) .... YES NO
   o. Persistent cough or cough up blood .... YES NO
   p. Veneral disease .... YES NO
   q. Epilepsy .... YES NO
   r. Sickle Cell disease .... YES NO
   s. Thyroid disease .... YES NO
   t. AIDS .... YES NO
   u. Emphysema .... YES NO
   v. Psychiatric treatment .... YES NO
   w. Cleft lip/palate .... YES NO
   x. Cerebral palsy .... YES NO
   y. Mental retardation .... YES NO
   z. Hearing disability .... YES NO
   aa. Developmental disability .... YES NO
      If yes, explain: _____
   bb. Was your child premature? .... YES NO
      If yes, how many weeks _____
   cc. Other: _____
9. Does your child have to urinate (pass water) more than six times a day? .... YES NO
10. Is your child thirsty much of the time? .... YES NO
11. Has your child had abnormal bleeding associated with previous surgery, extractions or accidents? .... YES NO
12. Does he/she bruise easily? .... YES NO

13. Has he/she ever required a blood transfusion? ..... YES NO
14. Does he/she have any blood disorders such as anemia, etc? .... YES NO
15. Has he/she ever had surgery, x-ray or chemotherapy for a tumor, growth, or other condition? .... YES NO
16. Does your child have a disability that prevents treatment in a dental office? .... YES NO
17. Is he/she taking any of the following?
   a. Antibiotics or sulfa drugs .... YES NO
   b. Anticoagulants (blood thinners) .... YES NO
   c. Medicine for high blood pressure .... YES NO
   d. Cortisone or steroids .... YES NO
   e. Tranquilizers .... YES NO
   f. Aspirin .... YES NO
   g. Dilantin or other anticonvulsant .... YES NO
   h. Insulin, tolbutamide, Orinase, or similar drug ... YES NO
   i. Any other? _____
18. Is he/she allergic to, or has he/she ever reacted adversely to, any of the following?
   a. Local anesthetics .... YES NO
   b. Penicillin or other antibiotics .... YES NO
   c. Sulfa drugs .... YES NO
   d. Barbituates, sedatives, or sleeping pills .... YES NO
   e. Aspirin .... YES NO
   f. Any other? _____
19. Has he/she any serious trouble associated with any previous dental treatment? .... YES NO
   If so, please explain: _____
20. Has your child been in any situation which could expose him/her to x-rays or other ionizing radiators? ...... YES NO
21. Last date of dental examination: _____
22. Has he/she ever had orthodontic treatment (worn braces)? .... YES NO
23. Has he/she ever been treated for any gum diseases (gingivitis, periodontitis, trenchmouth, pyorrhea)? ..... YES NO
24. Does his/her gums bleed when brushing teeth? .... YES NO
25. Does he/she grind or clench teeth? .... YES NO
26. Has he/she often had toothaches? .... YES NO
27. Has he/she had frequent sores in his/her mouth? .. YES NO
28. Has he/she had any injuries to his/her mouth or jaws? YES NO
   If yes, explain: _____
29. Does he/she have any sores or swellings of his/her mouth or jaws? .... YES NO
30. Have you been satisfied with your child's previous dental care? .... YES NO

ADOLESCENT WOMEN:
31. Are you pregnant now, or think you may be? .... YES NO
32. Do you anticipate becoming pregnant? .... YES NO
33. Are you taking the pill? .... YES NO

To the best of my knowledge, all of the preceding answers are true and correct. If my child ever has a change in his/her health or his/her medicines change, I will inform the doctor at the next appointment without fail.

Parent's Signature: _____ Date _____

MEDICAL HISTORY / PHYSICAL EXAMINATION REVIEW

Date   Addition   Student/Faculty Signatures

Figure 4.2 Pediatric medical history questionnaire. (From Malamed SF: Medical emergencies in the dental office, ed 6, St Louis, 2007, Mosby.)

use the multilanguage health history with a patient who speaks French. With the uniform health history question sequence, these health history translations can serve patients and dentists all around the world.

The health history is divided into sections related to signs and symptoms ("Have you experienced?"), diagnosed diseases ("Do you have or have you had?"), medical treatments (including drugs and other physiologically active compounds), and several other questions.

Although both long- and short-form medical history questionnaires are valuable in determining a patient's physical condition, a criticism of most available health history questionnaires is the absence of questions relating to the patient's attitudes toward dentistry. It is recommended that one or both of the following questions that relate to this all-important subject be included:

(1) *Do you feel very nervous about having dentistry treatment?*
(2) *Have you ever had a bad experience in the dental office?*

MetLife

Historia Médica
Spanish

University of the Pacific

Nombre del paciente: _____   No. de Ident. del Paciente: _____

Fecha de nacimiento: _____

I. MARQUE CON UN CÍRCULO LA RESPUESTA CORRECTA (Deje en BLANCO si no entiende la pregunta):

1. Sí   No   ¿Está en buena salud general?
2. Sí   No   ¿Han habido cambios en su salud durante el último año?
3. Sí   No   ¿Ha estado hospitalizado/a o ha tenido de una enfermedad grave en los últimos tres años?

   ¿Si Sí, por qué? _____

4. Sí   No   ¿Se encuentra actualmente bajo tratamiento médico? ¿Para qué? _____

   Fecha de su último examen médico: _____   Fecha de su última cita dental: _____

5. Sí   No   ¿Ha tenido problemas con algún tratamiento dental en el pasado?
6. Sí   No   ¿Tiene algún dolor ahora?

II. HA NOTADO:

7. Sí   No   ¿Dolor de pecho (angina)?
8. Sí   No   ¿Los tobillos hinchados?
9. Sí   No   ¿Falta de aliento?
10. Sí   No   ¿Reciente pérdida de peso, fiebre, sudor en la noche?
11. Sí   No   ¿Tos persistente o tos con sangre?
12. Sí   No   ¿Problemas de sangramiento, moretes?
13. Sí   No   ¿Problemas nasales (sinusitis)?
14. Sí   No   ¿Dificultad al tragar?
15. Sí   No   ¿Diarrea, estreñimiento, sangre en las heces?
16. Sí   No   ¿Vómitos con frecuencia, náuseas?
17. Sí   No   ¿Dificultad al orinar, sangre en la orina?

18. Sí   No   ¿Mareos?
19. Sí   No   ¿Ruidos o zumbidos en los oídos?
20. Sí   No   ¿Dolores de cabeza?
21. Sí   No   ¿Desmayos?
22. Sí   No   ¿Vista borrosa?
23. Sí   No   ¿Convulsiones?
24. Sí   No   ¿Sed excesiva?
25. Sí   No   ¿Orina con frecuencia?
26. Sí   No   ¿Boca seca?
27. Sí   No   ¿Ictericia?
28. Sí   No   ¿Dolor o rigidez en las articulaciones?

III. TIENE O HA TENIDO:

29. Sí   No   ¿Enfermedades del corazón?
30. Sí   No   ¿Infarto de corazón, defectos en el corazón?
31. Sí   No   ¿Soplos en el corazón?
32. Sí   No   ¿Fiebre reumática?
33. Sí   No   ¿Apoplejía, endurecimiento de las arterias?
34. Sí   No   ¿Presión sanguínea alta?
35. Sí   No   ¿Asma, tuberculosis, enfisema, otras enfermedades pulmonares?
36. Sí   No   ¿Hepatitis, otras enfermedades del hígado?
37. Sí   No   ¿Problemas del estómago, úlceras?
38. Sí   No   ¿Alergias a remedios, comidas, medicamentos látex?
39. Sí   No   ¿Familiares con diabetes, problemas de corazón, tumores?

40. Sí   No   ¿SIDA?
41. Sí   No   ¿Tumores, cáncer?
42. Sí   No   ¿Artritis, reuma?
43. Sí   No   ¿Enfermedades de los ojos?
44. Sí   No   ¿Enfermedades de la piel?
45. Sí   No   ¿Anemia?
46. Sí   No   ¿Enfermedades venéreas (sífilis o gonorrea)?
47. Sí   No   ¿Herpes?
48. Sí   No   ¿Enfermedades renales (riñón), vejiga?
49. Sí   No   ¿Enfermedades de tiroides o glándulas suprarrenales?
50. Sí   No   ¿Diabetes?

IV. TIENE O HA TENIDO:

51. Sí   No   ¿Tratamiento psiquiátrico?
52. Sí   No   ¿Tratamientos de radiación?
53. Sí   No   ¿Quimioterapia?
54. Sí   No   ¿Válvula artificial del corazón?
55. Sí   No   ¿Articulación artificial?

56. Sí   No   ¿Hospitalizaciones?
57. Sí   No   ¿Transfusiones de sangre?
58. Sí   No   ¿Cirugías?
59. Sí   No   ¿Marcapasos?
60. Sí   No   ¿Lentes de contacto?

V. ESTÁ TOMANDO:

61. Sí   No   ¿Drogas de uso recreativo?
62. Sí   No   ¿Remedios, medicamentos, medicamentos sin receta (incluyendo aspirina)?

63. Sí   No   ¿Tabaco de cualquier tipo?
64. Sí   No   ¿Alcohol (bebidas alcohólicas)?

Liste por favor: _____

VI. SÓLO PARA MUJERES:

65. Sí   No   ¿Está o podría estar embarazada o dando pecho?   66. Sí   No   ¿Está tomando pastillas anticonceptivas?

VII. PARA TODOS LOS PACIENTES:

67. Sí   No   ¿Tiene o ha tenido alguna otra enfermedad o problema médico que NO está en este cuestionario?

Si la respuesta es afirmativa, explique: _____

Que yo sepa, he respondido completamente y correctamente todas las preguntas. Informaré a mi dentista si hay algún cambio en mi salud y/o en los medicamentos que tomo.

Firma del Paciente _____ Fecha _____

REVISIÓN SUPLEMENTARIA:

1. Firma del Paciente _____ Fecha _____
2. Firma del Paciente _____ Fecha _____
3. Firma del Paciente _____ Fecha _____

The Health History is created and maintained by the University of the Pacific School of Dentistry, San Francisco, California.
Support for the translation and dissemination of the Health Histories comes from MetLife Dental Care.

Figure 4.3 Spanish-language health history questionnaire. (Reprinted with permission from University of the Pacific Arthur A. Dugoni School of Dentistry in San Francisco, CA.)

MetLife   **HEALTH HISTORY INTERVIEW**   **University of the Pacific**

Patient Name:_____

SIGNIFICANT MEDICAL FINDINGS	DENTAL MANAGEMENT CONSIDERATIONS	DATE

Record below the number and details of any YES
response noted on the Health History, plus details
of any YES response to questions A through F.

A.	yes/no	Cardiovascular
B.	yes/no	Infectious diseases
C.	yes/no	Allergy to medicines
D.	yes/no	Hematologic, bleeding
E.	yes/no	Medications
F.	yes/no	Other medical problems not asked?

_____   _____
Date   Doctor's Signature

This Health History Interview form is created and maintained by the University of the Pacific School of Dentistry, San Francisco, California.
Support for the translation and dissemination of the Health Histories comes from MetLife Dental Care.

Figure 4.4 Health history interview sheet. (Reprinted with permission from University of the Pacific
Arthur A. Dugoni School of Dentistry in San Francisco, CA.)

MetLife **MEDICAL CONSULTATION REQUEST** **University of the Pacific**

To: Dr._____

_____

_____

RE: _____

_____

Date of Birth

Please complete the form below and return it to

Dr._____

_____

_____

Phone # _____

Fax # _____

Our patient has presented with the following medical problem(s):_____

_____

_____

The following treatment is scheduled in our clinic:_____

_____

Most patients experience the following with the above planned procedures:

bleeding: • minimal (<50ml)   • significant (>50ml)
stress and anxiety: • low   • medium   • high

_____   _____
Dentist signature   Date

PHYSICIAN'S RESPONSE

Please provide any information regarding the above patient's need for antibiotic prophylaxis, current cardiovascular condition, coagulation ability, and the history and status of infectious diseases. Ordinarily, local anesthesia is obtained with 2% lidocaine, 1:100,000 epinephrine. For some surgical procedures, the epinephrine concentration may be increased to 1:50,000 for hemostasis. The epinephrine dose NEVER exceeds 0.2 mg total.

CHECK **ALL** THAT APPLY

- **OK** to **PROCEED** with dental treatment; **NO** special precautions and **NO** prophylactic antibiotics are needed.

- Antibiotic prophylaxis **IS** required for dental treatment according to the current American Heart Association and/or American Academy of Orthopedic Surgeons guidelines.

- Other precautions are required (please list):_____

_____

- **DO NOT** proceed with treatment. (Please give reason.)_____

_____

Treatment may proceed on (Date)_____

- Patient has an infectious disease:
  - AIDS (please provide current lab results)
  - TB (PPD+/active)
  - Hepatitis, type _____(acute/carrier)
  - Other (explain)_____

- Requested relevant medical and/or laboratory information is attached.

_____   _____
Physician signature   Date

PATIENT CONSENT

I agree to the release of my medical information to the University of the Pacific School of Dentistry.

_____   _____
Patient signature   Date

This Medical Consultation form is created and maintained by the University of the Pacific School of Dentistry, San Francisco, California. Support for the translation and dissemination of the health histories comes from MetLife Dental Care.

Figure 4.5 Medical consultation form. (Reprinted with permission from University of the Pacific Arthur A. Dugoni School of Dentistry in San Francisco, CA.)

Following is the UOP medical history questionnaire with a discussion of the significance of each question:

Medical History Questionnaire (see Fig. 4.1)

I. **CIRCLE APPROPRIATE ANSWER** (leave blank if you do not understand the question):

   1. **Is your general health good?**

> **COMMENT:** A general survey question seeking the patient's general impression of his or her health. Studies have demonstrated that a YES response to this question does not necessarily correlate with the patient's actual state of health.[6]

   2. **Has there been a change in your health within the last year?**

   3. **Have you been hospitalized or had a serious illness in the last 3 years?**

   If YES, why?

   4. **Are you being treated by a physician now? For what?**

   Date of last medical examination?

   Date of last dental examination?

> **COMMENT:** Questions 2, 3, and 4 seek information regarding recent changes in the patient's physical condition. In all instances of a positive response, an in-depth dialog history must follow to determine the precise nature of the change in health status, type of surgical procedure or illness, and the names of any medications the patient may now be taking to help manage the problem.

   5. **Have you had problems with prior dental treatment?**

> **COMMENT:** I have found that many adults are reluctant to verbally admit to the dentist, hygienist, or assistant their fears about treatment for fear of being labeled a "baby." This is especially true of young men in their late teens or early twenties; they attempt to "take it like a man" or "grin and bear it" rather than admit their fears. All too often, such macho behavior results in an episode of vasodepressor syncope. Whereas many such patients do not offer verbal admissions of fear, I have found that these same patients may volunteer the information in writing. (Additional ways a dentist can determine a patient's anxiety are discussed later in this chapter.)

   6. **Are you in pain now?**

> **COMMENT:** The primary aim of this question is related to dentistry. Its purpose is to determine what prompted the patient to seek dental care. If pain is present, the dentist may need to treat the patient immediately on an emergency basis, whereas in the more normal situation treatment can be delayed until future visits. This may affect the use of sedation because many sedation techniques require the patient to fast (NPO status) before administration of the drugs.

II. **HAVE YOU EXPERIENCED:**

   7. **Chest pain (angina)**

> **COMMENT:** A history of angina (defined, in part, as chest pain brought on by exertion and alleviated by rest) usually indicates the presence of a significant degree of coronary artery disease with attendant ischemia of the myocardium. The risk factor for the typical patient with stable angina is ASA 3.* Stress reduction is strongly recommended in these patients. In the presence of dental fears, sedation is absolutely indicated in the anginal patient. Inhalation sedation with N_2O-O_2 is preferred. Patients with unstable or recent-onset angina represent ASA 4 risks.

   8. **Swollen ankles?**

> **COMMENT:** Swollen ankles (pitting edema or dependent edema) indicate possible heart failure (HF). However, varicose veins, pregnancy, and renal dysfunction are other possible causes of ankle edema. Healthy persons who stand on their feet for long periods (e.g., mail carriers and dental staff members) also may develop ankle edema that is not life threatening, but merely esthetically unpleasing.

   9. **Shortness of breath?**

> **COMMENT:** Although the patient may respond negatively to the specific questions (questions 29 to 35) in Section III regarding the presence of various heart and lung disorders (e.g., angina, HF, pulmonary emphysema), clinical signs and symptoms of heart or lung disease may be evident. A positive response to this question does not always indicate that the patient suffers such a disorder. To more accurately determine the patient's status before the

---

*The ASA physical evaluation system is discussed in detail later in this chapter.

start of dental care, further evaluation is suggested. Because many CNS-depressant drugs are also (to varying degrees) potential respiratory depressants, respiratory function of the prospective sedation patient must be fully evaluated.

10. Recent weight loss, fever, night sweats?

COMMENT: The question refers primarily to an unexpected gain or loss of weight, not intentional dieting. Unexpected weight change may indicate HF, hypothyroidism (increased weight), hyperthyroidism, widespread carcinoma, uncontrolled diabetes mellitus (weight loss), or a number of other disorders. The presence of fever and/or night sweats should be pursued to determine whether they are innocent or perhaps clues to the presence of a more significant problem, such as tuberculosis.

11. Persistent cough, coughing up blood?

COMMENT: A positive response mandates in-depth dialog history to determine the cause of the persistent cough or hemoptysis (blood-tinged sputum). The most common causes of hemoptysis are bronchitis and bronchiectasis, neoplasms, and tuberculosis.

A chronic cough can indicate active tuberculosis or other chronic respiratory disorders, such as chronic bronchitis. Cough associated with an upper respiratory infection confers an ASA 2 classification on the patient, whereas chronic bronchitis in a patient who has smoked more than one pack of cigarettes daily for many years may indicate chronic lung disease and confer on the patient an ASA 3 risk. The dentist must weigh carefully the risks before administering CNS depressants—especially those, such as opioids and barbiturates, that depress respiration more than others—to patients who exhibit signs of diminished respiratory reserve (ASA 3 and 4).

12. Bleeding problems, bruising easily?

COMMENT: Bleeding disorders, such as hemophilia, are associated with prolonged bleeding or frequent bruising and can lead to modification of certain forms of dental therapy (e.g., surgery, technique of local anesthetic administration, and venipuncture) and must therefore be made known to the dentist before treatment is begun. Modifications in the planned dental treatment plan may be necessary when excessive bleeding is likely to be present.

13. Sinus problems?

COMMENT: Sinus problems can indicate the presence of an allergy (ASA 2), which should be pursued in the dialog history, or upper respiratory tract infection (URI) (ASA 2), such as a common cold. The patient may experience some respiratory distress when placed in a supine position; distress may also be present if a rubber dam is used. Specific treatment modifications—postponing treatment until the patient is able to breathe more comfortably, limiting the degree of recline in the dental chair, and foregoing use of a rubber dam—are advisable.

The occurrence of clinically significant respiratory problems during sedation and general anesthesia is increased in patients who have URIs and within the following 2 weeks.[7]

14. Difficulty swallowing?

COMMENT: Dysphagia, or the inability to swallow, can have many causes. Before the start of any dental treatment, the dentist should seek to determine the cause and severity of the patient's complaint.

15. Diarrhea, constipation, blood in stools?

COMMENT: This is an evaluation to determine whether gastrointestinal (GI) problems are present, many of which require patients to be medicated. Causes of blood in feces can range from benign, self-limiting events to serious life-threatening disease. Some common causes include anal fissures, aspirin-containing drugs, bleeding disorders, esophageal varices, foreign body trauma, hemorrhoids, neoplasms, use of orally administered steroids, the presence of intestinal polyps, and thrombocytopenia.

16. Frequent vomiting, nausea?

COMMENT: A multitude of causes can lead to nausea and vomiting. Medications, however, are among the most common causes.[8–10] Opiates, digitalis, levodopa, and many cancer drugs act on the chemoreceptor trigger zone in the area postrema to induce vomiting. Drugs that frequently induce nausea include nonsteroidal antiinflammatory drugs (NSAIDs), erythromycin, cardiac antidysrhythmics, antihypertensive drugs, diuretics, oral antidiabetic agents, oral contraceptives, and many GI drugs, such as sulfasalazine.[8–10]

GI and systemic infections, viral and bacterial, are the second most common cause of nausea and vomiting.

17. **Difficulty urinating, blood in urine?**

COMMENT: Hematuria, the presence of blood in the urine, requires evaluation to determine the cause, potentially indicative of urinary tract infection or obstruction.

18. **Dizziness?**

COMMENT: A positive response may indicate a patient's chronic postural (orthostatic) hypotension, symptomatic hypotension or anemia, or transient ischemic attack (TIA), a form of prestroke. In addition, patients with certain types of seizure disorders, such as the "drop attack," may report fainting or dizzy spells. The dentist may be advised to perform further evaluation, including a consultation with the patient's primary care physician. A TIA represents an ASA 3 risk, whereas chronic postural hypotension normally presents as an ASA 2 or 3 risk.

19. **Ringing in ears?**

COMMENT: Tinnitus (an auditory sensation in the absence of sound heard in one or both ears, such as ringing, buzzing, hissing, or clicking) is a common side effect of certain drugs, including salicylates, indomethacin, propranolol, levodopa, aminophylline, and caffeine. It may also be seen with multiple sclerosis, tumor, and ischemic infarction.

20. **Headaches?**

COMMENT: The presence of headache should be evaluated to determine the cause. Common causes include chronic daily headaches, cluster headaches, migraine headaches, and tension-type headaches. If necessary, consultation with the patient's primary care physician is warranted. Determine the drug(s) used by the patient to manage his or her symptoms, because many of these agents can have an influence on clotting.

21. **Fainting spells?**

COMMENT: See *Comment* for question 18.

22. **Blurred vision?**

COMMENT: Blurred vision is a common finding as persons age. Leading causes of blurred vision and blindness include glaucoma, diabetic retinopathy, and macular degeneration. Double vision, or diplopia, usually results from extraocular muscle imbalance, the cause of which must be sought. Common causes include damage to third, fourth, or sixth cranial nerves secondary to myasthenia gravis, vascular disturbances, and intracranial tumors.

23. **Seizures?**

COMMENT: Seizures are common dental emergencies. The most likely candidate to have a seizure is the epileptic patient. Even people with epilepsy that is well controlled with antiepileptic drugs may suffer seizures in stressful situations, such as might occur in the dental office. The dentist must determine the type, frequency of occurrence, and drug(s) used to prevent the seizure before the start of dental treatment. Treatment modification using the SRPs (discussed later in this chapter) is desirable for patients with known seizure disorders. Sedation is highly recommended in the fearful epileptic dental patient as a means of preventing a seizure from developing during treatment. People with epilepsy whose seizures are under control (infrequent) are ASA 2 risks; those with more frequent occurrence of seizures represent an ASA 3 or 4 risk.

24. **Excessive thirst?**

COMMENT: Polydipsia, or excessive thirst, is oftentimes seen in diabetes mellitus, diabetes insipidus, and hyperparathyroidism.

25. **Frequent urination?**

COMMENT: Polyuria, or frequent urination, may be benign (too much fluid intake) or a symptom of diabetes mellitus, diabetes insipidus, Cushing syndrome, or hyperparathyroidism.

26. **Dry mouth?**

COMMENT: Fear is a common cause of a dry mouth, especially in the dental environment. There exist many other causes of xerostomia, however, including Sjögren syndrome.

27. **Jaundice?**

COMMENT: Jaundice, or a yellowness of skin, whites of the eyes, and mucous membranes, is due to a deposition of bile pigment resulting from an excess of bilirubin in the blood (hyperbilirubinemia). It is frequently caused by obstruction of bile ducts, excessive destruction of red blood cells (hemolysis), or disturbances in the functioning of liver cells. Jaundice is a sign that might be indicative of a benign problem, such as a gallstone obstructing the common bile duct, or it might be due to pancreatic carcinoma involving the opening of the common bile duct into the duodenum. Because most drugs used in sedation undergo primary transformation in the liver, the presence of significant hepatic dysfunction will represent either a relative or absolute contraindication to the drug's administration.

28. Joint pain, stiffness?

COMMENT: A history of joint pain and stiffness (arthritis) may be associated with chronic use of salicylates (aspirin) or other NSAIDs, some of which may alter blood clotting. Arthritic patients who are receiving long-term corticosteroid therapy may suffer an increased risk of acute adrenal insufficiency, especially for the patient who has recently stopped taking the steroid. Such patients may require reinstitution of steroid therapy or a modification (increase) in corticosteroid doses during dental treatment so that their body will be better able to respond to any additional stress that might be associated with the treatment.

Because of possible difficulties in positioning the patient comfortably, modifications may be necessary to accommodate the patient's physical disability. Most patients receiving corticosteroids are categorized as an ASA 2 or 3 risk, depending on the reason for the medication and the degree of disability present. Patients with significantly disabling arthritis are ASA 3 risks. Positioning problems secondary to arthritis may negatively affect the use of sedation techniques.

III. **DO YOU HAVE OR HAVE YOU HAD:**
  29. **Heart disease?**

COMMENT: This represents a survey question seeking to detect the presence of any and all types of heart disease. In the presence of a YES answer, the dentist must seek more specific detailed information as to the nature and severity of the problem and a list of any medications taken by the patient to manage the condition. Because many forms of heart disease are exacerbated in the presence of stress, consideration of the SRP becomes increasingly important.

30. Heart attack, heart defects?

COMMENT: *Heart attack* is the lay term for myocardial infarction (MI). The dentist must determine the time that has elapsed since the patient suffered the MI, the severity of the MI, and the degree of residual myocardial damage to decide whether or not treatment modifications are indicated. Elective dental care should, in most instances, be postponed 6 months after an MI.[11] Most post-MI patients are considered ASA 3 risks; however, a patient who has experienced an MI fewer than 6 months before the planned dental treatment should be considered an ASA 4 risk. Where little or no residual damage to the myocardium is present, the patient may be considered an ASA 2 risk after 6 months.

Heart failure: The degree of heart failure (weakness of the "pump") present must be assessed through the dialog history. When a patient has a more serious condition, such as congestive heart failure (CHF) or dyspnea (labored breathing) at rest, specific treatment modifications are warranted. In this situation, the dentist must consider whether the patient requires supplemental O_2 during treatment. Whereas most HF patients are classified according to the American Society of Anesthesiologists' (ASA's) physical status classification system as an ASA 2 (mild HF without disability) or ASA 3 (disability developing with exertion or stress) risk, the presence of dyspnea at rest is an ASA 4 risk. Sedation is indicated in the ASA 2 and 3 HF patient, but care must be taken in selecting the appropriate drugs and technique to prevent additional respiratory depression.

Congenital heart lesions: An in-depth dialog history is required to determine the nature of the lesion and the degree of disability present. Patients can represent an ASA 2, 3, or 4 risk. The dentist may recommend medical consultation, especially for the pediatric patient, to judge the lesion's severity. Some dental treatments will require prophylactic antibiotics.

31. Heart murmurs?

COMMENT: Heart murmurs are common, and not all murmurs are clinically significant. The dentist should determine whether a murmur is functional (nonpathologic, or ASA 2) or whether clinical signs and symptoms of either valvular stenosis or regurgitation are present (ASA 3 or 4) and whether antibiotic prophylaxis is warranted. A major clinical symptom of a significant (organic) murmur is undue fatigue. Table 4.1 provides guidelines for antibiotic prophylaxis. These were most recently revised in 2007 and adopted in both the United

	Table 4.1	**Antibiotic Prophylaxis 2007. Regimen-Single Dose 30 to 60 Minutes Before Procedure**		
SITUATION		**AGENT**	**ADULTS**	**CHILDREN**
Oral		Amoxicillin	2 g	50 mg/kg
Unable to take oral medication		Ampicillin OR	2 g IM or IV*	50 mg/kg IM or IV
		Cefazolin or ceftriaxone	1 g IM or IV	50 mg/kg IM or IV
Allergic to penicillins or ampicillin		Cephalexin††	2 g	50 mg/kg
		OR		
		Clindamycin	600 mg	20 mg/kg
		OR		
		Azithromycin or clarithromycin	500 mg	15 mg/kg
Allergic to penicillins or ampicillin and		Cefazolin or ceftriaxone†	1 g IM or IV	50 mg/kg IM or IV
unable to take oral medication		OR		
		Clindamycin	600 mg IM or IV	20 mg/kg IM or IV

*IM, Intramuscular; IV, intravenous.
†Or other first- or second-generation oral cephalosporin in equivalent adult or pediatric dosage.
†Cephalosporins should not be used in an individual with a history of anaphylaxis, angioedema, or urticaria with penicillins or ampicillin.Wilson W, Taubert KA, Gewitz Mf D et al: Prevention of infective endocarditis: guidelines from the American Heart Association: a guideline from the American Heart Association Rheumatic Fever, Endocarditis, and Kawasaki Disease Committee, Council on Cardiovascular Disease in the Young, and the Council on Clinical Cardiology, Council on Cardiovascular Surgery and Anesthesia, and the Quality of Care and Outcomes Research Interdisciplinary Working Group, *Circulation* 116(15):1736–1754, 2007.

Box 4.1	**Cardiac Conditions Associated With the Highest Risk of Adverse Outcome From Endocarditis for Which Prophylaxis With Dental Procedures Is Recommended**

- Prosthetic cardiac valve
- Previous infective endocarditis
- Congenital heart disease (CHD)*
  - Unrepaired cyanotic CHD, including palliative shunts and conduits
  - Completely repaired congenital heart defect with prosthetic material or device, whether placed by surgery or by catheter intervention, during the first 6 months after the procedure†
  - Repaired CHD with residual defects at the site or adjacent to the site of a prosthetic patch or prosthetic device (which inhibit endothelialization)
- Cardiac transplantation recipients who develop cardiac valvulopathy

*Except for the conditions listed previously, antibiotic prophylaxis is no longer recommended for any form of CHD.
†Prophylaxis is recommended because endothelialization of prosthetic material occurs within 6 months after the procedure.

States and United Kingdom.[12–14] Box 4.1 categorizes cardiac problems as to their requirements for antibiotic prophylaxis, and Box 4.2 addresses prophylaxis and dental procedures specifically. As noted, there are fewer cardiac indications for prophylactic antibiotic administration before dental procedures.

Box 4.2	**Dental Procedures for Which Endocarditis Prophylaxis Is Recommended for Patients**

All dental procedures that involve manipulation of gingival tissue or the periapical region of teeth or perforation of the oral mucosa*

The following procedures and events do not need prophylaxis: routine anesthetic injections through noninfected tissue, taking dental radiographs, placement of removable prosthodontic or orthodontic appliances, adjustment of orthodontic appliances, placement of orthodontic brackets, shedding of deciduous teeth, and bleeding from trauma to the lips or oral mucosa.

Guidelines for antibiotic prophylaxis in orthopedic patients receiving joint replacements (e.g., knee, hip, elbow) were last updated in 2013.[15] The joint American Dental Association–American Academy of Orthopedic Surgeons (ADA–AAOS)[16] report cited a study showing that dental procedures are not risk factors for subsequent implant infection and that antibiotic prophylaxis does not reduce the risk of subsequent infection.[17] Furthermore, evidence exists that the perceived benefits to be gained are clearly outweighed by the risks (allergy, increased microbial resistance, cost) attendant with prophylactic antibiotics in both cardiovascular and orthopedic situations.[18]

32. **Rheumatic fever?**

COMMENT: A history of rheumatic fever should prompt the dentist to perform an in-depth dialog history for the presence of rheumatic heart disease (RHD). In the presence of RHD, antibiotic prophylaxis may be indicated as a means of minimizing the risk of developing subacute bacterial endocarditis (SBE). Depending on the severity of the disease and the presence of a disability, RHD patients can be an ASA 2, 3, or 4 risk. Additional treatment modifications may be advisable.

33. Stroke, hardening of arteries?

COMMENT: The dentist must pay close attention to stroke, cerebrovascular accident (CVA), or "brain attack" (the term increasingly used to confer on the lay public and health care professionals the urgency needed in prompt management of the victim of a CVA[19]). A patient who has suffered a CVA is at greater risk of suffering another CVA or a seizure should they become hypoxic. If the dentist employs sedation in patient management, only minimal to moderate levels, such as those provided through inhalation sedation or intravenous (IV) sedation, are recommended. The dentist should be especially sensitive to the presence of transient cerebral ischemia (TCI), a precursor to CVA; TCI represents an ASA 3 risk. The post-CVA patient is an ASA 4 risk within 6 months of the CVA, becoming an ASA 3 risk 6 or more months after the incident (if the recovery is uneventful). In rare cases, the post-CVA patient can be an ASA 2 risk.

34. High blood pressure?

COMMENT: Elevated blood pressure (BP) measurements are frequently encountered in the dental environment secondary to the added stress (e.g., situational anxiety; the "white coat" syndrome) many patients associate with a visit to the dental office. With a history of HBP, the dentist must determine the drugs the patient is taking, the potential side effects of those medications, and any possible interactions with other drugs that might be used during dental treatment. Guidelines for clinical evaluation of risk (ASA categories) based on adult BP values are presented later in this chapter. The SRP is a significant factor in minimizing further elevations in BP during treatment.

35. Asthma, tuberculosis, emphysema, other lung disease?

COMMENT: Determining the nature and severity of respiratory problems is an essential part of patient evaluation. Many acute problems developing in the dental environment are stress related, increasing the workload of

the cardiovascular system and the O_2 requirements of many tissues and organs in the body. The presence of severe respiratory disease can greatly influence the planned dental treatment and the choice of drugs and technique for sedation.

Asthma (bronchospasm) is marked by a partial obstruction of the lower airway. The dentist must determine the nature of the asthma (intrinsic [allergic] versus extrinsic [nonallergic]), frequency of acute episodes, causal factors, method of management of acute episodes, and drugs the patient may be taking to minimize the occurrence of acute episodes. Stress is a common precipitating factor in acute asthmatic episodes. The well-controlled asthmatic patient represents an ASA 2 risk, whereas the well-controlled but stress-induced asthmatic patient is an ASA 3 risk. Patients whose acute episodes are frequent and/or difficult to terminate (requiring hospitalization) are ASA 3 or 4 risks.

With a history of *tuberculosis*, the dentist must first determine whether the disease is active or arrested. (Arrested tuberculosis represents an ASA 2 risk.) Medical consultation and dental treatment modification are recommended when such information is not easily determined. Inhalation sedation with nitrous oxide (N_2O) and O_2 is not recommended for patients with active tuberculosis (ASA 3 or 4) because of the likelihood that the rubber goods (reservoir bag and conducting tubing) may become contaminated and the difficulty in their sterilization. However, for dentists who treat many patients with tuberculosis and other infectious diseases, disposable rubber goods for inhalation sedation units are recommended.

Emphysema is a form of chronic obstructive pulmonary disease (COPD), also called *chronic obstructive lung disease* (COLD). The emphysematous patient has a decreased respiratory reserve from which to draw if the body's cells require additional O_2, which they do in stressful situations. Supplemental O_2 therapy during dental treatment is recommended in severe cases of emphysema; however, the severely emphysematous (ASA 3, 4) patient should not receive more than 3 L of O_2 per minute.[20] This flow restriction helps to ensure that the dentist does not eliminate the patient's hypoxic drive, which is the emphysematous patient's primary stimulus for breathing. The emphysematous patient is considered an ASA 2, 3, or 4 risk depending on the degree of disability present.

36. Hepatitis, other liver disease?

COMMENT: These diseases or problems either are transmissible (hepatitis A and B) or indicate the presence of hepatic dysfunction. A history of blood transfusion or of past or present drug addiction should alert the dentist to a probable increase in the risk of hepatic dysfunction. (Hepatic dysfunction is a common finding in the parenteral drug abuse patient.) Hepatitis C is responsible for more than 90% of cases of posttransfusion hepatitis, but only 4% of cases are attributable to blood transfusions; up to 50% of cases are related to IV drug use. Incubation of hepatitis C averages 6 to 7 weeks. The clinical illness is mild, usually asymptomatic, and characterized by a high rate (>50%) of chronic hepatitis.[21] Because most drugs are biotransformed in the liver, care must be taken when selecting specific drugs and techniques of administration in the patient with significant hepatic dysfunction. Inhalation sedation with N_2O-O_2 is not contraindicated in these patients.

37. Stomach problems, ulcers?

COMMENT: The presence of stomach or intestinal ulcers may be indicative of acute or chronic anxiety and the possible use of medications such as tranquilizers, H_1 inhibitors, and antacids. Knowledge of which drugs are taken is important before additional drugs are administered in the dental office. A number of H_1 inhibitors are now over-the-counter drugs. Because many patients do not consider such drugs "real" medications, the dentist must specifically question the patient about them. The presence of ulcers does not itself represent an increased risk during treatment. In the absence of additional medical problems, the patient may represent an ASA 1 or 2 risk.

38. Allergies to drugs, foods, medications, latex?

COMMENT: The dentist must evaluate a patient's allergies (real and alleged) thoroughly before administering dental treatment or drugs. The importance of this question and its full evaluation cannot be overstated. A complete and vigorous dialog history must be undertaken before the start of any dental treatment, especially when a presumed or documented history of drug allergy is present. Adverse drug reactions are not uncommon. Many, if not most, are labeled as "allergy" by the patient and also on occasion by his or her physician. However, despite the great frequency with which allergy is reported, true documented and reproducible allergic drug reactions are relatively rare. All adverse drug reactions must be evaluated thoroughly, especially when the dentist plans to administer or prescribe closely related medications for the patient during dental treatment.

Two essential questions that must be asked for each alleged allergy are (1) describe your reaction, and (2) how was it managed?

The presence of allergy alone represents an ASA 2 risk. No emergency situation is as frightening to health care professionals as the acute, systemic allergic reaction known as *anaphylaxis*. Prevention of this life-threatening situation is more gratifying than treatment of anaphylaxis once it develops.

39. Family history of diabetes, heart problems, tumors?

COMMENT: Knowledge of family history can assist in determining the presence of a number of disorders that have some hereditary component.

40. AIDS?

COMMENT: Patients who have a positive test result for human immunodeficiency virus (HIV) are representative of every area of the population. The usual barrier techniques should be employed to minimize risk of cross infection to both the patient and staff members. Patients who are HIV positive are considered an ASA 2, 3, 4, or 5 risk depending on the progress of the infection.

41. Tumors, cancer?

COMMENT: The presence or prior existence of cancer of the head or neck may require specific modification of dental therapy. Irradiated tissues have decreased resistance to infection, diminished vascularity, and reduced healing capacity. However, no specific contraindication exists to the administration of drugs for the management of pain or anxiety in these patients. Many persons with cancer may also be receiving long-term therapy with CNS depressants, such as antianxiety drugs, hypnotics, and opioids. Consultation with the patient's oncologist is recommended before dental treatment. A past or current history of cancer does not necessarily increase the ASA risk status. However, patients who are cachectic or hospitalized or are in poor physical condition may represent an ASA 4 or 5 risk.

42. Arthritis, rheumatism?

COMMENT: See *Comment* for question 28.

43. Eye diseases?

COMMENT: For patients with *glaucoma*, the need to administer a drug that diminishes salivary gland secretions will need to be addressed. Anticholinergics, such as atropine, scopolamine, and glycopyrrolate, are contraindicated in patients with acute narrow angle glaucoma because these drugs produce an increase in intraocular pressure. Patients with glaucoma are usually ASA 2 risks.

44. Skin diseases?

COMMENT: Skin represents an elastic, rugged, self-regenerating, protective covering for the body. The skin also represents our primary physical presentation to the world and as such displays a myriad of clinical signs of disease processes, including allergy, cardiac, respiratory, hepatic, and endocrine disorders.[22]

45. Anemia?

COMMENT: Anemia is a relatively common adult ailment, especially among young adult women (iron-deficiency anemia). The dentist must determine the type of anemia present. The ability of the blood to carry O_2 or to give up O_2 to other cells is decreased in anemic patients. This decrease can become significant during procedures in which hypoxia is likely to develop.

Though rare, hypoxia is more likely to occur with the use of deep sedation. It can develop with intramuscular (IM), intranasal (IN), or IV drug administration in the absence of the concomitant administration of supplemental O_2. Hypoxia can become even more of a problem if the patient is anemic. ASA risk factors vary from 2 to 4 depending on the severity of the O_2 deficit.

Sickle cell anemia is seen exclusively in black patients. Periods of unusual stress or of O_2 deficiency (hypoxia) may precipitate sickle cell crisis. The administration of supplemental O_2 during treatment is strongly recommended for patients with sickle cell disease. Persons with sickle cell trait represent ASA 2 risks, whereas those with sickle cell disease are 2 or 3 risks.

In addition, congenital or idiopathic methemoglobinemia, though rare, is a relative contraindication to the administration of the amide local anesthetic prilocaine.[23]

46. VD (syphilis or gonorrhea)?

47. Herpes?

COMMENT: When treating patients with sexually transmitted diseases (STDs), dentists and staff members are at risk of infection. In the presence of oral lesions, elective dental care should be postponed. Standard barrier techniques—protective gloves, eyeglasses, and masks—provide operators with a degree of (but not total) protection. Such patients usually represent ASA 2 and 3 risks but may be a 4 or 5 risk in extreme situations.

48. Kidney, bladder disease?

COMMENT: The dentist should evaluate the nature of the renal disorder. Treatment modifications, including antibiotic prophylaxis, may be appropriate for several chronic forms of renal disease. Functionally anephric patients are an ASA 3 or 4 risk, whereas patients with most other forms of renal dysfunction are either an ASA 2 or 3 risk. Box 4.3 shows a sample dental referral letter for a patient on long-term hemodialysis treatment because of chronic kidney disease.

49. Thyroid, adrenal disease?

COMMENT: The clinical presence of thyroid or adrenal gland dysfunction—either hyperfunction or

Box 4.3	Hemodialysis Letter

Dear Doctor:

The patient who bears this note is undergoing long-term chronic hemodialysis treatment because of chronic kidney disease. In providing dental care to this patient, please observe the following precautions:

1. Dental treatment is most safely done 1 day after the last dialysis treatment or at least 8 hours thereafter. Residual heparin may make hemostasis difficult. (Some patients are on long-term anticoagulant therapy.)
2. We are concerned about bacteremic seeding of the arteriovenous shunt devices and heart valves. We recommend prophylactic antibiotics before and after dental treatment. Antibiotic selection and dosage can be tricky in renal failure.

We recommend 3 g of amoxicillin 1 hour before the procedure and 1.5 g 6 hours later. For patients with penicillin allergies, 1 g of erythromycin 1 hour before the procedure and 500 mg 6 hours later is recommended.

Sincerely,

hypofunction—should prompt the dentist to use caution in the administration of certain drug groups (e.g., epinephrine to hyperthyroid patients and CNS depressants to hypothyroid patients). In most instances, however, the patient has previously seen a physician and undergone treatment for thyroid disorder by the time he or she seeks dental treatment. In this case the patient is likely to be in a euthyroid state (normal blood levels of thyroid hormone) because of surgical intervention, irradiation, or drug therapy. The euthyroid state represents an ASA 2 risk, whereas clinical signs and symptoms of hyperthyroidism or hypothyroidism represent an ASA 3 or, in rare instances, ASA 4 risk.

Patients with hypofunctioning adrenal cortices have Addison disease and receive daily replacement doses of glucocorticosteroids. In stressful situations, their body may be unable to respond appropriately, leading to loss of consciousness. Hypersecretion of cortisone, Cushing syndrome, rarely results in a life-threatening situation.

50. **Diabetes?**

> **COMMENT:** A patient who responds positively to this question requires further inquiry to determine the type, severity, and degree of control of the diabetic condition. A patient with type 1 (insulin-dependent diabetes mellitus, or IDDM) or type 2 (non–insulin-dependent diabetes mellitus, or NIDDM) diabetes mellitus is rarely at great risk from dental care or commonly administered dental drugs (e.g., local anesthetics, epinephrine, antibiotics, CNS depressants). The NIDDM patient is usually an ASA 2 risk; the well-controlled IDDM patient, an ASA 3 risk; and the poorly controlled IDDM patient, an ASA 3 or 4 risk.

The greatest concerns during dental treatment relate to the possible effects of the dental care on subsequent eating and development of hypoglycemia (low blood sugar). Patients leaving a dental office with residual soft tissue anesthesia, especially in the mandible, usually defer eating until sensation returns, a period potentially of 3 to 5 (lidocaine, mepivacaine, articaine, prilocaine with vasoconstrictor) or more (up to 12) hours (bupivacaine with vasoconstrictor). Patients with diabetes have to modify their insulin doses if they do not maintain normal eating habits. Administration of the local anesthesia reversal agent, phentolamine mesylate, at the conclusion of dental treatment can minimize residual soft tissue anesthesia by up to 50%.[24]

IV. **DO YOU HAVE OR HAVE YOU HAD:**
  51. **Psychiatric care?**

> **COMMENT:** The dentist should be aware of any nervousness (in general or specifically related to dentistry) or history of psychiatric care before treating the patient. These patients may be receiving a number of drugs to manage their disorders that might interact with drugs the dentist uses to control pain and anxiety (Table 4.2). Medical consultation should be considered in such cases. Extremely fearful patients are ASA 2 risks, whereas patients receiving psychiatric care and drugs represent an ASA 2 or 3 risk.

  52. **Radiation treatments?**
  53. **Chemotherapy?**

> **COMMENT:** Therapies for cancer. See *Comment* for question 41.

  54. **Prosthetic heart valve?**

> **COMMENT:** Patients with prosthetic (artificial) heart valves are no longer uncommon. The dentist's primary concern is to determine whether antibiotic prophylaxis is required. Antibiotic prophylactic protocols were presented earlier in this chapter.[12–14] The dentist should be advised to consult with the patient's physician (e.g., the cardiologist or cardiothoracic surgeon) before treatment. Patients with prosthetic heart valves usually represent an ASA 2 or 3 risk.

  55. **Artificial joint?**

> **COMMENT:** Approximately 450,000 total joint arthroplasties are performed annually in the United States. An expert panel of dentists, orthopedic surgeons, and infectious disease specialists convened by the ADA and the AAOS performed a thorough review of the available data to determine the need for antibiotic prophylaxis to prevent hematogenous prosthetic joint infections in dental patients who have undergone total joint arthroplasties. The panel concluded that antibiotic prophylaxis is not recommended for dental patients with pins, plates, and screws or those who have undergone total joint replacements. However, dentists should consider premedication in a small number of patients who may be at increased risk for the development of hematogenous total joint infection (Box 4.4).[15–18]

text continued on p. 45

Table 4.2   Dental Drug Interactions

DENTAL DRUG	INTERACTING DRUG	CONSIDERATION	ACTION
Local anesthetics (LAs)	Cimetidine, β-adrenergic blocker (propranolol)	Hepatic metabolism of amide LA may be depressed	Use LAs cautiously, especially repeat dosages
	Antidysrhythmics (mexiletine, tocainide)	Additive CNS, CVS depression	Use LAs cautiously—keep dose as low as possible to achieve anesthesia
	CNS depressants; alcohol, antidepressants, antihistamines, benzodiazepines, antipsychotics, centrally acting antihypertensives, muscle relaxants, other LAs, opioids	**Possible additive or supraadditive CNS, respiratory depression**	**Consider limiting maximum dose of LAs, especially with opioids**
	Cholinesterase inhibitors: antimyasthenics, antiglaucoma drugs	Antimyasthenic drug dosage may require adjustment because LA inhibits neuromuscular transmission	MD consultation
Vasoconstrictors Epinephrine	α-Adrenergic blockers (phenoxybenzamine, prazosin) Antipsychotics (haloperidol, entacapone)	Possible hypotensive response after large dose of epinephrine	Use vasoconstrictor cautiously—as low a dose as possible
	Catecholamine-O methyltransferase inhibitors (tolcapone, entacapone)	May enhance systemic actions of vasoconstrictors	Use vasoconstrictor cautiously—as low a dose as possible
	CNS stimulants (amphetamine, methylphenidate); ergot derivatives (dihydroergotamine, methysergide)	↑ effect of stimulant or vasoconstrictor may occur	Use vasoconstrictor cautiously—as low a dose as possible
	Cocaine	**↑ effects of vasoconstrictors; can result in cardiac arrest**	**Avoid use of vasoconstrictor in patient under influence of cocaine**
	Digitalis glycosides (digoxin, digitoxin)	↑ risk of cardiac dysrhythmias	MD consultation
	Levodopa, thyroid hormones (levothyroxine, liothyronine)	Large doses of either (beyond replacement doses) may ↑ risk of cardiac toxicity	Use vasoconstrictor cautiously—as low a dose as possible
	Tricyclic antidepressants (amitriptyline, doxepin, imipramine)	**May enhance systemic effect of vasoconstrictor**	**Avoid use of levonordefrin or norepinephrine; use epinephrine cautiously—as low a dose as possible**
	Nonselective β-blockers (propranolol, nadolol)	May lead to hypertensive responses, especially to epinephrine	Monitor BP after initial LA injection

Continued

Table 4.2   Dental Drug Interactions—cont'd

DENTAL DRUG	INTERACTING DRUG	CONSIDERATION	ACTION
Benzodiazepines, zolpidem, zaleplon	**Alcohol or CNS depressants**	**Concurrent use may ↑ depressant effects of either drug**	**Observe for ↑ response to CNS depression; ↓ dose of BZD if necessary**
	Chlorpromazine	**With zolpidem, zaleplon:** concurrent use may prolong elimination half-life of chlorpromazine	
	Cimetidine	May enhance certain actions of BZD, especially sedation	Monitor for enhanced BZD response
	Disulfiram	May increase CNS-depressant action of certain BZD	Monitor for enhanced BZD response
	Erythromycin, clarithromycin, troleandomycin	May ↓ metabolism of certain BZD, ↑ CNS-depressant effect	Monitor for enhanced BZD response
	Imipramine	**With zolpidem, zaleplon:** concurrent use may ↑ drowsiness and risk of anterograde amnesia; may also ↓ peak concentrations of imipramine	
	Oral contraceptives	May inhibit metabolism of BZD that undergo oxidation	Monitor for enhanced BZD response
	Theophyllines	May antagonize sedative effects of BZD	Monitor for ↓ BZD response
Barbiturates	Acetaminophen	Risk of ↑ hepatotoxicity may exist with large or chronic barbiturate dose	Monitor liver enzyme; Avoid prolonged high dosage use
	Alcohol	Concurrent use may ↑ CNS-depressant effects of either agent	Monitor patient for CNS-depressant effects
	Anticoagulants	May ↑ metabolism of anticoagulants, resulting in a ↓ response	Barbiturate therapy should not be started or stopped without considering the possibility of readjustment of the anticoagulant dose
	Oral contraceptives	Reliability may be reduced because of accelerated estrogen metabolism caused by barbiturate's induction of hepatic enzymes	Suggest alternative form of birth control
	Doxycyclines	Phenobarbital ↓ doxycycline's half-life and serum levels	Dose of doxycycline may have to be increased
	MAO-I	MAO-I may enhance sedative effects of barbiturates	Consider reduced dosage of barbiturate
	Metronidazole	Antimicrobial effectiveness of metronidazole may be decreased	Dose of metronidazole may have to be increased
	Narcotics	May ↑ toxicity of meperidine and ↓ effect of methadone	Monitor for excessive meperidine effect; dosage of methadone may have to be increased
	Theophylline	Barbiturates ↓ theophylline levels possibly resulting in ↓ effects	MD consult
	Valproic acid	**Concurrent use may ↓ metabolism of barbiturates resulting in ↑ plasma concentrations**	**Monitor for excessive phenobarbital effect**

Drug	Interacting drug	Effect	Management
Opioids (used for minimal or moderate sedation)	**Benzodiazepines**	↑ **respiratory depression** ↑ **recovery time** ↑ **risk of hypotension**	Titrate dosages and monitor for excessive sedation
	Cimetidine	Actions of opioids may be enhanced resulting in toxicity	If significant
	CNS depressants Diuretics/antihypertensives	↑ **CNS depression** ↑ hypotensive effects	**Monitor for excess sedation** Monitor BP
	MAO inhibitors	With meperidine: agitation, seizures, fever, coma, apnea, death	Avoid this combination
	Phenothiazines	↑ or ↓ effects of opioid analgesic drugs Hypotension may occur when phenothiazine administered with meperidine	Avoid concurrent use of meperidine and phenothiazines
Chloral hydrate	CNS depressants	Concurrent use may ↑ CNS depressant effects of either drug	Monitor for excess CNS depression
	Anticoagulants, coumarin or indanedione derivative	Displacement of anticoagulants from its plasma protein ↑ anticoagulant effect	**Avoid use**
	Catecholamine	Large CH doses may sensitize myocardium to catecholamine	Avoid treating CH overdose with catecholamine
Standard opioids (used for postoperative pain management)	Agonist-antagonist drugs (nalbuphine, butorphanol, pentazocine)	Can lead to withdrawal syndrome or loss of analgesia with hypertension, tachycardia	Never prescribe agonist-antagonist opioids with conventional agonist opioids
	Alcohol	Sedative side effects	Advise patients never to drink alcohol when taking opioids
	Amphetamines	With meperidine: hypotension, respiratory collapse	Do not prescribe meperidine to a patient taking amphetamines
	Anticholinergics	Constipation	Prescribe opioids only for short periods of time; consider MD consultation
	Antidiarrheals	Constipation	Prescribe opioids only for short periods of time; consider MD consultation
	Antihypertensives and vasodilators	Potentiation of hypotensive effects	Advise patients to notify dentist if hypotension or dizziness occurs
	Barbiturates	Sedative side effects	Alert patient to possible additive side effects and to notify dentist if not tolerated
	CNS depressants	Sedative side effects	Alert patient to possible additive side effects and to notify dentist if not tolerated
	Hydroxyzine	Sedative side effects	Alert patient to possible additive side effects and to notify dentist if not tolerated
	Hypnotics (sedative)	Sedative side effects	Alert patient to possible additive side effects and to notify dentist if not tolerated
	MAO inhibitors Metoclopramide	With meperidine: severe hypertension Can antagonize metoclopramide	Avoid prescribing meperidine to patients taking MAO inhibitors; prescribe opioids for only short periods of time; consider MD consultation
	Other opioids	Sedative side effects	Avoid prescribing two opioids at one time, unless for chronic pain

Continued

Table 4.2　Dental Drug Interactions—cont'd

DENTAL DRUG	INTERACTING DRUG	CONSIDERATION	ACTION
NSAIDs	Alcohol	↑ risk of ulceration	Advise patient to avoid if possible
	Oral anticoagulants	↑ risk of bleeding	Advise patient that concurrent use is contraindicated
	Antihypertensives	Effect ↓ by NSAIDs	Monitor BP
	Aspirin	↑ risk of ulceration and bleeding	Advise patient that concurrent use is contraindicated
	NSAIDs other than aspirin	↑ risk of ulceration and bleeding	Avoid this combination
	Corticosteroids	↑ risk of bleeding	Avoid combination, if possible
	Cyclosporin	Can cause nephrotoxicity	Avoid combination, if possible
	Digitalis	↑ digitalis levels	Avoid combination, if possible
	Diuretics (especially triamterene)	Effects ↓ by NSAIDs	Monitor BP/excessive fluid retention
	Heparin	↑ risk of bleeding	Advise patient that concurrent use is contraindicated
	Oral hypoglycemics	Effect ↓ by NSAIDs	Advise patient to monitor blood glucose carefully
	Lithium	Concentration by NSAIDs	Contraindicated unless approved by MD, so avoid concurrent use
	Potassium supplements	↑ risk of ulceration	Avoid combination, if possible
	Valproic acid	↑ risk of ulceration and bleeding	Avoid combination, if possible
Penicillins and cephalosporins	Allopurinol	Concurrent use with ampicillin, amoxicillin, or amoxicillin with clavulanic acid incidence of rashes	Monitor for signs of rash and need to change to other antibiotic
	Oral contraceptives, combined with estrogen and progestin	Sporadic reports of ↓ oral contraceptive effectiveness resulting in unexplained pregnancies	Patient should be advised of the possible ↓ in effectiveness and encouraged to use alternate or additional method of birth control while taking these penicillins
	Probenecid	May ↓ renal tubular secretion of penicillin and cephalosporins resulting in and prolonged antibiotic blood levels	Monitor patient for any need in adjustment of antibiotic dose
Macrolides	Alfentanil	Prolonged or enhanced respiratory depression with concurrent use of erythromycin	Chronic preoperative and postoperative use of erythromycin contraindicated
	Carbamazepine	↑ risk of ataxia, vertigo, drowsiness, and confusion with concurrent use of erythromycin or clarithromycin	If used concurrently, must be done with great caution
	Cyclosporine	↑ immunosuppression and nephrotoxicity with concurrent use of erythromycin or clarithromycin	Concurrent use of these drugs is contraindicated
	Digoxin	Erythromycin can lead to digoxin blood levels leading to digitalis toxicity with resulting cardiac dysrhythmias	Concurrent use of these drugs is contraindicated
	Felodipine	↑ risk of hypotension, tachycardia and edema with concurrent use of erythromycin	Concurrent use of these drugs is contraindicated
	Lovastatin	Muscle pain and skeletal muscle lysis with concurrent use of erythromycin	Concurrent use of these drugs is contraindicated

Oral contraceptives with estrogen and progestin	Sporadic reports of ↓ oral contraceptive effectiveness resulting in unexplained pregnancies	Patient should be advised of the possible ↓ in effectiveness and encouraged to use alternate or additional method of birth control while taking these macrolides
Theophylline	↑ risk of tachycardia, cardiac dysrhythmias, tremors, and seizures reported with concurrent use of erythromycin or clarithromycin	**Concurrent use of these drugs is contraindicated**
Triazolam or midazolam	Marked ↑ in blood levels of both BZDs leading to ↑ depth of sedation and duration reported with concurrent use of erythromycin	**Concurrent use of these drugs is contraindicated**
Warfarin	Erythromycin and clarithromycin ↓ metabolism of warfarin and may significantly ↑ prothrombin and/or INR times and ↑ risk of serious bleeding in patients receiving anticoagulation therapy	Warfarin dosage adjustments may be necessary during and after therapy, and prothrombin or INR times should be monitored closely
Tetracyclines Combinations containing any of the following: antacids, calcium, magnesium, aluminum, iron supplements, sodium bicarbonate	Tetracycline molecules chelate divalent and trivalent cations, impairing absorption	Advise patients against taking these medications within 1–3 hr of taking oral tetracycline
Digoxin	**Tetracyclines may lead to ↑ digoxin blood levels, leading to digitalis toxicity with resulting cardiac dysrhythmias**	**Concurrent use of these drugs is contraindicated**
Oral contraceptives, estrogen and progestin combined	Reports of ↓ oral contraceptive effectiveness in women taking tetracyclines resulting in unplanned pregnancy	Patients should be advised of the possible reduction in the effectiveness and encouraged to use an alternative or additional method of contraception while taking tetracyclines
Warfarin	Tetracycline may ↓ metabolism of warfarin and may significantly prothrombin and/or INR times and ↑ risk of serious bleeding in patients receiving anticoagulation therapy	Warfarin dosage adjustments may be necessary during and after therapy, and prothrombin or INR times should be monitored closely
Clindamycin Antidiarrheals	Concurrent use of clindamycin and antidiarrheals containing kaolin or attapulgite may delay absorption of oral clindamycin	Concurrent use is contraindicated; otherwise patients should be advised to take absorbent antidiarrheals not less than 2 hr before or 3–4 hr after taking oral clindamycin
Narcotic analgesics	Concurrent use with clindamycin may lead to ↑ or prolonged respiratory depression apnea	If concurrent use of these drugs is necessary, caution and careful monitoring of respiration are indicated
Neuromuscular blocking agents	Concurrent use with clindamycin may enhance neuromuscular blockade, resulting in skeletal muscle weakness and respiratory depression or apnea	Avoid concurrent use; if use is necessary, carefully monitor patient for muscle weakness or respiratory depression

Continued

Table 4.2   Dental Drug Interactions—cont'd

DENTAL DRUG	INTERACTING DRUG	CONSIDERATION	ACTION
Metronidazole	Alcohol	Combination may produce a disulfiram effect, leading to facial flushing, headache, palpitations, and nausea	Concurrent use is contraindicated, and use should be delayed at least 1 day after ingestion of alcohol
	Anticoagulants	Coumarin or indanedione-derived anticoagulants may be potentiated by metronidazole resulting in ↑ prothrombin or INR times	Anticoagulant adjustments may be necessary in consultation with MD
	Cimetidine, phenobarbital, phenytoin	Hepatic clearance rates may be affected by concurrent use of metronidazole	Concurrent use of these drugs is contraindicated
	Disulfiram	In alcoholic patients, psychotic reactions have been reported in concurrent use to within 2 wk of use of disulfiram	Concurrent use of these drugs is contraindicated
Ciprofloxacin	Aminophylline, oxtriphylline, or theophylline	Concurrent use of these drugs and ciprofloxacin may result in ↑ risk of theophylline-related toxicity with serious life-threatening reactions	Concurrent use of these drugs is contraindicated
	Antacids containing aluminum, calcium, or magnesium; laxatives containing magnesium	Absorption of ciprofloxacin may be ↓ through chelation by these drugs	Concurrent use of these drugs is contraindicated
	Caffeine	Concurrent use of caffeine and ciprofloxacin may ↓ the metabolism of caffeine resulting in CNS stimulation	Concurrent use of these drugs is contraindicated
	Cyclosporine	Concurrent use of ciprofloxacin has been reported to ↑ serum creatinine and serum cyclosporine concentrations	Cyclosporine concentrations should be monitored, and dosage adjustments may be required
	Vitamin or mineral supplements containing ferrous sulfate or zinc	Absorption of ciprofloxacin may be ↓ through chelation by these agents	Concurrent use of these agents is contraindicated
	Warfarin	Concurrent use of warfarin and ciprofloxacin has been reported to ↑ the anticoagulant effect of warfarin, ↑ the risk of bleeding	The prothrombin time or INR of patients receiving warfarin and ciprofloxacin should be carefully removed
Trimethoprim and sulfamethoxazole	Coumarin or indanedione-derived anticoagulants	Concurrent use may prolong the patient's prothrombin time or INR and lead to bleeding	Prothrombin time or INR of patients concurrently taking these drugs should be monitored carefully
	Hydantoin anticonvulsants	Concurrent use may lead to excessive phenytoin serum levels	Concurrent use of these drugs is contraindicated
	Thiazide diuretics	Elderly patients taking thiazide diuretics have an ↑ risk of thrombocytopenia if these drugs are taken concurrently	If these drugs are taken concurrently, platelet counts and clinical signs of purpura should be carefully monitored

From Ciancio SG: ADA/PDR guide to dental therapeutics, ed 5, Chicago, 2012, American Dental Association.
CVS, Cardiovascular system; CNS, central nervous system; BP, blood pressure; BZD, benzodiazepine; CH, chloral hydrate; INR, international normalized ratio. Drug-drug interactions of greater clinical significance are emboldened for emphasis.

Box 4.4	Orthopedic Prophylaxis

Immunocompromised or Immunosuppressed Patients

Patients with inflammatory arthropathies: rheumatoid arthritis, systemic lupus erythematosus

Other Patients

Patients with insulin-dependent (type 1) diabetes

Patients who have had joint replacement within last 2 years

Patients who have had previous prosthetic joint infections

Malnourished patients

Hemophiliacs

Data from American Dental Association, American Academy of Orthopaedic Surgeons. Antibiotic prophylaxis for dental patients with total joint replacements, JADA 134(7):895–899, 2003.

56. **Hospitalization?**
57. **Blood transfusions?**
58. **Surgeries?**

> **COMMENT:** Determine the cause of the hospitalization, the duration of stay in the hospital, and any medications prescribed that the patient may be taking.

Determine the reason for the blood transfusion (e.g., prolonged bleeding, accident, type of surgery).

Determine the nature (elective, emergency) and type of surgery (cosmetic, GI, cardiac, etc.) and the patient's physical status at the present time.

59. **Pacemaker?**

> **COMMENT:** Cardiac pacemakers are implanted beneath the skin of the upper chest or the abdomen with pacing wires extending into the myocardium. The most frequent indication for the use of a pacemaker is the presence of a clinically significant dysrhythmia. Fixed-rate pacemakers provide a regular, continuous heart rate, regardless of the heart's inherent rhythm, whereas the much more common demand pacemaker is activated only when the heart rate falls into a predetermined/preprogrammed abnormal range. Although there is little indication for the administration of antibiotics in these patients, medical consultation is suggested before the start of treatment to obtain the specific recommendations of the patient's physician. The patient with a pacemaker is commonly an ASA 2 or 3 risk during dental treatment.

In recent years, persons who represent a significant risk of sudden unexpected death (e.g., cardiac arrest) as a result of electrical instability of the myocardium (e.g., ventricular fibrillation) have had implantable cardioverter-defibrillators placed below the skin of their chest. Medical consultation is strongly recommended for these patients.

60. **Contact lenses?**

> **COMMENT:** Contact lenses are commonly worn by persons with visual disturbances. Dental considerations for patients with contact lenses include removal of the lenses during the administration of any sedation technique. Sedated patients may not close their eyes as frequently as unsedated patients, thereby increasing the likelihood of irritating the sclera and cornea of the eye.

V.   **ARE YOU TAKING:**

61. **Recreational drugs?**

> **COMMENT:** Though some patients may not admit to the use of recreational drugs, it is important to ask the question. This becomes particularly important when the dentist is considering the use of CNS-depressant drugs for sedation or local anesthetics with or without a vasoconstrictor, such as epinephrine.

62. **Drugs, medications, over-the-counter medicines (including aspirin), natural remedies?**

> **COMMENT:** Because many patients make a distinction between the terms *drug* and *medication*, questionnaires should use both terms to determine what drugs (pharmaceutically active substances) a patient has taken. Unfortunately, in today's world, the term *drug* often connotes the illicit use of medications (e.g., opioids). In the minds of many patients, people "do" drugs, but "take" medications for the management of medical conditions. Natural remedies contain many active substances, some of which may interact with drugs commonly used in dentistry.[25,26]

The dentist must be aware of all medications and drugs that their patients take to control and treat medical disorders. Frequently, patients take medications without knowing the condition the medications are designed to treat; many patients do not even know the names of drugs that they are taking. It becomes important therefore for dentists to have available one or more means of identifying these medications and of determining their indications, side effects, and potential drug interactions. Many excellent sources are available, including online services, such as ClinicalKey[†] and Epocrates[‡]. The *Physicians' Desk Reference* (PDR),[27] both in hard copy and online, offers a picture section that aids in identification of commonly prescribed drugs. The PDR also offers *Physicians' Desk Reference for Herbal Medicines*.[28] The *ADA/PDR Guide to Dental Therapeutics* is also an invaluable reference to those drugs commonly employed in dentistry and to the medications most often prescribed by physicians. Potential complications and drug interactions are stressed.[29]

Knowledge of the drugs and medications their patients are taking permits dentists to identify medical disorders, possible side effects—some of which may be of significance in dental treatment (e.g., postural hypotension)—and possible interactions between those medications and the drugs administered during dental treatment (see Table 4.2).

63. **Tobacco in any form?**
64. **Alcohol?**

COMMENT: Chronic use of tobacco and/or alcohol over prolonged periods can lead to the development of potentially life-threatening problems, including neoplasms, hepatic dysfunction, and, in females, complications during pregnancy.

VI. WOMEN ONLY:

65. **Are you or could you be pregnant or nursing?**
66. **Taking birth control pills?**

COMMENT: Pregnancy represents a relative contraindication to extensive elective dental care, particularly during the first trimester. Consultation with the patient's obstetrician-gynecologist (OBGYN) is recommended before the start of any dental treatment. Although administration of local anesthetics with or without epinephrine is acceptable during pregnancy,[§] the dentist should evaluate the risk versus the benefits to be gained from the use of most sedative drugs. Of the available sedation techniques, inhalation sedation with

---

[†]ClinicalKey: *www.clinicalkey.com.*
[‡]Epocrates: *www.epocrates.com.*
[§]FDA pregnancy risk categories for local anesthetics: 'B'—lidocaine, prilocaine; 'C'—articaine, bupivacaine, mepivacaine; source: epocrates.com.

Box 4.5	FDA Pregnancy Categories

A	Studies have failed to demonstrate a risk to the fetus in any trimester
B	Animal reproduction studies fail to demonstrate a risk to the fetus; no human studies available
C	Only given after risks to the fetus are considered; animal reproduction studies have shown adverse effects on fetus; no human studies available
D	Definite human fetal risks; may be given in spite of risks if needed in life-threatening conditions
X	Absolute fetal abnormalities; not to be used any time during pregnancy because risks outweigh benefits

---

N_2O and O_2 is most recommended. Use of oral, IM, IN, or IV routes is not contraindicated, but should be reserved for those patients for whom other techniques are unavailable and then only following medical consultation. Food and Drug Administration (FDA) pregnancy categories are presented in Box 4.5, and known fetal effects of drugs are presented in Table 4.3.

VII. ALL PATIENTS:

67. **Do you have or have you had any other diseases or medical problems not listed on this form?**

COMMENT: The patient is encouraged to comment on specific matters not previously mentioned. Examples of several possibly significant disorders include acute intermittent porphyria, methemoglobinemia, atypical plasma cholinesterase, and malignant hyperthermia.

To the best of my knowledge, I have answered every question completely and accurately. I will inform my dentist of any change in my health and/or medication.

COMMENT: This final statement is important from a medical-legal perspective because although instances of purposeful lying on health histories are rare, they do occur. This statement must be accompanied by the date on which the history was completed and the signatures of

Table 4.3	Known Fetal Effects of Drugs
DRUG	EFFECT
Anesthetics, local	No adverse effects in dentistry
Atropine	Sympathomimetic effects
Barbiturates	Concentration is greater in fetus than in mother because fetal kidneys are unable to eliminate barbiturate
Bupivacaine	Does not cross placenta readily; no adverse effects in dentistry
Chlordiazepoxide	In initial 42 days of pregnancy, congenital abnormalities more frequent
Diazepam	In first trimester, cleft lip and palate increased fourfold
Epinephrine	No adverse effects reported for dental use
Hydroxyzine	Hypotonia reported
Lidocaine	No adverse effects reported in dentistry
Meperidine	Decreased neonatal respiration
Mepivacaine	No adverse effects reported in dentistry
Morphine	With chronic use, smaller newborns; withdrawal symptoms noted
N$_2$O	With few exposures, no adverse effects reported when a 30% O2 level is maintained and employed as an anesthetic for dental procedures; evidence suggests an increase in spontaneous abortion among wives of heavily exposed (>9 hr/wk) dental chairside assistants
Promethazine	Congenital hip dislocation
Prilocaine	No adverse effects reported in dentistry
Scopolamine	No adverse effects reported

Modified from Council on Dental Therapeutics: *J Am Dent Assoc* 107:857, 1983.

the patient (or the parent or guardian if the patient is a minor or is not legally competent) and of the dentist who reviews the history. This in effect becomes a contract obliging the patient, parent, or guardian to report any changes in the patient's health or medications. Brady and Martinoff demonstrated that a patient's analysis of personal health frequently is overly optimistic and that pertinent health matters sometimes are not immediately reported.[6]

The medical history questionnaire must be updated on a regular basis, approximately every 3 to 6 months or after any prolonged lapse in treatment. In most instances, the entire medical history questionnaire need not be redone. The dentist need only ask the following questions:

1. Have you experienced any change in your general health since your last dental visit?
2. Are you now under the care of a physician? If so, what is the condition being treated?
3. Are you currently taking any drugs, medications, or over-the-counter products?

If any of these questions elicits a positive response, a detailed dialog history should follow. For example, a patient may answer that no change has occurred in general health but may want to notify the dentist of a minor change in condition, such as the end of a pregnancy (It's a girl!) or of the recent diagnosis of NIDDM or asthma.

In either situation, a written record of having updated the history should be appended to the patient's progress notes or on the health history form. When the patient's health status has changed significantly since the last history was completed, the entire history should be redone (e.g., if a patient was recently diagnosed with cardiovascular disease and is managing it with a variety of drugs they were not previously taking).

In reality, most persons do not undergo significant changes in their health with any regularity. Thus one health history questionnaire can remain current for many years. Therefore the ability to demonstrate that a patient's medical history has been updated on a regular basis becomes all the more important.

The medical history questionnaire should be completed in ink. The dentist makes a correction or deletion by drawing a single line through the original entry without obliterating it. The change is then added along with the date of the change. The dentist initials the change. A written notation should be placed in the chart whenever a patient reveals significant information during the dialog history. As an example, when a patient answers affirmatively to the question about a "heart attack," the dentist's notation may read "2006" (the year the MI occurred).

Physical Examination

The medical history questionnaire is quite important to the overall assessment of a patient's physical and psychological status. There are, however, limitations to the questionnaire. For the questionnaire to be valuable, the patient must (1) be aware of the presence of any medical condition and (2) be willing to share this information with the dentist.

Most patients will not knowingly deceive their dentist by omitting important information from the medical history questionnaire, although cases in which such deception has occurred are on record. A patient seeking treatment for an acutely inflamed tooth decides to withhold from the dentist that he had an MI 2 months earlier because he knows that to tell the dentist would mean that he would not receive treatment.

The other factor, a patient's knowledge of his or her physical condition, is a much more likely cause of misinformation on the questionnaire. Most "healthy" persons do not visit their physician regularly for routine check-ups. Information has suggested that annual physical examination be discontinued in the younger healthy patient because it has not proven to be as valuable an aid in preventive medicine as was once thought.[30] In addition, most patients, primarily males, simply do not visit their physician on a regular basis, doing so instead only when they become ill. From this premise, it stands to reason that the true state of the patient's physical condition may be unknown to the patient. Feeling well, although usually a good indicator of health, is not a guarantor of good health.[6] Many disease entities may be present for a considerable length of time without exhibiting overt signs or symptoms that alert the patient of their presence (e.g., HBP, diabetes mellitus, cancer). When signs and symptoms are present, they are frequently mistaken for other, more benign problems. Although they may answer questions on the medical history questionnaire to the best of their knowledge, patients cannot give a positive response to a question unless they are aware that they have the condition. The first few questions on most histories refer to the length of time since the patient's last physical examination. The value of the remaining answers, dealing with specific disease processes, can be gauged from the patient's responses to these initial questions.

Because of these problems, which are inherent in the use of a patient-completed medical history questionnaire, the dentist must look for additional sources of information about the physical status of the patient. Physical examination of the patient provides much of this information. This consists of the following:

1. Monitoring of vital signs
2. Visual inspection of the patient
3. Function tests, as indicated
4. Auscultation of heart and lungs and laboratory tests, as indicated

Minimal physical evaluation for all potential patients should consist of (1) measurement of vital signs and (2) visual inspection of the patient.

The primary value of the physical examination is that it provides the dentist with important information concerning the physical condition of the patient immediately before the start of treatment, as contrasted with the questionnaire, which provides historical information. The patient should undergo a minimal physical evaluation at the initial visit to the office before the start of any dental treatment. Readings obtained at this time, called *baseline vital signs,* are recorded on the patient's chart.

Vital Signs

The six vital signs are as follows:
1. Blood pressure (BP)
2. Heart rate (pulse) and rhythm
3. Respiratory rate
4. Temperature
5. Height
6. Weight
   a. Body mass index (BMI)

Baseline vital signs should be obtained before the start of dental treatment. Although the screaming 3-year-old and the difficult-to-manage disabled adult may present difficulties, the doctor should make every effort to monitor and record baseline vital signs for each patient.

BP and heart rate and rhythm always should be recorded when possible. Respiratory rate also should be evaluated whenever possible, but usually must be assessed surreptitiously. Temperature recording may be part of the routine evaluation, but more commonly is done in situations in which it is deemed necessary (e.g., when infection is present or the patient appears febrile). Height and weight may be obtained in most instances by asking the patient, but should be measured when the response appears inconsistent with visual appearance. Weight is of considerable importance when parenteral (IM or IN) or enteral (oral) sedation is to be used. BMI provides a simple numeric measure of a person's thickness or thinness, allowing health professionals to discuss overweight and underweight problems more objectively with their patients. Moderately obese (BMI between 30 and 35), severely obese (BMI between 35 and 40), and morbidly obese (BMI greater than 40) individuals are at greater risk of many chronic and acute medical problems, including cardiac and respiratory conditions. It is this author's opinion that a BMI greater than 35 represents a contraindication to the administration of parenteral sedation (e.g., IV, IM, IN).

The following information describes the recommended techniques for the recording and interpretation of vital signs.

Blood Pressure

Technique. The following technique is recommended for the accurate manual determination of BP.[31] A stethoscope and sphygmomanometer (BP cuff) are the required equipment. The most accurate and reliable of these devices is the mercury-gravity manometer. The aneroid manometer, probably the most frequently used, is calibrated to be read in millimeters of mercury (mm Hg, or torr) and is also quite accurate if well maintained. Rough handling of the aneroid manometer may lead to erroneous readings. It is recommended that the aneroid manometer be recalibrated at least annually by checking it against a mercury manometer. Automatic BP monitors are today commonplace, as their accuracy has increased, while their cost has decreased, ranging from well under $100 to several thousand dollars. Likewise, their accuracies vary. The use of automatic monitors simplifies the monitoring of vital signs, but dentists should be advised to check the accuracy of these devices periodically (comparing values with those of a mercury manometer).

Though the most accurate, use of mercury manometers has become increasingly rare because they are too bulky for easy carrying and mercury spills are potentially dangerous.[32]

Aneroid manometers are easy to use, somewhat less accurate than the mercury manometer, and are more delicate, requiring recalibration at least annually or when dropped or bumped.[32]

Automatic devices containing all equipment in one unit negate the need for a separate stethoscope and manometer. Most are easy to use, whereas more expensive devices have automatic inflation and deflation systems and readable printouts of both BP and heart rate. As with the aneroid manometer, automatic BP systems are somewhat fragile, requiring recalibration on a regular schedule or when bumped or dropped. Body movements may influence accuracy, and even the most accurate devices do not work on certain people.[32]

Automatic BP monitors that fit on the patient's wrist are also available and easy to use. However, BP measurements at the wrist may not be as accurate as those taken at the upper arm, and systematic error can occur as a result of differences in the position of the wrist relative to the heart (see later discussion and Chapter 5).[33,34]

For routine preoperative monitoring of BP, the patient should be seated in the upright position. The arm should be at the level of the heart—relaxed, slightly flexed, and supported on a firm surface (e.g., the armrest of the dental chair). The patient should be permitted to sit for at least 5 minutes before the blood pressure recording is taken. This will permit the patient to relax somewhat so that the recorded pressure will be closer to the patient's baseline reading. During this time, other nonthreatening procedures may be carried out, such as review of the medical history questionnaire.

The BP cuff should be deflated before it is placed on the arm. The cuff should be wrapped evenly and firmly around the arm, with the center of the inflatable portion over the brachial artery and the rubber tubing lying along the medial aspect of the arm. The lower margin of the cuff should be placed approximately 2 to 3 cm (1 inch) above the antecubital fossa (the patient should still be able to flex the elbow with the cuff in place). A BP cuff is too tight if two fingers cannot be placed under the lower edge of the cuff. Too tight a cuff will decrease venous return from the arm, leading to erroneous measurements. A cuff is too loose (a much more common problem) if it may be easily pulled off of the arm with gentle tugging. A slight resistance should be present when a cuff is properly applied.

The radial pulse in the wrist should be palpated and the pressure in the cuff increased rapidly to a point approximately 30 mm Hg above the point at which the pulse disappears. The cuff should then be slowly deflated at a rate of 2 to 3 mm Hg/sec until the radial pulse returns. This is termed the *palpatory systolic pressure*. Residual pressure in the cuff should be released to permit venous drainage from the arm.

Determination of BP by the more accurate auscultatory method requires palpation of the brachial artery, located on the medial aspect of the antecubital fossa. The earpieces of the stethoscope should be placed facing forward, firmly in the recorder's ears. The diaphragm of the stethoscope must be placed firmly on the medial aspect of the antecubital fossa over the brachial artery. To reduce extraneous noise, the stethoscope should not touch the blood pressure cuff or rubber tubing.

The blood pressure cuff should be rapidly inflated to a level 30 mm Hg above the previously determined palpatory systolic pressure. Pressure in the cuff should be gradually released (2 to 3 mm/sec) until the first *sound* (a tapping sound) is heard through the stethoscope. This is referred to as the *systolic blood pressure*.

As the cuff deflates further, the sound undergoes changes in quality and intensity. As the cuff pressure approaches the diastolic pressure, the sound becomes dull and muffled and then ceases. The diastolic BP is best indicated as the point of complete cessation of sound. In some instances, however, complete cessation of sound does not occur, with the sound gradually fading out. In these instances, the point at which the sound became muffled is the diastolic pressure. The cuff should be slowly deflated to a point 10 mm Hg beyond the point of disappearance and then totally deflated.

Should additional recordings be necessary, a wait of at least 15 seconds is recommended before reinflating the BP cuff. This permits blood trapped in the arm to leave, providing more accurate readings.

BP is recorded on the patient's chart or sedation-anesthesia record as a fraction: 130/90 R or L (arm on which recorded).

Common errors in technique. Some common errors associated with recording BP lead to inaccurate readings (too high or too low). Lack of awareness of these may lead to unnecessary referral for medical consultation, added financial burden to the patient, and a loss of faith in the dentist.

1. Applying the BP cuff too loosely produces falsely elevated readings. This probably represents the most common error in recording BP.[35]
2. Use of the wrong cuff size can result in erroneous readings. A "normal adult" BP cuff placed on an obese arm will produce falsely elevated readings. This same cuff applied to the very thin arm of a child or adult will produce falsely low readings. Sphygmomanometers are available in a variety of sizes. The "ideal" cuff should have a bladder length that is 80% and a width that is at least 40% of the arm's circumference.[33] Recommended cuff sizes are presented in Table 4.4.[32]
3. An auscultatory gap may be present (Fig. 4.6), representing a loss of sound (a period of silence) between systolic and diastolic pressures, with the sound reappearing at a lower level. For example, systolic sounds are noticed at 230 mm Hg;

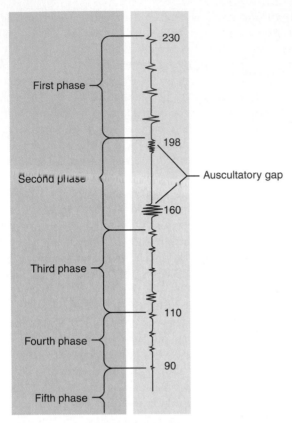

Blood pressure 230/110/90 mm Hg

Figure 4.6 Auscultatory gap.

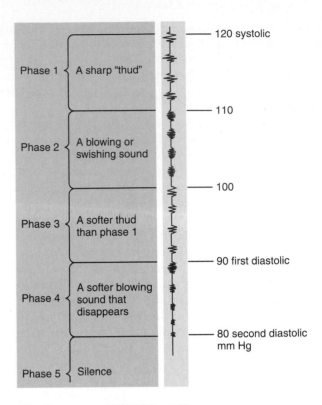

Blood pressure = 120/90/80 mm Hg

Figure 4.7 Korotkoff sounds.

Table 4.4	Recommended Blood Pressure Cuff Sizes	
ARM CIRCUMFERENCE	**CUFF**	**CUFF SIZE**
22–26 cm	Small adult	12 × 22 cm
27–34 cm	Adult	16 × 30 cm
35–44 cm	Large adult	16 × 36 cm
45–52 cm	Adult thigh	16 × 42 cm

Pickering TG, Hall JE, Appel LJ et al: Recommendations for blood pressure measurement in humans and experimental animals: Part 1: blood pressure measurement in humans: a statement for professionals from the subcommittee of professional and public education of the American Heart Association Council on High Blood Pressure Research, *Hypertension* 45:142–161, 2005.

however, the sound then disappears at 198 mm Hg, reappearing at approximately 160 mm Hg. All sound is lost at 90 mm Hg. An auscultatory gap occurred between 160 and 198 mm Hg. In this situation, if the person recording the BP had not palpated (estimated) the systolic BP before auscultation, the cuff might be inflated to some arbitrary pressure (e.g., 165 mm Hg). At this level, the recorder would pick up no sound because this lies within the auscultatory gap. Sounds would first be noted at 160 mm Hg, with their

disappearance at 90 mm Hg, levels well within therapy limits (see guidelines for BP, next subsection). In reality, however, this patient has a BP of 230/90 mm Hg, a significantly elevated BP that represents a greater risk to the patient during treatment (this patient is not considered to be a candidate for elective dental care). Although the auscultatory gap occurs only infrequently, the possibility of error may be eliminated by using the palpatory technique. A palpable pulse will be present throughout the gap (appearing in our example at 230 mm Hg), although the sound is not present. Although there is no pathologic significance to its presence, the auscultatory gap is found most often in patients with HBP.

4. The patient may be anxious. Having one's BP recorded may produce anxiety,[36] causing transient elevations in BP, primarily the systolic pressure (up to 6.3–7.9 mm Hg[37]). This is a result of situational anxiety or the "white coat" syndrome. This is even more likely to be noted in a patient who is to receive sedation for management of his or her dental fear. For this reason, it is recommended that baseline measurements of vital signs be obtained at a visit before the start of treatment, perhaps the first office visit when the patient will only be completing various forms. Measurements are more likely to be within normal limits (WNL) for the particular patient at this time.

5. BP is based on the Korotkoff sounds (Fig. 4.7) produced by the passage of blood through occluded, partially occluded,

Table 4.5	Guidelines for Blood Pressure (Adult)	
BLOOD PRESSURE (MM HG, OR TORR)	**ASA CLASSIFICATION**	**DENTAL THERAPY CONSIDERATION**
<140 and <90	1	1. Routine dental management 2. Recheck in 6 mo, unless specific treatment dictates more frequent monitoring
140–159 and/or 90–94	2	1. Recheck BP before dental treatment for three consecutive appointments; if all exceed these guidelines, medical consultation is indicated 2. Routine dental management 3. SRP as indicated
160–199 and/or 95–114	3	1. Recheck BP in 5 min 2. If BP is still elevated, a medical consultation before dental therapy is warranted 3. Routine dental therapy 4. SRP
200+ and/or 115+	4	1. Recheck BP in 5 min 2. Immediate medical consultation if still elevated 3. No dental therapy, routine or emergency,* until elevated BP is corrected 4. Refer to hospital if immediate dental therapy indicated

*When the BP of the patient is slightly above the cutoff for category 4 and anxiety is present, the use of inhalation sedation may be employed in an effort to diminish the BP (via the elimination of stress).

or unoccluded arteries. Watching a mercury column or needle on an aneroid manometer for "pulsations" leads to falsely elevated systolic pressures. Pulsations of the dial are noted approximately 10 to 15 mm Hg before the first Korotkoff sounds are heard.

6. Use of the left or right arm will produce differences in recorded BP. A difference of greater than 10 mm Hg may occur in readings between arms in approximately 20% of subjects.[38] There is no clear pattern. The difference does not appear to be determined by whether the subject is right- or left-handed.[38]

Guidelines for clinical evaluation. The University of Southern California (USC) School of Dentistry's physical evaluation system is based on the ASA's physical status classification system.[39] It details four risk categories based on a patient's medical history and physical evaluation. The ASA categories for BP recordings in adults are presented in Table 4.5.[40,41]

For the adult patient with a baseline BP in the ASA 1 range (<140/, <90 mm Hg), it is suggested that the BP be recorded every 6 months unless specific dental procedures demand more frequent monitoring. The parenteral administration of any drug (local anesthesia; IM, IV, IN, or inhalation sedation; or general anesthesia) mandates the more frequent recording of vital signs (see Chapter 5).

Patients with BPs in the ASA 2, 3, or 4 category should be monitored more frequently (e.g., at every appointment), as outlined in the guidelines. Patients with known HBP should also have their BP monitored at each visit to determine whether their BP is adequately controlled. It is impossible to gauge a BP by "looking" at a person or by asking, "How do you feel?" The routine monitoring of BP in all patients according to the treatment guidelines will effectively minimize the occurrence of acute complications of HBP (e.g., hemorrhagic CVA).

When parenteral or inhalation sedation techniques or general anesthesia is employed, there is a greater need for obtaining baseline vital signs. One factor that will be used to evaluate a patient's recovery from sedation and ability to be discharged from the office will be a comparison of the posttreatment vital signs with their baseline values.

Still another reason for routine monitoring of BP relates to the management of medical emergencies. After the basic steps of management (P → C → A → B) in each emergency, certain specific steps are necessary for definitive treatment (D). Primary among these is monitoring of vital signs, particularly BP. BP recorded during an emergency situation provides an important indicator of the status of the cardiovascular system. However, unless a baseline or nonemergency BP measurement has been recorded earlier, the value of the blood pressure obtained during the emergency is less significant. A recording of 80/50 mm Hg is less ominous in a patient with a preoperative reading of 100/60 mm Hg than if the pretreatment recording was 190/110 mm Hg. The absence of BP is always an indication for cardiopulmonary resuscitation.

The normal range for BP in younger patients is somewhat lower than that in adults. Table 4.6 presents a normal range of BP in infants and children.

Heart Rate and Rhythm

Technique. Heart rate (pulse) and rhythm may be measured at any readily accessible artery (Fig. 4.8). Most commonly used for routine measurement are the brachial artery, located on the medial aspect of the antecubital fossa, and the radial artery, located on the radial and ventral aspects of the wrist.

Table 4.6	Normal Blood Pressure for Various Ages	
AGES	MEAN SYSTOLIC ±2 SD	MEAN DIASTOLIC ±2 SD
Newborn	80 ± 16	46 ± 16
6 mo-1 yr	89 ± 29	60 ± 10*
1 yr	96 ± 30	66 ± 25*
2 yr	99 ± 25	64 ± 25*
3 yr	100 ±25	67 ± 23*
4 yr	99 ± 20	65 ± 20*
5–6 yr	94 ± 14	55 ± 9
6–7 yr	100 ± 15	56 ± 8
7–8 yr	102 ± 15	56 ± 8
8–9 yr	105 ± 16	57 ± 9
9–10 yr	107 ± 16	57 ± 9
10–11 yr	111 ± 17	58 ± 10
11–12 yr	113 ± 18	59 ± 10
12–13 yr	115 ± 19	59 ± 10
13–14 yr	118 ± 19	60 ± 10

*In this study, the point of muffling was taken as the diastolic pressure.
From: National High Blood Pressure Education Program Working Group on High Blood Pressure in Children and Adolescents. The fourth report on the diagnosis, evaluation, and treatment of high blood pressure in children and adolescents, *Pediatrics* 114(2 Suppl 4th Report):555–576, 2004.

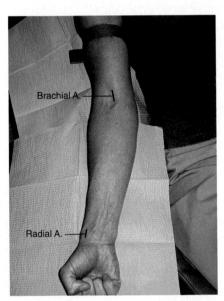

Figure 4.8 Pulse may be measured at any accessible artery. (From Malamed SF: Medical emergencies in the dental office, ed 7, St Louis, 2015, Mosby, p 41.)

When palpating an artery, one should use the fleshy portions of the index and middle fingers. Gentle pressure must be applied to feel the pulsation. Do not press so firmly that the artery is occluded and no pulsation is felt. The thumb ought not to be used to monitor pulse because it contains a fair-sized artery.

Automatic BP devices and pulse oximeters provide a measurement of the heart rate.

Guidelines for clinical evaluation. Three factors should be evaluated while the pulse is monitored:
1. The heart rate (recorded as beats per minute)
2. The rhythm of the heart (regular or irregular)
3. The quality of the pulse (thready, weak, bounding, full)

Heart rate should be evaluated for a minimum of 30 seconds, ideally for 1 minute. The normal resting heart rate for an adult ranges from 60 to 110 beats per minute. It is often lower in a well-conditioned athlete and elevated in the fearful individual. However, clinically significant disease may also produce slow (bradycardia [<60 per minute]) or rapid (tachycardia [>110 per minute]) heart rates. It is suggested that any heart rate below 60 or above 110 beats per minute (adult) be evaluated (initially via dialog history). Where no obvious cause is present (e.g., endurance sports, anxiety, prescription drugs [e.g., beta-blockers]), medical consultation should be considered.

The healthy heart maintains a relatively regular rhythm. Irregularities in rhythm should be confirmed and evaluated via dialog history and/or medical consultation before the start of treatment. The occasional *premature ventricular contraction (PVC)* is so common that it is not necessarily considered abnormal. PVCs may be produced by smoking, fatigue, stress, various drugs (e.g., epinephrine), and alcohol. Frequent PVCs are usually associated with a damaged or an ischemic myocardium. However, when PVCs are present at a frequency of five or more per minute, especially if they appear at irregular intervals, medical consultation should definitely be sought. Patients with five or more PVCs per minute are considered to be at greater risk for sudden cardiac death (ventricular fibrillation) and are more likely to have implanted automatic defibrillators.[42,43] Clinically, PVCs detected by palpation appear as a break in a generally regular rhythm in which a longer-than-normal pause (a "skipped beat") is noted ("felt") followed by the resumption of a regular rhythm.

A second disturbance of the pulse is termed *pulsus alternans.*[44] It is not truly a dysrhythmia, but a regular heart rate that is characterized by a pulse in which strong and weak beats alternate. It is produced by the alternating contractile force of a diseased left ventricle. Pulsus alternans is observed frequently in severe left ventricular failure, severe arterial HBP, and coronary artery disease. Medical consultation is indicated.

Many other dysrhythmias may be noted by palpation of the pulse. The "irregular irregularity" of *atrial fibrillation* is noted in hyperthyroid patients and warrants pretreatment consultation. *Sinus dysrhythmia* is detected frequently in healthy adolescent patients. It is noted as an increase in the heart rate followed by a decrease in rate that correlates with the breathing cycle (the heart rate increases during inspiration, decreases with expiration). Sinus dysrhythmia is not indicative of any cardiac abnormality and therefore does not require pretreatment consultation.

Table 4.7	Average Pulse Rate at Different Ages		
AGE	LOWER LIMITS OF NORMAL	AVERAGE	UPPER LIMITS OF NORMAL
Newborn	70	120	170
1–11 mo	80	120	160
2 yr	80	110	130
4 yr	80	100	120
6 yr	75	100	115
8 yr	70	90	110
10 yr	70	90	110

From Kliegman RM, Stanton BF, St. Geme JW, Schor NF, editors: *Nelson textbook of pediatrics*, ed 20, St Louis, 2016, Elsevier.

Table 4.8	Respiratory Rate by Age
AGE	RATE/MIN
Neonate	40
1 wk	30
1 yr	24
3 yr	22
5 yr	20
8 yr	18
12 yr	16
21 yr	12

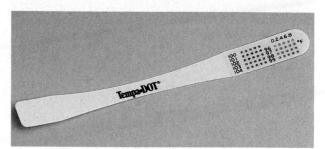

Figure 4.9 Disposable thermometer. (From Potter PA, Perry AG: *Fundamentals of nursing*, ed 7, St. Louis, 2009, Mosby.)

The quality of the pulse is commonly described as full, bounding, thready, or weak. These adjectives relate to the subjective "feel" of the pulse and are used to describe situations such as a "full bounding" pulse (as noted in severe arterial HBP) or a "weak thready" pulse (often noted in hypotensive patients with signs of shock). Table 4.7 presents the range of normal heart rates in children of various ages.

Respiratory Rate

Technique. Determination of respiratory rate must be made surreptitiously. Patients aware that their breathing is observed will not breathe normally. It is recommended therefore that respiration be monitored immediately after the heart rate. The observer's fingers are left on the patient's radial or brachial pulse after the heart rate has been determined; however, the observer counts respirations (by observing the rise and fall of the chest) instead for a minimum of 30 seconds, ideally for 1 minute.

Guidelines for clinical evaluation. Normal respiratory rate for an adult is 14 to 18 breaths per minute. Bradypnea (abnormally slow rate) may be produced by, among other causes, opioid administration, whereas tachypnea (abnormally rapid rate) is seen with fever, fear (e.g., hyperventilation), and alkalosis. The most common change in ventilation noted in the dental environment will be hyperventilation, an abnormal increase in the rate and depth of respiration. It is also seen, but much less frequently in the dental environment, in diabetic acidosis. The most common cause of hyperventilation in dental and surgical settings is extreme psychological stress.

Any significant variation in respiratory rate should be evaluated before treatment. The absence of spontaneous ventilation is always an indication for controlled ventilation (aka "rescue breathing") (P → C → A→ B). Table 4.8 presents the normal range of respiratory rate at different ages.

BP, heart rate and rhythm, and respiratory rate provide information about the functioning of the cardiorespiratory system. It is recommended that they be recorded as a part of the routine physical evaluation for all potential patients. Recording of the remaining vital signs—temperature, height, weight, and BMI—although desirable, may be considered optional. However, when parenteral drugs are to be administered, especially in lighter weight, younger, or older patients, recording of a patient's weight and determination of their BMI becomes considerably more important.

Temperature

Technique. Temperature should be monitored orally. The thermometer, sterilized and shaken down, is placed under the tongue of the patient, who has not eaten, smoked, or had anything to drink in the previous 10 minutes. The thermometer remains in the closed mouth for 2 minutes before removal. Disposable thermometers (Fig. 4.9) and digital thermometers (Fig. 4.10) are equally accurate and easy to use. Forehead thermometers are effective when the patient's behavior will not permit use of an oral thermometer (Fig. 4.11).

Guidelines for clinical evaluation. The "normal" oral temperature of 37.0°C (98.6°F) is only an average. The true range of normal is considered to be from 36.11°C to 37.56°C (97°F to 99.6°F). Temperatures vary during the day (from 0.5°F to 2.0°F), with the lowest in the early morning and highest in the late afternoon.

Fever represents an increase in temperature beyond 37.5°C (99.6°F). Temperatures in excess of 38.33°C (101°F) usually indicate the presence of an active disease process. Evaluation

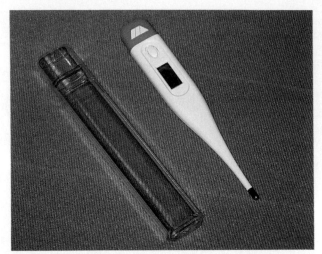

Figure 4.10 Digital thermometer. (Courtesy Sedation Resource, Lone Oak, TX, www.sedationresource.com.)

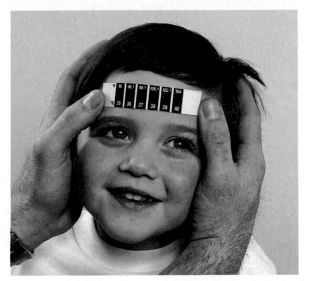

Figure 4.11 Forehead thermometers are effective when the patient's behavior will not permit use of an oral thermometer. (From Gerdin J: *Health careers today*, ed 7, St Louis, 2007, Mosby.)

	Table 4.9	Acceptable Weights (in Pounds) for Men and Women*	
Height	AGE 19–34 Years	AGE 35 Years and Older
5 in 0 ft	97–128	108–138
5 in 1 ft	101–132	111–143
5 in 2 ft	104–137	115–148
5 in 3 ft	107–141	119–152
5 in 4 ft	111–146	122–157
5 in 5 ft	114–150	126–162
5 in 6 ft	118–156	130–167
5 in 7 ft	121–160	134–172
5 in 8 ft	125–164	138–178
5 in 9 ft	129–169	142–183
5 in 10 ft	132–174	146–188
5 in 11 ft	136–179	151–194
6 in 0 ft	140–184	155–199
6 in 1 ft	144–189	159–205
6 in 2 ft	148–195	164–210

*Weights based on weighing in without shoes or clothes.
Department of Health & Human Services (HHS) and Department of Agriculture (USDA) Dietary Guidelines for Americans, 2005.

companies. New guidelines of range of normal height and weight have been published (Table 4.9).

Guidelines for clinical evaluation. Grossly obese or excessively underweight patients may have an active disease process. Obesity will be noted in various endocrine disorders, such as Cushing syndrome, whereas extreme loss of weight may be noted in pulmonary tuberculosis, malignancy, and hyperthyroidism. Anorexia nervosa should also be considered in extremely underweight individuals. In all instances where gross obesity or extreme loss of weight is noted, pretreatment medical consultation is recommended.

Excessively tall persons are referred to as *giants,* whereas persons who are decidedly shorter than average are called *dwarfs.* In both instances, endocrine gland dysfunction may be present. Medical consultation is usually not necessary for these patients.

Whenever a pharmacosedative technique is employed in which titration is not possible (IM, IN, or submucosal [SM]), the weight of the patient must be obtained. One method used to determine the appropriate dose of drug for the patient is the patient's lean body weight (see Chapters 9 and 35). It is suggested that the patient be weighed on a scale in the dentist's office rather than relying on the patient to tell you his or her weight.

Body Mass Index

BMI is a number calculated based on the weight and height of a person. BMI is a fairly reliable indicator of body fatness

of the cause of the fever is necessary before treatment. When dental or periodontal infection is considered to be a probable cause of elevated temperature, immediate treatment (e.g., incision and drainage [I & D], pulpal extirpation, or extraction) and antibiotic and antipyretic therapy are indicated. If the patient's temperature is 40.0° C (104° F) or higher, pretreatment medical consultation is indicated. The planned treatment, especially any treatment involving the administration of CNS depressants, should be postponed, if possible, until the cause of the elevated temperature is determined and treated.

Height and Weight

Technique. Patients should be asked to state their height and weight. The range of normal height and weight is quite variable and is available on charts developed by various insurance

Box 4.6	Comorbidities Associated With Overweight and Obesity in Adults

High blood pressure
Dyslipidemia (e.g., elevated LDL cholesterol; low HDL)
Type 2 diabetes
Coronary artery disease
Sleep apnea and respiratory problems
Cerebrovascular accident
Gallbladder disease
Osteoarthritis
Some cancers (endometrial, breast, and colon)

Table 4.10	Interpretation of BMI for Adults (Age 20 Years and Above)	
BMI	**WEIGHT STATUS**
18.5–25	Normal range
26–30	Overweight
31–35	Class 1 obesity
36–40	Class 2 obesity
40–49	Morbid obesity
50 and above	Super morbid obesity

for most people and is used primarily as a screening device for weight categories that may be associated with health problems.[45] BMI does not measure body fat directly, but research has demonstrated that BMI correlates to direct measures of body fat, such as underwater weighing and dual energy x-ray absorptiometry (DXA).[46,47] BMI is used as a screening tool, not as a diagnostic tool, to identify possible weight problems for adults and children. If BMI indicates excessive weight, the health care provider would perform additional evaluations—such as skinfold thickness measurements, dietary and physical activity evaluations, and family history—to determine if the excessive weight represents a health risk.

Overweight and obese individuals are at increased risk for many diseases (comorbidities) and health conditions[48] (Box 4.6).

BMI ranges (Table 4.10) are based on the relationship between body weight and disease and death.[49] BMI is calculated in the same way for both adults and children and is based on the following formulas:

With the metric system the formula for BMI calculation is:

$$\text{Weight (kg)} \div [\text{Height (m)}]^2$$

Using pounds and inches the formula for BMI calculation is:

$$\text{Weight (lb)} \div [\text{Height (in)}]^2 \times 703$$

For example: a patient weighing 70 kg, 170 cm in height the calculation is:

$$70 \div (1.7)^2 = 24.22$$

For example: a patient weighing 154 lb, 5'6" (66") in height, the calculation is:

$$154 \div (66)^2 \times 703 = 24.85$$

Guidelines for clinical evaluation. For both female and male adults (age 20 years and above), the standard weight categories are included in Table 4.10. A BMI calculator is presented in Table 4.11.

It is estimated that between 5 million and 11 million Americans are morbidly obese—about 1 in 20 people.[50]

The correlation between BMI and body fatness is fairly strong; however, the correlation does vary by sex, race, and age.[51,52] At the same BMI value women tend to have more body fat than men; older people tend to have more body fat than younger adults; and highly trained athletes may have a high BMI because of increased muscle mass rather than increased body fat.[52]

BMI is useful in dentistry as a means of determining a patient's potential risk of developing acute medical problems. Persons with BMI values of 30 to 39.9 (obese) would be considered an ASA 2 risk, whereas those with values of 40 and above would be considered either ASA 3 or 4 after further evaluation of their medical history to determine the presence and severity of the comorbidities associated with obesity (see Box 4.6). Patients with a BMI of 35 or greater are not acceptable candidates for parenteral sedation due to the increased incidence of comorbidities associated with obesity (see Box 4.6)[48].

Visual Inspection of the Patient

Visual observation of the patient provides the dentist with valuable information concerning the patient's medical status and level of apprehension toward the planned treatment. Observation of the patient's posture, body movements, speech, and skin can assist in a diagnosis of possibly significant disorders that may previously have been undetected. Management of many of these patients is discussed in Chapters 37 and 38.

Posture. Patients with CHF and other chronic pulmonary disorders may be forced to sit in a more upright position in the dental chair because of significant orthopnea. The arthritic patient with a rigid neck may need to rotate his or her entire trunk when turning toward the dentist to view an object from the side. Recognition of these factors will better enable the dentist to determine necessary treatment modifications.

Body movement. Involuntary body movements occurring in conscious patients may connote significant disorders. Tremor is noted in disorders such as fatigue, multiple sclerosis,

Table 4.11   BMI Calculator

Height	100	110	120	130	140	150	160	170	180	190	200	210	220	230	240	250
													Weight			
5'0''	20	21	23	25	27	29	31	33	35	37	39	41	43	45	47	49
5'1''	19	21	23	25	26	28	30	32	34	36	38	40	42	43	45	47
5'2''	18	20	22	24	26	27	29	31	33	35	37	38	40	42	44	46
5'3''	18	19	21	23	25	27	28	30	32	34	35	37	39	41	43	44
5'4''	17	19	21	22	24	26	27	29	31	33	34	36	38	39	41	43
5'5''	17	18	20	22	23	25	27	28	30	32	33	35	37	38	40	42
5'6''	16	18	19	21	23	24	26	27	29	31	32	34	36	37	39	40
5'7''	16	17	19	20	22	23	25	27	28	30	31	33	34	36	38	39
5'8''	15	17	18	20	21	23	24	26	27	29	30	32	33	35	36	38
5'9''	15	16	18	19	21	22	24	25	27	28	30	31	32	34	35	37
5'10''	14	16	17	19	20	22	23	24	26	27	29	30	32	33	34	36
5'11''	14	15	17	18	20	21	22	24	25	26	27	28	30	32	33	35
6'0''	14	15	16	18	19	20	22	23	24	26	27	28	30	31	33	34
6'1''	13	15	16	17	18	20	21	22	24	25	26	28	29	30	32	33
6'2''	13	14	15	17	18	19	21	22	23	24	26	27	28	30	31	32
6'3''	12	14	15	16	17	19	20	21	22	24	25	26	27	29	30	31
6'4''	12	13	15	16	17	18	19	21	22	23	24	26	27	28	29	30

parkinsonism, hyperthyroidism, and, of great importance to dentistry, hysteria and nervous tension.

Speech. The character of a patient's speech may also be significant. For example, a CVA may cause muscle paralysis leading to speech difficulties. Anxiety over impending treatment may also be noted by listening to a patient's speech. Rapid response to questions or a nervous quiver in the voice may indicate the presence of increased anxiety and the possible need for sedation during treatment.

Other disorders may be uncovered by the detection of odors on the patient's breath. A sweet, fruity odor of acetone is present in diabetic acidosis and ketosis. The smell of ammonia is noted in uremia. Probably the most likely odor to be on the breath of a fearful dental patient is that of alcohol. Detection of alcohol on a patient's breath should lead the dentist to consider the possibility of heightened anxiety or drug abuse. It is recommended that the planned pharmacosedative procedure be cancelled in a patient who has "self-medicated."

Skin. The skin is a vast source of information about the patient. It is my belief that the dentist should, as a matter of routine, shake hands on greeting the patient. Much information can be gathered from the feel of a patient's skin. For example, the skin of a very apprehensive person will feel cold and wet, that of a patient with a hyperthyroid condition will be warm and wet, and the skin of a patient with diabetic acidosis will be warm but dry, whereas the hypoglycemic individual is cold and wet to the touch.

Looking at skin is also valuable. The color of the skin is significant. Pallor (loss of normal skin color) may indicate anemia or heightened anxiety. Cyanosis, indicating HF, chronic pulmonary disease, or polycythemia, will be most notable in the nail beds and gingiva. Flushed skin may point to apprehension, hyperthyroidism, or elevated body temperature, whereas jaundice may indicate past or present hepatic disease.

Additional factors revealed through a visual examination of the patient include the presence of prominent jugular veins (in a patient seated upright), an indication of possible right-sided HF; clubbing of the fingers (cardiopulmonary disease); swelling of the ankles (seen in right HF, varicose veins, renal disease, and in the latter stages of pregnancy); and exophthalmos (hyperthyroidism).

For a more complete discussion of the art of observation and its importance in medical diagnosis, the reader is referred to a truly excellent textbook, *Mosby's Guide to Physical Examination.*[22]

Additional Evaluation Procedures

After completion of these three steps (medical history questionnaire, vital signs, and physical examination), it will occasionally be necessary to follow up with additional evaluation for specific medical disorders. This examination may include auscultation of the heart and lungs, testing for urinary or blood glucose levels, retinal examination, function tests for cardiorespiratory status (e.g., breath-holding test, match test), electrocardiographic examination, and blood chemistries. At present, many of these tests are used in dental offices but do not represent a standard of care in dentistry. However, when general anesthesia or certain sedation techniques are to be used, the level of routine pretreatment evaluation may require some or all of these evaluations.

Dialog History

After patient information has been collected, the dentist reviews with the patient any positive responses on the questionnaire, seeking to determine the severity of these disorders and any potential risk that they might represent during the planned treatment. This process is termed the *dialog history,* and it is an integral part of patient evaluation. The dentist must put to use all available knowledge of the disease to assess the degree of risk to the patient.

Several examples of dialog history are presented in the following sections. For a more in-depth description of dialog history for specific disease states, the reader is referred to *Medical Emergencies in the Dental Office,* seventh edition.[53]

In response to a positive reply to the question "Are you diabetic?" the dialog history that follows includes the following questions:

1. What type of diabetes do you have (insulin-dependent [type 1] or non–insulin-dependent [type 2])?
2. How do you control your diabetes (oral medications or injectable insulin)?
3. How often do you check your blood sugar level, and what are the measurements (monitoring the degree of control of the disease)?
4. Have you ever been hospitalized for your diabetic condition?

The following is a dialog history to be initiated with a positive reply to angina pectoris:

1. What precipitates your angina?
2. How frequently do you experience anginal episodes?
3. How long do your anginal episodes last?
4. Describe a typical anginal episode.
5. How does nitroglycerin affect the anginal episode?
6. How many tablets or sprays do you normally need to terminate the episode?
7. Are your anginal episodes stable (similar in nature), or has there been a recent change in their frequency, intensity, radiation pattern of pain, or response to nitroglycerin (seeking unstable or preinfarction angina)?

Dialog history should be completed for every positive response noted on the medical history. A written note should be included on the questionnaire that summarizes the patient's response to the questions. For example, "heart attack" is circled. Written by the dentist next to this on the questionnaire is the statement "June 2015," implying that the patient stated that the heart attack occurred in June 2015.

RECOGNITION OF ANXIETY

Thus far the primary thrust of our evaluation of the patient has been the medical history. Few, if any, questions have been directed at the patient's feelings toward the upcoming treatment. The typical medical history questionnaire (long form) has questions that ask "Do you have fainting spells or seizures?" and "Have you had any serious trouble associated with any previous dental treatment?" Most short-form histories contain no questions relating to this important area. Heightened anxiety and fear of dentistry or surgery are stresses that can lead to the exacerbation of medical problems, such as angina, seizures, or asthma, or other stress-related problems, such as hyperventilation or vasodepressor syncope. One of the goals of the physical evaluation is to determine whether the patient is psychologically able to tolerate the stress that is associated with the planned dental treatment. Two methods are available to recognize the presence of anxiety. First is the medical history questionnaire, and second is the art of observation.

Earlier in this chapter it was recommended that one or more questions relating to a patient's attitudes toward dentistry be included in the medical history questionnaire. It has been our experience at the USC School of Dentistry that patients who do not verbally admit their fears to their dentist will record such apprehension on the history questionnaire. A positive response to any of these questions should cause the dentist to begin a more in-depth interview with the patient, seeking to determine the reason for his or her fear of dentistry.

In the absence of such questions or in the absence of a positive response to such questions, careful observation of the patient will enable the dentist and staff members to recognize the presence of unusual degrees of anxiety. Some adult patients do volunteer to the dentist and staff that they are quite apprehensive; however, the vast majority of apprehensive adult patients (both sexes but males primarily) will do everything within their power to attempt to conceal their anxiety. The usual belief of patients is that their fear is irrational and probably even a bit childish and that they are the only persons who feel this way. They do not tell the dentist of their fear because they are afraid of being labeled "childish." Because this attitude exists in many adults, all members of the dental and medical office staff should be trained to recognize clinical signs and symptoms of heightened anxiety.

Although there are a number of levels into which anxiety may be subdivided, for the purposes of this discussion, two are discussed: moderate anxiety and severe (neurotic) anxiety.

Patients with severe anxiety usually do not attempt to hide this fact from their dentist. These persons usually do everything within their power to avoid becoming dental patients. It is estimated that between 14 million and 34 million adults in the United States avoid regular dental care because of their intense fears.[54] These persons constitute the severe anxiety group. When in the dental or medical office, they may be recognized by the following:

1. Increased BP and heart rate
2. Trembling
3. Excessive sweating
4. Dilated pupils

Severely apprehensive and fearful patients most often appear in the dental office suffering from a severe toothache or infection. On questioning, they state that they have had this problem for quite some time (e.g., months), not just a few days, and have exhausted every available means of home remedy (e.g., toothache drops and alcohol), which apparently worked for some time. The reason they are finally in the dental office is that for the past few nights they have been unable to sleep because of the intense pain that none of their home remedies could alleviate. These patients are driven by their pain to the dental office, where their usual expectation is to have the offending tooth removed. These patients frequently represent a significant management problem. Although they desire to have their dental problem treated, when the time comes for treatment to begin, their underlying fear of dentistry comes to the forefront, making it almost impossible for them to tolerate the procedure. In addition, and by no means of secondary importance, the dentist is often faced with the unpleasant prospect of either having to extract an acutely inflamed tooth or to extirpate the pulp of an acutely sensitive tooth—two situations in which achieving clinically adequate pain control can prove difficult, even in the best of circumstances.

Because of these factors, severely anxious patients will very often be candidates for the use of either IV moderate sedation or general anesthesia. Other techniques, such as oral, IM, or inhalation sedation, used as suggested will have a diminished likelihood of success, primarily because of their limited effectiveness or the constraints that are properly placed on their use. Younger children with severe anxiety and fear levels are candidates for IM, IN, or IV moderate or deep sedation or general anesthesia.

It is much more common to see patients with moderate degrees of dental anxiety. Most of these are adult patients who try to hide their fears from the dentist because they believe that, as adults, they should not admit to a fear of the dentist. Children, on the other hand, less inhibited and less mature than the typical adult, immediately let the office staff know their feelings toward dentistry. Assuming that adult patients may attempt to hide their fears, the dentist and staff should remain observant both before and during the planned treatment.

"Front-office" staff (e.g., the receptionist) will be able to overhear patients' conversations in the waiting room, or patients might ask important questions of the receptionist, such as "Is the doctor gentle?" or "Does the doctor use gas?" The receptionist should be trained to inform the dentist or chairside staff immediately whenever a patient makes statements that might indicate an increased degree of concern about upcoming treatment. This is also true for chairside personnel.

Shaking hands with the patient may lead to a presumption of anxiety when the patient's palms are cold and sweaty, especially when the office is not especially cool. Discussing a patient's prior dental experiences may give an indication of the dental anxiety status. The patient with a history of emergency care only (e.g., extractions or I & D) but who cancels or does not appear for subsequent (more routine) treatment may be a fearful individual. A patient with a history of multiple cancelled appointments may also be a fearful patient. This history should be discussed with the patient in an attempt to determine the reasons behind this pattern of treatment (or nontreatment).

The patient, once seated in the chair, should be listened to and watched. Apprehensive patients remain alert and on guard at all times. They sit at the edge of the chair, eyes roaming around the room, taking in everything. They exhibit an unnaturally stiff posture, their arms and legs tense. They may nervously play with a handkerchief or tissue, occasionally unaware that they are doing so. The "white-knuckle" syndrome may be observed, in which the patient clutches the armrest of the dental chair tightly enough that their knuckles become ischemic. Diaphoresis (sweating) of the palms and forehead may be noted, explained by the patient as "Gee, it's hot in here." The moderately apprehensive patient will be overly willing to aid the dentist. Actions are carried out quickly, usually without thinking. Questions to this patient are answered rapidly, usually too rapidly.

Once anxiety is recognized, be it through the questionnaire or by observation, the patient should be confronted with it. The straightforward approach is surprisingly successful, "Mr. Smith, I see from your medical history that you have had several unpleasant experiences in a dental office. Tell me about them." When the anxiety was determined visually, "Mrs. Smith, you appear to be somewhat nervous today. Is anything bothering you?" I have been truly amazed at how rapidly patients drop all pretenses at being calm once it is known that the dentist is aware of their fears. They usually say, "Doctor, I didn't think you could tell" or "I thought I could handle it." Now it is your job to determine the exact source of the patient's fears, such as injections or the drill. Once fears are made known, steps can be taken to minimize the development of adverse situations related to them.

The patient with moderate anxiety will usually prove to be manageable. In most cases, psychosedation will be effective in this patient. This may involve the administration of a drug (pharmacosedation) and/or a nondrug form of sedation (iatrosedation). General anesthesia will be needed only rarely for effective management of these patients.

With the information that has now been gathered concerning the patient's past and present medical and dental histories, vital signs, and physical examination, the basic goals of evaluation can now be completed.

DETERMINATION OF MEDICAL RISK

Having completed all of the components of the physical evaluation and a thorough dental examination, the dentist next takes all of this information and answers the following questions:

1. Is the patient capable, physically and psychologically, of tolerating in relative safety the stresses involved in the proposed treatment?

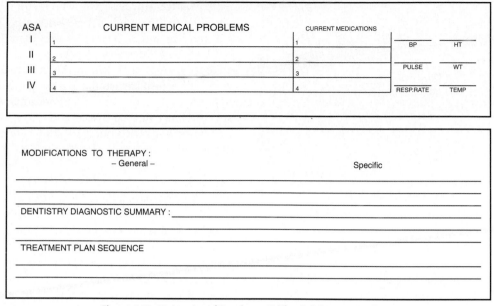

Figure 4.12 University of Southern California PE summary form.

2. Does the patient represent a greater risk (of morbidity or mortality) than normal during this treatment?
3. If the patient does represent an increased risk, what modifications will be necessary in the planned treatment to minimize this risk?
4. Is the risk too great for the patient to be managed safely as an outpatient in the medical or dental office?

In an effort to answer these questions, the USC School of Dentistry developed a physical evaluation system that attempts to assist the dentist in categorizing patients from the standpoint of risk factor orientation.[55,56] Its function is to assign the patient an appropriate risk category so that dental care can be provided to the patient in comfort and with increased safety. The system is based on the ASA physical status classification system, which is described next.

PHYSICAL STATUS CLASSIFICATION SYSTEM

In 1962 the American Society of Anesthesiology adopted what is now referred to as the *ASA physical status classification system*.[39] It represents a method of estimating medical risk presented by a patient undergoing a surgical procedure. The system was designed primarily for patients about to receive a general anesthetic, but since its introduction, the classification system has been used for all surgical patients regardless of anesthetic technique (e.g., general anesthesia, regional anesthesia, sedation). The system has been in continual use since 1962, virtually without change, and has proved to be a valuable method of determining surgical and anesthetic risk before the actual procedure.[57,58] The classification system follows**:

**If the procedure is performed as an emergency, an E is added to the previously defined ASA physical status (e.g., ASA E-3).

Class 1. A healthy patient (no physiologic, physical, or psychological abnormalities)
Class 2. A patient with mild systemic disease without limitation of daily activities
Class 3. A patient with severe systemic disease that limits activity but is not incapacitating
Class 4. A patient with incapacitating systemic disease that is a constant threat to life
Class 5. A moribund patient not expected to survive 24 hours with or without the operation
Class 6. A brain-dead patient whose organs are being removed for donor purposes

When this system was adapted for use in a typical outpatient dental or medical setting, ASA 5 and 6 were eliminated and an attempt was made to correlate the remaining four classifications with possible treatment modifications for dental treatment. Fig. 4.12 illustrates the USC physical evaluation form on which a summary of the patient's physical and psychological status is presented along with planned treatment modifications.

In the discussion of the ASA categories to follow, the term *normal or usual* activity is used along with the term *distress*. Definitions of these terms follow: *Normal* or *usual* activity is defined as the ability to climb one flight of stairs or to walk two level city blocks, and *distress* is defined as undue fatigue, shortness of breath, or chest pain. Fig. 4.13 illustrates the ASA classification system based on the ability to climb one flight of stairs. Each of the ASA classifications is reviewed with specific examples listed.

ASA 1

ASA 1 patients are considered to be "normal and healthy." They are able to carry out normal activity without distress. They are able to climb a flight of stairs or walk two level city

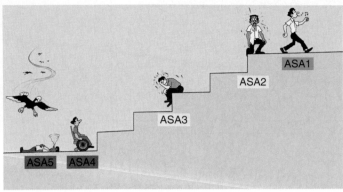

ASA CLASSIFICATION

Figure 4.13 ASA classification. (Courtesy Dr. Lawrence Day.)

blocks without distress (undue fatigue, shortness of breath, or chest pain).

Review of this patient's medical history, physical evaluation, and any other parameters that have been evaluated indicates no abnormalities (heart, lungs, liver, kidneys, and CNS are WNL). Physiologically, this patient should be able to tolerate the stresses associated with the planned treatment with no added risk of serious complications. Psychologically, this patient should encounter little or no difficulty in handling the proposed treatment. Healthy patients with little or no anxiety are classified as ASA 1. Treatment modifications are usually not warranted in this patient group. The ASA 1 patient is a candidate for any sedation technique or for outpatient general anesthesia. The ASA 1 patient represents a green traffic light (go) for treatment.

ASA 2

ASA 2 patients have "a mild systemic disease," or are healthy but have extreme anxiety and fear toward dentistry, or are pregnant. ASA 2 patients are able to complete normal activities but must rest because of distress. The ASA 2 patient can negotiate one flight of stairs or walk two level city blocks but must rest at the completion of the task because of distress (chest pain, undue fatigue, or shortness of breath).

ASA 2 patients are less stress tolerant than ASA 1 patients. However, they still represent a minimal risk during treatment. Elective treatment is in order, with consideration given for treatment modifications or special considerations, as warranted by the particular condition. Examples of such modifications include the use of sedative techniques, limiting the duration of treatment, and possibly obtaining medical consultation. There are no general limitations on the use of pharmacosedative procedures for the ASA 2 patient. Outpatient general anesthesia may be administered to ASA 2 patients. The ASA 2 patient represents a yellow traffic light (proceed with caution) for treatment. Treatment modifications should be considered.

Examples of ASA 2 patients are (1) the healthy, pregnant female; (2) the healthy but extremely phobic patient; (3) the

patient with a drug allergy or who is atopic (multiple allergies present); (4) the adult patient with a BP between 140 and 159 mm Hg and/or 90 and 94 mm Hg; (5) the patient with NIDDM (type 2 diabetes); (6) the patient with well-controlled epilepsy (no seizures within the past year); (7) the patient with well-controlled asthma; (8) the patient with a history of hyperthyroid or hypothyroid conditions who is under care and presently in a euthyroid condition; (9) ASA 1 patients presenting with URIs and (10) BMI between 30.0 and 39.9 (assess for the presence of comorbidities).

ASA 3

ASA 3 patients have "severe systemic disease that limits activity but is not incapacitating." An ASA 3 patient is able to climb a flight of stairs or walk two level city blocks but must stop at least once before reaching the goal because of distress.

The ASA 3 patient does not exhibit signs or symptoms of distress while at rest (e.g., in the reception room); however, in stressful situations (e.g., dental chair), signs and symptoms may develop.

ASA 3 patients are less able to tolerate stress than those classified as ASA 2. Elective dental care is still appropriate; however, the need for stress-reduction techniques and other treatment modifications is increased. Serious consideration must be given to treatment modifications in ASA 3 patients. Outpatient general anesthesia is not usually recommended for these patients; however, many of the pharmacosedation techniques may be used with some potential modification as to the length of procedure and the depth of sedation. ASA 3 patients represent a yellow traffic light (proceed with caution) for treatment.

Examples of ASA 3 patients include (1) the patient with well-controlled IDDM (type 1 diabetes); (2) the patient with symptomatic thyroid disease (hypothyroid or hyperthyroid); (3) the patient who had an MI more than 6 months ago with no residual complications; (4) the patient who had a CVA more than 6 months ago with no residual complications; (5) the adult patient with a BP between 160 and 199 mm Hg and/or 95 and 114 mm Hg; (6) the patient with epilepsy that is less well controlled (several seizures or more per year); (7) the asthmatic patient, less well controlled, stress or exercise induced, and/or a history of hospitalization because of status asthmaticus; (8) the patient with angina pectoris (stable angina [e.g., angina of exertion]); (9) the patient with HF, with orthopnea (more than two pillows), and/or ankle edema; (10) the patient with COPD (emphysema or chronic bronchitis); (11) patients who are functionally anephric (renal dialysis patients); and (12) BMI of 40.0 or greater (may represent ASA 3 or ASA 4 depending on the presence and severity of comorbidities).

ASA 4

ASA 4 patients have "an incapacitating disease that is a constant threat to life." ASA 4 patients are unable either to negotiate a flight of stairs or walk two level city blocks.

ASA 4 patients exhibit signs and symptoms of their medical problem(s) at rest. Seated in the reception room of the dental or medical office, such patients exhibit undue fatigue, shortness of breath, or chest pain. Patients in this category have a medical problem that is of greater significance than the planned dental treatment. Elective care should be postponed until the patient's medical condition has improved to at least an ASA 3. The ASA 4 patient represents a significant risk during treatment.

The management of dental emergencies, such as infection and pain, in the ASA 4 patient should be treated as conservatively as possible until the patient's physical condition improves. When possible, emergency care should be noninvasive, consisting of the prescription of drugs, such as analgesics for pain and antibiotics for infection. If sedation is necessary, inhalation sedation with N_2O-O_2 is preferred. In situations in which it is believed that immediate intervention is required (I & D, extraction, pulpal extirpation), it is recommended that, when possible, the ASA 4 patient receive such care within the confines of an acute care facility (e.g., hospital). Although the risk to the patient is still significant, the chance of survival should an acute medical emergency arise is likely increased.

The ASA 4 patient represents a red traffic light (stop; do not proceed) for treatment. Examples of ASA 4 patients include (1) the patient with unstable angina pectoris (preinfarction angina), (2) the patient who had an MI less than 6 months ago, (3) the patient who had a CVA less than 6 months ago, (4) the adult patient who has a BP of 200 mm Hg and/or 115 mm Hg or higher, (5) the patient with uncontrolled dysrhythmias (requires medical consultation before the start of treatment), (6) the patient with severe HF or COPD who is confined to a wheelchair and/or requires supplemental O_2 therapy, (7) the patient with uncontrolled epilepsy, (8) the patient with uncontrolled IDDM, and (9) the patient with a BMI of 40.0 or greater (may represent ASA 3 or ASA 4 depending on the presence and severity of comorbidities).

ASA 5

An ASA 5 patient is "a moribund patient not expected to survive 24 hours with or without operation." The ASA 5 patient is almost always a hospitalized patient with an end-stage disease. The ASA 5 patient is not a candidate for elective dental care. However, dental treatment is frequently required for the management of any intraoral and dental problems that arise. The nature of the dental care rendered is palliative—the relief of pain and/or infection. The physical condition of the ASA 5 patient is fragile at best. The use of local anesthetics and other CNS depressants should be undertaken with as much care as possible. ASA 5 patients should be monitored throughout the procedure.

The ASA 5 patient represents a red traffic light (stop; do not proceed) for elective treatment. Examples of ASA 5 patients include (1) the patient with end-stage cancer, (2) the patient with end-stage heart and/or lung disease, (3) the patient with end-stage hepatic disease, and (4) the patient with end-stage infectious disease.

The ASA physical evaluation system is quite simple to employ when a patient has an isolated medical problem. However, many patients are seen with histories of several significant diseases. On these occasions, the dentist must weigh the significance of each disease and make a judgment as to the appropriate ASA category. The system is not meant to be inflexible, but to function as a relative value system based on the dentist's clinical judgment. When the dentist is unable to determine the clinical significance of one or more disease processes, consultation with the patient's physician or other medical or dental colleagues is recommended. In all cases, however, the ultimate decision of whether to treat or to postpone treatment must be made by the treating dentist. Responsibility and liability rest solely in the hands of the dentist who treats, or does not treat, the patient.

STRESS-REDUCTION PROTOCOLS

At this point in our pretreatment evaluation of the patient, we have reviewed all of the history and physical evaluation data and assigned a physical status classification. Most patients will be assigned an ASA 1 or ASA 2 status (85% in most private dental practices), with fewer still categorized as ASA 3 (about 14%) and ASA 4.[59]

As has been discussed, every dental or surgical procedure is potentially stress inducing. Such stress may be of a physiologic nature (pain, strenuous exercise) or of a psychological nature (anxiety, fear). In both types, however, one of the responses of the body involves an increased release of catecholamines (epinephrine and norepinephrine) from the adrenal medulla into the cardiovascular system. This results in an increased workload on the cardiovascular system (increased rate and strength of myocardial contraction and an increased myocardial oxygen requirement). Although the ASA 1 patient may be quite able to tolerate such changes in cardiovascular activity, ASA 2, 3, and 4 patients are increasingly less able to safely tolerate this increased workload. The patient with stable angina (ASA 3) may respond with an episode of chest discomfort, and various dysrhythmias may develop. Pulmonary edema may develop in patients with HF. Patients with noncardiovascular disorders may also respond adversely when faced with increased levels of stress. For example, the patient with asthma may develop an acute episode of breathing distress, whereas the epileptic patient may suffer a seizure. Unusual degrees of stress in the ASA 1 patient may be responsible for several psychogenically induced emergency situations, such as hyperventilation or vasodepressor syncope.

Interviews with fearful dental patients have demonstrated that many begin to worry about their upcoming dental or surgical treatment 1 day or more before the appointment. These persons may be unable to sleep well the night before their appointment, thus arriving for the procedure fatigued and even more stress intolerant. The risk presented by this patient during treatment is further increased.

The SRPs are two series of procedures that, when used either individually or collectively, act to minimize stress during treatment and thereby decrease the risk presented by the patient.[2,60] These protocols are predicated on the belief that the prevention or reduction of stress ought to begin before the start of treatment and continue throughout the treatment period and, if indicated, into the postoperative period.

Stress-Reduction Protocol: Normal, Healthy, but Anxious Patient (ASA 1 or 2)

1. Recognition of anxiety
2. Premedication with CNS depressant (anxiolytic, hypnotic) the night before the scheduled appointment, as needed
3. Premedication with CNS depressant (anxiolytic, hypnotic) immediately (e.g., 1 hour) before the scheduled appointment, as needed
4. Appointment scheduled in the morning
5. Minimization of office waiting time
6. Psychosedation during treatment, as needed
7. Adequate pain control during treatment
8. Length of appointment variable
9. Postoperative pain and anxiety control

Stress-Reduction Protocol: Medical Risk Patient (ASA 3 and 4)

1. Recognition of medical risk
2. Medical consultation before treatment, as needed
3. Appointment scheduled in the morning
4. Preoperative and postoperative vital signs monitored and recorded
5. Psychosedation during treatment, as needed
6. Adequate pain control during treatment
7. Length of appointment variable, but not to exceed patient's limits of tolerance
8. Postoperative pain and anxiety control

Recognition of Medical Risk and Anxiety

Recognition of these factors represents the starting point for the management of stress in the dental or surgical patient. Medical risk assessment will be accurately determined by strict adherence to the measures previously described in this chapter. The recognition of anxiety is often a more difficult task. As has been described, visual observation of the patient and verbal communication can provide the dentist with clues to the presence of anxiety.

Medical Consultation

Medical consultation should be considered in those situations in which the dentist is uncertain about the degree of risk represented by the patient. Medical consultation is neither required nor recommended for all medically compromised patients. In all cases, it must be remembered that a consultation is but a request for additional information concerning a specific patient or disease process. The dentist is seeking information that will aid him or her in determining the degree of risk and

which therapy modifications might be beneficial. The ultimate responsibility for the care and safety of the patient rests solely with the person who treats the patient.

Premedication

Many apprehensive patients state that their fear of dentistry or surgery is so great that they are unable to sleep well the night before their appointment. Fatigued the next day, these patients are less able to tolerate any additional stresses placed on them during their treatment. Should the patient be medically compromised, the risk of an acute exacerbation of the patient's medical problem is significantly increased. In the ASA 1 patient, such additional stress might provoke a psychogenically induced response. A clinical manifestation of increased fatigue includes a lowered pain reaction threshold, whereby the patient is more likely to respond to a nonpainful stimulus as being painful than is a well-rested patient.

Whenever it has been determined that heightened anxiety exists, it should also be determined whether this anxiety interferes with the patient's sleep. Restful sleep the night before a scheduled morning appointment is desirable. The administration of an oral sedative is one method of achieving this goal. An antianxiety or sedative-hypnotic drug, such as diazepam, triazolam, flurazepam, zaleplon, or zolpidem, may be prescribed for administration 1 hour before sleep (e.g., 1 hour hs). Appropriate dosages of these and other drugs are discussed in Chapter 7. As the scheduled appointment approaches, the patient's anxiety level will heighten. In many cases the administration of an antianxiety or sedative-hypnotic drug approximately 1 hour before the scheduled appointment will decrease the patient's anxiety level to a degree such that the thought of dental or surgical treatment is no longer as frightening. Oral drugs should be administered approximately 1 hour before the scheduled start of treatment to permit a therapeutic blood level of the agent to develop. Though it is highly recommended that oral sedatives be administered to the patient in the dental office, oral drugs may be taken by the patient at home. Whenever a CNS-depressant drug has been prescribed to be taken by the patient at home, the dentist *must* advise the patient against driving a car or operating other potentially hazardous machinery. The appropriate use of oral antianxiety or sedative-hypnotic drugs is an excellent means of diminishing preoperative stress. Premedication might also include the need for preoperative antibiotic prophylaxis. Indications and protocols are found in Table 4.1 and Boxes 4.1 and 4.2.

Appointment Scheduling

Apprehensive or medically compromised patients are best able to tolerate stress when well rested. For most of these patients, the ideal time to schedule dental treatment is early in the day. This is also the case for apprehensive or medically compromised children.

If treatment is scheduled for the afternoon, the apprehensive patient must contend for many hours with the ominous specter of the dental or surgical appointment, casting a pall over everything the patient does before it, allowing more time to think and to worry about it. The patient becomes more anxious, thereby increasing the likelihood of adverse psychogenic reactions. A morning appointment permits this patient to "get it over with" and to then continue with their usual activities unfettered by anxiety.

For the medically compromised patient, the situation is somewhat similar. As fatigue sets in, the patient becomes less and less able to tolerate any further increase in stress. An appointment scheduled later in the day after hours at work and perhaps a drive through traffic will present the dentist with a medically compromised patient with little or no ability to handle adequately the additional stress of dental care. An early appointment provides the dentist and the patient with a degree of flexibility in patient management.

Minimization of Waiting Time

Once in the dental or medical office setting, the fearful patient should not be made to remain in the reception area or dental chair for extended periods before treatment begins. It is well known that anticipation of a procedure can induce more fear than the actual procedure.[61] Sitting and waiting allow the patient to smell dental smells, hear dental sounds, and fantasize about the "horrible things" that are going to happen. Cases of serious morbidity and death have occurred in the reception room of dental offices before the start of treatment.[62,63] This factor is of greater significance in the apprehensive patient.

Vital Signs (Preoperative and Postoperative)

Before treatment is started on a medically compromised patient, it is recommended that the dentist monitor and record the patient's vital signs. (Vital signs may be recorded by a trained auxiliary.) Signs monitored should include BP, heart rate and rhythm, and respiratory rate. Comparison of these preoperative vital signs with the baseline values recorded at a previous (nontreatment) visit can serve as an indicator of the patient's physical and emotional status on the day of treatment. Although especially relevant to patients with cardiovascular disease, it is recommended that preoperative vital signs be recorded on all medically compromised (all ASA 4 and 3 and appropriate ASA 2) patients. Postoperative vital signs should also be monitored and recorded in the dental chart for these same patients. Preoperative vital signs must be recorded for all patients receiving pharmacosedation.

Psychosedation During Therapy

Should additional stress reduction be deemed appropriate during treatment, any technique of sedation or general anesthesia may be considered. The means of selecting the appropriate technique for a given patient are discussed in subsequent sections of this book. Nondrug techniques include iatrosedation and hypnosis, whereas the more commonly used pharmacosedation procedures include oral, inhalation, IM, IN, and IV sedation. The primary goal of all these techniques is the same: the decrease

or elimination of stress in a conscious patient. When used as described in this book, this goal may readily be achieved without added risk to the patient.

Adequate Pain Control During Therapy

For stress reduction to be successful, it is essential that adequate pain control be obtained. The successful management of pain is of greater importance in the medically compromised patient than in the ASA 1 patient. The potentially adverse actions of endogenously released catecholamines on cardiovascular function in the patient with clinically significant heart or blood vessel disease warrant the inclusion of vasoconstrictors in the local anesthetic solution.[64] Without adequate control of pain, sedation and stress reduction are impossible to achieve.

Duration of Treatment

The duration of treatment is of significance to both medically compromised and fearful patients. In the absence of any medical factors indicating the need for shorter appointments, the length of the appointment should be determined by the dentist after consideration of the patient's desires. In many instances, a healthy but apprehensive patient (ASA 1) may prefer to have as few dental appointments as possible, regardless of their length. Appointments 3 hours or longer may constitute the preferred management for this otherwise healthy patient (assuming, of course, that the dentist too is an ASA 1 or 2). However, attempting to satisfy the patient's (or parents' or guardians') desires for longer appointments is inadvisable when the dentist believes that there are appropriate reasons for shorter appointments. Cases of serious morbidity and of death have occurred when the dentist complied with parents' wishes to complete their child's dental treatment in one long appointment. It is recommended that moderate or deep sedation procedures ideally not exceed 2 hours in length, unless absolutely necessary, but under no circumstances should the procedure exceed 4 hours.[65,66]

Unlike the fearful ASA 1 patient, the medically compromised patient should not be permitted to undergo longer appointments. In a dental chair, 1 hour of treatment is stressful for many persons. Even an ASA 1 patient may have difficulty tolerating 2- or 3-hour appointments. To permit the higher-risk patient to undergo extended treatments may unnecessarily increase risk. Dental appointments in the medically compromised patient should be shorter and not exceed the limit of the patient's tolerance. Signs that this limit has been reached include evidence of fatigue, restlessness, sweating, and evident discomfort by the patient. The most prudent means of managing the patient at this time is to terminate the procedure as expeditiously as possible and to reschedule their treatment.

Postoperative Control of Pain and Anxiety

Of equal importance to preoperative and intraoperative pain and anxiety control is their management in the posttreatment period. This is especially relevant for the patient who has undergone a potentially traumatic procedure (i.e., endodontics, periodontal or oral surgery, extensive oral reconstruction, or restorative procedures). The dentist must carefully consider any possible complications that could arise during the 24 hours immediately following treatment, discuss these with the patient, and then take steps to assist the patient in managing them. These steps include any or all of the following, when indicated:

1. Availability of the dentist via telephone around the clock
2. Pain control: prescription for analgesic drugs, as needed
3. Antibiotics: prescription for antibiotics, if the possibility of infection exists
4. Antianxiety agents, if in the dentist's opinion the patient may require them
5. Muscle relaxant drugs after prolonged therapy or multiple injections into one area (i.e., inferior alveolar nerve block)

The availability of the dentist by telephone around the clock has become a standard of care in the health professions. With answering services and mobile phones universally available, patients should be able to contact their dentist whenever necessary.

Pain Control

Several studies have demonstrated that unexpected pain is rated as being more uncomfortable than expected pain.[61] Should the possibility of discomfort (pain) following a procedure exist, the patient should be forewarned and an analgesic drug made available. When the possibility of posttreatment pain has not been discussed and it does develop, the patient immediately assumes that something has gone wrong. Such pain is recorded as more intense and anxiety provoking than pain that is expected (e.g., the patient has been advised of its likelihood) because of the emotional component of unexpected pain, which is not found in pain that is expected.[54] Should posttreatment pain, which has been discussed, fail to materialize, the patient will be all the more relaxed and confident in their dentist's abilities.

Through the use of the steps included in the SRP, patient management has been enlarged to include the preoperative and postoperative periods and the intraoperative period. These protocols have made it possible to manage the dental health needs of a broad spectrum of fearful and medically compromised patients with a minimal complication rate. Specific procedures included in the protocols are expanded throughout this book.

REFERENCES

1. Goldberger E: *Treatment of cardiac emergencies*, ed 5, St Louis, 1990, Mosby.
2. McCarthy FM: Stress reduction and therapy modifications. *J Calif Dent Assoc* 9:41–47, 1981.
3. McCarthy FM, Malamed SF: Physical evaluation system to determine medical risk and indicated dental therapy modifications. *J Am Dent Assoc* 99:181–184, 1979.
4. Berthelsen CL, Stilley KR: Automated personal health inventory for dentistry: a pilot study. *J Am Dent Assoc* 131:59–66, 2000.
5. Chestnutt IG, Morgan MZ, Hoddell C, Playle R: A comparison of a computer-based questionnaire and personal interviews in determining oral health-related behaviours. *Community Dent Oral Epidemiol* 32(6):410–417, 2004.
6. Brady WF, Martinoff JT: Validity of health history data collected from dental patients and patient perception of health status. *J Am Dent Assoc* 101:642–645, 1980.
7. Oofuvong M, Geater AF, Chongsuvivatwong V, et al: Excess costs and length of hospital stay attributable to perioperative respiratory events in children. *Anesth Analg* 120(2):411–419, 2015.
8. Jeske AH, editor: *Mosby's dental drug reference*, ed 10, St Louis, 2011, Mosby.
9. Fukuda K: Intravenous anesthetics. In Miller RD, editor: *Miller's anesthesia*, ed 6, Philadelphia, 2005, Elsevier.
10. Skidmore-Roth I: *Mosby's 2013 nursing drug reference*, ed 26, St Louis, 2013, Mosby.
11. Little J, Falace D, Miller C, et al: *Little and Falace's Dental management of the medically compromised patient*, ed 8, St Louis, 2012, Mosby.
12. Wilson W, Taubert KA, Gewitz M, et al: Prevention of infective endocarditis: guidelines from the American Heart Association: a guideline from the American Heart Association Rheumatic Fever, Endocarditis, and Kawasaki Disease Committee, Council on Cardiovascular Disease in the Young, and the Council on Clinical Cardiology, Council on Cardiovascular Surgery and Anesthesia, and the Quality of Care and Outcomes Research Interdisciplinary Working Group. *Circulation* 116(15):1736–1754, 2007.
13. National Institute for Health and Clinical Excellence: Prophylaxis against infective endocarditis. Antimicrobial prophylaxis against infective endocarditis in adults and children undergoing interventional procedures. Clinical guideline 64, London: NICE, 2008.
14. Joint Formulary Committee: *British National Formulary 55*, 2008, British Medical Association and Royal Pharmaceutical Society of Great Britain.
15. Rethman MP, Watters W, 3rd, Abt E, et al: The American Academy of Orthopaedic Surgeons and the American Dental Association clinical practice guideline on the prevention of orthopaedic implant infection in patients undergoing dental procedures. *J Bone Joint Surg Am* 95(8):745–747, 2013.
16. Watters W, 3rd, Rethman MP, Hanson NB, et al: Prevention of orthopaedic implant infection in patients undergoing dental procedures. *J Am Acad Orthop Surg* 21(3):180–189, 2013.
17. Berbari EF, Osmon DR, Carr A, et al: Dental procedures as risk factors for prosthetic hip or knee infection: a hospital-based prospective case-control study. *Clin Infect Dis* 50(1):8–16, 2010.
18. Sollecito TP, Abt E, Lockhart PB, et al: The use of prophylactic antibiotics prior to dental procedures in patients with prosthetic joints. *J Am Dent Assoc* 146(1):11–16, 2015.
19. http://neurosurgery.ucla.edu/body.cfm?id=231. (Accessed 30 July 2015).
20. National Collaborating Centre for Chronic Conditions, Chronic Obstructive Pulmonary Disease: National clinical guideline on management of chronic obstructive pulmonary disease in adults in primary and secondary care. *Thorax* 59(Suppl 1):1–232, 2004.
21. Yakahane Y, Kojima M, Sugai Y, et al: Hepatitis C virus infection in spouses of patients with type C chronic liver disease. *Ann Intern Med* 120(9):748–752, 1994.
22. Seidel HM, Ball JW, Dains J, editors: *Mosby's guide to physical examination*, St Louis, 2006, CV Mosby.

23. Wilburn-Goo D, Lloyd LM: When patients become cyanotic: acquired methemoglobinemia. *J Am Dent Assoc* 130:826–831, 1999.

24. Malamed SF: Reversing local anesthesia. *Inside Dent* 4(7):2–3, 2008.

25. DerMarderosian A, Beutler JA, editors: *The review of natural products*, St Louis, 2015, Facts and Comparisons.

26. Fetrow CH, Avila JR: *Professional's handbook of complementary and alternative medicine*, ed 3, Philadelphia, 2003, Lippincott Williams & Wilkins.

27. *2015 Physicians' desk reference,* ed 69, Oradell, NJ, 2015, Medical Economics.

28. Gruenwald J, Brendler T, Jaenicke C, editors: *2007 Physicians' desk reference for herbal medicines*, ed 4, Oradell, NJ, 2008, Medical Economics.

29. American Dental Association: *ADA/PDR guide to dental therapeutics*, ed 5, Chicago, 2012, The Association.

30. Smith DM, Lombardo JA, Robinson JB: The preparticipation evaluation. *Prim Care* 18:777–807, 1991.

31. American Heart Association: *Recommendations for human blood pressure determination by sphygmomanometry*, Dallas, 1967, The Association.

32. Pickering TG, Hall JE, Appel LJ, et al: Recommendations for blood pressure measurement in humans and experimental animals: Part 1: blood pressure measurement in humans: a statement for professionals from the subcommittee of professional and public education of the American Heart Association Council on High Blood Pressure Research. *Hypertension* 45:142–161, 2005.

33. Mitchell PT, Parlin RW, Blackburn H: Effect of vertical displacement of the arm on indirect blood pressure measurement. *N Engl J Med* 271:72–74, 1964.

34. Wonka F, Thummler M, Schoppe A: Clinical test of a blood pressure measurement device with a wrist cuff. *Blood Press Monit* 1:361–366, 1996.

35. Manning DM, Kuchirka C, Kaminski J: Miscuffing: inappropriate blood pressure cuff application. *Circulation* 68:763–766, 1983.

36. Manning G, Rushton L, Millar-Craig MW: Clinical implications of white coat hypertension: an ambulatory blood pressure monitoring study. *J Hum Hypertens* 13:817, 1999.

37. La Batide-Alamore A, Chatellier G, Bobrie G, et al: Comparison of nurse- and physician-determined clinic blood pressure levels in patients referred to a hypertension clinic: implications for subsequent management. *J Hypertens* 18:391–398, 2000.

38. Lane D, Beevers M, Barnes N, et al: Inter-arm differences in blood pressure: when are they clinically significant? *J Hypertens* 20:1089–1095, 2002.

39. American Society of Anesthesiologists: New classification of physical status. *Anesthesiology* 24:111, 1963.

40. Malamed SF: Blood pressure evaluation and the prevention of medical emergencies in dental practice. *J Prev Dent* 6:183, 1980.

41. Malamed SF: Prevention. In *Handbook of medical emergencies in the dental office*, ed 7, St Louis, 2015, CV Mosby, p 43.

42. Ryan TJ, Antman EM, Brooks NH, et al: 1999 update: ACC/AHA guidelines for the management of patients with acute myocardial infarction: a report of the American College of Cardiology/American Heart Association Task Force on Practice Guidelines (Committee on Management of Acute Myocardial Infarction). *J Am Coll Cardiol* 34:890–911, 1999.

43. Gregoratos G, Abrams J, Epstein AE, et al: ACC/AHA/NASPE 2002 Guideline update for implantation of cardiac pacemakers and antiarrhythmic devices: summary article: a report of the American College of Cardiology/American Heart Association Task Force on Practice Guidelines (ACC/AHA/NASPE Committee to Update the 1998 Pacemaker Guidelines). *Circulation* 106:2145–2161, 2002.

44. Weber M: Pulsus alternans. A case study. *Crit Care Nurse* 23(3):51–54, 2003.

45. Centers for Disease Control and Prevention: Body mass index. Available at http://www.cdc.gov/healthyweight/assessing/bmi/. (Accessed 30 July 2015).

46. Mei Z, Grummer-Strawn LM, Pietrobelli A, et al: Validity of body mass index compared with other body-composition screening indexes for the assessment of body fatness in children and adolescents. *Am J Clin Nutr* 75:978–985, 2002.

47. Garrow JS, Webster J: Quetelet's index (W/H2) as a measure of fatness. *Int J Obes* 9:147–153, 1985.

48. National Heart Lung and Blood Institute: Clinical guidelines on the identification, evaluation, and treatment of overweight and obesity in adults: the evidence report, Bethesda, MD, NHLB Institute, 1996.

49. World Health Organization Technical Report Series: *Physical status: the use and interpretation of anthropometry*, Geneva, Switzerland, 1995, World Health Organization.

50. Sturm R: Increases in morbid obesity in the USA: 2000–2005. *Public Health* 121:492–496, 2007.

51. Prentice AM, Jebb SA: Beyond body mass index. *Obes Rev* 2:141–147, 2001.

52. Gallagher D, Visser M, Sepulveda D, et al: How useful is BMI for comparison of body fatness across age, sex and ethnic groups? *Am J Epidemiol* 143:228–239, 1996.

53. Malamed SF: *Medical emergencies in the dental office*, ed 7, St Louis, 2015, CV Mosby.

54. Milgrom P, Weinstein P: *Treating fearful dental patients*, Seattle, 1996, University of Washington in Seattle, Continuing Dental Education.

55. McCarthy FM, Malamed SF: *Physical evaluation manual*, Los Angeles, 1975, University of Southern California School of Dentistry.

56. McCarthy FM, Malamed SF: Physical evaluation system to determine medical risk and indicated dental therapy modifications. *J Am Dent Assoc* 99:181–184, 1979.

57. Fleisher LA: Risk of anesthesia. In Miller RD, Fleisher LA, Johns RA, editors: *Miller's anesthesia*, ed 8, 2014, Churchill Livingstone.

58. Lagasse RS: Anesthesia safety: model or myth? A review of the published literature and analysis of current original data. *Anesthesiology* 97:1609–1617, 2002.

59. Malamed SF: ASA physical status, unpublished data, 2006.

60. Malamed SF: The stress reduction protocols: a method of minimizing risk in dental practice, paper presented at the fifth annual Continuing Education Seminar in Practical Considerations in IV and IM Dental Sedation, Miami, 1979, Mt Sinai Medical Center.

61. Corah NL, Gale EN, Illig SJ: Assessment of a dental anxiety scale. *J Am Dent Assoc* 97:816–819, 1981.

62. Matsuura H: Analysis of systemic complications and deaths during dental treatment in Japan. *Anesth Prog* 36:223–225, 1989.

63. Atherton GJ, McCaul JA, Williams SA: Medical emergencies in general dental practice in Great Britain. Part 1: their prevalence over a 10-year period. *Br Dent J* 186:72–79, 1999.

64. Haas DA: An update on local anesthetics in dentistry. *J Can Dent Assoc* 68(9):546–551, 2002.

65. Oregon Academy of General Dentistry – Oregon Health Sciences University School of Dentistry: Guidelines for intravenous moderate sedation, syllabus, August 2015.

66. Herman Ostrow School of Dentistry of USC: Guidelines for intravenous moderate sedation, syllabus, July 2014.

chapter 5

Monitoring During Sedation

CHAPTER OUTLINE

ROUTINE PREOPERATIVE MONITORING
- Pulse (Heart Rate and Rhythm)
- Blood Pressure
- Electrocardiography
- Ventilation
- Pulse Oximetry
- Carbon Dioxide Monitoring

- Bispectral Electroencephalographic Monitoring (BIS Monitoring)
- Temperature
- Other Monitoring Devices and Techniques

RECORDKEEPING
- Sedation Record
- General Anesthesia Record

The improvement of monitoring techniques and adoption of practice guidelines have advanced the safety of anesthesia and decreased mortality and morbidity.[1,2] A study of 359 preventable anesthesia incidents concluded that human error contributed to 82% of negative outcomes.[3] Many of these errors are caused by inadequate attention to details. Anesthesia—in all its clinical forms—is an art that encompasses collecting and analyzing information, then discerning and carrying out appropriate interventions. Careful attention and adequate understanding of how to monitor a patient can reduce human errors and adverse effects.

Monitoring is an essential aspect of sedation care. The word *monitor* comes from the Latin *monere,* meaning "to remind, admonish." It is an active process of identifying changes in physiological effects. Early recognition of pathologic physiological effects can reduce the likelihood of poor outcomes through early intervention.

Patients receiving anesthesia must be carefully monitored for its effects on the central nervous system (CNS), cardiovascular system, and respiratory system. Anesthesia suppresses many of the body's normal automatic functions and may significantly affect the patient's breathing, heart rate, blood pressure, and other vital functions. Early detection of adverse side effects allows corrective measures to be instituted in a timely fashion when they are more likely to be effective and prevent serious complications from arising. Early recognition and treatment of an anesthesia urgency can prevent it from becoming an anesthesia emergency.

Monitoring standards in dentistry derive from state laws, regulatory agencies, and professional societies. Standards for basic anesthetic monitoring are set by the Subcommittee of Standards and Practice Parameters of the American Society of Anesthesiologists (ASA). These standards were established in 1986 and have evolved with the implementation of new technology and practices. Last affirmed October 28, 2015, today's standards center on behaviors necessary to provide maximum possible warning of untoward events.[4] These standards highlight the importance of quality patient care, frequent measurements, and incorporating clinical judgment and expertise.

The ASA requires that two standards be met[4]:

Standard I – Mandates that qualified anesthesia personnel shall be present in the room throughout the delivery of general anesthesia, regional anesthesia, and monitored anesthesia care.

Standard II – Requires continually evaluating the patient's oxygenation, ventilation, circulation, and temperature.

It is important to note that continuous is defined as "prolonged without any interruption in time" and continual is defined as "repeated regularly and frequently in steady rapid succession." The ASA monitoring standards allow, under extenuating circumstances, the responsible anesthesiologist to waive certain requirements if absolutely necessary, but this event must be stated in a note in the patient's medical record and must include the reason for the waiver.[4] The ASA guidelines are listed in Box 5.1.

Box 5.1   Standards for Basic Anesthetic Monitoring[4]

These standards apply to all anesthesia care although, in emergency circumstances, appropriate life support measures take precedence. These standards may be exceeded at any time based on the judgment of the responsible anesthesiologist. They are intended to encourage quality patient care, but observing them cannot guarantee any specific patient outcome. They are subject to revision from time to time, as warranted by the evolution of technology and practice. They apply to all general anesthetics, regional anesthetics, and monitored anesthesia care. This set of standards addresses only the issue of basic anesthetic monitoring, which is one component of anesthesia care. In certain rare or unusual circumstances, 1) some of these methods of monitoring may be clinically impractical, and 2) appropriate use of the described monitoring methods may fail to detect untoward clinical developments. Brief interruptions of continual[†] monitoring may be unavoidable. These standards are not intended for application to the care of the obstetrical patient in labor or in the conduct of pain management.

1.   Standard I

Qualified anesthesia personnel shall be present in the room throughout the conduct of all general anesthetics, regional anesthetics, and monitored anesthesia care.

1.1   Objective

Because of the rapid changes in patient status during anesthesia, qualified anesthesia personnel shall be continuously present to monitor the patient and provide anesthesia care. In the event there is a direct known hazard, e.g., radiation, to the anesthesia personnel which might require intermittent remote observation of the patient, some provision for monitoring the patient must be made. In the event that an emergency requires the temporary absence of the person primarily responsible for the anesthetic, the best judgment of the anesthesiologist will be exercised in comparing the emergency with the anesthetized patient's condition and in the selection of the person left responsible for the anesthetic during the temporary absence.

2.   Standard II

During all anesthetics, the patient's oxygenation, ventilation, circulation, and temperature shall be continually evaluated.

2.1   Oxygenation

2.1.1 Objective

To ensure adequate oxygen concentration in the inspired gas and the blood during all anesthetics.

2.2   Methods

2.2.1 Inspired gas: During every administration of general anesthesia using an anesthesia machine, the concentration of oxygen in the patient breathing system shall be measured by an oxygen analyzer with a low oxygen concentration limit alarm in use.*

2.2.2 Blood oxygenation: During all anesthetics, a quantitative method of assessing oxygenation such as pulse oximetry shall be employed.* When the pulse oximeter is utilized, the variable pitch pulse tone and the low threshold alarm shall be audible to the anesthesiologist or the anesthesia care team personnel.* Adequate illumination and exposure of the patient are necessary to assess color.*

3.   Ventilation
3.1   Objective

To ensure adequate ventilation of the patient during all anesthetics.

3.2   Methods

3.2.1 Every patient receiving general anesthesia shall have the adequacy of ventilation continually evaluated. Qualitative clinical signs such as chest excursion, observation of the reservoir breathing bag, and auscultation of breath sounds are useful. Continual monitoring for the presence of expired carbon dioxide shall be performed unless invalidated by the nature of the patient, procedure, or equipment. Quantitative monitoring of the volume of expired gas is strongly encouraged.*

3.2.2 When an endotracheal tube or laryngeal mask is inserted, its correct positioning must be verified by clinical assessment and by identification of carbon dioxide in the expired gas. Continual end-tidal carbon dioxide analysis, in use from the time of endotracheal tube/laryngeal mask placement, until extubation/removal or initiating transfer to a postoperative care location, shall be performed using a quantitative method such as capnography, capnometry, or mass spectroscopy.* When capnography or capnometry is utilized, the end tidal CO_2 alarm shall be audible to the anesthesiologist or the anesthesia care team personnel.*

3.2.3 When ventilation is controlled by a mechanical ventilator, there shall be in continuous use a

---

[†]Note that "continual" is defined as "repeated regularly and frequently in steady rapid succession," whereas "continuous" means "prolonged without any interruption at any time."

*Under extenuating circumstances, the responsible anesthesiologist may waive the requirements marked with an asterisk (*); it is recommended that when this is done, it should be so stated (including the reasons) in a note in the patient's medical record.

From the American Society of Anesthesiologists, Committee on Standards and Practice Parameters: Standards for Basic Anesthetic Monitoring, Park Ridge, IL, October 28, 2015, American Society of Anesthesiologists.

Box 5.1	From the Standards for Basic Anesthetic Monitoring[4]—cont'd

device that is capable of detecting disconnection of components of the breathing system. The device must give an audible signal when its alarm threshold is exceeded.

3.2.4 During regional anesthesia (with no sedation) or local anesthesia (with no sedation), the adequacy of ventilation shall be evaluated by continual observation of qualitative clinical signs. During moderate or deep sedation the adequacy of ventilation shall be evaluated by continual observation of qualitative clinical signs and monitoring for the presence of exhaled carbon dioxide unless precluded or invalidated by the nature of the patient, procedure, or equipment.

4. Circulation

4.1 Objective

To ensure the adequacy of the patient's circulatory function during all anesthetics.

4.2 Methods

4.2.1 Every patient receiving anesthesia shall have the electrocardiogram continuously displayed from the beginning of anesthesia until preparing to leave the anesthetizing location.*

4.2.2 Every patient receiving anesthesia shall have arterial blood pressure and heart rate determined and evaluated at least every 5 minutes.*

4.2.3 Every patient receiving general anesthesia shall have, in addition to the above, circulatory function continually evaluated by at least one of the following: palpation of a pulse, auscultation of heart sounds, monitoring of a tracing of intraarterial pressure, ultrasound peripheral pulse monitoring, or pulse plethysmography or oximetry.

5. Body Temperature

5.1 Objective

To aid in the maintenance of appropriate body temperature during all anesthetics.

5.2 Methods

Every patient receiving anesthesia shall have temperature monitored when clinically significant changes in body temperature are intended, anticipated, or suspected.

Guidelines that specify requirements for monitoring patients during various levels of sedation and general anesthesia in dentistry have been published by the American Dental Association (ADA) and several other dental specialty organizations.[5,6] In general, all are consistent with guidelines suggested by the ASA[4] and take into account the unique aspects of sedative and anesthetic care delivery in a dental office setting.[6] These guidelines stress the triad of oxygenation, ventilation, and circulation (the airway, breathing, and circulation of basic life support). The American Society of Dentist Anesthesiologists (ASDA) has published parameters of care, as has the American Academy of Pediatric Dentistry (AAPD) and American Association of Oral and Maxillofacial Surgery (AAOMS).

According to ADA guidelines, the following functions must be continually assessed[7]:

- Consciousness
- Oxygenation
- Ventilation
- Circulation

An apparatus that measures a physiologic function may correctly be termed a monitor only if it delivers an audible and/or visual warning when the measured function falls outside of predetermined parameters (e.g., systolic blood pressure <90 mm Hg or >200 mm Hg). In the absence of a warning system, the device is more a measuring instrument than a monitor. The effectiveness of the monitor usually rests with the person administering the sedation or general anesthesia.

Many devices are available to assist in monitoring the sedated or anesthetized patient. In general, these devices are designed to measure the functioning of the following:

- CNS
- Respiratory system
- Cardiovascular system
- Temperature

Monitors can range from noninvasive to fully invasive as patient need dictates based on anticipated patient risk. Although fully invasive monitors have been shown to provide the highest accuracy, there is an increased risk associated with their placement and use, with complications more likely to develop because of the very nature of the techniques. In addition, invasive monitors are often quite time consuming to prepare for use. For outpatient sedation and anesthesia as used in dentistry and medicine, noninvasive devices have proven over the years to be highly reliable for monitoring patients before, during, and after treatment.[8]

The requirements of the ideal monitoring device are as follows[9]:

1. Safe
2. Reliable
3. Noninvasive

4. Easily interpretable
5. Easy to calibrate
6. Stable
7. Portable
8. Easily integrated with other monitoring equipment
9. No technical aid required
10. Inexpensive

There have been numerous advancements in technology and equipment over the last two decades. Although higher costs can be a deterrent, there are many benefits to using newer electronic monitors versus standard methods. Electronic monitors may improve a provider's response time in critical situations by alerting of a possible adverse situation more quickly. Because they measure at frequent and repetitive intervals, without fatigue or distraction, a portion of the human error element is removed. Additionally, many new devices contain Bluetooth components, providing even more versatility and ease of use. No longer are monitors and practitioners tethered to the patient during treatment, limiting access and mobility. Despite these perceived benefits, however, there is little substantiated evidence proving that electronic monitors, by themselves, reduce actual mortality and/or morbidity.[10] Ultimately, monitors are one of many means for a practitioner to gather perioperative patient information for interpretation and eventual response.

Monitor alarms have sometimes been found to present a challenge for clinicians by paradoxically impairing clinical vigilance, as they may have difficulty differentiating an alarm tone from regular frequencies.[11] Known as *alarm fatigue,* practitioners may adjust to the stimulation of constant sounds of monitors by tuning out, causing them to miss a crucial alarm. One study reported 80 monitor-related deaths over the course of 3.5 years, with alarm fatigue identified as the most frequently contributing factor.[12] In 2014 the ECRI Institute, a nonprofit that researches patient care improvement, identified alarm fatigue as the number-one health technology hazard in patient care.[13] Adjusting parameters to match the individual patient's traits and status can help counteract this problem.

ROUTINE PREOPERATIVE MONITORING

Before treating any dental or medical patient, baseline vital signs should be established as a part of the routine pretreatment patient evaluation (see Chapter 4). Vital signs recorded at this pretreatment visit include blood pressure, heart rate and rhythm, and respiratory rate. Additional vital signs to be monitored as indicated include temperature, height, and weight. Baseline SpO_2 (oxygen saturation levels) should be recorded in patients with respiratory issues and those with congenital cardiac defects.

These values should be recorded in the patient's chart (Fig. 5.1) to serve as a point of reference against which subsequent values obtained during treatment may be compared. Baseline vital signs should be recorded at a nonthreatening time when they are likely to represent "normal" for that patient. A patient's initial visit to the dental office, a time when no invasive dental care is planned, is more likely to provide reliable vital sign values.

Pulse (Heart Rate and Rhythm)

Monitoring of the pulse is recommended for all patients as a part of their routine preoperative evaluation (see Chapter 4). During general anesthesia, circulatory function must be continually evaluated. Preoperative values below 60 or greater than 110 beats per minute (in adult patients) should be evaluated before treatment is started. Preoperative recording of the heart rate and rhythm should be made whenever any drug is to be administered.

In adult patients, heart rate and rhythm should be monitored at regular 5-minute intervals during intramuscular (IM), intranasal (IN), and intravenous (IV) moderate sedation. In techniques of deep sedation or general anesthesia in which a more profound level of CNS depression is sought (such as IV sedation), continuous monitoring is mandatory.

The heart rate and rhythm can be measured manually or electronically. When measuring manually, the fleshy portions of two fingers are gently placed over a superficial artery for 30 seconds. Arteries that are accessible for monitoring of the pulse are listed in Table 5.1. The radial and brachial arteries are most frequently used during routine procedures, whereas the facial or labial arteries are accessible when working in or around the oral cavity. Palpation of the carotid artery is usually reserved for emergency situations. Locations of arteries are listed in Fig. 5.2.

It is suggested that the provider palpate a large artery on the patient at the start of a procedure so that he or she will know its precise location at a later time when perhaps conditions

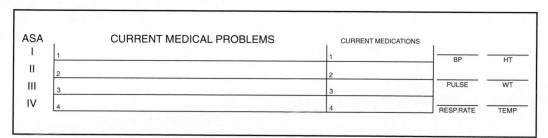

Figure 5.1 Baseline vital signs are recorded on the patient's dental chart.

Table 5.1	Arteries Employed for Pulse Determination

ARTERY	LOCATION
Radial	Ventrolateral wrist
Brachial	Medial antecubital fossa
Carotid	Groove between trachea and sternocleidomastoid muscle in neck
Labial	Upper lip
Facial	Cheek
Superficial temporal	Anterior to tragus of ear

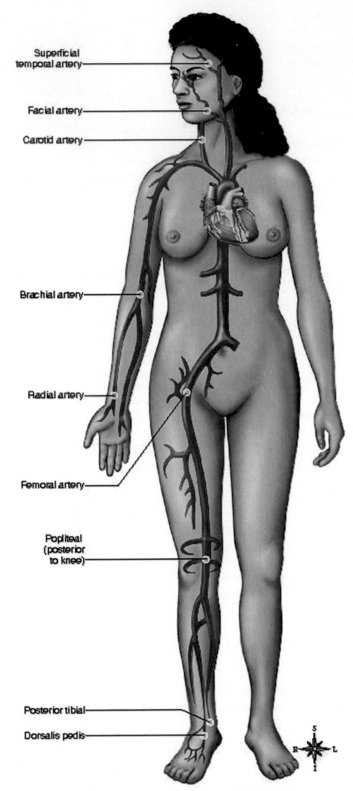

Figure 5.2 Pulse pressure points. (From Patton KT, Thibodeau GA: *Anatomy & physiology*, ed 9, St Louis, 2016, Elsevier.)

have deteriorated and the pulse may be weak or absent or the monitor malfunctions.

A rough but consistent estimate of systolic blood pressure may be obtained via palpation of three of the aforementioned arteries. When a radial artery pulse is palpable, the systolic blood pressure is at least 80 mm Hg. A brachial artery pulse will be palpable at a systolic pressure of 70 mm Hg, and a carotid artery pulse is present at a systolic reading of 60 mm Hg.[14] Therefore, if both the carotid and brachial pulses are present but the radial pulse is absent, it can be stated that (barring anatomic anomalies) the systolic blood pressure is greater than 70 mm Hg (brachial), but less than 80 mm Hg (radial). This technique is used almost exclusively in emergency situations in which a blood pressure monitoring apparatus is not immediately available or in which it is impossible to hear the sounds produced.

Pulse monitors provide a continuous measurement of the heart rate. These devices usually involve a simple electromechanical or optical transducer that is placed on a patient's fingertip or earlobe. A photoelectric beam is interrupted by the flow of blood through the finger following each contraction of the heart. This interruption produces a visual and/or audio signal.

In addition to their primary function(s), many monitoring devices, such as the pulse oximeter, automatic vital signs monitor, and the electrocardiograph (ECG), also measure the heart rate. Either a digital display or a graph on an oscilloscope is provided.

Blood Pressure

Along with heart rate and rhythm, monitoring blood pressure gauges the status of a patient's cardiovascular system (see Chapter 4). Blood pressure should be determined for all prospective dental patients as part of a pretreatment physical evaluation.

When moderate sedation techniques are implemented, particularly those in which more profound levels of CNS depression are expected, such as the parenteral moderate sedation techniques (IM, IN, IV), blood pressure must be monitored more frequently. Specifically, it is recommended that blood pressure be recorded every 5 minutes for the duration of the procedure, as well as immediately following the administration of any drug. The deeper the level of sedation and the less able the patient is to respond appropriately to verbal command, the more crucial it becomes for frequent blood pressure monitoring. During deep sedation and general anesthesia, blood pressure is monitored and recorded at 5-minute intervals.

Several methods exist to monitor blood pressure. A preferred method involves auscultation through the use of a stethoscope and sphygmomanometer (blood pressure cuff). An appropriately sized blood pressure cuff, encompassing 80% or more of the patient's upper arm circumference,[15] is typically applied for the duration of the procedure. It should be placed on the arm closest to the examiner. However, when an IV infusion is in place, the blood pressure cuff should, whenever possible, be placed on the opposing arm to prevent a temporary occlusion of the IV line whenever the cuff is inflated. The same is true when a pulse oximeter is used on a finger, as inflation of the blood pressure cuff results in obstruction of the underlying blood flow into the distal extremity, thus causing a deceptive drop in peripheral capillary oxygen saturation. This perceived fall in oxygen saturation frequently results in activation of the monitor's alarm system and thus presents the need for a practitioner to assess accuracy.

Korotkoff sounds result from turbulent blood flow from a compressed artery by a blood pressure cuff. Auscultation for Korotkoff sounds will allow for an approximate measurement of both systolic and diastolic blood pressure. The appearance of the first Korotkoff sounds represents the systolic pressure, whereas muffling or disappearance of the sound indicates the diastolic blood pressure.[10]

Concerns with auscultation of Korotkoff sounds include falsely high blood pressure estimates when the blood pressure cuff is too small, applied too loosely, or when the extremity is below heart level. Conversely, falsely low estimates can occur when the cuff is too large, when the extremity is above heart level, or after quick deflations.[10] This technique requires palpation and auscultation of pulsatile blood flow and can be problematic during conditions of low blood pressure.

In some situations, particularly with markedly obese individuals, it may be extremely difficult, if not impossible, to determine blood pressure accurately using auscultation. If this is the case, a palpatory blood pressure may be employed. After locating the radial artery in the wrist, the examiner should rapidly inflate the blood pressure cuff until the pulse disappears, continuing to inflate for an additional 20 to 30 mm Hg. While keeping his or her fingers over the radial artery, the examiner slowly decreases the pressure in the cuff until a pulse is felt. A relatively accurate systolic blood pressure may be obtained in this manner; however, no diastolic pressure is obtainable using this method. When this technique is used, a note should be entered in the anesthesia record, such as SYS BP: 130 mm Hg (palpation). Alternatively, altering the placement of the cuff to the wrist or ankle may be effective.

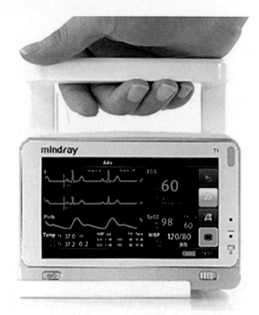

Figure 5.3 Mindray T1 monitor (ECG, SpO$_2$, temp, BP).

Blood pressure may also be monitored using automatic devices. In the late 1970s these microprocessor-controlled oscillotonometers largely replaced auscultatory and palpatory techniques for perioperative blood pressure monitoring. These devices measure mean arterial pressure (MAP) by sensing the point of maximal fluctuations in cuff pressure while deflating. Some devices simply require the inflation of the blood pressure cuff, after which the cuff's deflation becomes automatic. Pressure is released slowly, and auditory (beeping) and visual (flashing light) displays announce the systolic and diastolic pressures (and in many cases the heart rate, too). The cuff pressure is then sent to a transducer whose output is digitized for processing. The cuff is inflated and pressure is held while oscillations are sampled. If no oscillations are sensed, the microprocessor switches open a deflation valve and proceeds to the next pressure level for sampling. The microprocessor then compares the amplitude of oscillation pairs and numerically displays the blood pressure estimate. Digital readouts are available on most of these devices, and many also provide a printed record.

In recent years, second-generation blood pressure monitoring devices appear to be more reliable than earlier models. In addition, the cost of these instruments has become significantly more reasonable. Most of the newer blood pressure monitors can be programmed to record blood pressure at regular intervals (e.g., every 5 minutes). Some devices combine several functions. The device shown in Fig. 5.3 integrates blood pressure, heart rate, ECG, O$_2$ saturation, and temperature into one unit. The size and weight of monitors have also dramatically decreased in recent years. More manufacturers are emphasizing portability and modularity in new models.

It is strongly recommended that providers utilize authentic medical device blood pressure monitors and not those that are marketed for retail sales. The over-the-counter versions have been shown to be less accurate in cases of hypotension and are unreliable in instances of cardiac dysrhythmia.

Continuous noninvasive arterial blood pressure measurement (CNAP) is the latest development in noninvasive blood pressure monitoring. CNAP measures blood pressure continuously in real time and monitors without latency, much like a fully invasive arterial catheter system (not routinely used in dental sedation), yet it is completely noninvasive. It provides an accurate display of the arterial blood pressure trace with beat-to-beat blood pressure monitoring. Studies have shown accuracy even in instances of rapidly fluctuating hemodynamics.[9]

Electrocardiography

The ECG (Fig. 5.4) monitors both the heart rate and rhythm and provides a warning of the development of changes in the electrical activity of the myocardium. Patients with cardiac history or symptoms should have an ECG before sedation. Although 12 leads may be used, lead II (right arm → left leg) is most commonly used during anesthesia because it readily permits detection of dysrhythmias.

Textbooks on basic electrocardiography are available, enabling the reader to become proficient in the interpretation of ECG tracings. Normal sinus rhythm is illustrated in Fig. 5.5 and premature ventricular contractions (PVCs) in Fig. 5.6.

Although not required for use in all levels of sedation, the ECG does increase one's ability to detect possibly significant changes in functioning of the myocardium at a time when corrective treatment may usually restore a normal rhythm.

The appearance of dysrhythmias is more likely during general anesthesia than during moderate sedation.

Three common causes of dysrhythmias are:
1. Hypoxia, leading to myocardial ischemia
2. Endogenous catecholamine release, secondary to inadequate pain control or too light a level of CNS depression
3. Hypercapnia, resulting from poor ventilation

Management of dysrhythmias secondary to these causes, which are usually readily correctable, is done through:
1. Ensuring airway management and ventilation
2. Providing adequate pain control (e.g., local anesthesia)
3. Increasing the level of anesthesia (greater CNS depression)

Recommendations for the use of the ECG during sedation and anesthesia are found in Tables 5.2 and 5.3.

Ventilation

Of equal, if not greater, importance to monitoring cardiovascular function during sedative and general anesthetic procedures is monitoring the patient's respiratory status. Because all sedative and general anesthetic agents are CNS and respiratory

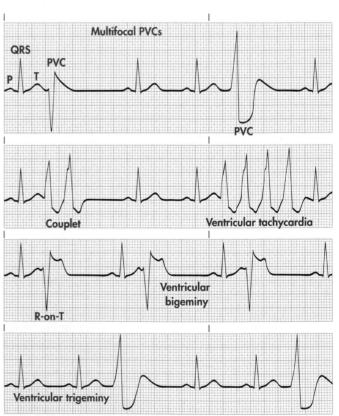

Figure 5.6 Premature ventricular contractions. (From Lewis SL et al: *Medical-surgical nursing: assessment and management of clinical problems*, ed 7, St Louis, 2007, Mosby.)

Figure 5.4 Vital signs monitor, includes ECG *(arrow)*.

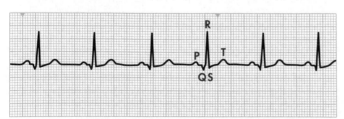

Figure 5.5 Normal sinus rhythm. (From Lewis SL et al: *Medical-surgical nursing: assessment and management of clinical problems*, ed 7, St Louis, 2007, Mosby.)

Table 5.2 — Recommended Monitoring for Adult Patients

Monitor	Local Anesthesia			Oral			IM/IN			Inhalation			IV			Outpatient			Inpatient		
	Pr	In	Po	Pr	In	Po	Pr	In	Po	Pr	In	Po	Pr	In	Po	Pr	In	Po	Pr	In	Po
Heart rate	**	0	*	**	0	*	**	**	**	**	**	**	**	**	**	**	**	**	**	**	**
								q 5 min			q 5 min			Cont.			Cont.			Cont.	
Blood pressure	**	*	*	**	*	*	**	**	**	**	*	**	**	**	**	**	**	**	**	**	**
								q 5 min			q 5 min			q 5 min			q 5 min			q 5 min	
ECG respiration	0	0	0	0	0	0	*	*	0	0	0	0	*	*	*	**	**	**	**	**	**
	**	0	0	**	0	0	**	**	**	**	*	**	**	**	**	**	**	**	**	**	**
	V			V			V	PT	V	V	V	V	V	PT	V	V	PT	V	V	PT/E	V
Oximetry	0	0	0	0	*	0	*	**	**	0	0	0	*	**	**	**	**	**	**	**	**
Temperature	*	0	0	*	0	0	*	0	0	*	0	0	*	0	0	**	*	*	**	**	*

0, Not essential; *, optional; **, recommended, *Pr*, preoperative; *In*, intraoperative; *Po*, postoperative; *Cont.*, continuous; *V*, visual; *PT*, pretracheal stethoscope; *E*, esophageal stethoscope.

Heart rate: Heart rate may be monitored by palpation in both the preoperative and postoperative periods; however, it is suggested that when the heart rate is monitored intraoperatively, an electrical monitor providing a continuous reading be used. Devices such as a pulse meter, pulse oximeter, capnograph, and ECG provide continuous heart monitoring.

Blood pressure (BP): When the recommendation for monitoring BP is **, I suggest that the BP cuff be kept on the patient's arm throughout the entire procedure.

Electrocardiograph (ECG): The ECG provides continuous monitoring of the electrical activity of the heart and the heart rate.

Respiration: Visual monitoring implies a casual observation of the movements of the patient's chest for 30–60 seconds. *PT*, pretracheal stethoscope, provides instantaneous evaluation of breath sounds and respiratory rate. *E*, the esophageal stethoscope, is inserted into the esophagus during general anesthesia, providing excellent sound quality for both heart and lung sounds.

Oximetry: Oximetry provides continuous monitoring of arterial O_2 saturation.

Temperature: Preoperative temperature monitoring may be done manually, but if intraoperative monitoring of body temperature is required, it is more readily achieved continuously via rectal or esophageal probe.

Table 5.3 — Recommended Monitoring for Pediatric Patients

Monitor	Local Anesthesia			Oral			IM/IN			Inhalation			IV			Outpatient			Inpatient		
	Pr	In	Po	Pr	In	Po	Pr	In	Po	Pr	In	Po	Pr	In	Po	Pr	In	Po	Pr	In	Po
Heart rate	**	0	*	**	**	**	**	**	**	**	**	**	**	**	**	**	**	**	**	**	**
					Cont.			Cont.			Cont.			Cont.			Cont.			Cont.	
Blood pressure	**	*	*	**	**	**	**	**	**	**	**	**	**	**	**	**	**	**	**	**	**
					q 5 min			q 5 min			q 5 min			q 5 min			q 5 min			q 5 min	
ECG respiration	0	0	0	0	0	0	*	*	0	0	0	0	*	*	*	**	**	**	**	**	**
	**	0	0	**	**	**	**	**	**	**	**	**	**	**	**	**	**	**	**	**	**
	V			V	PT		V	PT	V	V	V/PT	V	V	PT	V	V	PT	V	V	PT/E	V
Oximetry	0	0	0	**	**	**	*	**	**	0	0	0	*	**	**	**	**	**	**	**	**
Temperature	*	0	0	*	0	0	*	*	*	*	0	0	*	*	*	**	**	**	**	**	**

Refer to footnotes in Table 5.2.

depressants to a greater degree than they are cardiovascular depressants, respiratory changes are usually observed well before cardiovascular changes. Alterations in cardiac rhythm (dysrhythmias) observed on the ECG in the ASA 1 or 2 patient are likely to be produced by myocardial ischemia, which is most often secondary to respiratory depression or inadequate ventilation directly related to the drugs that have been administered.

Morbidities and mortalities occur secondary to respiratory depression (or arrest) that goes unrecognized for too long, followed by an ineffective response when finally recognized. Casual monitoring of respiratory adequacy by observation of the rise and fall of the patient's chest or by observation of the color of oral mucous membranes is unreliable and cannot be used as the sole method of monitoring respiratory status.

Respiratory adequacy may be crudely monitored by:
1. Determining the respiratory rate
2. Observing chest wall motion
3. Observing the color of the mucous membranes (oral membranes and fingernail beds)
4. Observing the inflation and deflation of the reservoir bag on the inhalation sedation unit—if inhalation sedation or O_2 is administered (and if the patient is breathing through his or her nose, not breathing through the mouth)

It must always be remembered that movement of the chest wall is not an absolute guarantee of air exchange between the lungs and the external environment. Chest wall movement indicates that a mechanical effort is being made to exchange air and that respiratory arrest has not occurred. The practitioner should be aware that the airway may be completely obstructed (e.g., tongue, foreign body) with no air exchange in the presence of spontaneous respiratory efforts. In addition, respiratory efforts normally indicate that cardiac arrest has not yet occurred because the primary cause of cardiac arrest during sedation and general anesthesia is the occurrence of acute dysrhythmias resulting from ischemia of the myocardium secondary to either respiratory arrest or airway obstruction. Respiratory arrest usually appears before cardiac arrest.

Similarly, observing the color of mucous membranes as a respiratory monitor is unreliable because cyanosis is not observed until some time after the patient has become hypoxic. In addition, placement of a rubber dam is indicated during many dental procedures, especially in patients receiving parenteral moderate or deep sedation or general anesthesia. The rubber dam conceals the lips and intraoral soft tissues, preventing this as a means of monitoring.

A valid method of determining air exchange is through visualization of the reservoir bag on an inhalation sedation unit or anesthesia machine, provided that an airtight seal of the mask is maintained. If leakage occurs around the sides of the nasal hood or if the patient begins to mouth breathe, the reservoir bag will cease to inflate and deflate during breathing.

While operating in the patient's oral cavity, the dental provider or assistant is able to determine whether air is being

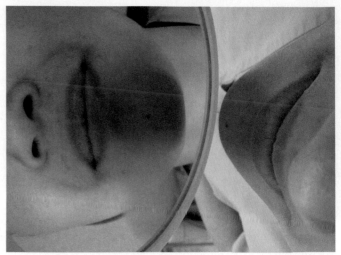

Figure 5.7 Fogging of mirror indicates exchange of air.

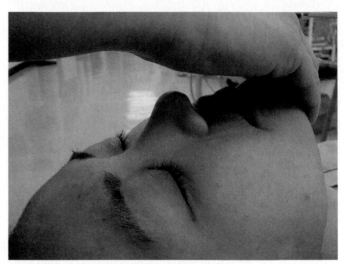

Figure 5.8 Hand held in front of patient's mouth and nose to feel exchange of air.

exchanged by the patient. A mirror held in the patient's mouth or in front of his or her nose will fog over if air is actively exchanged (Fig. 5.7). More effective is holding a hand in front of the patient's mouth and nose so that air is felt on the palm of the hand during exhalation if breathing is occurring (Fig. 5.8).

The precordial/pretracheal stethoscope is an inexpensive and extremely valuable monitoring device during anesthesia and sedation; it provides constant information concerning upper airway patency, continuous monitoring of heart sounds and ventilation, and a quality assessment of both ventilation efforts and respiration rate. Also, it is the only monitor that allows for detection of fluids in the airway. A weighted stethoscope head (also known as a *chest piece* or *bell*) is secured with double-sided adhesive tape (Fig. 5.9) to either the precordial (Fig. 5.10) or pretracheal region (Fig. 5.11) on the patient's chest.

When used as a pretracheal stethoscope, the weighted head is placed in the midline of the neck over the trachea just superior to the sternal notch (see Fig. 5.11). It lies above the lower end of the trachea at or just slightly above its bifurcation into the right and left main stem bronchi. Tubing connects this stethoscope to a binaural or monaural earpiece. The custom monaural earpiece is preferred because of its comfort and because it permits the user to carry on normal conversation while continually listening for the sounds associated with the exchange of air. Custom earpieces can usually be obtained from companies that manufacture hearing aids (e.g., Miracle Ear, *www.miracle-ear.com*). A Bluetooth version of a pretracheal stethoscope is also available. Placement in the pretracheal region allows for easy recognition of respiratory sounds, with diminished intensity of heart sounds, which may overwhelm the softer respiratory outputs when placed in the precordial region. It should also be noted that a softening of heart sounds is often indicative of a drop in blood pressure. The weighted stethoscope head is available in adult and pediatric sizes. When placed in the pretracheal region with double-sided adhesive disks, the pediatric head is adequate for both children and adults. The heavier adult stethoscope head is often uncomfortable for both children and adults.

When monitoring breathing, two elements must be considered:
1. Rate of breathing
2. Quality of breath sounds

Counting breaths for 15 or 30 seconds and multiplying by 4 or 2, respectively, will calculate the rate in breaths per minute. The most frequent disturbances in respiratory rate are an overly rapid rate (tachypnea) and an unusually slow rate (bradypnea). Tachypnea may indicate the presence of anxiety (e.g., hyperventilation), a pathologic condition (e.g., diabetic acidosis and ketosis), or elevated CO_2 levels; bradypnea is noted

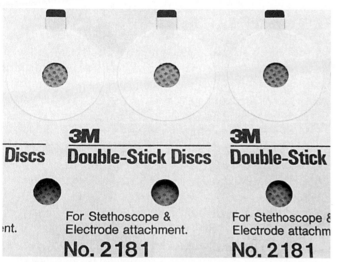

Figure 5.9 Double-sided tape for pretracheal stethoscope.

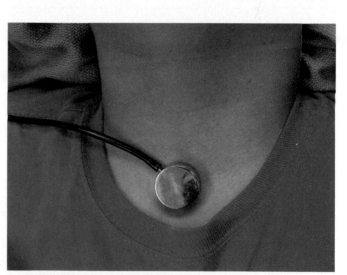

Figure 5.11 Pretracheal stethoscope on patient's neck.

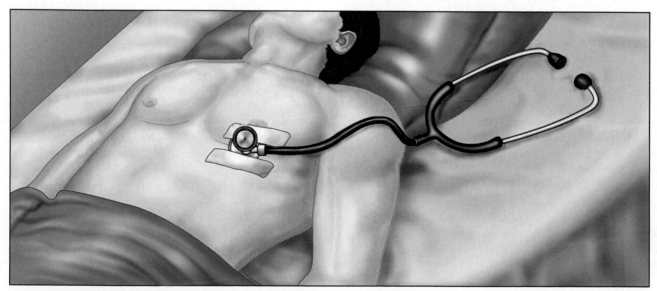

Figure 5.10 Precordial stethoscope provides an excellent monitor of both heart and respiratory sounds.

Table 5.4	Causes of Partial Airway Obstruction	
SOUND HEARD	PROBABLE Cause	MANAGEMENT
Snoring	Hypopharyngeal obstruction by the tongue	Repeat head tilt–chin lift
Gurgling	Foreign matter (blood, water, vomitus) in airway	Suction airway
Wheezing	Bronchospasm	Bronchodilator (via inhalation, only if conscious; IM, IV if unconscious)
Crowing (high-pitched)	Laryngospasm (partial)	Suction airway; + pressure O$_2$

after the administration of larger doses of an opioid (see Chapter 25).

The desired quality of breath sounds is relatively quiet "whooshing" sounds heard within the earpiece, indicating normal, unobstructed airflow and a patent airway.

Silence in the earpiece is ominous and must trigger an immediate response. Respiratory obstruction (in the presence of exaggerated ventilatory movements) or respiratory arrest (no chest movements) may have developed and must be immediately corrected, or it may merely be that the stethoscope chest piece has become inadvertently disconnected from the patient. Examples of airway obstruction are found in Table 5.4. Use of the pretracheal/precordial stethoscope decreases the time required for recognition of a potentially serious problem, allowing corrective measures to be implemented more expeditiously.

Wheezing indicates partial obstruction in the lower airways (e.g., bronchioles) and is termed *bronchospasm* (see Chapter 34). Management is required, but bronchospasm is not an immediate, acutely life-threatening situation, unlike complete airway obstruction.

Snoring or gurgling (sound of fluid) indicates the presence of a partial obstruction of the upper airway. Snoring most often results when the base of the tongue or the soft palate falls against the posterior pharyngeal wall; oftentimes during treatment dentists inadvertently push the tongue, causing an obstruction. *Bubbling, gurgling,* or *crackling sound of fluid* indicates the presence of a liquid (e.g., blood, saliva, water, or vomitus) in the airway. Management of snoring requires elevation of the mandible (head tilt/chin lift), which elevates the base of the tongue off of the posterior pharyngeal wall.

When foreign matter is present in the airway of a sedated or unconscious patient, three problems may develop:
1. Aspiration
2. Complete or partial obstruction of the airway
3. Laryngospasm

When the presence of fluid (or other foreign matter) is suspected, immediate management requires suctioning of the posterior pharynx. Normal breath sounds should return once the fluid is removed.

Other means of monitoring respiration include impedance pneumography, in which a high-frequency, low-amplitude current is injected across the chest cavity and the resulting voltage is measured. Current flows less easily through the chest as lungs fill, so an increased resistance in voltage indicates an increased lung volume.

Similarly, the acoustic respiration rate device uses an adhesive sensor with an integrated acoustic transducer that displays a continuous respiration rate, alerting providers at the first signs of an abnormal or compromised breathing pattern.

Pulse Oximetry

Monitoring breath sounds and the rate of respiration, although important to patient care during sedation and anesthesia, does not provide an absolutely accurate assessment of ventilatory efforts. ASA guidelines specifically require the use of an oxygen analyzer with a low concentration–limit audible alarm during general anesthesia and the quantitative assessment of blood oxygenation during any anesthesia care.[4] ADA guidelines indicate that when inhalation equipment is used, it must have a fail-safe system that is appropriately checked and calibrated. The equipment must also have either a functioning device that prohibits the delivery of less than 30% oxygen or an appropriately calibrated and functioning in-line oxygen analyzer with audible alarm.[7] The color of mucosa, skin, or blood must be continually evaluated, although these are late indicators of desaturation.

Pulse oximeters measure pulse rate and estimate oxygen saturation of hemoglobin (Fig. 5.12). They are noninvasive, continuous, autocalibrating, and provide quick response times. The pulse oximeter complements capnography to provide early warning of a desaturation event.[16]

The Closed Claims Project, established by the ASA to identify the source of complications during anesthesia, conducted an analysis in 1984 and determined that adverse respiratory events accounted for 34% of reported anesthesia claims, of which 85% resulted in brain damage or death. It was later determined that the use of pulse oximetry and capnography monitoring would have likely prevented many of these adverse events. Following the widespread adoption of pulse oximetry and capnography in the mid-1980s, respiratory adverse events decreased from 36% of claims in the 1970s to just 14% of the claims in the 1990s.[17]

A function of the pulse oximeter—indeed, its primary function during sedation and general anesthesia—is the detection and quantification of hypoxemia. Pulse oximeters measure the oxygen saturation of arterial blood. *Oxygen saturation* refers to the amount of oxygen carried by hemoglobin. Expressed as a percentage, oxygen saturation is the amount of oxygen carried compared with the total oxygen-carrying capacity of hemoglobin (100%). Breathing ambient air at sea level, an

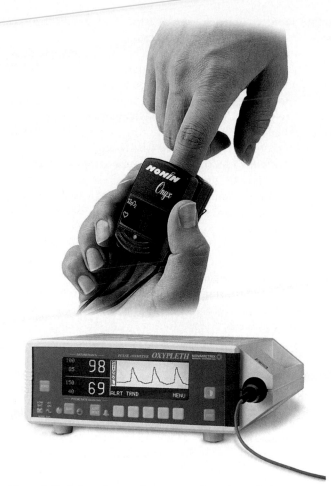

Figure 5.12 Pulse oximeter. (From Lewis SL et al: *Medical-surgical nursing: assessment and management of clinical problems,* ed 7, St Louis, 2007, Mosby.)

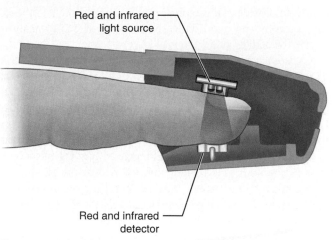

Red and infrared light source

Red and infrared detector

Figure 5.13 Pulse oximeter measures wavelengths of light passing through the finger.

acceptable normal SpO$_2$ range for a patient without pulmonary pathology is 95% to 99%; acceptable SpO$_2$ ranges decrease as elevation increases.[18]

The color of blood is a function of oxygen saturation, with a change in color resulting from the optical properties of hemoglobin and its interaction with oxygen. The ratio of oxygenated hemoglobin and reduced hemoglobin can be determined by absorption spectrophotometry—the process of passing two wavelengths of light through the body to a photodetector and measuring the changing absorbance of each of the wavelengths (Fig. 5.13). Pulse oximeters are able to perform a plethysmographic analysis to differentiate the pulsatile hemoglobin saturation from the nonpulsatile signal resulting from absorption and other matter such as skin, muscle, bone, and often nail polish.

The pulse oximeter measures the absorption of selected wavelengths of light (660 nm and 910 nm or 940 nm) as they pass through living tissue, such as the fingertip, toe, or earlobe. Oxygenated hemoglobin and hemoglobin absorb these wavelengths of light to differing degrees. The relative percentages

of these two hemoglobins are calculated within the oximeter, and the SpO$_2$ is displayed on the screen.[19]

Use of pulse oximetry has become the standard of care during moderate sedation, deep sedation, and general anesthesia for all patients. Where state regulation governs the administration of oral sedative drugs to pediatric patients, use of pulse oximetry is mandated.[20] Used in conjunction with the pretracheal/precordial stethoscope, pulse oximetry permits respiratory function of the sedated or anesthetized patient to be accurately and continuously evaluated, adding a level of increased safety to the procedure.

As mentioned previously, blood pressure monitoring occludes vascular flow of oxygenated hemoglobin, resulting in a false temporary desaturation. Newer technology has addressed this phenomenon. Massimo SET pulse oximetry utilizes advanced signal postprocessing techniques, which provides more accurate monitoring of arterial oxygen saturation and pulse rate, even during the most challenging conditions, such as times of low perfusion.[21]

Certain factors may cause inaccurate measurements, such as ill-fitting oximeter probes, excess ambient light, motion artifact (e.g., shivering), and cold extremities, so efforts should be made to minimize these factors.[18]

Carbon Dioxide Monitoring

Noninvasive CO$_2$ monitors have become increasingly popular. Measuring expiratory CO$_2$ is an important part of patient monitoring. The ASA guidelines specifically mandate continuously ensuring the adequacy of ventilation by physical diagnostic techniques during all anesthesia care. Quantitative monitoring of tidal volume and capnography are strongly encouraged in patients undergoing general anesthesia. When administering regional anesthesia or monitored anesthesia care, sufficient ventilation should be assessed by qualitative clinical signs and/or monitoring of exhaled carbon dioxide. Ensuring correct placement of an endotracheal intubation or laryngeal mask airway requires clinical assessment and qualitative identification of carbon dioxide in the expired gas. During general anesthesia, capnography and end-tidal carbon dioxide ($ETCO_2$) analysis are performed.[22]

Capnometry is the measurement and numeric representation of the CO_2 concentration during inspiration and expiration. A capnogram gives a continuous time display of the CO_2 concentration sampled at the patient's airway during ventilation. Using the principle of infrared absorption, these devices monitor the levels of inspired and $ETCO_2$, providing visual displays as a percentage (%) or millimeters of mercury (mm Hg). Response of the CO_2 monitor is virtually instantaneous, assessing every breath taken by the patient. Arterial O_2 saturation and respiratory rate are also provided in some models. Audible and visual alarms alert the operator if $ETCO_2$ values are less than or greater than the selected parameters or if apnea occurs. With a gas analyzer, when nitrous oxide (N_2O) is administered concurrently, the percentage of N_2O is also displayed.

Although still not considered the standard of care for moderate parenteral sedation, $ETCO_2$ monitoring has become increasingly recommended in outpatient general anesthesia because it provides yet another noninvasive means of monitoring the patient's ventilatory status and potentially increasing patient safety.

A proposed amendment to the ADA Guidelines for the Use of Sedation and General Anesthesia by Dentists supports the need for the use of capnography during moderate sedation in an open airway system, as well as the need for continual observation of qualitative clinical signs by monitoring for the presence of exhaled carbon dioxide.[23] With the development of future generations of CO_2 monitors, their use during moderate sedation, deep sedation, and general anesthesia for dentistry is likely to become standard of care.[22]

Bispectral Electroencephalographic Monitoring (BIS Monitoring)

According to ADA guidelines, the patient's level of consciousness must be continually monitored.[7] The bispectral index (BIS) is one of several technologies used to monitor depth of anesthesia. In the 1990s, medical device company Aspect Medical Systems began a research effort to develop the electroencephalogram (EEG) as a means of monitoring the depth of anesthesia, taking the complex EEG signal and processing the result into a single number, thus providing the anesthetist with a numeric indication of depth of anesthesia.[24,25] The Aspect EEG monitor quantitates anesthetic effects on the brain, specifically the hypnotic component of anesthesia.

The BIS index is a continuous EEG parameter that ranges from 0 (equivalent to EEG silence or flat line) to 100 (represents an awake CNS).[24] Loss of consciousness tends to occur at BIS values between 70 and 80. The manufacturer recommends that a BIS value between 40 and 60 indicates an appropriate level for general anesthesia.[25] Clinical correlations of the BIS index are shown in Fig. 5.14.

BIS monitoring allows the provider to adjust drugs to the specific needs of the individual patient, possibly resulting in a more rapid emergence from anesthesia and reducing the incidence of intraoperative awareness.[26]

Anesthetic techniques consisting of a low or moderate dose of an opioid analgesic and a hypnotic drug (e.g., volatile inhaled anesthetic, IV anesthetic) are the most accurately represented with BIS monitoring. Low opioid doses enable the BIS index to accurately reflect the pharmacodynamics of the hypnotic drugs on the CNS. BIS monitoring, however, has been shown to be less reliable in anesthetics involving higher-dose opioids and is insensitive to several commonly used anesthetic agents such as ketamine and nitrous oxide.[27]

Intraoperative awareness occurs at a rate of 1 to 2 incidents per 1000 general anesthesia cases,[24] thus making BIS monitoring an important dimension of monitoring general anesthesia and providing the anesthetist with the needed feedback to proactively adjust pharmaceutical components. However, in anxiolytic, moderate, and deep sedation cases, the current recommended standard for monitoring patient CNS function is through eliciting patient verbal responses or using physical stimulation to provoke a protective response.

Temperature

During all general anesthetics, the means for continuously measuring the patient's temperature must be available. When changes in body temperature are intended or anticipated, temperature should be continuously measured and recorded on the anesthesia record.[28] Monitoring of the patient's body temperature during parenteral sedation is not usually as critical as are the cardiovascular and respiratory parameters already discussed. However, it is important to determine whether a patient has elevated temperature before the start of the planned treatment. Fever increases the workload of the cardiovascular and respiratory systems. Heart and respiratory rates increase with an increase in body temperature. The patient's ability to tolerate stress decreases.

In the dental office, temperatures were once routinely monitored orally; however, with the newest advances in infrared light transmission, noninvasive arterial thermometers now provide accurate readings from the tympanic, axillary, and temporal regions. For oral monitoring, disposable or nondisposable traditional thermometers may be used. When a nondisposable thermometer is employed, it is placed in the sublingual area for 3 to 5 minutes before reading the temperature. The patient should not have had any hot or cold liquids or foods in his or her mouth immediately before temperature monitoring. Digital nondisposable thermometers are also available, providing a rapid assessment of body temperature.

Disposable thermometers using a system of chemicals that melt and recrystallize at specific temperatures have made the monitoring of temperature extremely simple and sanitary. When the unit is placed sublingually, the dots change color within approximately 30 seconds according to the patient's temperature. When patient compliance is lacking and it is desirable to record the temperature preoperatively, a chemical-dot thermometer may be used by holding the thermal-sensitive strip firmly

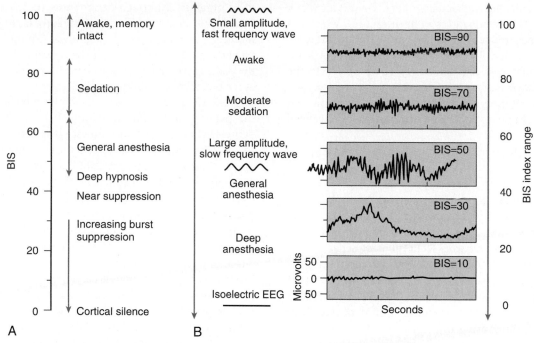

Figure 5.14 A, Clinical correlations of the BIS index. Maintaining the BIS index from 45 to 60 during general anesthesia appears to ensure unconsciousness with a hypnotic-opioid anesthetic technique while providing for rapid emergence. **B,** Electroencephalographic (EEG) changes observed with increasing depth of anesthesia. (Adapted from Johansen JW, Sebel PS: Development and clinical application of electroencephalographic bispectrum monitoring. *Anesthesiology* 93:1336, 2000.) (Redrawn from Kelley SD: Monitoring level of consciousness during anesthesia and sedation, Natick, MA, 2003, Aspect Medical Systems.)

against the patient's dry forehead for about 15 seconds. Color changes in the strips occur, indicating the patient's temperature. Because forehead temperatures are less than an actual core temperature reading, chemical-dot thermometers have been adjusted to accommodate for this difference (of about +4.5° F, or +2.5° C).

Noncontact infrared thermometers allow practitioners to measure temperature from a distance, providing a quick, noninvasive method of obtaining patient temperature by converting radiant power to an electrical signal that is displayed in units of temperature after compensating for ambient temperature (Fig. 5.15). This is a preferred method as it is non-disposable yet requires no sterilization between uses and has been shown to have the same accuracy as measurements taken via rectal mercury thermometers.[29]

The importance of monitoring temperature intraoperatively during general anesthesia is based on the need to prevent severe hypothermia, which develops as body heat is dissipated, and to monitor the possible development of malignant hyperthermia (hyperpyrexia), a serious complication during general anesthesia. Even minimal fluctuations (1.9° C) in core body temperature during the perioperative period have been shown to inhibit wound healing and increase postoperative complications.[30] Monitoring of the body temperature is a standard of care in pediatric general anesthesia.[28]

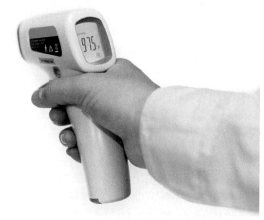

Figure 5.15 Noncontact infrared thermometer. (Photo © gettyimages.com.)

Other Monitoring Devices and Techniques

Other monitoring devices and techniques are available. However, the necessity of using them during the typical outpatient procedure on an ASA 1, 2, or 3 risk patient in the dental or medical office environment is questionable.

These additional procedures include monitoring of central venous pressure (CVP) as a measure of right-side heart filling pressures as a guide to intravascular volume. An elevated CVP indicates circulatory overload (as in heart failure), whereas a low CVP indicates reduced blood volume. Monitoring CVP necessitates the passage of a catheter from either the subclavian or internal jugular vein approximately 10 to 15 cm to the junction of the superior and inferior venae cavae and the right atrium. CVP monitoring is not recommended for use in ASA 1, 2, or 3 patients undergoing elective treatment under general anesthesia.

The level of CNS depression may be monitored through the use of the (noninvasive) EEG. Predictable changes are noted in the EEG with different anesthetic agents.[22] The need for EEG monitoring during sedative and most outpatient general anesthetic procedures is minimal, and it is not recommended.

Before reviewing the various techniques of sedation and general anesthesia with recommendations for monitoring for each, it must be emphasized that the most important system to monitor is the CNS, the one that is targeted for depression in our techniques. Therefore, the most important technique of patient monitoring during any sedation technique remains direct communication between the patient and the doctor. The ability of the moderately sedated patient to respond appropriately to command is an integral part of the definition of consciousness presented in Chapter 2. Lack of such an appropriate response is a call for immediate action to determine (and correct, if necessary) the cause of the lack of response. Direct communication with the patient is a means of determining the level of functioning of the CNS. Because virtually all drugs used in sedation and/or general anesthesia act primarily by depressing the CNS (this is their raison d'être), it is appropriate that the importance of monitoring the CNS be recognized. Monitoring of the respiratory and cardiovascular systems, though important, is considered secondary to CNS monitoring during minimal sedation (e.g., oral benzodiazepine or N_2O-O_2 inhalation sedation). As the level of CNS depression increases when moving from moderate to deep sedation, the patient's ability to respond appropriately is increasingly diminished, warranting an intensification of monitoring of "other systems"—respiratory and cardiovascular. Generalizing to a slight degree, most drugs used during sedation and general anesthesia (CNS depressants) depress breathing to a greater degree—often at sedative doses—than they depress the cardiovascular system, thus the emphasis on more intensive monitoring of respiratory function than of the cardiovascular system during moderate sedation. With the loss of consciousness, however, effective communication with the patient is lost, and the doctor must rely solely on respiratory and cardiovascular monitoring to assess the patient's clinical status.

Monitoring the pediatric patient proves to be somewhat more difficult if the patient presents a significant management problem. When oral, IN, or IM sedation is to be employed, the patient may be combative, crying, or screaming, making it virtually impossible for the recommended baseline vital signs

to be obtained. Although determining these parameters may be difficult or impossible, there actually is little necessity to monitor the vital signs of the patient during the immediate preoperative period when he or she is extremely active, because the patient's baseline vital signs have (hopefully) been recorded at the preoperative visit to the office. Monitoring of the patient, pediatric and adult, becomes increasingly more important when the patient, under the influence of the administered CNS depressant drugs, becomes quiescent and cooperative. Once this state is achieved (when dental care can commence), the doctor must become more vigilant in monitoring the parameters recommended (CNS, respiratory, cardiovascular). As with the sedated adult patient, monitoring of respiration becomes more critical as the level of sedation deepens. Some pediatric sedation techniques include the administration of opioid agonists, often in combination with other CNS depressants. Respiratory depression is a significant concern in these patients. The probability that the unmanageable pediatric patient has been placed into a physical restraint, such as the Pedi-Wrap or papoose board, increases the likelihood of respiratory depression while decreasing the team's ability to monitor respiration. A rubber dam used to isolate the oral cavity may also be in place, restricting mouth breathing and hindering visualization of oral mucous membranes. The use of a pretracheal stethoscope and pulse oximeter is therefore considered essential whenever parenteral pediatric sedation or more profound oral sedation is employed.

RECORDKEEPING

A written record must be prepared for each patient during the administration of sedative or anesthetic drugs. Such records serve several purposes:
1. As a trend plot of vital signs
2. As an aid to the clinician's memory
3. As documentation of a patient's response to the administration of drugs and the operative procedure
4. Nonclinically, as a legal document

Records maintained for sedative and general anesthetic procedures are essentially identical; however, a basic difference in these records is the frequency and the level of monitoring. Fig. 5.16 illustrates an example of a time-based record used in sedation and general anesthesia.

Sedation Record

In the sedation form (see Fig. 5.16) patient identification is presented on the top of the record followed by a summary of the patient's medical history and current medications. Baseline vital signs, NPO (nothing by mouth) status, and procedure are listed followed by a summation of monitors utilized, operator, assistant, start and stop times, premedications, and IV placements.

Intraoperative monitoring and drug administration data are found on the lower half of the chart (Fig. 5.17). Time is noted across the top column, and directly below are spaces for

Date			Pre-op Vitals	BP		HR		SpO₂		RR	

(form follows)

Date

Name

Pre-op Vitals | BP | HR | SpO₂ | RR

Age | Gender M   F | Weight   lbs. | Height | BMI | Mallampati | ASA

Medical History

NPO

NIBP   L   R
Pulse Oximeter

Solids   Hours   Clear Liquids   Hours

Precordial

Procedure(s):

ECG
EtCO₂

Medications

Operator: Assistants:

Drug Allergies

	Start	Finish	Premedication	IV 20G 22G
ANES				R L
SURG				Site

TIME

													Used	Wasted
Oxygen (LPM)														
Nitrous Oxide (LPM)														
Midazolam (mg)														
Diazepam (mg)														
Fentanyl (mcg)														
Meperidine (mg)														
Hydromorphone (mg)														
Sufentanil (mcg)														
Ketorolac (mg)														
NS (mL)														---
2% lidocaine 1:100K epi (mg)														---
4% articaine 1:100K epi (mg)														---
Response to Verbal Stimuli														
SpO₂														
Respiratory Rate														
EtCO₂ Present														
ECG Pattern														

Discharged to:

BP

HR   150

SpO₂

RR   100

☐ Awake   50

☐ Alert

☐ Ambulatory

Comments

Signature:

Figure 5.16 Anesthesia record, which may be used for sedation or general anesthesia.

Date			Pre-op Vitals	BP		HR		SpO₂		RR	
Name											
			Age	Gender	Weight	Height	BMI		Mallampati	ASA	
				M F	lbs.						
Medical History			NPO						NIBP L R		
									Pulse Oximeter		
			Solids Hours Clear Liquids Hours						Precordial		
			Procedure(s):						ECG		
Medications									EtCO₂		
			Operator:				Assistants:				
				Start	Finish		Premedication	IV	20G	22G	
Drug Allergies			ANES						R L		
			SURG						Site		

TIME															
Oxygen (LPM)															
Nitrous Oxide (LPM)														Used	Wasted
Midazolam (mg)															
Diazepam (mg)															
Fentanyl (mcg)															
Meperidine (mg)															
Hydromorphone (mg)															
Sufentanil (mcg)															
Ketorolac (mg)															
NS (mL)														---	
2% lidocaine 1:100K epi (mg)														---	
4% articaine 1:100K epi (mg)														---	
Response to Verbal Stimuli															
SpO₂															
Respiratory Rate															
EtCO₂ Present															
ECG Pattern															

Discharged to:

BP

HR   150

SpO₂

RR   100

☐ Awake   50

☐ Alert

☐ Ambulatory

Comments

Signature: _____

Figure 5.17 Intraoperative monitoring and drug administration data section.

recording vital signs and dosages of drugs administered. The names of all drugs administered, including local anesthetics, are listed, with the milligram dose or flow rate (liters per minute) of gases placed in the appropriate column. At the conclusion of the procedure, the final anesthesia and surgery times of the chart are completed, summarizing the drugs administered (used) and discarded (wasted) and additional comments (located at the bottom of the record).

The ADA recommends, minimally, that vital signs be recorded:
1. Preoperatively for baseline comparison
2. Intraoperatively after the administration of any drug
3. Interoperatively every 5 to 15 minutes during treatment (based on depth of sedative/anesthetic)
4. Immediately postoperatively
5. Just before discharge

The purpose of the comment section is to provide helpful hints that may improve the quality of subsequent sedation procedures on the same patient. For example, it might be noted that the only readily apparent site for venipuncture was the right antecubital fossa or that midazolam was somewhat ineffective in producing sedation but changing to diazepam markedly helped. The doctor and assistant then sign the form, which is placed into the patient's permanent dental or medical chart for future reference, if needed.

Many monitoring devices are supplied with an automatic printer that provides a chronologic record of vital signs; the reverse side of the monitoring sheet allows for a photocopy of this record to be attached. Because most of the monitor tapes record on thermal-sensitive paper, which fades over time, it is suggested that a photocopy of the tape be made and included on the sedation record. Many states require the use of time-based records, which detail the time that each medication was administered.

General Anesthesia Record

Because the patient receiving general anesthesia is unconscious and unable to respond to verbal or physical stimulation, intensified monitoring is an unconditional necessity. As described in the preceding section, the frequency and intensity of monitoring are increased as CNS depression increases. Several vital functions (e.g., heart rate and rhythm, respiration, SpO_2, temperature, and $ETCO_2$) are monitored continuously, whereas others, including blood pressure, are monitored at intervals of 5 minutes. Each of the small, thin vertical lines is an interval of 5 minutes; the thicker, darker lines represent 15 minutes (see Fig. 5.17). Drug administration is listed chronologically in addition to the performance of specific procedures, such as the start of anesthesia, the start of surgery (i.e., incision made), specific intraoperative procedures, the termination of surgery, and the termination of anesthesia.

Examples of completed sedation and general anesthesia records are presented in Fig. 5.18. The anesthesia record also provides an area for monitoring of the patient during the postoperative period in the anesthesia recovery room. The example record (see Fig. 5.17) lists the discharge information at the bottom left.

Recordkeeping is an important aid to the doctor in reconstructing events that occurred during a sedative or general anesthetic procedure. Review of records can also provide the doctor with information regarding a patient's prior response to certain drugs or procedures, possibly alerting the doctor to modify treatment or drug therapy at subsequent appointments. In addition, well-maintained written documentation can greatly assist in a doctor's defense, should a claim be made against the individual or facility.

Because of the potential value of the written sedation or anesthesia record, it is important that these records not be altered after the fact. In addition, it is essential that these records be completed using permanent ink. Should an error or omission be noted after the fact and it becomes necessary to add, change, or delete something from the written record, a single line should be drawn through the error (without obscuring it, which would only increase suspicion) and the correction entered and initialed. If this occurs at a later date, include both the time and date of the correction. The record should remain with the patient's medical or dental chart as a part of the permanent record.

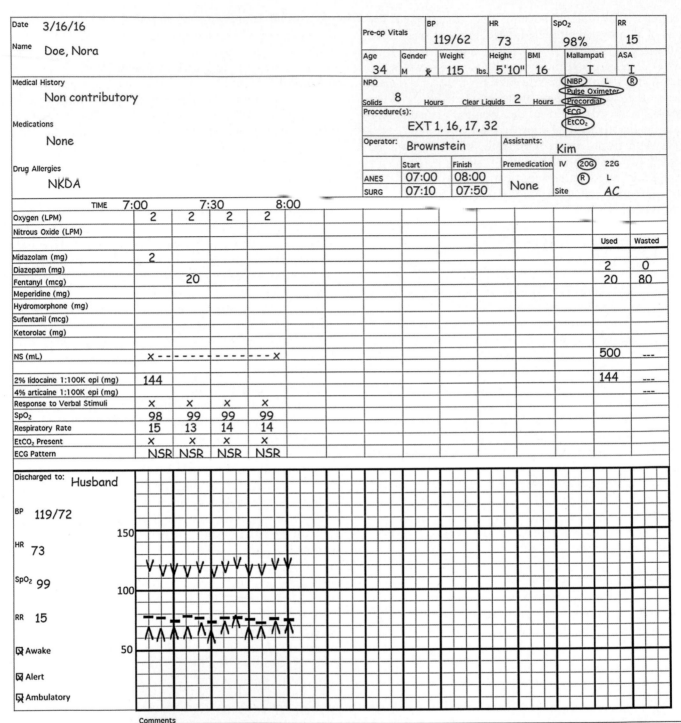

Comments

Pt. & responsible guardian ID, reviewed medical history, anesthetic plan established & reviewed with pt., all Q's answered, obtained written & verbal consents, supplemental O2, IV start, suctioned oropharynx, placed throat pack with safety floss attached, pt. tolerated anesthesia well throughout, end of surgery, removed throat pack, suctioned oropharynx, pt. awake, alert, and oriented x3, sustain SpO2 on RA, entered recovery phase, removed IV catheter, responsible party back for review of post op instructions. Addressed all Q's, pt. released into care of responsible party once all criteria for discharge fully met, instructed to contact anesthesia team with any post-op questions or concerns.

Figure 5.18 Completed anesthesia record.

REFERENCES

1. Lagasse RS: Anesthesia safety: model or myth? A review of the published literature and analysis of current original data. *Anesthesiology* 97(6):1609–1617, 2002.

2. Cooper JB, Gaba D: No myth: anesthesia is a model for addressing patient safety. *Anesthesiology* 97(6):1335–1337, 2002.

3. Cooper JB, Newbower RS, Long CD, McPeek B: Preventable anesthesia mishaps: a study of human factors. *Qual Saf Health Care* 11(3):277–282, 2002.

4. American Society of Anesthesiologists, Committee on Standards and Practice Parameters: Standards for basic anesthetic monitoring. Park Ridge, IL, 2015, American Society of Anesthesiologists.

5. Becker DE, Casabianca AB: Respiratory monitoring: physiological and technical considerations. *Anesth Prog* 56(1):14–22, 2009.

6. Rosenberg MB, Campbell RL: Guidelines for intraoperative monitoring of dental patients undergoing conscious sedation, deep sedation, and general anesthesia. *Oral Surg Oral Med Oral Pathol* 71(1):2–8, 1991.

7. American Dental Association, Council on Dental Education: Guidelines for the use of sedation and general anesthesia by dentists, adopted by the 2012 ADA House of Delegates, Chicago, 2012, The Association. Available at: https://www.ada.org/~/media/ADA/About%20the%20ADA/Files/anesthesia_use_guidelines.pdf?la=en. (Accessed 30 March 2016).

8. Janelle GM, Gravenstein M: An accuracy evaluation of the T-line tensymeter (continuous noninvasive blood pressure management device) versus conventional radial artery monitoring in surgical patients. *Anesth Analg* 102(2):484–490, 2006.

9. Lawler PG: Monitoring during general anesthesia. In Gray TC, Nunn JF, Utting JE, editors: *General anesthesia*, London, 1971, Butterworth.

10. Barash PG, Cullen BF, Stoelting RK, et al, editors: *Clinical anesthesia*, ed 7, Philadelphia, 2013, Lippincott Williams & Wilkins.

11. Loeb RG: A measure of intraoperative attention to monitor displays. *Anesth Analg* 76(2):337–341, 1993.

12. The Joint Commission Sentinel Event Alert: Medical device alarm safety in hospitals. Issue 50, April 8, 2013. Available at: http://www.jointcommission.org/sea_issue_50./. (Accessed 14 April 2016).

13. ECRI Institute: ECRI Institute announces top 10 health technology hazards report for 2015. Available at: https://www.ecri.org/press/Pages/ECRI-Institute-Announces-Top-10-Health-Technology-Hazards-for-2015.aspx. (Accessed 14 April 2016).

14. Casabianca AB, Becker DE: Cardiovascular monitoring: physiological and technical considerations. *Anesth Prog* 56(2):53–60, 2009.

15. Pickering TG, Hall JE, Appel LJ, et al; Council on High Blood Pressure Research Professional and Public Education Subcommittee, American Heart Association: Recommendations for blood pressure measurement in humans: an AHA scientific statement from the Council on High Blood Pressure Research Professional and Public Education Subcommittee. *J Clin Hypertens (Greenwich)* 7(2):102–109, 2005.

16. Cote CJ, Rolf N, Liu LM, et al: A single-blind study of combined pulse oximetry and capnography in children. *Anesthesiology* 74(6):980–987, 1991.

17. Domino KB, Lee LA: The Closed Claims Project: Has it influenced anesthetic practice and outcome? *Anesthesiol Clin North America* 20(3):485–501, 2002.

18. Luks AM, Swenson ER: Pulse oximetry at high altitude. *High Alt Med Biol* 12(2):109–119, 2011.

19. Severinghaus JW, Kelleher JF: Recent developments in pulse oximetry. *Anesthesiology* 76(6):1018–1038, 1992.

20. Barclays Official California Code of Regulations. Title 16. Professional and Vocational Regulations. Division 10. Dental Board of California. Chapter 2. Dentists. Article 5.5. Oral Conscious Sedation. Available at: www.dbc.ca.gov. (Accessed 14 April 2016).

21. Shah N, Ragaswamy HB, Govindugari K, Estanol L: Performance of three new-generation pulse oximeters during motion and low perfusion in volunteers. *J Clin Anesth* 24(5):385–391, 2012.

22. Vascello LA, Bowe EA: A case for capnographic monitoring as a standard of care. *J Oral Maxillofac Surg* 57(11):1342–1347, 1999.

23. ADA News: Comments sought on proposed sedation, anesthesia guideline revisions. June 16, 2014. Available at: http://www.ada.org/en/publications/ada-news/2014-archive/june/comments-sought-on-proposed-sedation-anesthesia-guideline-revisions. (Accessed 14 April 2016).

24. Stanski DR, Shafer SL: Measuring depth of anesthesia. In Miller RD, Fleisher LA, Johns RA, et al, editors: *Miller's anesthesia*, ed 6, London, 2005, Churchill Livingstone.

25. Kissin I: Depth of anesthesia and bispectral index monitoring. *Anesth Analg* 90(5):1114–1117, 2002.

26. National Institute for Healthcare Excellence: Depth of anaesthesia monitors – Bispectral Index (BIS), E-Entropy and Narcotrend-Compact M. NICE diagnostics guidance 6. Issued November 2012. Available at: www.nice.org.uk/dg6. (Accessed 15 April 2016).

27. Glass PS: Anesthetic drug interactions: an insight into general anesthesia—its mechanisms and dosing strategies. *Anesthesiology* 88(1):5–6, 1998.

28. Eichhorn JH, Cooper JB, Cullen DJ, et al: Standards for patient monitoring during anesthesia: Harvard Medical School. *JAMA* 256(8):1017–1020, 1986.

29. Sollai S, Dani C, Berti E, et al: Performance of a non-contact infrared thermometer in healthy newborns. *BMJ Open* 3:e008695, 2016.

30. Kurz A: Thermoregulation in anesthesia and intensive care medicine. *Best Pract Res Clin Anaesthesiol* 22(4):vii–viii, 2008.

chapter 6

Nondrug Techniques: Iatrosedation and Hypnosis

CHAPTER OUTLINE

Iatrosedation
Preparatory Communication
Euphemistic Language
Iatrosedation: Staff and Office
Clinical Demeanor
The Goal of Iatrosedation

Hypnosis
Hypnosis in Dentistry
The Success of Hypnosis
Education in Hypnosis

*I*n Chapter 3, the concept of sedation was described using the terms *psychosedation, iatrosedation,* and *pharmacosedation.* Definitions of these terms are presented at this time to provide groundwork for the remaining sections of this book.

The overall concept of *sedation* was originally defined as "the calming of a nervous, apprehensive individual, through the use of systemic drugs, without inducing the loss of consciousness."[1] Although this definition is essentially accurate, it requires further clarification. This is so because clinical techniques exist that act to diminish a patient's fears and anxieties toward dentistry and surgery that do not require the administration of drugs. In addition, the term *sedation,* implying relaxation of the mind, is too broad of a term because it is possible to specifically "relax" or "sedate" the function of other organs (e.g., the heart [through the use of β-blocking drugs]). Therefore the more specific term *psychosedation* is suggested when discussing the management of fear and anxiety. The term *psychosedative* describes a drug capable of producing relaxation of the patient's mind (e.g., central nervous system [CNS] depression). The two major categories of psychosedative techniques are *iatrosedative* techniques and *pharmacosedative* techniques.

Iatrosedation is defined in both a general and a more specific manner. The general definition of *iatrosedation* is those techniques of psychosedation not requiring drug administration. This chapter presents an introduction to these extremely valuable patient management techniques. The following are included in these techniques:

- Acupressure
- Acupuncture
- Audioanalgesia (e.g., music)
- Biofeedback
- Electronic dental anesthesia (EDA)
- Hypnosis
- Video

Iatrosedation and hypnosis are discussed in this chapter because they are both important components of the dentist's armamentarium against pain and anxiety. The reader interested in the other techniques previously listed is referred to specific references cited for each: acupressure,[2] acupuncture,[3] audioanalgesia,[4] biofeedback,[5,6] EDA,[4,7-8] and video.[9,10]

IATROSEDATION

Iatrosedation was defined in general terms as any technique of anxiety reduction in which no drug is given. At this point, a more specific definition of this same term is presented:

Iatrosedation: The relief of anxiety through the doctor's behavior.

This definition of the term *iatrosedation* was formulated by Dr. Nathan Friedman, for many years the chairman of the Section of Human Behavior at the University of Southern California School of Dentistry.[11-12] The word is derived from the Greek prefix *iatro,* meaning "pertaining to the doctor," and the word *sedation,* meaning "the relief of anxiety."[11]

The concept on which the technique of iatrosedation is based is rather simple: The behavior of the doctor and staff has a profound influence on the behavior of the patient.[11–13] Other names have been applied to this concept, including "suggestion," "chairside or bedside manner," and "the laying on of hands." The underlying premise of all these techniques is similar: One can use himself or herself to aid in relaxing the patient.

How important is iatrosedation in the overall concept of psychosedation? I have received extensive training in the administration of drugs for pharmacosedation and general anesthesia, yet I have received no formal training in any aspect of psychology or human behavior. It would appear, therefore, that I should have a strong bias toward the use of techniques requiring drug administration. When I first started my training in anesthesiology in 1969, this was true.

However, over these past 48 years, I have become sensitized to the fact that iatrosedation is an integral part of the success (or possible failure) of every procedure that we in medicine and dentistry attempt. The success or failure of every pharmacosedative procedure also hinges on the use of iatrosedation.

Two classic studies illustrate the importance of human behavior in the control of pain and anxiety. In the first, Egbert et al.[14] demonstrated the value of the preoperative visit by the anesthesiologist to patients about to undergo surgery the next day. Patients were placed into one of three groups.

Group 1 received a preoperative visit from the anesthesiologist but no preoperative drug for sedation before surgery. The purpose of the preoperative visit was to discuss the upcoming events with the patients and to answer any questions that they might pose to allay their fears. Group 2 received a sedative, pentobarbital, 1 hour preoperatively, but no preoperative visit from the anesthesiologist. Group 3 received both the visit from the anesthesiologist and the preoperative pentobarbital.

Results of the study demonstrated that patients in the first group were alert on arrival in the operating room, but were quite calm. They did not appear apprehensive. Patients in the second group were drowsy (the effect of the pentobarbital), but did not appear to be calm. They appeared quite concerned with the activities occurring around them. The third group, receiving both the visit and medication, were both drowsy and calm.

A second study by Egbert[15] once again demonstrated the value of iatrosedative techniques in patients undergoing surgery. Patients scheduled for abdominal surgery were placed in one of two groups.

Patients in group 1 were not told about postoperative discomfort (pain) following abdominal surgery. Patients were told that analgesics would be available if they were required. Patients in group 2 ("special care patients") were told that postoperative discomfort following abdominal surgery was quite usual and normal. The type of discomfort was described and its probable location. These patients were also told that analgesics would be available should they be required.

During the postoperative recovery period, patients in group 1 required twice the number of doses of analgesics for their discomfort as the patients who had been prepared for the discomfort. It appears that when pain is expected and is considered normal, the patient is better able to tolerate it. Put another way, it might be stated that pain that is expected by a patient simply does not hurt as much as unexpected pain. A significant anxiety component is noted with unexpected pain, a reaction that is not present with pain that is expected (normal). It is this anxiety (the fear that the presence of pain means that something is wrong) that makes the patient experience even more and greater discomfort. A second interesting finding in this study was that patients in the "special care" group recovered from their surgical procedure more rapidly and were discharged from the hospital an average of 2.7 days earlier than the patients in group 1. This may be because of the diminished requirement for analgesic drugs in the second group, leading to a reduction in drug-related side effects and complications that might impede recovery and discharge from the hospital.

These two studies by Egbert demonstrate the power of communication. I have been witness to many such demonstrations during the use of sedative drugs in dental practice. Unfortunately, not all communication works to the benefit of the doctor. This next case illustrates this point.

Case Study 6.1: The Power of Communication

A patient received inhalation sedation with nitrous oxide (N_2O) and oxygen (O_2) for root planing and curettage. The dentist performing the procedure was working with a dental assistant. The patient was receiving approximately 35% N_2O, was quite well sedated, and had a degree of soft tissue analgesia. Treatment was proceeding well despite the patient's earlier anxiety and sensitivity of the tissues. Approximately 20 minutes into the procedure, the dentist, who had been conversing casually with the dental assistant throughout the procedure, made the comment, "Gee, I haven't done one of these (root planing) in about 15 years." Almost immediately the patient grabbed the nasal hood, pulled it off his nose, sat up, and told the dentist he wanted to go home. The patient did not want to be treated by anyone in whom he did not have confidence (even a dentist who was quite capable of doing the procedure well). An offhand remark, meant for the ears of the dental assistant, had destroyed the patient's confidence in the dentist. This is an example of the power (albeit negative) of communication.

Case Study 6.2: Lack of Communication

Yet another example of the power of communication, or the lack of communication, is that of a young man, 26, who admits to being quite uncomfortable with dental treatment. He stated that his previous dentist would walk into the treatment room, tell him to open his mouth, and immediately start treatment, without ever saying hello. The patient was very aware of this and became uncomfortable with his overall care. This dentist suggested that perhaps the patient would be more comfortable if he took a sedative before his next appointment. The patient told us that his treatment was even more uncomfortable than it had been previously because under the influence of the medication he was more acutely aware of the dentist's lack of concern for him as a person. Following this treatment, the patient sought another dentist.

Communication is a powerful ally to the health professional. As these last cases illustrate, even when pharmacosedation is used, communication must never be ignored. Effective communication makes the drugs administered even more effective.

In the motion picture *The Doctor,*[16] a successful surgeon falls ill and enters into the contemporary health care system as a patient experiencing, as never before, the trials and tribulations that befall patients every day in the hospitals and medical centers of America. Through his negative experiences, the physician learns the value of communication and the importance of empathy in dealing with patients. This award-winning and highly successful film was based on a true story. Incoming residents in family practice medicine at the Long Beach (Calif.) Veterans Administration Hospital begin their hospital career as patients admitted to the hospital, undergoing the routines all patients face (hospital gowns, blood tests, impersonal attitudes by hospital staff).[17] Much of the commercial success of *The Doctor* was thought to be that audiences (all potential patients) believed that the message of the film struck home. The medical profession, to its credit, has recognized that the great emphasis placed in medical education on the "scientific process" leads to the isolation of the physician from the patient and has begun to take steps to right the perceived wrongs. In a 1992 paper, Spiro[18] states that "medical students lose some of their empathy as they learn science and detachment, and hospital residents lose the remainder in the weariness of overwork and in the isolation of the intensive care units that modern hospitals have become." Medical schools have begun to modify their curricula, including in them new programs on communication and human behavior, designed to prevent the impersonalization of the physician.[19-21]

Similar programs have been in place for years in many dental schools throughout the United States and other countries. Yet in the highly competitive world that is dentistry today, it is often the patient who gets lost in the shuffle. I detest the increasing use of the term *client* when discussing our *patients.* The importance of effective communication among the dentist and staff and patient can never be overemphasized. Interestingly, in the venue of continuing dental education, among the most popular programs offered are those in practice management— how to have a successful dental practice. The theme of communication is paramount in all these programs.

Preparatory Communication

In the studies by Egbert,[11,15] examples were presented of preparatory communication. Preparatory communication is aimed at minimizing or eliminating a patient's fear of the unknown, one of our most prominent fears. Within the realm of dentistry, patients possess many fears that are based on hearsay. Patients faced with the prospect of endodontic therapy become hysterical because of their mental picture of "root canal work." The thought of removing the "nerve" from a tooth is an unpleasant one to most persons. However, if the dentist spends but a few moments before the start of the endodontic treatment describing what is to be done or if educational pamphlets are available to the patient, such fears can be allayed. What is endodontic therapy? It may be described as the removal of tissue from the tooth followed by shaping and filling of the tooth (or canal) with an inert material. When root canal therapy is described in this manner, it appears much less traumatic to the patient.

A few moments spent with a patient describing the planned procedure before the start of a new mode of treatment serves to allay most of the patient's anxieties. Terms used to describe the treatment should be nonthreatening if preparatory communication is to be effective in decreasing fear. Explaining an endodontic procedure by stating that "we will give you a shot of anesthetic and then remove the nerve from the tooth" only succeeds in heightening a patient's fears. The art of semantics therefore plays an important role in communication between the dentist and patient. Friedman discusses the use of euphemistic language, which is the substitution of mild or inoffensive words for those that may offend or suggest something unpleasant.[11,12] The word *euphemism* is derived from the Greek *eu* (well) and *phanai* (to speak).

Euphemistic Language

The dental vocabulary is replete with threatening words, examples of which are presented here:
- Hurt, pain
- Needle, shot, injection
- Cut
- Cauterize
- Extract
- Drill
- Scalpel

- Operatory or surgery
- Nerve

Most health professionals, especially dentists, are acutely aware of the need to avoid using threatening words. However, occasions do arise when their use seems inescapable. For example, during the administration of a nasopalatine nerve block (perhaps the most difficult intraoral injection to administer atraumatically on a consistent basis), the patient might feel some pain (a negative word). Should the dentist tell the patient before the injection, "You will probably feel some *pain* during this injection," or "This *shot* will probably hurt a little"? The answer is "No," at least not in the manner described. When it is expected that there will be pain, a nonthreatening term, such as *discomfort*, can be substituted. The statement "I will be doing this slowly; if there should be some discomfort just raise your hand and I will stop immediately" relays the same information, but does not traumatize the patient psychologically, as did the preceding statement.

Examples of other terms that may be substituted for more traumatic ones are *discomfort* or *feel* in place of *hurt* or *pain,* as in, "I don't expect you to feel this" instead of "This won't hurt." The only word heard by the patient is "hurt." *Novocain* or *local anesthetic* in place of *needle, shot,* or *injection,* as in "We're going to give you a local anesthetic now," is preferable to "We're going to give you a shot (or injection) now." Canadian dentists have used the word *freeze* in this situation ("I am going to freeze you now") with great success. In essence the message delivered to the patient who is about to receive an injection of a local anesthetic is nonthreatening.

In pediatric dentistry, euphemistic language has always been an important means of describing to the younger, less mature patient the instruments and procedures used. The injection (administration) of a local anesthetic is described as "spraying sleepy water on a tooth," a saliva ejector is called a "vacuum cleaner," and preparation of a tooth with a drill is described as "tickling the tooth." Although the words used for adults may be different, the concept remains the same. Describe the procedure in a way that lessens, not heightens, a patient's anxiety. *Remove* may be substituted for *extract* or *extirpate* (i.e., "Tissue will be removed from the tooth" instead of "We will have to extirpate the nerve"). *Handpiece* is used in place of *drill*, and *treatment room* may be substituted for *operatory.*

Euphemistic Language in Sedation

Throughout this book, examples of euphemistic language are offered as they relate to the use of pharmacosedation. In describing the feelings a patient will experience during a sedative procedure or the equipment that is used to deliver the drugs to the patient, less threatening words or phrases are substituted for potentially more traumatic ones. An excellent example deals with the administration of diazepam, a drug used to obtain moderate levels of sedation via the intravenous (IV) route. Because diazepam is not water soluble, propylene glycol is used as a solvent. Propylene glycol can produce irritation of vein walls as the drug is injected. Some patients may experience this irritation only slightly or even not at all, whereas others may consider it quite uncomfortable. It is suggested that the person administering IV diazepam caution (e.g., advise) the patient before its administration that there is a possibility of discomfort. Should the dentist fail to tell the patient and a painful sensation does occur, the patient may become quite apprehensive, fearing that something is wrong. This possibility can be eliminated by forewarning the patient. The manner in which this potential "feeling" is described is important. Stating that the patient will experience a painful sensation or that there will be a burning sensation as the drug is injected is likely to put the patient on alert, increasing an already heightened anxiety level. A patient might ask himself or herself, "Why, if this drug is going to hurt when it is being injected, is the doctor using it at all?" I have found it best to tell the patient receiving IV diazepam: "You may experience a slight warmth in your arm as the drug is administered. This is entirely normal and will pass within a few seconds." In this manner, the patient is prepared but not frightened.

Inhalation sedation with N_2O-O_2 is commonly called *gas, laughing gas, sweet air,* or *medicated air* by dentists who believe that the chemical names may be too threatening to their patients.[22] Yet another euphemistic term relating to sedation comes to mind: With headlines concerning the illicit use of drugs, such as cocaine and narcotics, in newspapers and the electronic media seemingly daily, the very word *drug* has acquired a negative connotation. Use of the word *medication* relays the desired message in a more professional and less intimidating manner.

Iatrosedation: Staff and Office

The entire dental staff must be alert to the appropriate use of language, because much of a patient's contact in the office will be with persons other than the dentist. In addition, the demeanor of the receptionist, chairside personnel, and all others will either add to or detract from the environment in the office. Sedation does not just magically happen when a patient sits down in the dental chair. As demonstrated in the stress-reduction protocols (see Chapter 4), the recognition and management of anxiety must start before dental treatment commences. A receptionist is just as important in the management of anxiety as chairside personnel. The receptionist is trained to answer the telephone "with a smile," to help reassure the apprehensive patient and to relay such information to the dentist and other chairside personnel. The apprehensive patient is on the alert for clues on entering the dental office. A positive attitude on the part of the staff and a relaxed environment within the office will help allay the patient's fears. A busy, high-pressure office where staff members are constantly running about in a frenzy is not conducive to relaxation. The use of striking colors and loud rock music will also detract from a sedative environment (although patients' musical tastes do vary considerably). Conversely a low-pressure, relaxed office staff combined with a toned-down color scheme (earth colors) and a more moderate type of music provide a warm, cheerful environment that adds to the sedative effect of any drugs that may subsequently be administered.[23]

Once the patient arrives in the dental office, his or her presence should be acknowledged within a minute or two. Even when the dentist may be somewhat delayed in scheduling, the patient should be informed of this and not kept waiting for no apparent reason. The patient should be escorted to the (dental) treatment room (the term *operatory* or *surgery* is threatening to many patients) and seated in the dental chair. At this point, the dental assistant can aid the patient's level of comfort by simply adjusting the chair and headrest as may be desired by the patient or by offering the patient a facial tissue. An attitude of concern or empathy should be relayed by the assistant to the patient to help establish lines of communication. On entering the treatment room, the dentist should always greet the patient, shake hands (personal touches like this are greatly appreciated by the patient and are an aid in recognition of anxiety [cold, sweaty palms]), and spend a moment or two talking before starting treatment. I have been astounded by the number of fearful patients who have stated that the major reason they left a dentist was because "the doctor didn't care about me as a person." A few words spoken to the patient before and during treatment help establish a better working relationship between the treatment team and the patient.

I was present when a dental student was interviewing an apprehensive patient who he was seeing for the first time. The student had reviewed the patient's medical history questionnaire and was seeking to determine the causes of the patient's fear of dentistry. The audio portion of this taped interview demonstrated that the student was quite adept at obtaining the necessary information and at transmitting his desire to work with the patient to help him diminish his dental fear. However, when seen on video, the entire interview was considered a failure. The student dentist, asking all of the appropriate questions and expressing his concern for the patient, was standing with his back toward the patient and reading from a prepared list of questions. At no point during this 20-minute interview did the patient ever see the student's face for more than a few seconds at a time.

Clinical Demeanor

Why does a patient select one dentist over another? Most patients select a dentist after discussion with friends and relatives. Commonly expressed reasons for selection include the comments that this dentist "is good" or "is painless." It appears, therefore, that one of the primary considerations used in the selection process is a dentist's clinical demeanor.[24] This does not always mean that the technical quality of the dentistry is superior; it does, however, mean that the dentist "cares about the patients" and makes an effort to be gentle and to provide painless treatment.

Friedman[11,12] has stated that "the more threatening an instrument, the more significant your manner of wielding it" becomes to the patient. And what instrument is more threatening to a patient than the needle on the local anesthetic syringe?

De St. Georges opined that the two most important factors used when patients evaluate their dentist are: (2) the dentist does not hurt and (1) gives painless injections.[25]

A gentle touch is appreciated over a rough appearance. Expressions of concern, verbal or nonverbal, during treatment aid in allaying a patient's fears. A simple statement such as "If for any reason you would like me to stop, simply raise your hand and I will stop immediately" tells the patient of their dentist's concern. A new patient may test this system several times to be certain that the dentist was truthful, but once convinced will relax and permit treatment to continue.

The Goal of Iatrosedation

The ultimate goal of iatrosedation is to minimize the patient's requirement for pharmacosedation. Another goal is to open lines of communication so that the patient will not be inhibited from expressing true feelings or desires to the dentist or staff members. When patients are able to express their fears to the dentist before treatment begins, it becomes that much simpler to manage them during treatment.

Iatrosedation is an effective technique; however, it may not be adequate by itself to remove the fear of dentistry harbored by all patients. The use of supplemental pharmacosedation may be necessary in the initial phases of patient management. Iatrosedation effectively minimizes the depth of pharmacosedation required to reach a desired clinical level of relaxation, and/or it maximizes the effectiveness of the pharmacosedative technique used.

By communicating with our patients, we can begin the process of fear reduction during our initial contact. Through the establishment of rapport with the patient, we are able to determine the level of pharmacosedation (if any) required to manage the patient's dental fears and make more effective use of any drugs we might employ. The following case study serves to point out the objectives of iatrosedation.[26]

Case Study 6.3: Objectives of Iatrosedation

The patient, a 24-year-old college student, had purposely avoided dental treatment in the past until forced by pain to seek help. His anxieties were related to the sound of the dental handpiece and originated in childhood, when the patient was treated by a dentist who did not use local anesthesia. The patient associated the sound of the handpiece with the pain of "drilling." The patient arrived at the University of Southern California School of Dentistry emergency clinic with acute pulpitis of the mandibular right first molar.

The patient admitted to an extreme fear of dentistry and stated that despite his pain he could not tolerate dental treatment. At the first treatment visit, IV diazepam,

19 mg, was administered (via titration) to sedate the patient, and after mandibular anesthesia was obtained, the pulp was extirpated without incident. The patient later stated that he had "enjoyed" the dental appointment and wished to become a regular clinic patient.

At subsequent appointments, the patient did require the use of pharmacosedative techniques. However, at the end of eight dental visits, spanning a period of 3 months, the patient no longer required the use of pharmacosedation for his dental care. This is the goal. Through the combined use of iatrosedation and pharmacosedation, in many cases it is possible to achieve this goal of reeducating the fearful patient. This goal may easily be accomplished in those practices in which patients remain for many years, such as in general dental practice, pediatric dentistry, and periodontics. Because of the shorter treatment periods (e.g., fewer appointments) required in oral surgery and endodontics, this same goal is somewhat more elusive, although it is still achievable.

As stated in Chapter 2, the goal in initially using pharmacosedation as an aid in patient management is to eventually eliminate its need. The technique of iatrosedation will, of course, be used with each and every patient who appears in the office seeking treatment at each and every appointment.

HYPNOSIS

Hypnosis has been defined as a "special trancelike state in which the subject's attention is focused intensely on the hypnotist, while attention to other stimuli is markedly diminished."[27] Barber and Mayer[28] define hypnosis as "an altered state of consciousness characterized by narrowed, heightened attention, and the capacity for producing alterations in memory and perception."

Franz Anton Mesmer (1734–1815), a graduate of the University of Vienna School of Medicine, did a great deal of work on the subject of animal magnetism. His work became the subject of controversy throughout Europe, and his Magnetic Institute in Paris attracted many influential and rich persons. Banned from Paris, Mesmer moved his institute along with its ardent followers to Switzerland. Animal magnetism, or mesmerism as it came to be known, was an early form of hypnotism and as such was instrumental in the development of a new awareness of the possibilities of making people insensitive to pain. James Esdaile in India performed 73 painless surgical operations using mesmerism; however, the medical communities of the day remained unconvinced of its value, and mesmerism

remained a controversial topic within the medical community and among the public for many years to come.[29]

In 1837 the first reported case of a tooth extraction using mesmerism was published.[30] It was not until 1843 that the term *hypnotism* was introduced by James Braid.

At the end of the nineteenth century and the beginning of the twentieth century, the foundations of hypnosis were elucidated by Jean-Martin Charcot (1825–1893) and others. Sigmund Freud initiated the use of hypnosis as a therapeutic tool in psychoanalysis, a role that it still maintains today.[28]

Hypnosis in Dentistry

As with iatrosedation, hypnosis serves as a means of providing relaxation without the need for drug administration. In addition, hypnosis serves as a means of providing clinically acceptable pain control in some patients, making it a potentially valuable technique in dentistry.

Barber[31] lists the following possible uses of hypnosis in dentistry:
- Patient relaxation
- Anxiety reduction
- Orthodontics (aid in overcoming fear of orthodontics)
- Maintenance of comfort during prolonged treatments
- Modification of noxious dental habits (e.g., thumb sucking)
- Reduction of the need for anesthesia or analgesia
- Postoperative analgesia
- Substitution for premedication in general anesthesia
- Control of reflexes and autonomic processes (i.e., gagging, nausea, salivary flow, bleeding)
- Management of difficult patients

Hypnosis is an effective technique as an aid in helping patients overcome their fears of various procedures. Hypnotic suggestion has proven valuable in eliminating the fear of injections (both intraoral and IV or intramuscular) and the claustrophobic feeling some patients experience when the N_2O-O_2 inhalation sedation nasal hood is placed over their nose.[32] When venipuncture is difficult to achieve because of a patient's fear of needles, hypnosis may prove effective in eliminating or minimizing the fear.[33]

In many cases, hypnosis can be used in place of other, more conventional techniques of pain and anxiety control.[34] When hypnosis is successful, even local anesthetics for pain control may not be required, though their administration is still recommended for painful procedures. Postoperative complications and discomfort may be minimized through the effective use of posthypnotic suggestion, thereby decreasing a patient's requirement for analgesics and other drugs with their attendant side effects.[28]

The Success of Hypnosis

Although folklore acknowledges that only 25% of the population is "susceptible" to hypnosis, reports on the success of hypnosis in clinical practice are more positive. Beecher[35] reported that hypnosis is an effective substitute for anesthesia in all but approximately 20% of the surgical population tested. Barber and Mayer,[28] using a technique of hypnotic induction called *rapid induction analgesia,* reported that test subjects were able to "dramatically alter their awareness of experimental dental pain, irrespective of hypnotic susceptibility … Ninety-nine percent of unscreened dental patients were able to undergo normally painful dental procedures using only hypnosis, as induced by rapid induction analgesia."

Education in Hypnosis

Although some dental schools include training in hypnosis as a part of their curricula, most practicing dentists have not received training in the effective use of this potentially valuable technique. Two professional groups offer clinical workshops in hypnosis throughout the United States. The reader is referred to them for additional information and training in hypnosis.*

SUMMARY

In conclusion, I must restate the vital importance of iatrosedation in the everyday practice of medicine and dentistry. Iatrosedation must be employed by each of us whenever we are in contact with other human beings, be they our patients, staff, or simply other persons we come into contact with in our daily life. Our behavior and our appearance provide these persons with a sense of "like" or "dislike" toward us. For a practice of dentistry or medicine to be successful, an attitude of caring must become an integral part of office philosophy. In the absence of this caring attitude, patients feel isolated and alienated, increasing their own anxiety levels and producing additional management difficulties for the staff. The successful use of iatrosedation will enhance the effectiveness of the pharmacosedative techniques that will be discussed in the chapters to follow.

REFERENCES

1. Council on Dental Education: *Guidelines for teaching the comprehensive control of pain and anxiety in dentistry,* Chicago, 1993, American Dental Association.
2. Wang SM, Gaal D, Maranets I, et al: Acupressure and preoperative parental anxiety: a pilot study. *Anesth Analg* 101(3):666–669, table of contents, 2005.
3. Michalek-Sauberer A, Gusenleitner E, Gleiss A, et al: Auricular acupuncture effectively reduces state anxiety before dental treatment—a randomised controlled trial. *Clin Oral Investig* 16(6):1517–1522, 2012.

*American Society of Clinical Hypnosis, 130 East Elm Court, Suite 201 Roselle, IL 60172-2000; phone: 630-980-4740; fax: 630-351-8490; e-mail: info@asch.net; website: www.asch.net. Accessed August 7, 2015.
Society for Clinical and Experimental Hypnosis, SCEH Central Office, Washington State University, PO Box 642114, Pullman, WA 99164-2114; fax: 509-335-2097; e-mail: sceh@pullman.com; website: www.sceh.us. Accessed August 7, 2015.

4. Baghdadi ZD: Evaluation of audio analgesia for restorative care in children treated using electronic dental anesthesia. *J Clin Pediatr Dent* 25(1):9–12, 2000.
5. Elmore AM: Biofeedback therapy in the treatment of dental anxiety and dental phobia. *Dent Clin North Am* 32:735, 1988.
6. Little JW: Complementary and alternative medicine: impact on dentistry. *Oral Surg Oral Med Oral Pathol Oral Radiol Endod* 98(2):137–145, 2004.
7. Munshi AK, Hegde AM, Girdhar D: Clinical evaluation of electronic dental anesthesia for various procedures in pediatric dentistry. *J Clin Pediatr Dent* 24(3):199–204, 2000.
8. Pandit N, Gupta R, Chandoke U, Gugnani S: Comparative evaluation of topical and electronic anesthesia during scaling and root planing. *J Periodontol* 81(7):1035–1040, 2010.
9. Zhang G, Hou P, Zhou H, et al: Improved sedation for dental extraction by using video eyewear in conjunction with nitrous oxide: a randomized, controlled, cross-over clinical trial. *Oral Surg Oral Med Oral Pathol Oral Radiol* 113(2):188–192, 2012.
10. Ram D, Shapira J, Holan G, et al: Audiovisual video eyeglass distraction during dental treatment in children. *Quintessence Int* 41(8):673–967, 2010.
11. Friedman N: Iatrosedation. In McCarthy FM, editor: *Emergencies in dental practice,* ed 3, Philadelphia, 1979, WB Saunders.
12. Friedman N: Iatrosedation: the treatment of fear in the dental patient. *J Dent Educ* 47(2):91–95, 1983.
13. Taneja P: Iatrosedation: a holistic tool in the armamentarium of anxiety control. *SAAD Dig* 31:23–25, 2015.
14. Egbert L, Battit G, Turndoff H, et al: Value of the preoperative visit by an anesthetist. *JAMA* 195:553, 1963.
15. Egbert LD: Reduction of post-operative pain by encouragement and instruction of patients: a study of doctor-patient rapport. *N Engl J Med* 270:825, 1964.
16. Ziskin L: Producer: *The doctor,* Hollywood, 1991, Touchstone Films.
17. Long Beach Veterans Administration Hospital program, Long Beach, Calif.
18. Spiro H: What is empathy and can it be taught? *Ann Intern Med* 116:843, 1992.
19. Matthews DA, Feinstein AR: A review of systems for the personal aspects of patient care. *Am J Med Sci* 295:159, 1988.
20. Novack DH, Suchman AL, Clark W, et al: Calibrating the physician. Personal awareness and effective patient care. Working Group on Promoting Physician Personal Awareness, American Academy on Physician and Patient. *JAMA* 278(6):502–509, 1997.
21. Schattner A, Fletcher RH: Pearls and pitfalls in patient care: need to revive traditional clinical values. *Am J Med Sci* 327(2):79–85, 2004.
22. Shedlin M, Wallechinsky D: *Laughing gas, nitrous oxide,* Berkeley, 1973, And/Or Press.
23. Schmierer A: Use of relaxation sound tracks in the dental office. *Zahnarztl Prax* 42:286, 1991.
24. Friedman H: The doctor-patient relationship in an intravenous-sedation practice. *Anesth Prog* 23:48, 1976.
25. de St. Georges J: How dentists are judged by patients. *Dent Today* 23(8):96–99, 2004.
26. Malamed SF: A most powerful drug. *J Calif Acad Gen Dent* 4:17, 1979.
27. Patel B, Potter C, Mellor AC: The use of hypnosis in dentistry: a review. *Dent Update* 27(4):198–202, 2000.
28. Barber J, Mayer D: Evaluation of the efficacy and neural mechanism of a hypnotic analgesia procedure in experimental and clinical dental pain. *Pain* 4:41, 1977.
29. Lyons AS, Petrucelli RJ: *Medicine: an illustrated history,* New York, 1978, Harry N. Abrams.

30. Ring ME: *Dentistry: an illustrated history*, New York and St. Louis, 1985, Harry N. Abrams and Mosby.
31. Barber J: Acupuncture and hypnosis in dentistry. In Allen GD, editor: *Dental anesthesia and analgesia (local and general)*, ed 2, Baltimore, 1979, Williams & Wilkins.
32. DiBona MC: Nitrous oxide and hypnosis: a combined technique. *Anesth Prog* 26:17, 1979.
33. Morse DR, Cohen BB: Desensitization using meditation-hypnosis to control "needle" phobia in two dental patients. *Anesth Prog* 30:83, 1983.
34. Hilgard ER: Pain: its reduction and production under hypnosis. *Proc Am Philos Soc* 115:470, 1971.
35. Beecher HK: *Measurement of subjective responses*, New York, 1959, Oxford University Press.

Section III

ORAL, RECTAL, AND INTRAMUSCULAR SEDATION

In this, and in subsequent sections, the techniques of pharmacosedation are described in detail. Major sections are devoted to the inhalation and intravenous (IV) routes, two of the most useful pharmacosedative techniques. In this section, other routes of drug administration are discussed in depth: oral, rectal, and intramuscular (IM), each of which can prove to be quite effective within the practice of dentistry for the management of pain, fear, and anxiety. Three other potentially valuable routes of drug administration, sublingual, transdermal, and intranasal (IN), are presented in Chapter 9.

The oral route of drug administration has experienced an increased popularity within dentistry in the United States over the past 20 years. One drug, triazolam (Halcion), has become a very popular agent for the provision of minimal-to-moderate sedation.

The rectal route (see Chapter 8) has become less popular within dentistry, whereas the IN route of drug administration has become increasingly popular in recent years.

Each of these routes of drug administration may be used to produce sedation (minimal, moderate, or deep).

chapter 7

Oral Sedation

CHAPTER OUTLINE

The oral route is the oldest route of drug administration and still the most commonly used. It is also the most convenient and most economic method of drug administration. The oral route may be used quite effectively in dentistry for the reduction of stress before or during dental treatment and as a means of managing preoperative and postoperative pain. Although other routes of drug administration may be more reliable and more effective in producing a desired clinical effect, the oral route still maintains a valued place in dentistry's armamentarium against pain and anxiety.

ADVANTAGES

The oral route possesses several advantages over other routes of drug administration:
1. Almost universal acceptability
2. Ease of administration
3. Low cost
4. Decreased incidence of adverse reactions
5. Decreased severity of adverse reactions
6. No needles, syringes, or equipment

Most adults do not object to taking drugs by mouth. For better or worse, we have become a "pill-popping" society, a fact that makes the prescription of an anxiety-reducing (e.g., anxiolytic) drug before dental treatment all the more palatable to the patient. Many dentists in North America have been trained to provide anxiolysis (minimal sedation) or moderate sedation to their adult patients using oral central nervous system (CNS) depressants. An important exception to the acceptability of orally administered drugs is the young, immature child, who frequently proves unwilling to take any drugs by mouth.

Oral drugs are exceptionally easy for the dentist to administer. In some cases, the drug prescribed for sedation will be taken by the patient at home. It is more prudent, however, for the dentist to administer an oral CNS-depressant drug to the patient personally on their arrival in the dental office to better ensure proper dosage and time of administration. In either case, the administration of drugs via the oral route requires only that the dentist have knowledge of the pharmacologic action of the drug administered, its side effects, potential drug–drug interactions, and any contraindications to its administration. No special equipment or personnel is required for the safe use of the oral route in the adult patient.

The cost of most oral drugs is usually quite low, especially for the small number of doses employed in dentistry. Although there is significant variation in the cost of drugs, the oral form of a drug is usually less expensive than its parenteral counterpart.

Complications are possible whenever drugs are administered, regardless of the route of administration. Drug idiosyncrasy, allergy, and overdose, in addition to other adverse actions, can and do occur. Drug-related side effects are less likely to develop after enteral drug administration (i.e., oral, rectal) than after parenteral drug administration. In addition, adverse reactions following oral administration are often much less intense than those noted following parenteral administration of the same drug. This is not to imply that serious complications do not occur following oral drug administration. Berger, Green, and Melnick[1] reported cardiac arrest following oral diazepam intoxication, while Gill and Michaelides[2] described an anaphylactic response to oral penicillin. Other serious adverse reactions to orally prescribed drugs, including suicide, have been reported.[3–5]

The convenience of the oral route is a primary reason for its popularity. This technique can be employed with minimal risk if the dentist prescribing the drug(s) is knowledgeable of (1) the pharmacologic actions of the drug; (2) its indications, contraindications, precautions, side effects, and dosage; and (3) the medical history of the patient, especially as it relates to prior drug use, specific contraindications to the use of particular drugs, and prior reactions to the drug to be administered. No special equipment (e.g., needles, syringes) and no additional personnel are required when oral drugs are administered to adult patients.

The aforementioned advantages make the use of orally administered drugs quite compelling. However, there are, as with all routes of drug administration, some distinct disadvantages that effectively limit the clinical use of this route of drug administration.

DISADVANTAGES

Disadvantages associated with the oral route include the following:
1. Reliance on patient compliance
2. Prolonged latent period
3. Erratic and incomplete absorption of drugs from the gastrointestinal (GI) tract
4. Inability to titrate
5. Inability to readily lighten or deepen the level of sedation
6. Prolonged duration of action

When prescribing drugs for oral administration before coming to the dental office, the dentist must rely on the patient to take the drug as prescribed (the proper dose at the proper time). Although most patients will medicate themselves properly, some do not. This potential problem, termed *noncompliance,* is significant in medicine, especially in relation to long-term drug administration (e.g., antihypertensive drugs, HIV). The Council on Patient Information and Education estimates that 35% to 50% of all prescriptions dispensed by physicians are taken incorrectly by patients and that one in five patients never even bother to have the prescription filled.[6] One in seven stops taking the drug too soon. A noncompliance rate of 64.5% was found among patients on antihypertensive drug therapy.[7] Although noncompliance is not as critical a problem in the

dental situation, the administration of too small or too large a dose, too soon or too late, may significantly alter the drug's effectiveness during the treatment period. A common form of noncompliance is the taking of a dose larger than that prescribed; the patient's rationale is "if one (tablet or capsule) is good, then two or more will be better." This type of thinking leads to oversedation, overdose, and other unwanted and unpleasant dose-related complications. Fortunately (in this situation, at least), the erratic and incomplete absorption of orally administered drugs minimizes the development of serious problems from drug overadministration.

On many occasions, I have observed this phenomenon in pediatric dental patients: A parent or guardian administers a tablespoon of drug instead of a teaspoon or a larger dose than desired because the child did not take all of the first dose. Significant overdose, with attendant respiratory depression, can develop in this manner if the administered drug is a CNS depressant. The consequences of these actions are formidable, with potential morbidity or mortality as the result. This has led to the enactment of legislation in five states restricting the use of oral sedation in patients younger than 13 years of age to dentists who have received appropriate education and training in this patient population.[8] Oral sedation regulations vary considerably from state to state, province to province, and country to country.[8]

Oral Sedation in Adults. As of January 2017, 41 states had enacted legislation requiring a permit to administer oral sedation.[9]

The dentist prescribing oral drugs for the management of anxiety must never forget that these drugs are CNS depressants and that excessive CNS depression (e.g., oversedation or loss of consciousness [e.g., general anesthesia]) is always a possibility. To minimize concern over patient noncompliance, the dentist should (1) tell the patient, or the parent or guardian, exactly how much of the drug to take and at what time to take it; (2) write these instructions down and give them to the patient; (3) make sure that the prescription is clearly marked with these same instructions; (4) prescribe only the dose the patient is to take (this is warranted even though prescriptions for larger numbers of tablets or capsules are less expensive per item than are single doses); and (5) record the instructions given to the patient and the drug and its dose in the patient's chart.

When the patient or parent (or guardian) of a child is believed to be unreliable, the patient should be requested to appear in the dental office 1 hour before the scheduled treatment, where the drug can be administered to the patient by the dentist in a more controlled manner. As noted in Chapter 35, it is much preferred for a child to be premedicated in the dental office than at home.

A significant disadvantage of the oral route is its relatively long latent period (the period following administration before a clinical effect is observed). Most orally administered drugs have a latent period of approximately 30 minutes. At this time (30 minutes), the blood (plasma) level of the drug has reached the minimum (therapeutic) level required for clinical activity to be observed. Absorption of oral drugs occurs primarily from the small intestine with some absorption from the stomach (alcohol and aspirin are exceptions where significant absorption occurs from the stomach). Drug absorption into the cardiovascular system continues, and the blood level of the drug increases until a maximum level is reached. With most oral drugs, peak blood levels occur approximately 60 minutes following ingestion or 30 minutes following the onset of clinical activity. Peak blood level is equated clinically with maximal drug action (i.e., most intense analgesia or sedation).

In addition to a long latent period, most oral drugs are absorbed erratically and incompletely from the GI tract, which makes consistent clinical results difficult to achieve. A number of factors act to influence absorption of drugs from the GI tract as follows:
1. Lipid solubility
2. pH of the gastric tissues
3. Mucosal surface area
4. Gastric emptying time
5. Dosage form of the drug
6. Drug inactivation
7. Presence of food in the stomach
8. Bioavailability of the drug
9. Hepatic "first-pass" effect

Absorption

Both the lipid solubility of the drug and the pH of the gastric tissues affect drug absorption from the GI tract. Lipid-soluble drugs are absorbed more rapidly than non–lipid-soluble drugs. Gastric fluid has a pH of approximately 1.4. Drugs that are organic acids, such as aspirin, freely diffuse across the gastric mucosa into the circulatory system. Drugs that are bases (e.g., codeine) are poorly absorbed from the highly acid environment of the stomach. As gastric fluid leaves the stomach to enter the small intestine, its pH changes dramatically as a result of the addition of biliary, intestinal, and pancreatic secretions. In the intestinal environment, with its pH of approximately 4.0 to 6.0, the absorption of aspirin is slowed, whereas absorption of the more basic codeine is accelerated.

Primary absorption of most drugs occurs from the small intestine rather than the stomach. This is true even for drugs such as aspirin, because although the lower gastric pH favors its absorption, more than 90% of the absorption of aspirin occurs in the small intestine. The architecture of the small intestine is the primary reason for this. The process of absorption is facilitated by the small intestine's considerable surface area, consisting of microvilli, villi, and the folds of Kerckring. The stomach, by contrast, is a relatively smooth organ, poorly adapted for absorption.

Because the small intestine is the primary site for drug absorption, it is important to get the drug through the mouth, esophagus, and stomach and into the small intestine as rapidly as possible. The removal of foods and other substances from the stomach occurs by contraction of the antrum of the stomach.

The time required for a substance to be expelled from the stomach is the *gastric emptying time*. Liquids, when taken alone, require approximately 90 minutes to be removed, and a mixed meal of food and liquid requires about 4 hours to reach the duodenum. Liquids are discharged from the stomach into the duodenum at a rate of 10 mL/min. The presence of fat in the stomach significantly increases gastric emptying time. It is therefore recommended as a general rule that oral drugs be taken with a glass of water (approximately 8 oz) in the absence of food. In this manner, the drug's delivery to the duodenum is maximized, permitting more reliable absorption. Anxiety is another factor that delays gastric emptying. It is estimated that gastric emptying time can be delayed by as much as two times in the fearful patient,[10] thereby delaying the onset of action of antianxiety drugs. Thus a negative cycle is established. Oral antianxiety drugs are administered 1 hour before treatment to lessen the patient's fear of impending dental or surgical care, yet the very fear that we are seeking to manage inhibits absorption of the drug into the cardiovascular system. This helps explain why in the presence of extreme fear, orally administered drugs may prove ineffective despite having been administered as directed by the dentist.

Drugs administered in an aqueous solution are more rapidly absorbed than those given as an oily solution or in tablet or capsule form. The tablet or capsule must first dissolve in the gastric fluid before absorption can occur. Once it has dissolved, the size of the resulting particles of drug is important. The smaller the particle is, the greater the rate of drug absorption.[11] There is significant variation in the clinical effectiveness of different forms (i.e., liquid, capsule, tablet) of the same drug (see "Bioavailability").

Some drugs, such as morphine, cannot be administered orally because a significant level of drug inactivation occurs before they reach the cardiovascular system. Although the acidity of the stomach is the major cause of this, intestinal contents can also affect the actions of oral drugs. The *hepatic first-pass effect* is also involved. Drugs absorbed from the GI tract (stomach, intestine, colon) are first delivered to the liver via the hepatic portal system before entering into the systemic circulation. The liver is rich in enzymes that biotransform certain drugs into pharmacologically inactive by-products. A prime example of this is the antidysrhythmic drug lidocaine. Lidocaine is so completely transformed via the hepatic first-pass effect that the drug is essentially useless when administered orally.[12] However, modifying the chemical structure of lidocaine produced the chemical analog tocainide, which is clinically effective as an oral antidysrhythmic.[13] In the area of drugs used for anxiety reduction, there is a subtle (but not clinically significant) hepatic first-pass effect noted with the opioid analgesics.

The presence of food in the stomach decreases absorption of drugs into the cardiovascular system by increasing gastric emptying time, and if the drug is bound to food, it will not be available for absorption.[14] As mentioned previously, it is recommended that oral drugs be ingested with a full glass of water without food (unless a drug specifically requires that it be administered along with food as a means of minimizing gastric upset).

Bioavailability

Two tablets of the same dosage of the same drug from different manufacturers are said to be *chemically* equivalent. If the ensuing blood levels of the drugs are equivalent, they are said to be *biologically* equivalent. They are *therapeutically* equivalent if they are equally effective therapeutically. Drugs that are chemically equivalent are not necessarily biologically or therapeutically equivalent. These differences are termed *bioavailability*. Differences in bioavailability of drugs are most often seen with oral preparations. The difference in absorption of chemically equivalent drugs is related to differences in the size of particles or shape of crystals and to the rates of disintegration and dissolution of the drugs.

The slow onset of clinical activity of oral drugs prevents their titration. Ability to titrate a drug permits individualization of drug dosages for all patients. Undersedation or oversedation should not occur where titration is possible. The ability to titrate a drug to clinical effect is probably the greatest safety factors in drug administration. Unfortunately, the 30-minute latent period and 60-minute delay for the drug to reach peak blood level (for most oral drugs) preclude their titration. Care must be exacted to prevent underadministration or overadministration of orally administered CNS-depressant drugs.

Another disadvantage of orally administered drugs is the inability to either lighten or deepen the level of sedation rapidly. Should the effect of the drug prove inadequate, a second dose, though not recommended, may be given; however, the same time factors (30 and 60 minutes) will be required to achieve full benefit of the drug, making this option unattractive in the clinical setting. If, on the other hand, the effect of the initial dose proves too intense, there is no effective means of reversing it. This *lack of control* over the actions of the drug seriously impairs the usefulness of orally administered drugs in a typical outpatient dental environment.

The duration of clinical action of most oral drugs is approximately 3 to 4 hours. For the typical 1-hour dental appointment, this duration of action is entirely too long. Unfortunately, however, there is no means of reversing the clinical action of the orally administered drug. The patient will remain under the influence of the drug well into the postoperative period and be unable to leave the dental office unescorted. Patients receiving oral CNS depressants for stress reduction must always be cautioned against driving or operating potentially hazardous machinery. If patients receive oral sedative drugs at home before their dental appointment, they must be similarly cautioned.

RATIONALE FOR USE

When the advantages and disadvantages of the oral route are compared, it becomes obvious that a number of significant disadvantages are associated with this technique. These combine to produce a route of drug administration in which the administrator has little control over the ultimate clinical action of the drug.

This lack of control over drug action is a potential problem every time a drug is administered orally. This is particularly so when the drug is a CNS depressant, as are those used in the management of odontophobic patients. The potential for oversedation, respiratory depression, and loss of consciousness must always be considered when administration of an oral drug for anxiety relief is contemplated.

Despite the negative factors associated with oral sedation, there is considerable need in dentistry for orally administered drugs for stress reduction. The primary use of the oral route is in the management of anxiety before the dental procedure. However, because of the lack of control over the ultimate drug action, it is strongly suggested that only minimal-to-moderate sedation be sought via the oral route. Minimal sedation may prove adequate to reduce anxieties that develop before the dental appointment, but may prove inadequate in diminishing the fears occurring once the patient enters the dental office and commences treatment. It is possible to produce moderate-to-deep sedation with the oral route. However, the clinician must always keep in mind the lack of control over drug action and the wide range of individual responses to a given drug dose. The possibility of overdose, respiratory depression, impaired consciousness, or unconsciousness is increased as the degree of CNS depression increases. Persons untrained in the management of the unconscious airway ought not attempt to achieve deep sedation by the oral route. In addition, the dentist prescribing or administering oral drugs must possess a thorough knowledge of the drug's actions, contraindications, side effects, and precautions. The dentist must also be capable of prompt recognition and management of any adverse reaction that might develop (e.g., unconsciousness). This is the concept of "rescue" from a level of sedation beyond what is intended. If deep sedation is required, a more controllable technique of sedation (i.e., inhalation or IV) should be considered.

What then represents the rational use of the oral route in a typical dental practice? From the standpoint of safety, it is important that the clinician never seek to achieve a level of sedation beyond which he or she is comfortable (has been trained to use) and is capable of recognizing and managing any undesirable side effects that might develop. For these reasons, the rational use of oral sedation includes only minimal sedation or, in selected situations, moderate sedation. Deep sedation should be restricted to more controllable techniques.

The most common use of oral sedation is for the relief of anxiety in the hours immediately preceding a dental appointment. An antianxiety or sedative-hypnotic drug is used to reduce anxiety so that the patient will appear in the dental office for the scheduled appointment. More controllable techniques may be used at this time for intraoperative sedation, if necessary. When using oral drugs for this purpose, the clinician must remember to remind the patient of the absolute prohibition against driving a motor vehicle or operating hazardous machinery. If the patient has taken the drug at home, he or she should be advised against driving a car and should be accompanied to the office by (driven by) a responsible adult. For medicolegal purposes, this should also be noted in the patient's chart.

A second use for oral sedation is one that is often overlooked by a busy clinician. As noted earlier (see Chapter 4), not only do patients with fears of dentistry or surgery become apprehensive immediately before their appointment, often their anxieties start to build the *day before* the scheduled appointment. These persons might be unable to sleep the night before the appointment as they anticipate their upcoming "ordeal" and will be fatigued when they appear in the dental office the next day, a factor leading to a lowering of the pain reaction threshold. An antianxiety or hypnotic drug taken 1 hour before bedtime (1 hr hs) the night before the appointment can help ensure a restful night's sleep and a more stress-tolerant patient during treatment.

Other uses of the oral route in dentistry include the administration of drugs to inhibit salivary secretions (antisialagogues), drugs to prevent or to manage nausea (antiemetics), and antibiotics.

DRUGS

A large number of drugs may be administered orally in the management of anxiety. The overwhelming majority of these are classified as either antianxiety or sedative-hypnotic drugs. Other drug groups that may be used for this purpose are histamine blockers and opioids.

Before we discuss these drugs, a word is in order regarding the appropriate dosages to be used. The clinician must use as much information as is available to make an informed decision regarding the appropriate dose to administer, particularly when using the oral route. Information available to the clinician includes the patient's medical history, age, weight, and previous drug reactions. In addition, the clinician must determine the degree of anxiety present and the level of sedation sought. After consideration of these factors, a drug dose is determined.

A source of information regarding recommended dosages of drugs is the drug package insert or publications such as *Facts and Comparisons,*[15] *Physicians' Desk Reference,*[16] or *Mosby's Dental Drug Reference.*[17] Online sources of drug information, such as *ePocrates.com*[18] or *Mosby's ClinicalKey,*[19] are readily available for downloading onto a desktop computer, smart phone, or tablet device. An advantage of online drug data resources is that they are updated on a regular basis.

A common problem associated with the use of recommended doses is that they often lead to inadequate anxiety reduction in the dental or surgical setting. There is a reasonable explanation for this: the package insert recommends a certain dose of a drug to induce sedation or sleep in a nonstress situation,

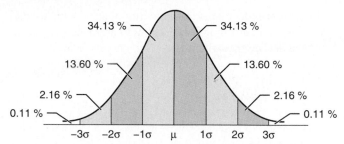

Figure 7.1 Normal distribution curve ("bell-shaped" curve). Persons will respond to drug dosages in dissimilar ways. Approximately 2.5% of persons will be extremely resistant to a "usual dose," and 2.5% will be quite sensitive to the same dose. (Data from Bennett CR: Jorgensen Memorial Lecture: drug interactions. *Anesth Prog* 30(4):106–112, 1983.)

such as the home environment. The dose of a drug that would effectively relax an apprehensive individual at home will possibly prove ineffective when the stresses of the dental office environment are added. For this reason, the doses recommended for oral sedation in this chapter and in many textbooks of pediatric dentistry may be somewhat higher than those in the drug package inserts.[20,21]

Many antianxiety and sedative-hypnotic drugs for oral administration are produced in three dosage forms. When a dosage is chosen for stress reduction in dental practice, these three dosage forms correlate with the normal distribution ("bell-shaped") curve (Fig. 7.1). The middle dosage form represents the "average" dose, producing clinically effective results (in nonstress situations) in approximately 70% (68.26%) of persons receiving it. The larger dosage form is for persons in whom the average dose proves to be ineffective or who have a greater degree of anxiety. The smaller dosage form is for persons in whom the average dose provides too intense a clinical effect, for persons with a lesser degree of anxiety, for elderly patients, or for debilitated patients. It must be remembered that the added stresses associated with dental or surgical treatment will increase the percentage of patients requiring larger-than-"usual" doses for management of their treatment-related fears.

Although titration (individualization of drug dosages) is not possible with orally administered drugs—a significant impediment to their safe use—it is possible in situations in which oral drugs are to be used over multiple appointments to *titrate by appointment*. This concept was introduced to me by Dr. Ronald Johnson, then chairman of the Department of Pediatric Dentistry at the University of Southern California.[22] Quite simply, titration by appointment means that the dentist will assess the efficacy of sedation achieved at the first appointment with a given drug dosage and, if necessary, increase or decrease the dosage of drug(s) administered at subsequent appointments. Therefore over a period of two to three visits, the appropriate dosage for that patient can be achieved (titrated). Titration by appointment is discussed more fully in the chapter on pediatric sedation (see Chapter 35).

In the remainder of this chapter, drugs that are administered orally for minimal-to-moderate sedation are reviewed. Drugs are discussed by their therapeutic category as follows:

1. Antianxiety drugs
2. Sedative-hypnotics
   a. Benzodiazepines
   b. Nonbenzodiazepines
3. Histamine blockers
4. Opioid analgesics

ANTIANXIETY DRUGS

Antianxiety drugs are used to manage mild-to-moderate daytime anxiety and tension. Drugs in this group share a similar CNS-depressant action: at therapeutic dosages they produce the level defined as minimal sedation, usually without impairing the patient's mental alertness or psychomotor performance. Groups of drugs that are commonly categorized as antianxiety drugs are as follows:

1. Benzodiazepines
   a. Diazepam
   b. Oxazepam
   c. Clorazepate
   d. Prazepam
   e. Halazepam
   f. Alprazolam
   g. Midazolam

For the management of mild-to-moderate levels of anxiety, the benzodiazepine antianxiety drugs are preferred. Benzodiazepine antianxiety drugs have a wide therapeutic dosage range and thus are less likely to produce undesirable side effects.

Although termed *antianxiety drugs*, a more appropriate name for these drugs might be *sedative-antianxiety drugs* because all drugs in this group possess sedative properties as well as antianxiety actions.

The antianxiety drugs have, in the past, been known by other names, such as *minor tranquilizers, anxiolytics, ataractics, anxiolytic sedatives,* and *psychosedatives.* The general category "antianxiety drugs" has become accepted for this group of drugs.

Benzodiazepine Antianxiety Agents

The benzodiazepines are the most effective drugs currently available for the management of anxiety. They also possess skeletal muscle–relaxant properties and are anticonvulsants. More than 2000 benzodiazepines have been synthesized since 1933. Chlordiazepoxide was the first benzodiazepine, introduced in 1960. In 2015, 53 benzodiazepines (Table 7.1) were available worldwide in oral formulations. Fifteen of the commonly used benzodiazepines are categorized as sedative-hypnotics, 15 as anxiolytics, 7 are indicated for use as antiepileptic drugs, and 1 as a skeletal muscle relaxant. (Some drugs are indicated for more than one group.)

The benzodiazepines represent *the* most popular class of drugs available today for the management of dental fear and

Table 7.1	Available Oral Benzodiazepines (August 2015)

Sedative-Hypnotic Benzodiazepines

- Brotizolam (Lendormin, Dormex, Sintonal, Noctilan)
- Cinolazepam (Gerodorm)
- Estazolam (ProSom, Nuctalon)
- Flunitrazepam (Rohypnol; Hipnosedon, Vulbegal, Fluscand, Flunipam, Ronal, Rohydorm)
- Flurazepam (Dalmane, Dalmadorm)
- Loprazolam (Dormonoct)
- Lormetazepam (Loramet, Noctamid, Pronoctan)
- Midazolam (Dormicum, Hypnovel, Dormonid)
- Nimetazepam (Ermin)
- Nitrazepam (Mogadon, Alodorm, Parisyn, Dumolid, Nitrazadon)
- Oxazepam (Seresta, Serax, Serenid, Serepax, Sobril, Oxabenz, Oxapax, Opamox)
- Quazepam (Doral)
- Temazepam (Restoril, Normison, Euhypnos, Temaza, Tenox)
- Triazolam (Halcion, Rilamir)

Anxiolytic Benzodiazepines

- Alprazolam (Xanax, Helex, Xanor, Onax, Alprox, Restyl, Solanex, Tafil)
- Bromazepam (Lexotan, Lexotanil, Lectopam, Bromam, Lexaurin)
- Chlordiazepoxide (Librium, Risolid, Elenium)
- Clonazepam (Rivotril, Klonopin)
- Cloxazolam (Rivatril, Rivotril, Klonopin, Iktorivil, Paxam)
- Clorazepate (Tranxene, Tranxilium)
- Diazepam (Antenex, Apaurin, Apzepam, Apozepam, Hexalid, Pax, Steslid, Vival, Valaxona)
- Halazepam (Paxipam)
- Ketazolam (Anxon)
- Lorazepam (Ativan, Temesta, Tavor, Lorenin, Lorsilan, Lorabenz)
- Medazepam (Nobrium, Ansilan, Mezapam, Rudotel, Raporan)
- Nordazepam (Madar, Stilny)
- Oxazepam (Serax, Serepax, Seresta, Serenid, Sobril, Oxabenz, Oxapax, Opamox)
- Pinazepam (Domar)
- Prazepam (Centrax, Lysanxia)

Anticonvulsants

- Clobazam
- Clonazepam
- Clorazepate
- Cloxazolam
- Diazepam
- Lorazepam
- Midazolam

Skeletal Muscle Relaxants

- Clonazepam
- Clonazolam
- Diazepam
- Etizolam (Etilaam, Etizest, Pasaden, Depas)
- Lorazepam
- Temazepam (Restoril, Normison, Euhypnos, Temaze, Tenox)
- Tetrazepam (Mylostan)

anxiety via the oral route of drug administration. Diazepam was, and in some cases still remains, a frequently prescribed drug in the United States since its introduction in 1977. Orally administered midazolam has become a very popular dental sedative, primarily in pediatrics, whereas in North America, triazolam has undergone a period of enthusiastic acceptance by many general dentists treating phobic adult patients.

Pharmacology

Mode of Action

The benzodiazepines have depressant effects on subcortical levels of the CNS. The specific anxiolytic effect of benzodiazepines is a result of their actions on the limbic system and the thalamus, those areas of the brain involved with emotions and behavior. Benzodiazepines have been called *limbic system sedatives* because they impair neuronal discharge in the amygdala and amygdala–hippocampus nerve transmission. Benzodiazepines depress the limbic system at doses smaller than those depressing the reticular activating system (RAS) and the cerebral cortex. Barbiturates and many other sedative-hypnotics, on the other hand, do not exhibit this selective depression, producing instead a more generalized CNS depression.

Specific receptors for benzodiazepines have been isolated within the spinal cord and the brain. The location of these receptors parallels that of γ-aminobutyric acid (GABA), the major inhibitory neurotransmitter in the brain, and of glycine, the major inhibitory neurotransmitter in the spinal cord.[23] Benzodiazepines act by intensifying the physiologic inhibitory effects of GABA by interfering with GABA reuptake.[24–26]

One of the most significant features of the benzodiazepines as a group is the very wide margin of safety between therapeutic and toxic doses. Ataxia and sedation develop only at doses beyond those required for antianxiety effects.

Central Nervous System

The principal behavioral effects of the benzodiazepines are the following:

1. Reduction of hostile and aggressive behavior (frequently termed *taming*)
2. Attenuation of the behavioral consequences of frustration, fear, and punishment (termed *disinhibition,* this is the most consistently observed behavioral action of the benzodiazepine antianxiety drugs)

It is interesting that when aggression and hostility are held in check by fear and anxiety, the ingestion of a benzodiazepine or other anxiolytic drug may produce a "paradoxical" increase in aggression. Other CNS depressants, such as the barbiturates, produce these same effects, but only at doses that produce drowsiness and motor incoordination. The benzodiazepines commonly achieve this action without these side effects.[27]

Other CNS actions of the benzodiazepines include skeletal muscle–relaxant properties and anticonvulsant effects.[28,29] The site of action of the muscle-relaxant properties of benzodiazepines is as yet undetermined; however, it is thought that the effect is central rather than peripheral. Skeletal muscle relaxation appears to be caused by a combination of central depression of the brainstem reticular formation and depression of polysynaptic spinal reflexes.[28,30] Anticonvulsant actions of benzodiazepines are produced by a depression of epileptiform discharge in the cerebral cortex and an enhancement of electrical activity of Purkinje cells. For effective anticonvulsant activity, the benzodiazepines must be administered intravenously (although intramuscularly[31] and intranasally[32] administered midazolam have terminated seizures). Diazepam and clonazepam are currently approved for anticonvulsant therapy.

Respiratory System

All sedative-hypnotics and antianxiety drugs (including benzodiazepines) are potential respiratory depressants. At usual therapeutic oral dosages in healthy normal-responding patients (middle of the bell-shaped curve), the benzodiazepines administered alone do not produce clinically significant respiratory depression and do not potentiate the depressant effects of opiates. Cases of significant respiratory depression and respiratory arrest following oral benzodiazepine ingestion have been reported.[33,34]

Cardiovascular System

Following oral administration to a healthy patient (American Society of Anesthesiologists [ASA] 1), benzodiazepines produce virtually no changes in cardiovascular function. Indeed, the benzodiazepines are frequently used in the management of anxiety and depression associated with cardiac disease. They are preferred to other sedative-hypnotics in this situation primarily because they do not produce unwanted degrees of CNS depression or restlessness and because they do not produce cardiovascular depression at therapeutic levels.[35]

Liver

The benzodiazepines undergo biotransformation in the liver (see following section); however, they do not stimulate the induction of hepatic microsomal enzymes. Potentially hazardous drug interactions, such as those observed between the barbiturates and coumarin anticoagulants, are not observed with benzodiazepines. In addition, patients with hepatic dysfunction may receive the benzodiazepines without increased risk of side effects, regardless of the cause of the hepatic dysfunction.

Absorption, Metabolism, Excretion

Following oral administration, all benzodiazepines are absorbed relatively rapidly and reliably from the GI tract. The rate at which maximum plasma levels develop exhibits significant variation among the different benzodiazepines and among individuals. Approximate time for peak plasma levels following oral administration of several benzodiazepines is shown in Table 7.2.

Benzodiazepines undergo biotransformation in the liver. There is considerable variation in the half-lives of these drugs: Diazepam's elimination half-life is 34 to 47 hours, whereas

Table 7.2	Onset of Peak Plasma Levels Following Oral Administration of Benzodiazepines

DRUG	PEAK PLASMA LEVEL (HR)
Flurazepam	1–1.5
Midazolam	0.5–1
Triazolam	0.5–2
Medazepam	1–1.5
Alprazolam	1–2
Oxazepam	3–4
Nitrazepam	0.5–3
Diazepam	1–1.5
Lorazepam	2–4
Halazepam	1–3
Temazepam	0.5–3
Chlordiazepoxide	1.5–4
Prazepam	2–6

Table 7.3	Properties of Benzodiazepines		
	PEAK PLASMA LEVEL (HR)	HALF-LIFE (HR)	ACTIVE METABOLITES
Alprazolam	1–2	10–20	No
Chlordiazepoxide	4	5–30	Yes
Clorazepate	Variable	35–152	Yes
Clonazepam	1–4	19.5–50	Yes
Diazepam	1–1.5	34–70	Yes
Flunitrazepam	0.5–3	18–26	Yes
Flurazepam	1–1.5	2.3	Yes
Halazepam	1–3	30–100	Yes
Lorazepam	2–4	3.3–14.8	No
Medazepam	1–1.5	36–200	–
Midazolam	0.5–1	1.5–2.5	No
Nitrazepam	0.5–3	17–48	No
Oxazepam	3–4	4–11	No
Prazepam	2–6	36–200	Yes
Temazepam	0.5–3	4–10.5	No
Triazolam	0.5–2	2	No

triazolam's is 2.0 hours. In addition, many of the benzodiazepines have biotransformation products that are pharmacologically as active as the parent drug (Table 7.3).

Chlordiazepoxide has a plasma half-life of between 5 and 30 hours and has as intermediate metabolites two pharmacologically active chemicals, desmethylchlordiazepoxide and demoxepam. The half-life of diazepam ranges between 34 and 70 hours (frequently quoted as "1 hour per year of age"). Pharmacologically active metabolites of diazepam include desmethyldiazepam (half-life of 96 hours), temazepam, and oxazepam. Flurazepam, with a plasma half-life of 2.3 hours, has an active metabolite with a half-life of 47 to 100 hours. Medazepam has three active metabolites: diazepam, desmethyldiazepam, and desmethylmedazepam; prazepam (half-life 36 to 200 hours) has among its metabolites desmethyldiazepam and oxazepam. Desmethyldiazepam is a metabolite of clorazepate.

Nitrazepam, oxazepam, lorazepam, midazolam, triazolam, temazepam, and alprazolam are biotransformed into pharmacologically inactive metabolites. The combination of rapid absorption from the GI tract (1 to 4 hours), short elimination half-life (4 to 11 hours), and inactive metabolites makes oxazepam an attractive drug for the management of anxiety within the dental or surgical environment. Lorazepam, on the other hand, with a slow rate of absorption (2 hours) and a half-life of 12 hours (range 3.3 to 14.8 hours), is less appealing. Triazolam, with a rapid onset of action and short half-life (2 hours), is ideally suited as a hypnotic in dentistry.[36–38]

All benzodiazepines are excreted in the feces and urine. The percentage of urinary excretion varies from 80% for flurazepam and oxazepam to 22% for prazepam.

Dependence

Psychological and physiologic dependence may develop to benzodiazepines.[39] The incidence of physiologic dependence is considerably less than that of psychological dependence. Physiologic dependence is unlikely to develop unless the patient takes doses much greater than therapeutically necessary over long periods of time. Within the dental setting, there is little likelihood of this occurring.

Oral Benzodiazepines in Dentistry

The benzodiazepines represent the most nearly ideal drugs for the management of anxiety. In the dental and surgical setting, benzodiazepines remain the drugs of choice via the oral route for the management of mild-to-moderate pretreatment anxiety and apprehension in the adult patient. These drugs provide a level of minimal-to-moderate sedation in most patients. Many benzodiazepines are currently available, and many more will surely become available in the future. Because there are significant differences in the onset of action and the duration of action among these drugs, the choice of a specific drug should be made only after consideration of the needs of both the patient and the dentist.

Although there are indications for the use of other drugs in specific instances, the drugs most ideally suited for pretreatment anxiolysis via oral administration in the dental and surgical setting are oxazepam and diazepam. For patients requiring sedation (hypnosis) to sleep restfully the evening before their treatment, flurazepam and triazolam are preferred. Oral triazolam has become a very popular drug for the provision of minimal-to-moderate sedation in dentistry in North America.[40–42] Triazolam will be reviewed in depth in the section of sedative-hypnotic benzodiazepines.

Contraindications

Allergy, psychoses, and acute narrow-angle glaucoma represent contraindications to the administration of benzodiazepines.[43] Benzodiazepines may be administered to patients with open-angle glaucoma who are receiving appropriate therapy.

Warnings

Patients must be advised against driving a motor vehicle or operating hazardous machinery. Other CNS depressants, such as alcohol, opioids, and barbiturates, should be avoided while benzodiazepines are used.[43] There is some evidence that the use of benzodiazepines (particularly chlordiazepoxide and diazepam) during the first trimester of pregnancy increases the risk of congenital malformations (e.g., cleft palate).[44] Benzodiazepines cross the placental barrier and are excreted in breast milk.

Benzodiazepines in Children

Use of oral diazepam tablets in children younger than 6 months of age is not recommended. Oral diazepam has been used successfully in pediatric dentistry. Recommended pediatric doses range from 0.15 to 0.3 mg/kg.[45,46] Midazolam, a sedative-hypnotic, is recommended in an oral dose of 0.2 to 0.5 mg/kg.[47,48] Oral forms of chlordiazepoxide and oxazepam are not recommended for children younger than 6 years. Clorazepate is not recommended in patients younger than 18 years. This is a common statement in the drug package insert of many drugs and is a reflection of an inadequate volume of research data on these age groups. A more in-depth discussion of the use of oral benzodiazepines in pediatrics can be found in Chapter 35.

Drug Interactions

Patients should be advised against the concurrent use of benzodiazepines and other CNS depressants. This includes alcohol; other psychotropic drugs, such as phenothiazines, opioids, barbiturates, and monoamine oxidase (MAO) inhibitors; and other antidepressants.[49]

Precautions

Drug dosages should be decreased in elderly or debilitated patients. Initial dosages should be small, with subsequent increases if warranted, as judged by the patient's response (titration by appointment). In this way, the adverse effects of drowsiness and ataxia may be minimized.

Adverse Reactions

The most frequently reported adverse reactions following oral benzodiazepine administration for anxiolysis include transient drowsiness (especially in the elderly or debilitated), fatigue, and ataxia.

Paradoxic reactions, although rare, may occur and consist of excitement, hallucinations, insomnia, and rage.[27,50] Discontinuance of drug administration leads to termination of these effects.

Chlordiazepoxide

Chlordiazepoxide was synthesized by Leo Sternbach in 1955.[51,52] When tested in 1957, it was demonstrated to possess hypnotic and sedative properties in addition to skeletal muscle–relaxant and anticonvulsant actions. The chemical is inactivated when exposed to ultraviolet light; thus it is marketed as a capsule. Chlordiazepoxide may also be used parenterally; however, because of its lack of stability, it must be prepared immediately before injection. Other benzodiazepines, such as diazepam, midazolam, and lorazepam, are more stable and are preferred to chlordiazepoxide when parenteral administration is required.

On February 24, 1960, the Food and Drug Administration (FDA) approved the marketing of the first benzodiazepine, chlordiazepoxide, under the brand name Librium.[51]

When administered orally, chlordiazepoxide is absorbed well from the GI tract; however, peak plasma levels of the drug do not develop for up to 4 hours. Although adequate anxiety reduction may develop within 1 to 2 hours, the slow onset of anxiolysis makes chlordiazepoxide less attractive than other, newer benzodiazepines in the management of mild-to-moderate anxiety in the pretreatment period in surgery and dentistry.

Diazepam

Diazepam was synthesized in 1959[53]; it was found to be equitoxic to chlordiazepoxide, but to have greater antianxiety, skeletal muscle–relaxing, and anticonvulsant properties. Marketed in December 1963 as Valium, diazepam quickly became one of the most prescribed drugs in the United States. By 1966, diazepam was one of the 50 most prescribed drugs, and by the 1970s, it was the leader among prescription drugs, a position it retained until recently.[54] In the United States, diazepam is only available in generic formulations, the proprietary name Valium having been retired in 1994.[55]

Following oral administration, diazepam is rapidly absorbed from the GI tract, achieving peak plasma levels within 2 hours. The drug may be administered 1 hour before treatment because 90% of the maximal clinical effect develops within this time. Because of its prolonged plasma half-life (20 to 70 hours) and the presence of active metabolites, cumulation of effect may develop with prolonged oral administration of diazepam. However, in the typical dental or surgical situation in which not more than one or two doses are prescribed, this effect does not occur. Diazepam is highly effective in the preoperative management of apprehension and mild-to-moderate anxiety. Its rapid onset of action makes it an appropriate drug for use in dental or surgical situations.

Patients receiving diazepam at home must be cautioned against operating a motor vehicle. They must be driven to the medical or dental facility by a responsible adult companion who can later drive them back home. Failure to warn a patient about this potential hazard may lead to legal action should a problem develop before or after treatment. That such problems do occur is seen in a study by Murray, in which 68 automobile drivers taking oral diazepam were monitored for a 3-month period. During this time, 16 of them were involved in accidents, an incidence 10 times greater than that expected.[56] Impaired motor function produced by the benzodiazepine was presumed to be the basis for the increase.

Dosage

The adult dosage for tension and anxiety states is 2 to 10 mg two to four times daily. For elderly patients or those with debilitating disease (ASA 3 or 4), recommended dosages are 2 to 2.5 mg once or twice daily to start; the dosage can then be increased if needed. The suggested dose for premedication is 5 to 10 mg 1 hour before bedtime or treatment.

Diazepam is not recommended for children younger than 6 months of age. For older children, the recommendation is 1 to 2.5 mg three to four times daily, with the dose increased if needed. Recommended pediatric doses range from 0.15 to 0.3 mg/kg.[57]

Availability

Diazepam (generic): 2-, 5-, and 10-mg tablets and as 5 mg/mL solution. Diazepam is a controlled substance in Schedule IV.[57]

Diazepam	
Pregnancy category	D
Lactation	NS
Metabolism	Liver
Excretion	Urine
DEA schedule	IV

Oxazepam

Oxazepam, synthesized in 1961, was marketed in 1965 under the proprietary name Serax. It possesses a short elimination half-life (5.7 to 10.9 hours) and no active metabolites. Oxazepam is therefore quite attractive in situations in which short-term anxiety control is required, such as during surgery or dentistry. The incidence of drowsiness is low, usually developing in persons receiving doses of 60 mg or more daily. Other side effects are similar to those for other members of this drug group.

Oxazepam is rapidly and reliably absorbed after oral administration, with peak plasma levels developing within 1 to 4 hours. This, in combination with the lack of active metabolites and a short half-life, makes oxazepam a preferred benzodiazepine for use as an antianxiety drug in dentistry.

Dosage

The adult dosage for mild-to-moderate anxiety and tension is 10 to 15 mg three to four times daily.[58] For elderly patients, the initial dosage is 10 mg three times daily, increased if needed to 15 mg three to four times daily.

An absolute dosage has not been established for children younger than 12 years. Oxazepam should not be taken by patients who are younger than 6 years.

Availability

Oxazepam (generic): 10-, 15-, and 30-mg capsules. Oxazepam is a controlled substance in Schedule IV.[58]

Oxazepam	
Pregnancy category	D
Lactation	NS
Metabolism	Liver
Excretion	Urine
DEA schedule	IV

Clorazepate

Clorazepate (also spelled chlorazepate) was available in the form of two salts: monopotassium and dipotassium salts. The dipotassium salt was marketed in 1972 as Tranxene, and clorazepate monopotassium was marketed in 1972 as Azene (no longer marketed). The dipotassium salt reaches peak plasma levels following oral administration in approximately 1 to 2 hours. The plasma half-life is approximately 48 hours.

Clorazepate itself cannot be absorbed from the GI tract. The chemical is hydrolyzed in the stomach to its active form, desmethyldiazepam, which is then absorbed, producing the clinical actions of the drug. The rate and extent of absorption of clorazepate from the GI tract depend on gastric pH. Antacid therapy significantly decreases the absorption of clorazepate. Clorazepate is useful in dental and surgical situations; however, oxazepam is preferred because it possesses a shorter half-life.

Dosage

The usual adult dosage is 15 to 60 mg daily, divided into two to four doses, or in one dose (15 mg) 1 hour before bedtime.[59] The dose for preoperative anxiety control is 15 mg of the dipotassium salt 1 hour before treatment.[59]

For elderly or debilitated patients, the initial dose of dipotassium salt is 7.5 to 15 mg. Adequate information is not available to establish a dosage in patients younger than 18 years.[59]

Availability

Clorazepate dipotassium: 3.75-, 7.5-, and 15-mg tablets. Clorazepate is a controlled substance in Schedule IV.[59]

Clorazepate	
Pregnancy category	D
Lactation	NS
Metabolism	Liver
Excretion	Feces and urine
DEA schedule	IV

Alprazolam

Alprazolam is another benzodiazepine derivative marketed as an antianxiety drug. It reaches peak plasma levels within 1 to

2 hours (orally) and has a half-life of 12 to 15 hours, with no active metabolites.

Dosage

The adult dosage for anxiety reduction is 0.25 to 0.5 mg three times a day.[60] Dosage for elderly or debilitated patients is 0.25 mg two or three times daily. Modification in dosage may be appropriate as based on patient response.

Availability

Xanax (Upjohn): 0.25-, 0.5-, 1.0-, and 2.0-mg tablets. Alprazolam is a controlled substance in Schedule IV.[60]

Alprazolam	
Pregnancy category	D
Lactation	NS
Metabolism	Liver
Excretion	Urine
DEA schedule	IV

Several other oral benzodiazepines have been mentioned, but they are unavailable at this time in the United States. These drugs include the following:

- **Nitrazepam** (Mogadon), discussed under sedative-hypnotics
- **Medazepam** (Nobrium), an antianxiety drug not available in the United States
- **Flunitrazepam** (Rohypnol), a hypnotic not available in the United States
- **Clonazepam** (Klonopin, Roche), available in the United States; however, it is indicated primarily as an anticonvulsant drug

For the management of milder degrees of anxiety (requiring minimal sedation) arising in the dental and surgical environment, there is probably no more effective group of drugs than the benzodiazepines. Pharmacologically, they offer significantly greater safety than other sedative-hypnotics. Although respiratory and cardiovascular depression are possible following oral administration of benzodiazepines, these are unlikely to develop. The most frequently observed side effect is a degree of sedation beyond what is being sought (moderate sedation).

As safe and as frequently administered as the benzodiazepines may be, it must be remembered that the patient must always be cautioned against driving a car when these drugs have been administered. Motor coordination may be subtly depressed, a condition that could have serious consequences for both the patient and the dentist.

SEDATIVE-HYPNOTICS

Sedative-hypnotics are drugs that produce either sedation or hypnosis, depending on the dosage of the drug administered and the patient's response to it. Lower dosages of these drugs produce a calming effect (sedation), usually associated with a degree of drowsiness and motor incoordination (ataxia), whereas higher dosages produce hypnosis (a state resembling physiologic sleep).

In previous editions of this textbook, a significant portion of the discussion of pharmacology of oral CNS-depressant drugs involved the barbiturates.[61] It is the belief of the author that there exists little to no indication for their administration orally for sedation in dentistry. The reader interested in the barbiturates for oral sedation in dentistry is referred to the discussion in prior editions.[61]

Benzodiazepine Sedative-Hypnotics

1. Benzodiazepines
   a. Flurazepam
   b. Temazepam
   c. Triazolam
   d. Lorazepam
   e. Midazolam
2. Nonbenzodiazepine sedative-hypnotics
   a. Zolpidem
   b. Zaleplon
   c. Eszopiclone
3. Chloral derivatives
   a. Chloral hydrate

Benzodiazepines

The benzodiazepines include some drugs categorized as sedative-hypnotics and others categorized as anxiolytics (see previous discussion). All benzodiazepines have hypnotic effects to a degree; however, the incidence of side effects and the duration of action of some benzodiazepines preclude their use in this area. The pharmacology of this important therapeutic drug group was reviewed in depth in the previous section on oral antianxiety drugs.

One of the primary benefits gained from using benzodiazepines instead of drugs such as the barbiturates as sedative-hypnotics is a decreased occurrence of the hangover effect that so often accompanies the barbiturates. Additional benefits include a minimal effect on the hepatic microsomal enzyme system and that pharmacologically the benzodiazepines present less of a risk to the patient than do the barbiturates. Six benzodiazepines have received significant attention as sedative-hypnotics: flurazepam, temazepam, triazolam, lorazepam, midazolam, and nitrazepam (not available in the United States) (Table 7.4).

Flurazepam

Flurazepam, like most other benzodiazepines, has been demonstrated to produce its clinical action on the hypothalamus and the amygdala. Because of the lack of hepatic microsomal enzyme induction, the dose of flurazepam required to induce sleep does not increase with prolonged administration. Following oral administration, flurazepam is rapidly absorbed and distributed; peak plasma levels develop within 30 to 60

Table 7.4	**Availability of Benzodiazepines (Oral)**			
GENERIC	PROPRIETARY (USA)	CLASS	AVAILABILITY (MG)	DOSE* (MG)
Alprazolam	Xanax, Niravam,	AA	0.25, 0.5, 1, 2	0.25–0.5
Chlorazepate with dipotassium	Generic only	AA	3.75, 7.5, 15	15–30
Chlordiazepoxide	Generic only	AA	5, 10, 25	5–10
Clonazepam	Klonopin	AC	0.5, 1, 2	0.25–0.5
Diazepam	Valium	AA	2, 5, 10	2–10
Flunitrazepam	Rohypnol	SH	2	0.25–2
Flurazepam	Generic only	SH	15, 30	15–30
Lorazepam	Ativan	SH, AA	0.5, 1, 2	2–4
Midazolam	Generic only	SH	2 mg/mL syrup	2 mg/mL
Oxazepam	Generic only	AA	10, 15, 30	10–30
Temazepam	Restoril	SH	7.5, 15, 22.5, 30	7.5–30
Triazolam	Halcion	SH	0.125, 0.25	0.25–0.5

AA, Antianxiety; *AC*, anticonvulsant; *SH*, sedative-hypnotic.
*For nighttime sedation or preoperative anxiety control.

minutes. Because flurazepam is biotransformed in the liver, the drug should be used with caution in patients with hepatic dysfunction. The half-life of flurazepam is 47 to 100 hours.

The incidence of side effects occurring with flurazepam administration is approximately 7%. The most frequently reported side effects include dizziness, drowsiness, lightheadedness, staggering, and ataxia. The hangover effect so often seen with barbiturates is infrequent with flurazepam.

The clinically effective dose of flurazepam has been demonstrated to be 15 to 30 mg administered 1 hour before the start of dental treatment.[62]

Contraindications

The use of flurazepam is contraindicated in patients with hypersensitivity (allergy) to benzodiazepines and in pregnant women.[63]

Warnings

Patients should be cautioned against operating motor vehicles or hazardous machinery and combining other CNS-depressant drugs, such as alcohol, with flurazepam.[63]

Drug Interactions

Additive CNS-depressant actions may develop when flurazepam is administered to patients taking other CNS depressants, such as alcohol, barbiturates, or opioids.[63]

Dosage

The usual dose of flurazepam is 30 mg taken 1 hour before bedtime. In elderly or debilitated patients, a 15-mg dose is recommended.[63]

Availability

Flurazepam (generic): 15- and 30-mg capsules. Flurazepam is a controlled substance in Schedule IV.[63]

Flurazepam	
Pregnancy category	X
Lactation	Safety unknown
Metabolism	Liver
Excretion	Urine (<1% unchanged)
DEA schedule	IV

Temazepam

Temazepam is absorbed slowly after oral administration. Onset occurs within 20 to 30 minutes; however, peak plasma levels require 2 to 3 hours (whereas flurazepam reaches peak levels at 30 minutes to 1 hour). The mean plasma half-life is 10 hours, and there are no significant active metabolites. The primary clinical use of temazepam is for patients having difficulty remaining asleep once they fall asleep. Because of its slow onset of action, temazepam is not effective in patients having difficulty falling asleep.

Contraindications, warnings, and drug interactions are similar to those for flurazepam (discussed previously).

Dosage

The usual dose is 30 mg 1 hour before bedtime.[64] The 15-mg dosage form should be used initially in elderly and debilitated patients.

Availability

Restoril (Sandoz): 7.5-, 15-, 22.5- and 30-mg capsules. Temazepam is a controlled substance in Schedule IV.[64]

Temazepam	
Pregnancy category	X
Lactation	Probably safe
Metabolism	Liver
Excretion	Urine 80%–90%, <1% unchanged
DEA schedule	IV

Triazolam

Triazolam is another benzodiazepine derivative. It was approved for marketing as a hypnotic in 1982 and has become the most prescribed psychoactive drug in the United States.[65] Triazolam is valuable in dentistry because of its short half-life of 1.5 to 5.5 hours and because it has no active metabolites.[66] Peak plasma levels develop at 1.3 hours (following oral administration). Very little residual drowsiness (hangover) is noted with triazolam.

Triazolam has been used extensively in dentistry as an effective oral drug in the management of pretreatment anxiety.[36,37,40–42,67–70] A number of trials have evaluated its effectiveness in pediatric populations.[38,71–72] The use of oral triazolam in pediatric anxiety control is discussed more fully in Chapter 35.

Triazolam has become a commonly used drug in dentistry in the United States. It is used in an incremental dosing regimen in which a patient receives multiple doses of the drug in an effort to reach the appropriate level of CNS depression.[73–75] Recent reports suggest that incremental dosing of triazolam may be an effective technique for producing moderate sedation in the dental setting; however, little laboratory or clinical data are available to evaluate the efficacy and safety of this approach.[73–75]

Contraindications

Triazolam is contraindicated in pregnant patients.[76]

Warnings

Overdose of triazolam may develop at four times the recommended therapeutic dosage. Patients receiving triazolam must be cautioned against operating machinery or driving a motor vehicle and against the simultaneous ingestion of alcohol and other CNS-depressant drugs.[76]

Anterograde amnesia of varying intensity and paradoxical reactions have been reported following therapeutic doses of triazolam.[77,78] Cases of "traveler's amnesia" have been reported by persons taking triazolam to induce sleep while traveling, such as during an airplane flight.[79] In some of these cases, insufficient time was allowed for the sleep period before awakening and before beginning activity. Triazolam (Halcion) has received some extremely negative press.[80,81] After reports of several serious complications, including suicide, Great Britain banned the prescription of triazolam.[82] It is still unavailable in Great Britain today (as of January 2017).[83] Following discussion of the safety and potential hazards posed by triazolam, the U.S. FDA decided against issuing any prohibitions on the prescription of this drug in the United States.[84]

Drug Interactions

Additive CNS-depressant actions may develop when triazolam is administered to patients receiving other CNS depressants, such as alcohol, barbiturates, or opioids.[76]

Adverse Reactions

The most common adverse side effects noted after triazolam administration are drowsiness (14.0%), headache (9.7%), dizziness (7.8%), and nervousness (5.2%).[76]

Dosage

A hypnotic dose of 0.25 mg 1 hour before bedtime or 1 hour before dental treatment is adequate for most patients, and a dose of 0.125 mg may be sufficient for selected patients. A dose of 0.5 mg should be reserved for patients who do not respond adequately to a smaller dose because the risk of several adverse reactions increases with the size of the dose administered.[76]

In elderly or debilitated patients, the recommended dose is 0.125 to 0.25 mg. The initial dose in this group should be 0.125 mg.[76]

Availability

Halcion (Upjohn): 0.125- and 0.25-mg tablets. Triazolam is a controlled substance in Schedule IV.[76]

Triazolam	
Pregnancy category	X
Lactation	Safety unknown
Metabolism	Liver
Excretion	Urine—minimally unchanged
DEA schedule	IV

Lorazepam

Lorazepam is absorbed slowly after oral administration; peak plasma levels develop in 2 hours, and the mean half-life is 12 hours. The drug was marketed in 1977 under the trade name of Ativan. Lorazepam is also available for parenteral administration. Orally the drug is effective as an antianxiety and hypnotic drug.[85] It is one of the few benzodiazepines not possessing active metabolites. Hepatic dysfunction (hepatitis, cirrhosis) does not alter the manner in which lorazepam is handled by the liver.

Several studies have evaluated lorazepam's utility in dentistry.[86,87] Because of its long duration of clinical action, its administration orally is recommended only for longer dental procedures (in excess of 2 hours).

Contraindications

Lorazepam is contraindicated in patients with known sensitivity to benzodiazepines and with narrow-angle glaucoma.[88]

Warnings

Lorazepam is not recommended for patients with a primary depressive disorder or psychosis. Patients receiving lorazepam must be cautioned against operating machinery or driving a motor vehicle and against the simultaneous ingestion of alcohol and other CNS-depressant drugs.[88]

Drug Interactions

Additive CNS-depressant effects develop with the concurrent administration of other CNS-depressant drugs, such as opioids, barbiturates, and alcohol.[88]

Adverse Reactions

The most frequently observed side effects of lorazepam are sedation (15.9%), dizziness (6.9%), weakness (4.2%), and ataxia (3.4%).[88]

Because of the greater possibility of unwanted sedation with lorazepam than with other benzodiazepines, its use in the immediate preoperative period should be discouraged unless the dentist desires this effect and if arrangements have been made for the patient to be escorted from the office by a responsible adult companion. The use of lorazepam the evening before treatment to ensure a restful night's sleep appears more reasonable.

Dosage

The usual adult dosage of lorazepam is from 2 to 6 mg in two or three divided doses.[88] The largest dose should be taken 1 hour before bedtime. For anxiety the initial dose is from 2 to 3 mg per day in two to three doses. Elderly or debilitated patients should receive an initial dose of 1 to 2 mg per day in divided dosages.[88] The safety and efficacy of lorazepam in patients younger than 12 years have not been established (as is true for most drugs). For preoperative anxiety control or as an aid to sleep before dental or surgical treatment, a single dose of 2 to 4 mg may be given 1 hour before sleep or 1 hour before the appointment.[88]

Availability

Ativan (Wyeth): 0.5-, 1-, and 2-mg tablets. Ativan is a controlled substance in Schedule IV.[88]

Lorazepam	
Pregnancy category	D
Lactation	Possibly unsafe
Metabolism	Liver
Excretion	Urine
DEA schedule	IV

Midazolam

Midazolam is available in an oral dosage form for use as a sedative-hypnotic. It is prepared in the United States as a syrup in a concentration of 2 mg/mL.[89]

The absorption and onset of clinical action of midazolam are more rapid than those of benzodiazepines, with which it has been compared.[90,91] Peak action after oral administration occurs within 30 minutes.[92] Monti et al[93] concluded that a 15-mg oral dose of midazolam was appropriate for patients demonstrating difficulty in falling asleep and that a 30-mg dose was appropriate in patients having difficulties in staying asleep. The actions of midazolam are less apparent after 8 hours than those of other benzodiazepines.[90] Hildebrand et al[94] concluded that absorption of midazolam is better with oral than with intramuscular (IM) administration. The clinical pharmacology of midazolam is discussed in more detail in Chapters 9 (IN), 10 (IM), and 25 (IV). Midazolam has been employed orally as premedication before surgical procedures in medicine[95] and in dentistry for adults[96,97] and children.[97–101]

The usual adult oral dosage of midazolam when used to help induce sleep is 15 mg taken 1 hour before bedtime. Wahlmann, Dietrich, and Fischer[96] administered a dose of 7.5 mg preoperatively for anxiety control in adults before oral surgery with little success, whereas Luyk and Whitley,[97] using the same dose, demonstrated significant anxiolysis, amnesia, and patient preference. Using a 10-mg dose of the parenteral form of midazolam orally, Turner and Paech[95] found the drug to be equal to a 20-mg dose of oral temazepam in anxiolysis and sedation preceding day-case gynecologic surgery. In pediatrics, oral doses of midazolam have proven effective in dosages ranging from 0.2 mg/kg[99] to 0.4 mg/kg[102,103] to 0.5 mg/kg[97,104–106] to 0.75 mg/kg.[102]

Contraindications

Contraindications are similar to those of other benzodiazepines and include narrow-angle glaucoma, severe respiratory disease (chronic obstructive pulmonary disease [COPD]), heart failure (HF), and impaired renal or hepatic function.[89]

Dosage

For procedural sedation in pediatric patients older than 6 months of age, the recommended dosage of midazolam syrup is 0.25 to 0.5 mg/kg. The maximum dose should not exceed 20 mg.[89]

Availability

Midazolam is available as a 2.0 mg/mL syrup. In other countries, midazolam is available as 7.5-mg tablets.[89]

Midazolam is no longer marketed under the proprietary name Versed in the United States.

Midazolam	
Pregnancy category	D
Lactation	Safety unknown
Metabolism	Liver
Excretion	Urine (<1% unchanged)
DEA schedule	IV

> **COMMENT:** The benzodiazepines are the preferred drugs for the management of preoperative anxiety in the dental setting. This is also the case in situations in which nighttime sedation is desirable. The primary advantage of the benzodiazepines over other sedative-hypnotics is their comparative safety. The benzodiazepines have proven to be relatively innocuous when taken alone in intentional or accidental overdose.[107] In addition, the benzodiazepines do not produce clinically significant hepatic microsomal enzyme induction, nor do they interact as significantly with other drugs, such as the coumarin anticoagulants.
>
> The benzodiazepines most preferred for their hypnotic effects, either for sleep the evening before treatment or for preoperative sedation, are flurazepam (30 or 15 mg) and triazolam (0.25 or 0.125 mg). With the introduction of an oral preparation, midazolam has become an attractive drug for preoperative sedation in children.

Nonbenzodiazepine Anxiolytics-Hypnotics

Zolpidem and zaleplon are pyrazolopyrimidines.[108] Known as the 'Z' drugs (along with zopiclone), they are used primarily for the treatment of insomnia.[109–111]

Zolpidem

Zolpidem tartrate is a nonbenzodiazepine sedative-hypnotic of the pyrazolopyrimidine class used for the short-term management of insomnia. It was approved for use in the United States in 1993.

Actions

Although zolpidem is unrelated structurally to benzodiazepines, it interacts with a GABA–benzodiazepine receptor complex and shares some of the pharmacologic properties of benzodiazepines. It is a strong sedative with only mild anxiolytic, myorelaxant, and anticonvulsant properties. It has been shown to be effective in inducing and maintaining sleep in adults.[109–112]

Following oral administration, zolpidem is rapidly absorbed from the GI tract, having an onset of action of 45 minutes and a peak effect seen in 1.6 hours. It is metabolized in the liver, with an elimination half-life of 2.6 hours. Zolpidem is converted into inactive metabolites eliminated primarily through renal clearance.[113]

Precautions

Respiratory depression is not usually seen in healthy patients receiving hypnotic doses of zolpidem. If it is used in patients with compromised respiratory function, the likelihood of depressed respiratory drive is increased.[114]

Contraindications

Contraindications include a history of hypersensitivity to zolpidem. Zolpidem should be used cautiously in patients with acute intermittent porphyria or impaired renal or hepatic function, in addiction-prone patients, and during pregnancy and lactation.[114]

Adverse Effects

Adverse effects most commonly observed (>3%) include dizziness, drugged feelings, headache, allergy, back pain, drowsiness, lethargy, nausea, dyspepsia, diarrhea, myalgia, arthralgia, and dry mouth.[114]

Availability

Zolpidem tartrate (Ambien, Searle): 5- and 10-mg tablets.[114]

Dosage

Adult: 5 to 10 mg PO hs (by mouth at bedtime).[114]

Dosage

Pediatric: The safety and efficacy of zolpidem have not been established in children.[114]

Dosage

Geriatric: Elderly and debilitated patients may be especially sensitive to the effects of zolpidem. An initial dose of 5 mg orally is recommended in these patients.[114]

Zolpidem	
Pregnancy category	C
Lactation	Possibly unsafe
Metabolism	Liver
Excretion	Urine primarily
DEA schedule	IV

Zaleplon

Zaleplon is another nonbenzodiazepine sedative-hypnotic of the pyrazolopyrimidine class used for the short-term management of insomnia.[113,115–117]

Actions

Pharmacologically and pharmacokinetically, zaleplon is similar to zolpidem.[113,115] Both are hypnotic agents with short half-lives, and both have been demonstrated to interact with GABA receptors. Zaleplon appears to be absorbed and eliminated more rapidly than zolpidem.[113,115]

Precautions

No precautions are known, according to the manufacturer.[118]

Contraindications

Use with caution in patients who demonstrate hypersensitivity to this class of drugs, in patients with impaired hepatic function, in elderly patients, in pregnant patients, in those with pulmonary disease, and in those with a history of drug abuse.[118–120]

Adverse Effects

Dependency and abuse are potential problems associated with prolonged administration. More common adverse reactions include drowsiness, amnesia, paresthesias, abnormal vision, dizziness, headache, hangover effect, rebound insomnia, and confusion.[118]

Dosage

Adult: 5 to 10 mg orally 1 hour before sleep.[118]

Dosage

Pediatric: The safety and efficacy of zaleplon have not been established in children.[118]

Availability

Zaleplon (Sonata): 5- and 10-mg capsules.[118]

Zaleplon	
Pregnancy category	C
Lactation	Probably safe
Metabolism	Liver
Excretion	Urine 70% (<1% unchanged)
DEA schedule	IV

Eszopiclone

Eszopiclone is a nonbenzodiazepine sedative-hypnotic indicated for the chronic treatment of insomnia. Although chemically unrelated to other hypnotics, such as the benzodiazepines, eszopiclone does share some pharmacologic actions with these drugs. Eszopiclone has a rapid onset of action and should only be taken immediately before going to sleep.[117,121,122] Eszopiclone has two primary metabolites with little or no activity at recommended therapeutic doses, which reduces the possibility of residual next-day effects from prolonged or excessive sedation. CNS depression with impairment of cognitive and motor function, commonly seen with long-acting benzodiazepines in the treatment for insomnia, is not common with eszopiclone.

Actions

The sedative, anticonvulsant, anxiolytic, and myorelaxant drug properties of sedative-hypnotics are thought to be induced by subunit modulation of the GABAA receptor chloride channel macromolecular complex. Although eszopiclone is chemically unrelated to the benzodiazepines, animal studies have shown that, similar to benzodiazepines, it nonselectively binds to all three GABAA receptor subtypes. Therefore eszopiclone shares the sedative effects normally seen with the benzodiazepines. Flumazenil, a benzodiazepine antagonist, antagonizes the sedative actions of eszopiclone. Eszopiclone is administered orally and is rapidly absorbed from the GI tract. Peak plasma concentrations occur within 1 hour of a single oral dose.[113,115,121] The presence of food reduces the amount of drug absorbed and increases the time to achieve maximum concentration, resulting in delayed sleep onset. Eszopiclone is 52% to 59% protein bound. Hepatic oxidation and demethylation occur via CYP3A4 and 2E1 metabolism; two primary metabolites are produced, one of which has substantially lower potency than eszopiclone, and the other is essentially inactive.[113,115,121] The elimination half-life is approximately 6 hours in patients with normal hepatic function. Up to 75% of an oral dose of eszopiclone is excreted as metabolites in the urine, and less than 10% is excreted as unchanged drug.[121]

Precautions

Timing of eszopiclone administration is important. Eszopiclone should be given immediately before retiring.[117,121-122] Taking a sedative-hypnotic while the patient is still up and about may induce short-term memory impairment, hallucinations, impaired coordination, dizziness, and lightheadedness.[117,121-122]

Contraindications

This medication should be avoided in those with a hypersensitivity to eszopiclone or any ingredient in the product. Reactions including anaphylaxis or angioedema may occur with sedative-hypnotics and may become evident as early as the initial dose.[121]

Adverse Effects

Sedative-hypnotic medications have the potential to cause sleep-related behaviors, such as sleep driving, a state of driving after ingestion of a sedative-hypnotic while not fully awake and having no memory of the event.[117,119-120] Other sleep-related behaviors may include sleepwalking (somnambulism) or making phone calls or eating while asleep.[119,120] The exact incidences among various sedative products are unknown; however, patients should be informed of the risks before receiving any medication from this class, including eszopiclone.[119-121]

Dosage

Adult: 1 to 3 mg orally immediately before retiring. At the present time (January 2017), there is no literature supporting the use of eszopiclone in dentistry.[123]

Dosage

Pediatric: The safety and efficacy of eszopiclone have not been established in children.[121]

Availability

Eszopiclone (Lunesta): 1-, 2-, and 3-mg tablets.[121]

Eszopiclone	
Pregnancy category	C
Lactation	Safety unknown
Metabolism	Liver
Excretion	Urine 75% (<10% unchanged)
DEA schedule	IV

Chloral Derivatives
Chloral Hydrate

Several drugs classified as chloral derivatives may be used for hypnosis or sedation. Within the practice of dentistry, one drug, chloral hydrate, was a popular drug for the management of anxiety, particularly in pediatric dentistry. Since the introduction of benzodiazepines, chloral hydrate has fallen into disfavor.[124] Both the FDA and the European Medicines Agency (EMA) have withdrawn approval of chloral hydrate, as well as the proprietary names of Aquachloral, Chloralum, and Somnote. Generic alternatives may be available through compounding pharmacies.[125,126]

Chloral hydrate, first synthesized in 1832, was the first member of the hypnotic group of drugs. With the introduction of the barbiturates, interest in chloral hydrate waned; however, starting in the 1950s, there was a renewed interest in it. Chloral hydrate available for oral administration as a syrup.

Chloral hydrate is quite irritating to skin and mucous membranes. It also produces GI irritation in a high percentage of patients.[23] Gastric upset may be minimized by diluting the drug or by following the drug immediately with a full glass (8 oz) of water or milk. In pediatric dentistry particularly, the syrup was used frequently. Unfortunately, the elixir has an unpleasant taste, which may be masked by mixing the drug with a suitable liquid, such as ginger ale or fruit juice.

Chloral hydrate does not possess any analgesic properties; therefore the drug should not be administered to patients who are in pain because their response may become quite exaggerated. The effects of a therapeutic dose of chloral hydrate on blood pressure and respiration are negligible, similar to those occurring in normal sleep.[127] Chloral hydrate is rapidly absorbed through the GI tract into the cardiovascular system and undergoes metabolic degradation in the liver and kidneys into its active form, trichloroethanol.[127] Other chloral derivatives, chloral betaine and triclofos sodium, undergo metabolic degradation into chloral hydrate and then into trichloroethanol. Trichloroethanol is thought to be the active metabolite responsible for the CNS-depressant effects of these three drugs. The chloral derivatives may be administered safely to patients with hepatic and renal dysfunction. The half-life of chloral hydrate is 7 to 9.5 hours.[127]

Among the untoward effects produced by the irritating properties of chloral hydrate are an unpleasant taste, gastric upset, nausea, vomiting, and flatulence. Other CNS effects considered uncomfortable are lightheadedness, ataxia, and nightmares.[128] Hangover occurs much less commonly than with barbiturates. Chloral hydrate, although not metabolized by the hepatic microsomal enzyme system, does accelerate the metabolism of drugs such as the coumarin anticoagulants. The toxic oral dose reported for chloral hydrate is 10 g, although death has been reported with as little as 4000 mg (4 g).[127] More important in clinical situations is the dose of chloral hydrate based on patient body weight. A commonly used oral dose of chloral hydrate is 50 mg/kg (or about 22.5 mg/lb) of body weight, with a suggested range of 40 to 60 mg/kg.[23,129–131]

In a 1992 survey of pediatric residency programs, it was determined that chloral hydrate in doses between 25 and 100 mg/kg was the most common drug used for sedation.[132]

Reports of overdose following chloral hydrate administration in pediatric dentistry are rare, but have included cases of life-threatening hypotension and respiratory arrest following estimated doses of 86 and 118 mg/kg.[129,133] The GI upset produced by chloral hydrate proves to be advantageous when accidental overdose occurs. With doses larger than 60 mg/kg, vomiting is frequently noted, thus diminishing the absorption of chloral hydrate from the GI tract and limiting the degree of overdose observed.[23]

Following oral administration, the onset of action of chloral hydrate is rapid; drowsiness or arousable sleep usually develops within 30 to 45 minutes. Duration of action is 2 to 5 hours.[127]

Chloral hydrate is useful as a sedative before dental care and to assist the patient in achieving a restful night's sleep before a scheduled treatment. It is an especially useful drug in debilitated, elderly, and younger patients. Chloral hydrate appears to be less effective when given in smaller doses or when used for dental care in older patients with disabilities.[134–136] A 2012 Cochrane Database review of sedatives in pediatric dentistry found chloral hydrate to be of minimal effectiveness,[102] whereas its use in pediatric ophthalmic surgery has high success rates.[137]

Contraindications

Allergy to chloral hydrate or other chloral derivatives, severe hepatic or renal dysfunction, severe heart disease, and gastritis are contraindications. Chloral hydrate should not be prescribed to nursing women because the drug does appear in breast milk.[127]

Warnings

Prolonged use of chloral hydrate may be habit forming. This is unlikely to occur in dental situations because of the manner in which the drug is prescribed.

Drug Interactions

Chloral hydrate must be used with caution in patients who are concurrently receiving the coumarin anticoagulants. Prothrombin times should be monitored on a more frequent basis. Doses of chloral hydrate should be decreased in patients receiving other CNS-depressant drugs, such as alcohol, opioids, and barbiturates, because additive CNS depression will develop.[127]

Precautions

Chloral hydrate should be used with caution in patients with severe cardiovascular disease because large doses (significantly greater than therapeutic) may further depress the myocardium.[127,129] In therapeutic dosages, there is no contraindication to the administration of this drug in patients with cardiovascular disease.

Adverse Reactions

The most frequently reported adverse effect of chloral hydrate is gastric irritability. The only other adverse reaction reported on occasion is the occurrence of a skin rash.[127]

Dosage

The dosages presented here are for the adult patient. The use of chloral hydrate in pediatric dentistry is presented in Chapter 35.

The hypnotic dose of chloral hydrate is 500 to 1000 mg taken 15 to 30 minutes before bedtime. The usual dose for sedation in a nondental setting is 250 mg, however, when chloral hydrate is administered for surgery or dental procedures, doses of 500 to 1500 mg may be required.[127]

When the capsule form of chloral hydrate is prescribed, the drug should be taken with a full (8-oz) glass of water. If administered as an elixir or syrup, chloral hydrate should be mixed in one-half glass of water, ginger ale, or fruit juice.

Availability

Chloral hydrate is no longer available in generic or proprietary forms in the United States and United Kingdom, though it may be available through compounding pharmacies in the United States.

Chloral Hydrate and Dentistry

Since the introduction of benzodiazepines, specifically diazepam, midazolam, and triazolam, the need for chloral hydrate has diminished significantly. Given that chloral hydrate is no longer an approved drug in the United States, the United Kingdom, and the European Union, its administration in dentistry cannot be recommended.[125,126]

Chloral Hydrate – Discontinued in United States and United Kingdom (Generic Not Available; May be Available Through Compounding Pharmacies in the United States)	
Pregnancy category	C
Lactation	Probably safe
Metabolism	Liver, plasma, kidney
Excretion	Urine
DEA schedule	IV

HISTAMINE (H₁) BLOCKERS (ANTIHISTAMINES)

CNS depression (sedation and hypnosis) is a known side effect of some drugs used primarily for other purposes. Such effects occur with many of the histamine blockers, drugs used primarily in the management of allergies, motion sickness, and parkinsonism. Several histamine blockers demonstrate this property and are marketed primarily as sedative-hypnotics. These drugs include methapyrilene, pyrilamine, diphenhydramine, promethazine, and hydroxyzine.

Methapyrilene and pyrilamine are available as nonprescription sedative-hypnotics, usually in combination with scopolamine. Diphenhydramine in 25-mg capsules has been approved by the FDA as a nonprescription preparation.

The two histamine blockers most frequently used for their sedative-antianxiety properties are promethazine and hydroxyzine. In dentistry, these drugs have proven quite useful, primarily in pediatric dentistry.

Promethazine

Promethazine is a phenothiazine derivative commonly used as an antiemetic for management of nausea and vomiting, for preoperative sedation, for sedation and the relief of apprehension and anxiety, to produce a light sleep from which the patient is easily aroused, and in the management of various forms of allergic reaction.

Promethazine was marketed in 1951 under the brand name Phenergan. Its first reported use in dentistry was in 1959, when it was used in conjunction with meperidine and chlorpromazine in the lytic cocktail DPT (Demerol, Phenergan, Thorazine). Its primary function in this cocktail was to serve as an antiemetic to control nausea and vomiting commonly produced by opioids.

In dentistry, promethazine is frequently used in pediatric sedation. In a 1973 survey of drug use in pediatric dentistry, promethazine was the fourth most frequently employed solo premedicant and the most commonly used combination drug (with meperidine),[138] and a 1987 survey found the use of promethazine remaining high, ranking third as a solo premedicant and remaining first (with meperidine) as a combination drug.[139]

Promethazine is a *phenothiazine,* a group of drugs classified as *antipsychotics.* The primary use of these drugs (Table 7.5) is to decrease agitation, hostility, combativeness, and hyperactivity. They are also useful in the management of nausea and vomiting, and some members have potent antihistaminic actions. Promethazine differs structurally from the antipsychotic phenothiazines by the presence of a branched side chain and no ring substitution. It is believed that this structural difference

Table 7.5	Phenothiazines	
GENERIC	**PROPRIETARY**	**SEDATIVE ACTION**
Chlorpromazine	Thorazine	High
Promethazine	Phenergan	High
Thioridazine	Mellaril	High
Prochlorperazine	Compazine	Moderate
Promazine	Sparine	Moderate
Trifluoperazine	Stelazine	Moderate
Perphenazine	Trilafon	Low to moderate

is responsible for the lack of antipsychotic action. Promethazine is an H_1 receptor–blocking drug, providing antihistaminic, antiemetic, and sedative effects.

All phenothiazines produce some degree of sedation (CNS depression). The action of these drugs is quite different from that of the barbiturates, benzodiazepines, and other sedative-hypnotics. Two major differences are that (1) phenothiazines, in large doses, do not produce unconsciousness or depress respiration or the cardiovascular system, and (2) the phenothiazines are not addictive.[140,141]

On the negative side, all phenothiazines are capable of producing extrapyramidal reactions.[142,143] They usually develop early in phenothiazine therapy and most often prove quite benign; however, they may require treatment. The incidence of extrapyramidal reactions is greatest with perphenazine, prochlorperazine, and trifluoperazine and lowest with promethazine and thioridazine.[143]

Four types of extrapyramidal reaction may be observed.[143] *Akathisia* (motor restlessness) refers to the compelling need of the patient to be in constant motion. The patient feels the need to get up and walk or continuously move about. *Acute dystonias* include perioral spasms (protrusion of the tongue), mandibular tics, facial grimacing, hyperextension of the neck and trunk, and clonic convulsions. These reactions may be accompanied by hyperhidrosis, pallor, fever, and increased anxiety. *Parkinsonism,* which consists of tremors, rigidity, shuffling gait, postural abnormalities, masklike facies, and hypersalivation, may also occur. *Tardive dyskinesia* represents a late-appearing neurologic syndrome associated with antipsychotic drug use. It is more common in older patients and is characterized by choreiform movements of the face, trunk, and extremities.

Management of extrapyramidal reactions involves the discontinuance of the offending drug and the possible administration of an antiparkinsonism drug, such as diphenhydramine (Benadryl 50 mg IM or IV in adults) or trihexyphenidyl (Artane 5 to 15 mg daily orally).[144]

Many phenothiazines act on the cardiovascular system to produce postural (orthostatic) hypotension and a reflex tachycardia. This is most common with chlorpromazine. The phenothiazines undergo metabolic degradation in the liver and are excreted in the urine and feces.

Contraindications

Known allergy to phenothiazines is a contraindication to the use of promethazine and other phenothiazines.

Warnings

Patients receiving other CNS depressants should be aware of the additive effects of the phenothiazines. These drugs should either be eliminated or their dosages reduced.

Precautions

Patients must be advised against operating a motor vehicle or potentially hazardous machinery. Phenothiazines must be used with caution in patients with a history of convulsive disorders because they may lower the seizure threshold.

Children with acute disease, such as chickenpox, measles, and gastroenteritis, appear much more susceptible to extrapyramidal reactions, especially dystonias, than do adults.

Adverse Reactions

The most frequently reported adverse reactions to phenothiazines include dryness of the mouth, blurring of vision, and, less commonly, dizziness. Oversedation is the most frequently observed side effect of promethazine. In general, the phenothiazines have a high therapeutic index and are remarkably safe drugs. Extrapyramidal reactions are the most significant side effects of these drugs.[144,145]

Dosage

The adult dose for sedation is 25 to 50 mg 1 hour before treatment; for preoperative sedation, the dose is 50 mg 1 hour before bedtime.[145] In children, the dose for sedation is 12.5 to 25 mg 1 hour before treatment.[145]

For preoperative sedation in pediatric dentistry, the traditional dose recommendation for promethazine is 2.2 mg/kg when used alone and 1.1 mg/kg when used in combination with other CNS depressants.[145]

Availability

Promethazine (generic): 12.5-, 25-, and 50-mg tablets and 6.25 mg/5 mL (1.5% alcohol) syrup.[145]

Promethazine	
Pregnancy category	C
Lactation	Possibly unsafe
Metabolism	Liver
Excretion	Urine and feces
DEA schedule	Rx

Hydroxyzine

Hydroxyzine is derived from a group of drugs called *diphenylethanes.* Although classified as a histamine (H_1) blocker, hydroxyzine also possesses sedative, antiemetic, antispasmodic, and anticholinergic properties. Two forms of the drug are available: hydroxyzine hydrochloride (Atarax) and hydroxyzine pamoate (Vistaril). Hydroxyzine is the most popular oral sedative in the practice of pediatric dentistry, with 50% of the responding pedodontists using one or both drugs.[138–140]

The sedative actions of hydroxyzine are not produced by cortical depression. It is thought to suppress some hypothalamic nuclei and to extend its actions peripherally into the sympathetic portion of the autonomic nervous system.

Following oral administration, hydroxyzine is rapidly absorbed from the GI tract, with clinical actions observed within 15 to 30 minutes. Maximal clinical actions develop in

2 hours, with an approximate duration of action of 3 to 4 hours.[146]

The oral liquid form of hydroxyzine hydrochloride is more pleasant tasting to most patients than the liquid form of hydroxyzine pamoate. This fact is of particular importance in pediatric dentistry.[146]

When these drugs are administered in combination with opioids, their dosage should be decreased by 50% because the depressant actions of opioids (and barbiturates) are potentiated by hydroxyzine.

Indications for the use of hydroxyzine include providing total management of long-term anxiety and tension, managing anxiety and tension in which the causative stress is temporary (e.g., dental or other surgical procedures), providing preoperative sedation, allaying of apprehension and anxiety in the cardiac-risk patient, and managing nausea and vomiting. Hydroxyzine is metabolized in the liver and excreted in urine.[146]

In dental practice, the use of hydroxyzine as a sole drug is limited to the management of children with mild-to-moderate fear. It is often used in combination with either meperidine or chloral hydrate for management of more fearful pediatric patients.[147–149]

The incidence of side effects is quite low, with transient drowsiness observed most commonly. Emergence delirium has also been reported following hydroxyzine administration.[150] Fatal overdose with hydroxyzine is extremely uncommon, and withdrawal reactions after long-term therapy have never been reported.

Contraindications

Contraindications include previous hypersensitivity to hydroxyzine.

Drug Interactions

Hydroxyzine will potentiate the CNS-depressant actions of drugs such as barbiturates, opioids, alcohol, sedative-hypnotics, and antianxiety drugs. Dosages of these drugs should be decreased by 50% when they are administered concurrently with hydroxyzine.

Precautions

Patients receiving hydroxyzine must be warned against operating a motor vehicle or hazardous machinery. Children receiving hydroxyzine should be kept under observation by their parent or guardian for the remainder of the day.[146]

Dosage

The adult dosage ranges from 25 mg three times a day to 100 mg four times a day. The dosage for children younger than 6 years is 2 mg/kg daily orally in divided doses every 6 to 8 hours.[146] The dosage for children 6 to 12 years is 12.5 to 25 mg orally every 6 to 8 hours. The dose for preoperative drug in adults is 50 to 100 mg 1 hour preoperatively.[146]

In pediatric dentistry, the oral dose of hydroxyzine is 1.1 to 2.2 mg/kg when it is used as a sole drug for anxiety control.

When it is administered in conjunction with other CNS depressants, such as meperidine or chloral hydrate, the dose of hydroxyzine should be reduced by 50%.[146]

Availability

Hydroxyzine hydrochloride (Atarax) has been discontinued in the United States. Hydroxyzine pamoate (Vistaril, Pfizer): 25- and 50-mg capsules.[146]

Hydroxyzine	
Pregnancy category	C
Lactation	Probably safe
Metabolism	Liver
Excretion	Urine
DEA schedule	Rx

OPIOIDS (NARCOTICS)

Opioids are classified as strong analgesics. Their primary indication is for the relief of moderate-to-severe pain. Beneficially, opioids alter a patient's psychological response to pain and suppress anxiety and apprehension. Many opioids are used parenterally as preanesthetic drugs because of their sedative, antianxiety, and analgesic properties. On the other hand, many anesthesiologists prefer to administer sedative-hypnotics or antianxiety drugs preoperatively unless pain is present. In the absence of pain, opioids administered alone frequently produce dysphoria instead of sedation. To achieve antianxiety and sedative effects, opioids ought not be administered via the oral route. Absorption following oral administration is not as consistent as with parenteral administration, and the incidence of unwanted side effects (postural hypotension, nausea, and vomiting) is considerably greater. The resulting sedative effect varies significantly from patient to patient. Respiratory and cardiovascular depression may be noted and, if present, can result in airway obstruction, hypoventilation, and hypotension. Oral opioid administration should be reserved for the management of *pain* when milder analgesics have proved ineffectual.

THE ORAL SEDATION APPOINTMENT—ADULT PATIENT

At a previous visit, the patient has been evaluated for suitableness for oral sedation. Their medical history has been reviewed and baseline vital signs recorded. Preoperative instructions are reviewed and a copy given to the patient.

On the day of the appointment, the patient is scheduled to appear at the dental office 1 hour before the scheduled start of dental treatment.

The oral sedative drug is administered to the patient with 8 oz of water in the dental office by the dentist or staff member.

The patient is kept in an area that is monitored constantly. Ideally, this would be the room in which dental treatment is done, but the reception room could also be appropriate, providing the patient remains under constant supervision.

At 45 minutes, the dentist should evaluate the efficacy of the oral sedative drug and, if an appropriate response has occurred, bring the patient back to the treatment room. The patient *must* be assisted when walking to the treatment room and never left to walk alone. If the patient is not yet adequately sedated, permit them an additional 15 or 20 minutes before reevaluating them and bring them to the treatment room.

When a sedated patient is standing or walking, a member of the dental office staff *must* be with them at all times.

The appropriate monitors are applied as per state or provincial regulation. Commonly, these include pulse oximetry (or, increasingly, capnography) and a blood pressure cuff. Preoperative vital signs are monitored and recorded on the anesthesia-sedation record.

Oxygen may be administered via nasal mask or nasal cannula if desired by the dentist.

The patient should be placed in a supine position in the dental chair or as close to supine as they will allow.

In the event that the level of sedation provided by the orally administered drug is less than desired, the dentist may carefully *titrate* the flow of nitrous oxide-oxygen (N_2O-O_2) to the desired level of moderate sedation. The dentist must check with his or her state or provincial dental regulatory agency to determine whether the addition of N_2O-O_2 to a patient receiving oral sedation is permissible.

Vital signs are monitored continuously and recorded every 5 minutes (or as mandated by the appropriate state/provincial regulatory agency) on the anesthesia-sedation record.

Local anesthesia is administered to the patient exactly as it would be administered had the patient not received sedation. Sedation is *not* a substitute for local anesthesia.

If N_2O-O_2 has been administered, the flow of N_2O is terminated at the conclusion of the traumatic part of the dental procedure and the patient is permitted to breathe 100% oxygen for a minimum of 5 minutes.

At the conclusion of the dental treatment, postoperative vital signs are recorded onto the anesthesia-sedation record.

The patient is positioned comfortably in the dental chair, and recovery is assessed.

If deemed capable of being discharged in the company of a responsible adult, the escort is brought into the treatment room where the postoperative instructions are read to, and then a copy is given to, both the patient and the escort.

When the sedated patient stands, a member of the dental office staff must be with them at all times until they are placed into the passenger or back seat of the car and the seat belt fastened.

Later that afternoon or early that evening the dentist should make the postoperative telephone call to the patient. Determine how he or she is doing and review with him or her the postoperative instructions. Because some patients may experience retrograde amnesia with some of the oral CNS depressants (e.g., triazolam, midazolam), reviewing these instructions may be the first time that they are actually hearing them.

SUMMARY

The oral route of drug administration may be used successfully to provide minimal-to-moderate levels of sedation appropriate for the relief of mild-to-moderate degrees of apprehension and anxiety. Because of inherent difficulties attendant in achieving precise levels of sedation (the inability to titrate), it is recommended that only minimal-to-moderate levels of sedation be sought by the oral route.

A large number of drugs are presently available for the relief of anxiety via oral administration. This chapter describes only commonly used drugs in dentistry and surgery and those that appear most applicable in the outpatient environment. In general, these drugs belong to a small number of drug groups: the benzodiazepines, the nonbenzodiazepine sedative-hypnotics, and the histamine blockers.

Although all drugs may be employed by the knowledgeable, well-trained dentist, the more prudent will restrict prescribing habits to a limited number of drugs with which he or she is familiar. From the practical point of view, the benzodiazepines are the drugs of choice for preoperative management of anxiety in dentistry and surgery. Although many benzodiazepines are available, midazolam, oxazepam, and diazepam are the most frequently employed and are highly recommended for management of milder levels of anxiety in dentistry. Triazolam and flurazepam, classified as sedative-hypnotics, are useful for moderate anxiety and are administered the evening before treatment and frequently on the day of treatment.

Two newer drugs, zolpidem and zaleplon, appear efficacious in the management of pretreatment anxiety. At present, their use in dentistry is minimal. Other drug groups should be considered for use where the benzodiazepines are contraindicated or have proved ineffective and when other more controllable techniques of pharmacosedation are unavailable.

Ease of drug prescription is a minor factor in selection of a suitable drug for premedication, but one that must be considered. Among the drugs discussed in this chapter, the benzodiazepines and chloral hydrate are placed in Schedule IV on the controlled substances schedule.

REFERENCES

1. Berger R, Green G, Melnick A: Cardiac arrest caused by oral diazepam intoxication. *Clin Pediatr* 14:842–844, 1975.
2. Gill CJ, Michaelides PL: Dental drugs and anaphylactic reactions: report of a case. *Oral Surg* 50:30–32, 1980.
3. Johnson AG, Seideman P, Day RO: Adverse drug interactions with nonsteroidal anti-inflammatory drugs (NSAIDs): recognition, management and avoidance. *Drug Saf* 8:99–127, 1993.

4. Centini F, Fiore C, Riezzo I, et al: Suicide due to oral ingestion of lidocaine: a case report and review of the literature. *Forensic Sci Int* 171(1):57–62, 2007.

5. Papadopoulos J, O'Neil MG: Utilization of a glucagon infusion in the management of a massive nifedipine overdose. *J Emerg Med* 18(4):453–455, 2000.

6. National Council on Patient Information and Education (NCPIE). Available at <http://www.talkaboutrx.org/index.jsp>. (Accessed 10 August 2015).

7. Ghembaza MA, Senoussaoui Y, Tani MK, Meguenni K: Impact of patient knowledge of hypertension complications on adherence to antihypertensive therapy. *Curr Hypertens Rev* 10(1):41–48, 2011.

8. Gosnell E, Tor S, Thikkurissy S, Smiley M: Pediatrics: an update of sedation monitoring guidelines. In Boynes SG, editor: *Dental anesthesiology: a guide to the rules and regulations of the United States of America*, ed 4, Chicago, 2011, No-No Orchard Publishing, pp 44–52.

9. LaPointe L, Guelmann M, Primosch R: State regulations governing oral sedation in dental practice. *Pediatr Dent* 34(7):489–492, 2012.

10. Magni G, Cadamuro M, Borgherini G, et al: Psychological stress and gastric emptying time in normal subjects. *Psychol Rep* 68:739–746, 1991.

11. Sugito K, Ogata H, Goto H, et al: Gastric emptying rate of drug preparations. III. Effects of size of enteric micro-capsules with mean diameters ranging from 0.1 to 1.1 mm in man. *Chem Pharm Bull* 40:3343–3345, 1992.

12. Wedlund PJ, Wilkinson GR: Hepatic tissue binding and the oral first-pass effect. *J Pharm Sci* 73:422–425, 1984.

13. Lucas WJ, Maccioli GA, Mueller RA: Advances in oral anti-arrhythmic therapy: implications for the anaesthetist. *Can J Anaesth* 37:94–101, 1990.

14. Zimmermann T, Leitold M: The influence of food intake on gastrointestinal pH and gastric emptying time: experience with two radiotelemetering methods (Heidelberg pH capsule system and Flexilog 1010). *Int J Clin Pharmacol Ther Toxicol* 30:477–478, 1992.

15. *Drug facts and comparisons (pocket edition) 2014*, ed 68, Philadelphia, 2014, Lippincott Williams & Wilkins.

16. Physicians' desk reference, 2015, ed 69. Available at <www.PDR.net>.

17. Jeske A: *Mosby's dental drug reference*, ed 11, St Louis, 2013, Mosby.

18. Epocrates.com: Available at <www.ePocrates.com>.

19. ClinicalKey: Available at <www.ClinicalKey.com>.

20. Wilson S: Minimal and moderate sedation agents. In Wright GZ, Kupietzky A, editors: *Behavior management in dentistry for children*, ed 2, Ames, 2014, John Wiley & Sons.

21. Wilson S, Ganzberg S: Pain reaction control: sedation. In Casamassimo PS, Fields HW, Jr, McTigue D, Nowak A, editors: *Pediatric dentistry: infancy through adolescence*, ed 5, Philadelphia, 2013, Elsevier Saunders.

22. Johnson R: Personal communications, 1992.

23. Moore P, Haupt M: Sedative drugs in pediatric dentistry. In Dionne RA, Phero JC, Becker DE, editors: *Management of pain and anxiety in dental practice*, Philadelphia, 2002, WB Saunders.

24. Aitkenhead AR, Moppett IK, Thompson JP: Sedative and hypnotic drugs. In Aitkenhead AR, Moppett IK, Thompson JP, editors: *Smith and Aitkenhead's textbook of anaesthesia*, ed 6, London, 2013, Elsevier Limited, pp 110–115.

25. Proekt A, Hemmings HC: Mechanisms of drug action. In Hemmings HC, Egan TD, editors: *Pharmacology and physiology for anesthesia*, Philadelphia, 2013, Saunders/Elsevier, pp 3–19.

26. Bonisch H: The pharmacology of benzodiazepines. *Pharm Unserer Zeit* 36(3):186–194, 2007.

27. Greenblatt DJ, Miller LG, Shader RI: Benzodiazepine discontinuation syndromes. *J Psychiatr Res* 24(Suppl):73–79, 1990.

28. Oreland L: The benzodiazepines: a pharmacological overview. *Acta Anaesthesiol Scand* 88(Suppl):13–16, 1988.

29. Asmussen S, Maybauer DM, Maybauer MO: Intramuscular versus intravenous benzodiazepines for status epilepticus. *N Engl J Med* 366(20):1943–1944, 2012.

30. Simiand J, Keane PE, Biziere K, et al: Comparative study in mice of tetrazepam and other centrally active skeletal muscle relaxants. *Arch Int Pharmacodyn Ther* 297:272–285, 1989.

31. Rogalski R, Rogalski A: Benzodiazepine selection in the management of status epilepticus: a review. *Adv Emerg Nurs J* 37(2):83–94, 2015.

32. Mula M: The safety and tolerability of intranasal midazolam in epilepsy. *Expert Rev Neurother* 14(7):735–740, 2014.

33. Classen DC, Pestotnik SL, Evans RS, et al: Intensive surveillance of midazolam use in hospitalized patients and the occurrence of cardiorespiratory arrest. *Pharmacotherapy* 12:213–216, 1992.

34. Daneshmend TK, Bell GD, Logan RF: Sedation for upper gastrointestinal endoscopy: results of a nationwide survey. *Gut* 32:12–15, 1991.

35. Greenblatt DJ, Shader RI: *Benzodiazepines in clinical practice*, New York, 1974, Raven Press.

36. Gordon SM, Shimizu N, Shlash D, Dionne RA: Evidence of safety for individualized dosing of enteral sedation. *Gen Dent* 55(5):410–415, 2007.

37. Lieblich SE, Horswell B: Attenuation of anxiety in ambulatory oral surgery patients with oral triazolam. *J Oral Maxillofac Surg* 49:792–796, 1991.

38. Raadal M, Coldwell SE, Kaakko T, et al: A randomized clinical trial of triazolam in 3- to 5-year-olds. *J Dent Res* 78(6):1197–1203, 1999.

39. Edwards JG, Cantopher T, Olivieri S: Benzodiazepine dependence and the problems of withdrawal. *Postgrad Med* 66(Suppl 2):S27–S35, 1990.

40. Goodchild JH, Feck AS, Silverman MD: Anxiolysis in general dental practice. *Dent Today* 22(3):106–111, 2003.

41. Feck AS, Goodchild JH: Rehabilitation of a fearful dental patient with oral sedation: utilizing the incremental oral administration technique. *Gen Dent* 53(1):22–26, 2005.

42. Flanagan D, Goodchild JH: Comparison of triazolam and zaleplon for sedation of dental patients. *Dent Today* 24(9):64–66, 2005.

43. Richa S, Yazbek JC: Ocular adverse effects of common psychotropic agents: a review. *CNS Drugs* 24(6):501–526, 2010.

44. Laegreid L, Olegard R, Conradi N, et al: Congenital malformations and maternal consumption of benzodiazepines. *Dev Med Child Neurol* 32:432–441, 1990.

45. Badalaty MM, Houpt MI, Koenigsberg SR, et al: A comparison of chloral hydrate and diazepam sedation in young children. *Pediatr Dent* 12:33–37, 1990.

46. Palma-Aguirre JA, Rodriguez-Palomares C: Indications and contraindications for analgesics and antibiotics in pediatric dentistry. *Practica Odontol* 10:11–12, 14, 16, 1989.

47. Azevedo ID, Ferreira MA, da Costa AP, et al: Efficacy and safety of midazolam for sedation in pediatric dentistry: a controlled clinical trial. *J Dent Child (Chic)* 80(3):133–138, 2013.

48. Damle SG, Gandhi M, Laheri V: Comparison of oral ketamine and oral midazolam as sedative agents in pediatric dentistry. *J Indian Soc Pedod Prev Dent* 26(3):97–101, 2008.

49. Hines LE, Murphy JE: Potentially harmful drug-drug interactions in the elderly: a review. *Am J Geriatr Pharmacother* 9(6):364–377, 2011.

50. Rothschild AJ: Disinhibition, amnestic reactions, and other adverse reactions secondary to triazolam: a review of the literature. *J Clin Psychiatry* 53(Suppl):69–79, 1992.

51. Sternbach LH: The discovery of Librium. *Agents Actions* 2(4):193–196, 1972.

52. Sternbach LH: The benzodiazepine story. *Prog Drug Res* 22:229–266, 1978.

53. Sternbach LH, Sancilio FD, Blount JF: Quinazolines and 1,4-benzodiazepines. 64. Comparison of the stereochemistry of diazepam with that of close analogs with marginal biological activity. *J Med Chem* 17(3):374–377, 1974.

54. <http://www.medscape.com/viewarticle/834578>. (Accessed 24 August 2015).

55. <http://www.pharmacyreviewer.com/forum/overcoming-anxiety-and-all-about-anti-anxiety-drugs-and-sedatives/43801-roche-discontinue-making-valium.html>. (Accessed 24 August 2015).

56. Murray JB: Effects of Valium and Librium on human psychomotor and cognitive functions. *Genet Psychol Monogr* 109:167, 1984.

57. Diazepam drug monograph, ClinicalKey. Available at <www.ClinicalKey.com>. (Accessed 2 April 2015).

58. Oxazepam drug monograph, ClinicalKey. Available at <www.ClinicalKey.com>. (Accessed 8 January 2015).

59. Clorazepate drug monograph, ClinicalKey. Available at <www.ClinicalKey.com>. (Accessed 16 July 2015).

60. Alprazolam drug monograph, ClinicalKey. Available at <www.ClinicalKey.com>. (Accessed 16 April 2014).

61. Malamed SF: *Sedation: a guide to patient management*, ed 4, St Louis, 2003, CV Mosby, pp 95–98.

62. Loeffler PM: Oral benzodiazepines and conscious sedation: a review. *J Oral Maxillofac Surg* 50:989, 1992.

63. Flurazepam drug monograph, ClinicalKey. Available at <www.ClinicalKey.com>. (Accessed 17 October 2013).

64. Temazepam drug monograph, ClinicalKey. Available at <www.ClinicalKey.com>. (Accessed 16 April 2014).

65. Greenblatt DJ: Pharmacology of benzodiazepine hypnotics. *J Clin Psychiatry* 53(Suppl):7–13, 1992.

66. Garzone PD, Kroboth PD: Pharmacokinetics of the newer benzodiazepines. *Clin Pharmacokinet* 16:337–364, 1989.

67. Berthold CW, Schneider A, Dionne RA: Using triazolam to reduce dental anxiety. *J Am Dent Assoc* 124(11):58–64, 1993.

68. Flanagan D: Oral triazolam sedation in implant dentistry. *J Oral Implantol* 30(2):93–97, 2004.

69. Berthold C: Enteral sedation: safety, efficacy, and controversy. *Compend Contin Educ Dent* 28(5):264–271, 2007.

70. Gordon SM, Shimizu N, Shlash D, Dionne RA: Evidence of safety for individualized dosing of enteral sedation. *Gen Dent* 55(5):410–415, 2007.

71. Meyer ML, Mourino AP, Farrington FH: Comparison of triazolam to a chloral hydrate/hydroxyzine combination in the sedation of pediatric dental patients. *Pediatr Dent* 12:283–287, 1990.

72. Raadal M, Coldwell SE, Kaakko T, et al: A randomized clinical trial of triazolam in 3- to 5-year-olds. *J Dent Res* 78(6):1197–1203, 1999.

73. Donaldson M, Goodchild JH: Maximum cumulative doses of sedation medications for in-office use. *Gen Dent* 55(2):143–148, 2007.

74. Dionne RA, Yagiela JA, Cote CJ, et al: Balancing efficacy and safety in the use of oral sedation in dental outpatients. *J Am Dent Assoc* 137(4):502–513, 2006.

75. Goodchild JH, Donaldson M: Calculating and justifying total anxiolytic doses of medications for in-office use. *Gen Dent* 54(1):54–57, 2006.

76. Triazolam drug monograph, ClinicalKey. Available at <www.ClinicalKey.com>. (Accessed 11 February 2015).

77. Greenfield DP: What about Halcion? *N J Med* 88:889, 1991. (editorial).

78. Goodchild JH, Donaldson M: Hallucinations and delirium in the dental office following triazolam administration. *Anesth Prog* 52(1):17–20, 2005.

79. Bixler EO, Kales A, Manfredi RL, et al: Next-day memory impairment with triazolam. *Lancet* 337:827–831, 1991.

80. Medawar C, Rassaby E: Triazolam overdose, alcohol, and manslaughter. *Lancet* 338:1515–1516, 1991.

81. Schneider PJ, Perry PJ: Triazolam: an "abused drug" by the lay press? *Drug Intell Clin Pharm* 24:389–392, 1990.

82. Myrhed M: Background and current status. Halcion (triazolam) banned in England-Sweden investigates. *Lakartidningen* 88(4035):4038, 1991.

83. Personal communication, Dr. Nigel Robb. August 15, 2015.

84. Wysowski DK, Barash D: Adverse behavioral reactions attributed to triazolam in the Food and Drug Administration's spontaneous reporting system. *Arch Intern Med* 151:2003–2008, 1991.

85. Moroz G: High-potency benzodiazepines: recent clinical results. *J Clin Psychiatry* 65(Suppl 5):13–18, 2004.

86. Rubin J, Schweggmann I, Uys P: Lorazepam as a premedicant in dental surgery. *SAMJ* 58(3):124–126, 1980.

87. Merin RL: Adult oral sedation in California: what can a dentist do without a special permit or certificate from the Dental Board of California? *J Calif Dent Assoc* 34(12):959–968, 2006.

88. Lorazepam drug monograph, ClinicalKey. Available at <www.ClinicalKey.com>. (Accessed 16 April 2014).

89. Midazolam drug monograph, ClinicalKey. Available at <www.ClinicalKey.com>. (Accessed 25 March 2015).

90. Castleden CM, Allen JG, Altman J, et al: A comparison of oral midazolam, nitrazepam, and placebo in young and elderly subjects. *Eur J Clin Pharmacol* 32:253–257, 1987.

91. Jochemsen R, van Rijn PA, Hazelzet TG, et al: Comparative pharmacokinetics of midazolam and loprazolam in healthy subjects after oral administration. *Biopharm Drug Dispos* 7:53–61, 1986.

92. Langlois S, Kneeft JH, Chouinard G, et al: Midazolam: kinetics and effects on memory, sensorium, and haemodynamics. *Br J Clin Pharmacol* 23:273–278, 1987.

93. Monti JM, Alterwain P, Debellis J, et al: Short-term sleep laboratory evaluation of midazolam in chronic insomniacs: preliminary results. *Arzneimittelforschung* 37:54–57, 1987.

94. Hildebrand PJ, Elwood RJ, McClean E, et al: Intramuscular and oral midazolam: some factors influencing uptake. *Anaesthesia* 38:1220–1221, 1983.

95. Turner GA, Paech M: A comparison of oral midazolam solution with temazepam as a day case premedicant. *Anaesth Intensive Care* 19:365–368, 1991.

96. Wahlmann UW, Dietrich U, Fischer W: The question of oral sedation using midazolam in outpatient dental surgery. *Deut Zahnarzt Z* 47:66–68, 1992.

97. Luyk NH, Whitley BD: Efficacy of oral midazolam prior to intravenous sedation for the removal of third molars. *Int J Oral Maxillofac Surg* 20:264–267, 1991.

98. Parnis SJ, Foate JA, vander Walt JH, et al: Oral midazolam is an effective premedicant for children having day-care anaesthesia. *Anaesth Intensive Care* 20:9–14, 1992.

99. Payne KA, Coetzee AR, Mattheyse FJ: Midazolam and amnesia in pediatric premedication. *Acta Anaesthesiol Belg* 42:101–105, 1991.

100. Hennes HM, Wagner V, Bonadio WA, et al: The effect of oral midazolam on anxiety of preschool children during laceration repair. *Ann Emerg Med* 19:1006–1009, 1990.

101. Alcaino EA: Conscious sedation in paediatric dentistry: current philosophies and techniques. *Ann R Australas Coll Dent Surg* 15:206–210, 2000.

102. Lourenco-Matharu L, Ashley PF, Furness S: Sedation of children undergoing dental treatment. *Cochrane Database Syst Rev* (3):CD003877, 2012.

103. Tolksdorf W, Eick C: Rectal, oral and nasal premedication using midazolam in children aged 1-6 years: a comparative clinical study. *Anaesthetist* 40:661–667, 1991.

104. Molter G, Altmayer P, Castor G, et al: Oral premedication with midazolam in children. *Anaesthesiol Reanim* 16:75–83, 1991.

105. Feld LH, Negus JB, White PF: Oral midazolam preanesthetic drug in pediatric outpatients. *Anesthesiology* 73:831–834, 1990.

106. Weldon BC, Watcha MF, White PF: Oral midazolam in children: effect of time and adjunctive therapy. *Anesth Analg* 75:51–55, 1992.

107. Miller NS, Gold MS: Benzodiazepines: a major problem: introduction. *J Subst Abuse Treat* 8:3–7, 1991.

108. George CF: Pyrazolopyrimidines. *Lancet* 358(9293):1623–1626, 2001.

109. Langtry HD, Benfield P: Zolpidem. A review of its pharmacodynamic and pharmacokinetic properties and therapeutic potential. *Drugs* 40(2):291–313, 1990.

110. Huedo-Medina TB, Kirsch I, Middlemass J, et al: Effectiveness of non-benzodiazepine hypnotics in treatment of adult insomnia: meta-analysis of data submitted to the Food and Drug Administration. *BMJ* 345:e8343, 2012.

111. Richey SM, Krystal AD: Pharmacological advances in the treatment of insomnia. *Curr Pharm Des* 17(15):1471–1475, 2011.

112. Salva P, Costa J: Clinical pharmacokinetics and pharmacodynamics of zolpidem: therapeutic implications. *Clin Pharmacokinet* 29:142–153, 1995.

113. Drover DR: Comparative pharmacokinetics and pharmacodynamics of short-acting hypnosedatives: zaleplon, zolpidem and zopiclone. *Clin Pharmacokinet* 43(4):227–238, 2004.

114. Zolpidem drug monograph, ClinicalKey. Available at <www.ClinicalKey.com>. (Accessed 8 October 2014).

115. Drover D, Lemmens H, Naidu S, et al: Pharmacokinetics, pharmacodynamics, and relative pharmacokinetic/pharmacodynamic profiles of zaleplon and zolpidem. *Clin Ther* 22:1443–1461, 2000.

116. Zaleplon. *Am J Health Syst Pharm* 57:430, 2000.

117. Stranks EK, Crowe SF: The acute cognitive effects of zopiclone, zolpidem, zaleplon, and eszopiclone: a systematic review and meta-analysis. *J Clin Exp Neuropsychol* 36(7):691–700, 2014.

118. Zaleplon drug monograph, ClinicalKey. Available at <www.ClinicalKey.com>. (Accessed 2 May 2013).

119. Gunja N: In the Zzz zone: the effects of Z-drugs on human performance and driving. *J Med Toxicol* 9(2):163–171, 2013.

120. Kapil V, Green JL, Le Lait C, et al: Misuse of benzodiazepines and Z-drugs in the UK. *Br J Psychiatry* 205(5):407–408, 2014.

121. Eszopiclone drug monograph, ClinicalKey. Available at <www.ClinicalKey.com>. (Accessed 17 February 2015).

122. Owen RT: Eszopiclone: an update on its use in insomnia. *Drugs Today (Barc)* 47(4):263–275, 2011.

123. McKenzie WS, Rosenberg M: What every dentist should know about the "z-sedatives.". *J Mass Dent Soc* 56(3):44–45, 2007.

124. Braham RL, Bogetz MS, Kimura M: Pharmacologic patient management in pediatric dentistry: an update. *J Dent Child* 60(4-5):270–280, 1993.

125. <http://www.ashp.org/menu/DrugShortages/DrugsNoLongerAvailable/bulletin.aspx?id=902>. (Accessed 24 August 2015).

126. Meadows M: The FDA takes action against unapproved drugs. *FDA Consum* January-February 2007.

127. Chloral hydrate drug monograph, ClinicalKey. Available at <www.ClinicalKey.com>. (Accessed 15 July 2015).

128. Greenberg SB, Faerber EN, Aspinall CL, et al: High-dose chloral hydrate sedation for children undergoing MR imaging: safety and efficacy in relation to age. *Am J Roentgenol* 161:639–641, 1993.

129. Nordenberg A, Dalisle G, Izukawa T: Cardiac arrhythmias in a child due to chloral hydrate ingestion. *Pediatrics* 47:134–135, 1971.

130. Judish GF, Andreasen S, Bell EB: Chloral hydrate sedation as a substitute for examination under anesthesia in pediatric ophthalmology. *Am J Ophthalmol* 89:560–563, 1982.

131. Thompson JR, Schneider S, Ashwal S, et al: The choice of sedation for computed tomography in children: a prospective evaluation. *Neuroradiology* 143:475–479, 1982.

132. Cook BA, Bass JW, Nomizu S, et al: Sedation of children for technical procedures: current standard of practice. *Clin Pediatr* 31:137–142, 1992.

133. Troutman KC: Misuse of chloral hydrate in sedating a pediatric patient, ADSA Mortality and Morbidity Conference, ADSA Annual Meeting, Boston, 1984.

134. Moore PA: Therapeutic assessment of chloral hydrate premedication for pediatric dentistry. *Anesth Prog* 31:191–196, 1984.

135. Smith RC: Chloral hydrate sedation for handicapped children: a double-blind study. *Anesth Prog* 24:159–162, 1977.

136. Barr ES, Wynn RL, Spedding RH: Oral premedication for the problem child: placebo and chloral hydrate. *J Pedod* 1(4):272–280, 1977.

137. Wilson ME, Karaoui M, Al Djasim L, et al: The safety and efficacy of chloral hydrate sedation for pediatric ophthalmic procedures: a retrospective review. *J Pediatr Ophthalmol Strabismus* 51(3):154–159, 2014.

138. Wright GZ, McAulay DJ: Current premedicating trends in pedodontics. *J Dent Child* 40:185–187, 1973.

139. Wright GZ, Chiasson RC: The use of sedation drugs by Canadian pediatric dentists. *Pediatr Dent* 9:308–311, 1987.

140. Jones KF: Preoperative drugs in operative dentistry for children. *J Dent Child* 36:93, 1969.

141. Pautola A, Elomaa M: The use of promethazine and diazepam in dental treatment of apprehensive children. *Suom Hammaslaak Toim* 67:226–234, 1971.

142. Skorin L, Jr, Onofrey BE, DeWitt JD: Phenothiazine-induced oculogyric crisis. *J Am Optom Assoc* 58:316–318, 1987.

143. Jellinger KA: Neuropathology of movement disorders. In Winn HR, editor: *Youman's neurological surgery*, ed 6, Philadelphia, 2011, Saunders, Elsevier, pp 871–898.

144. Lopez-Rois F, Couce Pico M, Calvo Fernandez J, et al: Drug-induced extrapyramidal syndrome: apropos of 22 cases. *Anales Esp Pediatr* 26:91–93, 1987.

145. Promethazine drug monograph, ClinicalKey. Available at <www.ClinicalKey.com>. (Accessed 30 July 2015).

146. Hydroxyzine drug monograph, ClinicalKey. Available at <www.ClinicalKey.com>. (Accessed 24 August 2015).

147. Faytrouny M, Okte Z, Kucukyavuz Z: Comparison of two different dosages of hydroxyzine for sedation in the paediatric dental patient. *Int J Paediatr Dent* 17(5):378–382, 2007.

148. Torres-Perez J, Tapia-Garcia I, Rosales-Berber MA, et al: Comparison of three conscious sedation regimens for pediatric dental patients. *J Clin Pediatr Dent* 31(3):183–186, 2007.

149. Soares F, Britto LR, Vertucci FJ, et al: Interdisciplinary approach to endodontic therapy for uncooperative children in a dental school environment. *J Dent Educ* 70(12):1362–1365, 2006.

150. Dahmani S, Delivet H, Hilly J: Emergence delirium in children: an update. *Curr Opin Anaesthesiol* 27(3):309–315, 2014.

chapter 8

Rectal Sedation

Interest in the rectal route of drug administration has increased in anesthesiology and, to a lesser extent, in dentistry in recent years.[1–3] Historically the rectal route of drug administration was used for the administration of smoke ("fumigation") for resuscitation[4] and the administration of anesthetics. An ether boiler for rectal application was developed in 1847 by Pirogoff.[1,5] With the advent of more reliable routes of drug administration (e.g., intravenous [IV] and inhalation), use of the rectal route decreased.

Certain situations remain in which rectal drug administration may be valuable. These include the administration of a drug to a patient who is unwilling or unable to take drugs orally. In most instances, this is a child or an adult with a disability requiring sedation either to permit treatment to proceed[6–8] or as a preliminary to the induction of general anesthesia.[9–11] Another situation in which rectal drugs are warranted is the administration of antiemetics to patients with nausea and vomiting.[12] Although parenteral administration is preferred (if the patient is present in the office where the drug may be injected), rectal administration can be used if the patient objects to injection or if the patient is at home. Another indication for rectal administration of drugs is analgesics for postoperative control of pain.[13]

ADVANTAGES

Advantages of the rectal route include a relatively rapid onset of clinical activity; a decreased incidence and intensity of drug-related side effects; the lack of a needle, syringe, or other potentially threatening equipment; the avoidance of an injection; ease of administration (many children who vehemently object to the oral route will not object to this route); and its low cost.

In the past, it was thought that rectally administered drugs were absorbed directly into the systemic circulation via the vena cava, bypassing the enterohepatic circulation and thereby eliminating the hepatic first-pass effect that influences the clinical activity of most drugs administered enterally.[14] The superior rectal vein empties into the inferior mesenteric vein and then into the portal system. The middle and inferior rectal veins empty into the internal iliac vein and the inferior vena cava.[15,16] However, it has been demonstrated that hepatic clearance is *the* main factor affecting bioavailability of rectally administered drugs.[1] This may be because blood flow occurs through anastomoses that interconnect the superior, middle, and inferior rectal venous systems, thereby producing a hepatic first-pass effect with rectally administered drugs. Other potential factors, such as adsorption by feces, intraluminal degradation by microorganisms, metabolism within the mucosal cell, and lymphatic drainage, do not significantly affect the fate of rectally administered drugs.

Comparing the oral, nasal, and rectal administration of the water-soluble benzodiazepine midazolam, Tolksdorf[9] found that children aged 1 to 6 years accepted the oral drug better than rectal or nasal, but that the rectally administered midazolam had the most rapid onset of action and fewest side effects in the postoperative period. In several studies, peak levels of clinical action were noted rapidly after rectal administration. Roelofse et al[6] noted good anxiolysis, sedation, and cooperation

30 minutes after rectal administration of midazolam, whereas Kraus et al[17] noted peak plasma levels of midazolam at 7.5 minutes.

DISADVANTAGES

Disadvantages of the rectal route include inconvenience to the administrator and the patient, variable absorption of some drugs from the large intestine, possible irritation of the intestines by some drugs, inability to reverse the action of the drug easily, prolonged recovery with some drugs, and an inability to titrate precise individual doses.

The primary use of rectal drug administration in both medicine and dentistry is management of uncooperative patients, whether children or adults. It is strongly advised that rectally administered central nervous system (CNS) depressants be administered in the medical or dental office by the dentist or a staff person (or parent, if the patient is a child). Signs and symptoms of sedation develop rapidly with many rectal drugs; clinical sedation is evident at 15 to 30 minutes.[6,17] Because the possibility of oversedation exists, it would be beneficial for the patient to be in an environment where oversedation could be easily recognized and the patient managed ("rescued"). An automobile en route to the dentist's office is not a desirable location.

Because of the lack of control over the clinical actions of the drug, rectal administration ought not to be used in an effort to achieve deep sedation unless the dentist has been well trained in general anesthesia and is able to manage the airway of an unconscious patient. The recommended use of rectal sedation is for the induction of minimal-to-moderate sedation when other, more controllable methods of anxiety control (IV, inhalation) may be added, if needed, during treatment. Rectally administered drugs may provide a level of patient management adequate for many procedures, such as root planing and curettage[7] and restoration or extraction of primary teeth,[8] but it may prove inadequate for procedures such as radiographs, which require a patient to remain immobile during exposure,[18] though more recent studies do demonstrate considerable success with rectal sedation for radiologic examination.[19,20]

The administration of rectal drugs is often considered difficult for the administrator and uncomfortable for the patient. Of 80 children receiving rectal premedication, deWaal, Huisman, and Veerman reported that 66 (82.5%) accepted rectal instillation well, 12 (15%) moderately well, and 2 (2.5%) poorly.[21]

The patient receiving rectal drugs for sedation should receive supplemental oxygen and be monitored via pulse oximetry and pretracheal stethoscope. Personnel and equipment for resuscitation must always be available.

DRUGS

Many drugs have been administered rectally. Ideally a rectally administered drug will be available as a suppository, although in several cases (e.g., midazolam), drug formulations designed for parenteral administration have been successfully employed. Historically the two major drug groups that have been employed rectally are the barbiturates and opioids. More recently, the rectal administration of the benzodiazepine midazolam has received considerable attention. Because barbiturates are no longer recommended for clinical use in sedation, the discussion to follow will focus on nonbarbiturates. Full discussion of the rectal administration of barbiturates may be found in prior editions of this textbook.[22]

1. Opioids
   a. Hydromorphone
   b. Oxymorphone
2. Promethazine
3. Chloral hydrate
4. Benzodiazepines
   a. Diazepam
   b. Midazolam
5. Ketamine

Hydromorphone

Hydromorphone is an opioid analgesic whose primary indication is the relief of pain. One of the advantages of hydromorphone is a low incidence of nausea and vomiting. Sleep occurring after its administration is a result of the relief of pain, not hypnosis.

Hydromorphone administered rectally provides long-lasting pain relief. The onset of action of the drug occurs within 30 minutes, and it has a duration of action of 4 to 5 hours.

Dosage

Adults: 3 mg suppository PR (per rectum) every 6 to 8 hours. Titrate to pain relief.[23]

Availability

Dilaudid (Knoll): 3-mg suppositories. Hydromorphone is classified as a Schedule II drug.

Oxymorphone

Oxymorphone is a rapid-acting opioid analgesic used primarily for the management of pain. It also produces sedation and is therefore indicated for use in preoperative sedation. Following oral or rectal administration, the onset of action occurs within 30 minutes; the duration of action is approximately 6 hours.

Dosage

Adults: 5 mg PR every 4 to 6 hours. Doses may be cautiously increased as needed. Geriatric or debilitated adults may require lower doses or extended dosing intervals.[24] The safe use of oxymorphone in children younger than 12 years has not been established.

Availability

Numorphan (DuPont): 5-mg suppositories. Oxymorphone is classified as a Schedule II drug.

Promethazine

The pharmacology of promethazine, a phenothiazine derivative, has been discussed in the section on oral sedation (see Chapter 7). Promethazine may also be administered rectally for preoperative sedation and in the management of nausea and vomiting.

Dosage

The usual adult dose is 25 to 50 mg 1 hour before bedtime. For preoperative sedation of adults, the dose is 50 mg 1 hour before treatment. For sedation of children ≥2 years, the usual dose is 12.5 to 25 mg 1 hour before treatment.[25]

Availability

Phenergan (Wyeth): 12.5-, 25-, and 50-mg suppositories.

Chloral Hydrate

Chloral hydrate, a nonbarbiturate sedative-hypnotic, no longer available in the United States and the United Kingdom, has been reviewed in Chapter 7. Chloral hydrate is also used rectally for preoperative sedation.

Dosage

For adults for preoperative sedation or to aid in falling asleep the night before dental treatment, the usual dose is 650 to 1300 mg 1 hour before treatment or bedtime. The dosage for children is discussed in Chapter 35.

Availability

Rectules (Fellows): 650- and 1300-mg suppositories. Chloral hydrate is classified as a Schedule IV drug. Chloral hydrate is no longer available in the United States, United Kingdom and European Union.

Diazepam

Diazepam has been used rectally for two specific purposes in medicine: management of seizures[26] and management of anxiety in a variety of clinical settings, including in terminal cancer patients[27] and in adults for sedation during oral surgery.[28] The pediatric use of rectal diazepam has been well received.[29] Mattila et al[30] stated that the rectal solution of diazepam is a faster and more effective and reliable alternative to either tablets or suppositories and to the uncertain intramuscular (IM) injection of diazepam. Diazepam is not available at this time in the United States in a rectal formulation; however, it is available in this form in many countries, where its administration rectally has been well accepted.

Flaitz, Nowak, and Hicks[31] reported on the effective use of rectally administered diazepam for pediatric sedation in dentistry. Using the IV formulation of diazepam, a dose of 0.6 mg/kg was administered rectally. Effective levels of both sedation and anterograde amnesia were found in most patients. A potential complication of the rectal administration of diazepam is intestinal irritation, the incidence of which is thought to be quite low.[32]

Midazolam

Midazolam, a water-soluble benzodiazepine, has received considerable attention as a rectally administered drug for premedication or sedation.[6,8,9,11,17,18,21,33–38] Various doses of rectal midazolam have been used, ranging from 0.2 to 5.0 mg/kg. It appears that a rectal dose of approximately 0.35 mg/kg[6,17,39] to 0.5 mg/kg[9,21] provides a rapid onset of action and a high level of successful sedation, with minimal intraoperative or postoperative complications. Roelofse et al[6,39] observed that 23% of the 60 patients receiving rectal midazolam exhibited disinhibition reactions, particularly those receiving a dose of 0.45 mg/kg. Reactions observed included agitation-excitement, restlessness-irritation, disorientation-confusion, and emotional-crying responses.

Midazolam is not available in a rectal formulation. The parenteral formulation of midazolam has been used, with 2 mL of midazolam diluted with 8 mL of distilled water.[21] This volume is then instilled behind the anal sphincter with a suitable plastic applicator. Unlike diazepam, midazolam has not been observed to produce irritation of the rectal mucosa.

Studies in which vital signs and other physiologic parameters were monitored after the rectal administration of midazolam show no clinically significant changes in arterial blood pressure, heart rate, oxyhemoglobin saturation, or end-tidal carbon dioxide concentrations.[11,40]

Availability

Midazolam is not available as a rectal formulation, nor is it recommended for rectal administration in the United States. Several European countries (e.g., France and Switzerland) have approved the pediatric use of midazolam via rectal administration.[41] Midazolam is classified as a Schedule IV drug.

Ketamine

Ketamine, a cyclohexane derivative, is classified as a dissociative anesthetic. First reported in 1969, ketamine produces a surgical-depth anesthesia by interrupting afferent impulses reaching the cerebral cortex.[42] During dissociative anesthesia, patients appear to be awake—their eyes may be open, their mouths moving—yet they are incapable of purposefully reacting to environmental stimulation with appropriate motor responses.[43] The pharmacology of ketamine is discussed in greater detail in Chapter 31. Although used primarily via the IM and IV routes, ketamine has also been administered rectally for premedication or sedation.[1,35,38] Holm-Knudsen, Sjogren, and Laub[35] used 10 mg/kg ketamine and 0.2 mg/kg midazolam for induction of general anesthesia in healthy 2- to 10-year-olds and reported that no cases of rectal irritation or unpleasant dreams occurred and that postoperative analgesia was good. Vander Bijl, Roelofse, and Stander[38] also administered rectal ketamine (5 mg/kg) and midazolam (0.3 mg/kg) to patients 2 to 9 years old. They reported that 30 minutes after administration of the two drugs, good anxiolysis, sedation, and cooperation were obtained in most patients. The group that received midazolam alone appeared to have more efficacious results and fewer adverse effects than the group that received ketamine alone (but no statistical difference was noted).[38]

A commonly reported side effect of ketamine via any route of administration is vivid dreams or hallucinations.[42] Such adverse events are rarely noted in pediatric patients, who generally tolerate ketamine anesthesia quite well. Ketamine should not be used by dentists who are not trained in general anesthesia and in the management of the airway of the unconscious patient.

Lytic Cocktail

The lytic cocktail is a combination of meperidine (Demerol), promethazine (Phenergan), and chlorpromazine (Thorazine), also known as *DPT*.[43] Used intramuscularly, DPT was frequently used in hospitals (especially in the emergency room) during painful procedures. The efficacy of this mixture is poor, especially when compared with alternative approaches, and it has been associated with a high frequency of adverse effects.[44,45] It has been used rectally in pediatric patients. A dose of 0.07 mL/kg was administered to patients ranging in age from 1 to 12 years.[46] One milliliter of lytic cocktail contains 28 mg meperidine, 7 mg promethazine, and 7 mg chlorpromazine. Satisfactory sedation was achieved before operation in most patients, but following the procedure, rectally premedicated patients were less sedated than a control group that received IM DPT.

The lytic cocktail has fallen into disfavor, and this is noted in the U.S. Department of Health and Human Services' *Clinical Practice Guideline on Acute Pain Management*.[47] They conclude that the lytic cocktail "is not recommended for general use and should be used only in exceptional circumstances."

COMPLICATIONS OF RECTAL ADMINISTRATION

Several complications are associated with rectal administration of drugs. Primary among these is the initiation of a bowel movement by instillation of a large volume of fluid into the rectum.[14] The incidence of this complication is not documented, but it is estimated to occur in 5% to 10% of patients receiving rectal drugs.[14]

Irritation of rectal mucosa, even to the extent of ulceration, is possible with certain drugs and with prolonged rectal administration.[48] Long-term rectal administration of acetylsalicylic acid has produced rectal ulceration. However, even single-dose rectal instillation has produced rectal irritation.

The potential for oversedation or the loss of consciousness (general anesthesia), both with attendant risk of airway obstruction produced by the relaxed tongue, must be considered whenever rectally administered drugs are intended to provide deep sedation. This risk is increased when opioid agonists or ketamine are used. The occurrence of oversedation, inadvertent general anesthesia, or airway obstruction is decreased when rectal benzodiazepines are employed.

SUMMARY

The use of rectally administered drugs has increased in popularity in many countries, especially since the introduction of midazolam. Clinical trials have demonstrated that drugs administered rectally are usually well accepted, are well tolerated, and provide a relatively rapid onset of action with a minimum of adverse effects or complications. Rectally administered drugs provide an alternative to the oral and parenteral routes, which might prove difficult to employ or be contraindicated in certain populations, such as pediatric patients and patients with disabilities.

Rectal sedation should be considered only by dentists who are knowledgeable in the pharmacology of the drug(s) to be administered and in the potential side effects and complications of the technique and drug(s) and who are adept in the management of the unconscious patient and airway. In addition, I strongly recommend that (1) supplemental oxygen be administered to all patients receiving sedation via rectal drugs; (2) an IV infusion be maintained throughout the procedure; and (3) continuous monitoring of the patient, to include pulse oximetry, capnography (where required by state or provincial mandate), and a pretracheal stethoscope, be employed.

When rectal sedation is used, the drug should be administered in the dental office to ensure proper dosing and monitoring following administration. Whenever possible, the use of benzodiazepines, midazolam or diazepam, should be considered. Opioids, ketamine, and especially the barbiturates or lytic cocktail ought not to be given rectally. Adequately trained personnel must be available to manage the patient during and after sedation.

State and provincial regulations for enteral sedation (oral) govern the use of rectal sedation in most jurisdictions.

REFERENCES

1. Jantzen JP, Diehl P: Rectal administration of drugs: fundamentals and applications in anesthesia. *Anaesthesist* 40:251, 1991.
2. Jannin V, Lemagnen G, Gueroult P, et al: Rectal route in the 21st century to treat children. *Adv Drug Deliv Rev* 73:34–49, 2014.
3. Standing JF, Tibboel D, Korpela R, Olkkola KT: Diclofenac pharmacokinetic meta-analysis and dose recommendations for surgical pain in children aged 1-12 years. *Paediatr Anaesth* 21(3):316–324, 2011.
4. American Heart Association: National Academy of Sciences and National Research Council standards for cardiopulmonary resuscitation (CPR) and emergency cardiac care (ECC). *JAMA* 227(Suppl):833, 1974.
5. Sykes WS: *Essays on the first hundred years of anaesthesia*, Edinburgh, 1960, ES Livingstone.
6. Roelofse JA, vander Bilj P, Stegmann DH, et al: Preanesthetic medication with rectal midazolam in children undergoing dental extractions. *J Oral Maxillofac Surg* 48:791, 1990.
7. Berthold C: Enteral sedation: safety, efficacy, and controversy. *Compend Contin Educ Dent* 28(5):264–271, 2007.

8. Kraemer N, Krafft T, Kinzelmann KH: Treatment of deciduous teeth under rectal midazolam sedation. *Deut Zahnarzt Z* 46:609, 1991.

9. Tolksdorf W, Eicj C: Rectal, oral and nasal premedication using midazolam in children aged 1-6 years: a comparative clinical study. *Anaesthesist* 40:661, 1991.

10. Kasaba T, Nonoue T, Yanagidani T, et al: Effects of rectal premedication and the mother's presence on induction of pediatric anesthesia. *Masui Jpn J Anesth* 40:552–556, 1991.

11. Spear RM, Yaster M, Berkowitz ID, et al: Preinduction of anesthesia in children with rectally administered midazolam. *Anesthesiology* 74:670–674, 1991.

12. Layeeque R, Siegel F, Kass R, et al: Prevention of nausea and vomiting following breast surgery. *Am J Surg* 191(6);767–772, 2006.

13. Maunuksela EL, Ryhaenen P, Janhunen L: Efficacy of rectal ibuprofen in controlling postoperative pain in children. *Can J Anaesth* 39:226, 1992.

14. Giovannitti JA, Trapp LD: Adult sedation: oral, rectal, IM, IV. In Dionne RA, Phero JC, editors: *Management of pain and anxiety in dental practice*, New York, 1991, Elsevier.

15. De Boer A, De Leede L, Breimer D: Drug absorption by sublingual and rectal routes. *Br J Anaesth* 56:69, 1984.

16. De Boer A, Moolenaar F, Leede LG, et al: Rectal drug administration: clinical pharmacokinetic considerations. *Clin Pharmacokinet* 7:285–311, 1982.

17. Kraus GB, Gruber RG, Knoll R, et al: Pharmacokinetic studies following intravenous and rectal administration of midazolam in children. *Anaesthesist* 38:658–663, 1989.

18. Coventry DM, Martin CS, Burke AM: Sedation for paediatric computerized tomography: double-blind assessment of rectal midazolam. *Eur J Anaesthesiol* 8:29, 1991.

19. Glasier CM, Stark JE, Brown R, et al: Rectal thiopental sodium for sedation of pediatric patients undergoing MR and other imaging studies. *AJNR Am J Neuroradiol* 16(1):111–114, 1995.

20. Alp H, Guler I, Orbak Z, et al: Efficacy and safety of rectal thiopental: sedation for children undergoing computed tomography and magnetic resonance imaging. *Pediatr Int* 41(5):538–541, 1999.

21. deWaal FC, Huisman J, Veerman AJ: Rectal premedication with midazolam in children: a comparative clinical study. *Tijdschr Kindergeneesk* 56:82, 1988.

22. Malamed SF: Rectal sedation. In Malamed SF, editor: *Sedation: a guide to patient management*, ed 4, St Louis, 2002, Mosby.

23. Dilaudid drug monograph, ClinicalKey. Available at www.ClinicalKey.com. Accessed 17 August 2015.

24. Numorphan drug monograph, ClinicalKey. Available at www.ClinicalKey.com. Accessed 9 July 2015.

25. Promethazine drug monograph, ClinicalKey. Available at www.ClinicalKey.com. Accessed 30 July 2015.

26. Dhillon S, Ngwane E, Richens A: Rectal absorption of diazepam in epileptic children. *Arch Dis Child* 57:264, 1982.

27. Ehsanullah RS, Galloway DB, Gusterson FR, et al: A double-blind crossover study of diazepam rectal suppositories, 5 mg and 10 mg, for sedation with advanced malignant disease. *Pharmatherapeutica* 3:215–220, 1982.

28. Lundgren S: Serum concentration and drug effect after intravenous and rectal administration of diazepam. *Anesth Prog* 34:128, 1987.

29. Knudsen F: Plasma-diazepam in infants after rectal administration in solution and by suppository. *Acta Paediatr Scand* 66:563, 1977.

30. Mattila MA, Ruoppi MK, Ahlstrom-Bengg E, et al: Diazepam in rectal solution as premedication in children, with special reference to serum concentrations. *Br J Anaesth* 53:1269–1272, 1981.

31. Flaitz CM, Nowak AJ, Hicks MJ: Evaluation of anterograde amnesic effect of rectally administered diazepam in the sedated pedodontic patient. *J Dent Child* 53:17, 1986.

32. Lundgren S, Rosenquist J: Comparison of sedation, amnesia, and patient comfort produced by intravenous and rectal diazepam. *J Oral Maxillofac Surg* 42:646, 1984.

33. Piotrowski R, Petrow N: Anesthesia induction in children: propofol in comparison with thiopental following premedication with midazolam. *Anaesthesist* 39:398, 1990.

34. Molter G, Castor G, Altmayer P: Psychosomatic, sedative and hemodynamic reactions following preoperative administration of midazolam in children. *Klin Padiatr* 202:328, 1990.

35. Holm-Knudsen R, Sjogren P, Laub M: Midazolam and ketamine for rectal premedication and induction of anesthesia in children. *Anaesthesist* 39:255, 1990.

36. Tolksdorf W, Bremerich D, Nordmeyer U: Midazolam for premedication of infants. A comparison of the effect between oral and rectal administration. *Anasthesiol Intensivmed Notfallmed* 24:355, 1989.

37. Saint-Maurice C, Esteve C, Holzer J, et al: Better acceptance of measures for induction of anesthesia after rectal premedication with midazolam in children: comparison of results of an open and placebo-controlled study. *Anaesthesist* 36:629–633, 1987.

38. vander Bijl P, Roelofse JA, Stander IA: Rectal ketamine and midazolam for premedication in pediatric dentistry. *J Oral Maxillofac Surg* 49:1050, 1991.

39. Roelofse JA, de V Joubert JJ: Arterial oxygen saturation in children receiving rectal midazolam as premedication for oral surgical procedures. *Anesth Prog* 37:286, 1990.

40. Roelofse JA, Stegmann DH, Hartshorne J, et al: Paradoxical reactions to rectal midazolam as premedication in children. *Int J Oral Maxillofac Surg* 19:2–6, 1990.

41. Moore PA: Pediatric medication with rectal midazolam in children undergoing dental extractions. Discussion. *J Oral Maxillofac Surg* 48:797, 1990.

42. Becsey L, Malamed S, Radnay P, et al: Reduction of the psychotomimetic and circulatory side effects of ketamine by droperidol. *Anesthesiology* 37:536–542, 1972.

43. Anonymous: Reappraisal of lytic cocktail/Demerol, Phenergan, and Thorazine (DPT) for the sedation of children. American Academy of Pediatrics Committee on Drugs. *Pediatrics* 95(4):598–602, 1995.

44. Benusis KP, Kapaun D, Furnam LJ: Respiratory depression in a child following meperidine, promethazine, and chlorpromazine premedication: report of a case. *J Dent Child* 46:50, 1979.

45. Nahata N, Clotz M, Krogg E: Adverse effects of meperidine, promethazine, and chlorpromazine for sedation in pediatric patients. *Clin Pediatr* 24:558, 1985.

46. Laub M, Sjogren P, Holm-Knudsen R, et al: Lytic cocktail in children: rectal versus intramuscular administration. *Anaesthesia* 45:110–112, 1990.

47. U.S. Department of Health and Human Services: Clinical practice guideline: acute pain management: operative or medical procedures and trauma, publication no. 92-2, Rockville, MD, 1992, U.S. Department of Health and Human Services, Public Health Service, Agency for Health Care Policy and Research.

48. van Hoogdalem E, de Boer AG, Breimer DD: Pharmacokinetics of rectal drug administration, part I. General considerations and clinical applications of centrally acting drugs. *Clin Pharmacokinet* 21:11, 1991.

chapter 9

Sublingual, Transdermal, and Intranasal Sedation

CHAPTER OUTLINE

SUBLINGUAL SEDATION
Nitroglycerin
Opioids
Oral Transmucosal Fentanyl Citrate
(Fentanyl "Lollipop")
Sedatives

TRANSDERMAL SEDATION
Opioids
Antiemetics
INTRANASAL SEDATION
Midazolam
Sufentanil

$\mathcal{E}$fforts have been directed at seeking alternative routes of drug administration for use where traditional routes are unavailable or where patient cooperation is lacking. Such situations include younger children or infants (the "precooperative patient"), where cooperation does not exist; older patients requiring long-term drug therapy, where noncompliance with administration recommendations is a significant problem; and victims of burns, trauma, or life-threatening emergencies, where other routes of administration are not present, yet rapid onset of drug action is necessary.

Three routes of drug administration—sublingual (SL), transdermal, and intranasal (IN)—are discussed. These techniques are becoming increasingly popular in many areas of medicine. The IN route, in particular, has seen a dramatic increase in popularity in medicine and, to an increasing degree, in dentistry.[1–3] IN midazolam has become a commonly employed drug in the management of status epilepticus in infants and smaller children,[4-6] and the IN administration of nonsteroidal antiinflammatory (NSAID) drugs has gained popularity.[7,8] The recently FDA-approved (June 2016) nasal local anesthetic mist (tetracaine HCl and oxymetazoline – Kovanaze) allows for pain-free dental treatment of maxillary non-molar teeth.[9,10]

Transdermal drug administration is most often used for sustained-action drug administration (e.g., scopolamine as an anti–motion sickness therapy), whereas *SL* and *IN* drug administration provide a considerably more rapid onset of clinical action.

SUBLINGUAL SEDATION

SL drug administration has a long history.[11,12] Indeed, SL administration of nitroglycerin tablets has been the recommended route for management of anginal pain for decades.[13,14] SL placement of nitroglycerin tablets usually provides relief from anginal discomfort within 2 minutes.

An advantage of SL drug administration is that the drug enters directly into the systemic circulation, almost entirely bypassing the enterohepatic circulation. This avoids the hepatic first-pass effect, in which a percentage of the drug is biotransformed before ever having the opportunity to enter the general circulation and to reach its target organ (e.g., brain).[15-17] Harris and Robinson[18] have stated that SL drug delivery provides rapid absorption and good bioavailability for some drugs, although this site is not well suited to sustained-delivery systems. Patient cooperation is important to the success of the SL route of administration, which minimizes its use in many pediatric and other uncooperative patients.[19]

Among the drugs that have been used sublingually are nitroglycerin in the management of angina pectoris, acute pulmonary edema, and acute myocardial infarction[20]; heparin in the prophylaxis of atherosclerotic disease[21]; nifedipine, a calcium channel blocker, for the management of acute hypertensive urgencies and emergencies[22–28]; opioids, such as meperidine and buprenorphine, for relief of pain in cancer[29,30] or after abdominal or gynecologic surgery[19,31]; and sedatives for premedication and sedation.[32–34]

Nitroglycerin

Nitroglycerin is administered sublingually in the management of anginal discomfort. Rapid SL absorption provides venodilation within 2 minutes. Epicardial coronary arteries demonstrate a 28% increase in normal luminal area, whereas in severely stenotic coronary arteries the increase is 29%.[14] The rapidity of onset and degree of vasodilation observed make nitroglycerin the drug of choice for the management of angina pectoris. Side effects of SL nitroglycerin are few and usually not severe. However, in certain individuals, SL nitroglycerin has provoked severe side effects. Brandes, Santiago, and Limacher[35] report on 35 cases of nitroglycerin-induced hypotension, bradycardia, apnea, and unconsciousness and conclude that this is a drug-induced effect of nitroglycerin that is independent of the route of administration and is unpredictable. They recommend close monitoring whenever nitroglycerin is administered.

Therapeutic advantage may be taken of the hypotensive side effect of nitroglycerin in the management of acute hypertensive episodes. Acute hypertensive episodes are classified as either "urgencies" or "emergencies," with the level of blood pressure elevation determining the classification. Hypertensive emergencies involve significantly greater blood pressure elevations and require more aggressive and immediate treatment than do hypertensive urgencies.[22] Although nitroglycerin has been used effectively sublingually, the calcium channel blocker nifedipine has received considerably more attention in the management of both hypertensive urgencies and emergencies. SL nifedipine is rapidly absorbed, leading to improved myocardial perfusion, increased coronary blood flow, and decreased coronary vascular resistance.[23] A capsule of nifedipine is punctured several times (in the dental office, an explorer or small round bur will be sufficient for this purpose), placed under the tongue, and sucked on by the patient. Nifedipine SL has been used in the management of clonidine overdose, which produces severe hypertension and altered mental status. SL nifedipine (20 mg) produces a rapid decline in blood pressure and improved mental status.[24] As with nitroglycerin, SL nifedipine used for management of acute hypertensive episodes may produce symptomatic hypotension in some patients.[27] Vital signs should be monitored closely whenever SL nifedipine is used. SL nifedipine may cause serious dose-dependent adverse effects.[28]

Opioids

Many studies have reported on the efficacy of SL administration of opioids in palliative care in cancer pain[36,37] and for preanesthetic sedation.[31] Korttilla and Hovorka[31] compared SL buprenorphine with intramuscular (IM) oxycodone as a preanesthetic medication. Preoperatively the SL opioid produced less drowsiness and sedation and alleviated patients' apprehension significantly less than oxycodone. However, in the recovery room, moderate-to-severe pain was more common with oxycodone than with SL buprenorphine. SL buprenorphine was as effective as IM oxycodone for pain relief. However, two patients receiving SL opioids developed severe respiratory depression postoperatively. The authors concluded that SL opioids can provide good postoperative pain relief for gynecologic procedures performed under anesthesia, but that patients must be monitored because of the potential for respiratory depression. In a similar study, Carl et al[19] compared SL and IM buprenorphine and IM meperidine for pain control after major abdominal surgery. Patients receiving SL buprenorphine were significantly more conscious in the immediate postoperative period than either IM group, yet all three groups demonstrated equal pain relief. Sedation and nausea were the most common complications in all three groups. Three cases of IM meperidine and one of IM buprenorphine required intermittent positive-pressure ventilation (IPPV) for respiratory depression. They concluded that SL opioids are useful for postoperative pain and exhibited administrative advantages when patients were able to cooperate. Several studies have looked at the use of opioids for the long-term relief of cancer pain, concluding that SL morphine has enabled patients whose cancer pain is refractory to traditional methods of drug delivery to obtain satisfactory control of their symptoms.[29,30,36,37]

Oral Transmucosal Fentanyl Citrate (Fentanyl "Lollipop")

Fentanyl has also been formulated as a lozenge or lollipop (Fentanyl Oralet, Abbott Laboratories). Originally designed for use in long-term pain management in cancer patients,[38,39] oral transmucosal fentanyl citrate (OTFC) has demonstrated advantages in the management of moderate-to-severe postoperative pain[40] and as a preoperative sedative in children.[41,42] The use of OTFC has been studied as an alternative to oral and parenteral medication in younger or older patients who are unwilling or unable to tolerate orally administered drugs.[43–50] Although several doses have been evaluated, most studies indicated that a dose of 15 to 20 µg/kg provides the optimal sedation and anxiolysis preoperatively.[43,44] Acceptance of the lollipop was reported as universal in most studies, a significant advantage over most other forms of drug administration.[43–47] The objective onset of sedation was noted to develop from 10 minutes[45] to 30 minutes[43] following administration of the lollipop. After beginning OTFC, 60% of patients became drowsy or sedated in 12 to 30 minutes.[47] When volunteers were asked to rapidly suck the lollipop (as opposed to allowing it to passively dissolve), a more rapid onset of a pleasant feeling (the first subjective sensation) was observed. However, the onset of subjective sedation or analgesia was no more rapid than with passive dissolution.[44]

The use of fentanyl lollipops is not without the potential for side effects. Significant decreases in respiratory rate and arterial oxygen saturation (SpO_2) have been reported.[16,43,45,49] Management of these episodes of opioid-induced respiratory depression was simple: reminding the patient to breathe.[43] Other side effects noted with some frequency included pruritus[43,46,49] in 80%[43] to 90%[46] of patients preoperatively and 33% to 70% postoperatively,[43] postoperative nausea (30% to 58%[43]), and vomiting (50% to 83%),[43,46,48–49] which was not significantly reduced by the prophylactic administration of the antiemetic droperidol.[48]

The conclusion reached by most authors is that OTFC is a reliable means of inducing rapid, noninvasive preoperative sedation for pediatric outpatients undergoing short operations[48,50] or in the emergency room.[44] They further observe that OTFC use is associated with potentially significant reductions in respiratory rate and SpO_2 and a high incidence of postoperative nausea and vomiting and pruritus.[45] In the absence of controlled clinical trials in dental outpatients that have not occurred since publication of the previous edition (2010), it seems prudent to withhold recommendation of this method of opioid administration for preoperative sedation in dentistry.

Sedatives

Several studies have reported on the use of the SL route for preoperative sedation. Two have compared the SL administration of a benzodiazepine with oral administration. Gram-Hansen and Schultz,[32] administering 2.5 mg lorazepam either orally or sublingually before gynecologic surgery, found a maximal plasma concentration at 40 minutes orally and 60 minutes after SL administration. Garzone and Kroboth,[33] looking at alprazolam and triazolam, found peak concentrations that occurred earlier and were higher following SL versus oral administration. SL lormetazepam (2.5 mg) followed in 35 minutes by intravenous (IV) diazepam (10 mg) was compared with SL placebo followed in 35 minutes by IV diazepam (10 mg) in patients undergoing surgical removal of impacted third molars.[34] A rapid onset of sedation was noted after SL lormetazepam administration, whereas the course and duration of postoperative sedation, measured using standard psychometric tests, were similar following both treatments. Surgeons' ratings indicated that SL lormetazepam was comparable with IV diazepam, but patients' ratings indicated greater satisfaction with and preference for IV diazepam. Significant anterograde amnesia was found following both treatments. The authors indicate that SL lormetazepam may have a role in anesthesia as a premedicant and for minimal or moderate sedation. Studies with triazolam have shown that SL administration results in peak triazolam concentrations that are higher and occur earlier than with the oral route.[51] Similar findings have been seen with SL midazolam.[51-53]

SUMMARY (SUBLINGUAL SEDATION)

The SL route of drug administration possesses possible uses in dentistry in two distinct areas. First, for the management of preoperative fears and anxiety, the use of certain drugs, such as benzodiazepines, appears to provide a level of sedation comparable with that achieved with orally administered drugs. The onset of action also appears comparable with that of oral drugs. The second possible use for SL administration in dentistry is in management of postoperative pain. SL opioid administration appears to provide adequate pain relief with less sedation

than IM opioids. The potential for opioid-induced respiratory depression is still present; therefore the usual postoperative monitoring practices must be continued when SL opioids are used. Patient cooperation is essential for SL delivery of drugs to be effective. Therefore the use of SL administration in younger children or any uncooperative patient is not recommended.

TRANSDERMAL SEDATION

The administration of drugs through the skin (transdermally) has existed for a long time. In the past, the most commonly applied systems were topically applied creams and ointments for dermatologic disorders. The occurrence of systemic side effects with some of these formulations is indicative of absorption through the skin. In a broad sense, the term *transdermal delivery system* includes all topically administered drug formulations intended to deliver the active ingredient into the general circulation.[54] Serious consideration for the transdermal delivery of drugs for systemic therapy began with a number of revolutionary ideas in the early 1970s.[55] Modern transdermal therapeutic systems (TTSs) have been successfully marketed since the 1980s.[56] Drugs such as nitroglycerin (angina),[57] scopolamine (anti–motion sickness),[58,59] clonidine (high blood pressure),[60] estradiol (postmenopause),[61] and nicotine (smoking cessation)[62] are the current prominent representatives that have met expectations regarding therapeutic benefits based on TTS applications. The use of opioids, primarily fentanyl, via TTS for pain management has also met with considerable clinical success.[63–65]

A major advantage of TTS is the avoidance of the hepatic first-pass effect. Other advantages include simplified dosage regimens, enhanced compliance, reduced side effects, and improved disease therapy.[66]

The intact skin provides an efficient barrier against percutaneous absorption of drugs.[67] This barrier function can be ascribed to the structure of the stratum corneum, which consists of alternating lipoidal and hydrophilic regions, making intact skin relatively impermeable. This impermeability of skin is associated with its dual functions as a protective barrier against invasion by microorganisms and the prevention of the loss of physiologically essential substances, such as water. Elucidation of factors that contribute to this impermeability has made the use of skin as a route for controlled systemic drug delivery possible.[54] For drugs used for systemic therapy to be delivered through the skin, permeability must be enhanced by either modifying the drug molecules or applying skin permeation enhancers to reduce the barrier property of the skin.[68] Traditionally, enhancement of skin permeability is achieved by either improvement of drug lipophilicity and the partition of drugs into the skin or through direct actions of skin permeation enhancers on the chemical structure and/or composition of lipids and proteins in the stratum corneum.

A number of transdermal delivery systems are currently employed that allow for effective absorption of drugs of low molecular mass across the skin.[69] The most widely used system is the membrane-permeation–controlled system. A second system is the microsealed system, a partition-controlled delivery system that contains a drug reservoir with a saturated suspension of the drug in a water-miscible solvent homogeneously dispersed in a silicone elastomer matrix. A third system is the matrix-diffusion–controlled system, and a fourth system is the gradient-charged system. Nitroglycerin TTS is based on a multilayered laminated polymeric structure. A layer of vinyl chloride copolymer or terpolymer containing the drug is sandwiched between two or more layers of polymeric films. Nitroglycerin is released from the device at a controlled rate by a process of diffusion through the reservoir and one of the outer layers, which can function as a rate-controlling membrane.[70] Advanced transdermal systems are being developed, including iontophoretic and sonophoretic systems, thermosetting gels, prodrugs, and liposomes.[54] Penetration enhancers, such as Azone, may allow the delivery of larger molecules, such as proteins and polypeptides.

Systemic and localized side effects may be noted with the use of transdermal drug delivery systems. These have included skin inflammation and allergy[56,68,71,72] and drug tolerance.[57,72] Side effects produced by the drug are similar to those noted with other routes of drug delivery.

The onset of clinical activity of TTS-administered drugs is slow, hence the primary use of this technique for sustained-release drug therapy. After application of a transdermal fentanyl patch, fentanyl is absorbed into the skin beneath the patch, where a depot forms in the upper skin layers. Plasma fentanyl concentrations are barely detectable for about 2 hours after patch placement. From 8 to 12 hours after patch placement, however, plasma fentanyl concentrations approximate those achieved with equivalent IV doses.[65]

Opioids

Interest in the use of transdermal drug delivery systems in dentistry centers on postoperative pain management. Opioids, particularly fentanyl, have received attention in the management of both chronic (cancer) and acute (postoperative) pain.

Mosser[73] describes the unique pharmacokinetics of the transdermal system, including a prolonged time to peak analgesic effect, a long elimination half-life, and the skin depot concept, and recommends fentanyl over parenterally administered opioids in the treatment of cancer pain. Calis, Kohler, and Corso[65] also recommend fentanyl TTS for management of chronic cancer-related pain. The use of TTS for acute postoperative pain is not as well accepted. Although Clotz and Nahata[74] state that the transdermal fentanyl patch seems to provide the same degree of analgesia as a continuous IV infusion, Calis, Kohler, and Corso[65] state that the overall efficacy and safety of the transdermal fentanyl system for the treatment of postoperative pain has not been adequately evaluated.

Antiemetics

A second area in which TTS drug delivery systems have potential utility in dentistry is in the delivery of antiemetics. Swallowed blood is a potent emetic following surgical procedures. In addition, the administration of opioid analgesics during the surgical procedure or postoperatively is associated with an increased likelihood of nausea and vomiting.

Scopolamine was one of the first drugs employed transdermally in the management of motion sickness.[75] When it is administered transdermally, its duration of effect is 72 hours compared with a 3- to 6-hour duration when administered orally or parenterally. Transdermal administration is associated with a lower incidence of dose-related side effects than orally or parenterally administered scopolamine. The most commonly observed side effects following transdermal administration have been dry mouth, drowsiness, and impairment of ocular accommodation, including blurred vision and mydriasis. Systemic side effects, such as adverse central nervous system (CNS) effects, difficulty in urinating, rashes, and erythema, have been reported only occasionally. Schuh, Tolksdorf, and Hucke evaluated the efficacy of transdermal scopolamine in preventing nausea and vomiting in postsurgical patients.[76] Scopolamine has a well-documented postoperative antiemetic effect. One study has demonstrated a 50% reduction of emetic symptoms compared with placebo.[77] In this study of cholecystectomy patients (a procedure with a high incidence of postoperative emesis), the antinausea and antiemetic effect of scopolamine TTS was insufficient and significantly less than that seen with IV droperidol (7.5 mg).[76] In the droperidol group, 45% of patients did not have nausea, and vomiting occurred in only 25%, whereas in the scopolamine TTS group, only 15% did not become nauseous and 50% vomited. Further study is warranted to determine the efficacy of transdermal scopolamine as an antiemetic following oral surgical procedures.

SUMMARY (TRANSDERMAL SEDATION)

Transdermal drug delivery systems provide an easy, reliable mechanism of administering drugs when rapid onset is not important. Transdermal drug delivery bypasses the enterohepatic circulation, thereby providing a more reliable clinical action. With many drugs, the efficacy of transdermal delivery is equivalent to that of a continuous IV infusion, yet in a noninvasive system.

It appears that the transdermal use of opioids might prove advantageous in dental situations in which long-term pain control is required but patient compliance is suspect. Drug-related side effects following transdermal delivery, although less common, are the same as those noted when other administration techniques are used. Oversedation and respiratory depression must be considered whenever opioids are employed. Use of transdermal opioids should be reserved for clinical situations in which patient monitoring can be ensured throughout the drug's delivery. The use of transdermal scopolamine as an antiemetic following dental surgery requires additional research before its use can be recommended.

INTRANASAL SEDATION

A relatively recent addition to the drug administration armamentarium, IN drugs have been used primarily in pediatric patients as a way to circumvent the need for injection or oral drug administration in unwilling patients.[78,79] Absorption of IN drugs occurs directly into the systemic circulation, avoiding the enterohepatic circulation.[80,81] Clinical trials have demonstrated that rates of absorption and bioavailability of IN drugs are close to those with IM administration, with peak plasma levels of the agent occurring approximately 10 minutes after administration.[81-87] Midazolam, a water-soluble benzodiazepine,[78,79,81-88] and sufentanil,[87,88] an opioid analgesic, have received the most attention regarding administration via the IN route.

Midazolam

Midazolam has been demonstrated to provide a consistent level of CNS activity following IN administration.[79,82-88] A dose of 0.2 mg/kg appears to be the most effective in pediatric patients for premedication before general anesthesia,[84,85,87,89] with somewhat larger doses recommended for sedation adequate to permit treatment.[90]

The mean IN absorption rates (t_{max}) of flurazepam, midazolam, and triazolam were 1.7, 2, and 2.6 times faster, respectively, than those achieved with oral dosing.[91] When children accept oral administration at all, they appear to accept it better than drugs administered intranasally.[89] IN drugs are administered by either the parent or the dentist using a 1- or 3-mL syringe with an aerosolizing adapter attached (Fig. 9.1) and with the child seated on the parent's lap. Some children are temporarily distressed at the instillation of the fluid (drug) into the nose,

but all rapidly settled down again in the presence of their parents.[78] An undiluted solution of the drug should be used to prevent large volumes of liquid instilled into the nose and possibly entering the pharynx and producing coughing or sneezing, with attendant expulsion of the drug and decreased absorption. Rose, Simon, and Haberer[86] found IN midazolam to be slightly more effective than oral diazepam as preanesthetic medication in children, producing anxiolysis and sedation with rapid onset. Buenz and Gossler[84] suggest that with the advent of a more concentrated solution of midazolam (>5 mg/mL), IN application is also conceivable as a premedication in adults.

The IM and IN routes of midazolam administration have been compared. There were no significant differences in the onset of sedation (12.42 ± 4.07 minutes for IM; 15.26 ± 7.99 minutes for IN), the degree of sedation, and the response to venipuncture.[85] Theissen et al[92] compared IM and IN midazolam for sedation in adults before endoscopy of the upper gastrointestinal tract. Sedation was equivalent in both groups, with three patients ($n = 10$) in the IM group experiencing retrograde amnesia (0 in the IN group). No significant differences in the degrees of anterograde amnesia were noted in either group. IN administration of midazolam was concluded to be a simple, nontraumatic, well-tolerated alternative to the IM route of sedation for bronchoscopy in adults.

Several studies have compared IN midazolam with IV midazolam. The half-life of midazolam is similar (2.2 hours IN vs. 2.4 hours IV) following IM and IV administration in children ages 1 to 5 years.[82] At 10 minutes following IN administration, the mean plasma concentration of midazolam was 57% of that in the IV group.[83]

An additional finding noted by one observer was the association of IN instillation of midazolam with a sense of euphoria

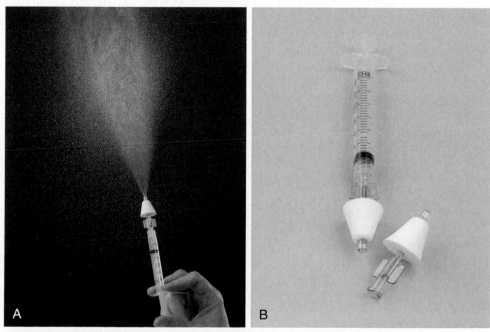

Figure 9.1 A-B, Aerosol spray on IN syringe. (Courtesy www.intranasal.net.)

that occurred almost immediately. This effect was not observed when midazolam was administered by other routes.[89]

Two studies used IN midazolam for procedures akin to dental care. In one, IN midazolam was employed in adults for sedation during upper gastrointestinal endoscopy, and it compared well with IM midazolam.[92] Only two patients (n = 20) receiving IM or IN midazolam had a bad opinion of their experience, compared with four of the nine receiving placebo. IN midazolam was used for sedation before ophthalmologic examination in children ranging in age from 3.5 months to 10 years.[90] An IN midazolam dose of 0.35 to 0.5 mg/kg provided a rapid onset of sedation that was adequate in all cases to permit ocular examination. In all of the IN midazolam studies reported, oxygen saturation was monitored throughout the procedure, including recovery. No instances of significant desaturation were reported.

IN midazolam in a dose of approximately 0.2 mg/kg appears to be an acceptable alternative to both oral and IM administration of midazolam for premedication before additional IV sedation or general anesthesia. A larger dose, 0.35 to 0.5 mg/kg, may be necessary if the IN drug is the sole route of sedative administration. It may be of significant value as an alternative in cases in which IM sedation is necessary, such as venipuncture in the uncooperative child or adult. When more profound and more controllable levels of sedation are desired, the IV route is recommended. IN midazolam provides the level of sedation adequate to permit separation of the child from the parent and to enable the patient to tolerate venipuncture with minimal distress.

My own clinical experience using IN midazolam (a dose of 0.2 mg/kg) in a pediatric population has shown that use of an aerosol spray (similar to a nasal decongestant spray) is better tolerated by patients than a syringe (Fig. 9.2).[93] Use of a syringe often results in the fluid leaking into the patient's throat, precipitating crying and coughing. The clinical efficacy of IN midazolam appears to be similar to that of IM midazolam in both speed of onset and ability to separate the patient from

his or her parent.[93] Primosch and Guelmann, using IN midazolam administered by either drops or spray, found that spray administration of IN midazolam produced significantly less aversive behavior than administering drops in 2- to 3-year-old dental patients of similar behavioral characteristics.[94] The effectiveness of the conscious sedation technique was not influenced by the method of nasal administration.[94] However, as with other nontitratable techniques, there were occasions when IN midazolam demonstrated little or no clinical effect.[93]

Recent studies in pediatric dentistry have confirmed the success of IN midazolam.[94–99] as well as in adults undergoing implant surgery.[100] Several authors recommended the use of IN midazolam only by dentists who have been trained in pediatric sedation and who are well prepared to recognize and treat hypoventilation, as noted by pulse oximetry.[94–96,98,100]

Sufentanil

Sufentanil, an opioid analgesic, was one of the first drugs to receive attention for preoperative sedation by IN administration.[87,88] Both IV and IN sufentanil (IV and IN dose of 15 μg) had rapid onset of action and limited duration.[101] At 10 minutes, all patients (n = 8) in the IV group were sedated, compared with only two in the IN group. However, no significant differences in sedation were observed in either group at 20 to 60 minutes. These findings are in agreement with measured plasma levels of sufentanil, which are significantly lower following IN than IV administration at 5 and 10 minutes, 36% and 56%, of those after IV dosing, respectively. From 30 minutes on, plasma concentrations were virtually identical following both IN and IV sedation. An important finding was a clinically significant decrease in arterial oxygen pressure (PaO_2) at 5 minutes after IV administration of sufentanil that was not observed following IN administration.[79] In a pediatric trial (including children ages 6 months to 7 years) for premedication, doses of 0.15, 0.30, and 0.45 μg/kg of sufentanil were administered intranasally before induction of general anesthesia.[102] Patients receiving sufentanil were more likely to separate willingly from their parents and to be judged as calm at or before 10 minutes compared with placebo-treated patients. However, patients receiving 0.45 μg/kg had a higher incidence of vomiting in the recovery room and during the first postoperative day. Relative to IN midazolam, IN sufentanil was accepted more readily by children but produced a significantly greater incidence of decreased PaO_2.[101]

IN sufentanil produces a euphoric effect in addition to anxiolysis and sedation.[102] IN sufentanil has been used in the management of acute pain associated with traumatic injury[103,104] and with ketamine in preoperative sedation before general anesthesia.[105] Its onset of action is similar to that of IN midazolam. However, the potential decrease in PaO_2 and the increased potential for nausea and vomiting following IN sufentanil administration call for intensified monitoring (oximetry and visual observation) during both the perioperative and postoperative periods. The use of IN midazolam does not appear to be associated with either of these two clinical actions.

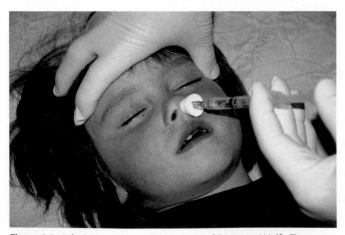

Figure 9.2 Administration via the IN route. (Courtesy Wolfe Tory Medical, Inc., www.wolfetory.com.)

SUMMARY (INTRANASAL SEDATION)

The IN route of drug administration has become increasingly valuable in dentistry. A rapid onset of action enables IN drugs to be used when speed is of the essence, such as for premedication of the uncooperative child. Although some degree of cooperation is necessary, IN drugs are more readily administered than oral drugs when no patient cooperation is available. Use of an aerosol spray for drug administration is preferred to a syringe. As a noninvasive technique, IN administration has few of the potential side effects and complications that are associated with IM drug administration (see Chapters 3 and 10).

Two drugs, sufentanil and midazolam, have received the most study to date and have been demonstrated to be quite effective intranasally. The IN use of sufentanil is associated with the potential development of significant opioid-related side effects, such as nausea, vomiting, and respiratory depression. The benzodiazepine midazolam provides clinical actions that are similar to sufentanil's, but is not associated with its side effects. Intensive monitoring should be used whenever IN drugs are administered.

REFERENCES

1. Chopra R, Mittal M, Bansal K, Chaudhuri P: Buccal midazolam spray as an alternative to intranasal route for conscious sedation in pediatric dentistry. *J Clin Pediatr Dent* 38(2):171–173, 2013.
2. Wood M: The safety and efficacy of using a concentrated intranasal midazolam formulation for paediatric dental sedation. *SAAD Dig* 27:16–23, 2011.
3. Johnson E, Briskie D, Majewski R, et al: The physiologic and behavioral effects of oral and intranasal midazolam in pediatric dental patients. *Pediatr Dent* 37(3):229–238, 2010.
4. Kyrkou M, Harbord M, Kyrkou N, et al: Community use of intranasal midazolam for managing prolonged seizures. *J Intellect Dev Disabil* 31(3):131–138, 2006.
5. Wolfe TR, Macfarlane TC: Intranasal midazolam therapy for pediatric status epilepticus. *Am J Emerg Med* 24(3):343–346, 2006.
6. Mahmoudian T, Zadeh MM: Comparison of intranasal midazolam with intravenous diazepam for treating acute seizures in children. *Epilepsy Behav* 5(2):253–255, 2004.
7. Bacon R, Newman S, Rankin L, et al: Pulmonary and nasal deposition of ketorolac tromethamine solution (SPRIX) following intranasal administration. *Int J Pharm* 431(1–2):39–44, 2012.
8. Bullingham R, Juan A: Comparison of intranasal ketorolac tromethamine pharmacokinetics in younger and older adults. *Drugs Aging* 29(11):899–904, 2012.
9. Giannakopoulos H, Levin LM, Chou JC, et al: The cardiovascular effects and pharmacokinetics of intranasal tetracaine plus oxymetazoline: preliminary findings. *J Am Dent Assoc* 143(8):872–880, 2012.
10. Ciancio SG, Hutcheson MC, Ayoub F, et al: Safety and efficacy of a novel nasal spray for maxillary dental anesthesia. *J Dent Res* 92(7 Suppl):43S–48S, 2013.
11. Wang Z, Chow MS: Overview and appraisal of the current concept and technologies for improvement of sublingual drug delivery. *Ther deliv* 5(7):807–816, 2014.
12. Sattar M, Sayed OM, Lane ME: Oral transmucosal drug delivery—current status and future prospects. *Int J Pharm* 471(1-2):498–506, 2014.
13. Kosmicki MA: Long-term use of short- and long-acting nitrates in stable angina pectoris. *Curr Clin Pharmacol* 4(2):132–141, 2009.
14. Brown BG: Response of normal and diseased epicardial coronary arteries to vasoactive drugs: quantitative arteriographic studies. *Am J Cardiol* 56(9):23E–29E, 1985.
15. Aliberti G, D'Erasmo E, Oddo CM, et al: Effect of the acute sublingual administration of ketanserin in hypertensive patients. *Cardiovasc Drugs Ther* 5:697–699, 1991.
16. DeBoer A, DeLeede L, Breimer D: Drug absorption by sublingual and rectal routes. *Br J Anaesth* 56:69, 1984.
17. Motwani JG, Lipworth BJ: Clinical pharmacokinetics of drug administered buccally and sublingually. *Clin Pharmacokinet* 21:83–94, 1991.
18. Harris D, Robinson JR: Drug delivery via the mucous membranes of the oral cavity. *J Pharm Sci* 81:1–10, 1992.
19. Carl P, Crawford ME, Masden NB, et al: Pain relief after major abdominal surgery: a double-blind controlled comparison of sublingual buprenorphine, intramuscular buprenorphine, and intramuscular meperidine. *Anesth Analg* 66:142–146, 1987.
20. Schneider W, Bussmann WD, Hartmann A, et al: Nitrate therapy in heart failure. *Cardiology* 79(Suppl 2):5–13, 1991.
21. Kanabrocki EL, Bremner WF, Sothern RB, et al: A quest for the relief of atherosclerosis: potential role of intrapulmonary heparin-a hypothesis. *Q J Med* 83:259–282, 1992.
22. Gonzalez-Ramallo VJ, Muino-Miguez A: Hypertensive crises and emergencies: the concept and initial management. *Ann Intern Med* 7:422–427, 1990.
23. Cohn PF: Effects of calcium channel blockers on the coronary circulation. *Am J Hypertens* 3(Pt 2):2995–3045, 1990.
24. Dire DJ, Kuhns DW: The use of sublingual nifedipine in a patient with clonidine overdose. *J Emerg Med* 6:125–128, 1988.
25. Garcia JY, Jr, Vidt DG: Current management of hypertensive emergencies. *Drugs* 34:263–278, 1978.
26. Bauer JH, Reams GP: The role of calcium entry blockers in hypertensive emergencies. *Circulation* 75(Pt 2):V174–V180, 1987.
27. Wachter RM: Symptomatic hypotension induced by nifedipine in the acute treatment of severe hypertension. *Arch Intern Med* 147:556–558, 1987.
28. Ishibashi Y, Shimada T, Yoshitomi H, et al: Sublingual nifedipine in elderly patients: even a low dose induces myocardial ischaemia. *Clin Exp Pharmacol Physiol* 26:404–410, 1999.
29. Ripamonti C, Bruera E: Rectal, buccal, and sublingual narcotics for the management of cancer pain. *J Palliative Care* 7:30–35, 1991.
30. Shepard KV, Bakst AW: Alternate delivery methods for morphine sulfate in cancer pain. *Cleve Clin J Med* 57:48–52, 1990.
31. Korttilla K, Hovorka J: Buprenorphine as premedication and as analgesic during and after light isoflurane-N2O-O2 anaesthesia: a comparison with oxycodone plus fentanyl. *Acta Anaesthesiol Scand* 31:673–679, 1987.
32. Gram-Hansen P, Schultz A: Plasma concentrations following oral and sublingual administration of lorazepam. *Int J Clin Pharmacol Ther Toxicol* 26:323–324, 1988.
33. Garzone PD, Kroboth PD: Pharmacokinetics of the newer benzodiazepines. *Clin Pharmacokinet* 16:337–364, 1989.

34. O'Boyle CA, Barry H, Fox E, et al: Controlled comparison of a new sublingual lormetazepam formulation and IV diazepam in outpatient minor oral surgery. *Br J Anaesth* 60:419–425, 1988.

35. Brandes W, Santiago T, Limacher M: Nitroglycerin-induced hypotension, bradycardia, and asystole: report of a case and review of the literature. *Clin Cardiol* 13:741–744, 1990.

36. Kestenbaum MG, Vilches AO, Messersmith S, et al: Alternative routes to oral opioid administration in palliative care: a review and clinical summary. *Pain Med* 15(7):1129–1153, 2014.

37. Leppert W, Krajnik M, Wordliczek J: Delivery systems of opioid analgesics for pain relief: a review. *Curr Pharma Des.* 19(41):7271–7293, 2013.

38. Portenoy RK, Payne R, Coluzzi P, et al: Oral transmucosal fentanyl citrate (OTFC) for the treatment of breakthrough pain in cancer patients: a controlled dose titration study. *Pain* 79:303–312, 1999.

39. Rhiner M, Kedziera P: Managing breakthrough cancer pain: a new approach. *Home Healthc Nurse* 17(Suppl):1–12, quiz 13–15, 1999.

40. Lichtor JL, Sevarino FB, Joshi GP, et al: The relative potency of oral transmucosal fentanyl citrate compared with intravenous morphine in the treatment of moderate to severe postoperative pain. *Anesth Analg* 89:732–738, 1999.

41. Ginsberg B, Dear RB, Margolis JO, et al: Oral transmucosal fentanyl citrate as an anaesthetic premedication when dosed to an opioid effect vs. total opioid consumption. *Paediatr Anaesth* 8:413–418, 1998.

42. Dsida RM, Wheeler M, Birmingham PK, et al: Premedication of pediatric tonsillectomy patients with oral transmucosal fentanyl citrate. *Anesth Analg* 86:66–70, 1998.

43. Streisand JB, Stanley TH, Hague B, et al: Oral transmucosal fentanyl citrate premedication in children. *Anesth Analg* 69:28–34, 1989.

44. Stanley TH, Hague B, Mock DL, et al: Oral transmucosal fentanyl citrate (lollipop) premedication in human volunteers. *Anesth Analg* 69:21–27, 1989.

45. Stanley TH, Leiman BC, Rawal N, et al: The effects of oral transmucosal fentanyl citrate premedication on preoperative behavioral responses and gastric volumes and acidity in children. *Anesth Analg* 69:328–335, 1989.

46. Nelson PS, Streisand JB, Mulder SM, et al: Comparison of oral transmucosal fentanyl citrate and an oral solution of meperidine, diazepam, and atropine for premedication in children. *Anesthesiology* 70:616–621, 1989.

47. Lind GH, Marcus MA, Mears SL, et al: Oral transmucosal fentanyl citrate for analgesia and sedation in the emergency department. *Ann Emerg Med* 20:1117–1120, 1991.

48. Friesen RH, Lockhart CH: Oral transmucosal fentanyl citrate for preanesthetic medication of pediatric day surgery patients with and without droperidol as a prophylactic anti-emetic. *Anesthesiology* 76:46–51, 1992.

49. Feld LH, Champeau MW, van Steennis CA, et al: Preanesthetic medication in children: a comparison of oral transmucosal fentanyl citrate versus placebo. *Anesthesiology* 71:374–377, 1989.

50. Ashburn MA, Streisand JB, Tarver SD, et al: Oral transmucosal fentanyl citrate for premedication in paediatric outpatients. *Can J Anaesth* 37:857–866, 1990.

51. Garzone PD, Kroboth PD: Pharmacokinetics of the newer benzodiazepines. *Clin Pharmacokinet* 16(6):337–364, 1989.

52. Nordstrom K, Allen MH: Alternative delivery systems for agents to treat acute agitation: progress to date. *Drugs* 73(16):1783–1792, 2013.

53. Zhang H, Zhang J, Streisand JB: Oral mucosal drug delivery: clinical pharmacokinetics and therapeutic applications. *Clin Pharmacokinet* 41(9):661–680, 2002.

54. Ranade VV: Drug delivery systems. 6. Transdermal drug delivery. *J Clin Pharmacol* 31:401–418, 1991.

55. Merkle HP: Transdermal delivery systems. *Methods Find Exp Clin Pharmacol* 11:135–153, 1989.

56. Asmussen B: Transdermal therapeutic systems: actual state and future developments. *Methods Find Exp Clin Pharmacol* 13:343–351, 1991.

57. Todd PA, Goa KL, Langtry HD: Transdermal nitroglycerin (glyceryl trinitrate): a review of its pharmacology and therapeutic use. *Drugs* 40(6):880–902, 1990.

58. Scopoderm: transdermal hyoscine for motion sickness. *Drug Ther Bull* 27:91–92, 1989.

59. Parrott AC: Transdermal scopolamine: a review of its effects upon motion sickness, psychological performance, and physiological functioning. *Aviat Space Environ Med* 60:1–9, 1989.

60. Lowenthat DT, Matzek KM, MacGregor TR: Clinical pharmacokinetics of clonidine. *Clin Pharmacokinet* 14:287–310, 1988.

61. Balfour JA, Heel RC: Transdermal estradiol: a review of its pharmacodynamic and pharmacokinetic properties, and therapeutic efficacy in the treatment of menopausal complaints. *Drugs* 40:561–582, 1990.

62. Simon JA, Carmody TP, Hudes ES, et al: Intensive smoking cessation counseling versus minimal counseling among hospitalized smokers treated with transdermal nicotine replacement: a randomized trial. *Am J Med* 114(7):555–562, 2003.

63. Chiou TJ, Liu CY, Tzeng WF, et al: The use of transdermal fentanyl in cancer pain—a compliance study of outpatients in Taiwan. *Am J Hosp Palliat Care* 27(1):31–37, 2010.

64. Samala RV, Bloise R, Davis MP: Efficacy and safety of a six-hour continuous overlap method for converting intravenous to transdermal fentanyl in cancer pain. *J Pain Symptom Manage* 48(1):132–136, 2014.

65. Calis KA, Kohler DR, Corso DM: Transdermally administered fentanyl for pain management. *Clin Pharm* 11:22–36, 1992.

66. Geraets D, Burke T: Sustained-release dosage forms. *Iowa Med* 80:141–146, 1990.

67. Wiechers JW: The barrier function of the skin in relation to percutaneous absorption of drugs. *Pharm Weekbl (sci ed)* 11:185–198, 1989.

68. Xu P, Chien YW: Enhanced skin permeability for transdermal drug delivery: physiopathological and physiochemical considerations. *Crit Rev Ther Drug Carrier Syst* 8:211–236, 1991.

69. Karzel K, Liedtke RK: Mechanisms of transcutaneous absorption: pharmacologic and biochemical aspects. *Arzneimittelforschung* 39:1487–1491, 1989.

70. Shah KR, Ng S, Zeoli L, et al: Hercon technology for transdermal delivery of drugs. *J Biomater Appl* 1:239–273, 1986.

71. Hogan DJ, Maibach HI: Adverse dermatologic reactions to transdermal drug delivery systems. *J Am Acad Dermatol* 22:811–814, 1990.

72. Anderson KA: A practical guide to nitrate use. *Postgrad Med* 89(1):67–70, 75–76, 78, 1991.

73. Mosser KH: Transdermal fentanyl in cancer pain. *Am Fam Physician* 45:2289–2294, 1992.

74. Clotz MA, Nahata MC: Clinical uses of fentanyl, sufentanil, and alfentanil. *Clin Pharm* 10:581–593, 1991.

75. Clissold SP, Heel RC: Transdermal hyoscine (scopolamine): a preliminary review of its pharmacodynamic properties and therapeutic efficacy. *Drugs* 29:189–207, 1985.

76. Schuh R, Tolksdorf W, Hucke H: Transdermal scopolamine or droperidol in the prevention of postoperative nausea and vomiting in cholecystectomy patients. *Anaesthesiol Intensivmed Notfallmed* 22:261–266, 1987.

77. Palazzo MG, Strunin L: Anaesthesia and emesis. I: etiology. *Can Anaesthet Soc J* 31:178–187, 1984.

78. Wilton NCT, Leigh J, Rosen DR, et al: Preanesthetic sedation of preschool children using intranasal midazolam. *Anesthesiology* 69:972–975, 1988.

79. Saint-Maurice C, Landais A, Delleur MM, et al: The use of midazolam in diagnostic and short surgical procedures in children. *Acta Anaesthes Scand* 92(Suppl):39–41, 1990.

80. Sarkar MA: Drug metabolism in the nasal mucosa. *Pharmaceut Res* 9(1):1–9, 1992.

81. Fukuta O, Braham RL, Yanase H, et al: Intranasal administration of midazolam: pharmacokinetic and pharmacodynamic properties and sedative potential. *ASDC J Dent Child* 64(2):89–98, 1997.

82. Rey E, Delaunay L, Pons G, et al: Pharmacokinetics of midazolam in children: comparative study of intranasal and intravenous administration. *Eur J Clin Pharmacol* 41:355–357, 1991.

83. Walbergh EJ, Wills RJ, Eckhert J: Plasma concentrations of midazolam in children following intranasal administration. *Anesthesiology* 74(2):233–235, 1991.

84. Buenz R, Gossler M: Intranasal premedication of young children using midazolam (Dormicum): clinical experience. *Anaesthesiol Intensivmed Notfallmed Schmerzther* 26(2):76–78, 1991.

85. de Santos P, Chabas E, Valero R, et al: Comparison of intramuscular and intranasal premedication with midazolam in children. *Rev Esp Anesthesiol Reanimac* 38:12–15, 1991.

86. Rose E, Simon D, Haberer JP: Premedication with intranasal midazolam in pediatric anesthesia. *Ann Fr Anesth Reanim* 9(4):326–330, 1990.

87. Karl HW, Keifer AT, Rosenberger JL, et al: Comparison of the safety and efficacy of intranasal midazolam and sufentanil for preinduction of anesthesia in pediatric patients. *Anesthesiology* 76:209–215, 1992.

88. Vercauteren M, Boech E, Hanegreefs H, et al: Intranasal sufentanil for pre-operative sedation. *Anaesthesia* 43:270–273, 1988.

89. Tolksdorf W, Eick C: Rectal, oral and nasal premedication using midazolam in children aged 1-6 years: a comparative clinical study. *Anaesthetist* 40(12):661–667, 1991.

90. Gobeaux D, Sardnal F, Cohn H, et al: Intranasal midazolam in pediatric ophthalmology. *Cah Anesthesiol* 39:34–36, 1991.

91. Lui CY, Amidon GL, Goldberg A: Intranasal absorption of flurazepam, midazolam, and triazolam in dogs. *J Pharm Sci* 80(12):1125–1129, 1991.

92. Theissen O, Boileau S, Wahl D, et al: Sedation with intranasal midazolam for endoscopy of the upper digestive tract. *Ann Fr Anesth Reanim* 10:450–455, 1991.

93. Lam C, Udin RD, Malamed SF, et al: Midazolam premedication in children: a pilot study comparing intramuscular and intranasal administration. *Anesth Prog* 52(2):56–61, 2005.

94. Primosch RE, Guelmann M: Comparison of drops versus spray administration of intranasal midazolam in two- and three-year-old children for dental sedation. *Pediatr Dent* 27(5):401–408, 2005.

95. Wood M: The safety and efficacy of intranasal midazolam sedation combined with inhalation sedation with nitrous oxide and oxygen in paediatric dental patients as an alternative to general anaesthesia. *SAAD Dig* 26:12–22, 2010.

96. Johnson E, Briskie D, Majewski R, et al: The physiologic and behavioral effects of oral and intranasal midazolam in pediatric dental patients. *Pediatr Dent* 32(3):229–238, 2010.

97. Heard C, Smith J, Creighton P, et al: A comparison of four sedation techniques for pediatric dental surgery. *Paediatr Anaesth* 20(10):924–930, 2010.

98. Wood M: The safety and efficacy of using a concentrated intranasal midazolam formulation for paediatric dental sedation. *SAAD Dig* 27:16–23, 2011.

99. Chopra R, Mittal M, Bansal K, Chaudhuri P: Buccal midazolam spray as an alternative to intranasal route for conscious sedation in pediatric dentistry. *J Clin Pediatr Dent* 38(2):171–173, 2013.

100. Manani G, Facco E, Cordioli A, et al: Bispectral Index in the sedation with intranasal midazolam and intravenous diazepam in dental practice. *Minerva Stomatol* 56(3):85–104, 2007.

101. Helmers JH, Noorduin H, van Peer A, et al: Comparison of intravenous and intranasal sufentanil absorption and sedation. *Can J Anaesth* 36:494–497, 1989.

102. Henderson JM, Brodsky DA, Fisher DM, et al: Pre-induction of anesthesia in pediatric patients with nasally administered sufentanil. *Anesthesiology* 68:671–675, 1988.

103. Steenblik J, Goodman M, Davis V, et al: Intranasal sufentanil for the treatment of acute pain in a winter resort clinic. *Am J Emerg Med* 30(9):1817–1821, 2012.

104. Stephen R, Lingenfelter E, Broadwater-Hollifield C, Madsen T: Intranasal sufentanil provides adequate analgesia for emergency department patients with extremity injuries. *J Opioid Manag* 8(4):237–241, 2012.

105. Nielsen BN, Friis SM, Romsing J, et al: Intranasal sufentanil/ketamine analgesia in children. *Paediatr Anaesth* 24(2):170–180, 2014.

chapter 10

Intramuscular Sedation

The intramuscular (IM) route of drug administration is a parenteral technique in which the drug enters the cardiovascular system (CVS) without first passing through the gastrointestinal (GI) tract. Parenteral techniques possess an advantage over enteral techniques (oral, rectal) in that the drug does not first have to pass through the enterohepatic circulation before entering the systemic circulation. This eliminates several disadvantages of enteral routes, including the hepatic first-pass effect, presence of food in the stomach, and delayed gastric emptying. The advantages and disadvantages of the IM route were discussed in Chapter 3 and are summarized in Box 10.1.

Probably the most significant negative aspect of using the IM route is an inability to titrate the drug to a desired clinical effect. The dentist is unable to consistently predict the proper dose to administer in any given patient, leading to the use of an "educated guesstimate" based on a number of factors to be discussed shortly. Although the dose is often appropriate, situations occur in which the calculated dose proves ineffective, leading to an inability to treat the patient. More significant,

however, are those occasions when the calculated dose has proven too great for the patient, leading to possibly dire consequences for both the patient and the dentist.[1-5]

The IM route of drug administration is indicated for use in almost any patient; however, several factors must be considered in determining the depth of sedation that can (and should) safely be sought via this route. As mentioned, inability to titrate is a prime negative consideration, as is the inability to rapidly reverse the actions of the drug.

Suggested uses of the IM route in the dental office include the following:

1. The adult patient when other, more controllable, parenteral routes (intravenous [IV], inhalation) are unavailable
2. The precooperative pediatric patient in whom other routes have proven ineffective
3. The disruptive handicapped adult or child patient in whom other routes have proven ineffective
4. The disruptive pediatric patient or adult or child with a disability, for use as premedication before the use of IV sedation or general anesthesia

Box 10.1	Advantages/Disadvantages of Intramuscular Drug Administration
Advantages	**Disadvantages**
Rapid onset of action (10–15 min)	Inability to titrate (10–15 min onset)
Maximal clinical effect (30 min)	Inability to reverse drug action
More reliable absorption than oral, rectal	Prolonged duration of drug effect
Patient cooperation not as essential	Injection needed
	Possible needle-stick injury

5. The administration of emergency drugs to any patient in whom the IV route is unavailable

The last factor, the administration of emergency drugs, is the reason I believe that all dental personnel should be trained to administer drugs intramuscularly. Although IV drug administration is more rapidly effective, in an emergency situation, the IM route may be the only practical route immediately available.

The level of central nervous system (CNS) depression sought via the IM route will vary considerably, from minimal sedation in a frightened but otherwise healthy adult, to moderate or deep levels of sedation in the unmanageable child or adult or patient with a disability in whom the only alternative to IM sedation is general anesthesia. It must be stated here (as it is repeatedly throughout this text) that the dentist administering drugs to a patient must know his or her limitations in drug usage. Important factors in deciding the depth of sedation to which a patient may safely be brought include (1) the physical status of the patient, (2) the training of the dentist and staff, and (3) the availability of trained personnel and equipment for the prompt and effective management of any emergency situation that might conceivably arise as a result of the use of a drug or coincident with its use—the concept of "rescue" from a more profound level of CNS depression than that sought. Deep sedation must not be employed by a dentist who is not well versed in the art and science of anesthesiology and in the management of the unconscious airway.

All 50 states in the United States and most provinces in Canada require a dentist employing parenteral (IM/intranasal [IN]/IV) sedation to obtain a specific parenteral sedation permit from their state or provincial dental board. Requirements for parenteral sedation permits vary from jurisdiction to jurisdiction, but all take into account the degree of education in the technique, preparedness for emergencies, and demonstrated clinical proficiency.[6]

In the healthy adult, there are few indications for IM sedation. Most adults, although not "liking it," will tolerate an IM injection of a drug. If the patient can psychologically tolerate this traumatic event (the "sticking of a needle into the skin

[muscle]"), the IV route of administration is preferred. The IV route is more controllable than is the IM route. If a needle is to be inserted into a patient's body for the purpose of administering a CNS-depressant drug, it is much preferred, for reasons of safety and effectiveness, to administer such drugs intravenously. IV administration offers immensely more control over the drug's actions, and in many cases, unwanted reactions to the drug can be quickly reversed (e.g., with the IV administration of naloxone or flumazenil). In the absence of superficial veins, elective venipuncture and IV moderate sedation are contraindicated; the inability to breathe through the nose or adverse clinical experience in the past with inhalation sedation contraindicates nitrous oxide–oxygen (N_2O-O_2). In these situations, IM moderate sedation in an adult patient should receive serious consideration.

In the child, the IM route is more frequently indicated. Both IV and inhalation moderate sedation require a degree of patient cooperation to be successful. The overtly disruptive child will neither permit a venipuncture nor allow a nasal hood to be placed and maintained over his or her nose, thereby dooming these two valuable techniques to failure. In such a situation, the IM (or IN—see Chapter 9) route may be the only sedative route with a likelihood of success. Failure of the IM technique most likely means that the patient will have to receive dental care under general anesthesia.

Some patients with physical or mental disabilities, both pediatric and adult, are unable to tolerate dental care in the usual manner and are therefore candidates for sedative techniques. Although many of these patients are manageable with oral, inhalation, or IV moderate sedation, disruptive patients with disabilities may require IM drug administration as a means of calming them before the use of other, more controllable sedation techniques.

Another use of the IM route in dentistry is the administration of nonsedative drugs. These drugs may also be administered orally or rectally; however, because of the greatly increased reliability of absorption and greater efficacy noted with the IM route, this technique should be considered when these drugs are used. Drugs commonly administered via this route are the anticholinergics (atropine, scopolamine, glycopyrrolate), nonsteroidal antiinflammatory drugs (NSAIDs, e.g., ketorolac), and the antiemetics (ondansetron [Zofran], promethazine). These drugs are discussed later in this chapter. The suggested uses of IM drug administration in dentistry are presented in Box 10.2.

SUBMUCOSAL SEDATION

A variation on IM drug administration called *submucosal (SM) administration* has been used in pediatric dentistry.[7] In the SM technique, a CNS-depressant drug is injected into the mucous membrane in either the maxillary or mandibular buccal fold. An advantage of SM administration over IM administration is a slightly more rapid—but not clinically significant—onset of clinical action.[8,9] However, this same rapid onset of action may

Box 10.2 **Recommended Use of the Intramuscular Route**

For Sedation in the Following Types of Patients
1. The adult patient, when inhalation and IV routes are unavailable
2. The disruptive pediatric or adult patient in whom other routes have proven ineffective
3. The disruptive child or adult with disabilities in whom other routes have proven ineffective

Uses of the Intramuscular Route
1. Premedication before IV sedation or general anesthesia in the precooperative pediatric patient or adult or pediatric patient with disabilities
2. Administration of antiemetics, NSAIDs, or anticholinergics
3. Administration of emergency drugs when IV administration is not available

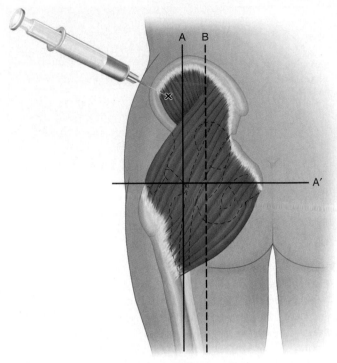

Figure 10.1 Gluteal region, divided into quadrants. The upper outer quadrant is the recommended site for IM injection. Lines A and A′ represent boundaries in classic IM technique. Line B demonstrates the ease with which a landmark may be displaced, increasing the risk of sciatic nerve injury.

also be associated with a more rapid appearance of undesirable drug actions, such as respiratory depression. As originally developed, the SM route was used for the administration of opioid agonists (OAs), such as alphaprodine.[10] The technique has fallen into disrepute because of a significant number of serious adverse reactions that were noted in conjunction with the SM administration of alphaprodine.[1–3,7] The SM route is discussed in greater detail in Chapter 35.

SITES OF INTRAMUSCULAR DRUG ADMINISTRATION

Four sites are available for IM drug administration.[11-13] Proper site selection varies from patient to patient and is an important factor in the safety of this technique. The sites most commonly chosen for the administration of IM drugs are the following:
1. Gluteal area
2. Ventrogluteal area
3. Vastus lateralis
4. Deltoid area

Each potential site for IM drug administration has specific advantages and disadvantages that must be considered before final site selection is made.

Gluteal Area

The upper outer quadrant of the gluteal region is the most commonly used site for IM drug administration in adults.[14] The gluteus maximus is the muscle most commonly used.

The gluteal region extends superiorly to the anterior superior iliac spine (Fig. 10.1). With this as a landmark, the region is divided into quadrants. The upper outer quadrant is the most anatomically safe because it is distant from the sciatic nerve

and the superior gluteal artery.[15] The lower inner aspect of the upper outer quadrant is the preferred site within this quadrant.

The gluteal region in the adult can accept 4 to 8 mL of solution.[12,15] In addition, the skin of this region is relatively thin and is more easily penetrated by the needle.

The upper inner quadrant is unacceptable as an IM injection site because it contains the roots of the sacral plexus. The lower inner quadrant contains the sciatic nerve. Ceravolo et al[14] report a nerve injury rate of up to 8% following IM injection into the gluteal region.

For injection into the upper outer quadrant, the patient should be lying face down on a bed or examining table with the toes in and arms hanging off the table.[16] This permits maximal relaxation. Although this site is also used with the patient standing, it is not as highly recommended because the muscles do not relax as well in this position. Muscle tissue that is contracted does not accommodate the injected fluid, forcing it upward into the subcutaneous tissues, where absorption is less reliable and slower and where certain drugs are more likely to produce tissue irritation and damage. In addition, the administration of IM drugs into contracted muscle is thought to be more uncomfortable than IM injection into relaxed muscle.[13]

Of the four available IM injection sites, the gluteal region is the least well perfused, having 20% lower perfusion than

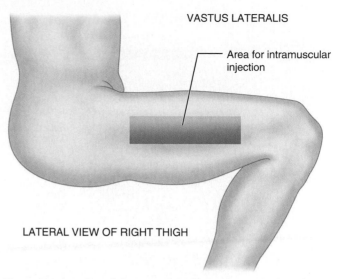

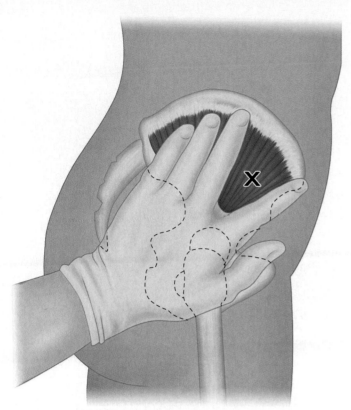

Figure 10.2 Ventrogluteal region. Index finger locates anterior iliac spine; index and middle fingers spread apart forming a V. Needle puncture occurs between fingers (X) and is aimed toward the iliac crest.

Figure 10.3 Location of the vastus lateralis site on anterior lateral aspect of thigh, the preferred site for IM drug administration in infants and children.

the deltoid.[17] Because perfusion is the rate-limiting step in the absorption of IM drugs, the rate of onset of action of drugs administered in the gluteal region is somewhat slower than when alternative sites are used.[12,15]

The gluteal region requires a degree of patient disrobing for the injection to be properly administered. This may, in some instances, limit the utility of the gluteal region in the adult patient within the dental office; however, with assistance from the parent or guardian, this site may readily be employed in the pediatric patient with little or no loss of modesty.

Ventrogluteal Region

The ventrogluteal region lies in close proximity to the gluteal region. Its primary use is for IM injection in patients who are bedridden and unable to lie face down.[15]

The site is located among three bony landmarks that are usually quite readily palpated. These are the anterior superior iliac spine, the iliac crest, and the greater trochanter of the femur. Anatomically, this region lies at some distance from the sciatic nerve and other anatomically important structures.[16]

For this site to be properly used, the anterior superior iliac spine is located with the tip of the index finger (Fig. 10.2). The left hand is pressed onto the hip with the palm of the hand over the greater trochanter and the fingers pointed toward

the patient's head. The index and middle fingers are spread as far as possible, forming a V, with the tip of the ventrally placed finger pressed down on the soft tissue over the anterior superior iliac spine, preventing movement of the skin. The needle puncture is made between these fingers and aimed just below the iliac crest.

The ventrogluteal region in an adult is capable of managing 4 to 8 mL of solution. This site is rarely used in the typical dental office situation. Where bedridden patients are treated, this IM site warrants consideration.

Vastus Lateralis

The anterior aspect of the thigh is probably the safest region in which to deposit IM drugs. Although not of consequence in the typical dental situation, the vastus lateralis can accommodate volumes of solution up to 15 mL, whereas the gluteal and ventrogluteal can accommodate approximately 4 to 8 mL each before muscle distortion and dissection occur, leading to increased pain during and after injection.

The site for injection in the vastus lateralis muscle is a narrow rectangular band running along the anterior lateral aspect of the thigh (Fig. 10.3). The region begins approximately one handbreadth above the knee and runs to the same distance below the greater trochanter of the femur.[16]

Anatomically the vastus lateralis site contains no structures of importance (Fig. 10.4). Overly deep penetration of the needle may strike the femur, resulting in discomfort and possible needle breakage. All significant anatomic structures are located on the medial and posterior aspects of the thigh (the femoral artery and vein and the sciatic nerve).

This site is strongly recommended for use in small children.[12] Injection in the gluteal muscles is contraindicated in children who have not yet begun to walk because of the lack of maturity

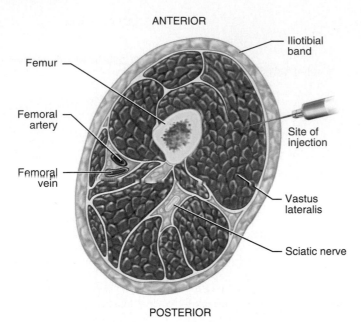

Figure 10.4 Cross-section through vastus lateralis injection site, illustrating location of anatomically significant structures.

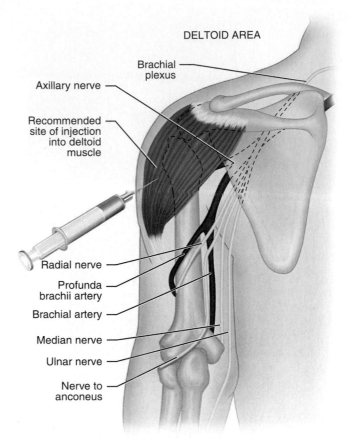

Figure 10.5 Middeltoid injection site in upper third of arm.

and development of their gluteal musculature. The gluteal region ought not to be chosen until at least 1 full year after the child has begun to walk.[18]

Some degree of disrobing is required when the vastus lateralis site is used. The site is more readily accessible in the woman wearing a skirt or dress, but it is of absolute importance that a female assistant be present with the dentist in the treatment room throughout the time that the injection is given. In any patient wearing pants or slacks, a greater degree of disrobing is required, a fact that might discourage use of this site. In the pediatric patient, the vastus lateralis may readily be employed with assistance from the patient's parent or guardian.

In adult or larger pediatric patients who are unmanageable (e.g., combative) and when IM drug administration is considered mandatory, IM injection into the vastus lateralis muscle through the patient's clothing is appropriate. Although sterile technique cannot be maintained in this situation, it is unlikely that complications will be noted. This consideration is of special importance when a life-threatening situation develops (e.g., anaphylaxis) and immediate drug therapy is warranted (e.g., epinephrine).

The vastus lateralis muscle is capable of receiving 8 to 15 mL of injected drug (in adults) without distortion or dissection of muscle fibers. This represents the largest available reservoir for IM drugs in the adult body.

Deltoid

The deltoid muscle is easily accessible in the upper third of the arm. The injection is given between the upper and lower portions of the deltoid muscle (Fig. 10.5), thereby avoiding the radial nerve.

The boundaries of the deltoid region form a rectangle. The superior border is formed by the lower edge of the acromion (the outward extension of the spine of the scapula). The inferior boundary lies opposite the axilla or armpit. The side boundaries are two lines drawn parallel to the arm, about one third to two thirds of the way around the lateral aspect of the upper arm.

Advantages of the deltoid region include easy access in most patients. It is important that the patient not be permitted to simply roll up the shirt sleeve to expose the injection site because if the sleeve is tight, it may not permit visualization of the entire site, in which case the injection might be administered inferior to the desired area and in too close proximity to the radial nerve. The patient should be required to remove the shirt or blouse to expose the entire injection site. A female assistant must be with the dentist (male or female) if the patient is female. Another positive factor in the deltoid region is more rapid absorption of the injected drug into the CVS than is seen with any of the other IM injection sites. Perfusion is 20% greater in the deltoid region than in the gluteal region.[15] The deltoid region is not recommended for use in the infant or child who has not yet begun to walk.[12]

Table 10.1	Comparison of Intramuscular Injection Sites				
IM INJECTION SITE	PERFUSION*	ADULT (ML)	INFANT	CHILD	ADULT
Vastus lateralis	2	8–15	+	+	+
Gluteal/ventrogluteal	3	4–8	–	–	+/–
Deltoid	1	4	–	–	+
*1, Most vascular; 2, moderate vascular; 3, least vascular.					

The degree of disrobing required to visualize the injection site is not usually of significance in the deltoid region, making this the most easily used IM injection site in dentistry. This site may be used with the patient lying down, sitting, or standing.

Probably the only negative feature of this site, other than the anatomy, is its lack of size; it is able to accommodate only up to 4 mL of solution (adult). However, this is not of significance in dentistry because it is rare to ever administer more than 3 mL intramuscularly. Giovannitti and Trapp[19] suggest the deltoid muscle as the preferred site for IM sedation in the dental environment.

Site Selection

Selection of the site for IM injection in dentistry is predicated on several factors, including the size (age) of the patient, degree of patient cooperation, and volume of solution to be injected. In the younger (smaller) pediatric patient, the preferred site for IM injection is the vastus lateralis, whereas in older children the vastus lateralis and the deltoid regions are recommended. In the adult, the preferred sites for IM injection are the deltoid region, vastus lateralis, and both gluteal injection sites. Table 10.1 compares the four IM injection sites.

ARMAMENTARIUM

Very few items are required for IM drug administration. Included in this list are the following:
1. Sterile, disposable syringe (1 to 2 mL) with needle (18, 20, or 21 gauge) of appropriate length
2. Alcohol sponges
3. Sterile gauze
4. Band-Aid type of bandage
5. Desired drug

TECHNIQUE

The appropriate injection site for the IM injection must be selected. After disrobing the patient, if necessary, the dentist must carefully palpate the site on every patient to determine the precise anatomic landmarks. Visual examination alone should never be relied on to determine landmarks. From the point of view of propriety (and medicolegally), it is important that the dentist have another staff member present in the treatment room during the injection, especially if the patient

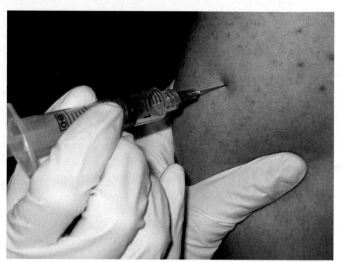

Figure 10.6 Area to be injected is grasped with one hand, holding tissue taut, while the syringe, held in a dartlike grasp, is inserted to the proper depth. (From Malamed SF: *Medical emergencies in the dental office*, ed 7, St Louis, 2015, Elsevier Mosby.)

is of the opposite sex from the dentist. The following are step-by-step instructions for the administration of an IM injection.[12,16,20]

1. Cleanse the skin thoroughly using a suitable antiseptic (e.g., isopropyl alcohol). Apply friction while cleansing the area with a circular motion from the injection site outward. The antiseptic should be permitted to dry before injection. Injection into a moistened area may introduce antiseptic into the tissues, which will lead to discomfort and possibly to tissue irritation.
2. Grasp the tissue to be injected with one hand, keeping the tissue taut. Holding the syringe in a dartlike grasp, introduce the needle to its appropriate depth (deep within muscle tissue) with one quick motion. Although the depth of insertion will vary from patient to patient, the needle should not be inserted, for safety reasons, more than approximately three-fourths of its length into tissue (Fig. 10.6).
3. With the needle at its proper depth, aspirate, pulling the plunger of the syringe back slightly to determine whether the needle tip lies within the lumen of a blood vessel. Rotate the syringe a quarter turn and reaspirate to ensure that the needle tip was not lying against the wall of a vessel. If blood appears in the syringe at any time, withdraw the syringe

from the tissue and prepare a different injection site. In the uncooperative pediatric or adult patient, it may prove difficult or impossible to perform this step as described. Aspiration should be performed whenever possible before IM injection.

4. Following negative aspiration, inject the drug slowly. In most IM injections, the solution flows quite easily into the tissues. Rapid injection produces increased patient discomfort and should be avoided. Release the pressure that has been maintained on the tissues during needle insertion. Maintaining the pressure during injection of the drug may force solution to backtrack along the path of needle insertion into the subcutaneous tissues, where tissue irritation may occur, or out of the tissue through the injection site. Release of pressure prevents this from occurring.

5. Holding a dry, sterile gauze in the other hand (non–syringe-holding hand), slowly withdraw the needle from the tissue. Place the dry gauze over the puncture point for approximately 2 minutes to prevent bleeding. A bandage can be placed over the site after this time. Care must be taken with the now-contaminated needle to prevent accidental percutaneous puncture of the treating staff. The used needle and syringe should be disposed of in a sharps container.

6. Massage or rub the injection site to increase the blood flow through the area and speed up drug absorption.

7. Record in the patient's chart the date, time of injection, site of injection, drug used, and dose.

8. Observe the patient during the post-IM injection period for the onset of sedation and/or undesirable actions (e.g., syncope, overdose, allergy).

COMPLICATIONS

Although rare, complications can arise after IM drug administration. In most cases, the complication appears to be directly related to the site of needle entry and drug deposition.[21,22]

The needle itself produces injury to structures through which it passes. Nerve damage, consisting of paralysis (usually of the sciatic nerve in gluteal injection), hyperesthesia, or paresthesia, has been reported after IM injection. In addition, inadvertent IV and intraarterial (IA) drug administration have occurred, as well as air embolism, periostitis, and hematoma. Many of these complications have potentially serious consequences, and, of course, steps should be taken to prevent their occurrence. Knowledge of anatomy and proper injection technique will minimize these complications.

The drugs that are administered intramuscularly are, in some cases, capable of producing injury to the tissues into which they are deposited. Injuries such as *abscess, cyst* and *scar formation,* and *necrosis* and *sloughing of skin* at the injection site may occur. Although these are potential complications with all drugs, there are a few drugs that, because of their pH or viscosity, are more apt to produce these problems. These drugs include diazepam and hydroxyzine. Improper injection technique, specifically when the drug has not been injected

deep into the muscle or when the tissue is kept taut following the injection of the drug with leakage of the drug into the subcutaneous tissues as the needle is withdrawn, is a common cause of this problem.

Nerve injury of any type is managed conservatively. In many cases, the injury may not be noted by the patient for several days following the IM injection or, in the case of a younger patient or a patient with a disability, possibly for several months, thus emphasizing the importance of precise recordkeeping. The site of injection should always be recorded when an IM drug is given. When injury is detected, the patient should return to the office so that the nature and extent of the injury may be noted on the chart. Unless the injury is severe, the management of choice for most nerve injury is "tincture of time." Most minor traumatic nerve injuries resolve with time. In most instances, normal function returns within 6 months. The patient should be advised of this time factor at the onset. A few cases of nerve injury do not resolve completely within 6 months and require additional time (an unknown duration) or may never return completely to normal function. Periodic examination of the patient during this time span (e.g., once every month) is recommended to keep the dentist informed of any progress and to keep the patient aware of the dentist's concern.

Discomfort secondary to the injury should be manageable with mild analgesics, such as aspirin, or another NSAID such as ibuprofen. If more potent analgesics are required, consultation with a physician is recommended because this might indicate a greater degree of injury.

If the injury appears more severe at the onset, the patient should be referred to a physician, preferably a neurologist, for examination. Medical management usually is consistent with that described. Referral to a physician should also be given serious consideration if the patient appears to be dissatisfied with the progress of his or her recovery or with the management of the injury by the "dental doctor." Before referral of the patient to the physician, a telephone call from the dentist explaining the circumstances surrounding the case is appropriate.

Although legal action following nerve injury does occur, the number of such cases is extremely small. A patient who is satisfied with their treatment is less likely to initiate a legal action than the patient who believes that the care rendered is below the usual standard.

Inadvertent IV or *IA* drug administration ought to never occur. Proper IM technique requires aspiration before injection of the drug. The presence of blood in the syringe indicates a positive aspiration. The dentist should remove the syringe from the injection site, apply pressure to the site to prevent hematoma, and inject the patient at a different location.

Because the drugs administered for sedation are CNS depressants, clinical signs and symptoms attending this complication (accidental IV or IA administration) are related to the degree of CNS depression that develops. This may range from a slightly oversedated patient—one who is conscious but sedated to a degree beyond which the dentist feels comfortable—to the patient who may be unconscious but breathing (requiring airway management), to the unconscious patient whose breathing is quite depressed or who may be apneic. These latter patients require "rescue": airway management with assisted or controlled ventilation. The pharmacology and the cerebral blood level of the drug(s) injected determine the severity of the reaction that develops. Some sedative drugs, such as benzodiazepines (e.g., midazolam) and hydroxyzine, although capable of producing significant CNS depression, are less likely to than barbiturates (no longer recommended) and opioids.

Management (rescue) of an oversedated patient consists primarily of airway maintenance (A, airway) and, when necessary, assisted or controlled ventilation (B, breathing). In addition, some drugs, such as the opioids and benzodiazepines, have pharmacologic antagonists that may be administered in these circumstances. Their use and a more detailed discussion of the management of the oversedated patient are found in Chapters 27 and 34.

Air embolism has been reported after IM drug administration. With proper technique in loading a drug into a syringe, there ought not to be any air remaining in its barrel. In addition, avoidance of inadvertent intravascular injection (see previous discussion) will prevent this occurrence.

Periostitis is an inflammation of the periosteum. If acute, it may be associated with severe pain and suppuration. It occurs frequently secondary to infection. The condition usually becomes chronic in nature and is characterized by tenderness and swelling of the tissues overlying the bone. It can also be produced by the inadvertent striking of the needle against the periosteum during insertion. Proper technique involves grasping the tissue being injected between the fingers, pulling it away from the bone, and inserting the needle to the proper depth (varying from patient to patient and from site to site). This technique minimizes the development of periostitis.

If the patient complains of soreness, tenderness, and swelling at the site of an IM injection 2 days or more following injection, the complaint should be evaluated by bringing the patient to the office, examining the area, and, if necessary, seeking a medical consultation. Management of milder degrees of periostitis involves "tincture of time" and the maintenance of good relations with the patient. If signs of suppuration and swelling appear, antibiotics are indicated (usually penicillin). Medical consultation should be sought in this situation.

Hematoma is, by definition, a tumor consisting of effused blood. It develops following puncture of a blood vessel, either an artery or a vein. Clinically a small but gradually enlarging swelling, bluish in color, will be observed at the site of needle insertion, either during injection or, more commonly, after withdrawal of the needle from the tissues. Management consists of pressure applied directly to the site of bleeding for a minimum of 2 to 5 minutes. If the site subsequently becomes sore, heat can be applied to it (but not less than 4 hours after the bleeding ceases) and mild analgesics (e.g., NSAIDs) administered. The effused blood is gradually resorbed into the CVS, a process

requiring 7 to 10 days. Heat should not be applied to the site of a hematoma within the first few hours because heat produces vasodilation, which may restart the bleeding.

An *abscess* may occur after IM injection if either the needle or the solution injected was contaminated. Management consists of antibiotics (penicillin) and immediate medical consultation. Prevention consists of sterile technique in handling both drugs and equipment.

Cyst formation, *scarring*, and *necrosis* and *sloughing* of tissues may also occur. Although several factors may be responsible for these, many are produced by the tissues' reaction to the injected drug. Drugs that are irritating to the tissues are more commonly involved in these complications. Superficial injection of drugs is another possible cause of this problem. Management should consist of referral to a physician, preferably a dermatologist. Complications of IM injections are listed in Box 10.3.

DETERMINATION OF DOSAGE

The factors that influence the way in which a drug acts in a given patient were discussed in Chapters 3 and 7. With IM administration of CNS depressants, the influence of these various factors becomes quite important. How can the informed clinician safely determine the appropriate IM dose of the drug or drugs that are to be administered to a patient for intraoperative sedation?

Most IM drugs have their dosages determined, in large part, by the body weight of the patient. Although this is far from an absolute guarantee of proper dosage, in most cases, a therapeutically effective result will occur. Other factors that must be considered in determining dosage include the degree of anxiety, the level of sedation desired, the patient's age and health status, prior response of the patient to CNS-depressant drugs, and the education and experience of the drug's administrator.

For the adult patient, dosages for the drugs discussed are based primarily on body weight, expressed in milligrams per

---

Box 10.3   Complications of Intramuscular Injections

Nerve injury
Paralysis
Paresthesia
Hyperesthesia
Intravascular injection
Intravenous
Intraarterial
Air embolism
Periostitis
Hematoma
Abscess
Cyst and scar formation

kilogram (mg/kg) or milligrams per pound (mg/lb). From this calculated dose, the dentist will decrease or increase the actual dosage administered as determined from the other factors mentioned. For example, a patient weighing 70 kg is to receive a drug, the recommended dose of which is 1.0 mg/kg. The calculated dose of this drug for the patient is therefore 70 mg. If the patient were a healthy individual (American Society of Anesthesiologists [ASA] 1), this dose would be appropriate; however, if this patient is older, has a history of cardiovascular or other serious systemic disorders, or has a history of over-reaction to average drug dosages (is a hyperresponder), a smaller dose (e.g., 50 mg) might be administered. The level to which the drug dosage is decreased is left to the clinical judgment of the dentist administering it. Conversely, an ASA 1 patient demonstrating high levels of anxiety, with a history of hypo-responding to CNS-depressant drugs, might be administered a dose somewhat greater than that determined strictly by body weight.

In the pediatric patient, the same factors must be considered in determining drug dosage. The patient's age is often considered in determining the dosage of a drug. For example, for a given drug, the dose for a 3-year-old patient may be 12.5 mg, whereas the dose for a 4-year-old is 25 mg. Dosages based solely on the patient's age are apt to lead to inaccuracies because patients of the same age will vary considerably in physical stature and body weight. The patient's age should not be the primary factor by which the dose of a drug is determined.

Several rules have been used for years in the determination of pediatric drug dosages. *Clark's rule* takes the weight of the child in pounds and divides it by 150 (the weight of the average adult in pounds). The resultant fraction is multiplied by the adult dosage of the drug.

Clark's rule:

Pediatric dose $= (Weight\ of\ child\ [lb] \div 150) \times$ adult dose

Young's rule divides the age of the child in years by the age of the child plus 12 and then multiplies this number by the adult dose.

Young's rule:

$$Pediatric\ dose = (Age\ of\ child\ [yr] \div age\ of\ child + 12) \times$$
$$adult\ dose$$

A factor that has proven even more accurate in determining effective pediatric dosages is the body surface area of the patient. Table 10.2 permits a determination of the approximate surface area of the patient. The pediatric dosage is determined as a percentage of the usual adult dosage, based on the average adult surface area of 1.73 m^2.

Most of the drugs discussed in this chapter have their dosages presented on a milligram per kilogram (or pound) of body weight basis. Although not the most accurate method available, this remains the most frequently employed method of determining IM drug dosage. The reader may employ the surface area

Table 10.2	Determination of Children's Doses From Adult Doses on the Basis of Surface Area		
WEIGHT APPROXIMATE		**APPROXIMATE SURFACE AREA (M²)**	**PERCENTAGE OF ADULT DOSE***
(kg)	**(lb)**		
2	4.4	0.15	9
4	8.8	0.25	14
6	13.2	0.33	19
8	17.6	0.40	23
10	22.0	0.46	27
15	33.0	0.63	36
20	44.0	0.83	48
25	55.0	0.95	55
30	66.0	1.08	62
35	77.0	1.20	69
40	88.0	1.30	75
45	99.0	1.40	81
50	110.0	1.51	87
55	121.0	1.58	91

*Based on average adult surface area of 1.73 m².
From Modell W: *Modell's drugs in current use and new drugs*, ed 34, New York, 1988, Springer.

method of determining pediatric dosages for any drug listed in this book by simply referring to Table 10.2.

Dosages based on body weight (e.g., 1 mg/kg or 0.5 mg/lb) are determined by the middle of the "bell-shaped" curve (see Fig. 7.1). Approximately 70% of patients respond appropriately to this dose, with 15% undersedated. Unfortunately, another 15% respond in an exaggerated manner—oversedation.

The degree of education and experience of the drug administrator has a significant bearing on the level of CNS depression to which the patient may safely be taken, which will obviously influence the dosage of drug administered. Doctors who have completed residency training in anesthesiology (dentist anesthesiologists) will be better able to administer larger doses of drugs to patients in a safe manner than those who have completed a short postgraduate program (e.g., continuing education). All dental personnel involved in patient management should be adept in monitoring vital signs and in recognizing and managing life-threatening emergencies, including the ability to rescue the patient from an unintended lapse into a deeper level of CNS depression (e.g., perform basic life support).

DRUGS

A myriad of drugs are available for the management of anxiety via IM administration. The level of sedation may vary from lighter levels (minimal-to-moderate sedation) to levels

<table>
<tr><td>Box 10.4</td><td>Frequently Used Drugs via Intramuscular Administration</td></tr>
</table>

Antianxiety Drugs and Sedative-Hypnotics
Diazepam
Lorazepam
Midazolam

Histamine Blockers (Antihistamines)
Promethazine
Hydroxyzine

Opioid Analgesics
Morphine
Meperidine
Fentanyl

Opioid Agonist-Antagonists
Butorphanol
Nalbuphine

Dissociative Anesthetic
Ketamine hydrochloride

Anticholinergics
Atropine
Scopolamine
Glycopyrrolate

approaching unconsciousness (deep sedation). Although certain drugs are more apt to produce more profound sedation than others, any of the following drugs listed can produce overly deep sedation in certain patients (e.g., hyperresponders). When IM drug dosage is determined, it must always be remembered that the administrator cannot control the drug's action and that titration is not possible via this route. Care and prudence must be exercised whenever IM drugs are administered to all patients, but especially to pediatric, geriatric, or medically compromised patients. Box 10.4 lists drugs that are commonly given via IM administration in dentistry. As will be noted with specific drugs, different levels of training are recommended for their safe use. In some situations, the dentist should have received training in general anesthesia and be capable of managing the unconscious airway before ever considering the use of the drug in question.

Antianxiety Drugs and Sedative-Hypnotics

In this group of drugs—antianxiety and sedative-hypnotics—I have included the benzodiazepines and histamine blockers, drugs commonly used for minimal-to-moderate levels of sedation when given as solo agents. However, it is not uncommon to combine one of the drugs in this category with an opioid analgesic to provide deeper levels of sedation. When this is

done, it is necessary for the dentist and all staff members to have been thoroughly trained in general anesthesia and patient monitoring. The barbiturates were eliminated from discussion of IM drugs in the fifth edition of this textbook (2010). Negatives associated with their IM administration outweigh, in my mind, any benefit gained from their administration. Primary among these is the degree of respiratory depression seen at therapeutic levels of barbiturates. The reader is referred to previous editions of this textbook for any discussion of IM barbiturates.

Diazepam

Before the introduction of midazolam, diazepam (Valium) was commonly administered via the IM route in preoperative anxiety control in the hospital setting. It may also be given in dentistry via this route, but because of the availability of the IV route and the advantages of IM midazolam, diazepam is only rarely used IM in dentistry.

Another reason for the infrequent use of diazepam IM was the results of early studies on the absorption of diazepam from IM injection sites. Diazepam injectable is an extremely lipophilic drug, and early studies on absorption of IM diazepam were conflicting.[23-26] Peak plasma levels were noted 60 minutes after oral dosing, whereas IM dosing required 90 minutes.[26] Absorption of diazepam from IM injection sites may be slow or incomplete, or both, because of its lipophilic nature. However, another report indicates that IM diazepam absorption appears to be more rapid when the drug is injected into the deltoid rather than the gluteal or vastus lateralis muscle groups.[27] The most likely explanation is the higher blood flow per gram of tissue in the deltoid muscle group.[25] In the gluteal area, the depth of injection may be a factor in the completeness of absorption of diazepam. Given equal doses of diazepam via the oral and IM routes, the oral dose will be absorbed more completely than the IM dose, and in many cases, the rate of onset will be shorter via the oral route than with the IM route.[26] However, diazepam deposited deeply into muscle (preferably the deltoid) can produce satisfactory sedation in most patients.

Contraindications

Parenteral diazepam should be avoided in patients with known hypersensitivities to it or other benzodiazepines, in patients with acute narrow-angle glaucoma, and in patients with narrow-angle glaucoma unless they are receiving appropriate therapy.[28]

Warnings

When used in combination with other CNS depressants, particularly opioid analgesics, the dosage of the opioid should be decreased by approximately one third to minimize the occurrence of oversedation or of other more serious complications.

Diazepam should not be given during the first trimester of pregnancy because an increased risk of congenital malformations has been observed. Diazepam crosses the placental barrier, potentially producing depression of the fetus. Its use in pregnancy is not recommended (pregnancy category D).[28]

Injectable diazepam doses should be decreased when patients are receiving other CNS depressants, such as barbiturates, phenothiazines, opioids, and alcohol. Elderly and debilitated patients usually require decreased doses of diazepam to achieve a desired clinical effect.

Dosage

The IM route is usually not recommended due to slow and erratic absorption. Inject deeply into a large muscle mass. Aspirate before injection to avoid injection into a blood vessel.[28] The usual adult dose for preoperative sedation is 10 mg 30 minutes to 1 hour before treatment.[28] The preferred injection site for diazepam is the deltoid muscle. Regardless of the IM injection site, diazepam should be deposited deep into muscle to prevent discomfort and provide more reliable absorption. The dose for elderly or debilitated patients is 2 to 5 mg 30 minutes to 1 hour before treatment. The dose of parenteral diazepam for children should not exceed 0.25 mg/kg of body weight, administered deep into the gluteal or deltoid regions.[28] For example, a child weighing 20 kg (44 lb) will receive a dose of 5 mg IM diazepam. Since the introduction of midazolam, the IM use of diazepam has greatly diminished.

Availability

Diazepam: 5 mg/mL in 2-mL ampules and 10-mL vials; 5 mg/mL in 2-mL preloaded syringes. Injectable diazepam also contains 40% propylene glycol, 10% ethyl alcohol, 5% sodium benzoate, benzoic acid, and 1.5% benzyl alcohol. Diazepam is classified as a Schedule IV drug.

Diazepam	
Pregnancy category	D
Lactation	NS
Metabolism	Liver
Excretion	Urine
DEA schedule	IV

Lorazepam

Lorazepam (Ativan) is another benzodiazepine available for parenteral administration. Its action following parenteral administration is primarily that of sedation rather than anxiolysis. A potential benefit of IM lorazepam is that it frequently provides a degree of amnesia. This lack of recall is maximal within 2 hours of IM injection.

Because the agent is virtually insoluble in water, its onset of action may prove to be prolonged in some patients, although, as with diazepam, the onset of action will be about 15 minutes in most patients. Peak plasma levels of lorazepam are seen in 60 to 90 minutes.[29] The duration of action of lorazepam following IM administration is approximately 6 to 8 hours. The major side effects are excessive sleepiness and a prolonged amnesic period.

Odugbesan and Magbagbeola[30] recommend that the IV route be preferred to IM for administration of lorazepam, providing a somewhat more rapid onset of activity. Patients receiving lorazepam IM must not be permitted to leave the dental office unescorted and must be advised of the possibly enhanced CNS-depressant actions of other agents, such as opioids, alcohol, and barbiturates. Because of the prolonged duration of action of lorazepam, it is seldom used in the outpatient practice of dentistry.

Warnings

Lorazepam should not be administered to pregnant patients because it may increase the risk of congenital malformation. Patients must be advised against driving a car or operating hazardous machinery for a period of 24 to 48 hours, a period of time that may severely limit the usefulness of this agent in an ambulatory dental patient.[29]

Precautions

Additive CNS depression is observed when lorazepam is administered concurrently with barbiturates, alcohol, opioids, phenothiazines, antidepressants, scopolamine, and monoamine oxidase inhibitors (MAOIs). When scopolamine is used concurrently with lorazepam, the incidence of hallucinations and irrational behavior is increased. The use of IM lorazepam has resulted in discomfort at the injection site, including a sensation of burning, or observed redness. The overall incidence of burning and pain is about 17% immediately after the injection and 1.4% 24 hours later. Of patients receiving IM lorazepam, 2% had redness immediately after the injection and 0.5% noted redness after 24 hours.[29]

Dosage

The usual adult dose of lorazepam for preoperative sedation is 0.05 mg/kg (0.025 mg/lb) to a maximum of 4 mg. The drug should be administered undiluted deep into the muscle mass. If dilution is desired (it is not recommended for IM injection), sterile water for injection, sodium chloride injection, and 5% dextrose injection are compatible solutions. The use of lorazepam in patients younger than 18 years is not recommended because of insufficient data.[29]

Availability

Ativan (Wyeth): 2 and 4 mg/mL in 10-mL vials. The drug should be stored in a refrigerator. Lorazepam is classified as a Schedule IV drug.[29]

Lorazepam	
Pregnancy category	D
Lactation	NS
Metabolism	Liver
Excretion	Urine
DEA schedule	IV

Midazolam

Midazolam (Versed, Dormicum, Hypnovel) is a water-soluble benzodiazepine approved for use in the United States in 1986. It is well absorbed following IM administration and is frequently administered as an alternative to opioid agonists as a means of managing pretreatment anxiety. In my clinic, IM midazolam has been used with great success as a sole agent or in conjunction with IV midazolam in the management of patients with disabilities (adult and pediatric) and in the management of behavioral problems in pediatric dentistry.[31,32] These techniques are described in detail in Chapters 35 and 38. Midazolam provides a degree of retrograde amnesia in many patients following IM administration.[33]

Warnings

Midazolam, like other CNS depressants, may produce respiratory depression. This is especially likely to occur in patients who are receiving other CNS depressants (opioids, barbiturates) concurrently and in patients with preexisting cardiopulmonary disease. Special care must be taken whenever midazolam is administered to these patients.[34]

Dosage

For use in the extremely fearful pediatric or handicapped patient, I have employed an IM dose of 0.15 mg/kg.[32,33] Dosages should be decreased in the presence of cardiorespiratory disease or other indicators of increased responsiveness to benzodiazepines.[34] Continuous monitoring of the patient is essential once the drug is administered.

Availability

Midazolam: 1 and 5 mg/mL in 2- and 5-mL ampules. Midazolam is classified as a Schedule IV drug. The proprietary form of midazolam – Versed – has been discontinued. Midazolam is available as a generic.

Midazolam	
Pregnancy category	D
Lactation	unknown
Metabolism	Liver
Excretion	Feces and urine
DEA schedule	IV

Lorazepam is seldom used in dentistry via the IM route. The primary dental indication for the use of lorazepam IM might be a patient about to undergo a long dental appointment (lasting longer than 3 hours) or one in whom a degree of amnesia is desired. Diazepam has received considerable use as an IM agent for preoperative sedation, although primarily in hospital situations rather than in outpatient dentistry. When injected deep into muscle, especially the deltoid, it appears to be an effective preoperative sedative. Midazolam, a water-soluble benzodiazepine, has proved to be a very effective IM sedative agent, especially in the pediatric and handicapped population.

Histamine Blockers (Antihistamines)

Two drugs classified as histamine blockers are commonly administered via the IM route for sedation before dental treatment. Although used primarily in pediatric dentistry, they may also be used effectively in the adult patient.

The pharmacology of these drugs, promethazine and hydroxyzine, is reviewed in Chapter 7 because these drugs are also effective anxiolytics when administered orally. In this chapter, the clinical pharmacology of these drugs following IM administration is presented.

Promethazine

Promethazine hydrochloride, a phenothiazine derivative, is frequently employed via the IM or IV route for the management of anxiety. Other indications for use of promethazine include the management of allergic reactions and motion sickness, as an antiemetic, and as a preoperative sedative.[35]

Subcutaneous (SC) injection is contraindicated because promethazine produces localized tissue irritation that could lead to necrosis and sloughing. Deep IM injection is preferred to SC administration. The risk of this complication is considerably diminished with IM administration because of the superior vascularity of muscle. Onset of action following IM administration is rapid (10 to 15 minutes). Duration of action, however, is quite long, with the patient usually "feeling" the effects of the drug for up to 24 hours. If the patient is a child, a parent must be cautioned to watch the child during this time, not permitting bicycle riding or participation in any hazardous activities. The adult patient must also be cautioned and advised not to drive a car or operate hazardous machinery for 24 hours.

Because the degree of sedation produced by IM promethazine as a sole IM agent will be mild, it is common to administer an opioid along with promethazine when more profound sedation is desired. Promethazine was frequently administered in combination with a barbiturate and an atropine-like agent. This latter combination was commonly used as premedication for the hospitalized patient about to undergo surgery and general anesthesia. It is extremely important to remember that when promethazine is combined with an opioid, the dose of the opioid must be decreased by 25% to 50%; if combined with a barbiturate, the barbiturate dose must be reduced by 50%. Promethazine may produce additive effects with other CNS depressants, or the effect may be one of potentiation. In either case, the administration of "average" doses of both CNS depressants is likely to result in excessive degrees of CNS and possible respiratory depression.

In addition to its H1-receptor–blocking actions, sedative, and antiemetic effects, promethazine has anticholinergic properties. Promethazine is therefore not recommended for patients with narrow-angle glaucoma, prostatic hypertrophy, stenosing peptic ulcer, pyloroduodenal obstruction, or bladder neck obstruction. Because these medical problems are rarely mentioned on the typical medical history questionnaire, the dentist considering the use of promethazine must question the patient specifically about these conditions.

When used as a sole drug in pediatric dentistry, promethazine is effective in the management of children with lesser degrees of anxiety. It is not, however, usually effective in the management of children with extreme apprehension or of the disruptive, unmanageable child. In these situations, promethazine will be combined with other CNS depressants, most commonly opioids, such as meperidine. A discussion of the use of these drugs in combinations is presented in Chapter 35.

Dosage

The usual dose of promethazine for adults for preoperative sedation is 25 to 50 mg 1 hour before treatment. The dose as an antiemetic is 12.5 to 25 mg every 4 hours. The dose for children for preoperative sedation is 1.0 mg/kg or 0.5 mg/lb, not to exceed 50 mg.[35]

Availability

Phenergan (Wyeth-Ayerst): 25 and 50 mg/mL.

Promethazine	
Pregnancy category	C
Lactation	NS
Metabolism	Liver
Excretion	Feces and urine
DEA schedule	Not controlled

Hydroxyzine

Hydroxyzine hydrochloride is available for parenteral administration. The drug is not recommended for IV, IA, or SC administration because of adverse reactions that have occurred after its administration via these routes.[36]

Advantages of hydroxyzine in dentistry include its antiemetic and sedative actions and that it potentiates the CNS-depressant actions of opioids and barbiturates, permitting their dosages to be decreased by as much as 50%.

As with promethazine, hydroxyzine as a sole agent will prove effective in the management of lesser degrees of anxiety (e.g., minimal sedation); however, unless combined with opioids or inhalation sedation (N_2O-O_2) to provide moderate sedation, hydroxyzine will be ineffective in more severe anxiety. Patients must be cautioned not to drive a car or to operate hazardous machinery for up to 24 hours following administration of IM hydroxyzine hydrochloride.

Because of possible tissue irritation following hydroxyzine injection, the preferred IM injection site in adults is the upper outer quadrant of the buttock or the vastus lateralis; in children, the vastus lateralis is preferred.[37] The deltoid region should not be used until it is well developed (adults and teenagers),

and the lower and middle third of the upper arm should never be used because of the risk of radial nerve injury.

Dosage

The usual adult dose of hydroxyzine for preoperative sedation is 25 to 100 mg 1 hour before treatment. The dose for use as an antiemetic is 25 to 50 mg. The dose for children for preoperative sedation is 1.0 mg/kg (0.5 mg/lb) 1 hour before treatment. The antiemetic dose for children is 1.0 mg/kg (0.5 mg/lb).[37]

Availability

Vistaril (Pfizer): 25 and 50 mg/mL in 1-mL ampules and 10 ml multiple-dose vials.

Hydroxyzine	
Pregnancy category	C
Lactation	NS
Metabolism	Liver
Excretion	Urine
DEA schedule	Not controlled

Promethazine and hydroxyzine are effective drugs for IM minimal-to-moderate sedation. Used primarily in pediatric dentistry and usually in conjunction with opioids, promethazine and hydroxyzine can be employed with success in the adult patient. Although the dosage range is wide, the dentist will select the appropriate dose of the drug after consideration of the factors discussed previously in this section. When used as sole drugs, their greatest efficacy is in the patient exhibiting milder levels of anxiety or one in whom only minimal sedation is desired.

Opioid Agonists

The OAs, although classified as strong analgesics, are commonly used to aid in the management of anxiety in both medicine and dentistry. Although opioids may be employed as solo agents in this regard, this is uncommon; more often they are administered conjointly with nonopioid CNS depressants, such as benzodiazepines or histamine blockers, to provide a greater depth of sedation than the latter drugs can produce by themselves.

The administration of opioids by any route of administration, particularly parenterally, must be approached with caution. As discussed under the pharmacology of these potent drugs, a significant number of potentially serious side effects and drug–drug interactions may be observed following opioid administration. Although the incidence of most side effects is dose related, many serious problems have been encountered following dosages well within the "normal" range. Because OAs are quite potent, the dentist is cautioned to be absolutely certain, beyond any degree of doubt, that his or her entire staff is fully prepared, both mentally and technically, to recognize and manage any opioid-induced complications. Without this preparation, parenteral opioid analgesics should not be used.

There is a need for opioids in dentistry. OAs are, to a degree, valuable in the management of severe postoperative discomfort following surgical procedures. In this regard, the most practical route of administration often is the oral route, although most OAs possess a significant hepatic first-pass effect and are more effective following parenteral administration. However, it may be more prudent to forgo parenteral administration of OAs in the ambulatory outpatient setting. If a drug-related problem develops following patient discharge, assistance might not be immediately available. Parenteral administration of OAs for postoperative discomfort in the hospitalized, monitored, nonambulatory patient is much more practical and is indeed the most common method of administration.

Another use of OAs in dentistry is in the management of more intense degrees of anxiety and fear. All OAs, as CNS depressants, possess the ability to produce a state of sedation, and advantage may be taken of this to aid in patient management. The use of OA analgesics as solo drugs for the management of anxiety is not always the most rational approach. Larger doses of the OAs must be administered to achieve a desired level of sedation when they are administered alone than when OAs are administered concurrently with other nonopioid CNS depressants. Adverse effects of the OAs are potentially more serious than those of nonopioids (although even nonopioids may produce morbidity and mortality) and are dose related. It simply makes sense (1) to avoid the use of OAs unless there is a definite reason for their use and (2) to use the smallest clinically effective dose of the OA.

An ever-growing number of OAs has been introduced into clinical practice. However, a small group of these drugs probably represents 99% of all OAs used in medicine and dentistry. These include meperidine and fentanyl and its congeners alfentanil and sufentanil. To these must be added the opioid agonist-antagonists (OAAns) exemplified by pentazocine, butorphanol, and nalbuphine.

Pharmacology

Morphine, although not commonly used in dentistry because of its long duration of action, is recognized as the prototypical OA. Its pharmacology is reviewed in some depth as representative of the entire group. Other OAs used in dentistry are discussed later, and the differences in their actions from those of morphine are pointed out.

Mechanism of Action

A significant body of research exists concerning the mechanisms of action of OAs. Four major stereospecific receptors for OAs and opioid antagonists have been located within the CNS, the spinal cord, the trigeminal nucleus, the brainstem solitary nuclei and area postrema of the medulla, the medial thalamus, the limbic system (amygdala), and the periaqueductal gray matter of the mesencephalon (brainstem).[38] The periaqueductal gray matter has been identified as a site important

to opioid-induced analgesia and to the perception of pain. In addition to the discovery of these receptors, endogenous opioid-like substances called *enkephalins* and *endorphins* have been isolated.[39] Both possess potent opioid-like properties and have received extensive examination as to their role in the management of pain.

μ-receptors are thought to be responsible for supraspinal analgesia, respiratory depression, euphoria, and physical dependence; κ-receptors are associated with alterations in affective behavior; σ-receptors are involved in the dysphoria, hallucinations, and vasomotor stimulation associated with some opioids; and δ-receptors appear to modulate the actions of the μ-receptors.[40-42] Table 10.3 summarizes the actions of these four opioid receptors. OAs are drugs that bind with the μ-, κ-, and δ-fibers. OAAns (opioid agonist-antagonists) possess either agonist or antagonist actions at the various receptors, and opioid antagonists (OAns) possess antagonist actions at the receptors.

It is likely that OAs and the endogenous opioids (endorphins and enkephalins) act to alter pain perception and pain reaction by inhibiting neuronal activity at their receptor sites through a decrease in sodium conductance through ion channels in nerve membranes. That opioid receptors are found in certain areas of the CNS in greater abundance than in others lends credence to this theory. OAs modify both components of the pain experience: the perception of pain and the reaction of the patient to pain. The presence of opioid receptors within the substantia gelatinosa of the spinal cord, the trigeminal nucleus, and the periaqueductal gray matter provides a reasonable explanation of the effect of OAs on pain perception, and the identification of opioid receptors located within the amygdala of the limbic system and the medial thalamus aids in explaining their effects on the reaction to pain. Patients receiving OAs may still perceive pain, but their reaction to it is usually diminished. OAs separate pain from suffering. ("It hurts, but I don't care!"). The side effect of nausea and vomiting is explained by the presence of opioid receptors within the area postrema of the medulla, and their presence within the solitary nuclei explains the antitussive, hypotensive, and GI effects of OAs. The two primary areas influenced by morphine are the CNS and the GI tract, the only areas in which opioid receptors have been found.

Central Nervous System Effects

Morphine produces analgesia, drowsiness, mood changes, and mental clouding. Of significance is the fact that morphine produces analgesia without inducing the loss of consciousness. Following a therapeutic dose of morphine (10 to 15 mg) to patients in pain or feeling anxiety or fear, any or all of these may disappear. Pain may be diminished in intensity or eradicated completely, accompanied frequently by drowsiness. The extremities become quite heavy, the body becomes warm, itching develops on the face (most frequently the nose or upper lip), and the mouth becomes dry. Some patients may become euphoric.

Table 10.3	Classification of Opioid Receptors		
RECEPTOR	EFFECT	AGONIST	ANTAGONIST
μ1	Supraspinal analgesia	β-Endorphin	Naloxone
		Morphine	Pentazocine
μ2	Depression of ventilation	Morphine	Naloxone
		Meperidine	
	Indifference or euphoria	Sufentanil	
		Alfentanil	
	Miosis	Fentanyl	
	Bradycardia		
	Hypothermia		
	Physical dependence		
δ	Modulates μ	Leu-enkephalin	Met-enkephalin
κ	Miosis	Dynorphin	
	Sedation	Pentazocine	
	Analgesia	Butorphanol	
σ	Dysphoria	Ketamine	Naloxone
	Tachycardia	Pentazocine	
	Tachypnea		
	Mydriasis		

Interestingly, when the same dose of morphine is administered to a pain-free patient, the reaction may not be as pleasant. Many patients report dysphoria rather than euphoria, consisting of increased anxiety or fear and frequently of nausea or vomiting.

With increased doses (15 to 20 mg), the subjective effects of morphine are increased. Drowsiness is increased, euphoria (when present) is accentuated, and patients in severe pain not relieved by smaller doses report relief. The side effects of nausea, vomiting, and respiratory depression are also accentuated.

Morphine and other OAs appear to be much more effective in the relief of dull, aching, continuous pain than that of a sharp, intermittent nature. Patients often report that they still feel the pain but that it no longer bothers them. It appears that the OAs primarily affect those systems responsible for the affective responses to noxious stimuli. Therefore, when patients no longer respond to pain in the usual manner, their ability to tolerate the noxious stimulus may be dramatically increased, although their ability to perceive the pain is relatively unaltered.

Pupillary Responses

Morphine and many other OAs produce a dose-related constriction (miosis) of the pupil. Although the pupil still responds to changes in light, miosis produced by morphine is evident even in total darkness. Marked miosis and pinpoint pupils are considered pathognomonic of OA overdose. Atropine (and related agents) administered concurrently with OAs counteracts morphine-induced miosis.

Respiratory Responses

Morphine and other OAs produce a dose-related respiratory depression. Respiratory depression is observed even at therapeutic doses of morphine and is the most significant undesirable effect of the OAs. Opioid-induced respiratory depression is a major factor in many instances of morbidity and mortality occurring following IM or IV sedation.[19]

Morphine depresses the responsiveness of the medullary respiratory centers to carbon dioxide (CO_2) in addition to depressing the pontine and medullary centers that regulate respiratory rhythm and rate. Clinically, it is observed that the rate, minute volume, and tidal exchange are all depressed by OAs. Normal respiratory rates of 16 to 20 breaths per minute may decrease to as few as 3 to 4 breaths per minute following overdose. Maximal respiratory depression following morphine administration develops 7 minutes after IV administration, 30 minutes after IM administration, and 90 minutes after SC administration. Respiratory depression may be present for up to 4 to 5 hours after morphine administration.

All OAs are capable of producing respiratory depression. When equianalgesic doses are administered, the degree of respiratory depression is not significantly different from that produced by morphine.[43]

Nausea and Emetic Actions

Nausea and vomiting produced by morphine and other OAs result from direct stimulation of the chemoreceptor zone for emesis, located in the area postrema of the medulla. This emetic effect is counteracted by OAns.

It is significant that the incidence of nausea and vomiting is considerably greater in ambulatory patients than in recumbent patients. Nausea occurs in approximately 40% and vomiting in 15% of ambulatory patients receiving 15 mg morphine subcutaneously. It is probable that the emetic effect is produced in part by a peripheral effect on the vestibular apparatus of the ear and by orthostatic hypotension.[44]

Because most dental patients are ambulatory, the potential for nausea and vomiting following OA administration in dentistry is increased. Reversal of the OA with an antagonist before discharge of the patient might be considered as a means of minimizing this occurrence, but it must be remembered that the continued presence of the OA in the blood in the immediate postoperative period will aid in the management of any pain that might develop. In addition, it has been found that reversal of OAs not only reverses their adverse actions (respiratory depression, nausea, vomiting), but also reverses their analgesic actions. Routine reversal of OAs with OAns before patient discharge is not recommended. Use of OAns should be reserved for those few situations in which their administration is essential to a patient's safety. Probably the most effective means of minimizing the occurrence of nausea and vomiting following opioid administration is to minimize the dose administered to the patient, as this complication is dose related.

Cardiovascular Effects

Morphine in therapeutic doses has virtually no effect on blood pressure (BP) and heart rate or rhythm when patients are in the supine position.[43] Actions on the CVS do not develop until doses well into the overdose range are administered, and even then, the CVS is not affected to a great degree. The most significant factor in hypotension developing following OA overdose is hypoxia. In the presence of opioid overdose with adequate oxygenation, the BP usually is maintained within normal limits.

Postural (orthostatic) hypotension does increase in incidence and severity with increasing doses of morphine and other OAs, a factor to be considered in the usual ambulatory dental office environment. This is thought to be a result of peripheral vasodilation occurring as a result of histamine release associated with OA administration. Whenever the patient is shifted from a recumbent to a more upright position, the ability of the CVS to respond to the effect of gravity will be depressed by the OA. Slower changes in patient positioning are essential to prevent or minimize postural hypotension. Minimizing OA doses further diminishes the incidence of this dose-related situation. Postural hypotension is most likely to be noted with morphine and meperidine (which provoke the greatest release of histamine).

Another result of OA histamine release is the possible development of pruritus at the site of administration. This effect is responsible for the flushed feeling and itching that develop in some patients following IV administration. This is discussed in detail in the section on IV sedation.

OAs have little or no effect on the myocardium, producing either an increase in heart rate or no change. The cerebral circulation, likewise, is little affected by therapeutic doses of morphine. However, in the presence of respiratory depression and elevated CO_2 levels, cerebral blood vessels dilate and intracranial pressure increases.

Gastrointestinal Tract Effects

Morphine produces constipation by decreasing motility of the stomach, duodenum, and colon in addition to diminishing both pancreatic and biliary secretions. Because morphine increases biliary tract pressure, its use in patients with biliary colic may produce an increase in pain rather than relief.

Smooth Muscle Effects

Morphine and other OAs increase smooth muscle tonus throughout the body, such as in the ureter, urinary bladder, uterus, and bronchioles. Although therapeutic doses of OAs do not produce significant bronchospasm, their administration to patients with asthma may aggravate this condition, possibly precipitating bronchospasm. OAs ought to be avoided in patients with a history of asthma (a relative contraindication).

Tolerance, Physical Dependence, and Abuse Potential

The development of tolerance and physical dependence following repeated use is a characteristic of all OAs. This represents one of the limiting factors in the use of these drugs. Within dentistry the potential for producing addiction in a patient through use of OAs for sedation is quite unlikely to develop; however, the presence of OAs within the office does increase the potential for unauthorized use of the drugs by persons unassociated with the dental office (after-hours robbery) or, unfortunately, by dental personnel themselves. Although it is not as significant a problem in dentistry as within the medical community, opioid abuse by health care professionals does occur and must be scrupulously guarded against.

Because OAs are Schedule II drugs, they must be stored in a locked cabinet or storage area. Precise records as to the use of these drugs are mandatory so that anyone can determine the fate of a package of OAs. These records are reviewed in the section on IV sedation.

Absorption, Distribution, Biotransformation, and Excretion

OAs are rapidly absorbed following SC, SM, or IM injection (Table 10.4). Because of a significant hepatic first-pass effect, parenteral doses of OAs are considerably more effective than equal doses administered orally (only 30% of an oral dose of morphine reaches the systemic circulation).

Morphine leaves the blood rapidly and is distributed to the kidney, liver, lungs, and spleen. The major portion of the drug is found in skeletal muscle. Accumulation of the drug in tissues is rare, and within 24 hours, the tissue concentration of morphine is quite low.

Table 10.4	Comparison of Opioid Agonists and Opioid Agonist-Antagonists via Intramuscular or Submucosal Injection				
	ONSET (MIN)	PEAK ACTION (MIN)	DURATION (HR)	ADULT DOSE	PEDIATRIC DOSE (MG/KG)
Opioid Agonists					
Morphine	20	30–90	Up to 7	5–15 mg	0.1–0.2
Meperidine	10–15	30–60	2–4	50–100 mg	1–2
Fentanyl	5–15	30	1–2	0.05–0.1 mg	—
Opioid Agonist-Antagonists					
Butorphanol	10	30–60	3–4	2–4 mg	—
Nalbuphine	15	—	3–6	10 mg/70 kg	

The OAs undergo biotransformation within the liver and are excreted in urine. Only a small fraction of the administered dose is found unmetabolized in urine.

Contraindications

The only absolute contraindication to the use of morphine is the presence of allergy.

Warnings

OAs should not be administered to patients with head injury or increased intracranial pressure because of the respiratory-depressant actions of these drugs and their ability to increase intracranial pressure.[45] Within the typical dental environment, this is an unlikely occurrence.

Morphine and other OAs should be used cautiously, if at all, in patients with asthma; chronic obstructive pulmonary disease (COPD); or any degree of respiratory depression, hypoxia, or hypercarbia.[45] Even usual therapeutic doses of OAs in these patients may significantly decrease respiratory drive while simultaneously increasing airway resistance to the point of producing apnea.

Patients receiving OAs must be cautioned against operating motor vehicles or other hazardous machinery. Orthostatic hypotension, nausea, and vomiting are more likely to develop in ambulatory patients receiving OAs.[45]

OAs cross the placenta and may produce fetal respiratory depression. The use of OAs in the pregnant patient should be considered only following consultation with the patient's physician and only if other techniques and drugs are unavailable. The benefit versus the risk of drug administration should always be considered.[45]

Drug Interactions

OAs must be used with caution in patients who are receiving other CNS depressants, such as other OAs, phenothiazines, benzodiazepines, sedative-hypnotics, tricyclic antidepressants, and alcohol. Exaggerated clinical effects, including respiratory depression, hypotension, profound sedation, and unconsciousness, may and have developed.

The use of meperidine in patients receiving MAOIs is contraindicated because patients have experienced unpredict-able, severe, and occasionally fatal reactions.[45] Because the therapeutic actions of the MAOIs may continue for 14 days after their discontinuance, meperidine should not be used until at least 2 weeks following the last dose of the MAOI. The reactions are of two types. Some responses involve unconsciousness, severe respiratory depression, cyanosis, and hypotension, resembling acute opioid overdose. Other responses are characterized by hyperexcitability, convulsions, tachycardia, hyperpyrexia, and hypertension. The use of OAns in the management of these reactions has not always proved effective.

Precautions

Doses of OAs must be decreased in patients who are elderly or debilitated or are known to be sensitive to CNS depressants. Among these are patients with cardiovascular, pulmonary, or hepatic disease. Doses should also be decreased in patients with hypothyroid conditions, alcoholism, convulsive disorders, asthma, Addison disease, and prostatic hypertrophy or urethral stricture.[45]

OAs may aggravate preexisting convulsions in patients with seizure disorders. Convulsions may develop in patients without a history of seizures if the OA is administered in a dose considerably above that recommended because of the development of tolerance.[45]

Adverse Reactions

The most significant adverse reaction associated with the administration of OAs is respiratory depression. Respiratory depression is dose dependent; however, some degree of depression is usually present even with therapeutic doses of most OAs. All aspects of respiration are depressed, but probably the most observable change is respiratory rate, which will be reduced significantly from the normal adult range of 16 to 20 breaths per minute to as little as 3 to 4 breaths per minute. Respiratory rates below 8 breaths per minute following administration of OAs should be evaluated carefully and, if necessary, treatment instituted to correct the situation. In addition to respiratory depression, respiratory arrest, cardiovascular depression, and cardiac arrest have been noted following OA administration.

Among the more common side effects of the OAs are lightheadedness, dizziness, nausea, vomiting, and diaphoresis (sweating). These appear to be more common in ambulatory patients. Because most of these effects are dose related, the use of smaller doses, as recommended in this text, should minimize the development of these undesirable effects. If side effects develop despite use of smaller doses, the ambulatory patient should be advised to lie down and avoid unnecessary positional changes, a maneuver that often alleviates the symptoms.

Other adverse reactions associated with OAs include euphoria, dysphoria, headache, insomnia, agitation, tremor, uncoordinated muscular movements, transient hallucinations, disorientation, visual disturbances, dry mouth, constipation, biliary tract spasm, flushing of the face, tachycardia, bradycardia, palpitation, faintness, syncope, urinary retention, reduced libido, pruritus, urticaria, skin rashes, and edema.[45] In other words, the OAs are capable of producing just about any and every side effect that most other drugs (or even nondrugs) may produce.[46,47]

Overdose

Overdose produced by opioids is manifested by respiratory depression, primarily a decrease in the rate and tidal volume of breathing. In more profound overdose, the patient may lose consciousness, with pupils becoming constricted (miosis), muscles flaccid, and skin cold and clammy. Bradycardia or hypotension or both may be present. Respiratory arrest may develop.

The primary goal in the management of overdose from any OA is airway maintenance (A, airway) and the delivery of oxygen to the lungs, CVS, and brain (B, breathing). Ventilation may need to be assisted or indeed controlled by the person managing the patient. Once a patent airway is established and oxygenation ensured, the administration of an OAns may be considered (D, definitive care). Naloxone is the drug of choice, administered by the IV route, if possible, or IM, if necessary. Other drugs and measures that may be considered are oxygen, IV fluids, and vasopressors. More specific details of management of drug-related overdose are discussed in Chapter 27.

Morphine

The pharmacology of morphine has been discussed at great length in the preceding section. Morphine is used as the sulfate (frequently abbreviated as MS). Following IM or SC administration, the onset of action develops within 20 minutes, with a peak effect noted between 30 and 90 minutes. Unfortunately, for most dental situations, the average duration of clinical effect of morphine sulfate is approximately 7 hours. Approximately 90% of the dose administered is excreted within 24 hours, primarily in the urine.

Morphine is employed primarily as an analgesic, but it is also used commonly as a preoperative sedative before surgery and general anesthesia. Morphine is absorbed more reliably following parenteral administration than oral administration, primarily because of a significant hepatic first-pass effect.

Dosage

The usual adult dose of morphine for preoperative sedation is 5 to 15 mg 30 minutes preoperatively. The usual dose for children for preoperative sedation is 0.1 to 0.2 mg/kg (0.05 to 0.1 mg/lb).[45]

Availability

Morphine sulfate: 8, 10, and 15 mg/mL in 1-mL ampules; 15 mg/mL in 20-mL vials. Morphine is classified as a Schedule II drug.[45]

Morphine	
Pregnancy category	C
Lactation	Probably safe
Metabolism	Liver
Excretion	Urine
DEA schedule	II

Meperidine

Meperidine was first synthesized in 1939 and was studied as an atropine-like agent.[43] Its analgesic properties quickly became recognized, and its atropine-like properties are today listed as side effects of the drug.

Following IM or SC administration, the onset of action of meperidine is more rapid than that of morphine (10 to 15 minutes), and its duration of action is somewhat shorter (2 to 4 hours). Maximal effectiveness develops between 30 and 60 minutes. Before the introduction of fentanyl, meperidine was the most commonly used OA in dentistry. Its clinical onset and duration of action are quite amenable to the typical dental appointment.[48] At doses of 80 to 100 mg, meperidine is equianalgesic with 10 mg morphine sulfate. Meperidine is approximately half as effective orally as parenterally.[43]

Peak respiratory depression following IM administration of meperidine develops in 1 hour with a return toward normal at 2 hours, although measurable respiratory depression may be noted for up to 4 hours. OAns readily reverse opioid-produced respiratory depression. As with morphine sulfate, meperidine produces virtually no untoward effect on the CVS at therapeutic doses. Ambulatory patients are more likely to experience postural hypotension. Although IV meperidine may produce a tachycardia, IM meperidine seldom does. Meperidine produces less smooth muscle spasm, less constipation, and less depression of the cough reflex than equianalgesic doses of morphine sulfate.[43]

Dosage

The usual adult dose for preoperative sedation is 50 to 100 mg intramuscularly 30 to 90 minutes before treatment. The usual dose for children for preoperative sedation is 1 to 2 mg/kg

(0.5 to 1.0 mg/lb) intramuscularly 30 to 90 minutes before treatment.[49]

Availability

Meperidine: 25 mg/mL in 1-mL ampules; 50 mg/mL in 1-mL ampules and 30-mL vials; 75 mg/mL in 1- and 1.5-mL ampules; 100 mg/mL in 1-, 2-, 20-, and 30-mL ampules and vials. Demerol (Sanofi Winthrop): 25-, 50-, 75-, and 100-mg/mL ampules and vials. Meperidine is classified as a Schedule II drug.[49]

Meperidine	
Pregnancy category	C
Lactation	Safety unknown
Metabolism	Liver, mostly
Excretion	Urine
DEA schedule	II

> **COMMENT:** For IM administration of meperidine and other OAs, it is reasonable to employ one of the more concentrated dosage forms of the drug (e.g., 50 mg/mL) to minimize the volume of solution injected. On the other hand, when administered intravenously, more dilute concentrations of these same drugs are recommended to minimize the risk of mistakenly administering too large a dose.

Meperidine With Promethazine

Meperidine is combined with the phenothiazine–histamine blocker promethazine to produce a drug combination that was popular in pediatric dentistry and is still in use today, although in limited fashion. The pharmacology of the individual drugs has been discussed. This drug combination came into being because several clinical studies demonstrated that promethazine potentiated the analgesic and sedative properties of the OA meperidine. The dose of meperidine necessary to produce clinically effective sedation or analgesia could be reduced by almost 50% when promethazine was added.[48]

The combination is clinically useful in pediatric dentistry because the mixture produces more sedation than is seen with either drug alone. It is available in both oral and injectable forms, but its primary effectiveness has been in IM administration. Following IM administration, the combination produces a clinical effect within 15 to 30 minutes, with a duration of action of 3 to 4 hours.[50]

Dosage

The usual adult dose for preoperative sedation is 25 to 50 mg of each component (1 to 2 mL) 15 to 30 minutes before treatment. Although the recommended dose for children is listed as 0.5 mg/lb of body weight,[50] many pediatric dentistry textbooks indicate a smaller dose: 0.02 mg/kg (0.01 mg/lb) intramuscularly 15 to 30 minutes preoperatively.[51-53]

Availability

The proprietary name, Mepergan, is no longer available in the United States. Generic versions—25 mg meperidine and 25 mg promethazine per milliliter—may still be available.[54] The combination of meperidine and promethazine is classified as a Schedule II drug.[50]

Meperidine and Promethazine	
Pregnancy category	N/A
Lactation	NS
Metabolism	Liver
Excretion	Urine
DEA schedule	II

Fentanyl

Fentanyl is a rapid-onset, short-duration OA with qualitative clinical actions similar to those of morphine and meperidine. Fentanyl is significantly more potent, however, with a dose of 0.1 mg equianalgesic to 10 mg morphine and 75 mg meperidine. In other words, 1 mg of fentanyl is equianalgesic to 100 mg morphine or 750 mg meperidine.[55]

As do other OAs, fentanyl produces a dose-related respiratory depression. However, respiratory depression produced by fentanyl may be of longer duration than its analgesic action. Fentanyl appears to produce less nausea and vomiting than do most other OAs. Other OA actions are also observed: miosis, bradycardia, bronchoconstriction, and euphoria. A potentially serious reaction to fentanyl administration is muscular rigidity ("chest wall rigidity"), which is quite rare, developing primarily after IV administration and involving most muscles, but particularly the muscles of the chest wall and muscles of respiration.[56,57] Chest wall rigidity is discussed in depth in the section on IV sedation.

Fentanyl is used primarily via the IV route, either alone or as the opioid component of Innovar (consisting of fentanyl and droperidol), for the induction and maintenance of neuroleptanesthesia (see Section VI). In addition, fentanyl is used to provide sedation preoperatively or postoperatively as an analgesic.

The onset of action of fentanyl following IM administration is 5 to 15 minutes; maximal effect develops within 30 minutes, and the duration of action is approximately 1 to 2 hours. These figures demonstrate that fentanyl is an OA whose clinical actions are quite well suited to the typical, short (1-hour) dental or surgical appointment. Fentanyl, used by an appropriately trained dentist, is a useful drug for the management of pain and anxiety, via either the IV or IM route.

Dosage

The usual adult dose for preoperative sedation is 0.05 to 0.1 mg intramuscularly 30 to 60 minutes preoperatively. The dose must be decreased in elderly and debilitated patients and in patients who have received other CNS depressants. Fentanyl is recommended for IV administration, but there is no recommended dose for children via the IM route.[58]

Availability

Sublimaze (Janssen): 0.05 mg/mL in 2- and 5-mL ampules. Fentanyl is classified as a Schedule II drug.

Fentanyl	
Pregnancy category	C
Lactation	NS
Metabolism	Liver
Excretion	Urine
DEA schedule	II

Alfentanil, sufentanil, and remifentanil are congeners of fentanyl that have gained popularity for short dental procedures. They are similar to fentanyl in most properties. The primary route of administration of alfentanil, sufentanil, and remifentanil is intravenously. The fentanyl family is discussed in greater detail in Chapter 25.

The opioid agonist analgesics just presented are those most frequently given intramuscularly in both medicine and dentistry for the management of anxiety in the preoperative period. From the practical point of view, the most useful OAs for most dental procedures would be those possessing the shortest duration of action: fentanyl, sufentanil, and alfentanil. The IM administration of fentanyl and its congeners has not received much attention within dentistry. Their primary use is via IV administration, where a short duration makes them appropriate for many procedures. Fentanyl has replaced meperidine as the most used OA in dentistry. Meperidine, with its longer history of use and its longer duration of action, is administered either IM or IV. In pediatric dentistry, meperidine was used less often than the no-longer-available alphaprodine, primarily because of its longer duration of action, but it is much more commonly employed today. Morphine, although an excellent agent, is rarely used IM in outpatient dentistry and surgery because of its long duration of action.

Opioid Agonist-Antagonists

Three opioid agonist-antagonists are available for IM and IV use. These drugs differ from the OAs in that they possess not only opioid-like properties (agonist) but also OAn properties. The systemic effects described earlier for morphine, as the prototypical opioid, represent agonistic actions. Antagonistic actions include (1) prevention of agonist effects if administered before or simultaneously with the OA, (2) reversal of agonist effects if administered after the OA, and (3) precipitation of acute withdrawal syndrome almost immediately in the opioid-dependent individual. One compound, naloxone, is considered a pure antagonist and is an important drug in the management of opioid overdose. Its actions and use are described in Chapter 25. Pentazocine, butorphanol, and nalbuphine are drugs with mixed agonist and antagonist activities and are discussed next.

Pentazocine

Pentazocine was a product of research aimed at developing an effective analgesic with little or no abuse potential. It possesses agonistic properties and very weak antagonistic actions ($\frac{1}{50}$th as potent as nalorphine as an antagonist). Its actions mimic those of morphine, including a sense of euphoria. Since it was introduced in the 1960s, many instances of psychological and physical dependence to pentazocine have been documented. Because of its antagonistic properties, the administration of pentazocine to opioid-dependent persons may precipitate acute withdrawal syndrome, an action not produced by OAs.[59]

Today, pentazocine is rarely administered in dentistry as a sedative via either the IM or IV routes. For a more detailed description of the pharmacology, dosage, and administration technique for pentazocine, previous editions of this textbook should be consulted.[60]

Butorphanol

Butorphanol is a potent analgesic with an onset of action within 10 minutes following IM administration; it reaches a peak level of clinical activity at 30 to 60 minutes with a duration of analgesia of 3 to 4 hours. An OAAn, its antagonistic actions are approximately 30 times those of pentazocine and about $\frac{1}{40}$th those of naloxone. In analgesic properties, butorphanol is 3.5 to 7 times more potent than morphine (2 mg = 10 mg).[61]

Side effects of butorphanol are similar to those of other OAs, including the possibility of respiratory depression. Although 2 mg of butorphanol does produce respiratory depression equivalent to that produced by 10 mg of morphine, increasing the dose of butorphanol to 4 mg or greater does not appreciably increase the degree of respiratory depression (there is a "ceiling effect" on respiratory depression). This one factor should make butorphanol (and nalbuphine [see later]) an important drug in dentistry's armamentarium against anxiety and pain. Although the magnitude of respiratory depression observed with butorphanol appears not to be dose related (above the 2-mg dose), the duration of respiratory depression is dose related. Naloxone rapidly reverses respiratory depression produced by butorphanol.[62]

Cardiovascular effects of butorphanol include increased BP and heart rate. In addition, butorphanol increases cardiac workload by increasing pulmonary artery pressure, left ventricular end-diastolic pressure, and pulmonary vascular resistance. For these reasons, the use of butorphanol is contraindicated in patients with recent myocardial infarction, coronary insufficiency, or ventricular dysfunction.[61] These patients normally represent ASA IV risks and are not candidates for dental treatment.

Butorphanol has received attention in both medicine and dentistry as a drug for preoperative sedation. It may be administered intravenously, intranasally, or intramuscularly.

Dosage

The usual adult dose for preoperative sedation is 2 mg intramuscularly 15 to 30 minutes before treatment. Doses larger than 4 mg are not recommended because of a lack of sufficient information.[63]

Availability

Stadol (Mead Johnson): 1 and 2 mg/mL in 1- and 2-mL vials. Butorphanol is classified as a Schedule IV drug.

Butorphanol	
Pregnancy category	C
Lactation	S
Metabolism	Liver, extensively
Excretion	Urine
DEA schedule	IV

Nalbuphine

Nalbuphine is another analgesic possessing OAAns properties. Nalbuphine is equipotent with morphine on a milligram basis. Following IM administration, onset of action is noted within 15 minutes, with a duration of action from 3 to 6 hours. The plasma half-life of nalbuphine is 5 hours. The opioid antagonistic activity of nalbuphine is one-fourth that of nalorphine and 10 times that of pentazocine.[64]

As with butorphanol, the actions, side effects, contraindications, and warnings are similar to those of OAs. The one major difference in pharmacology between butorphanol and nalbuphine is the absence of any increased cardiovascular workload with nalbuphine. Its use is not contraindicated in cardiovascular-risk patients.[65]

At the usual IM therapeutic dose of 10 mg (for a 70-kg patient), nalbuphine produces respiratory depression equivalent to 10 mg morphine sulfate. Increasing the dosage of nalbuphine does not appreciably increase the degree of respiratory depression (as also seen with butorphanol, there is a ceiling effect with regard to respiratory depression). Naloxone readily reverses respiratory depression produced by nalbuphine.

Dosage

The usual adult dose of nalbuphine for preoperative sedation is 10 mg/70 kg 15 to 30 minutes before the procedure. The dose should be adjusted based on the patient's physical and emotional status, the depth of sedation desired, the patient's age, and the presence of other CNS depressants. Because of a lack of clinical experience, the administration of nalbuphine to patients younger than 18 years is not recommended.[65]

Availability

Nubain (DuPont): 10 mg/mL in 1-, 2-, and 10-mL ampules. Nalbuphine is not classified as a schedule drug.

Nalbuphine	
Pregnancy category	B
Lactation	Safety unknown
Metabolism	Liver
Excretion	Feces and urine
DEA schedule	Not controlled

OAAns offer the significant advantage over the OAs (morphine, meperidine, fentanyl) of a ceiling effect in dose-related respiratory depression. Although this action will not be of great significance in the doses usually employed for sedation in dentistry (up to 2 mg butorphanol or 10 mg nalbuphine), accidental overadministration of these drugs is less likely to result in serious respiratory depression or respiratory arrest. As with the OAs, the dentist using OAAns drugs must be prepared to both recognize and manage any unwanted side effects produced by these agents. Their presumed safety is not an excuse to forgo routine patient monitoring during the procedure. To do so is to invite disaster.

Nonsteroidal Antiinflammatory Drugs
Ketorolac

Ketorolac is an NSAID possessing appropriate solubility and which produces minimal tissue irritation, making it suitable for IM injection. Ketorolac, as a potent NSAID, relieves pain through inhibition of arachidonic acid synthesis at the cyclooxygenase level and possesses no central opioid effects.[66] Ketorolac has analgesic potencies comparable with those of morphine, with the following IM equivalence: 30 to 90 mg ketorolac equals 6 to 12 mg morphine.[67] Ketorolac is indicated for the short-term (up to 5 days) management of moderately severe acute pain that requires analgesia at the opioid level. It is not indicated for minor or chronic painful conditions. Increasing the dose beyond the label recommendations will not provide better efficacy, but will result in increasing risk of developing serious adverse events. It is useful by itself or in combination with opioids, decreasing the required dose of opioid by approximately 45%.[66,68] It is especially useful when opioids are contraindicated, especially to prevent respiratory depression and sedation. When ketorolac proves to be ineffective in pain management, opioids should be considered.[69]

Dosage

Following IM administration, onset occurs within 10 minutes, and peak blood levels are reached in 45 to 50 minutes, with a duration of approximately 6 hours.[68,70] Ketorolac is administered as a 30- to 60-mg IM loading dose followed by 15 or 30 mg IM every 6 hours, with a maximum first-day dose of 150 mg and 120 mg on subsequent days up to a recommended maximum of 5 days. The lower dose range is recommended for elderly patients, patients weighing less than 50 kg, and patients with impaired renal function.[70]

Availability

Toradol (Syntex): 15-mg/mL Tubex cartridge–needle unit, 1-mL syringe; 30 mg/mL 1- and 2-mL syringe.

Ketorolac	
Pregnancy category	C
Lactation	S
Metabolism	Liver, mostly
Excretion	Urine, primarily
DEA schedule	Not controlled

Dissociative Anesthetic
Ketamine

Ketamine, a phencyclidine derivative, is administered parenterally to produce a state called *dissociative anesthesia*.[71] Following administration, the patient becomes mentally dissociated from the environment. Phencyclidine is used in veterinary medicine and was a popular drug of abuse known as *angel dust*. Ketamine may be used to produce a state of general anesthesia (its primary use) or, in subanesthetic doses, to induce a state resembling sedation. Within 5 to 8 minutes following IM administration, the patient loses consciousness. Recovery of consciousness occurs within 10 to 20 minutes, but it is several hours before the patient has recovered fully. The state of unconsciousness produced by ketamine differs significantly from that produced by more traditional general anesthetics. Dissociative anesthesia is described in Chapters 25 and 31.

Pharmacology

Ketamine exerts its dissociative effects by interrupting the cerebral association pathways and by depression of the thalamocortical tracts. The reticular activating system, the limbic system, and the medulla are little affected.

The CVS is stimulated following ketamine administration (most general anesthetics depress the CVS). Increases occur in mean arterial pressure, heart rate, and cardiac output, brought about by direct stimulation by ketamine. The median elevation in BP following IM ketamine is about 20% to 25% above preanesthetic levels. Airway patency is normally easily maintained following ketamine administration because muscle tonus is actually increased, in direct contrast to decreased muscle tonus seen with other general anesthetics. Protective reflexes are also maintained, but there is some degree of diminution of their effectiveness. Administration of overly large doses of ketamine may produce apnea.[72] The administrator of ketamine must remain ever vigilant during patient treatment with this drug. Ketamine undergoes biotransformation in the liver into alcohols, which are excreted in urine.

The use of ketamine is contraindicated in patients with high BP, severe psychiatric disorders, increased intracranial pressure, epilepsy, arteriosclerotic heart disease, or cerebrovascular accident.[73]

Probably the major adverse action observed following ketamine administration is the development of unpleasant dreaming, confused states, and frightening or upsetting hallucinations during recovery. These are more likely to occur in adults than in children. When they do occur in children, they are usually less intense than those in adults.[74,75]

Ketamine should never be used, in either anesthetic or subanesthetic doses, by a dentist untrained in anesthesiology. The differences between a ketamine-induced state of general anesthesia and the more traditional stage III anesthesia may tempt unqualified persons to believe that they are able to safely employ this drug in their practice. Rest assured that this is not the case. I have had more than 1000 case experiences with ketamine and can attest to the fact that this drug can, although it is only on very rare occasions, produce some urgent and emergent situations. Dentists not fully prepared for these reactions will be unable to respond to them effectively, much to their patient's detriment. The reader is referred to Chapters 25 and 31 for a more complete discussion of ketamine, its dosages and availability, and the concept of dissociative anesthesia.

Ketamine	
Pregnancy category	D
Lactation	NS
Metabolism	Liver
Excretion	Kidney
DEA schedule	III

Anticholinergic Drugs

The anticholinergic drugs atropine, scopolamine, and glycopyrrolate are also called *cholinergic blocking agents, belladonna alkaloids,* and *antimuscarinic drugs.* Commonly employed in general anesthesia, anticholinergics are also frequently used in dentistry. Their primary use in dentistry is for the reduction of salivary flow. In addition, their vagolytic actions are effective in the prevention or management of clinically significant bradycardia. These drugs may be administered subcutaneously, intramuscularly, or intravenously. Anticholinergics act as competitive antagonists of the postganglionic receptor located at the neuroeffector junction of the parasympathetic nervous system.[76]

Pharmacology
Eye

The anticholinergics block parasympathetic receptors in the sphincter of the iris and the ciliary muscle, producing dilation of the pupil (mydriasis) and an inability of the eye to accommodate (cycloplegia). There is little effect on intraocular pressure, except in patients with narrow-angle glaucoma, in whom significant increases in intraocular pressure may result. Narrow-angle glaucoma represents a contraindication to the use of these agents.[76]

Respiratory System
Administration of anticholinergics removes the parasympathetic nervous system's control over bronchial smooth muscle, leaving it under sole control of the sympathetic nervous system, which produces bronchodilation. Secretion of all glands within the oral cavity, pharynx, and respiratory tract is inhibited. Anticholinergics are frequently used before the induction of general anesthesia to minimize the risk of laryngospasm. This desirable action is a result of the decrease in secretions within the respiratory tract.

Salivary Glands
All parasympathetically mediated salivary secretions are completely inhibited by these agents. It is not uncommon for the patient receiving an anticholinergic to complain to the dentist that his mouth is overly dry, making it difficult to swallow or to speak.

Gastrointestinal Tract
The anticholinergic agents inhibit GI motility.

Cardiovascular System
The actions of the vagus nerve on the heart are diminished when anticholinergics are administered. This is termed the *vagolytic effect* and is of importance during the induction and maintenance of general anesthesia. There is an increase in heart rate following administration of usual therapeutic doses (0.4 to 0.6 mg) of atropine and scopolamine. Clinically significant bradycardia is managed with a dose of 1.0 mg atropine. Glycopyrrolate does not produce this effect to the same degree.

Urinary Tract
Anticholinergic drugs inhibit contractions of the bladder and ureter and produce dilation of the pelvis of the kidney, all of which act to produce urinary retention. In the presence of prostatic hypertrophy, this retention is more likely to develop.

Body Temperature
The anticholinergics inhibit sweating through their action on the cholinergic fibers of the sympathetic nervous system that innervate sweat glands. Body temperature rises following their administration. Elevation in temperature is the most serious and potentially life-threatening result of overdose of these agents.

Motion Sickness
Anticholinergics have been used for centuries in the management of motion sickness. They appear to act on the vestibular end organs, the cerebral cortex, or both. Scopolamine is more effective as an anti–motion sickness agent than is atropine.

Scopolamine is available for this use in the form of a transdermal patch (see Chapter 9).

Absorption, Metabolism, and Excretion
Anticholinergics are rapidly absorbed following IM administration. The liver is primarily responsible for their biotransformation, and the kidney is the main route of excretion. The half-life of atropine is 4 hours.

Contraindications
Anticholinergics are contraindicated in patients with untreated glaucoma (acute narrow angle), adhesions between the iris and the lens of the eye, and asthma. Their use in patients with prostatic hypertrophy is contraindicated because of the risk of increased urinary retention.

Drug Interactions
Anticholinergics should be used with caution in patients receiving other drugs possessing anticholinergic actions. These include tricyclic antidepressants, antipsychotics, histamine blockers, and antiparkinsonism drugs.

Adverse Reactions
Although there is great potential for individual variation in response to these drugs, Table 10.5 shows the usual pattern of adverse response to atropine.

Atropine
Atropine sulfate is commonly used in general anesthesia, both preoperatively and during the surgical procedure. Its primary functions during this time are (1) the inhibition of secretions within the respiratory tract, thereby minimizing the risk of laryngospasm but not preventing it; and (2) the vagolytic action of the drug on the heart, minimizing the occurrence of vagally

Table 10.5	Adverse Response to Atropine
DOSE	**RESPONSE**
0.5 mg	Slight drying of mouth, bradycardia, inhibition of sweating
1.0 mg	Greater dryness of nose and mouth, increased thirst, slowing then acceleration of the heart, slight mydriasis
2.0 mg	Very dry mouth, tachycardia with palpitation, mydriasis, slight blurring of near vision, flushed dry skin
5.0 mg	Increase in previously listed symptoms, disturbance of speech, difficulty in swallowing, headache, hot dry skin, restlessness
10.0 mg and above	Previously listed symptoms to extreme degree, ataxia, excitement, disorientation, hallucinations, delirium, coma*

*"Red as a beet, dry as a bone, and mad as a hatter" describes the patient during an anticholinergic overdose.

induced bradycardia. Atropine is more effective than scopolamine as a vagolytic agent, but does not possess the CNS-depressant or amnesic actions of scopolamine; however, these actions of scopolamine are not observed following IM administration, but only after IV administration.

The recommended adult parenteral dose of atropine (0.4 to 0.6 mg) does not produce an increase in intraocular pressure and is not contraindicated in patients with glaucoma.[77] Should such an increase in pressure develop, it may be counteracted with topically applied pilocarpine. Following IM administration, atropine produces clinical actions within 10 to 15 minutes, with a duration of action of 90 minutes.

Dosage

The usual adult dose is 0.4 to 0.6 mg intramuscularly 10 to 20 minutes before treatment. For children, the following dosage schedule for parenteral atropine is recommended in the drug product insert.[77]

7–16 lb	0.1 mg
17–24 lb	0.15 mg
24–40 lb	0.2 mg
40–65 lb	0.3 mg
65–90 lb	0.4 mg
More than 90 lb	0.4–0.6 mg

Availability

Atropine sulfate: 0.3, 0.4, 0.5, 0.6, 1.0, and 1.3 mg/mL. Atropine is not classified as a schedule drug.

Atropine	
Pregnancy category	C
Lactation	S
Metabolism	Other
Excretion	Urine
DEA schedule	Not controlled

Scopolamine

Scopolamine hydrobromide possesses the same pharmacologic properties as atropine, but in some cases to differing degrees. The vagolytic action of scopolamine is less than that of atropine, as is its effect in producing mydriasis. In addition, whereas atropine produces a stimulation of the CNS, scopolamine depresses the cerebral cortex. Scopolamine possesses a more intense drying effect than atropine.

In dentistry, scopolamine is primarily used for its ability to produce sedation and a degree of amnesia (as a component of the original *Jorgensen technique* of IV sedation—see Chapter 26). Following IM administration, the onset of action is 10 to 15 minutes, with a duration of action of approximately 90 minutes.

A possible side effect of scopolamine is the occurrence of excitement, restlessness, disorientation, and delirium during the postoperative recovery period.[78] This does not occur with atropine or glycopyrrolate. *Emergence delirium,* as it is known, is more likely to be observed in the very young or older adult patient, and it may be treated effectively with physostigmine (1 to 3 mg IV or IM). Emergence delirium is more common following IV than IM scopolamine administration; it is discussed more fully in Chapter 27.

Dosage

The usual adult dose is 0.32 to 0.65 mg 10 to 15 minutes before the procedure. The dose for children 6 months to 3 years old is 0.1 to 0.15 mg; for children 3 to 6 years old, 0.15 to 0.2 mg; and for children 6 to 12 years old, 0.2 to 0.3 mg.[79]

Availability

Scopolamine hydrobromide: 0.3, 0.4, and 0.6 mg/mL. Scopolamine is not classified as a schedule drug.

Scopolamine	
Pregnancy category	C
Lactation	S
Metabolism	Liver
Excretion	Urine
DEA schedule	Not controlled

Glycopyrrolate

Glycopyrrolate (introduced in 1961) is similar in many ways to atropine and scopolamine. Following IM administration, glycopyrrolate acts within 10 to 15 minutes, exerts a maximal effect in 30 to 45 minutes, and has a duration of action of approximately 7 hours, considerably longer than that of the other anticholinergics.[80]

Because glycopyrrolate is a quaternary ammonium compound, it does not pass through lipid membranes, such as the blood–brain barrier, as do atropine and scopolamine (tertiary amines, which pass easily through lipid membranes). Glycopyrrolate does not produce sedation or emergence delirium.

The drying effect of a 0.2-mg dose of glycopyrrolate is equal to that of 0.4 mg atropine. Glycopyrrolate offers the same vagolytic action as atropine and scopolamine; however, importantly, glycopyrrolate does not produce tachycardia or dysrhythmias as frequently as the other anticholinergics. This action may be significant in the cardiac-risk patient receiving these drugs (a beneficial effect) or in situations in which the dentist wishes to increase a too-slow heart rate (glycopyrrolate would not be indicated). Glycopyrrolate offers an attractive alternative to atropine and scopolamine when long-duration drying action is desired during dental procedures.

Dosage

The usual adult dose is 0.1 to 0.2 mg intramuscularly 30 to 60 minutes before treatment. The dose for children is between 0.004 and 0.01 mg/kg 30 to 60 minutes before treatment.[80]

Table 10.6	Comparison of Anticholinergic Actions		
	ATROPINE	**SCOPOLAMINE**	**GLYCOPYRROLATE**
Effect on secretions	Effective	Effective	Effective
Vagolytic action	Effective	Less than atropine	Effective
Tachycardia, dysrhythmias	Yes	Yes	Less likely
Effect on eye	Mydriasis	Less than atropine	Mydriasis
Effect on central nervous system	Stimulates	Depresses cortex	Stimulates

Availability

Glycopyrrolate hydrobromide (Robinul, Robins): 0.2 mg/mL. Glycopyrrolate is not classified as a schedule drug.

Glycopyrrolate	
Pregnancy category	B
Lactation	NS
Metabolism	Unknown
Excretion	Feces, primarily
DEA schedule	Not controlled

The anticholinergics are most often used in conjunction with parenterally administered CNS depressants. The primary goal in their use is a reduction in salivary secretions, leading to the production of a dry operating field; a secondary goal during IM sedation is the vagolytic actions of the drug. CNS depression produced by scopolamine via the IM route is usually insignificant compared with the other drugs used. Although all three drugs are effective and safe when used in therapeutic dosages, scopolamine should not be used if the sole aim in using an anticholinergic is the production of a dry field or its vagolytic actions. Atropine or glycopyrrolate are more appropriate in this regard. Scopolamine is indicated for use when a degree of CNS depression or amnesia is desired, although IV administration produces a much more reliable effect than does IM administration. In addition, scopolamine has the disturbing ability to produce emergence delirium; the other anticholinergics do not. Table 10.6 compares the actions of the anticholinergics.

Intramuscular Sedation Techniques

The drugs discussed in this chapter are those most often used intramuscularly for sedation. Box 10.5 classifies them into therapeutic categories. Group A includes the most effective IM drugs when lesser degrees of anxiety are present.

Used alone, group A drugs provide minimal-to-moderate levels of sedation in most patients. The benzodiazepines diazepam, lorazepam, and midazolam are the preferred drugs. Promethazine and hydroxyzine are less often used intramuscularly.

Box 10.5	Drugs Used in Intramuscular Sedation		
	Group A	**Group B**	**Group C**
	Diazepam*	Morphine[†]	Atropine
	Lorazepam[†]	Meperidine	Scopolamine
	Midazolam	Fentanyl	Glycopyrrolate[†]
	Promethazine	Alfentanil	
	Hydroxyzine*	Sufentanil	
	Butorphanol		
	Nalbuphine		

*May irritate tissues at injection site unless deposited deep into tissues.
[†]Long duration of action limits outpatient use.

Lorazepam is long acting and thus rarely indicated for IM administration in the outpatient environment. Diazepam should be injected deeply into muscle to decrease tissue irritation and to maximize its absorption, which might still be inconsistent. Water-soluble midazolam has proven to be a highly effective rapid-onset IM agent in the benzodiazepine class. Midazolam is extremely effective in the initial management of both patients with disabilities and pediatric patients who are precooperative or uncooperative and will not voluntarily be seated in the dental chair. The use of midazolam in these situations is discussed fully in Chapters 35 and 38.

Promethazine is a reliable drug for IM administration, providing slightly longer durations than midazolam or diazepam. Hydroxyzine must be injected deep into muscle to prevent tissue irritation.

When administered as discussed, group A drugs usually provide a level of moderate sedation adequate to permit treatment of adult patients with milder degrees of anxiety or adequate to place the fearful pediatric or handicapped patient into the dental chair, where other, more controllable techniques of drug administration may be employed (i.e., IV and/or inhalation).

Group B drugs are the OAs and agonist-antagonists. Their most rational use is for pain control in the posttreatment period. Although they will also provide a variable degree of sedation, their primary use for this indication cannot be recommended. Group A drugs are more specific and effective in managing fear and anxiety and have the additional benefit of producing fewer adverse effects (specifically, respiratory depression).

Group B drugs are frequently administered in combination with a group A drug in the management of patients with greater degrees of dental or surgical fear. When combined, the dose of the group B drug must be decreased from its "normal" level (when they are administered alone) because of the very real possibility of additive or potentiating actions, specifically CNS and respiratory depression. Combinations of group A and B drugs are most often used to provide deep sedation in pediatric patients (see Chapter 35) and patients with disabilities (see Chapter 38) and in the management of the overtly disruptive or uncooperative patient. Use of any group B drug for sedation or analgesia requires that the dentist and staff closely monitor the patient and quickly recognize and manage any adverse reactions (to "rescue" the patient from a level of sedation deeper than that sought).

Group C drugs, the anticholinergics, may be administered alone or in combination with group A and/or B drugs. They function not to provide CNS sedation (although scopolamine, to a minor degree, may do so), but rather to provide a vagolytic action (glycopyrrolate does this to a lesser degree) and to reduce secretions in the oral cavity and respiratory tract. Doses of group C agents need not be reduced when they are used in combination with group A and/or B drugs.

For decreasing salivary flow only, atropine is most commonly recommended. Glycopyrrolate maintains this action for too long a period for most dental procedures. Scopolamine may produce CNS depression and emergence delirium, with the latter occurring more commonly in patients younger than 6 years and older than 65 years of age.

The IM administration of two drugs from the same therapeutic category (i.e., meperidine and fentanyl or diazepam and midazolam) is only rarely recommended. Table 10.7 summarizes the recommended use of the drug groups listed.

Commonly Used Intramuscular Drug Combinations
Midazolam or Diazepam and Opioid Agonist

The combination of a benzodiazepine and opioid is used in both medicine and dentistry in adult and pediatric patients. Because the clinical effect of both diazepam and midazolam lasts 3 to 4 hours following IM administration, the selection of an appropriate opioid is important. IM morphine, with a duration of up to 7 hours, is too long acting for most medical and dental procedures. Where a patient may be kept under continual observation for several hours immediately posttreatment and where posttreatment pain is a significant factor, IM morphine may be indicated. Shorter-acting opioids, such as meperidine and fentanyl, are more appropriate for administration with midazolam or diazepam. Another problem arises where diazepam is to be used. Because it is lipid soluble, diazepam cannot be mixed in the same syringe with any of the opioids (all of which are water soluble). Two IM injections must therefore be administered. Water-soluble midazolam, on the other hand, which may be combined in the same syringe with the opioids, usually represents the most reasonable choice for an intramuscularly administered benzodiazepine.

Promethazine Plus Opioid

Because of the moderate duration (2 to 4 hours) of promethazine, it may be combined with meperidine, fentanyl, and its congeners in the same syringe. The proprietary name, Mepergan, a premixed formulation of promethazine and meperidine, is no longer manufactured in the United States.[54] Generic formulations may still be available. This combination is rather popular in pediatric medicine and dentistry for management of the overtly disruptive patient. Promethazine functions both as an antiemetic to counter this action of the opioid and to provide an added degree of sedation. Each milliliter of Mepergan contains 25 mg promethazine and 25 mg meperidine. Giovannitti and Trapp[19] consider this combination to be the most ideal choice for IM sedation. Suggested doses are 0.7 mg/kg

Table 10.7	Recommended Use of Drug Groups		
Drug Group	**Recommendation**	**Level of Sedation***
A alone (benzodiazepines)	High	Light to moderate
A alone (nonbenzodiazepines)	Low (but better than B alone)	Moderate to deep
B alone	Low	Moderate to deep
C alone	High	For ↓ secretions
A and B	High	Moderate to deep
A and C	High	Light to moderate and ↓ secretions
B and C	Low	Moderate to deep and ↓ secretions
A, B, and C	High	Moderate to deep and ↓ secretions

*Level of sedation may vary considerably with the same milligram-per-kilogram dose from patient to patient. Level indicated is usual level sought. The training and ability of the sedation team to safely manage the patient ultimately determine the level of sedation that should be employed.

promethazine and 1.0 mg/kg meperidine. Each drug is drawn up individually into the same syringe and administered intramuscularly. If after 45 minutes sedation is inadequate, N_2O-O_2 sedation, titrated to effect, may be added.[19]

Hydroxyzine Plus Opioid

Similar to promethazine and opioid in depth and duration, hydroxyzine may be combined with meperidine or fentanyl. Hydroxyzine serves to minimize opioid-induced nausea and vomiting and to provide a degree of sedation. It is used primarily in the management of the acutely disruptive or uncooperative child. This technique and promethazine plus opioid may also be used in adults.

Meperidine, Promethazine, and Chlorpromazine

This combination is probably more familiar by the name *lytic cocktail* or by its abbreviation, DPT, taken from the proprietary names of the three agents Demerol, Phenergan, and Thorazine. DPT is rarely used today for sedation, primarily because of the chlorpromazine and its potentially significant side effects. It provides a long duration and a moderately deep level of sedation. Administration of this technique for IM sedation is actively discouraged.[81,82]

Monitoring During Intramuscular Sedation

A significant change in the use of IM-SM sedation since the initial publication of this book in 1985 has been the increased importance of monitoring whenever IM-SM agents are used. The greater the depth of sedation (CNS depression) obtained, the greater the level of monitoring required to ensure patient safety.

When moderate sedation is the goal, direct communication with the sedated patient is the most important monitor (CNS), although respiratory and cardiovascular monitoring are also mandatory. However, patient responsiveness is diminished when deep sedation is the goal, and monitoring of other systems must be intensified.

Vital signs must be checked continuously (heart rate, oxygen saturation, end tidal CO_2 [if required]) or at regular intervals (BP, respiratory rate), commonly every 5 minutes, throughout the period of sedation (which starts when the patient first receives a sedation drug [before the actual dental or surgical treatment] and extends into the posttreatment period). The use of the pretracheal stethoscope is highly recommended for IM-SM techniques. In pediatrics, placement of the stethoscope over the precordium is acceptable, although its placement over the trachea immediately superior to the sternal notch is preferred. In adults, pretracheal placement is preferred.

The use of pulse oximetry is considered standard of care for IM-SM moderate and deep sedation. The combination of a pretracheal stethoscope and pulse oximetry provides the dentist with an immediate and continuous "feel" as to the respiratory and ventilatory status of the patient, which is important because the respiratory system is the system most

readily influenced (after the CNS) by the IM-SM agents used for sedation.

Additional monitoring techniques, such as capnography and electrocardiography, are being mandated by an increasing number of dental regulatory agencies, but are not considered to be essential monitors during IM-SM moderate sedation, although the use of capnography during deep sedation has become increasingly popular. I do not consider monitoring of the electrical activity of the myocardium (ECG) during moderate sedation to be of as critical importance as respiratory monitoring. The doctor must check the mandated monitoring requirements established by his or her state or provincial regulatory agency.

The IM Sedation Appointment

The adult patient has been evaluated at a prior appointment, both dentally and medically, for the appropriateness of being sedated. For whatever reason, other routes of drug administration have been ruled out (inhalation sedation—patient cannot breathe through their nose; IV—lack of any obvious superficial veins; oral—simply did not work).

The dental treatment plan has been formulated, and preoperative instructions are discussed with and given to the patient. Preoperative instructions for IM sedation are the same as those for other parenteral techniques. An example of preoperative instructions is found in Chapter 26.

The patient is brought into the treatment area, placed in the dental chair, and appropriate monitors are applied (e.g., pulse oximeter, BP cuff). For recordkeeping, the time the patient is seated in the dental chair should be recorded as the sedation "start time." The IM drug(s) are administered by the dentist.

Oxygen delivery may be started at this time using either a nasal cannula or nasal hood.

Kept under continuous observation by a trained staff person (the definition of this "trained staff person" will vary from jurisdiction to jurisdiction—always consult your state or provincial board's regulations), the drug is permitted time to reach a maximal clinical effect. This usually occurs in approximately 20 to 30 minutes.

The level of sedation is assessed and, if appropriate, the dental treatment commenced.

If it is believed that the level of sedation is inadequate, it is prudent for the dentist to consider one of the following alternatives:

1. Attempt to carry out the dental treatment in this less-than-ideal environment.
2. Cancel the appointment and reschedule for another technique or other drug(s).
3. Titrate N_2O-O_2 until the desired level of moderate sedation is achieved (if permitted by your state or provincial dental regulatory agency).

Option No. 3 is the most appropriate.

A fourth option, though actually not a viable option, would be to administer an additional dose of the IM drug. Because IM drugs cannot be titrated, to administer a second dose intramuscularly increases the risk of "overshooting" the desired level of CNS depression, resulting in a "too deep" patient in whom dentistry cannot be carried out or in a patient who needs to be "rescued" until they return to a moderate level of sedation.

Continuous monitoring of O_2 saturation and heart rate is performed with periodic (e.g., every 5 min) recording of BP.

At the conclusion of the dental treatment, vital signs are recorded once again (postoperative vital signs) and the patient assessed for recovery and their ability to be discharged from the office.

Criteria for recovery from IM sedation are the same as those for IV sedation and are discussed in Chapter 26.

When the patient is deemed fit for discharge, the responsible adult escort is brought into the room and the postsedation instructions are both told to and given to the patient and the escort (see Box 26.2).

One final set of vital signs is recorded (discharge vital signs), and the patient is escorted from the dental office in the company of an office staff member, who will stay with the patient until he or she is safely buckled into the passenger seat or back seat of a car. The time recorded for the end of sedation is the time the patient leaves the dental chair.

A posttreatment telephone call is made to the patient either late in the afternoon or early in the evening (dependent on when the patient was discharged from the office) on the day of treatment, at which time the dentist seeks to determine (1) how the recovery is progressing, (2) if there are any questions from the patient, and (3) if any minor problems have developed. Additionally, it is good practice to fully review the postoperative instructions at this time.

SUMMARY

The IM route of drug administration has definite advantages compared with oral administration; however, compared with the inhalation and IV routes, IM fares poorly. In adults, the only rationale for the IM route is a lack of success with other, more controllable routes. In pediatrics or with patients with disabilities, however, the IM (or SM) route may prove to be the only effective patient management technique available aside from general anesthesia.

Drugs administered intramuscularly must have their doses carefully calculated. Once administered IM, it is difficult, if not impossible, to reverse the actions of most drugs. Basic management (rescue) of overly sedated patients must consist primarily of basic life support: airway maintenance, breathing (spontaneous, assisted, or controlled), and circulation. Dentists using the IM route must be adept at patient monitoring and be trained in management of the unconscious airway.

REFERENCES

1. Hine CH, Pasi A: Fatality after use of alphaprodine in analgesia for dental surgery: report of a case. *J Am Dent Assoc* 84:858–861, 1972.

2. Okuji DM: Hypoxic encephalopathy after the administration of alphaprodine hydrochloride. *J Am Dent Assoc* 103:50–52, 1981.

3. Goodson JM, Moore PA: Life-threatening reactions following pedodontic sedation: an assessment of narcotic, local anesthetic and antiemetic drug interaction. *J Am Dent Assoc* 107:239–245, 1983.

4. Moore PA, Goodson JM: Risk appraisal of narcotic sedation for children. *Anesth Prog* 32:129–139, 1985.

5. Lee HH, Milgrom P, Starks H, Burke W: Trends in death associated with pediatric dental sedation and general anesthesia. *Paediatr Anaesth* 23(8):741–746, 2013.

6. Council on Governmental Affairs, Chicago, April 2014 American Dental Association.

7. Alphaprodine. *Pediatr Dent* 4(special issue 1):156–206, 1982.

8. Trapp L, Goodson JM, Price DC: Evaluation of oral submucosal blood flow at dental injection sites by radioactive xenon clearance in beagle dogs. *J Dent Res* 56(8):889–893, 1977.

9. Hine CH, Pasi A: Fatality after use of alphaprodine in analgesia for dental surgery: report of a case. *J Am Dent Assoc* 84(4):858–861, 1972.

10. Metroka DC, Marchesani JR, Carrel R: A submucous technique utilizing a narcotic and a potentiator. *J Pedod* 4(2):124–138, 1980.

11. Jensen ST, Coke JM, Cohen L: Intramuscular injection technique. *J Am Dent Assoc* 100(5):700–702, 1980.

12. Zelman S: Notes on techniques of intramuscular injection: the avoidance of needless pain and morbidity. *Am J Med Sci* 241:563–574, 1961.

13. Evans E, Proctor J, Fratkin M, et al: Blood flow in muscle groups and drug absorption. *Clin Pharmacol Ther* 17(1):44–47, 1975.

14. Ceravolo FJ, Meyers HE, Michael JJ, et al: Full dentition periodontal surgery using intravenous conscious sedation: a report of 10,000 cases. *J Periodontol* 57(6):383–384, 1986.

15. Greenblatt D, Koch-Weser J: Intramuscular injection of drugs. *N Engl J Med* 295(10):542–546, 1976.

16. Grohar ME: *How to give an intramuscular injection*, New York, 1980, Pfizer Laboratories.

17. Greenblatt D, Shader R, Koch-Weser J: Serum creatinine phosphokinase concentration after intramuscular chlordiazepoxide and its solvent. *J Clin Pharmacol* 16(2–3):118–121, 1976.

18. Beyea SC, Nicoll LH: Administration of medications via the intramuscular route: an integrative review of the literature and research-based protocol for the procedure. *Appl Nurs Res* 8(1):23–33, 1995.

19. Giovannitti JA, Trapp LD: Adult sedation: oral, rectal, IM, IV. In Dionne RA, Phero JC, editors: *Management of pain and anxiety in dental practice*, New York, 1991, Elsevier.

20. Rodger MA, King L: Drawing up and administering intramuscular injections: a review of the literature. *J Adv Nurs* 31(3):574–582, 2000.

21. Hanson DJ: Intramuscular injection injuries and complications. *Gen Pract* 27:109, 1963.

22. Tsokos M, Puschel K: Iatrogenic *Staphylococcus aureus* septicaemia following intravenous and intramuscular injections: clinical course and pathomorphological findings. *Int J Legal Med* 112(5):303–308, 1999.

23. McCaughey W, Dundee JW: Comparison of the sedative effects of diazepam given by the oral and intramuscular routes. *Br J Anaesth* 44(8):901–902, 1972.

24. Baird ES, Hailey DM: Plasma levels of diazepam and its major metabolite following intramuscular administration. *Br J Anaesth* 45(6):546–548, 1973.

25. Kortilla K, Linnoila M: Absorption and sedative effects of diazepam after oral administration and intramuscular administration into the vastus lateralis muscle and the deltoid muscle. *Br J Anaesth* 47(8):857–862, 1975.

26. Moolenaar F, Bakker S, Visser J, et al: Biopharmaceutics of rectal administration of drugs in man. IX: comparative biopharmaceutics of diazepam after single rectal, oral, intramuscular and intravenous administration in man. *Int J Pharmaceut* 5:127, 1980.

27. Divoll M, Greenblatt DJ, Ochs HR, et al: Absolute bioavailability of oral and intramuscular diazepam: effect of age and sex. *Anesth Analg* 62(1):1–8, 1983.

20. Diazepam Drug Monograph, ClinicalKey April 2, 2015, www.clinicalkey.com. (Accessed 12 October 2015).

29. Lorazepam Drug Monograph, ClinicalKey, April 16, 2014, www.clinicalkey.com. (Accessed 12 October 2015).

30. Odugbesan CO, Magbagbeola JA: Parenteral premedication with lorazepam: a dose/response study. *Afr J Med Sci* 14:65–69, 1985.

31. Malamed SF, Quinn CL, Hatch HG: Pediatric sedation with intramuscular and intravenous midazolam. *Anesth Prog* 36:155–157, 1989.

32. Malamed SF, Gottschalk HW, Mulligan R, et al: Intravenous sedation for conservative dentistry for disabled patients. *Anesth Prog* 36:140–142, 1989.

33. Theissen O, Boileua S, Wahl D, et al: Sedation with intranasal midazolam for endoscopy of the upper digestive tract. *Ann Fr Anesth Reanim* 10:450–455, 1990.

34. Midazolam Drug Monograph, ClinicalKey, March 25, 2015, www.clinicalkey.com. (Accessed 12 October 2015).

35. Promethazine Drug Monograph, ClinicalKey, July 30, 2015, www.clinicalkey.com. (Accessed 26 October 2015).

36. Allen GD: *Dental anesthesia and analgesia*, ed 2, Baltimore, 1979, Williams & Wilkins.

37. Hydroxyzine Drug Monograph, ClinicalKey, August 17, 2015, www.clinicalkey.com. (Accessed 26 October 2015).

38. Chang KJ, Cuatrecasas P: Heterogeneity and properties of opiate receptors. *Fed Proc* 40(13):2729–2734, 1981.

39. Ossipov MH, Gebhart GF, Porreca F: Opioid analgesics and antagonists. In Yagiela JA, Dowd FJ, editors: *Pharmacology and therapeutics for dentistry*, ed 6, St Louis, 2011, Mosby, pp 307–323.

40. Phillips WJ: Central nervous system pain receptors. In Faust RJ, editor: *Anesthesiology review*, New York, 2002, Churchill Livingstone.

41. Shields SE: Pharmacokinetics of epidural narcotics. In Faust RJ, editor: *Anesthesiology review*, New York, 2002, Churchill Livingstone.

42. Way EL: Sites and mechanisms of basic narcotic function based on current research. *Ann Emerg Med* 15(9):1021–1025, 1986.

43. Yaksh TL, Wallace MS: Opioids, analgesia and pain management. In Brunton L, Chabner B, Knollman B, editors: *The pharmacological basis of therapeutics*, ed 12, New York, 2011, McGraw-Hill, pp 481–526.

44. Manzini JL, Somoza EJ, Fridlender HI: Oral morphine in the treatment of patients with terminal disease. *Medicina* 50(6):532–536, 1990.

45. Morphine Drug Monograph, ClinicalKey, June 9, 2015, www.clinicalkey.com. (Accessed 26 October 2015).

46. Reidenberg MM, Lowenthal DT: Adverse nondrug reactions. *N Engl J Med* 279(13):678–679, 1968.

47. Meyer FP, Troger U, Rohl FW: Adverse nondrug reactions: an update. *Clin Pharmacol Ther* 60(3):347–352, 1996.

48. Roberts SM, Wilson CF, Seale NS, et al: Evaluation of morphine as compared to meperidine when administered to the moderately anxious pediatric dental patient. *Pediatr Dent* 14(5):306–313, 1992.

49. Meperidine Drug Monograph, ClinicalKey, June 9, 2015, www.clinicalkey.com. (Accessed 26 October 2015).

50. Mepergan Drug Monograph, ClinicalKey, June 9, 2015, www.clinicalkey.com. (Accessed 22 October 2015).

51. Wilson S: Minimal and moderate sedation agents. In Wright GZ, Kupietzky A, editors: *Behavior management in dentistry for children*, ed 2, Philadelphia, 2014, WB Saunders, pp 159–176.

52. Dock M: Pharmacologic management of patient behavior. In Dean JA, Avery DR, McDonald RE, editors: *McDonald and Avery dentistry for the child and adolescent*, ed 9, 2011, Mosby Elsevier, pp 253–276.

53. Alcaino EA, McDonald J, Cooper MG, Mallii S. Pharmacological behaviour management. In Cameron A, Widner R, editors: *Handbook of pediatric dentistry*, St Louis, 2013, Mosby-Elsevier, pp 25–46.

54. Mepergan. http://www.rxlist.com/mepergan-drug.htm. (Accessed 22 October 2015).

55. Wiullens JS, Myslinski NR: Pharmacodynamics, pharmacokinetics, and clinical uses of fentanyl, sufentanil, and alfentanil. *Heart Lung* 22(3):239–251, 1993.

56. Ackerman WE, Phero JC, Theodore GT: Ineffective ventilation during conscious sedation due to chest wall rigidity after intravenous midazolam and fentanyl. *Anesth Prog* 37(1):46–48, 1990.

57. Coruh B, Tonelli MR, Park DR: Fentanyl-induced chest wall rigidity. *Chest* 143(4):1145–1146, 2013.

58. Fentanyl, Drug Monograph, ClinicalKey, June 4, 2015, www.clinicalkey.com. (Accessed 25 October 2015).

59. Hsu JY, Lian JD, Shu KH, et al: Pentazocine addict nephropathy: a case report. *Chung-hua I Hsueh Tsa Chih (Chin Med J)* 49(3):207–211, 1992.

60. Malamed SF: Intramuscular sedation. In *Sedation: a guide to patient management*, ed 5, St Louis, 2010, C.V. Mosby, Inc., p 152.

61. Vandam LD: Drug therapy: butorphanol. *N Engl J Med* 302(7):381–384, 1980.

62. Laffey DA, Kay NH: Premedication with butorphanol: a comparison with morphine. *Br J Anaesth* 56(4):363–367, 1984.

63. Butorphanol Drug Monograph. ClinicalKey, February 28, 2012, www.clinicalkey.com. (Accessed 25 October 2015).

64. Pinnock CA, Bell A, Smith G: A comparison of nalbuphine and morphine as premedication agents for minor gynaecological surgery. *Anaesthesia* 40(11):1078–1081, 1985.

65. Nalbuphine, Drug Monograph ClinicalKey, April 9, 2012, www.clinicalkey.com. (Accessed 25 October 2015).

66. Cataldo PA, Senagore AJ, Kilbride MJ: Ketorolac and patient controlled analgesia in the treatment of postoperative pain. *Surg Gynecol Obstet* 176(5):435–438, 1993.

67. Sinha VR, Kumar RV, Singh G: Ketorolac tromethamine formulations: an overview. *Expert Opin Drug Deliv* 6(9):961–975, 2009.

68. Lassen K, Epstein-Stiles M, Olsson GL: Ketorolac: a new parenteral nonsteroidal anti-inflammatory drug for postoperative pain management. *J Post Anesth Nurs* 7(4):238–242, 1992.

69. Acute Pain Management Guideline Panel: Acute pain management operative or medical procedures and trauma, clinical practice guideline, AHCPR Publication No. 92-2, Rockville, 1992, Agency for Health Care Policy and Research, Public Health Service, U.S. Department of Health and Human Services.

70. Ketorolac, Drug Monograph ClinicalKey, August 17, 2015, www.clinicalkey.com. (Accessed 25 October 2015).

71. Reich DL, Silvay G: Ketamine: an update on the first twenty-five years of clinical experience. *Can J Anaesth* 36(2):186–197, 1989.

72. White PF, Ham J, Way WL, et al: Pharmacology of ketamine isomers in surgical patients. *Anesthesiology* 52(3):231–239, 1980.

73. Ketamine, Drug Monograph ClinicalKey, December 20, 2013, www.clinicalkey.com. (Accessed 25 October 2015).

74. Roelofse JA, Vander-Bijl P: Adverse reactions to midazolam and ketamine premedication in children. *Anesth Prog* 38(2):73, 1992.

75. Folayan MO, Faponle AF, Oziegbe EO, Adetoye AO: A prospective study on the effectiveness of ketamine and diazepam used for conscious sedation in paediatric dental patients' management. *Eur J Paediatr Dent* 15(2):132–136, 2014.

76. Dietz NM: The pharmacology of atropine, scopolamine, and glycopyrrolate. In Murray MJ, Harrison BA, Mueller JT, et al, editors: *Faust's anesthesiology review*, ed 4, Philadelphia, 2015, Saunders-Elsevier, pp 187–188.

77. Atropine, Drug Monograph ClinicalKey, July 20, 2015, www.clinicalkey.com. (Accessed 25 October 2015).

78. Holzgrafe RE, Vondrell JJ, Mintz SM: Reversal of postoperative reactions to scopolamine with physostigmine. *Anesth Analg* 52(6):921–925, 1973.

79. Scopolamine hydrobromide, Drug Monograph ClinicalKey, March 24, 2015, www.clinicalkey.com. (Accessed 25 October 2015).

80. Glycopyrrolate Drug Monograph ClinicalKey, August 17, 2015, www.clinicalkey.com. (Accessed 25 October 2015).

81. U.S. Department of Health and Human Services: Management of postoperative and procedural pain in infants, children and adolescents. In *Clinical practice guideline: acute pain management: operative or medical procedures and trauma*, Rockville, MD, 1992, USDHHS.

82. Nahata M, Clotz M, Krogg E: Adverse effects of meperidine, promethazine, and chlorpromazine for sedation in pediatric patients. *Clin Pediatr (Phila)* 24(10):558–560, 1985.

Section IV

INHALATION SEDATION

In the technique of inhalation sedation, gaseous agents are absorbed from the lungs into the cardiovascular system. Although any number of inhalation anesthetics may be administered for the production of sedation (see Section VI), only one, nitrous oxide, is used by any appreciable number of health professionals (including, but not limited to, dentists, physicians, nurses, and podiatrists). This section is therefore devoted to a discussion of the use of nitrous oxide-oxygen (N_2O-O_2) inhalation sedation.

Inhalation sedation with nitrous oxide (N_2O) and oxygen (O_2) has significant advantages over other techniques of sedation, yet it possesses no disadvantages of consequence. This technique is an important part of the armamentarium for the management of fear and anxiety; indeed, the number of health professionals using N_2O-O_2 has risen steadily during the past decades. In the United States it is estimated that approximately 40% of practicing dentists and 90% of all pedodontists currently use N_2O-O_2,[1] and virtually all dental graduates today enter into dental practice proficient in its safe and effective use.[2] In addition, as of September 2015, 32 states have modified their dental practice acts to permit the registered dental hygienist to administer N_2O-O_2 (Table IV.1).[3] In fields other than dentistry, health professionals are beginning to use this valuable technique of sedation to their patients' benefit. In anesthesia, N_2O-O_2 has been used for more than 100 years as an important component of most general anesthetics, primarily as a means of permitting other, more potent, and potentially more dangerous general anesthetics to be used effectively in smaller doses and consequently in a safer manner. In the past 45 years, N_2O-O_2 has been used by emergency medical personnel, both in the hospital and in mobile coronary care units, to decrease or to eliminate pain caused by an acute myocardial infarction[4] and traumatic injuries.[5,6] Many dermatologists, plastic and reconstructive surgeons, urologists, radiologists, and ophthalmologists use N_2O-O_2 as an aid in

Table IV.1	Nitrous Oxide Administration by Dental Hygienists – State Chart		
STATE & YEAR IMPLEMENTED	**STATUTE OR RULES**	**EDUCATION REQUIRED**	**PERMIT OR CERTIFICATE**
AK 1997	Rules	3 hrs clinical; 3 hrs didactic CPR	No
AR 1994	Rules	Minimum of 4 hrs	No
AZ 1976	Rules	36 hrs; included in local anesthesia course	No
CA 1974	Rules	Board approved course	No
CO 1997	Statute	16 hrs	Yes
DC 2004	Rules	32 hrs	Yes
FL 2005 (Monitor only)	Rules	Two day course training; CPR	No
IA 2001	Rules	Board approved course or part of degree	No
ID 1979	Rules	Degree completion or accredited	No
IL 1999	Rules	14 hrs	No
KS 1994	Statute	Board approved course; 12 hrs	No
KY 2002	Statute	2 hrs clinical in addition to 32 hrs of local anesthesia courses and 12 hrs of practical demonstration	Yes
LA 2010	Statute	Board approved course; 8 hrs	Yes
MD 2016	Statute	6-hour Board-approved course; 4 hrs didactic; 2 hrs clinical	Yes
ME 2006	Rules	8 hrs didactic; 8 hours clinical; CODA/board approved course and exam	Yes
MI 2004	Statute	4 hrs didactic; 4 hrs clinical	Yes
MN 1995	Rules	12 hrs of clinical didactic CPR	No
MO 1994	Rules	Course that provides proof of compentence	Yes
MS 2012		Currently licensed dentist may instruct a dental auxiliary to monitor nitrous-oxide under their direct supervision. Dental auxiliary must be CPR certified.	No
MT	Rules	None	No
NH 2006	Statute	8 hrs didactic; 6 hrs clinical	Yes
NJ 2008 (Monitor only)	Rules	7 hrs didactic; 7 hrs clinical; CPR	Yes
NM 2005	Rules	CPR competence	No
NV 1982	Statute	Board approval course or part of degree	Yes
NY 2001	Statute	30 hrs didactic; 15 hrs clinical	Yes
OH 2010	Rules	4 hrs didactic; 2 hrs clinical; written exam; clinical evaluation	Yes
OK 1975	Rules	12 hrs completion in board approved course	No
OR 1975	Rules	14 hrs in N2O CPR	Yes
RI 2011	Rules	4 hrs didactic; 4 hrs clinical	Yes
SD 1992	Rules	Board approved course	Yes
TN 2000	Rules	Board approved course	Yes
UT 1983	Statute	Board approved course or part of degree	Yes
VA 2006 – On patients 18 or older only	Statute	8 hrs didactic; 8 hrs clinical	Yes
WA 1971	Rules	Didactic clinical competency	No
WI 2014	Statute	Certification program sponsored by an accredited dental or dental hygiene school or an approved ADA CERP or AGD PACE provider. Minimum of 8 hrs of didactic instruction.	Yes
WY 2008	Rules	Board approved course	Yes

patient management during minor surgical or diagnostic procedures.[7,8] In the practice of podiatric medicine, there has been a significant increase in interest in inhalation sedation.[9]

Much of the current interest in inhalation sedation has occurred following a change in the basic concept concerning the goals sought in the use of N_2O-O_2. Once used solely as a general anesthetic (1800s) and later as an analgesic (1940s to 1950s), N_2O-O_2 is now employed to produce sedation. Safety to the patient is significantly increased because the sedated patient remains conscious (and responsive) throughout the inhalation procedure. In addition, there have been important changes in the design of the inhalation sedation unit used to deliver these gases. Derived from the operating room general anesthesia machine, today's inhalation sedation unit has incorporated into it safety features that make the technique of inhalation sedation one that is virtually free of significant risk to the patient.

This section consists of a series of smaller chapters than the preceding section. It is hoped that this will enable the reader to more effectively locate material that is of importance to him or her. Subsequent chapters in this section will provide in-depth discussions of the development of inhalation sedation; the advantages, disadvantages, and indications for inhalation sedation; the pharmacology of the gases used and the mechanisms by which gaseous anesthetics produce their effect; the armamentarium for inhalation sedation; techniques for administration of N_2O-O_2; complications associated with its administration; and current concerns about N_2O, including chronic exposure, recreational abuse, and the occurrence of sexual phenomena. Concluding chapters discuss practical considerations concerning the use of inhalation sedation and educational guidelines established that relate to this important technique. Nitrous oxide was the first drug employed to achieve this magical state of anesthesia and sedation, which enables surgeons to successfully complete surgical procedures on patients without the dreaded presence of pain.

REFERENCES

1. Jones TW, Greenfield W: Position paper of the ADA ad hoc committee on trace anesthetics as a potential health hazard in dentistry. *J Am Dent Assoc* 95(4):751–756, 1977.
2. Commission on Dental Accreditation: *Accreditation standards for advanced education programs in general dentistry*, Chicago, 1998, American Dental Association.
3. States that permit dental hygienists to administer nitrous oxide. American Dental Hygienists Association. Chicago. www.adha.org 2014, (Accessed 1 November 2015).
4. Kerr F, Brown MG, Irving JB, et al: A double-blind trial of patient-controlled nitrous-oxide/oxygen analgesia in myocardial infarction. *Lancet* 1(7922):1397–1400, 1975.
5. Onody P, Gil P, Hennequin M: Safety of inhalation of a 50% Nitrous Oxide/Oxygen Premix: a prospective survey of 35,828 administrations. *Drug Saf* 29(7):633–640, 2006.
6. Faddy SC, Garlick SR: A systematic review of the safety of analgesia with 50% nitrous oxide: can lay responders use analgesic gases in the prehospital setting? *Emerg Med J* 22(12):901–906, 2005.
7. Corboy JM: Nitrous oxide analgesia for outpatient surgery. *J Am Intraocul Implant Soc* 10(2):232–234, 1984.
8. Cruickshank JC, Sykes SH: Office sedation. *Adv Dermatol* 7:291–313, 1992.
9. Harris WC, Jr, Alpert WJ, Gill JJ, Marcinko DE: Nitrous oxide and Valium use in podiatric surgery for production of conscious sedation. *J Am Podiatry Assoc* 72(10):505–510, 1982.

chapter 11

Inhalation Sedation: Historical Perspective

CHAPTER OUTLINE

It has been said that "the only thing new is the history we have not read." The history of inhalation sedation is quite remarkable and indeed colorful. This history is the story of the development of the art and science of anesthesiology. It is presented in part for the reader to better appreciate the benefits we enjoy today using nitrous oxide–oxygen (N_2O–O_2) sedation. The improvement in techniques, equipment, and administration of nitrous oxide has increased tremendously over the 245 years that have passed since the discovery of N_2O and the more than 173 years since it was first used as an agent for sedation.

BEGINNINGS (PRE-1844)

As difficult as it is to imagine, the gases oxygen (O_2) and N_2O were once unknown. It was not until 1771 that the German scientist Karl Scheele (1742–1786) and the Englishman Sir Joseph Priestley (1733–1804), working independently, discovered O_2. In 1727 O_2 had been prepared by Stephen Hales; however, he did not recognize that it was an element, and credit for the discovery of O_2 is given to Scheele and Priestley. The year following the discovery of O_2 Priestley discovered N_2O.[1,2]

During the late 1700s a branch of science known as *pneumatic medicine* came into being. Thomas Beddoes' Pneumatic Institute in Bristol, England, became one of the major centers of investigation of the newly discovered gaseous "vapors." It was at this time that Sir Humphrey Davy (1778–1829) became interested in the study of these gaseous agents. In 1795 at the age of 17, Davy had become an apprentice to the surgeon J. B. Borlase and, during his stay with Borlase, had experimented with N_2O and the effects of its inhalation. Davy became the superintendent of the Pneumatic Institute in 1798 and a year later published his book *Researches, Chemical and Philosophical; Chiefly Concerning Nitrous Oxide*. In this book Davy hinted that the inhalation of N_2O might be used to diminish pain during surgical procedures. He also provided the still commonly used nickname "laughing gas" (Fig. 11.1). The following is an excerpt from Davy's work on N_2O in which he explains the effects of the agent on himself following self-administration for a toothache and gingival inflammation:

On the day when the inflammation was the most troublesome, I breathed three large doses of nitrous oxide. The pain always diminished after the first four or five inspirations; the thrilling came on as usual, and uneasiness was for a few minutes swallowed up in pleasure. As the former state of mind returned, the state of organ returned with it; and I once imagined that the pain was more severe after the experiment than before. … As nitrous oxide in its extensive operation appears capable of destroying physical pain, it may probably be used with advantage during surgical operations in which no great effusion of blood takes place.[3]

Unfortunately, both Davy and the rest of the medical profession failed to take serious notice of N_2O or to administer it for the relief of pain during surgery. One of the reasons for this failure to even try these newer gaseous agents was the fact that during the late 1700s and early 1800s, "ether frolics" and "laughing gas demonstrations" were a popular source of entertainment and enjoyment among younger people (Fig. 11.2). Ether (ethyl ether) had been first described by Valerius Cordus in Germany in 1540, who called it *sweet vitriol*.[1] In

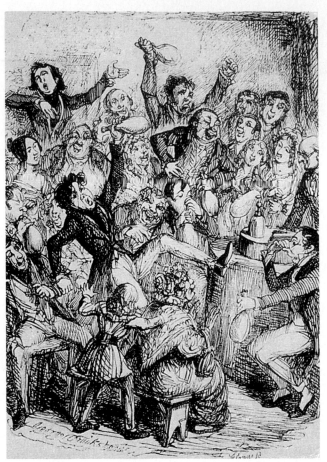

Figure 11.1 "Laughing gas." (From Scoffern: Chemistry No Mystery, 1839.)

1794 Beddoes[4] reported that ether produced a deep sleep. As with N_2O, however, ether had also been used as a source of entertainment in the late eighteenth and early nineteenth centuries. The thought that agents such as ether and N_2O, which were commonly used to produce intoxication, could ever be employed during surgery as a means of abolishing pain was offered serious consideration by very few persons.

One of these persons, Henry Hill Hickman (1800–1830), an English physician, experimented with the use of carbon dioxide (CO_2) for the creation of "suspended animation." Hickman successfully performed surgical procedures on animals using the inhalation of CO_2 to abolish pain during the procedure. In 1824 Hickman's paper, "A Letter on Suspended Animation," was published.[5] Unfortunately, the medical profession did not take notice, and Hickman's potentially important research was ignored and forgotten.

In 1831 yet another volatile agent, chloroform, was discovered. Working independently, Von Liebig (1803–1873) in Germany, Guthrie (1782–1848) in New York, and Soubeiran (1793–1858) in France are credited with its discovery.

In 1842 two other ambitious men took the great step forward and successfully administered ether to a patient during a surgical procedure. In Rochester, New York, Dr. W. E. Clark administered ether to a patient having a tooth extracted by a dentist, Dr. Elijah Pope. In Georgia, Dr. Crawford W. Long administered ether to John Venable for the removal of a tumor from his neck. It is interesting that neither of these persons thought this discovery important enough to write about it in the scientific journals. Dr. Long finally wrote about his use of the agent, stating that he had used it on three occasions in 1842 and on at least one occasion annually since that time.[6] The date of Long's paper was 1849, years after he had originally used ether clinically. The purpose of the paper was to lay claim to the title of the "Founder of General Anesthesia," which was at that time being contested among Morton, Wells, and Jackson, three men who are discussed shortly.

Thus for several more years patients requiring surgery were left with the same two options they had faced for centuries: endure the surgical procedure without benefit of any means of abolishing pain or elect not to have the surgery and face probable death.

However, as the 1840s progressed, things were about to change. It is interesting that one of these great changes occurred in a most unusual setting—a popular science lecture during which volunteers from the audience were permitted to experience the effects of N_2O.

THE EARLY DAYS (1844–1862)

On December 10, 1844, in the town of Hartford, Connecticut, Professor Gardner Quincy Colton presented a popular science lecture. Professor Colton was an itinerant medical school dropout from Columbia University, traveling around the countryside presenting his show of new scientific and quasi-scientific discoveries to eager audiences.[7] In his show, N_2O gas was discussed and demonstrated, and as a part of the demonstration, male volunteers were invited from the audience to partake of the effects of N_2O (Fig. 11.3). Women were also permitted to try N_2O, but not in the presence of the men. A private session was held for the women.

A Hartford dentist, Dr. Horace Wells (1815–1848), was in the audience on this particular evening (Fig. 11.4). Wells had a productive dental practice but, being an especially sensitive person, had difficulty in dealing with the terrible anguish and suffering of his patients. In the early 1840s, in dentistry, as in medicine, medications for the prevention and relief of pain were nonexistent. At the demonstration a store clerk by the name of Samuel Cooley, as well as several other men, volunteered to receive N_2O. Breathing 100% N_2O from a spigot attached to a bladder bag filled with the gas, Cooley quickly became intoxicated, running about the stage. During his running about, Cooley's leg hit the side of a table quite hard, yet Cooley continued to carry on as before, apparently oblivious of his injury. The skin had been broken, the wound bleeding, but there was no indication that Cooley either felt discomfort or was even aware of the injury. Wells spoke with Cooley after the incident and confirmed that he had been unaware of the injury.

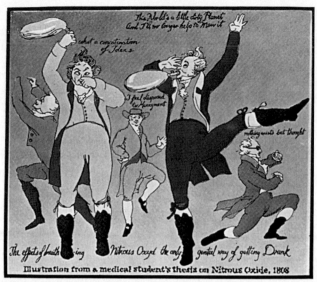

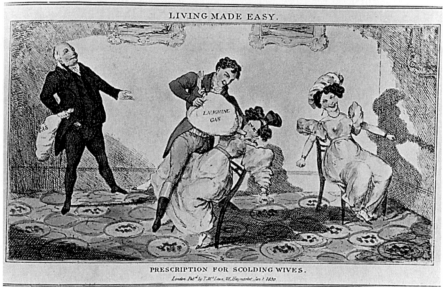

Figure 11.2 Nitrous oxide was used exclusively in a social setting in the early 1800s, as illustrated by these drawings from publications of that era. (From Shelden M, Wallechinsky D: *Laughing gas, nitrous oxide*, Berkeley, 1973, And/Or Press.)

Wells discussed this occurrence with Professor Colton and arranged for a demonstration of N₂O at Wells' dental office the next day. At the office, on December 11, 1844, a reluctant Colton served as the anesthesiologist as another dentist, Dr. John Riggs, extracted a wisdom tooth from Dr. Wells. After recovering from the effects of the N₂O, Wells stated that he had been totally unaware of the procedure and that there had been absolutely no pain associated with it.[8] Wells was taught the process of manufacturing N₂O by Professor Colton and shortly thereafter began using it in his dental practice with great success.

Through his association with William T. G. Morton, Wells was able to gain permission to demonstrate his newly found technique to the medical students and faculty at the prestigious Harvard Medical School. Morton, a dentist who became a student and later a partner of Dr. Wells in Hartford, eventually left dentistry, becoming a medical student at Harvard. Morton was present in the audience on this fateful day. Using a medical student volunteer as a patient, Dr. Wells administered N₂O to the patient through a newly developed inhaler. As the patient lapsed into unconsciousness, Wells had to remove the inhaler, pick up his instruments, and attempt to extract the volunteer's infected tooth. During the extraction attempt the patient cried out. The audience, assuming that the procedure had failed, proceeded to boo and hiss Wells until he was forced to leave the demonstration hall, thoroughly humiliated and his demonstration deemed a failure.[9]

On awakening, the patient stated that he was unaware that anything had happened, did not remember crying out, and had no memory of the attempted extraction. Unfortunately

EXHIBITION

OF THE EFFECTS PRODUCED BY INHALING

NITROUS OXIDE, EXHILERATING OR

LAUGHING GAS

WILL BE GIVEN AT *The Masonic Hall*
Saturday EVENING *15 April 1845*

30 GALLONS OF GAS will be prepared and administered to all in the audience who desire to inhale it.
MEN will be invited from the audience to protect those under the influence of the Gas from injuring themselves or others. This course is adopted that no apprehension of danger may be entertained.
Probably no one will attempt to fight.
THE EFFECT OF THE GAS is to make those who inhale it either

LAUGH, SING, DANCE, SPEAK OR FIGHT, &c. &c.

according to the leading trait of their character. They seem to retain consciousness enough not to say or do that which they would have occasion to regret.

N.B. The Gas will be administered only to gentlemen of the first respectability. The object is to make the entertainment in every respect, a genteel affair.

Those who inhale the Gas once, are always anxious to inhale it the second time. There is not an exception to this rule.

No language can describe the delightful sensation produced. Robert Southey, (poet) once said that "the atmosphere of the highest of all possible heavens must be composed of this Gas."

For a full account of the effect produced upon some of the most distinguished men of Europe, see Hooper's Medical Dictionary, under the head of Nitrogen.

The History and properties of the Gas will be explained at the commencement of the entertainment.

The entertainment will be accompanied by experiments in

ELECTRICITY

ENTERTAINMENT TO COMMENCE AT 7 O'CLOCK.
TICKETS 12½ CENTS,
For sale at the principal Bookstores, and at the Door

Figure 11.3 Nitrous oxide was discussed and demonstrated through exhibitions and shows that traveled around the countryside.

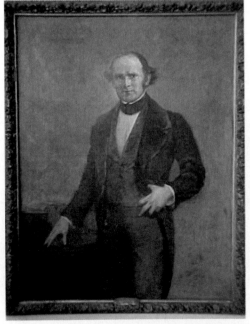

Figure 11.4 Horace Wells (1815–1848). (Courtesy the Horace Wells Museum, Hartford, Conn.)

for Wells, this admission came too late. Wells returned to Hartford and continued his practice of dentistry, as well as the use of N_2O.

There are several possible explanations for the "failure" of the demonstration given by Wells. The first and most likely reason is that Wells had to function in the dual capacity of both the anesthesiologist and surgeon. However, at the time of Wells' demonstration there was no experience to judge from, for this was the first time such a procedure had been attempted. Although the patient was anesthetized by the N_2O initially, at the point at which Wells began the extraction of the tooth he had to stop the administration of the gas to the patient. Breathing only room air, the patient would naturally begin to recover from the effects of the N_2O, gradually regaining consciousness. The pharmacokinetics of N_2O are such that the gas maintains a rapid onset of action and an equally rapid termination of action when its administration is discontinued.

A second possible explanation is the concept of biologic variability. As is well known today and has been stressed throughout this text, people respond differently when given the same dose of a drug. This concept is illustrated with the so-called *bell-shaped, or normal distribution, curve* (see Fig. 7.1).

Unfortunately for Wells, in 1844 this concept was unknown. The patient may have been what would today be called a *hyporesponder,* a patient requiring a larger dose of a medication to achieve a desired clinical action.

The third possible explanation for the so-called failure is the lack of knowledge of the various levels of anesthesia. After the patient recovered, he stated that he had been unaware of any discomfort or of his crying out. These responses of Wells' patient are associated with the type of anesthesia commonly known as *ultralight general anesthesia.* At this level the patient is indeed unconscious, although minimally. He is quite able to react to pain and move about in response to it; however, because of the level of central nervous system (CNS) depression, he is unable to remember anything occurring at this time.

Unfortunately for Wells, the medical profession, and the many patients requiring surgery at that time, this information was unknown. Surgery continued for a short while longer without the benefit of pain-relieving medications.

Within a year or so of his ill-fated demonstration of N_2O, a discouraged Wells abandoned the practice of dentistry. He ceased to publicize N_2O and to attempt to introduce it into clinical use, although he personally knew that it could be used successfully. He was able to earn a living by partaking in several strange occupations—buying pictures in Paris to sell in the United States and traveling around the countryside with a troupe of singing canaries. Wells continued to experiment with newer inhalation agents and soon became addicted to chloroform. Many of the founders of anesthesia became addicted to the chemicals they discovered, for they had no one to experiment on but themselves. The concept of addiction was unknown at the time and proved to be a terrible personal price to pay for the introduction of newer drugs and chemicals.[10]

In May 1848 a friend of Wells asked him to provide a vial of sulfuric acid so that he could throw it at a prostitute who earlier had damaged his clothes. Several days later, after Wells had inhaled some chloroform, he returned alone to Broadway in New York and, while under the influence of the chloroform, threw sulfuric acid at two other prostitutes. Arrested and placed in jail for these acts, Wells took his own life. The following are excerpts from the last letters written by Wells.[11]

Sunday, 7 o'clock pm

… I again take up this pen to finish what I have to say. … Before 12 tonight to pay the debt of Nature; yes, if I were free to go tomorrow I could not live and be called a villain. God knows I am not one. … Oh, what misery I shall bring on all my near relatives, and what still more distresses me is the fact that my name is familiar to the whole scientific world as being connected with an important discovery. And now, while I am scarcely able to hold my pen, I must to all say farewell! … Did I live I should become a maniac. The instrument of my destruction was obtained when the officer who had me in charge permitted me to go to my room yesterday.

Horace Wells

To my dear wife
I feel that I am fast becoming a deranged man, or I would desist from this act. I can't live and keep my reason, and on this account God will forgive the deed. I can say no more.

Horace Wells

On May 30, 1848, Horace Wells, later acknowledged as the founder of anesthesia, committed suicide while in jail by cutting the femoral artery in his left thigh with a razor. Before this act, Wells had inhaled some chloroform to produce insensibility to the pain.[12]

Interestingly, N_2O was reintroduced in 1863 by Professor Colton in New Haven, Connecticut.[13] The Colton Dental Association devoted the next 33 years to extracting teeth under N_2O. With 193,800 patients and no recorded fatalities, N_2O became the most commonly used inhalation anesthetic, a position it still maintains today.

William T. G. Morton (1819–1868) is the next major character in the story of the development of anesthesia. Morton learned of the idea of inhalation anesthesia from Wells, under whom he was a student of dentistry and then an associate in dental practice in Hartford. Morton later entered into medical school at Harvard, and it was through Morton's connections that Wells obtained the invitation to his ill-fated demonstration of N_2O anesthesia. Morton was a member of the audience at that demonstration. A more effective anesthetic gas was required, and Morton began to experiment with ether. How Morton came to work with ether became a topic of considerable discussion and controversy as the years passed. It is possible that he learned of ether through "ether parties" that were at the time a frequent entertainment of the medical students or that he was pushed into its use through a professor of his at Harvard, Charles Thomas Jackson (1805–1880), a physician and chemist.

Morton experimented to a small degree on animals (his family dog) and on himself before his first use of ether on a patient. That patient, Mr. Eben Frost, received ether for the extraction of a tooth on September 30, 1846. Morton recorded the incident as follows:

Toward evening a man residing in Boston came in, suffering great pain, and wishing to have a tooth extracted. He was afraid of the operation, and asked if he could be mesmerized. I told him I had something better, and saturating my handkerchief, gave it to him to inhale. He became unconscious almost immediately. It was dark, and Dr. Hayden held the lamp while I extracted a firmly rooted bicuspid tooth. There was not much alteration in the pulse and no relaxing of the muscles. He recovered in a minute and knew nothing of what had been done for him. He remained for some time talking about the experiment. This was the 30th of September 1846.[10]

Morton continued to experiment with ether, both on his own and with Dr. Henry J. Bigelow, for whom Morton administered ether for more than 37 operations. All of these cases were done before the famous demonstration of ether at the Massachusetts General Hospital in 1846.[14]

On October 16, 1846 (now called Ether Day), Morton administered ether to Gilbert Abbott (Fig. 11.5). The famous surgeon John Collins Warren excised a tumor from the jaw of Mr. Abbott. Although considered an absolute success, Morton's demonstration was actually little more successful than Wells' had been. Abbott later mentioned that when the incision was first made it felt as though his neck had been scratched by a hoe. However, unlike Wells, Morton was not hissed out of

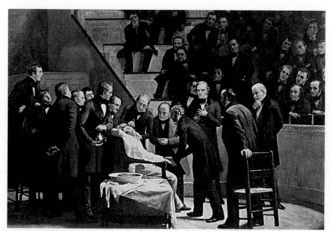

Figure 11.5 William T. G. Morton administering ether to Gilbert Abbott as John Collins Warren removes a tumor from the neck of Abbott in the famed Ether Dome at the Massachusetts General Hospital, October 16, 1846. (Courtesy Boston Medical Library in the F. A. Countway Library of Medicine, Boston.)

the operating theater. The reason for this is twofold: first, Dr. Bigelow had attested to Dr. Warren the success of ether; therefore, Warren was more inclined to believe that this new agent was not a fraud but, in fact, the real thing. Second, and of considerable importance, is the fact that Morton was a physician and not a dentist. At the time, dentistry was looked down on by the medical profession as a mere trade. That Wells should have even attempted to demonstrate his new technique to such an august group, including Warren, was, sad to say, quite laughable. His audience was filled with cynics and disbelievers. Morton, on the other hand, being a member of the "club," was more readily accepted. When the endorsement of Bigelow is added, it is readily seen why the less-than-absolutely successful procedure was proclaimed as the great event it truly was. In the words of John Collins Warren, "Gentlemen, you have witnessed a miracle. This is no humbug!"[14-16]

Ether had been for many years a popular agent for enjoyment. Ether follies were a popular form of entertainment, especially among medical students. Morton, acutely aware that if he were to suggest that this same agent be used for a serious purpose he might also be laughed at, modified the agent. He added a dye to it and called it *Letheon,* thus gaining acceptance for it among his colleagues.[17] The surgical amphitheater at the Massachusetts General Hospital in which this famed event took place has been preserved and is today known as the Ether Dome.

News of Morton's "etherization" spread rapidly throughout the United States and Europe, creating a degree of celebrity for Morton. On December 21, 1846, Dr. Robert Liston performed the first surgical procedure under "etherization" in England. Almost immediately following the introduction of etherization into surgery by Morton, Dr. Charles T. Jackson came forward to lay claim to its discovery, stating that it was he who had suggested its use to Morton, had advised him about the nature of the agent, and had advised him of the best manner in which to administer it. The controversy was only beginning. Soon Morton, Wells, and Jackson were engaging in bitter accusations and secret deals, each in an effort to prove that it was he in fact who was the sole founder of anesthesia. To complicate the matter still further, Crawford W. Long, who had first administered ether in 1842, came forward in 1849 to lay claim to this title.[18]

The name *etherization* was used for only a short time, and a more acceptable name for this new technique was being sought. Among the terms offered for this process were the following: *aethereal influence, aethereal inhalation, aetherealization, aetherization, anaestheticization, anaesthism, anodyne process, apathisation, ethereal state, etherification, hebetization, lethargic state, letheonization, narcotism, somniferous agent, sopor, soporization, soporized state,* and *stupefaction.*[14]

It was Dr. Oliver Wendell Holmes, the physician, author, and father of a Supreme Court justice, who suggested the name *anesthesia.* At the height of the controversy over the founding of anesthesia, Holmes wrote to Morton:

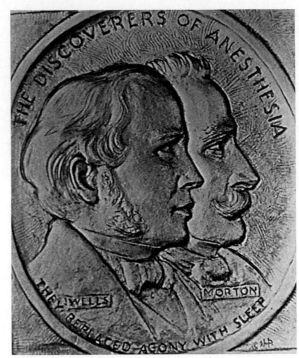

Figure 11.6 William T. G. Morton and Horace Wells, the discoverers of anesthesia.

Everybody wants to have a hand in the great discovery. All I will do is to give you a hint or two as to the names to be applied to the state produced and to the agent. The state should, I think, be called anesthesia. The adjective will be anesthetic. Thus we might say the "state of anesthesia" or the "anesthetic state."[7]

The name *anesthesia,* as suggested by Holmes, had been used by Plato in 400 BC to describe the absence of feelings in a philosophical sense. In the first century AD, Dioscorides also used the term to denote the absence of physical sensation.

Morton shortly gave up the practice of dentistry, devoting his time to the practice of anesthesia. He was thus the first person to specialize full time in the field of anesthesiology (Fig. 11.6). In addition, he was involved in the manufacture of anesthetic inhalers and other devices for the administration of anesthetic gases.

Morton fought bitterly, seeking to obtain recognition as the founder of anesthesia. Three times he petitioned the Congress of the United States for such recognition, and he spoke personally with President James Knox Polk, but during his lifetime Morton was never granted recognition as the father of ether anesthesia. Morton died of a cerebral hemorrhage in 1868, a discouraged and disappointed man. His tombstone reads: "Inventor and Revealer of Inhalation Anesthesia: Before Whom, in All Time, Surgery was Agony; By Whom, Pain in Surgery was Averted and Annulled; Since Whom, Science has Control of Pain."

As to the matter of who was the discoverer of anesthesia, the question is still debated. However, in 1864 the American Dental Association passed the following resolution:

Therefore Be It Resolved, by the American Dental Association, that to Horace Wells, of Hartford, Connecticut (now deceased), belongs the credit and honor of the introduction of anesthesia in the United States of America, and we do firmly protest against the injustice done to truth and the memory of Dr. Horace Wells, in the effort made during a series of years and especially at the last session of Congress, to award the credit to other persons or person.[18]

In 1870 the American Medical Association followed suit, and a resolution, introduced by Dr. H. R. Storer of Massachusetts, was passed recognizing the discovery of anesthesia by Horace Wells: "Resolved, that the honor of the discovery of practical anesthesia is due to the late Dr. Horace Wells of Connecticut."[19]

Despite the controversy surrounding the discovery of anesthesia, the use of both N_2O and Letheon, as Morton's ether was known, was quite slow in developing. Bitter opposition to these new drugs was found within both the medical and dental professions in the United States in the late 1840s. In 1848 the American Society of Dental Surgeons stated in regard to the use of ether and chloroform: "Hence, in all minor operations in surgery their administration is forbidden; and that their demand in the practice of dental surgery is small."[20] The *Dental News Letter* of July 1849, which was published in Philadelphia, stated "The Letheon is still used to considerable extent in Boston, for extraction of teeth; while in this city and in most other places, so far as we have been able to learn, it has been generally abandoned."[2] It was claimed that the use of ether encouraged charlatanism.

Meanwhile, in England in the late 1840s and early 1850s, the discoveries of Wells and Morton were well received. In addition, chloroform, which had been introduced in 1831, became widely used.[15] Two names—John Snow and James Young Simpson—must be mentioned. John Snow (1813–1858) became the first physician after Morton to specialize in anesthesia (Fig. 11.7). During his career he designed new inhalers for the delivery of anesthetics, primarily ether, which he used for extractions. In 1847 Snow published his classic textbook *On the Inhalation of Ether,* and in 1858, he published *On Chloroform and Other Anaesthetics.*[21,22]

James Young Simpson (1811–1870) was an English obstetrician. On January 19, 1847, Simpson introduced the use of ether into his obstetric practice. Although he liked the drug and the lessening of discomfort it brought his patients, Simpson disliked the disagreeable odor and the potential for nausea and vomiting associated with ether. He began to search for a better agent.

Simpson and his assistants, Keith and Matthew Duncan, began to experiment on themselves by inhaling various chemicals.[23] Although their research was not extensive, it did produce a very valuable clinical agent. In November 1847, at

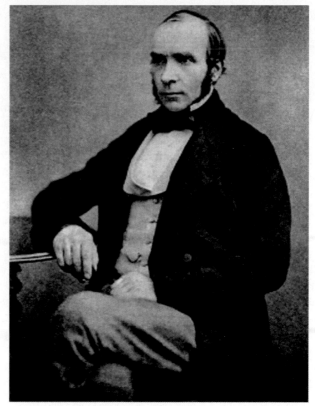

Figure 11.7 John Snow (1813–1858).

the suggestion of David Waldie, a pharmacist from Liverpool, Simpson and his assistants experimented with perchloride of formyl, or chloroform, as it is known today. They found that chloroform worked quite well, and Simpson almost immediately began to use it as a means of alleviating the pains of childbirth.

Immediately, Simpson found himself embroiled in controversy with the Church of England. The propriety of abolishing pain during childbirth was the major point of contention. The argument used by the anti-Simpson clergy came from the Bible (*Genesis* 3:16):

Unto the woman he said, I will greatly multiply thy sorrow and thy conception; in sorrow thou shalt bring forth children, and thy desire shall be to thy husband, and he shall rule over thee.

Simpson was quite able to cope with the controversy and continued to use chloroform as an analgesic to diminish labor pains. However, because of the controversy, other physicians were very slow to adopt chloroform. On April 7, 1853, John Snow administered chloroform analgesia to Queen Victoria at the birth of Prince Leopold, despite the fact that *The Lancet* had stated in no uncertain terms that the use of chloroform in normal labor is *never* justified. Nevertheless, Queen Victoria received chloroform analgesia for 53 minutes, the chloroform administered by a handkerchief. As mentioned by Snow in his subsequent book on chloroform, Queen Victoria expressed herself as greatly relieved by the administration.[22] Indeed, on

April 14, 1857, Snow again administered chloroform analgesia to the queen at the birth of Princess Beatrice.

The use of chloroform as an analgesic and the administration of anesthetics for the relief of pain during childbirth received a great boost by the actions of Queen Victoria. The field of anesthesia began to grow, as did its problems.

On November 10, 1847, Simpson published an account of his experiences with chloroform. This report was published only 6 days after Simpson first began to use chloroform, and it contained a glowing account of its anesthetic capabilities. Unfortunately, as is known today all drugs possess undesirable as well as desirable effects. At the time of publication of Simpson's report, the undesirable effects of chloroform were unknown (or unreported). Its ability to produce sudden cardiac arrest remained unknown for approximately 11 weeks, until January 28, 1848, when Dr. Meggison, an untrained country doctor, administered chloroform to a 15-year-old patient, Hannah Greener, who "died like a shot rabbit" upon receiving chloroform.[24] Today it is known that the effects of epinephrine on the myocardium and heart rhythm are exaggerated by chloroform, producing possibly fatal ventricular fibrillation.[25] Hannah Greener was, in the words of Dr. Meggison, "fretting all the day before 'crying continually and wishing she were dead rather than submit to it'."[26]

Simpson could not believe that chloroform could have been responsible for the death of Hannah Greener. He stated, in defense of chloroform, that the death of Hannah Greener had been caused by the brandy and water that had been poured into her mouth while she was unconscious (done in an attempt at resuscitation). He said that Greener had drowned from this fluid. The fact is we will never know what killed Hannah Greener. Deaths from light chloroform anesthesia continued to be reported, but the older generation of doctors and chloroform advocates refused to believe that a very small dose of chloroform could possibly kill a patient. It was not until 1911, when A. Goodman Levy published the results of his experiments on epinephrine and light chloroform anesthesia, that a possible mechanism of Hannah Greener's death was finally and satisfactorily explained—the propensity of chloroform to induce cardiac dysrhythmias, especially in the presence of elevated plasma epinephrine.[25]

During the ensuing 10 years (1850–1860), the use of ether and chloroform in dentistry became quite widespread and deaths continued to be reported. Controversy developed over the use of these agents within both medicine and dentistry. Thomas, in his interesting paper, "Some Early Papers on Dental Anaesthesia,"[26] cites two authors, Fowell[27] and Tomes,[28] regarding these agents. Fowell is quoted:

Some persons, I am sorry to say, have become so enamored of chloroform or ether ... as to refuse to permit the operation (of dental extraction) without its assistance ... but when it comes to the removal of a tooth, which is an act simple in its execution and quick in its effect, I must confess that I think it is indiscreet.

Tomes stated: "We surely use a great power to overcome a very trifling difficulty, when we give chloroform preparatory to extracting an ordinary tooth." Tomes was also aware of the advantages of analgesia as opposed to general anesthesia: "On many occasions the patient has been perfectly aware of the steps of the operation, has felt the instrument grasp the tooth ... and yet has felt little or no pain."

At the beginning of the 1860s, ether and chloroform were the dominant forms of anesthesia being used in the medical and dental professions. N_2O was used, but not as extensively, primarily because of the difficulties in its manufacture and storage.

ANESTHESIA DEVELOPS (1863–1898)

In July 1863 Gardner Quincy Colton, the man who had given Horace Wells the idea of using N_2O as an anesthetic in 1844, reintroduced it to the dental profession. N_2O had not been in very common use since the death of Wells and the introduction of ether and chloroform. Colton established "dental institutes" in cities throughout the United States. These institutes specialized in tooth extractions under N_2O general anesthesia. One hundred percent N_2O was administered with the patient's nose held closed by the administrator as the patient inhaled through his or her mouth. Colton soon became the most renowned figure in the world of N_2O. By 1881, 18 years after his reintroduction of N_2O, Colton had administered it to 121,709 persons without a death. Each of these cases has subsequently been documented.[29] That Colton was able to obtain such an outstanding record using an anesthetic gas without supplemental O_2 is truly outstanding. Yet Colton would have argued that the use of 100% N_2O was perfectly safe because the oxygen molecule attached to the nitrogen (N_2) would provide the cells of the body with whatever oxygen they required. It is now known that this oxygen is not available for use by the body. Fortunately, the vast majority of cases reported by Colton were of only 1 or 2 minutes in duration (tooth extraction); however, some did last for as long as 16 minutes without adverse effect, according to Colton. In addition, such was the clinical experience and technical excellence of Colton that he was able to administer this drug to more than 120,000 persons without a single death, despite the fact that his entire practice was based on an incorrect principle!

Dr. Edmund W. Andrews (1824–1904), a physician born in Vermont, was one of the founders of the Chicago Medical College, the forerunner of the Northwestern School of Medicine. However, Andrews' major claim to fame, and indeed a most significant one in the history of anesthesia, was the addition of 20% O_2 to N_2O. Andrews published his findings in an 1868 article in the *Chicago Medical Examiner,* titled "The Oxygen Mixture; A New Anesthetic Combination."[30] Andrews claimed this combination to be safer and more pleasant than any anesthetic mixture then known. In 1862 Joseph T. Clover (1825–1882) had introduced the mixture of chloroform and air. Clover also sought to make ether anesthesia safer by inducing anesthesia with N_2O and then maintaining anesthesia by adding ether to it. Indeed, Andrews was right in his thoughts about the combination of 20% O_2 and 80% N_2O. His concept of the use of this agent, as well as all other anesthetics, still holds true today, 155 years later.

In 1868 Paul Bert, a student of the great Claude Bernard, wrote that the use of 100% N_2O for more than 2 minutes would bring about signs and symptoms of asphyxia. Bert designed an apparatus capable of delivering 25% O_2 and 75% N_2O.[31,32]

Shortly thereafter, in 1872 in England, liquid N_2O became commercially available to the dental and medical professions, making its use much more practical and considerably safer. No longer did physicians and dentists have to manufacture their own N_2O with the risk of including impurities in the gas.

In 1881 two developments that had profound effects on the use of N_2O occurred in widely separate parts of the world. In St. Petersburg, Russia, an obstetrician, S. Klikovitsch, first used N_2O as an analgesic to relieve the pains of labor. As the years passed, the production of analgesia was to become a primary indication for the use of N_2O.

In the same year in Philadelphia, the S. S. White Manufacturing Company began to supply liquefied N_2O to the medical and dental professions. It also introduced an apparatus that permitted the delivery of the gas from the cylinder to the patient. This device revolutionized and simplified the administration of N_2O and provided a great boost to its use.

Sir Frederick Hewitt (1857–1916) invented the first practical anesthesia machine for administering N_2O and O_2 in fixed proportions in 1887. By 1889 N_2O-O_2 analgesia was being used in dentistry during cavity preparation in Liverpool, England. Several problems were associated with the use of N_2O-O_2 analgesia at that time. The use of very-low-speed handpieces, with no local anesthesia (by 1890 cocaine injection into the gums was becoming an accepted method of pain control) or poor local anesthesia, plus the fact that much of the N_2O and O_2 being used was impure, led to a significant number of side effects (e.g., nausea, vomiting, and excitement). As the 1890s continued, the use of N_2O-O_2 analgesia gradually declined.

THE TWENTIETH CENTURY

By 1898 both Hewitt in England and White in the United States had developed new devices for the administration of N_2O-O_2. In 1902 the Cleveland Dental Manufacturing Company introduced a machine designed by Charles K. Teter, DDS. This machine could deliver O_2, N_2O, and other anesthetic gases. Eight years later (in 1910), two of the major manufacturers of anesthesia equipment entered into the marketplace. J. A. Heidbrink, of Minneapolis, modified the 1902 Teter machine and introduced a new model for the administration of N_2O and O_2. Heidbrink's interest in anesthesia began while he was a dental student. He had suffered such excruciating pain during

the extraction of his third molars without the benefit of anesthesia that he decided to correct the situation. Also in 1910, E. I. McKesson, MD, introduced the first intermittent-flow machine with accurate percentage control for N_2O-O_2. McKesson soon became the undisputed international authority on N_2O anesthesia and a leader in its development.

Teter, Heidbrink, and McKesson, by virtue of the many papers they wrote and lectures and clinical demonstrations they presented, were largely responsible for the increased use of N_2O-O_2 anesthesia for surgical operations throughout the United States.[33,34]

Periods of interest in N_2O were invariably followed by periods of almost total neglect. Two such periods of heightened interest occurred between 1913 and 1918 and between 1932 and 1938. Failures and side effects with the technique were not uncommon, even with the advent of newer machines and the increasing purity of the gases. The technique of N_2O anesthesia was not taught at any dental school or in any postgraduate program during this time; thus it was difficult for a dentist to learn the technique. The manufacturers of the anesthesia machines provided courses for doctors, but the quality of these courses was uniformly poor by modern standards.

A good description of the use of N_2O-O_2 analgesia in dentistry in 1923 is provided by Nevin and Puterbaugh:

For its administration the patient is seated comfortably in the dental chair and the nasal inhaler adjusted carefully in order to avoid leakage about its margin and waste of the anesthetic. Since the patient does not lose consciousness at any time the mouth is left uncovered, no prop between the teeth being required. Before the anesthetic is started it is explained to the patient that he is to administer his own anesthetic. He is directed to breathe through his nose until a sense of numbness and stiffness comes over him which is felt extending to his finger tips, at which time his teeth, when snapped sharply together, will feel like wooden pegs set in wooden jaws. He is told that in this state he will feel no pain; that he need not go to sleep but that when he feels he is about to lose consciousness he is then to breathe through his mouth and by so doing he will remain awake.

He is repeatedly reminded that while he will feel the vibration of the bur and be conscious of everything that is going on, the sense of pain will be entirely obtunded; that should he feel the slightest indication of pain he is to breathe entirely through his nose until the pain disappears. Nitrous oxid [sic] and oxygen are then turned on in proportion of twenty per cent oxygen and eighty per cent nitrous oxid. This mixture is administered throughout and, being of the same oxygen percentage as atmospheric air, there are no asphyxial symptoms exhibited at any time during the administration. Patients take quite an interest in this type of anesthesia for they feel that they are a part of its administration and willingly endeavor to cooperate for its success. This method may be safely employed for periods up to one half hour; if continued longer it is occasionally followed by nausea and slight headache, which, of course, should be avoided by arranging for a greater number of sittings of shorter periods each.

The types of procedures best suited for analgesia are the excavation of hypersensitive dentin, the preparing of roots for the adaptation of crowns and bridges, the scaling of deep pyorrhea pockets, etc. It will not obtund pain sufficiently to permit the removal of vital pulps or the extraction of teeth or the lancing of abscesses, all of which require complete anesthesia for their performance.[35]

Throughout the 1930s, and into the 1940s, most dentists who used N_2O worked with N_2O-O_2 in a ratio of 80% to 20% described previously, although many still employed 100% N_2O general anesthesia. The number of dentists using N_2O increased as the 1940s passed, the purity of the gases improved, and the quality of the machines for gas delivery increased, yet the success rate of N_2O-O_2 analgesia still remained low.[36]

During the 1940s, fundamental changes in pain control in dentistry occurred. The use of local anesthesia as the primary means of pain control became more accepted. In 1945 lidocaine, the first of the newer, more effective amide-type local anesthetics, was introduced into clinical use. N_2O, which had been introduced in 1844 as a means of eliminating pain, was no longer the "ideal" drug for this task. Over the next few years the manner in which N_2O was used was modified. Rather than seeking the elimination of pain as its primary goal, N_2O could now be used for the management of anxiety and the production of relaxation (sedation). With this change in the goal being sought came changes in technique, dosage, and the approach to the patient.

In 1947 the third edition of Dr. Harry M. Seldin's classic textbook, *Practical Anesthesia for Dental and Oral Surgery: Local and General,* was published.[37] In Chapter 22, "The Administration of Nitrous Oxide and Its Mixtures," Dr. Seldin describes the ways in which the drug was used in the 1940s:

The administration of nitrous oxide is no longer limited to the use of the gas by itself. In order to obviate the haphazard technique of "straight" nitrous oxide anesthesia, to reduce the possibility of unfavorable sequelae, and to extend the operating time, oxygen has been added. … Nitrous oxide is given in one of three ways:

1. *Pure nitrous oxide, with the exclusion of air or oxygen, usually referred to as "straight nitrous oxide."*
2. *Nitrous oxide with air.*
3. *Nitrous oxide with oxygen.*

Straight nitrous oxide. Pure nitrous oxide without the addition of air or oxygen was the first form in which the gas was employed for the purpose of producing unconsciousness. Today, despite the tremendous advances in the art of anesthesia, some, few, practitioners still persist in the use of so-called "straight nitrous oxide."

The technique is simplicity itself. The pure gas is delivered to the patient from … the tank. … As soon as the patient shows the classical signs of asphyxia (thirty to sixty seconds):

dilated pupils, absence of all reflexes, cyanosis, clonic muscular spasms, and jactitation, the inhaler is removed, a gauze pack forced into the posterior part of the mouth, and the operation commenced. The exodontist must work at top speed, usually with little regard for the oral tissues. It is evident that lacerations and sharp bony processes are inevitable when extensive exodontia must be completed in the 2 minutes or so available before consciousness returns. … Many of the pioneers in dental anesthetics developed unusual speed and dexterity, and could accomplish an unbelievable amount of work with a single administration. … The phrase "turn them black, then bring them back" was commonly used to describe this technique.

There are certain limitations to this method. The period of anesthesia is very short, being frequently less than thirty seconds and rarely longer than 1 minute. … When the operation requires more time, the patient often recovers sufficiently to interfere with the procedure.

However, in light of the present knowledge of anesthetic gases, there is today no justification for use of the rather crude method described. The addition of oxygen to the nitrous oxide has immeasurably improved operative technique under anesthesia. Speed ceases to be the prime factor.[37]

The term *blue gassing* refers to this technique of administration of pure N_2O. Blue gassing was employed in dentistry for many years, even well into the 1950s and early 1960s. Seldin goes on to describe two other techniques of N_2O anesthesia:

Nitrous oxide-air mixtures. Although narcosis with gas and air has been employed, it can hardly be recommended. This method is extremely trying for the anesthetist, and the end result is not particularly gratifying. In addition to the prevalence of asphyxial symptoms … anesthesia is not smooth, and nausea appears almost routinely after anesthesias of more than five minutes' duration; the recovery of the patient is uncomfortably retarded. Most of these deleterious effects may be attributed to the high percentage of nitrogen (N_2) included in the anesthetic mixture.

Nitrous oxide-oxygen mixtures. Mixtures of nitrous oxide with oxygen have held and still hold a paramount and proved position in dental anesthesia.

Seldin describes two induction techniques. The first is the slow induction technique in which the patient is administered an N_2O-O_2 ratio of 93% to 7% for 1 minute. As signs of excitement develop, 100% N_2O is administered until the patient reaches the third stage of anesthesia. Sufficient O_2 is then added to maintain the desired plane of anesthesia. In the rapid induction technique, 100% N_2O is given for 45 to 60 seconds until the patient reaches the third stage of anesthesia, at which point 10% O_2 is added. The percentage of O_2 is changed to meet the needs of the patient:

The anesthetic level is a variable depending on the type of individual and may differ within the limits of 5% to 80% of oxygen and 20% to 95% of nitrous oxide. Any point within these rather widely divergent extremes may be required to maintain different subjects at an even keel in the normal plane in the third stage.

Seldin then recommends "setting the dial at 100% oxygen for several inhalations" at the end of the procedure. In discussing analgesia with N_2O, he states:

It is evident that analgesia with nitrous oxide and oxygen is an exceedingly safe procedure, because nitrous oxide is in itself the least harmful anesthetic known to the profession. ... Analgesia may be maintained without the slightest danger for periods of thirty minutes and longer on any patient, regardless of age. As a matter of fact, elderly patients frequently make the best cases.

The concepts of individual variation and titration are discussed by Seldin:

After the first few inhalations, each subject becomes a law unto himself, and his personal needs in respect to the proper mixture of these gases must be determined by the various symptoms of analgesia manifested by him from 1 minute to the next. In fact, considerable variations in the dial settings may be detected for the same person from day to day. This proves the falsity and irrationality of the recommendations made by gas-machine demonstrators that a standard percentage setting, consistently maintained, will induce and sustain perfect analgesia on all patients, irrespective of age or physical condition.

Many of the so-called modern concepts underlying the use of inhalation anesthetics and other parenterally administered drugs were discussed in Seldin's textbook. Much of the impetus for the use of N_2O-O_2 analgesia and sedation stems from his writings and lectures.

MODERN TIMES (1950–PRESENT)

The Development of Courses and Guidelines

In the 1950s and 1960s N_2O was becoming more frequently used in dentistry. The use of 100% N_2O was decreasing rapidly, and with the advent of newer, more effective, local anesthetics such as lidocaine and mepivacaine for operative pain control, N_2O-O_2 became a very popular agent for the management of the apprehensive dental patient. Interest in the field of anesthesiology in dentistry grew, and in 1953 the American Dental Society of Anesthesiology was formed. In the years that have followed, this organization has led the way in advancing the standards and practices in the use of anesthesia (general, local, and sedation) within dentistry in the United States.[2,38]

A few dental schools added courses in inhalation sedation to the dental curriculum as the 1950s gave way to the 1960s. Postgraduate programs in inhalation sedation increased in number; however, with but few exceptions, their quality remained low. One man, however, Dr. Harry Langa, presented

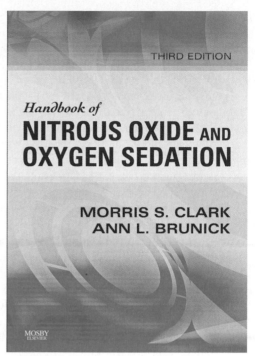

Figure 11.8 *Handbook of Nitrous Oxide and Oxygen Sedation,* by Morris Clark and Ann Brunick (2015).

postgraduate programs of quality throughout these years. Dr. Langa began using N_2O in 1936 and presented his first course in 1949. Between that time and the publication of the second edition of his classic textbook, *Relative Analgesia in Dental Practice: Inhalation Analgesia and Sedation with Nitrous Oxide,* in 1976, he had trained more than 6000 dentists to use this technique safely.[39] More recently *A Handbook of Nitrous Oxide and Oxygen Sedation,* by Morris Clark and Ann Brunick (1999),[40] represents the most comprehensive textbook devoted solely to inhalation sedation with N_2O. Its authors have trained more than 4500 dentists and hygienists in inhalation sedation in the United States and internationally (Fig. 11.8).

As schools and other organizations began to present courses in inhalation sedation, it became obvious that the level of training being offered and its quality varied considerably. It was decided that standards ought to be established for the teaching of the various techniques of pain and anxiety control in dentistry. In 1964 the American Dental Society of Anesthesiology held the first of four workshops, attended by representatives of 43 dental schools, out of which came the *Guidelines for Teaching the Comprehensive Control of Pain and Anxiety in Dentistry.*[41] Included within these guidelines is an outline for inhalation sedation courses. The most recent version of these recommendations is presented in Chapter 19.[42] With adoption of these guidelines, the overall quality of training in inhalation sedation was significantly improved. Three primary areas—the undergraduate dental student, the graduate dental student, and continuing education for the postgraduate student—were addressed by the guidelines. There remains a growing trend to learn more about the use of N_2O and how it can be more useful in today's dental and medical practice. The topic of teaching inhalation sedation is discussed in detail in Chapter 19.

The Early Anesthesia Machine

Another area requiring improvement was the inhalation sedation unit itself. Significant changes had been made in the method of delivering N_2O-O_2 to the patient since the first clinical use of the agent in 1844. Early in the history of inhalation anesthesia, a bladder bag filled with 100% N_2O was used. A spigot attached to the bag was placed into the patient's mouth, the patient inhaled the gas and lost consciousness, the spigot was removed, and the procedure was carried out as quickly as possible.

By 1846 Morton had improved on this method of delivering inhalation anesthetics to the patient. John Snow, in England, devised and first used an inhaler in 1847 that was quite similar to the full-face masks used today in anesthesia.[21]

As has been mentioned in this chapter, one of the major drawbacks to the use of N_2O was the need for the doctor to manufacture the agent himself. The process was cumbersome, and storage of the gas difficult. However, in 1872 the Johnson Brothers, in England, began to produce liquefied N_2O on a commercial basis. Approximately 5 years later, the S.S. White Company of Philadelphia began the marketing of liquefied N_2O cylinders in the United States. They also manufactured an anesthesia device that administered N_2O gas from the cylinder to the patient. The use of N_2O was greatly enhanced by this innovation.

In 1898 Sir Frederick Hewitt manufactured and sold the first devices for delivering N_2O-O_2 anesthesia. Shortly thereafter, the S. S. White Company patented their own similar device. Dr. Charles K. Teter introduced the second N_2O-O_2 anesthesia machine in the United States in 1902. E. I. McKesson perfected the first intermittent-flow N_2O-O_2 anesthesia machine with an accurate means of controlling the percentages of both gases and marketed it in 1910. Also in 1910, the third of the pioneers in the manufacture of anesthesia devices, J. A. Heidbrink, DDS, entered the marketplace. His model "OO" appeared, later followed by the model "T." This device included a reducing valve that served as a flowmeter. By 1918 the four major manufacturers of anesthesia devices in the United States were McKesson, Connell, von Foregger, and Heidbrink.

From the designs of these and other pioneers, the modern anesthesia machine has developed. The inhalation sedation apparatus used today for the administration of N_2O-O_2 is modified from this device (Fig. 11.9). The major change required to adapt the anesthesia machine for inhalation sedation was the removal from the unit of all but the O_2 and N_2O gas supplies and flowmeters. However, situations developed in which the cylinder of O_2 became depleted during a procedure, resulting in the delivery of 100% N_2O to the patient. In too many situations, serious morbidity and in some cases mortality occurred. In 1976 the American Dental Association's Council on Dental Materials, Instruments, and Equipment adopted standards for the manufacture of inhalation sedation units in the United States.[43] These standards required inhalation sedation devices to incorporate a series of failsafe devices into the unit. The primary goal of these devices was to prevent the administration of O_2 in a less-than-atmospheric concentration.

With more and more scientific information being gathered about the effects of the gases used in inhalation sedation, further modification of these units has occurred. For example, in recent years the nasal inhaler has undergone a change in design in order to minimize the chronic inhalation of trace amounts of N_2O by dental personnel.[44] The scavenging nasal hood has been introduced. Other refinements in the apparatus for the delivery of N_2O-O_2 will be forthcoming as knowledge of the technique and drugs increases.

Since the first edition of this book was published in 1985, I have noticed a significant change in the composition of enrollees in continuing education courses in inhalation sedation. Throughout the 1970s and early 1980s, course participants were almost exclusively dentists and other dental personnel. Only occasionally did other health professionals (physicians, podiatrists) enroll in these programs. Indeed, review of course rosters through 1984 reveals but three nondental health professionals (one physician, two podiatrists) of a total course enrollment of more than 800 "offices."

As mentioned, there is a tremendous growing interest among practitioners across all lines and disciplines of health care involving N_2O inhalation sedation. The use of inhalation sedation in dental hygiene has particularly grown in popularity. N_2O is currently being used by dental hygienists in 32 states with the physical presence of a dentist.[45] Hygienists are capitalizing on the comfort afforded patients with use of N_2O for procedures such as scaling and root planing. As we progress

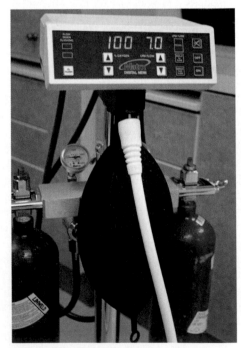

Figure 11.9 Modern inhalation sedation unit.

through these chapters on inhalation sedation, we review various aspects of nitrous oxide delivery. These include tangential information that will be offered to help the practitioner problem-solve and apply inhalation sedation even more creatively. The history of N_2O-O_2 sedation is colorful, interesting, insightful, and a source of pride for the dental profession inasmuch as we can gain an appreciation for the sacrifices made to make this first anesthetic available to humankind.

In the succeeding chapters in this section, we review the indications for inhalation sedation, the pharmacology of N_2O and O_2, techniques of their delivery to patients, complications associated with its use, and the components of the armamentarium. All of the material contained in these chapters was in large part first discovered or developed by the men discussed in this chapter. The history of anesthesia to a very large degree is the history of N_2O.

REFERENCES

1. Lee JA, Atkinson RS: *A synopsis of anesthesia*, ed 5, Baltimore, 1964, Williams & Wilkins.
2. Greenfield W: Anesthesiology in dentistry: past, present and future. *Anesth Prog* 23(4):104–110, 129–132, 1976.
3. Davy H: Researches, chemical and philosophical; chiefly concerning nitrous oxide, 1800. In Fullmer JZ, editor: *Sir Humphry Davy's published works*, Cambridge, MA, 1969, Harvard University Press.
4. Cartwright FF: *The English pioneers of anaesthesia (Beddoes, Davy, and Hickman)*, Bristol, 1952, J Wright.
5. Hickman HH: A letter on suspended animation, 1824 (pamphlet).
6. Long C: An account of the first use of sulphuric ether by inhalation as an anaesthetic in surgical operations. *South Med Surg J* 5(12):705–713, 1849.
7. Jacobsohn PH: Dentistry's answer to "the humiliating spectacle": Dr. Wells and his discovery. *J Am Dent Assoc* 125(12):1576–1581, 1994.
8. Raper HR: *Man against pain*, New York, 1945, Prentice Hall.
9. Fenster JM: *Ether day: the strange tale of America's greatest medical discovery and the haunted man who made it*, New York, 2001, HarperCollins.
10. Archer WH: Chronological history of Horace Wells, discoverer of anesthesia. *Bull Hist Med* 7:1140, 1939.
11. Wells H: Letter. *Br Med J* May 31:305, 1848.
12. Menczer LF, Mittleman M, Wildsmith JA: Horace Wells. *J Am Dent Assoc* 110(5):773–776, 1985.
13. Jacobsohn PH: What others said about Wells, memorials, tributes, affirmations. *J Am Dent Assoc* 125(12):1583–1584, 1994.
14. Bankoff G: *The conquest of pain: the story of anesthesia*, London, 1946, MacDonald.
15. Sykes WS: *Essays on the first hundred years of anaesthesia (vol I and II)*. Edinburgh, 1961, E & S Livingstone.
16. Driscoll EJ: Dental anesthesiology: its history and continuing evolution. *Anesth Prog* 25(5):143–152, 1978.
17. Smith WDA: *Under the influence: a history of nitrous oxide and oxygen anaesthesia*, Park Ridge, IL, 1982, Wood Library, Museum of Anesthesiology.
18. American Dental Association: *Transactions of the fourth annual meeting at Niagara Falls*, New York, 1864.
19. Archer WH: Life and letters of Horace Wells, discoverer of anesthesia. *J Am Coll Dent* 11:81, 1944.

20. American Society of Dental Surgeons: Resolutions adopted at eighth annual meeting. *Am J Dent Sci* 9:1848.
21. Snow J: *On the inhalation of ether*, London, 1858, J Churchill.
22. Snow J: *On chloroform and other anaesthetics*, London, 1858, J Churchill.
23. Chancellor JW: Dr. Wells' impact on dentistry and medicine. *J Am Dent Assoc* 125(12):1585–1589, 1994.
24. Sykes WS, Ellis RH, editors: *Essays on the first hundred years of anaesthesia (vol III)*. Edinburgh, 1982, Churchill Livingstone.
25. Levy AG: Sudden death under light chloroform anaesthesia. *J Physiol* 42:3, 1911.
26. Thomas KB: Some early papers on dental anaesthesia. *Br Dent J* 116:139, 1964.
27. Fowell S: *A treatise on dentistry*, ed 2, London, 1859, J Mitchell.
28. Tomes J: *A course of lecture notes on dental physiology and surgery*, London, 1848, John Parker.
29. Archer WH: *A manual of dental anesthesia: an illustrated guide for student and practitioner*, Philadelphia, 1952, WB Saunders.
30. Andrews E: The oxygen mixture: a new anesthetic combination. *Chic Med Exam* 9:656, 1868.
31. Bert P: Sur la possibilité d'obtenir, a l'aide du protoxyde de d'azote, une insensibilité de longue durée, et sur l'innocuité de cet anesthétique [Concerning the possibility of obtaining, by the aid of the protoxide of nitrogen, an insensibility of long duration and concerning the innocuousness of that anesthetic]. *C R Acad Sci (Paris)* 87:728, 1878.
32. MacAfee KA, 2nd: Nitrous oxide. I. Historical perspective and patient selection. *Compend Contin Educ Dent* 10(6):1989.
33. Archer WH: *The history of anesthesia, Proceedings of the dental centenary celebration*, Baltimore, 1940, Waverly Press.
34. Archer WH: The history of anesthesia. In Archer WH, editor: *A manual of dental anesthesia*, Philadelphia, 1958, WB Saunders.
35. Nevin M, Puterbaugh PG: *Conduction, infiltration and general anesthesia in dentistry*, New York, 1923, Dental Items of Interest Publishing.
36. Lippe HT: Nitrous oxide analgesia in cavity preparation. *Temple Dent Rev* 14:7, 1944.
37. Seldin HM: *Practical anesthesia for dental and oral surgery*, ed 3, Philadelphia, 1947, Lea & Febiger.
38. Allison ML, Kinney W, Lynch DF, et al: The American Dental Society of Anesthesiology: 1953–1978. *Anesth Prog* 25(1):9–30, 1978.
39. Langa H: *Relative analgesia in dental practice*, ed 2, Philadelphia, 1976, WB Saunders.
40. Clark M, Brunick A: *Handbook of nitrous oxide and oxygen sedation*, ed 4, St Louis, 2015, Mosby.
41. American Dental Association Council on Dental Education: Guidelines for teaching the comprehensive control of pain and anxiety in dentistry. *J Dent Educ* 36(1):62–67, 1972.
42. House of Delegates, American Dental Association Council on Dental Education: *Guidelines for teaching pain control and sedation to dentists and dental students*, Chicago, 2016, The Association.
43. American Dental Association, Council on Dental Materials, Instruments and Equipment: *Revised guidelines for the acceptance program for nitrous oxide-oxygen sedation machines and devices*, Chicago, 1986, The Association.
44. Whitcher C, Zimmerman DC, Piziali RL: Control of occupational exposure to nitrous oxide in the oral surgery office. *J Oral Surg* 36(6):431–440, 1978.
45. States that permit dental hygienists to administer nitrous oxide. American Dental Hygienists Association. Chicago. www.adha.org 2014 (Accessed 1 November 2015).

chapter 12

Inhalation Sedation: Rationale

CHAPTER OUTLINE

The technique of inhalation sedation with nitrous oxide (N$_2$O) and oxygen (O$_2$) possesses many significant advantages over other techniques of pharmacosedation. Inhalation sedation represents the most nearly "ideal" clinical sedative technique. This chapter discusses the indications for the use of N$_2$O-O$_2$ in dentistry and other branches of medicine (Fig. 12.1).

ADVANTAGES

1. The onset of action of inhalation sedation is the most rapid of all sedation techniques; more rapid than that of oral, rectal, intranasal (IN), or intramuscular (IM) sedation. The onset of action of intravenous (IV) medications is approximately, but not quite, equal to that of inhalation sedation.

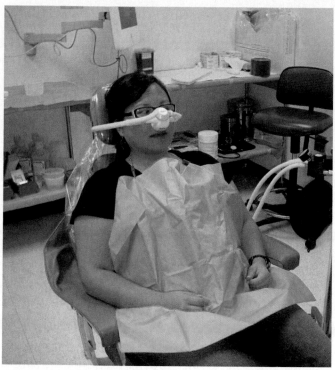

Figure 12.1 Patient receiving inhalation sedation with N_2O and O_2.

Oral	30-min onset
Rectal	30-min onset
IM, IN	10- to 15-min onset
IV	20-sec onset (approximate arm-to-brain circulation time); 1–2 min for clinical actions to develop
Inhalation	<20 sec pulmonary circulation to brain time; 2- to 3-min onset for clinical actions to develop

2. Peak clinical effect does not develop in most techniques for a considerable time. Although variations do exist, peak clinical actions do not develop for most orally, rectally, intranasally, and intramuscularly administered drugs for a period of time that makes their titration impossible. Only inhalation and IV drug administration provide peak clinical actions in a time span permitting titration. For the IV route, this time-to-peak effect varies with the drug administered, ranging from 1 minute to approximately 20 minutes (e.g., lorazepam).

Oral	60-min peak action
Rectal	60-min peak action
IM, IN	30-min peak action
IV	60-sec to 20-min peak action
Inhalation	3- to 5-min peak action

3. The depth of sedation achieved with inhalation sedation may be altered from moment to moment, permitting the drug administrator to increase or decrease the depth of sedation. With no other technique of sedation does the administrator have as much control over the clinical actions of the drugs. This degree of control represents a significant safety feature of inhalation sedation.

Oral	Cannot easily deepen or lighten sedation
Rectal	Cannot easily deepen or lighten sedation
IM, IN	Cannot easily deepen or lighten sedation
IV	Sedation level may easily be deepened; however, lessening of sedation is difficult to achieve
Inhalation	Sedation levels *easily* changed either way

4. The duration of action is an important consideration in the selection of a pharmacosedative technique in an outpatient. In situations in which a sedation technique has a relatively fixed duration of clinical activity, dental treatment must be tailored to this, whereas in those techniques with a flexible duration of action, the planned procedure may be of any length (e.g., a minute or so for the taking of radiographs or 3 to 4 hours [or longer] for preparation and impression of multiple abutments for fixed bridgework).

Oral	Fixed duration of action, approximately 2–3 hr
Rectal	Fixed duration of action, approximately 2–3 hr
IM, IN	Fixed duration of action, approximately 2–4 hr, with significant variation by drug
IV	Fixed duration of action, with significant variation by drug Diazepam, midazolam, 45 min Promethazine, 90 min
Inhalation	Duration variable, at discretion of administrator

5. Recovery time from inhalation sedation is rapid and is the most complete of any pharmacosedation technique. Because N_2O is not metabolized by the body, the gas is rapidly and virtually completely eliminated from the body within 3 to 5 minutes. In all other techniques, the recovery from sedation is considerably slower.[1]

Oral	Recovery not entirely complete even after 2–3 hr
Rectal	Recovery not entirely complete even after 2–3 hr
IM, IN	Recovery not entirely complete even after 2–3 hr
IV	Recovery not entirely complete even after 2–3 hr
Inhalation	Recovery usually complete after 3–5 min of inhalation of 100% O_2

6. As discussed, titration is the ability to administer small, incremental doses of a drug until a desired clinical action is obtained. In my opinion, the ability to titrate a drug represents the greatest safety feature a technique can possess because it permits the drug administrator virtually absolute control over the actions of the drug.[2] Significant drug overdose will not develop in techniques in which titration is possible as long as the administrator does indeed titrate the drug.

Oral	Titration not possible
Rectal	Titration not possible
IM, IN	Titration not possible
IV	Titration possible
Inhalation	Titration possible

7. In an outpatient setting, it is advantageous for the patient to be discharged from the office after a procedure with no prohibitions on activities. Unfortunately, because all of the drugs administered for the reduction of fear and anxiety are central nervous system (CNS) depressants, the patient may not be permitted to leave the office unescorted to operate a motor vehicle or to perform tasks requiring mental alertness for a number of hours after the administration of these drugs.[3] To do so is to increase the potential risk to both the patient (physical risk) and the dentist (legal risk). Recovery must be complete, with absolutely no doubt in the mind of the dentist that the patient is able to function normally; if not, the patient should not be permitted to leave the office unescorted.

Oral	Recovery not complete; patient always requires escort
Rectal	Recovery not complete; as usually used in pediatric dentistry, patient will be escorted by parent or guardian
IM, IN	Recovery not complete; patient always requires escort

| IV | Recovery not complete; patient always requires escort |
| Inhalation | Recovery almost always complete; patient usually may be discharged from office alone, with no admonitions about activities |

8. No injection is required for the administration of inhalation sedation. (Local anesthesia is still necessary.)
9. Inhalation sedation with N_2O-O_2 is safe. Very few side effects are associated with its use, as described in the following chapters.
10. The drugs used in this technique have no adverse effects on the liver, kidneys, brain, or cardiovascular and respiratory systems.
11. Inhalation sedation with N_2O-O_2 can be used instead of local anesthesia in certain procedures. N_2O does possess analgesic properties when given in the usual sedative concentrations. The analgesia produced by a 50% concentration of N_2O is equivalent to that of 10 to 15 mg of morphine. However, the degree of analgesia is quite variable from patient to patient and therefore cannot be relied on to provide all of the pain control required for a procedure. Certain procedures, such as those involving soft tissues (scaling, curettage), may be performed in many instances without using local anesthesia.

DISADVANTAGES

The following are disadvantages associated with N_2O-O_2 inhalation sedation.
1. The initial cost of the equipment required for inhalation sedation is high.
2. The continuing cost of the gases (O_2 and N_2O) used in inhalation sedation is high.
3. The equipment required for inhalation sedation occupies considerable space within the dental surgery suite. Placed in the usual small dental surgery office, a portable N_2O-O_2 unit can be quite cumbersome.
4. N_2O is not a potent agent. When it is used in combination with at least 20% O_2, there will be a small percentage of patients in whom the technique will fail to produce the desired clinical actions. In no circumstance should N_2O ever be administered with less than 20% O_2. Inhalation sedation units available in the United States (and increasingly worldwide) are designed so that they will not deliver less than 30% O_2, with a maximum limit of 70%. N_2O inhalation sedation with N_2O-O_2 is not a panacea. Failures will occur primarily because of the lack of potency of the agent or due to the administration and/or titration technique.
5. A degree of cooperation is required from the patient. For inhalation sedation to be effective, the patient must be able to inhale the gases through either the nose or the mouth.

Should the patient be unable or unwilling to do so, clinical failure will result.

6. All members of the sedation team employing N_2O-O_2 must receive training in its safe and effective use. Ideally, this training is acquired in dental, dental hygiene, or dental assisting school. Postgraduate continuing education courses are also available, but quality varies tremendously in these programs. The guidelines established by the American Dental Association (ADA), the American Dental Society of Anesthesiology (ADSA), and the American Dental Education Association (ADEA) recommend no fewer than 14 hours of training, including treatment of dental patients receiving inhalation sedation (see Chapter 19).[4]

7. There is a possibility that unscavenged trace nitrous oxide can be deleterious.

INDICATIONS

The primary indications for the use of inhalation sedation are the same as those for other sedative techniques: the management of fear and anxiety, the medically compromised patient, and the management of gagging.[5] Over and above these usual indications, N_2O-O_2 is readily controllable; this permits its use for aspects of dental care in which the use of moderate sedation might not usually be considered.

Many procedures that are generally considered nonthreatening or even innocuous might, however, prove to be extremely traumatic to some patients. Many of these procedures lend themselves quite readily to the use of N_2O-O_2.

Anxiety

The major indication for the use of N_2O-O_2 inhalation sedation in dentistry is, of course, the management of fear and anxiety related to the dental experience. As discussed in the preceding section on the advantages of inhalation sedation, N_2O-O_2 represents the most nearly ideal sedation technique. Were it not for the fact that some persons are not comfortable with the effects of N_2O-O_2, that some others will not achieve clinically adequate sedation at permissible percentages, and that still others are unable to breathe through their noses, inhalation sedation would be the only technique of sedation required for the management of dental anxieties.

Medically Compromised Patients

In recent years, the use of N_2O-O_2 has become increasingly important in the management of medically compromised patients. The general evaluation of these patients is discussed in Chapter 4; however, I believe that it is important to review some of these patients and discuss the relevance of their diseases to the use of N_2O-O_2.

Cardiovascular Disease

The use of N_2O-O_2 in patients with cardiovascular disease is one of the most valuable methods of minimizing risk to the patient during dental care. In most, if not all, significant cardiovascular disease states one factor likely to produce an exacerbation of clinical signs and symptoms is an O_2 deficit in the myocardium. Myocardial ischemia is produced in many patients by an increased cardiovascular workload—an increase in the heart rate and in the force of contraction of the heart. In the patient with an underlying cardiovascular disorder that may be asymptomatic while the patient is at rest (nonstressed), this increased workload of the myocardium, leading to ischemia, may precipitate an acute cardiovascular event.

Because O_2 deficit is responsible for the onset of most anginal episodes, an increased severity of heart failure, cardiac dysrhythmias, and possibly myocardial infarction, any sedative technique that decreases the myocardial O_2 requirement will decrease the risk to the patient during dental treatment.[6] Therefore any sedative procedure is appropriate for use in these patients. However, N_2O-O_2 inhalation sedation has several advantages over other techniques: in addition to providing a reduction of anxiety, it produces an elevation in the pain reaction threshold and provides the myocardium and entire body with a minimum of 30%, but more frequently 50% to 70%, O_2.[7] Therefore at its very worst, the patient is receiving approximately 50% more O_2 than he or she would from atmospheric air, which has an O_2 content of 20.9%.

I have employed N_2O-O_2 inhalation sedation as an emergency and preoperative agent with great success in patients with angina pectoris, heart failure, severe cardiac dysrhythmias, past myocardial infarction, and high blood pressure in addition to other cardiovascular disorders.[8,9]

The use of N_2O-O_2 in patients with severe cardiovascular disease has received considerable attention in the past 20 years. Emergency medical personnel in Wales and Great Britain have employed a premixed combination of N_2O and O_2 in a ratio of 40% to 60% (Entonox) for the management of pain during an acute myocardial infarction.[6,10] In the past, management of the pain of a myocardial infarction was achieved through the IV administration of opioid analgesics (commonly morphine). The success of N_2O-O_2 in this life-threatening situation was such that paramedical units in a growing number of areas throughout the United States are today incorporating its use into their armamentarium (Fig. 12.2).[11] In the United States the most commonly used concentration of N_2O to O_2 has been 50%. At this concentration (available under the proprietary name Dolonox), N_2O has analgesic properties, diminishing or eliminating pain; has sedative properties, helping the victim to relax and become more comfortable, thereby reducing the workload of the myocardium; and provides the patient with 50% O_2—two and a half times the volume found in atmospheric air. In a study by Thompson and Lown,[6] it was found that 75% of patients receiving 35% N_2O and 65% O_2 during acute myocardial infarction have either a distinct decrease in the severity of their pain (36%) or state that the pain was eliminated entirely (39%). Inhalation sedation with N_2O-O_2 has been found to be the most appropriate technique of sedation for the patient with preexisting cardiovascular disease.

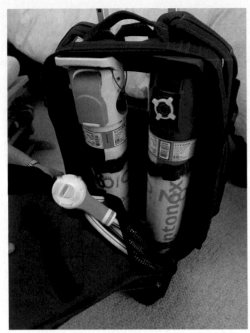

Figure 12.2 Portable N_2O-O_2 unit employed by paramedical personnel. (Courtesy Linde Healthcare.)

Respiratory Disease

The use of inhalation anesthetics is frequently contraindicated in patients with acute or chronic respiratory disease. However, N_2O-O_2 is used quite successfully and without untoward incident in many patients with respiratory disease.

Chronic obstructive pulmonary disease (COPD) represents a relative contraindication to the successful use of N_2O-O_2. Although it is possible for the patient to become apneic during the procedure as a result of the elevation of the O_2 level in the blood, this is rarely a clinical finding. In my involvement with the administration of N_2O-O_2 inhalation sedation since 1972, including many patients with respiratory disorders, this situation has never developed. The primary concern with patients with significant respiratory disease is the potential lack of sedative effect of the N_2O-O_2.

Occasionally the dentist will receive a medical consultation that states that the use of N_2O-O_2 is contraindicated in asthmatic patients. N_2O may be administered quite safely in patients such as these.[12] The reason behind this medical consultation is that anesthetic gases that are irritating to the respiratory mucosa may precipitate an acute episode of bronchospasm in patients with hyperactive airway disease (e.g., asthmatics). Many anesthetic gases are contraindicated in asthmatic patients. However, N_2O is a nonirritating vapor that does not exacerbate asthma. The use of sedation in the asthmatic patient is frequently warranted because increased stress is a potential cause of acute exacerbation of asthma. N_2O-O_2 represents a very effective and safe technique of sedation in these patients.

Patients with chronic nasal obstruction, either from anatomic abnormalities (deviated nasal septum) or pathologic conditions (allergy, upper respiratory tract infection), will be difficult to sedate adequately with gaseous agents. In addition, the potential for the infection of other patients through the use of a nasal hood that has become contaminated should be considered before N_2O-O_2 is administered to patients who are ill.

Cerebrovascular Disease

The patient who has had a cerebrovascular accident (CVA, "stroke," "brain attack") is unable to tolerate levels of O_2 below normal without an increased risk of developing seizure activity or additional neuronal damage. Deep sedation is contraindicated because of the increased (although unlikely) possibility of hypoxia. Whereas other techniques of sedation may be considered for these patients, the one most highly recommended for the patient who has had a CVA is N_2O-O_2 inhalation sedation. The major recommendation for this technique is the elevated level of O_2 that is routinely provided to the patient. As it is used in dentistry today, there is little or no likelihood of a hypoxic episode developing.

Hepatic Disease

Hepatic disease, such as cirrhosis or hepatitis, represents a contraindication (either relative or absolute) to the use of many of the drugs discussed in this text because most of them undergo biotransformation in the liver. In the presence of significant hepatic dysfunction (American Society of Anesthesiologists [ASA] 3 or 4), the rate of biotransformation (elimination half-life) of a drug is slowed, potentially resulting in higher plasma levels, which in turn leads to an increase in the drug effect and a prolongation of its clinical activity. However, N_2O does not undergo biotransformation anywhere within the body (see Chapter 13) and may therefore be used without additional risk and with a high probability of success in the patient with hepatic dysfunction.

Epilepsy and Seizure Disorders

As with patients who have had a CVA, patients with a history of chronic idiopathic seizure activity (epilepsy) are more sensitive to hypoxia than are healthy patients. Seizure activity is precipitated more readily in these patients; therefore hypoxia must be guarded against much more scrupulously. N_2O is not epileptogenic (it does not increase the risk of seizures developing) and therefore may be administered to these patients as long as hypoxia is prevented. Increased stress and anxiety have been demonstrated to be precipitating causes of seizures. With the sedation machines available today and adherence to the technique of administering N_2O-O_2 presented in Chapter 15, epilepsy does not represent a contraindication to the use of inhalation sedation.

Pregnancy

N_2O does cross the placenta to the fetus, producing the same degree of CNS depression as in the mother. If delivered in combination with adequate levels of O_2 (greater than 20%), N_2O-O_2 inhalation sedation represents the recommended sedation technique for use during pregnancy. Medical consultation with the patient's physician before its use is suggested.

Allergy

No allergies to N_2O have ever been reported.

Diabetes

Diabetes mellitus does not represent a contraindication to the use of N_2O-O_2.

Gagging

Gagging is a potential problem during many dental procedures, especially in the maxillary palatal and the posterior mandibular lingual regions. Although there is no absolute solution to this problem (other than general anesthesia), inhalation sedation with N_2O-O_2 has proven to be highly effective in eliminating or at least minimizing severe gagging. Patients are titrated with N_2O-O_2 to their sedation level, at which point impressions, radiographs, or other procedures may be completed. The use of N_2O-O_2 to diminish the gag reflex may require placing the patient in an upright position for some or all of the procedure. Although this position is not usually recommended during sedation (supine is preferred), some procedures, such as impressions in the maxilla, may require modification of position for increased patient safety. Where other sedation techniques (especially IV sedation) are also effective in decreasing gagging, only N_2O is practical to use for extremely short procedures, such as radiographs or impressions.

CONTRAINDICATIONS

There are relatively few absolute contraindications to the administration of N_2O-O_2 inhalation sedation as long as the percentage of O_2 administered with the N_2O is greater than 20% (atmospheric concentration).[13] However, there are several relative contraindications to this technique. A relative contraindication implies that there is an increased potential for an adverse reaction to develop in a certain patient. Although the technique in question may be used, if there exists another technique without this contraindication that would prove to be equally successful, it should be used in place of the contraindicated technique. The following are relative contraindications to N_2O-O_2 inhalation sedation.

Patients With a Compulsive Personality

The use of N_2O-O_2 sedation (or, for that matter, any sedation technique) in a person with a compulsive personality would result in a very low probability of success. Persons with compulsive personalities, or "take-charge" persons, are ones who would not like the feeling of "losing control" associated with the use of sedation. These patients will consciously, or more likely subconsciously, "fight" the effects of the drug(s).

Claustrophobic Patients

Inhalation sedation will have a very low success rate in patients who are unable to tolerate the nasal hood or face mask used in the administration of gaseous agents. This is not a problem in patients undergoing general anesthesia because anesthesia may be induced by IV drugs, with the face mask applied after unconsciousness is induced; however, sedated patients are, of course, conscious throughout the procedure and, if fearful of the mask, will be unable to become comfortable. The nasal cannula should not be used to administer N_2O because of its inability to be scavenged (see Chapters 13 and 17).

Children With Severe Behavior Problems

The use of N_2O-O_2 in children who are severely disruptive will usually prove to be futile. A degree of patient cooperation is required for this technique to be successful. Patients must accept the nasal hood and be willing and able to breathe through their nose. Precooperative or noncooperative children (or adult patients with disabilities) will breathe through their mouths, crying, screaming, or moving about in the chair, thus negating the effects of any N_2O that they may inhale. Management of these patients is discussed in Chapter 35.

Patients With Severe Personality Disorders

Patients who are under psychiatric care and are receiving psychotropic drugs, usually mood-elevating antidepressants, should be evaluated carefully before the administration of any form of sedation.[14] Although no serious drug–drug interactions develop between N_2O-O_2 and these psychotropic drugs, it may be prudent to avoid altering the consciousness of persons who have but a tenuous grip on reality.[15] Medical consultation before the use of any sedative technique is strongly indicated.

Upper Respiratory Tract Infection or Other Acute Respiratory Conditions

Because N_2O-O_2 must be inhaled through the nose during dental treatment, any respiratory problem preventing the use of the nose as a route of entry for the anesthetic gases represents a relative contraindication to this technique. The common cold, acute or chronic sinus problems, chronic mouth breathing, allergy, tuberculosis, and bronchitis represent situations in which the technique of inhalation sedation might best be avoided, if possible. Other techniques may be substituted effectively. Aside from the difficulty in achieving sedation when the patient is unable to inhale through the nose, there is the distinct possibility of contaminating the rubber goods of the inhalation sedation unit.

Sedation of patients with significant respiratory disorders with any technique is relatively contraindicated, as the incidence of airway complications is increased in these patients.[16]

Patients with chronic respiratory or other potentially contagious diseases (tuberculosis, human immunodeficiency virus/acquired immunodeficiency syndrome) who require inhalation sedation may be provided (at cost, of course) with their own "disposable" rubber goods for inhalation sedation. Such disposable systems, consisting of nasal hood, tubing, and reservoir bag, are available at relatively modest cost and will minimize the risk of cross contamination.

Chronic Obstructive Pulmonary Disease

COPD (e.g., emphysema, chronic bronchitis) represents a relative contraindication to inhalation sedation because of the potential effect of administering a gas mixture enriched with O_2 to these patients, many of whom have chronically elevated CO_2 blood levels. Whereas the usual stimulus for breathing in a healthy person is an increase in the blood CO_2 level, patients with COPD have a diminished or absent ability to respond to this stimulus. In its place, the stimulus for breathing in these patients is a lowered blood O_2 content. In the administration of inhalation sedation, an O_2-enriched mixture of gases is always provided, raising the O_2 saturation of the blood. The stimulus for involuntary breathing has now been removed, and the patient should be watched for apnea. In the unconscious patient during general anesthesia, the patient will be closely observed; however, in the conscious patient (e.g., during inhalation sedation), where voluntary control over breathing is maintained, prolonged apnea does not develop. These patients should be evaluated quite carefully before the planned dental treatment to assess their ability to tolerate dental therapy in general. Most of these patients represent ASA 3 or 4 risks during dental treatment.

The Patient Who Does Not Want N₂O-O₂

The nasal hood should never be forced onto a patient. Should the adult patient be uncomfortable with the nasal hood, it is often best to remove it. Discuss the reason for the discomfort and, if needed, employ a different sedation technique. Because of the light level of moderate sedation produced by N_2O-O_2, it is impossible to overwhelm a patient with the drug against his or her will.

Pregnancy

The use of sedation in the pregnant patient has been discussed in Chapter 4. It is desirable to avoid the use of any drugs (if possible) during the first trimester to prevent increasing the slight risk for spontaneous abortion or the development of a fetal malformation that might be related to a drug administered at this time. Drugs may be employed in the second trimester if necessary but, as always, with caution, especially CNS depressants, and only after consultation with the patient's primary care physician or OB-GYN. Of the techniques that might be used for the reduction of anxiety in the pregnant patient, the safest and most recommended is inhalation sedation with N_2O-O_2. N_2O is not metabolized in the body and has virtually no effect on most organ systems, and it is rapidly and almost entirely removed from the body within 3 to 5 minutes; these facts provide ample evidence of its superiority over other techniques. In the third trimester of pregnancy, the major consideration in determining whether to treat the patient must be the possibility of the patient giving birth during the dental appointment. As the patient nears term, it might be prudent to postpone any nonemergency treatment. However, should emergency care be necessary and if the patient requires sedation, the use of inhalation sedation is suggested. Prior consultation with the patient's obstetrician is advisable whenever sedation is considered for a pregnant patient.[17,18]

Besides the three major indications for the use of inhalation sedation—anxiety, medically compromised patient, and gagging—there are a multitude of uses for this technique in other areas of dentistry, including procedures that are usually considered too minor or too short to employ sedation. Very often the dentist or hygienist will advise a patient that the procedure will "hurt just a little." It is this type of procedure that is appropriate for the use of inhalation sedation.

RESTORATIVE DENTISTRY

Initial Dental Examination

Patients who have come to the dental office in pain may be extremely uncomfortable during the initial examination because of the sensitivity of their soft tissues or teeth. Sedation with N_2O-O_2 and the elevation in pain threshold accompanying it will make this potentially traumatic procedure more tolerable for the patient.

Removal of Provisional Crowns or Bridges

The removal of provisional crowns or bridges from vital teeth is often done without the benefit of local anesthesia because the procedure is short and associated with minimal discomfort. This discomfort may be eliminated or minimized through the use of N_2O-O_2. The drying and cleansing of the prepared vital teeth for the cementation of crowns or bridges is also an appropriate area for the use of N_2O-O_2 sedation.

Occlusal Adjustment

Occlusal adjustment of crowns, bridges, or natural teeth rarely requires the use of local anesthesia. There are patients, however, who are quite uncomfortable during this procedure. The sound of the drill or the vibration of the bur on the tooth makes some patients extremely tense. Sedation with N_2O-O_2 can eliminate this response in most patients.

Insertion of Matrix Bands or Wedges

The insertion of matrix bands or wedges between teeth before the placement of a restoration may be uncomfortable for the patient if soft tissue anesthesia is not present. Sedation with N_2O-O_2 provides soft tissue analgesia in many patients, thus making this procedure less traumatic.

PERIODONTICS AND DENTAL HYGIENE

Within the specialty of periodontology, there is a need for sedation. Surgical procedures in general are more anxiety producing than more routine nonsurgical procedures. The use of inhalation sedation with N_2O-O_2 is especially recommended in periodontics, primarily in its nonsurgical aspect, because in a significant percentage of patients, a degree of soft tissue analgesia will be noted, helping make the procedure less traumatic.

Initial Periodontal Examination

The initial periodontal examination and probing can be quite traumatic to patients, especially patients in whom significant periodontal disease is present. Inflamed, swollen soft tissues and teeth with deep periodontal pockets will be extremely sensitive during this examination. Inhalation sedation provides both a relaxed patient and a degree of soft tissue analgesia, which ranges from the total loss of sensation in these tissues to decreased sensitivity so that, although the patient still feels the pain, it no longer bothers him or her (Nitrous oxide, similar to narcotics, separates pain from suffering).

Scaling, Curettage, and Root Planing

One of the most important uses of N_2O-O_2 within periodontics is for scaling, curettage, and root planing. As mentioned, most patients receiving N_2O-O_2 at sedative levels will develop a degree of soft tissue analgesia. Scaling, curettage, and root planing are three procedures that, although not normally traumatic, may be so on occasion. The administration of local anesthesia is one means of alleviating this discomfort; however, N_2O-O_2 offers the patient and dentist or hygienist a more pleasant means of achieving essentially the same goal with a technique that is almost immediately reversible on completion of the procedure. As of June 2016, 32 states in the United States permit trained registered dental hygienists to administer N_2O-O_2 to their patients.[19] The response from hygienists, dentists, and patients has been almost universally positive.

Use of Ultrasonic Instruments

Ultrasonic instruments are commonly used during periodontal procedures to aid in the removal of calculus from teeth. Some patients may find the use of these devices threatening and uncomfortable. Sedation with N_2O-O_2 is a means of eliminating this fear for most patients.

Periodontal Surgery

Patients facing periodontal surgery often request the use of sedation because of the nature and length of the surgical procedure. Inhalation sedation with N_2O-O_2 is an appropriate procedure for many of these patients, although IV sedation is also commonly used during periodontal surgery.

ORAL AND MAXILLOFACIAL SURGERY

Lengthy Surgical Procedures

As discussed in the preceding paragraph, N_2O-O_2 sedation is an acceptable technique for use in the patient undergoing any lengthy procedure as a means of helping make the procedure more tolerable and for providing analgesia.

Management of Abscesses

When an incision and drainage (I&D) procedure is planned to help relieve the discomfort of an abscess, it is often difficult to achieve adequate pain control through the administration of local anesthetics, primarily because of the change in tissue pH brought about by the formation of purulent material within the infected area. Inhalation sedation with N_2O-O_2 may be used to advantage in this situation because of its ability to provide a degree of soft tissue analgesia.[13] Titration of the patient to the usual sedative level will almost always provide a degree of soft tissue analgesia sufficient to permit the I&D procedure to be completed in comfort or with minimal discomfort.

Management of Postoperative Complications

Inhalation sedation can be of great benefit in the management of localized osteitis (dry socket). Localized osteitis most commonly occurs following extraction of third molars, and its management requires irrigation of the socket and placement of medicated packs into the socket to cover the exposed bone. Local anesthesia is not always used for this procedure, which may produce some patient discomfort. Inhalation sedation can provide a degree of sedation and analgesia for the brief period necessary to complete the irrigation and packing of the extraction site.

Suture Removal

Another potential postoperative use for N_2O-O_2 is as an aid in the removal of sutures, although it is not normally required for this procedure. However, there are occasions when sutures are difficult to locate, and there also is a potential for the scissors to irritate the soft tissues as the sutures are sought. Inhalation sedation is an excellent means of minimizing potential discomfort.

ENDODONTICS

Clinically, adequate pain control in endodontically involved teeth, although less of a problem since the introduction of intraosseous local anesthesia, articaine HCl, and local anesthetic buffering, may occasionally prove to be difficult to achieve. Unfortunately, there are no panaceas. An aid to achieving adequate pain control in such cases, however, is N_2O-O_2 sedation. Although the discomfort involved in the opening into the pulp chamber of a "hot" tooth may not be entirely eliminated, N_2O will raise the pain reaction threshold, thereby modifying the patient's response to it so that the patient, although still aware of his or her pain, is no longer bothered by it.

Rubber Dam Clamps

The placement of a rubber dam clamp on the neck of an endodontically involved tooth is almost always entirely atraumatic. However, when the clinical crown of a tooth is inadequate to support the clamp, tissue clamping may be required. Either local anesthesia or N_2O-O_2 inhalation sedation may be employed to alleviate patient discomfort in this procedure.

Gaining Access to the Pulp Chamber

On extremely rare occasions (e.g., mandibular molars), it may be difficult to achieve adequate pulpal anesthesia in the vital tooth about to undergo pulpal therapy. As the endodontic access preparation nears the pulp chamber, the patient experiences greater and greater discomfort. Once the pulp chamber has been entered, an intrapulpal injection may be administered that will usually eliminate, once and for all, any further discomfort. However, the greatest problem may be in reaching the point at which an intrapulpal injection can be administered. Should the patient experience great discomfort as the preparation approaches the pulp chamber, N_2O-O_2 inhalation sedation may be administered to raise the pain reaction threshold, thereby modifying (although not usually eliminating) the discomfort experienced by the patient.

Instrumenting Canals

Following extirpation of pulpal tissues, the endodontically involved tooth must be prepared for filling. During instrumentation, local anesthetics might not be used because there should be no discomfort or, at the most, minimal discomfort. Some patients, however, may be quite uncomfortable, and the administration of local anesthesia and/or N_2O-O_2 is recommended.

Filling of Root Canals

As in the instrumentation of the root canal, discomfort is usually nonexistent or, at most, only minimal during the filling of root canals; therefore local anesthesia is rarely used. Should patient discomfort or anxiety be present, N_2O-O_2 administration is recommended.

FIXED PROSTHODONTICS

Impression Taking

Inhalation sedation may be valuable in two parts of the impression-taking process. First, if local anesthesia has not been administered, N_2O-O_2, through its ability to elevate the pain reaction threshold, will enable the patient to better tolerate any discomfort associated with the procedure. Second, N_2O-O_2 will aid in diminishing the gag reflex, so there will be little or no difficulty in placing the impression materials and trays.

Gingival retraction cord is placed into the sulcus of abutment teeth before taking impressions to aid in visualizing and gaining access to the margins of the impression. In the absence of local anesthesia, packing of retraction cord may prove to be uncomfortable for the patient, a situation that can be minimized or eliminated by N_2O-O_2.

Removal of Provisional Crowns and Bridges

It is not uncommon for provisional crowns and bridges to be removed without local anesthesia. This will precede the taking of impressions, the trying in of crowns and bridges, and their cementation. The removal of excess cement from a vital tooth and its drying before impressions or cementation may be associated with a degree of discomfort. This sensitivity may be decreased or eliminated with N_2O-O_2.

Adjustment of Castings

After provisional crowns and bridges are removed, the cast crowns and bridges will be tried in and, if necessary, adjusted. This process may be uncomfortable for some patients, especially if the abutment teeth are vital and if local anesthesia has not been administered (as may often be the case). Occlusal adjustment of these castings may produce intense vibration and noise, which may bother the patient. Sedation with N_2O-O_2 is recommended in these situations.

REMOVABLE PROSTHODONTICS
Preparation of Abutment Teeth

Unlike fixed prosthodontics, in which pain control with local anesthetics is normally required for the preparation of abutment teeth, there is usually minimal discomfort associated with the preparation of teeth for removable prostheses. Local anesthesia is rarely required for this process, yet some patients will experience a degree of tooth sensitivity or anxiety related to this procedure. Inhalation sedation with N_2O-O_2 is an appropriate means of managing any anxiety or discomfort associated with preparing teeth for removable prosthodontic appliances.

Determination of Centric Relationships

Although it is not a muscle-relaxing drug combination, N_2O-O_2 can aid in determining the centric relationship in a patient having difficulty relaxing his or her muscles by helping the patient relax psychologically, thereby taking his or her mind off the procedure and permitting a more accurate tracing of the centric relationship.

Occlusal Adjustments and Impression Taking

As in fixed prosthodontics, N_2O-O_2 inhalation sedation may prove to be a valuable aid in adjusting occlusion and taking impressions for removable prostheses.

Fitting of Immediate Dentures

Immediate dentures are placed into the patient's mouth immediately after the extraction of teeth. The tissues in the oral cavity at that time are usually well anesthetized, and there is no discomfort during this procedure. However, at subsequent visits, the removal of the immediate full denture may prove to be quite uncomfortable because the underlying soft tissues may have not yet fully healed and there may be areas of tissue irritation from the denture itself. When used at this time, N_2O-O_2 sedation can benefit both the patient and the dentist.

ORAL RADIOLOGY

Although N_2O-O_2 is not historically used in oral radiology, there are some scenarios during which its use may prove beneficial. The use of N_2O with the placement of intraoral films can be highly effective in eliminating or at least minimizing the gag reflex. Patients with limiting anatomy, such as shallow palates, exostosis, or trauma, can also benefit from reduced pain. The previously mentioned indications such as anxiety and managing appropriate medically compromised patients also apply to oral radiology. It is worth noting that proper film placement and tubing adjustment must be monitored to prevent shadowing in radiographs. New nasal hoods do not contain metal, obviating this concern.

ORTHODONTICS

The need for sedation and pain control is minimal in most orthodontic procedures, so much so that many orthodontists rarely, if ever, administer local anesthetics. However, there are occasions when the use of sedation for a brief time may prove to be quite beneficial. These include impression taking, in which excessive gagging can be minimized, and the placement or removal of bands and wires, in which soft tissue analgesia produced by the N_2O-O_2 can eliminate or modify any discomfort.

PEDIATRIC DENTISTRY

Inhalation sedation with N_2O-O_2 is one of the most valuable sedative techniques available for use in children.[20,21] The range of procedures in which the use of this technique is appropriate is unlimited. The indications for inhalation sedation in children are the same as those for adults. One complicating factor to be considered is that for inhalation sedation to be effective, the patient must be willing to accept the nasal hood and to breathe through his or her nose. Unfortunately, the pediatric patient who is a more severe behavior management problem may be unwilling to accept the nasal hood, minimizing the success of inhalation sedation. The use of N_2O-O_2 inhalation sedation in pediatric dentistry is discussed in Chapters 15 and 35.

N_2O-O_2 inhalation sedation is rapidly expanding in use around the globe. Practitioners across disciplines of health care are increasingly recognizing the benefits of its pain and anxiety reduction. As seen by the comparisons with other methods of pharmacosedation, N_2O-O_2 inhalation sedation is superior in many ways.

REFERENCES

1. Faddy SC, Garlick SR: A systematic review of the safety of analgesia with 50% nitrous oxide; can lay responders use analgesic gases in the prehospital setting? *Emerg Med J* 22(12):901–908, 2005.
2. Stewart RD: Nitrous oxide sedation/analgesia in emergency medicine. *Ann Emerg Med* 14(2):139–148, 1985.
3. Ayer WA, Jr, Domoto PK, Gale EN, et al: Overcoming dental fear: strategies for its prevention and management. *J Am Dent Assoc* 107(1):18–27, 1983.
4. House of Delegates, American Dental Association: Guidelines for teaching pain control and sedation to dentists and dental students, Chicago, Oct. 2016, American Dental Association.
5. Chidiac JJ, Domoto PK, Gale EN, et al: Gagging prevention using nitrous oxide or table salt: a comparative pilot study. *Int J Prosthodont* 14(4):364–366, 2001.
6. Thompson PL, Lown B: Nitrous oxide as an analgesic in acute myocardial infarction. *JAMA* 235(9):924–927, 1976.
7. Keer F, Irving JB, Ewing DJ, Kirby BJ: Nitrous oxide analgesia in myocardial infarction. *Lancet* 1(7741):63–66, 1972.
8. Flomenbaum N, Gallagher EJ, Eagen K, Jacobson S: Self-administered nitrous oxide: an adjunct analgesic. *JACEP* 8(3):95–97, 1979.
9. Hayes GB: Relief of cardiac chest pain in the field. *Emerg Care Q* 3:49, 1987.
10. Pons PT: Nitrous oxide analgesia. *Emerg Med Clin North Am* 6(4):777–782, 1988.
11. O'Leary U, Puglia C, Friehling TD, Kowey PR: Nitrous oxide anesthesia in patients with ischemic chest discomfort: effect on beta-endorphins. *J Clin Pharmacol* 27(12):957–961, 1987.
12. Rogers MC, Tinker JH, Covino BG, et al: *Principles and practice of anesthesiology*, St Louis, 1993, Mosby.
13. Clark M, Brunick A: *Handbook of nitrous oxide and oxygen sedation*, ed 4, St Louis, 2015, Mosby.
14. Gillman MA: Analgesic nitrous oxide as a therapeutic and investigative tool in neurological conditions. In Sinha KK, editor: *Progress in clinical neurosciences* (vol 2). Ranchi, India, 1985, Neurological Society of India.
15. deWet J, Lichtigfeld FJ, Gillman MA: Psychotropic analgesic nitrous oxide (PAN) for hyperactivity. *Aust N Z J Psychiatry* 35(4):543–544, 2001.
16. Canet J, Gallart L: Predicting postoperative pulmonary complications in the general population. *Curr Opin Anaesthesiol* 26(2):107–115, 2013.
17. Minnett RJ: Self-administered anaesthesia in childbirth. *Br Med J* 1:501, 1934.
18. Santos AC, Pedersen H: Current controversies in obstetric anesthesia. *Anesth Anal* 78(4):753–760, 1994.
19. States that permit dental hygienists to administer nitrous oxide. American Dental Hygienists Association. Chicago. www.adha.org 2016 (Accessed 8 December 2016).
20. Gamis AS, Knapp JF, Glenski JA: Nitrous oxide analgesia in a pediatric emergency department. *Ann Emerg Med* 18(2):177–181, 1989.
21. Haupt M: Project USAP 2000-use of sedative agents by pediatric dentists: a 15-year follow-up survey. *Pediatr Dent* 24:289–294, 2002.

chapter 13

Pharmacology, Anatomy, and Physiology

CHAPTER OUTLINE

Pharmacology

NITROUS OXIDE

Preparation

Nitrous oxide (N_2O, dinitrogen monoxide) is prepared commercially through the heating of ammonium nitrate crystals to $240°C$, at which point the ammonium nitrate decomposes into N_2O and H_2O.

The gas is then chemically scrubbed to remove any alkaline and acid substances and is then compressed in stages so that the less easily liquefied gases, such as nitrogen (N_2) and oxygen (O_2), are separated out. Finally, it is compressed and stored in metal cylinders, in which approximately 30% of the N_2O in the full cylinder is liquefied. According to the *U.S.*

Pharmacopeia, N_2O must be 97% pure; however, with the manufacturing processes in use today, the gas usually approaches a purity of 99.5% (Fig. 13.1).[1]

The most common impurities associated with the manufacture of N_2O are N_2, nitric oxide (NO), nitrogen dioxide (NO_2), ammonia (NH_4), water vapor, and carbon monoxide (CO). NO is the most dangerous impurity because, like CO, it may combine with hemoglobin and prevent the absorption of O_2, or it may react with water vapor to form acids that may damage the pulmonary epithelium and produce pulmonary edema. NO is formed when N_2O is heated above $450°C$.

As prepared, N_2O is anhydrous. The absence of water in the gas is of importance because water vapor would freeze as it passes through the reducing valve (see Chapter 14), leading to a drop in the gas pressure.

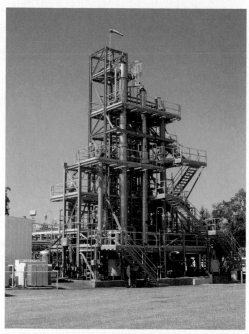

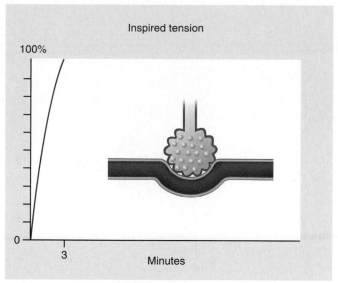

Figure 13.2 Primary saturation of a gaseous agent with a blood–gas solubility coefficient of 0.00 (totally insoluble) occurs within a very brief period. Both onset and recovery are extremely rapid.

Figure 13.1 A typical manufacturing plant in which N_2O is prepared. (Courtesy Airgas Nitrous Oxide Corp.)

Properties
Physical Properties

N_2O is a nonirritating, sweet-smelling, colorless gas. It is the only nonorganic compound other than carbon dioxide (CO_2) that has any central nervous system (CNS)-depressant properties and is the only inorganic gas used to produce anesthesia in humans. The molecular weight of N_2O is 44, and its specific gravity is 1.53, compared with that of air, which is 1.

N_2O gas is converted to a clear and colorless liquid at 288°C at 50 atm of pressure. The boiling point of N_2O is −89°C. Its oil–water solubility coefficient is 3.2, and the blood–gas solubility coefficient is 0.47.

Chemical Properties

N_2O is stable under pressure at usual temperatures. However, NO is formed when N_2O is heated above 450°C. Marketed in cylinders as a liquid under pressure (vapor pressure at room temperature is 50 atm), N_2O returns to the gaseous state as it is released from the cylinder. An interesting phenomenon occurs as the N_2O exits the cylinder. The walls of the cylinder become cold, and in some instances, frost may be evident around the exit portal of the gas. This occurs because the liquid N_2O requires heat for vaporization into the gaseous state. The heat required for vaporization is obtained from the walls of the metal cylinder and from the surrounding air, with the result that the cylinder becomes cool to the touch.

Solubility

N_2O is relatively insoluble in the blood (its blood–gas solubility coefficient is 0.47 at 378°C) and is carried in the blood in physical solution only, not combining with any blood elements. The oxygen in the N_2O molecule is not available for use by the tissues because N_2O does not break down in the body.

Solubility is a term used to describe how a gas is distributed between two media (e.g., gas and blood). If the concentration of an anesthetic gas in blood is 2 volumes percent and this is in equilibrium with a concentration in the alveolus of 1 volume percent, the blood–gas solubility would be 2.

When an anesthetic gas is first inspired, blood entering the alveolus by the pulmonary artery contains none of it. When reaching the pulmonary capillary, the blood is suddenly exposed to the tension of the gas present in the alveolus. If the gas is totally insoluble in the blood (blood–gas partition coefficient of 0), none of the agent will be taken up by the circulation, and the alveolar concentration will rise rapidly and will soon equal the inspired concentration (Fig. 13.2).

If, on the other hand, the anesthetic is slightly soluble in blood, only small quantities will be carried by the bloodstream. Alveolar concentration will again rise rapidly (Fig. 13.3).

Because alveolar concentration determines the tension of the anesthetic in the arterial circulation, the tension will also rise rapidly, even though only a small volume of the agent is present in the blood. As the blood travels through the various tissues of the body, the anesthetic is given up and the venous blood returns to the lungs with a decreased anesthetic gas tension.

N_2O and desflurane are examples of anesthetic gases with low blood solubility (Table 13.1). On inhalation, these gases rapidly diffuse across the alveolar membrane into the blood. Because of their low blood solubility, only a small quantity is absorbed and the alveolar tension rises rapidly so that the tension of the gas in the blood is also increased

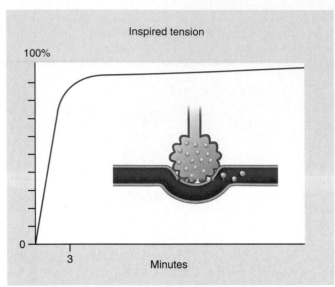

Figure 13.3 N$_2$O, with a blood–gas solubility coefficient of 0.47 (relatively insoluble), demonstrates both rapid onset and rapid recovery. Primary saturation of blood occurs within 3 to 5 minutes.

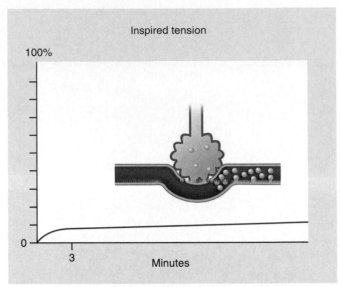

Figure 13.4 Primary saturation of a gaseous agent with a high blood–gas solubility coefficient (quite soluble) occurs quite slowly. Both onset and clinical recovery are prolonged. Methoxyflurane is an example of a very soluble agent.

Table 13.1	Blood–Gas Partition Coefficients of Inhalation Anesthetics
AGENT	**BLOOD–GAS SOLUBILITY COEFFICIENT**
Desflurane	0.42
Nitrous oxide	0.47
Sevoflurane	0.068
Isoflurane	1.40
Enflurane	1.91
Halothane	2.36
Chloroform	10.30
Diethyl ether	12.10
Methoxyflurane	13.00

quickly (see Fig. 13.3). Because of the rich cerebral blood supply, the tension of these gases within the brain also rises rapidly, and the onset of clinical actions is quickly apparent. Likewise, the rate of recovery from sedation or anesthesia produced by these gases is equally rapid once delivery of the anesthetic ceases.[2,3]

Conversely, gases with high blood solubility require longer periods of time for the onset of action to develop. Large volumes of the gas are absorbed by the blood (as by a piece of absorbent paper) so that the alveolar tension rises quite slowly (Fig. 13.4). Tension of the gas within the blood also rises slowly in this case, and the induction of sedation or anesthesia is noticeably slower, as is the return to the preanesthetic state after termination of drug administration.

N$_2$O is not flammable. However, it does support combustion of other agents, even in the absence of O$_2$, because at temperatures above 450°C, N$_2$O breaks down into N$_2$ and O$_2$.

Potency

N$_2$O is the least potent of the anesthetic gases; however, it remains the most frequently administered inhalation anesthetic. At one time, it was thought that any anesthetic effects of N$_2$O were a result of the exclusion of O$_2$ from cells in the brain because N$_2$O is 35 times more soluble in plasma than N$_2$ and 100 times more soluble than O$_2$.[4] It has since been demonstrated that N$_2$O can, in the presence of adequate O$_2$, produce CNS depression. Guedel classification stage II anesthesia (delirium) is often produced if the patient is not monitored properly.

With a MAC (the minimal alveolar concentration of an anesthetic that prevents movement in 50% of subjects in response to a standard surgical incision) of 105%, N$_2$O is unable to produce adequate anesthesia unless it is administered under hyperbaric conditions. More realistically, surgical-depth anesthesia is usually not obtainable unless a more potent inhalation or intravenous (IV) anesthetic is combined with N$_2$O. Such IV agents include propofol, opioids, and inhalation anesthetics include sevoflurane, isoflurane, and desflurane. These are discussed in Section VI.

That N$_2$O in subanesthetic doses produces analgesia, a change in the patient's perception of pain, is no longer doubted. It is estimated that a 50%:50% mixture of N$_2$O-O$_2$ produces the analgesic effectiveness of 10 to 15 mg of morphine.[5] However, biologic variability can significantly alter these figures in individual patients.

Pharmacology

After N$_2$O is inspired through the mouth and/or nose, the gas is transported through the respiratory tract into alveolar sacs, where it is rapidly absorbed into the pulmonary circulation. Because of the high inspired concentration of N_2O and the large gradient of N_2O between the alveolar sacs and the blood, up to 1000 mL of N_2O may be absorbed every minute. N_2O replaces N_2 in the blood; the N_2 is eliminated as the N_2O-O_2 mixture is inhaled. Because N_2O is 35 times as soluble in the blood as the N_2 it replaces, large volumes of N_2O may be absorbed over prolonged periods of administration.[4,6]

Potential changes may occur within air-filled body cavities during the administration of N_2O because of the extent of its absorption. During the induction of N_2O-O_2 sedation or anesthesia and during long procedures, N_2O enters a closed air-filled space 35 times more rapidly than N_2 leaves the cavity. This produces an increase in the pressure or volume of that cavity or space. Specific examples of this include increased intestinal distention if bowel obstruction is present, increased pressure in the pleural space aggravating a pneumothorax, and expansion of the middle ear airspace to the point of actually displacing a tympanoplasty graft.[7]

Because of its rapid uptake, two interesting phenomena—the so-called concentration effect and the second-gas effect—are seen when N_2O is administered. The *concentration effect* occurs when high concentrations of a gas are administered. The higher the concentration of the gas inhaled, the more rapidly the arterial tension of the gas increases. For example, a patient receiving N_2O-O_2 in a ratio of 75%:25% will absorb up to 1000 mL/min of N_2O during the initial stages of induction. As the volume of N_2O is removed from the lungs into the blood, fresh gas is literally sucked up into the lung from the anesthesia machine, thereby increasing the rate at which the N_2O arterial tension increases. If, however, a patient receives only 10% N_2O (a figure more appropriate in dentistry than 75%), the uptake of N_2O by the blood will be only 150 mL/min, which results in no significant change in the rate at which the agent is absorbed or the rate of rise of N_2O arterial tension.[8]

The *second-gas effect* occurs when a second inhalation anesthetic is administered along with N_2O-O_2. The second-gas effect is also related to the rapid uptake of as much as 1000 mL/min of N_2O-O_2 during the induction of anesthesia. Because of the extremely rapid uptake of a large volume of N_2O, a form of vacuum develops in the alveoli that forces even more fresh gas (N_2O-O_2 plus other inhalation anesthetics) into the lungs. For example, if halothane (1%) is administered along with N_2O-O_2 in a ratio of 75%:25%, its uptake will be more rapid than predicted. This is the second-gas effect.[9]

N_2O is absorbed rapidly from the alveolar sacs into the pulmonary circulation. Primary saturation of the blood and brain with N_2O is accomplished by the displacement of N_2 from the alveoli and the blood and occurs within 3 to 5 minutes of the onset of N_2O-O_2 administration.[6] Clinically, this is significant because the patient should be permitted to remain (ideally) at a given level of N_2O for 3 to 5 minutes before the inspired N_2O concentration is increased. This permits the full

clinical effect of the given concentration of N_2O to develop before additional gas is added. In actual clinical practice, the 3- to 5-minute wait is not necessary. A thorough discussion is presented in Chapter 15. Tissues with a greater blood flow, including the brain, heart, liver, and kidneys, will receive more N_2O and consequently absorb greater volumes of the gas. The remaining tissues, with a relatively poor blood supply, fat, muscle, and connective tissues, absorb only a small portion of N_2O until primary saturation is completed. At this time, these tissues play a major role in N_2O absorption. Because the uptake and absorption of N_2O by these tissues is slow (denitrogenation may require 6 to 7 hours), there is no reservoir of N_2O present in them to impede recovery when N_2O delivery is terminated.

For years it was believed that N_2O did not undergo biotransformation in the body. However, it is demonstrated that anaerobic bacteria in the bowel metabolize N_2O through a reductive pathway with the production of free radicals. There is no convincing evidence that these free radicals cause any specific organ damage.[10] Despite this, the vast majority of inhaled N_2O is exhaled through the lungs within 3 to 5 minutes after termination of its delivery. Approximately 1% of the inhaled N_2O will be eliminated more slowly (over 24 hours) through the lungs and skin.[6]

At the completion of the procedure, the N_2O flow is terminated. N_2O diffuses out of the blood and into the alveoli as rapidly as it diffused into the blood during induction. If the patient is allowed to breathe atmospheric air at this time, a phenomenon known as *diffusion hypoxia* (and the Fick principle) may develop.[11] Diffusion hypoxia is responsible for most reports of headache, nausea, and lethargy occurring after N_2O administration—a hangover effect. The alveoli of the patient breathing atmospheric air become filled with a mixture of N_2, O_2, CO_2, water vapor, and N_2O. During the first few minutes the patient breathes atmospheric air, large volumes of N_2O diffuse through the blood into the lungs and are exhaled. As much as 1500 mL of N_2O may be exhaled in the first minute by a patient having breathed N_2O-O_2 in a ratio of 75%:25%. This figure falls to 1200 mL in the second minute and 1000 mL in the third. The concentration effect, discussed previously, is now reversed, and gases rush out of the lungs. More CO_2 is removed from the blood than usual because of this effect, lowering the CO_2 tension of the blood. Decreased CO_2 tension of the blood reduces the stimulus for breathing and produces a depression of respiration.

More important, the rapid diffusion of large volumes of N_2O into the alveoli produces a significant dilution of the O_2 present. In the normal alveolus, approximately 14% O_2 is present. This may be reduced to as little as 10% during the first few minutes after termination of N_2O flow. Hypoxia results, producing headache, nausea, and lethargy.

The adverse effects of diffusion hypoxia may be prevented through the routine administration of 100% O_2 for a minimum of 3 to 5 minutes at the termination of the procedure.[12] After

N_2O-O_2 inhalation sedation as usually employed in dentistry, diffusion hypoxia is unlikely to develop, and when it does, it is usually clinically insignificant.

Recovery from the effects of N_2O is usually rapid and complete. If, in the opinion of the drug administrator, the patient has fully recovered, the patient may be permitted to leave the office unescorted, to drive his or her motor vehicle, and to return to normal activities with no prohibitions. This vitally important aspect of N_2O-O_2 sedation is discussed thoroughly in Chapter 15.

N_2O is nonallergenic. There has never been a reported allergic reaction to N_2O. It is less toxic than any other inhalation anesthetic.

Central Nervous System

The actual mechanism of action of N_2O is unknown, but almost all forms of sensation are depressed (sight, hearing, touch, and pain). Memory is affected to a minimal degree, as is the ability to concentrate or perform acts requiring intelligence.[13] When administered in conjunction with physiologic levels of O_2 (greater than 20%), N_2O produces a mild depression of the CNS, primarily the cerebral cortex. At therapeutic levels, N_2O does not exert any other actions on the CNS. The area postrema (the vomiting center) of the medulla is not affected by N_2O unless hypoxia or anoxia is present. Nausea and vomiting occurring after the administration of N_2O are uncommon in the absence of anoxia or hypoxia.[14]

Cardiovascular System

A slight depression of myocardial contraction is produced at a ratio of 80% N_2O:20% O_2 through a direct action of the drug on the heart.[15] The response of vascular smooth muscle to norepinephrine is slightly increased at this level. At levels below this ratio, there is no clinically significant effect on the cardiovascular system.

No changes in the heart rate or cardiac output are directly attributable to N_2O. In the absence of hypoxia or hypercarbia, blood pressure remains stable with an insignificant drop as sedation continues.[16] Cutaneous vasodilation is observed, which produces a degree of flushing and perspiration.[17] The vasodilation can be used to clinical advantage to facilitate venipuncture in patients who are apprehensive or in whom superficial veins are difficult to locate.

Respiratory System

N_2O is not irritating to the pulmonary epithelium; it may therefore be administered to patients with asthma with no increased risk of bronchospasm.[18] Changes in respiratory rate or depth are more likely to result from the sedative relief of anxiety (slower, deeper) or the approach of the excitement stage (Guedel anesthesia stage 2) (rapid, shallow) rather than through a direct action of N_2O on the respiratory system. The resting respiratory minute volume is slightly elevated at a ratio of N_2O-O_2 of 50%:50% with no effect on the respiratory response to CO_2.[19]

Gastrointestinal Tract

N_2O has no clinically significant actions on the gastrointestinal tract or any organs. In the presence of hepatic dysfunction, N_2O may still be used to effect with no increased risk of overdose or adverse reaction.[20]

Kidneys

N_2O exerts no significant effects on the kidneys or on the volume and composition of urine.[3]

Hematopoiesis

Nitrous oxide inactivates methionine synthase by oxidizing the cobalt in vitamin B_{12}. Methionine synthase is a ubiquitous cytosolic enzyme that plays a crucial role in the synthesis of DNA, RNA, myelin, catecholamines, and other products. Decreased methionine synthase activity can result in both genetic and protein aberrations. Liver biopsies have demonstrated a 50% reduction in methionine synthase activity at 45 to 90 min in patients administered 70% N_2O.[21] This can affect DNA synthesis, producing a picture similar to pernicious anemia in laboratory animals exposed to N_2O for prolonged periods. Long-term exposure to N_2O (as in the management of tetanus) can produce transient bone marrow depression. All reported cases have involved exposure to N_2O for more than 24 hours.[22,23]

The effects of repeated short-term exposure to N_2O are of greater concern. A neuropathy resembling vitamin B12 deficiency has been reported in dentists using N_2O regularly in their practices and in persons abusing the drug.[24] It is thought that this is a result of the combination of N_2O's actions on methionine synthetase and of the long-term exposure to unusually high N_2O concentrations as the dental team operates in the oral cavity.[6] In addition, there is a consistent finding in retrospective epidemiologic studies that the incidence of spontaneous abortion is increased among women working in operating rooms.[25] To date, no cause-and-effect relationship has been proven. Wynn has indicated that fertility is decreased in women exposed to N_2O for long periods.[26] The important subject of the safety of N_2O use in a dental office to the dental staff is discussed in depth in Chapter 17.

Skeletal Muscle

N_2O does not produce relaxation of skeletal muscles. Any observed effect of this nature during inhalation sedation is attributable to the relief of anxiety rather than to a direct action of N_2O.

Uterus and Pregnancy

N_2O-O_2 are commonly used as an aid in the management of discomfort during labor and delivery.[27] Uterine contractions are not inhibited in either amplitude or frequency.[28] N_2O passes easily across the placenta into the fetus, where the O_2 concentration of fetal blood may fall dramatically if less than 20% O_2 is delivered with the N_2O.[29] Pregnancy does not pose a contraindication to the use of N_2O-O_2 inhalation sedation (see

Chapters 4 and 12 for a more complete discussion of the use of sedation during pregnancy).

Physiologic Contraindications

"There are no contraindications to the use of nitrous oxide in combination with an adequate percentage of oxygen."[30]

"If administered with a minimum of 25% oxygen, it is a safe agent."[31]

"Nitrous oxide is a very safe anesthetic if oxygen is supplied in sufficient concentration."[32]

In the past few years, it has become apparent that N_2O is not an innocuous vapor, as it was once considered. Chronic exposure of dental personnel to low levels of N_2O has been associated (though not definitively proved) with increased risk of spontaneous abortion, fetal malformation, and other types of disease.[33–35] On the other hand, chronic exposure of dental personnel (or others) to high levels of N_2O has been demonstrated beyond a doubt to be capable of producing a sensory neuropathy that is extremely debilitating to the professional.[36,37] The occurrence of N_2O neuropathy is usually limited to persons who have purposefully abused the drug. These two very important subjects are discussed in depth in Chapter 17.

OXYGEN

O_2 is the second component of the inhalation sedation technique. First prepared in 1727 by Stephen Hales (who did not recognize it as an element), it was discovered as an element in 1771 by Joseph Priestley (the same man who discovered N_2O 5 years later) and almost simultaneously by Karl Scheele (1771).[3]

Preparation

O_2 is most commonly prepared by the fractional distillation of liquid air. N_2 is the first gas to boil off, with O_2 remaining as a liquid. This method of preparation was first employed in 1895 by Linde. Other methods of preparation of O_2 include the following:
1. Heating of barium peroxide (BaO_2) to 800° C, at which point it forms $BaO + O_2$
2. The electrolysis of water: $2 H_2O = 2 H_2 + O_2$
3. The reaction between sodium peroxide and water: $2 Na_2O_2 + 2 H_2O = 4 NaOH + O_2$

Properties

O_2 is a clear, colorless, odorless gas with a molecular weight of 32. It comprises 20.93% of atmospheric air. Its specific gravity is 1.105, whereas that of air is 1. It is stored in compressed gas cylinders in a gaseous state. A full cylinder has 2000 lb of pressure per square inch (psi) at room temperature. Its solubility in water is 2.4 volumes percent at 37° C and 4.9 volumes percent at 0° C. The cylinder of O_2 is green in the United States and white internationally, as per World Health Organization standards.[3]

O_2 is not flammable (cannot be ignited), but does support combustion. Under high pressure in the presence of oil or grease, O_2 may cause an explosion.[38,39] Therefore the use of oil and grease should be strictly avoided in and around O_2 cylinders, reducing valves, wall outlets, and cylinder outlets.[38,39]

Effects of 100% Oxygen
Central Nervous System
The inhalation of 100% O_2 has no effect on the cerebral cortex. Electroencephalographic (EEG) tracings are unchanged.[3,40–42] Cerebral blood flow may be decreased by as much as 10% as a result of constriction of the cerebral blood vessels occurring with 100% O_2 inhalation.[3,40–42]

Cardiovascular System
The inhalation of 100% O_2 is associated with a slight fall in both the heart rate (3 to 4 beats/min) and cardiac output (10% to 20%).[43] Coronary artery blood flow may be decreased up to 10% at this time. There is a slight increase in diastolic, but no change in the systolic, blood pressure with inhalation of 100% O_2.[44] This is a result of increased peripheral resistance secondary to a generalized vasoconstriction that occurs in the systemic, cerebral, renal, and retinal vessels on inhalation of 100% O_2.[45]

The inhalation of more than 40% O_2 in premature infants may produce retrolental fibroplasia many months later.[46]

Respiratory System
After 2 minutes of inhaling 100% O_2, minute volume is slightly depressed (3%). This occurs because ambient air (20.93% O_2) produces a continuous tonic stimulation of respiration through the chemoreceptors that are located in the carotid and aortic bodies. Inhalation of 100% O_2 abolishes this reflex stimulation, resulting in a decrease in minute volume. After 6 to 8 minutes of 100% O_2, minute volume exchange actually increases by 7.6%. This increase is produced through stimulation of the lower respiratory passages by O_2, which acts as an irritant, or by dilation of the pulmonary capillaries by O_2 with the production of reflex respiratory stimulation from mild pulmonary congestion.

Anatomy
RESPIRATORY SYSTEM

The anatomy of the respiratory system is reviewed here so that those involved in the use of inhalation sedation will possess a better knowledge of the processes involved in producing the observed state of relaxation.

The respiratory system is composed of a number of parts. These may be divided into two groups: (1) those parts of the respiratory system involved in the transport of gases to and from the outside of the body to and from the respiratory zone of the lungs and (2) those parts involved with the exchange of gases between the blood and the air, variously called the *exchange portion of the lung* and the *respiratory zone*. The portion of the respiratory system involved in conduction of gases is termed *anatomic dead space* because there is no exchange of O_2 and CO_2 between the air and the blood.

Structures included in the conducting portion of the respiratory system are as follows (Fig. 13.5):

Nose
Pharynx
- Nasopharynx
- Oropharynx
- Hypopharynx

Larynx
Trachea
Bronchi
Bronchioles

The mouth is considered to be an accessory respiratory passage. Structures included in the respiratory zone are as follows:

Respiratory bronchioles
Alveolar ducts
Alveolar sacs
Alveoli

Nose

The nose, or nasal cavity, is anatomically the most superior part of the respiratory system. It starts as two flexible, flared, rubbery entryways termed *wings* or *alae,* enclosing a space on either side called the *vestibule*. The nasal cavities continue posteriorly as paired airspaces. The right and left sides are separated by the bony nasal septum. At its posterior aspect above and behind the soft palate, the septum ends and the right and left nasal cavities unite to form the uppermost portion of the pharynx, the nasopharynx.

The nose has several functions in respiration.[47,48] Its primary function is to warm and humidify air. The process of warming air is readily accomplished by the mucous membranes of the nose, which are well endowed with an excellent blood supply. This large blood flow through the mucous membranes of the nose is responsible for warming of the air, a process that continues throughout the respiratory tract.

The nose also serves as (1) a defense against organisms and foreign materials, a function carried out by cilia found throughout the nose and by the mucous film found throughout the respiratory tract—submucosal glands and goblet cells are responsible for the formation of this mucinous lining; (2) a conduit for air to travel to and from the external environment to the lungs; (3) vocal resonance, a function of both the nose and sinuses (empty airspaces found within the skull, emptying into the nasal cavity); and (4) an organ involved in the sense of smell.

In inhalation sedation as practiced in dentistry, the nose is, of necessity, the prime route of entry of the anesthetic gases into the patient. Situations in which the patient becomes unable to breathe through their nose, such as a deviated septum and chronic or acute sinusitis, will complicate or contraindicate the inhalation sedation procedure.

Mouth

The mouth is considered an accessory respiratory passage. Most people will breathe through the mouth at times, especially during speech and whenever their nasal passages are occluded, such as in respiratory infections. As with the nose, the mouth, because of its mucosal surface and its rich blood supply, serves to warm and humidify the air as it enters the body. The mouth ends at the posterior palatine pillars. These pillars extend superiorly to meet the uvula, a fleshy tab of soft tissue located in the midline at the posterior border of the soft palate.

The base of the tongue rises out of the hypopharynx to occupy the floor of the mouth. Using the other passive structures of the oral cavity for support, the tongue and the oropharyngeal reflexes actively protect against threats to the airway.[49]

Because the mouth is the region in which dentistry is performed, this area is not involved in the routine administration of N_2O and O_2; however, the mouth is available for the administration of gases, especially O_2, during emergencies. In such cases, both the mouth and nose may be used for the purposes of ventilation.

Pharynx

The pharynx extends from the posterior portion of the nose to the level of the lower border of the cricoid cartilage, where it becomes continuous with the esophagus and the respiratory tract through the larynx.[48] The word *pharynx* is derived from the Greek word for "throat." For anatomic purposes, the pharynx is divided into three regions: the nasopharynx, oropharynx, and hypopharynx. The nasopharynx extends from the back of the nasal cavity to the level of the soft palate. The eustachian tubes open into the nasopharynx and connect with the middle ear. The oropharynx starts superiorly at the level of the soft palate to the level of the cricoid cartilage and the base of the tongue inferiorly. The hypopharynx, also known as the *laryngopharynx*, starts superiorly at the epiglottis to the division of the esophagus and larynx. It is the shortest of the three divisions. The major functions of the pharynx are the conduction, warming, and humidification of air and the removal of foreign materials. The junction of the pharynx and the esophagus represents the narrowest part of the alimentary canal. Foreign bodies trapped at this level may produce aspiration or significant decreases in airflow.[50,51]

Epiglottis

Although not an integral part of the respiratory system, the epiglottis, a platelike structure extending from the base of the tongue backward and upward, must be mentioned. It functions as a flaplike covering over the larynx that closes during swallowing, covering the airway so that swallowed materials enter the esophagus, not the trachea.[47]

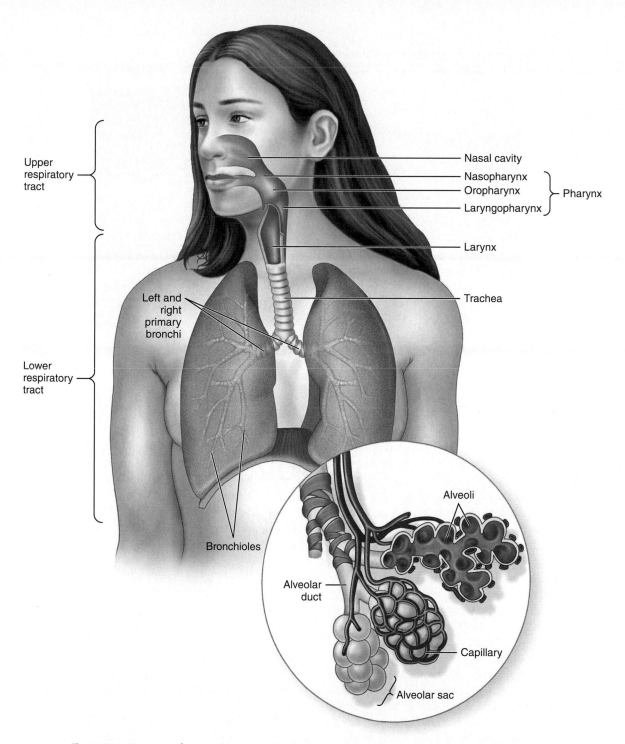

Figure 13.5 Structures forming the conducting portion of the respiratory system. The inset shows the alveolar sacs where the interchange of O_2 and CO_2 takes place through the walls of the grapelike alveoli. Capillaries surround the alveoli.

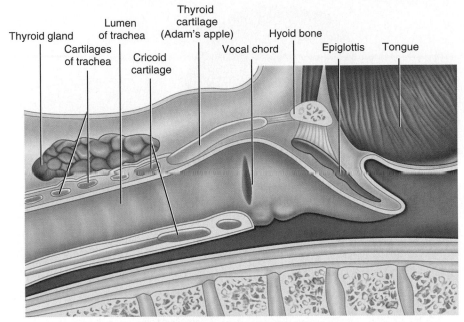

Figure 13.6 Sagittal section of the larynx.

Larynx

The adult larynx is found at the level of the first through the fifth cervical vertebrae, consisting of a number of articulated cartilages surrounding the upper end of the trachea (Fig. 13.6).[52] "Adam's apple" is another common name for the larynx (more accurately, Adam's apple denotes the thyroid cartilage). The laryngeal cavity extends from just below the epiglottis to the lower level of the cricoid cartilage, where it becomes continuous with the trachea.

The primary function of the larynx is phonation, but it also has a protective function because the airway becomes quite narrow at this point. Structures found within the laryngeal cavity include the vestibular folds (i.e., the false vocal cords) and the vocal cords (i.e., the true vocal cords), which are two pearly white folds of mucous membrane.

The narrowest portion of the larynx in the adult is located at the true vocal cords.[47] Larger aspirated objects will become lodged at this site. They can usually be dislodged by the abdominal thrust or chest thrust. In the child younger than 10 years, the narrowest portion of the larynx occurs at the level of cricoid cartilage.[47,48] Should material be small enough to pass between the vocal cords, in the adult and in larger children, it will usually enter either the right or left main stem bronchus, a situation that is serious but not acutely life threatening.

Trachea

The trachea is a tubular structure that begins at the cricoid cartilage. The tube of the trachea is formed with approximately 16 to 22 C-shaped cartilaginous rings that are incomplete on their posterior surface. A thin muscle band extends between the incomplete posterior ends of the U-shaped cartilages. The trachea extends through the neck into the mediastinum to a point behind the junction of the upper and middle thirds of the sternum, where it divides into the right and left main stem bronchi. The *carina* is the name given to the cartilage located at the point of bifurcation. The carina is located approximately 5 cm below the suprasternal notch.[47] The trachea is about 10 to 13 cm long and has an outer diameter of 2.5 cm and an inner diameter of 1.0 to 1.5 cm. This dimension is enlarged in elderly persons and decreased during pregnancy because of edema.

Bronchi

At the level of the carina, the right and left main stem bronchi branch off from the trachea. Because of the position of the heart in the left side of the mediastinum, the angle formed by the left main stem bronchus (45 to 55 degrees) is somewhat greater than that formed by the right main stem bronchus (20 to 30 degrees). This is of importance, as aspirated objects will have a greater tendency to enter into the right lung than the left.[47,48]

Each of the main stem bronchi divides into branches that supply each of the lobes of the lung. The right main stem bronchus is wider and shorter than the left, giving branches to the upper and middle lobes and then continuing to become the branch to the right lower lobe. The right upper lobe bronchus has its origin about 2 cm from the carina, whereas the left arises about 5 cm from the carina.[48] Each of these bronchi in turn gives off branches.[53] The right upper lobe bronchus gives rise to three main divisions, the right middle lobe bronchus to two divisions, and the right lower lobe bronchus to five or six divisions. The left main stem bronchus is somewhat longer and narrower than the right. It ends at the origin of the left upper lobe bronchus and continues to become the main bronchus to the left lower lobe. The left upper lobe main bronchus originates at the bifurcation of the left main stem bronchus and gives off three branches. The left lower lobe main bronchus, the direct continuation of the left main stem bronchus, gives rise to four branches.[53,54]

Bronchioles

The bronchi continue to bifurcate and trifurcate well into the periphery of each lung. As these divisions occur, the number of bronchi increases significantly, as does the total surface area of the lung. As the bronchi continue to divide, they become smaller, and their cartilaginous rings gradually recede, becoming irregular plates. Cartilage is found in bronchioles until their diameter is approximately 0.66 to 1 mm, at which point cartilage disappears entirely.[55]

The first 17 divisions of the tracheobronchial tree make up the **conducting zone** because the exchange of O_2 and CO_2—the primary function of the lungs—cannot occur here. This is also termed *dead space*. Approximately 150 mL of air is found in the conducting zone in the average-sized adult.[56] From divisions 17 to 23, changes occur in the walls and linings of the airway that dramatically increase their surface area. These airways comprise what is called the **respiratory zone** and include respiratory bronchioles, alveolar ducts, alveolar sacs, and alveoli (see Fig. 13.7). The alveolus represents the final airspace and is the unit in which the exchange of gases occurs.

Alveolus

The alveolus is essentially a pocket of air surrounded by a thin membrane containing capillaries (Fig. 13.7). The distance between the air within the alveolus and the capillary is approximately 0.35 to 2.5 mm. This thin wall is essential for the rapid exchange of gases between air and blood. Gases within the alveoli are separated from blood by four thin layers:
1. Mucinous covering
2. Alveolar epithelium (incomplete)
3. Interstitial layer
4. Endothelial cells lining pulmonary capillaries

Blood remains within the pulmonary capillaries for approximately 0.5 seconds, yet gas exchange is so swift that it is completed by the time the blood has completed only one fourth of its journey through the capillary.

Physiology
RESPIRATION

Gases are inhaled through the nose and/or mouth and are transported to the respiratory zone of the lungs, the more than 300 million alveoli in which the interchange of gases between the alveolus and the pulmonary capillaries occurs. The exchange of gases in the alveoli depends entirely on diffusion of gases across membranes and is controlled by the partial pressure of the respective gases on either side of the alveolar membrane.

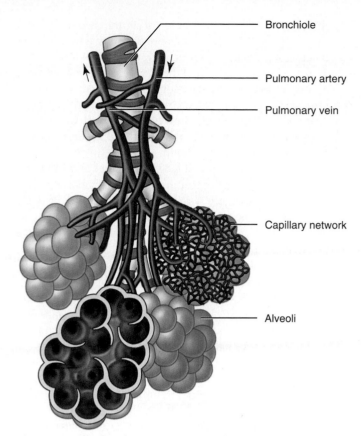

Figure 13.7 Alveoli and surrounding vasculature. The capillary bed in this area is the densest vascular network in the entire body.

Pulmonary capillaries are unique in that they form the densest capillary network in the entire body. It is estimated that pulmonary capillaries are approximately 10 mm long and 7 mm wide. So finely interlaced are they that they may be considered more of a pool of blood vessels than a series of pipes. In adults, the surface area of the pulmonary capillary–alveolar interface is about 70 m^2, or approximately 40 times the surface area of the body.[57] At any given moment, there is approximately 100 to 300 mL of blood within these pulmonary capillaries. George et al have compared this with the spreading of a teaspoon of blood over 1 m^2 of surface area.[55]

The gases within the alveoli are separated from the capillaries by approximately 1 to 2 mm of tissue: the mucinous covering of the alveolus; the alveolar epithelium, which in some places is incomplete; an interstitial layer; and the endothelium covering the pulmonary capillary.

Mechanics of Respiration

How do gases get into the alveolus from outside the body? Air moves from the external environment to the level of the alveolar capillary membrane because of differences of pressure within the respiratory system. Gases move from a zone of higher pressure to one of lower pressure.

The typical respiratory cycle can be divided into five phases: preinspiration, peak inspiration, end inspiration, peak expiration, and end expiration.

At preinspiration, the pressure within the pleural cavity is negative: -5 cm H_2O, the pressure of the normal resting lung. This negative pressure is produced by the natural tendency of the lung to recoil inward and of the chest wall to recoil outward.

As inspiration begins, the muscles of inspiration contract and the chest cavity (thorax) expands, increasing the negative pressure within the thorax to even more than it was at rest. This results in an expansion of the alveoli and the development of negative pressure within them.

With the development of negative pressure within the alveoli—a pressure negative to atmospheric pressure—air begins to flow into the respiratory system through the nose and mouth. As air enters the system, a tidal volume develops, resulting in the end of inspiration. Pleural pressure reaches its most negative point, alveolar pressure returns to zero as gases enter the alveoli, airflow into the lung ceases, and the maximum inspiratory volume is reached. Expiration now begins.

Pleural pressure begins to return to its original value (-5 cm H_2O), resulting in the creation of positive pressure within the alveoli during expiration and maximal expiratory flow out of the respiratory system. At the end of expiration, pleural pressure has returned to baseline, alveolar pressure has returned to zero, flow has ceased, and the expiratory volume has been delivered, returning the lung to its resting capacity. Under normal respiratory conditions (quiet breathing), most of the pressure that is generated occurs as a result of the elastic characteristics of the lungs.

Muscles are involved in the process of breathing, helping produce the increases in negative pressures that draw air into the respiratory system. These muscles are as follows:

1. Diaphragm (primary)
2. Intercostals (primary)
3. Abdominals (accessory)
4. Scalenes (accessory)
5. Sternocleidomastoid (accessory)
6. Some back muscles (accessory)

The diaphragm is the primary muscle involved in quiet breathing. In normal breathing, a 1-cm downward movement of the diaphragm causes 350 mL of air to enter the lung. The normal 500-mL tidal volume will therefore require approximately a 1.5-cm downward movement of the diaphragm. In quiet breathing, the diaphragm is probably the only muscle of respiration working. Intercostal muscles do not participate in quiet breathing. Abdominal muscles do not participate in quiet breathing or in ventilation up to about 40 L/min (lpm). The abdominal muscles take a more active part as the volume of air inspired increases, and above 90 lpm (as seen in strenuous exercise), the abdominals are actively contributing by forceful contraction. The scalenes do contract during quiet breathing; however, their contribution to the total volume of air inspired is not great. The sternocleidomastoids do not participate in quiet respiration; however, their actions do become more forceful as ventilation increases. All of the muscles that participate in respiration are attached to the thoracic cage.

Table 13.2	Composition of the Major Gases Found in the Respiratory System (Percentages)		
GAS	INSPIRED AIR	ALVEOLAR AIR	EXPIRED AIR
O_2	20.94	14.2	16.3
CO_2	0.04	5.5	4.0
N_2	79.02	80.3	79.7

Table 13.3	Partial Pressures of Gases			
GAS (MM HG)	AIR (MM HG)	ALVEOLUS (MM HG)	ARTERIAL BLOOD (MM HG)	VENOUS BLOOD (MM HG)
O_2	158.2	103	100	40
CO_2	0.3	40	40	46
N_2	596.5	570	573	573
H_2O vapor	5.0	47	47	47

Composition of Respiratory Gases

The composition of the major gases found in the respiratory system is shown in Table 13.2. Water vapor constitutes less than 1% of atmospheric air, whereas alveolar air, fully saturated with water vapor, contains 6.2%. The pressure exerted by the water vapor is 47 mm Hg and must be taken into account in determining the partial pressures of the gases within the alveoli.

Barometric pressure − water vapor pressure = alveolar partial pressure

$$760 \, mm \, Hg - 47 \, mm \, Hg = 713 \, mm \, Hg$$

The partial pressure of gases within the alveolus is determined as follows:

$$Alveolar \; O_2 \; tension = 713 \times 14.2/100 = 103 \, mm \, Hg$$

$$Alveolar \; CO_2 \; tension = 713 \times 5.5/100 = 40 \, mm \, Hg$$

$$Alveolar \; N_2 \; tension = 713 \times 80.3/100 = 570 \, mm \, Hg$$

$$Water \; vapor = 47 \, mm \, Hg$$

$$Total \; pressures = 760 \, mm \, Hg$$

The speed at which gases diffuse across membranes is controlled by several factors, the most important of which is their partial pressure in each compartment (Table 13.3). For example, the partial pressure of O_2 within the alveolus is 103 mm Hg, whereas in the pulmonary capillary its tension is only 40 mm Hg. O_2 is therefore forced into the capillary from the alveolus.

When arterial blood arrives at the tissues in the body, it still has an O_2 tension of 100 mm Hg, whereas the O_2 tension within the tissues is only 40 mm Hg. The O_2 therefore travels from the plasma into the tissues because of this pressure gradient. The O_2 tension within the plasma falls. In a resting state, the tissues remove approximately 30% of the available O_2. Venous blood leaving the tissues still contains quite a bit of O_2; however, during violent exercise, the tissues may remove almost all of the available O_2. On returning to the lungs, venous blood quickly surrenders its CO_2 (partial pressure 46 mm Hg) to the alveolus (partial pressure 40 mm Hg), and O_2 diffuses from the alveolus into the capillary blood (capillary PO_2 40 mm Hg; alveolar PO_2 103 mm Hg).

Disease states may alter the rate at which the exchange of gases occurs within the lungs. For example, in emphysema the total surface area of the alveolar membranes is decreased; in pneumonia the alveolar walls become thickened, thereby inhibiting diffusion; and in asthma the increase in bronchial secretions also acts to impede the exchange of gases. In methemoglobinemia the O_2-carrying capacity of the blood is decreased.

When inhaled into the lungs, N_2O will act in the same manner as the gases described previously. When N_2O is first inhaled, its partial pressure within the alveolus will be quite high, whereas that within the capillary will be zero. N_2O flow will occur rapidly from the alveolus to the capillary, and the same response will develop within tissues. As the blood becomes saturated with N_2O (3 to 5 minutes), the rate of diffusion into the cardiovascular system decreases. At the termination of the procedure, the patient is administered 100% O_2, and N_2O is eliminated. The alveolus now contains little or no N_2O, whereas venous blood returning to the lung is rich in N_2O, so N_2O now diffuses out of the blood into the alveolus and out of the body through the respiratory tract.[58]

REFERENCES

1. The National Formulary: *The US pharmacopeia*, Rockville, 2015, US Pharmacopeial Convention. www.usp.org. (Accessed November 6, 2015).
2. Wood M, Wood AJ: *Drugs and anesthesia: pharmacology for anesthesiologists*, Baltimore, 1982, Williams & Wilkins.
3. Patel PM, Patel HH, Roth DM: General anesthetics and therapeutic gases. In Brunton L, Chabner B, Knollman B, editors: *Goodman & Gilman's pharmacological basis of therapeutics*, ed 12, New York, 2001, McGraw Hill, pp 527–565.
4. Farber NE, Stuth Ekehard AE, Stucke AG, Pagel PS: Inhaled anesthetics: pulmonary pharmacology. In Miller R, Erikkson LI, Fleisher L, et al, editors: *Miller's anesthesia*, ed 8, Philadelphia, 2015, Saunders Elsevier, pp 670–705.
5. Gillman MA: Analgesic (sub anesthetic) nitrous oxide interacts with the endogenous opioid system: a review of the evidence. *Life Sci* 39(14):1209–1221, 1986.
6. Longnecker DE, Miller FL: Pharmacology of inhalational anesthetics. In Longnecker DE, Tinker JH, Morgan G, Jr, editors: *Principles and practice of anesthesiology*, ed 2, St Louis, 1998, Mosby.
7. Taylor E, Feinstein R, White PF, Soper N: Anesthesia for laparoscopic cholecystectomy: is nitrous oxide contraindicated? *Anesthesiology* 76(4):541–543, 1992.
8. Severinghaus JW: The rate of uptake of nitrous oxide in man. *J Clin Invest* 33(9):1183–1189, 1954.
9. Epstein RM, Rackow H, Salanitre E, Wolf GL: Influence of the concentration effect on the uptake of anesthetic mixtures. *Anesthesiology* 25:364–371, 1964.
10. Eger EI, II: *Nitrous oxide*, New York, 1985, Elsevier.
11. Jeske AH, Whitmire CW, Freels C, Fuentes M: Noninvasive assessment of diffusion following administration of nitrous oxide-oxygen. *Anesth Prog* 51(1):10–13, 2004.
12. Quarnstrom FC, Milgrom P, Bishop MJ, DeRouen TA: Clinical study of diffusion hypoxia after nitrous oxide analgesia. *Anesth Prog* 38(1):21–23, 1991.
13. Ramsey DS, Leonesio RJ, Whitney CW, et al: Paradoxical effects of nitrous oxide on human memory. *Psychopharmacology (Berl)* 106(3):370–374, 1992.
14. Smiley BA, Paradise NF: Does the duration of N_2O administration affect postoperative nausea and vomiting? *Nurse Anesth* 2(1):13–18, 1991.
15. Stowe DF, Monroe SM, Marijic J, et al: Effects of nitrous oxide on contractile function and metabolism of the isolated heart. *Anesthesiology* 73(6):1220–1226, 1990.
16. Hornbein TF, Martin WE, Bonica JJ, et al: Nitrous oxide effects on the circulatory and ventilatory responses to halothane. *Anesthesiology* 31(3):250–260, 1969.
17. Moore PA: Nitrous oxide: oxygen sedation: induction and recovery. *Curr Rev Nurse Anesth* 4:35, 1981.
18. Pasternak LR: Outpatient anesthesia. In Rogers MC, Tinker JH, Covino BG, et al, editors: *Principles and practice of anesthesiology*, St Louis, 1993, Mosby.
19. Yacoub O, Doell D, Kryger MH, Anthonisen NR: Depression of hypoxic ventilatory response by nitrous oxide. *Anesthesiology* 45(4):385–389, 1976.
20. Ross JA, Monk SJ, Duffy SW: Effect of nitrous oxide on halothane-induced hepatotoxicity in hypoxic, enzyme-induced rats. *Br J Anaesth* 56(5):527–533, 1984.
21. Caswell RD: Nitrous oxide. In Murray MJ, Harrison BA, Mueller JT, et al, editors: *Faust's anesthesiology review*, ed 4, Philadelphia, 2015, Saunders Elsevier, pp 150–152.
22. Henry RJ: Assessing environmental health concerns associated with nitrous oxide. *J Am Dent Assoc* 123(12):41–47, 1992.
23. Franco G: Occupational exposure to anaesthetics: liver injury, microsomal enzyme induction and preventive aspects. *Ital Med Lavoro* 11(5):205–208, 1989.
24. Layzer RB: Myeloneuropathy after prolonged exposure to nitrous oxide. *Lancet* 2(8102):1227–1230, 1978.
25. Eger EI, II: Fetal injury and abortion associated with occupational exposure to inhaled anesthetics. *AANA J* 59(4):309–312, 1991.
26. Wynn RL: Nitrous oxide and fertility, part I. *Gen Dent* 41(2):122–123, 1993.
27. Marx GF, Katsnelson T: The introduction of nitrous oxide analgesia into obstetrics. *Obstet Gynecol* 80(4):715–718, 1992.
28. Arai M, Nishijima M, Tatsuma H: Analgesia and anesthesia during labor in Japan and developed countries. *Asia Oceania J Obstet Gynaecol* 15(3):213–221, 1989.
29. Landon MJ, Toothill VJ: Effect of nitrous oxide on placental methionine synthase activity. *Br J Anaesth* 58(5):524–527, 1986.
30. Wylie WD, Churchill-Davidson HC: *A practice of anesthesia*, ed 4, Philadelphia, 1978, WB Saunders.
31. Lichtiger M, Moya F: *Introduction to the practice of anesthesia*, New York, 1974, Harper & Row.
32. Snow JC: *Manual of anesthesia*, Boston, 1977, Little, Brown.
33. Baden JM, Fujinaga M: Effects of nitrous oxide on day 9 rat embryos grown in culture. *Br J Anaesth* 66(4):500–503, 1991.

34. Schumann D: Nitrous oxide anaesthesia: risks to health personnel. *Int Nurs Rev* 37(1):214–217, 1990.

35. Littner MM, Kaffe I, Tamse A: Occupational hazards in the dental office and their control. IV. Measures for controlling contamination of anesthetic gas: nitrous oxide. *Quintess Intern* 14(4):461–464, 1983.

36. Stacy CB, DiRocco A, Gould RJ: Methionine in the treatment of nitrous oxide-induced neuropathy and myeloneuropathy. *J Neurol* 239(7):401–403, 1992.

37. Chanarin I: The effects of nitrous oxide on cobalamins, folates, and on related events. *Crit Rev Toxicol* 10(3):179–213, 1982.

38. Mishra D: Oxygen gas cylinder explosion. *J Indian Med Assoc* 93(3):114–115, 1995.

39. Sues B Clinton FD put out fire at dental office. WBRZ Television. September 1, 2014. http://www.wbrz.com/news/firefighters-put-out-fire-at-clinton-dental-office. Accessed 6 November 2015.

40. Robiolio M, Rumsey WL, Wilson OF: Oxygen diffusion and mitochondrial respiration in neuroblastic cells. *Am J Physiol* 256(6 Pt 1):C1207–C1213, 1989.

41. Bleiberg B, Kerem D: Central nervous system oxygen toxicity in the resting rat: postponement by intermittent oxygen exposure. *Undersea Biomed Res* 15(5):337–352, 1988.

42. Bryan RM, Jr: Cerebral blood flow and energy metabolism during stress. *Am J Physiol* 259(2 Pt 2):H269–H280, 1990.

43. Ward JP, McMurtry IF: Mechanisms of hypoxic pulmonary vasoconstriction and their roles in pulmonary hypertension: new findings for an old problem. *Curr Opin Pharmacol* 9(3):287–296, 2009.

44. Martindale W: *Extra pharmacopoeia*, ed 29, London, 1989, Pharmaceutical Press.

45. Rothe CF, Maass-Moreno R, Flanagan AD: Effects of hypercapnia and hypoxia on the cardiovascular system: vascular capacitance and aortic chemoreceptors. *Am J Physiol* 259(3 Pt 2):H932–H939, 1990.

46. Weiss NS: Oxygen and retrolental fibrodysplasia: did epidemiology help or hinder? *Epidemiology* 2(1):60, 1991.

47. Morris IR: Functional anatomy of the upper airway. *Emerg Med Clin North Am* 6(4):639–669, 1988.

48. Devereux G, Douglas G: The respiratory system. In Graham D, Nicol F, Robertson C, editors: *MacLeod's clinical examination*, ed 13, London, Churchill Livingstone Elsevier, 2013, pp 137–163.

49. Block C, Vrechner V: Unusual problems in airway management. II. The influence of the temporomandibular joint, the mandible, and associated structures on endotracheal intubation. *Anesth Analg* 50(1):115–123, 1971.

50. Daniilidis J, Symeonidis B, Triaridis K, Kouloulas A: Foreign body in the airways: a review of 90 cases. *Arch Otolaryngol* 103(10):570–573, 1977.

51. Kim IN, Brummitt WM, Humphry A, et al: Foreign body in the airway: a review of 202 cases. *Laryngoscope* 83(3):347–354, 1973.

52. Roberts JT: Functional anatomy of the larynx. *Int Anesthesiol Clin* 28(2):101–105, 1990.

53. Ellis H, Feldman S: *Anatomy for anesthetists*, ed 4, Oxford, 1983, Blackwell Scientific.

54. Clemente CD, editor: *Gray's anatomy of the human body*, ed 30, Philadelphia, 1984, Lea & Febiger.

55. George RB, Chesson AL, Rennard SI: Functional anatomy of the respiratory system. In George RB, Matthay MA, Light RW, et al, editors: *Chest medicine: essentials of pulmonary and critical care medicine*, Baltimore, 1995, Williams & Wilkins.

56. Stoelting RD: *Pharmacology and physiology in anesthetic practice*, ed 2, Philadelphia, 1991, JB Lippincott.

57. Light RW: Mechanics of respiration. In George RB, Matthay MA, Light RW, et al, editors: *Chest medicine: essentials of pulmonary and critical care medicine*, Baltimore, 1995, Williams & Wilkins.

58. Clark M, Brunick A: *Handbook of nitrous oxide and oxygen sedation*, ed 4, St Louis, 2015, Mosby.

chapter 14

Inhalation Sedation Equipment

CHAPTER OUTLINE

The equipment for the delivery of nitrous oxide-oxygen (N_2O-O_2) inhalation sedation is quite simple. Primary equipment consists of a supply of the gases and an apparatus for their delivery to the patient. The modern inhalation sedation unit is a compact, continuous-flow machine used for the administration of compressed gases under controlled conditions. This sedation unit is a modification of the machines used to administer inhalation general anesthesia. These machines (Fig. 14.1) are capable of delivering a number of inhalation anesthetic agents (Fig. 14.2), whereas the inhalation sedation unit has been altered to deliver only two gases: N_2O and O_2.

TYPES OF INHALATION SEDATION UNITS

There exist two basic types of inhalation sedation unit. Only one is recommended for use. These are the continuous-flow machine and the intermittent- or demand-flow unit. Although these devices are similar in design, there are some very significant differences in their operation. The demand-flow unit is no longer used in dentistry in North America; however, it is mentioned here for the sake of completeness. The reader should then be better able to understand the mechanism and reasons why the continuous-flow unit is more popular and recommended for use in dentistry.

Demand-Flow Units

The demand-flow type of N_2O-O_2 inhalation sedation unit does not deliver gas continuously to the patient, but varies the rate and volume of delivered gas according to the patient's respiratory demands and requirements. In this sense, the demand-flow type of inhalation sedation unit may be compared with the face mask employed by SCUBA (Self-Contained Underwater Breathing Apparatus) divers, which operates on the same principle. A major advantage of the demand-flow

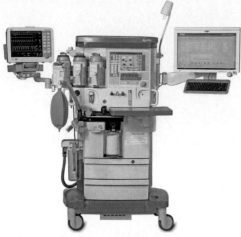

Figure 14.1 General anesthesia machines can deliver multiple anesthetic gases and contain multiple monitoring devices. Apollo Anesthesia Workstation with Omega widescreen solution and Innovian Anesthesia (anesthesia information management). (Courtesy Draeger Medical, Inc.)

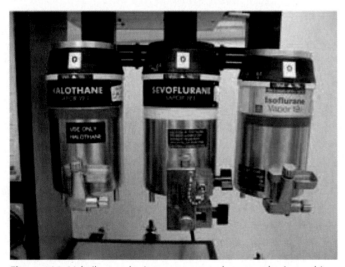

Figure 14.2 Volatile anesthetic gases mounted on anesthesia machine.

type of unit is the economy obtained from the decreased volume of compressed gases used.

In operation, the gases delivered are proportioned by the machine. Only one dial, which changes the percentages of gases delivered, need be adjusted. This dial provides a direct indication of the percentage of O_2 delivered in the mixture (the remainder of gas is N_2O). The mechanism involved in the demand-flow unit is much more complex than the flowmeter and in clinical practice has been subject to a greater percentage of error. Demand-flow units show only what was set, not what is actually delivered. If a discrepancy develops between the dial and the actual gas flow, there is no warning while the unit is in operation.[1]

Several disadvantages are associated with demand-flow units. One is that the volume flow of anesthetic gases per minute is

not visible or registered anywhere on the machine. In place of this, there is a dial on which the percentages of the gases delivered are recorded and another on which the pressure at which they are delivered is visible. The lack of ability to visually monitor the flow of gases to the patient is a major disadvantage of the demand-flow unit.

A second disadvantage of the demand-flow unit is the lack of accuracy of the mixer valve. The percentage of gas delivered is not accurate over the full range of delivery (0% to 100% N_2O). Gauert and Husted[2] and Allen[3] demonstrated the lack of accuracy of two demand-flow units: the McKesson Nargraf and Narmatic. At an indicated O_2 percentage of 75%, the actual delivered O_2 percentage ranged from 80% to 45%, whereas at 50% indicated O_2, the actual delivered percentage ranged from 75% to 22%. Having to rely on a mixer valve that is inaccurate in a machine in which the flow of the individual gases cannot be visualized provides two significant disadvantages to the use of demand-flow units.

The gas circuit followed by the N_2O and O_2 in the demand-flow machine is as follows:

1. Compressed-gas cylinders
2. Pressure-reducing valves
3. Mixing valve with percentage of N_2O or O_2
4. Pressure regulator (to vary flow of gases)
5. Demand valve
6. Conducting tubes
7. Nasal hood
8. Expiratory valve

Clinical examples of demand-flow inhalation sedation-anesthesia units include the following:

1. Jectaflow
2. Walton (primarily used in the United Kingdom)
3. McKesson Euthesor
4. McKesson Nargraf
5. McKesson Narmatic

Allen stated that fatalities have resulted from misunderstanding the use of the demand-flow machine.[3] In light of this and the distinct advantages of the continuous-flow machines (see discussion later), primarily their greater accuracy and that the flow of gases can be visualized, demand-flow inhalation sedation units are obsolete and their use falls below the current standard of care. A demand-flow unit known as Nitronox is used in the hospital and ambulatory setting. This demand-flow unit is unique in that the percentage is not adjustable (fixed at 50/50, O_2 and N_2O) and extremely accurate. In dentistry as practiced in North America, this type of unit would fall below the standard of care because it prevents the important practice of titration from occurring.

Continuous-Flow Units

In stark contrast to demand-flow units are the continuous-flow units. These units contain flowmeters and are characterized by the continuous flow of gases, regardless of the respiratory pattern of the patient. Gas continues to be delivered through the machine even as the patient exhales. Whereas continuous-flow machines use a greater volume of gas over a given period of time than the demand-flow unit, this minor disadvantage is more than compensated for by the significantly greater accuracy and safety of continuous-flow units. The two major disadvantages of the demand-flow unit are eliminated in continuous-flow machines. The inability to visualize the flow of gases and the inaccuracy of the mixer valve are eliminated through the incorporation of a flowmeter. Accuracies to within plus or minus 2% can be achieved in gas flow with the flowmeters available today.

The gas circuit used in the typical continuous-flow unit consists of the following:

1. Gas cylinders
2. Reducing valves
3. Flowmeters
4. Reservoir bag
5. Conducting tubing
6. Nasal hood

All inhalation sedation units contain the same basic components (Figs. 14.3 to 14.5):

1. Compressed-gas cylinders
2. Reducing valves (regulators)
3. Pressure gauges
4. Flowmeters

5. Reservoir bag
6. Conducting tubing
7. Full face mask, nasal hood, or nasal cannula

In addition to these, the central storage systems contain manifolds and wall outlets. Modern inhalation sedation equipment is also equipped with multiple safety features that are designed to prevent the inadvertent or accidental administration

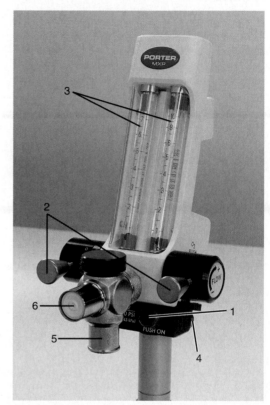

Figure 14.4 Continuous-flow sedation unit (portable, side view). *1,* master control (on-off); *2,* control knobs for N₂O and O₂; *3,* flowmeters; *4,* O₂ flush button; *5,* tee (attachment) for reservoir bag; *6,* one-way valve to patient. (Courtesy Porter Instrument, Parker Hannifin Corporation.)

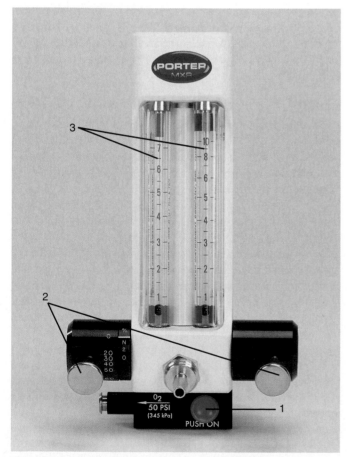

Figure 14.3 Continuous-flow sedation unit (portable, front view). *1,* master control (on-off); *2,* control knobs for N₂O and O₂; *3,* flowmeters. (Courtesy Porter Instrument, Parker Hannifin Corporation.)

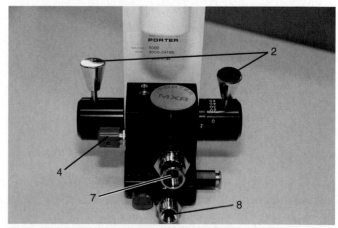

Figure 14.5 Continuous-flow inhalation sedation unit (portable, from behind). *2,* control knobs for N₂O and O₂; *4,* O₂ flush button; *7,* N₂O low-pressure tube connector; *8,* O₂ low-pressure tube connector.

of less than 20% O_2. These safety features are discussed in the following paragraphs.

Among the continuous-flow inhalation sedation units, there are three subgroups. Although each is the same basic unit, the differences among them are the manner in which compressed gases are delivered to the unit and their portability.

Portable System

In the portable system (Fig. 14.6), rolling stand compressed-gas cylinders are attached to the inhalation sedation unit at the yoke assembly. This system is used in offices where the frequency of N_2O-O_2 use is low or in situations in which the expense of a central storage system is prohibitive.

The primary drawback to long-term use of a portable system lies in its economics. Portable systems require use of smaller

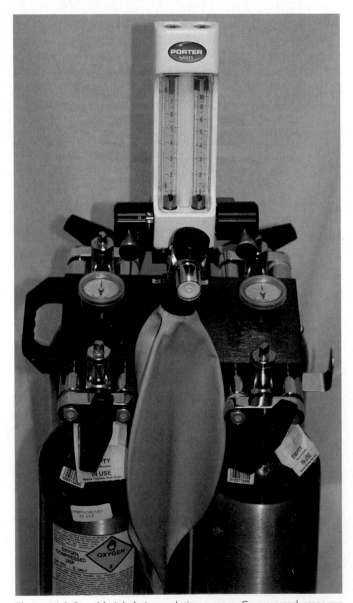

Figure 14.6 Portable inhalation sedation system. Compressed gases are attached to the unit at the yoke assembly.

compressed-gas cylinders ("E"), which consequently require replacement more frequently than the larger "G" and "H" cylinders used in central systems. The lower cost of larger, nonportable cylinders more than justifies their use, especially where N_2O-O_2 is used more frequently.

Central Storage System

In the central storage system, the supply of N_2O and O_2 is located at a distance from the area in which the gases are delivered to patients. In the treatment area, the inhalation sedation unit (also called the *head*) will be present along with the accessory equipment required for the delivery of the gases. The head is usually mounted on a wall or bracket. Heads are available in numerous versions from entry-level, pneumatic-type systems to modern digital gas delivery systems. Gas cylinders are maintained in a storage area, and gases are delivered to the treatment area through copper pipes. Because these cylinders are stored in a separate location at a distance from the treatment area, larger cylinders are used in the central storage systems. These cylinders are not portable, but they contain significantly more compressed gas than do the smaller cylinders used on portable systems. Multiple treatment areas may be connected through copper piping to this storage area and operated from this bank of cylinders.

The central system is most advantageous in offices that use inhalation sedation on a more regular basis. The greater initial cost of a central storage system is quickly made up in savings obtained from the use of the larger gas cylinders.

Central Storage System With Mobile Heads

Representing a compromise between the portable and central storage systems, the central storage system with mobile heads permits the use of larger compressed-gas cylinders, whereas the inhalation sedation unit sits on a portable stand (without the yoke apparatus), which may be moved from treatment area to treatment area as the need for inhalation sedation arises. Quick-connect tubing attaches the unit to the O_2 and N_2O outlets on the wall in each treatment area.

This system is recommended for offices in which the economics of central storage warrant its installation but the frequency of use of inhalation sedation does not justify the purchase of heads for all treatment areas. One head may be used throughout the office, with others added to the system as increased demand dictates.

Only the continuous-flow unit is considered in our discussion of inhalation sedation. Major components of this system are discussed in depth so that the administrator of inhalation sedation will become knowledgeable about this equipment and comfortable in its clinical use.

Compressed-Gas Cylinders

Gases dispensed at a pressure greater than 25 lb per square inch (25 psig [pounds per square inch gauge pressure]) at 25°C (70°F) are considered compressed gases, according to the hazardous materials regulations of the U.S. Department of Transportation (DOT). Such gases are used in the health professions and in nonhealth professions (e.g., construction, automobile racing). Because of the potential for serious injury from improper handling of these cylinders, the DOT has promulgated regulations for these gases, some of which are discussed in the following paragraphs.[4]

Cylinders that are used to store and transport compressed gases are manufactured from $\frac{3}{8}$ -inch-thick steel. Some cylinders of N_2O have been made from aluminum.

All compressed-gas cylinders are tested in accordance with DOT regulations every 5 years to ensure their integrity. Testing is performed by internal hydrostatic pressure, the pressure to which the cylinder is tested based on the size of the cylinder. The shoulder of the cylinder is marked with a metal stamp indicating the date the cylinder was commissioned, dates of testing in accordance with DOT regulations, the pressure for which the cylinder is designed, the insignia of the testing facility, and the identification of the manufacturer of the cylinder (Fig. 14.7).

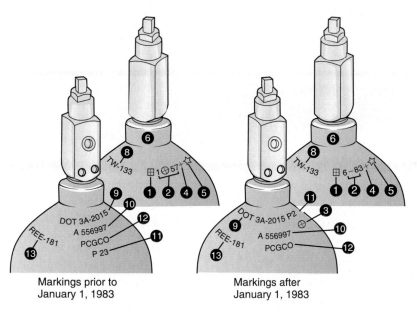

Markings prior to
January 1, 1983

Markings after
January 1, 1983

Item	Description
1	Brand identification
2	Manufacturer's test date
3	Manufacturer's registered symbol
4	Cylinder meets 10% overfill specification
5	Cylinder meets 10-year hydrostatic test exemption
6	Collar
7	Cylinder (label not shown)
8	Tare weight
9	DOT specification and service pressure
10	Manufacturer's serial number
11	Inspector's mark
12	Registered owner (PCGCO = Nellcor Puritan Bennett)
13	Rejection elastic expansion limit in cubic centimeters

Figure 14.7 Cylinder shoulder markings detailing various information. (From Clark MS, Brunick AL: *Handbook of nitrous oxide and oxygen sedation*, ed 4, St Louis, 2015, Mosby.)

Cylinders are designed to handle 1.66 times the usual pressure. For example, an O_2 cylinder usually under 2000 psig is designed to hold up to 3400 psig.

In addition, the American Society of Anesthesiologists, the American Hospital Association, and the medical gas industry have adopted a uniform color code that is used on all compressed-gas cylinders (Table 14.1, Fig. 14.8). The agents used in inhalation sedation, N_2O and O_2, are color-coded light blue and green, respectively, in the United States.

The following are important considerations for handling compressed gas cylinders:

1. Use no grease, oil, or lubricant of any type to lubricate cylinder valves, gauges, regulators, or other fittings that may come into contact with gases. This is extremely dangerous.

Table 14.1	Cylinder Color Codes for Various Countries	
COUNTRY	**N_2O**	**O_2**
Argentina	Blue	White with green cross
Australia	Blue	White
Canada	Blue	White
China	Gray	Blue
India	Blue	Black with white shoulders
Germany	Gray	Blue
Japan	Black	White
South Africa	Blue	Black with white shoulders
Sweden	Blue	White
United Kingdom	Blue	White
United States	Blue	Green

From Clark MS and Brunick AL: *Handbook of nitrous oxide and oxygen sedation*, ed 4, St Louis, 2015, Mosby.

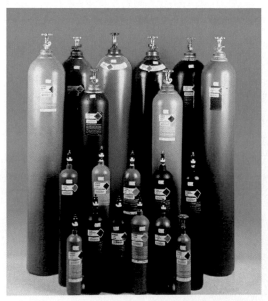

Figure 14.8 Various gas cylinder sizes. (Copyright © 2017 Medtronic. All rights reserved. Used with the permission of Medtronic.)

2. Store full cylinders in the vertical position.
3. Store cylinders in an area in which the temperature does not fluctuate; heat in particular should be avoided.
4. Handle cylinders with care: especially avoid dropping them.
5. Open cylinder valves slowly in a counterclockwise direction. Valves must be fully opened to prevent gas leakage from the valve stems.
6. Close all cylinder valves tightly when not in use. This is important to prevent contamination from water or dirt, regardless of whether the cylinder contains gas or is empty.
7. Cylinders should be "cracked" before attached to the sedation or anesthesia machine. The term *cracked* signifies opening the cylinder just slightly, allowing some gas to escape, thereby blowing out any particles of dust that may have lodged in the orifice of the cylinder.

The importance of keeping grease and oil away from compressed gases is so great that additional comment is required. Grease or oil in the presence of a compressed gas forms a potentially explosive mixture. When a cylinder is opened, high-pressure gas (e.g., O_2 at 2000 psig) is reduced suddenly to approximately 50 psig and to atmospheric pressure by the reducing valve. Sudden expansion of the compressed gas as it exits the cylinder cools the gas to subzero temperatures. The cylinder valve will become cool, with frost possibly forming. However, almost immediately, as more gas rushes from the cylinder into the restricted space of the reducing valve, both the pressure and temperature are increased. The temperature may increase sufficiently, albeit for only a few seconds, to ignite any combustible materials that may be present (e.g., grease or oil). Temperatures in excess of 815°C (1500°F)—well above the ignition temperature of grease or oil—can be produced at this time.

Once the grease or oil ignites, either N_2O or O_2, although nonflammable, will support combustion. Temperature and pressure within the cylinder increase even further, producing two grave problems: (1) the rapid increase in pressure will soon exceed the limits of the cylinder, leading to an explosion; and (2) as the temperature within the cylinder increases, the valve stem of the cylinder, composed of an alloy with a melting point of 93°C, will melt, thereby releasing the contents of the cylinder. These processes may occur within 1 to 2 seconds. Death and serious injuries to the dentist, staff, and patients have occurred in this manner.[5]

Compressed-gas cylinders are manufactured in a variety of sizes. They are classified by letter, with the "A" cylinder the smallest and the "HH" the largest (Fig. 14.9). In inhalation sedation with N_2O-O_2, the cylinder sizes used are the "E," "G," and "H." E cylinders are used for both N_2O and O_2 in portable units, whereas larger cylinders are used in central storage systems—G cylinders for N_2O and H cylinders for O_2. The physical characteristics of these and other compressed-gas cylinders are compared in Table 14.2, and the gas capacities of the E, G, and H cylinders are compared in Table 14.3.

Safety features incorporated in the compressed-gas cylinders include color coding (N_2O, blue; O_2, green) and the pin index

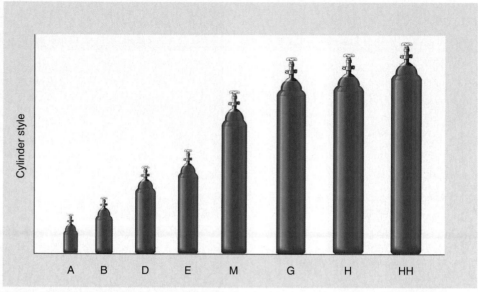

Figure 14.9 Various sizes of compressed-gas cylinders. (Redrawn from Williams RH: *Textbook of endocrinology*, ed 6, Philadelphia, 1982, WB Saunders.)

Table 14.2	Characteristics of Compressed-Gas Cylinders	
CYLINDER	**DIMENSIONS (IN)**	**WEIGHT OF EMPTY CYLINDER (LB)**
A	3.0 × 10	2.75
B	3.5 × 17	8
D	4.25 × 20	12
E	4.25 × 29.5	21
M	7.12 × 46	74
G	8.5 × 55	130
H	9.0 × 55	130
HH	9.25 × 59	136

Table 14.3	Comparison of E, G, and H Cylinders	
N_2O CYLINDER SIZE	**E**	**G**
Dimensions	4.5 in wide	8.5 in wide
	29.5 in high	55 in high
	21 lb weight	130 lb weight
Color of cylinder (USA)	Light blue	Light blue
(International)	Blue	Blue
Psi—full	750–800	750–800
Capacity (L)	159	13,839
(gal)	420	3200
Physical state of contents	Gas and liquid	Gas and liquid
O_2 CYLINDER SIZE	**E**	**H**
Dimensions	4.5 in wide	9 in wide
	29.5 in high	55 in high
	21 lb weight	130 lb weight
Color of cylinder (USA)	Green	Green
(International)	White	White
Psi—full	2000	2200
Capacity (L)	625	6909
(gal)	165	1400
Physical state of contents	Gas	Gas

safety system (see Fig. 14.36). The pin index safety system is designed to make it physically impossible for an N_2O cylinder to be inadvertently attached to the O_2 portion of the delivery system and vice versa. This is achieved through a series of holes in the stem of the cylinder that have a unique configuration permitting attachment only to the correct yoke on the sedation unit. Fig. 14.10 illustrates the pin index safety system for N_2O and O_2. The large hole on the top of the stem is the orifice through which the compressed gas exits the cylinder. The two holes beneath the orifice accept pins found on the yoke of the sedation machine. They are countersunk approximately 0.25 inch. On the yoke of the inhalation sedation unit are found pins that will permit the attachment of the appropriate compressed-gas cylinder (Fig. 14.11). These pins are welded into the unit. The pin index safety system is designed to prevent the inadvertent attachment of a gas cylinder to the wrong yoke and thus the accidental delivery of 100% N_2O when 100% O_2 is desired, a situation with potentially catastrophic

consequences. Errors have been noted in pin indexing of cylinders.[6–8] Careful checking of all compressed-gas cylinders before their use is essential to safety.

Oxygen Cylinder and Contents

Oxygen (O_2) in a compressed-gas cylinder is present in a gaseous state. The gas pressure in a full E cylinder is

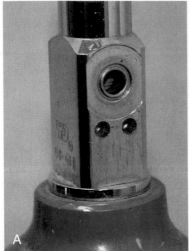

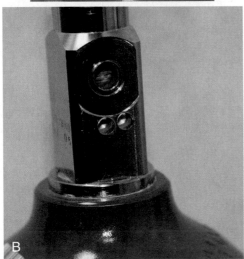

Figure 14.10 Pin index safety system for O_2 **(A)** and N_2O **(B).** Large orifice on top of cylinder permits gas to exit cylinder. Smaller holes below are pin indexed for specific compressed gas.

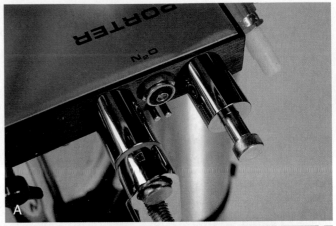

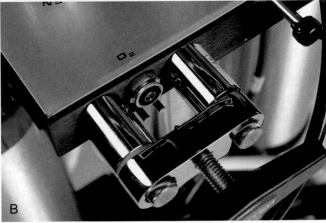

Figure 14.11 Pins, which are located on yoke of inhalation sedation unit, are aligned to permit attachment of only one compressed gas.

approximately 1900 psig[8] at 70°F (25°C) (Fig. 14.12, A), whereas the pressure within the larger H cylinder is approximately 2200 psig.[9] O_2 cylinders are color-coded white internationally and green in the United States. One ounce of O_2 liquid is equivalent to 5.22 gal of O_2 gas.

Because the O_2 cylinder contains only gas, the pressure gauge on the machine yoke reflects the actual contents of the cylinder. In other words, as O_2 leaves the cylinder, the pressure within the cylinder will drop accordingly. Therefore if an O_2 cylinder records a pressure of 1000 psig (Fig. 14.13), the cylinder is 1000/1900, or 52% full. A full E cylinder of O_2 will produce 660 L of gaseous O_2. At a flow rate of 6 L/min, this tank would empty in 110 minutes (660/6 = 110 minutes). This is an important factor in the safety of inhalation sedation because if an O_2 cylinder became empty during a procedure while the N_2O cylinder still contained gas, it would be potentially possible to administer 100% N_2O. Although there are additional safety features designed to prevent this occurrence,

the administrator of the N_2O-O_2 can see the "fuel gauge" for the O_2, thus allowing a new cylinder to be opened before the nearly empty cylinder is depleted. If the sedation machine is equipped with two E cylinders of O_2, only one should be open and in use at any one time so that both tanks are not emptied simultaneously.[10]

Nitrous Oxide Cylinder and Contents

N_2O in compressed-gas cylinders is present in both the liquid and gaseous states. N_2O cylinders are factory filled to 90% to 95% capacity with liquid N_2O.[10] Above the liquid in the tank is N_2O gas. The gas pressure within the cylinder of N_2O is approximately 750 psig at 25°C (70°F) (see Fig. 14.12, B) within both the E and G cylinders. N_2O compressed-gas cylinders are color-coded blue internationally and light blue in the United States. One ounce of N_2O liquid provides 3.88 gal of N_2O gas. A full E cylinder of N_2O produces approximately 1600 L of gaseous N_2O at sea level and room temperature, whereas the larger H cylinder provides approximately 16,000 L of N_2O gas.[11]

Because of the presence of liquid N_2O in the cylinder, the gas pressure gauge on the cylinder will record "full" (approximately 750 psig) as long as any liquid remains in the cylinder.

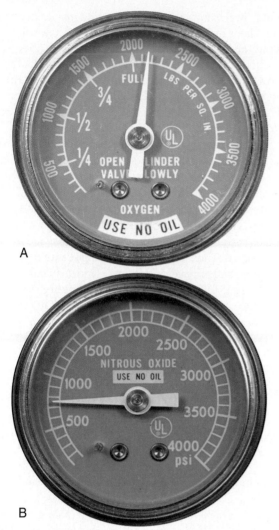

A

B

Figure 14.12 Pressure gauges on inhalation sedation unit. **A,** O$_2$ pressure gauge. **B,** N$_2$O pressure gauge. (From Darby ML, Walsh MM: *Dental hygiene: theory and practice*, ed 3, St Louis, Saunders, 2010.)

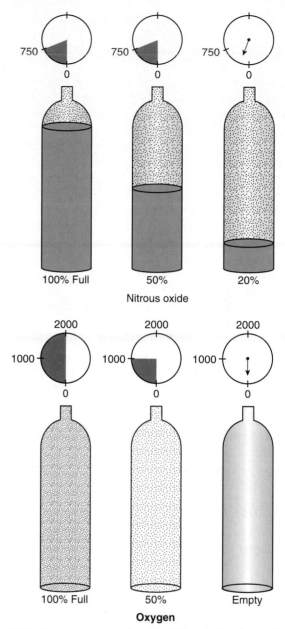

Figure 14.13 Pressure gauge readings for N$_2$O and O$_2$ cylinders. (From Clark MS, Brunick AL: *Handbook of nitrous oxide and oxygen sedation*, ed 4, St Louis, 2015, Mosby.)

The pressure of the N$_2$O vapor floating above the liquid N$_2$O is 750 psig (see Fig. 14.13). As the gaseous N$_2$O exits from the cylinder, liquid N$_2$O vaporizes to replace it. The pressure of this "new" gas is 750 psig. This process continues, liquid N$_2$O converting to gaseous N$_2$O, with the gas pressure remaining at 750 psig, until no more liquid remains to replace the gas. The pressure gauge for N$_2$O therefore cannot be used as an accurate measurement of the contents of the cylinder. Once all of the liquid N$_2$O is gone and only gaseous N$_2$O remains, the pressure gauge will fall in relation to the pressure of gas now remaining (acting now like an O$_2$ pressure gauge). In normal clinical usage of inhalation sedation, it has been our experience that 2.5 O$_2$ cylinders are used for every N$_2$O cylinder of the same size. The presence of N$_2$O in a liquid state is the reason for the increased volume of gas within the N$_2$O cylinder compared with the O$_2$ cylinders.

In central storage systems, it is recommended that there be no fewer than two H cylinders of O$_2$ and one G cylinder of N$_2$O. In portable systems, on the other hand, one or two E cylinders of N$_2$O and two E O$_2$ cylinders are recommended.

Regulators

Regulators, also called *reducing valves*, are located between the compressed-gas cylinder and the flowmeter. In central storage systems, regulators are commonly placed on the cylinder itself. The regulator functions to reduce the high-pressure gas coming from the cylinder (750 [N$_2$O] to 2200 psig [O$_2$]) to a pressure that is safe for both the patient and the sedation unit. Regulators function to maintain a constant gas pressure to flowmeters and to the patient regardless of the pressure of gas contained within the cylinder. Maintaining a constant, relatively low pressure within the body of the N_2O unit minimizes the potential for damage to the machine produced by high-pressure gases. The actual delivery pressure of the gas is set by the manufacturer of the equipment at 45 to 55 psig. When gases enter directly from cylinders, the pressure is reduced to 45 psig, whereas gases entering through a pipeline (central systems) maintain a pressure of 50 to 55 psig.

Regulators on portable units are located between the cylinders of gas and the flowmeters on the yoke (see Fig. 14.4). Central systems commonly have a regulator attached directly to the cylinder, in which case it often has a gas pressure gauge combined with it. This type of system, with individual regulators for each cylinder of compressed gas, requires that the cylinders be switched on and off each day. In addition, when a cylinder of gas empties, there is no automatic system for switching to a reserve tank (as is present with the more expensive manifold system; see next section).

It is within the reducing valve that the recompression of gases produces a tremendous increase in temperature to about 815°C to 1093°C (1500°F to 2000°F). This happens when a cylinder of O_2 at 2200 psig is quickly opened and the high-pressure gas is forced into a reducing valve. Although the reducing valve lowers this pressure to approximately 50 psig, gas backs up in the reducing valve, producing a recompression of gas that leads to a temperature increase. Temperature increases can ignite oil, grease, or Teflon that might be found in this area, leading to explosion and fire. Proper care and handling of cylinders (see previous discussion) will prevent this potentially disastrous consequence.

Manifolds (Central System Only)

A manifold joins multiple compressed-gas cylinders (Fig. 14.14). For example, 12 N_2O cylinders may be attached to a single

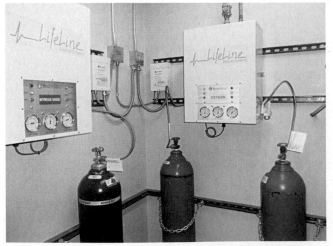

Figure 14.14 Manifold connecting N_2O and O_2 cylinders for use in a central system. Manifold provides automatic switch over from the cylinder in use. (From Clark MS, Brunick AL: *Handbook of nitrous oxide and oxygen sedation*, ed 4, St Louis, 2015, Mosby.)

manifold. Twelve hoses will enter into the manifold, one from each regulator on the cylinder; but only one hose will exit the manifold, carrying the gas under low pressure (50 psig) to each station outlet in the individual treatment rooms. The National Fire Protection Agency (NFPA) allows for only a level 3 system in dental offices. This allows for the equivalent of two H cylinders of O_2 and two G cylinders of N_2O in use and an additional two of each cylinder to be in storage.

A nonautomatic manifold is most commonly used. When a cylinder is empty, it must physically be turned off and a new cylinder opened by a staff member. Automatic manifolds are also available. The advantage of these more expensive devices is that they automatically activate a full reserve cylinder of gas when the cylinder in use empties. Other items found on all manifolds include a safety pressure-relief valve and an alarm monitor gauge. The latter monitors the pressure of gas in the line (50 psig) and activates a high-low alarm should the pressure exceed 75 psig or fall below 40 psig. A typical manifold in a dental office will operate two O_2 cylinders, and a second manifold operates either one or two N_2O cylinders.

Yokes (Portable System Only)

The yoke assembly holds the cylinder of compressed gas tightly in contact with the nipples of the portable sedation unit (see Fig. 14.6). Metal pins below the collar of the nipple are situated in such a way that they will accept only one specific type of compressed gas (see Fig. 14.11). This constitutes the pin index safety system.

In the portable inhalation sedation unit, the circuit of gases to this point has been from the cylinder through the yoke and into the reducing valve, the portion of the circuit termed the *high-pressure system;* the circuit from the reducing valve to the patient is called the *low-pressure system.* From the reducing valve the gas enters low-pressure tubing (color-coded for specific gases) that conducts the gas to attachments at the rear of the inhalation sedation unit. It is here that another safety feature of inhalation anesthetic systems is found. The diameter index safety system (DISS) (Fig. 14.15; see also Fig. 14.37 later) is designed to ensure that the correct medical gas enters the correct part of the anesthesia (sedation) machine.[12,13] Accidental attachment is prevented in two ways: First, the diameter of the attachments differs considerably (see Fig. 14.15, *A*); and second, the threading of the attachments differs (see Fig. 14.15, *B*), making it physically impossible to inadvertently attach tubing to the wrong inlet on the sedation or anesthesia machine. Once in the machine, the gases are directed to the appropriate flowmeters, where precise volumes may be delivered to the patient.

The circuit thus far in the central system is similar, with a few important differences. Gas leaving the cylinder enters the reducing valve and the manifold directly, from which it is directed from the storage area through specially prepared copper tubing to the individual treatment areas in the dental office. This tubing may be found in the walls, ceilings, or floors and leads to outlets in the individual treatment rooms. The outlet station

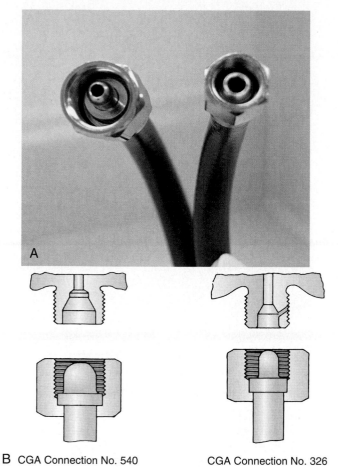

Figure 14.15 A and **B,** Diameter index safety system. Connectors attaching low-pressure tubing to inhalation sedation unit are of different diameters. O_2 (green) is of smaller diameter than nitrous oxide (blue), thus preventing accidental crossing of attachments. (From Clark MS, Brunick AL: *Handbook of nitrous oxide and oxygen sedation,* ed 4, St Louis, 2015, Mosby.)

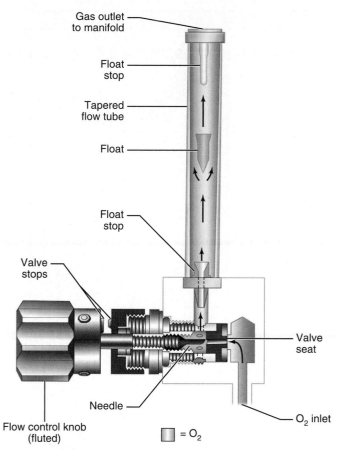

Figure 14.16 O_2 flowmeter and flow control valve.

possesses attachments for N_2O and O_2 hoses that are quick connects, permitting rapid attachment and disconnection of the hoses.[10] To prevent accidental crossing of these hoses, the DISS is incorporated into the quick connect for N_2O and O_2.

Flowmeters

From the reducing valves, the individual gases are carried through low-pressure tubing into the back of the sedation unit. The gases are then directed to the flowmeters (see Fig. 14.3), which permit the administrator to deliver a precise volume of either gas to the patient. Flowmeters are calibrated only for the gas that will flow through them (N_2O or O_2).[11] Gas flows are calibrated to be read at 25°C at 76 cm Hg (atmospheric pressure). Flowmeters measure the actual quantity of gas in motion rather than static cylinder pressure (as measured by the pressure gauges). If the flow of gas is interrupted, the flowmeter will read zero.

The flowmeter is actually a very simple device. Gas enters a tube formed with a tapering lumen that grows wider from the gas inlet at the bottom to the outlet at its top. A float used for measuring the volume is found inside the flowmeter. The float is either a ball or a rotameter. When a ball is used, the precise flow volume of gas is read using the middle of the ball, whereas with the rotameter, the flow is read at the top of the bobbin.

Once the flow of gas is started, gas enters the bottom of the flowmeter. The gas forces the float up into the flowmeter tube. Because the flowmeter is tapered, the area surrounding the float increases in size as the increased flow of gas causes the float to bob at a higher level; the flow rate is proportional to the size of the space surrounding the float.

The calibrations on the flowmeter tubes indicate the flow of gas in liters per minute (L/min). Adjustment of the gas flow is accomplished by means of a fine-needle valve for each flowmeter. The knobs that control the gases are both touch-coded and color-coded. In the United States the O_2 control knob is green in color and fluted, whereas the N_2O control knob is blue and not fluted (Fig. 14.16).[14] The characteristics of the knobs may vary with dental mixers. In North America, the O_2 flowmeter is positioned on the right side of the bank of flowmeters.[15]

Three types of devices—the rotameter, ball, and rod—are used inside the flowmeter to measure gas flow. The rod type of flowmeter is seldom used any longer, primarily because its

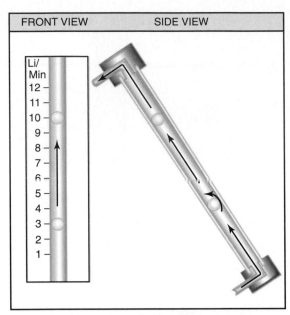

Figure 14.17 Ball type of flowmeter.

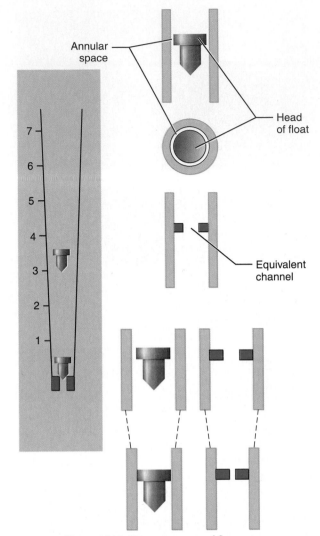

Figure 14.18 Rotameter type of flowmeter.

accuracy is not as great as that of the ball or rotameter. Accuracy for the rod type of flowmeter is ±7%.

In the ball type of flowmeter, a ball is forced up into the flowmeter by the gas entering the meter. For best accuracy, this type of flowmeter is placed on an inclined plane (Fig. 14.17). The ball type of flowmeter is the most commonly used today. Its accuracy is ±5%, and it is least accurate at very low flow rates.

The rotameter type of flowmeter is the most accurate, with an accuracy of ±2%. A metal bobbin, usually aluminum, is pushed upward in the flowmeter by the force of the gas passing through the meter. This stream of gas also causes the rotameter to rotate. Flowmeters in this type of unit must be vertical (Fig. 14.18). The three types of flowmeters are compared in Table 14.4.

As the anesthetic gases leave through the top of their respective flowmeters, they are combined in the mixing chamber, which is found within the head of the sedation unit. From this point, a combination of the gases flows through the machine. These gases now exit the sedation unit through the outflow tube, which is also known as a *bag-tee* (Figs. 14.6 and 14.19), and are carried to the patient.

Flowmeter Advancements

Although the old flow tube flowmeter technology is still available today, it is being replaced by state-of-the-art digital electronic flow-control devices on all major N_2O-O_2 sedation devices manufactured in the United States: Accutron and Matrx (Fig. 14.20). The devices have resolution of the gas flow in increments of 0.1 L/min, and the total flow and percentage O_2 are displayed digitally, eliminating the guesswork or calculations required with simple flow tube devices. The ability to clean the front panel with just a "wipe" reduces the potential of cross-infection

Table 14.4	**Characteristics of Flowmeters**		
	ROTAMETER	**BALL**	**ROD**
Accuracy	±2%	±5%	±7%
Current use	Intermediate use	Most common	Least common
Flowmeter angle	Vertical	Inclined	Vertical
Material	Aluminum	Plastic	Metal

among patients, an issue associated with crevasses created by knobs and levers. Patient safety is ensured with built-in alarms for all gas depletion conditions, along with servo control of the gas delivery (what you see is what you get). Continuous internal self-monitoring of all operational parameters by the device frees the practitioner to concentrate on the patient's needs. The device alerts the practitioner or staff to unusual

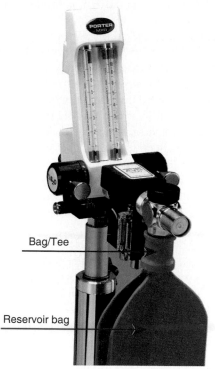

Figure 14.19 Sedation machine – reservoir bag (arrow). (Courtesy Porter Instrument, Parker Hannifin Corporation.)

parameters requiring attention, similar to those seen in larger hospital-based systems.

The digital units deliver pure O_2 during the "flush" function by electronically shutting off the N_2O flow, as opposed to the flow tube units, which only dilute the N_2O delivered. The removal of extra steps in shutting down the N_2O supply before pressing the "flush" button greatly simplifies the practitioner's tasks.

The units contain flashing light-emitting diodes (LEDs) to afford the practitioner a simple method of ensuring that the individual component gas is flowing and that the relative ratio and amount of flow are correct. In addition, the digital unit provides the capability of displaying the flow rate of either of the constituent gases. The nonsilenceable alarm function for O_2 depletion ensures adequate patient safety. The air intake valve located on the bag-tee provides room air to the patient whenever the patient's breathing demand is greater than the combined output of the mixer head's settings and reservoir bag volume.

Various models of the electronic gas-mixing head allow mounting as a wall unit, portable unit, countertop unit, or a flush mount unit in modern cabinetry. Digital heads have the most flexibility, especially when combined with various remote bag-tee options provided by the manufacturer. The units are fully compatible with central gas supply systems, such as the popular Flo-Safe Manifold, Centurion Gas Manifold, and all existing scavenging systems. It is available with the American Dental Association (ADA) recommended 45 L/min[16] scavenging control valve in various mounting configurations.

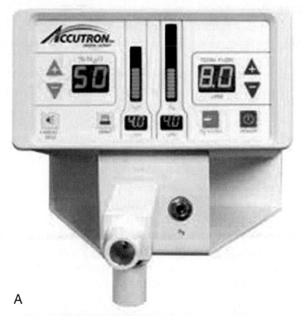

A

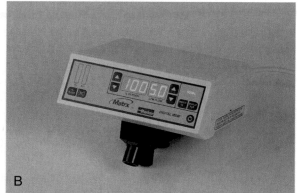

B

Figure 14.20 (A) Accutron N_2O-O_2 machine, **(B)** Porter N_2O-O_2 machine. (A, © 2017 Accutron, Inc., a subsidiary of Crosstex International, Inc. B, Courtesy Porter Instrument, Parker Hannifin Corporation.)

Electronic digital administration heads for delivery of inhalation sedation advance the art of dentistry. The digital heads, once considered the wave of the future, are the de facto "standard" today. The digital accuracy and exacting control are highly recommended for patient comfort and safety.

Emergency Air Intake Valve

An emergency air intake valve is located on the bag-tee above the reservoir bag. It provides the patient with a supply of atmospheric air in the event that the sedation unit ceases to function and gas flow from the machine is terminated. During normal use, the emergency air valve remains shut, but it opens automatically once gas flow through the machine is terminated. This prevents the patient from experiencing a feeling of discomfort or suffocation as he or she attempts to breathe through the nasal hood when the unit is not working and the reservoir bag is deflated.[17]

Latex-Free Accessory Equipment

All equipment used in N_2O-O_2 administration is latex free. Hence, the term *rubber goods* is obsolete. From the outlet tube, the anesthetic gases are carried to the patient. In addition to the reservoir bag, the latex-free equipment consists of conducting tubes and a face mask, nasal hood, or nasal cannula.

Reservoir Bag

Reservoir bags are bladder-type bags, made of latex-free material or silicone, ranging in size from 1 L to 8 L. The 3-L reservoir bag is the most frequently used in dentistry (Fig. 14.21). Although commonly used, latex-free bags deteriorate more rapidly than silicone bags, especially in areas in which high levels of atmospheric pollutants are found (the planet Earth).

The reservoir bag attaches to the base of the bag-tee, usually immediately below the emergency air inlet valve (see Figs. 14.19 and 14.21). A portion of the gas(es) delivered through the unit to the patient is diverted into the reservoir bag, where it may be used for any of several purposes.

The primary function of the reservoir bag during inhalation sedation is to provide a reservoir from which additional gas may be drawn should the respiratory demands of the patient exceed the gas flow delivered from the machine. During normal (quiet) respiration, the patient receives only fresh gases delivered from the sedation unit, with little or none taken from the reservoir bag. However, should the patient take an especially deep breath, the machine will be unable to accommodate the necessary volume; in the absence of the reservoir bag, the patient will experience a feeling of difficulty breathing. The reservoir bag prevents or minimizes this occurrence.

A second use of the reservoir bag during sedation is to serve as a monitoring device for respiration. Assuming an airtight seal of the nasal hood and no mouth breathing, the reservoir bag will inflate slightly with every exhalation and deflate slightly with each inhalation, permitting the operator to easily determine respiratory rate.

A third potential use for the reservoir bag is its use as a means of providing O_2 during assisted or controlled ventilation. Provided that a full-face mask is properly positioned with an airtight seal and a patent airway, the reservoir bag is squeezed and its contents are forced into the patient's lungs (Fig. 14.22). It is quite a bit more difficult to ventilate the patient with the reservoir bag when the nasal hood is used. Adequate ventilation can be accomplished with the nasal hood, but this is not likely to be effective in the hands of an inexperienced person (a person who is not trained in anesthesiology). Controlled and assisted ventilation are impossible with a nasal cannula because the reservoir bag is removed from the sedation machine when a cannula is used.

The reservoir bag is of considerable importance in general anesthesia because during this time the patient is unconscious and unable to respond to the commands of the anesthesiologist. Other means of determining the physical status of the patient must be used. Monitoring vital signs becomes quite important. Respiratory rate and depth can be monitored easily by observing and feeling the reservoir bag. Should respiratory depth become shallow, the anesthesiologist can assist a patient's breathing by gently squeezing the bag as the patient begins to breathe spontaneously. Should spontaneous respiration cease, controlled respiration can be started, with the anesthesiologist squeezing the reservoir bag once every 5 seconds for an adult and every 3 seconds for the child and infant.

The reservoir bag was, in the past, called a rebreathing bag. Years ago it was possible for the patient to exhale into the

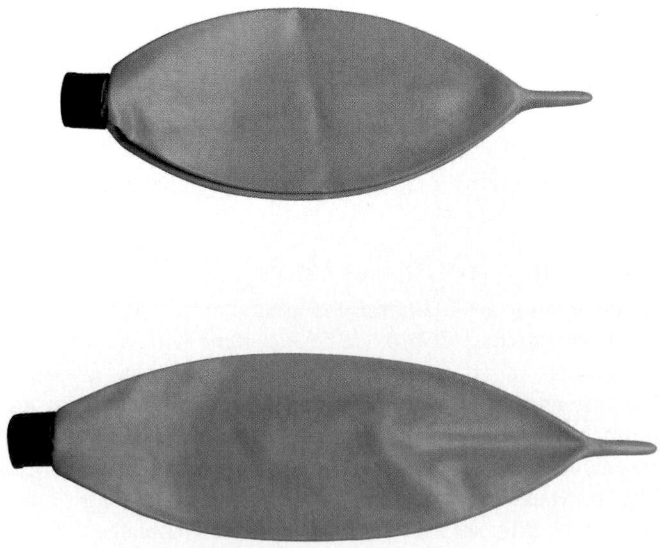

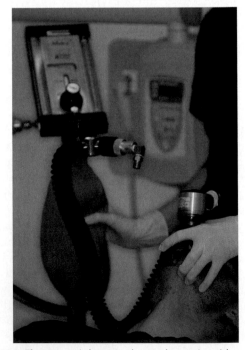

Figure 14.22 The reservoir bag may be used to assist with patient ventilation in the event of a respiratory emergency.

Figure 14.21 Two- and three-liter reservoir bags are most commonly used in dentistry.

nasal hood, and if the total flow of gas from the sedation unit was low, the exhaled gases could be forced backward through the conducting tubing to reach the reservoir bag. On inhalation these same gases, now containing elevated concentrations of carbon dioxide (CO_2), would be rebreathed. Rebreathing gas containing elevated CO_2 levels can lead to undesirable consequences if permitted to continue for extended periods. One-way valves have been placed into the bag-tee of contemporary machines to prevent the possibility of rebreathing.

For the adult patient receiving moderate sedation, the 3- or 5-L reservoir bag is used. In pediatric procedures, smaller (1-, 2-, or 3-L) reservoir bags are used.

Conducting Tubes

A variable length of hose, called either *conducting tubing* or a *breathing tube,* connects the bag-tee to the nasal hood. The hose is of large diameter, is corrugated, and is usually made of a non-latex material (Fig. 14.23). The large diameter minimizes any resistance to the flow of gases from the machine through the tubes to the patient, and the corrugation prevents inadvertent kinking or occlusion of its lumen. In moderate sedation procedures, the corrugated tubing is less essential than it is during general anesthesia. During N_2O-O_2 sedation, should a hose conducting gas to the patient become occluded by some means, the patient, still conscious, would comment on the increased difficulty of obtaining an adequate gas supply through the nosepiece. During general anesthesia, however, with the patient unconscious and unable to reply, occlusion of the tube carrying gas from the anesthesia machine would produce little or no immediate outward change in appearance, the lack of O_2 producing a deeper level of "general anesthesia." Only after possibly irreversible brain damage has occurred will changes be noticed by the less-than-expert observer. Thus the corrugated tubing present on all sedation units is a remnant of the general anesthesia machine from which the modern sedation unit evolved.

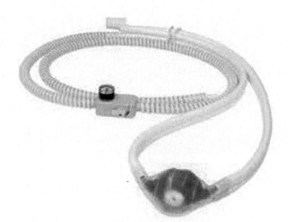

Figure 14.23 Corrugated conducting tubing. Large diameter minimizes resistance to gas flow. (© 2017 Accutron, Inc., a subsidiary of Crosstex International, Inc.)

The corrugated tubing is attached to one or two noncorrugated tubes that attach directly to the breathing apparatus (e.g., nasal hood) on the patient. Called the *breathing circuit,* these tubes are of smaller diameter than the corrugated tubing; however, they do not add significantly to the resistance to gas flow to the patient (Fig. 14.24, *A* and *B*). Commonly, two tubes are attached to the corrugated tubing. These tubes come around the sides of the dental chair and are attached to the breathing apparatus. In both cases, the tubing must be secured so that the patient remains comfortable and so that leakage will not occur around the sides of the breathing apparatus. With double tubing, there is the possibility that the tubing will be kinked as it comes around the side of the dental chair (see Fig. 14.24, *C*). Care is required when securing the tubing to prevent this from occurring.

Breathing Apparatus
Full-Face Mask

Three types of breathing apparatus may be used to deliver N_2O-O_2 to the patient. The face mask covers both the mouth and nose of the patient (Fig. 14.25, *A* and *B*). Although the face mask is the most effective method of delivering gases to the patient, in dentistry the face mask is impractical because the mouth must remain available for the dental procedure to occur. However, the presence of a face mask in the dental office is important in emergency situations because the face mask provides the optimal means of delivering O_2 to the patient (provided the person delivering the O_2 has received training in emergency airway management).

Nasal Cannula

The nasal cannula (Fig. 14.26) is quite different from the face mask. Made from a softened plastic, the two short ($\frac{1}{8}$-inch-long) prongs are placed into the nostrils of the patient. The device is used primarily to provide hospitalized patients with supplemental O_2. It is impossible to obtain an airtight seal with the nasal cannula, a fact that is detrimental to its use during N_2O-O_2 sedation because it leads to a significant degree of dilution of the gases delivered from the machine. To compensate for this air dilution, greater volumes of gases must be delivered to the patient. This is especially relevant for N_2O because significantly greater volumes of N_2O will be needed to produce a desired sedation level. It is often impossible to obtain clinically adequate sedation with the cannula even when maximum volumes of N_2O are delivered. Because of air dilution and the greater volumes of gases used, there is considerably greater contamination of the clinical environment with N_2O than is present when a nasal hood is used.

The primary advantages of the nasal cannula include its usefulness in patients with a fear of the face mask or the nasal hood and in claustrophobic patients. These persons are unable to tolerate the face mask or nasal hood comfortably, whereas the nasal cannula invariably proves satisfactory to them. A second advantage of the cannula is during treatment of maxillary anterior teeth. With a traditional nasal hood that rests over

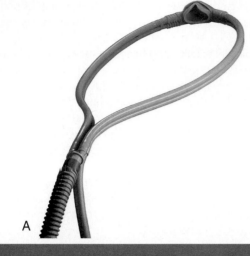

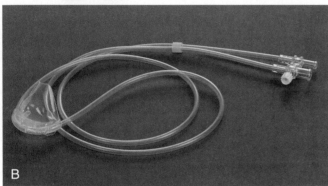

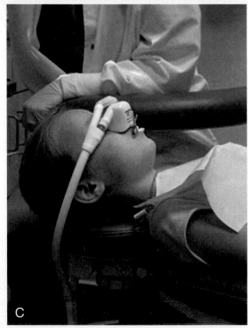

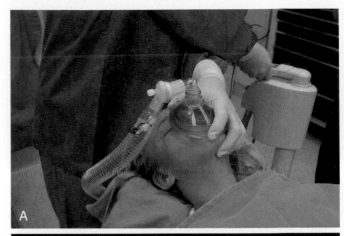

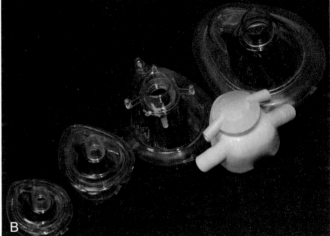

Figure 14.25 A, Face mask covers both nose and mouth of patient. Although inconvenient during dental care, it is appropriate for use in emergency situations. **B,** Face masks are available in a variety of sizes.

Figure 14.24 A and **B,** N₂O-O₂ breathing circuits. **C,** Noncorrugated tubing can become occluded as it bends around the sides of the dental chair.

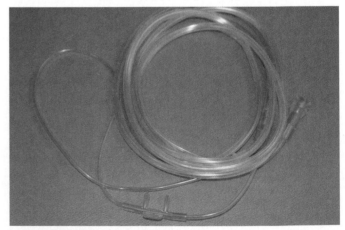

Figure 14.26 Nasal cannula. Two short plastic prongs are placed in the nares of the patient.

the patient's upper lip and against his or her maxillary anterior teeth, treatment involving the labial soft tissues or the teeth themselves may prove difficult because the nasal hood compresses the upper lip against the soft and hard tissues in this region. One way to minimize this potential difficulty is to place cotton rolls under the patient's upper lip before placing the nasal hood. The cannula, however, does not interfere with dental treatment in this area (Fig. 14.27).

A disadvantage of the nasal cannula is the necessity to remove the reservoir bag from the sedation unit, thereby negating its usefulness as a monitoring or ventilatory device. In its place is a plug, directing all gases from the machine into the cannula.

Because the gases delivered from the sedation unit (O_2 and N_2O) are both anhydrous, they are directed through a humidifier before they are sent to the patient when a cannula is used (Fig. 14.28). The humidifier is placed on the end of the outlet tube, to which is attached the nasal cannula.

The tubing of the nasal cannula is narrow. Gases delivered to the cannula through the outlet tube and humidifier will therefore gain considerable velocity as they pass from the wider bore of the outlet tube to the narrower space of the cannula. The force of the gas exiting the cannula may prove uncomfortable for the patient.

With today's concern about the potential hazards of trace contamination of the environment with N_2O, the use of the nasal cannula cannot be recommended except in those very few cases in which inhalation sedation must be used and other methods of delivering the gases to the patient are unacceptable.

Nasal Hood

The nasal hood, a device designed to fit comfortably and securely over the patient's nose, comes in two types. The traditional nasal hood (commonly called a *nosepiece*) has one or two tubes entering into it (Fig. 14.29). These tubes deliver gases from the inhalation sedation unit. Exhaled gases are eliminated into the surrounding environment through an exhaling valve located on top of the nasal hood. Along with the exhaling valve, the nasal hood may possess an air-dilution valve.

The second type of delivery system is the scavenging nasal hood. The prototypical scavenging nasal hood has four tubes entering it. Two tubes deliver fresh gases from the sedation unit; the other tubes carry exhaled gases away from the treatment area to a safe repository (Fig. 14.30). Concern about the possible deleterious effects on dental staff of prolonged exposure to low levels of N_2O has made use of the scavenging nasal hood the standard of care.

The nasal hood is made of nitrile or silicone, which readily adapts to the contours of the patient's face, providing an airtight seal (Fig. 14.31). Nasal hoods are designed in a variety of sizes, and it is important that several sizes be available (Fig. 14.32).

The traditional nasal hood contains one or two inlets through which fresh gases are delivered from the sedation unit to the patient. On the top of the mask is an opening into which has

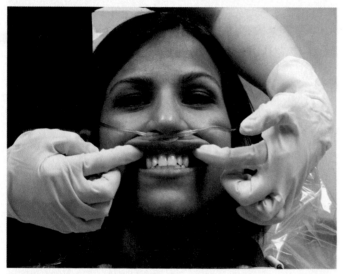

Figure 14.27 Nasal cannula does not interfere with dental treatment in maxillary anterior region. (Courtesy Dr. Morris Clark.)

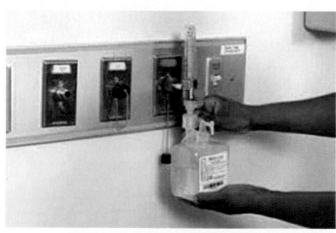

Figure 14.28 Nasal cannula with humidifier.

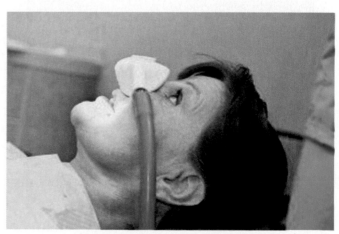

Figure 14.29 Traditional nasal hood.

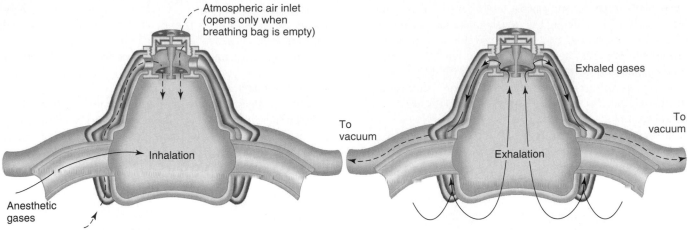

Figure 14.30 Diagram of scavenging nasal hood.

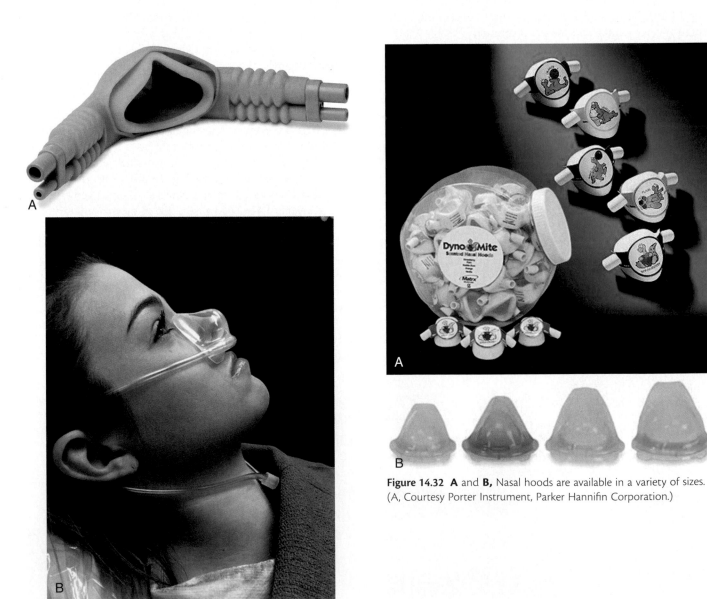

Figure 14.31 A, Scavenging nasal hood. **B,** Silhouette scavenging nasal hood. (Courtesy Porter Instrument, Parker Hannifin Corporation.)

Figure 14.32 A and **B,** Nasal hoods are available in a variety of sizes. (A, Courtesy Porter Instrument, Parker Hannifin Corporation.)

been placed one or more valves. When only one valve is present, it is an exhaling or one-way valve, permitting the patient to eliminate all exhaled gases into the environment and to inhale only fresh gases from the machine. The exhaling valve contains a thin wafer (Fig. 14.33, *A*) that sits over the opening in the valve. On exhalation, the wafer is lifted by the force of the

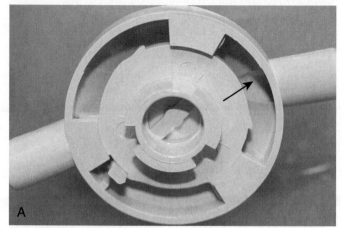

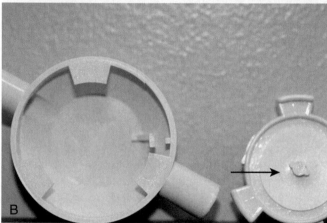

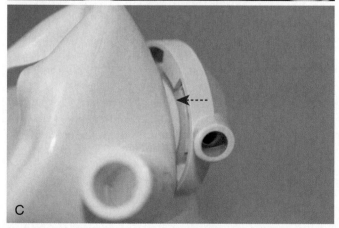

Figure 14.33 A, Internal view of nasal hood. **B,** Air dilution valve is opening below exhaling valve *(arrow)*, which permits entry of atmospheric air during inhalation. **C,** Exhaling valve on nasal hood. Thin wafer *(dotted arrow)* seals orifice while patient inhales, but is forced off orifice when patient exhales.

gases, and the gases are eliminated. On inhalation, the negative pressure created within the nosepiece forces the wafer down into the hole, sealing it shut and thus allowing the patient to inhale only the gases from the machine.

A second valve, present on some nasal hoods, is called the *inhaling* or *air-dilution valve.* It consists of an opening from the inside of the nasal hood directly to the atmosphere (see Fig. 14.33, *B*). As the patient exhales, gases escape from this valve (as in the exhaling valve); however, on inhalation, this valve remains open, permitting the patient to breathe in an unknown quantity of ambient air along with the fresh gases from the sedation unit. It has been estimated that the inspired percentage of N_2O may be diluted by 50% if the air-dilution valve is fully opened. The value of the air-dilution valve is that it permits the patient to breathe comfortably regardless of the volume of gas delivered from the machine; however, because of dilution, the volume of N_2O must be increased significantly, producing considerably higher concentrations of N_2O in the ambient air, which is undesirable.

The air-dilution valve can be opened or closed, whereas the exhaling valve cannot be closed. (see Fig. 14.33, *C*). If two valves are present on the nasal hood, it is recommended that the air-dilution valve be kept closed. There are virtually no indications for the use of an opened air-dilution valve. Newer nasal hoods are manufactured without the air-dilution valve.

The conventional nasal hood is no longer recommended for use with inhalation sedation. Although the absolute risk of chronic inhalation of low concentrations of N_2O is as yet undetermined, evidence indicates that there are no desirable attributes to its inhalation by health professionals. The scavenging nasal hood should be used whenever N_2O is administered and is today considered the standard of care.

Scavenging Nasal Hood

With concern over the possible long-term effects of trace levels of N_2O on chairside personnel (see Chapter 17), it has become mandatory to attempt to eliminate exhaled N_2O from the ambient air: To this end, the scavenging nasal hood was developed (see Figs. 14.30 and 14.31). Many such devices are available, but the principle behind their effectiveness is essentially the same.

Scavenging nasal hoods are, quite simply, double nosepieces: a smaller inner mask receiving gases from the anesthesia machine and a slightly larger outer mask that sits directly over the first, which removes exhaled gases from the treatment area. The outer nosepiece is connected to the suction device in the dental operatory, permitting exhaust gases to be vented from the dental operatory through the vacuum system (see Fig. 14.31). The effectiveness of this system is in part responsible for the 50 ppm standard for ambient levels of N_2O currently in use today. The scavenging system is discussed in Chapter 17, but at present, the scavenging mask represents the most effective means of minimizing N_2O contamination in the dental or surgical environment and has become the standard of care.

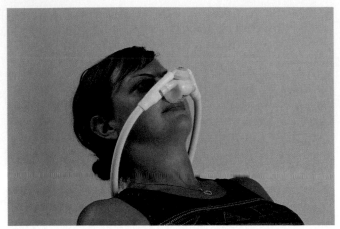

Figure 14.34 Matrx breathing circuit.

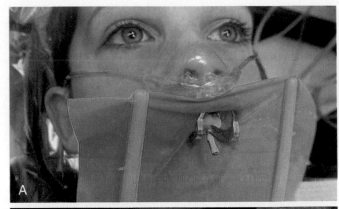

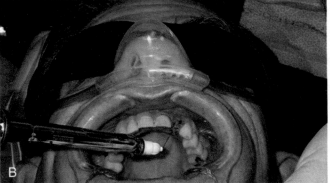

Figure 14.35 The Silhouette scavenging nasal hood is transparent, contains no metal, and is smaller than conventional nasal hoods. (Courtesy Porter Instrument, Parker Hannifin Corporation.)

Most scavenging nasal hoods include a scavenging cone that sits atop the nasal hood (Fig. 14.34). This type of mask has the additional advantage of scavenging the treatment room when not scavenging the patient's exhalation. Scavenging nasal hoods are considered to be the standard of care and should always be employed during the administration of N_2O-O_2 inhalation sedation.

Modern nasal hoods do not contain any metal. The recently introduced Silhouette scavenging nasal hood is transparent, contains no metal, and is of smaller size than previous scavenging systems, leading to ease of access during dental treatment (Figs. 14.31, B and 14.35). This contrasts dramatically with older nasal hoods in which the valves very often contained metal springs or clips. The disadvantage of nasal hoods containing metal became apparent when radiographs were taken. Invariably the metal would be superimposed directly above a critical portion of the film. With modern nasal hoods, radiographs may be taken without removing the nasal hood.

SAFETY FEATURES

All inhalation sedation units available in the United States incorporate a series of safety features. The primary purpose of these features is to prevent the delivery, either accidental or intentional, of less than atmospheric levels of O_2 (20.9%).

The Council on Dental Materials, Instruments, and Equipment of the ADA has issued guidelines for inhalation sedation units.[17] Although these safety features work well to minimize the occurrence of accidents, it must be emphasized that all mechanical devices are capable of failing, so the administrator of inhalation sedation should never rely entirely on them for a patient's safety.[5-7] Visual and verbal monitoring of the patient and visual monitoring of the sedation unit are essential at all times.

Pin Index Safety System

The pin index safety system makes it physically impossible to attach an N_2O–compressed-gas cylinder to the yoke attachment for O_2 (or any other compressed-gas yoke except N_2O), which could result in the inadvertent administration of 100% N_2O instead of 100% O_2. The pin index safety system consists of a series of pins, the configuration of which differs for each compressed gas (Fig. 14.36), on the yoke of the sedation unit and a matching series of holes on the compressed-gas cylinders. However, I have seen a blue cylinder (presumably N_2O) with the pin index system for O_2.[6] Beware!

Diameter Index Safety System

The DISS makes it impossible to attach a low-pressure hose to the wrong outlet on the sedation unit (Fig. 14.37).[18] The diameter of the couplings differs significantly (the coupling for N_2O is larger than that for O_2). In addition, the threading of the attachments differs, making it physically impossible to accidentally cross the low-pressure hoses and deliver the wrong gas to the patient. This system also exists as a safeguard on the larger G and H cylinders.

Minimum Oxygen Liter Flow

Inhalation sedation units are designed so that once turned on the unit delivers a preset minimum liter flow of O_2 through the flowmeter. In most units, this minimum flow is 2.5 or 3.0 L/min of O_2. The flow of N_2O cannot start until a flow of O_2 has been established.

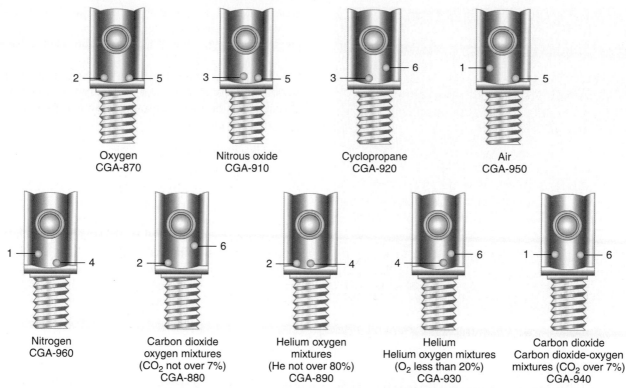

Figure 14.36 Pin index safety system for compressed-gas cylinders.

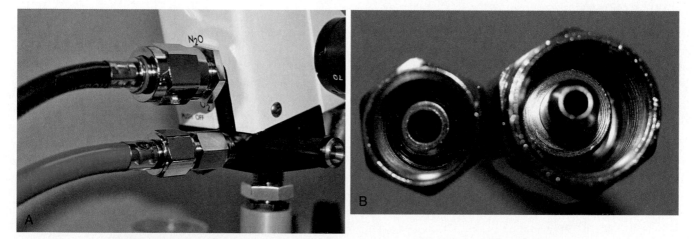

Figure 14.37 **A,** Back of inhalation sedation unit. Note different diameters of N_2O *(right)* and O_2 *(left)* connectors. **B,** Diameter index safety system. Diameter and threading of N_2O coupling *(right)* differ from those of O_2 coupling *(left)*, thus preventing accidental attachments to wrong side of inhalation sedation unit. (Part A from Clark MS, Brunick AL: *Handbook of nitrous oxide and oxygen sedation,* ed 4, St Louis, 2015, Mosby.)

Minimum Oxygen Percentage

Similar to the minimum O_2 liter flow, this safety feature sets a minimum percentage of O_2 that may be delivered to the patient. This minimum O_2 percentage is 30% (some units provide a minimum of 25%, others 50%). This allows for a possible error in calibration of the flowmeters of approximately ±5% while still delivering more than 20% O_2 to the patient.

The ball type of flowmeter has a ±5% accuracy rating, and the rotameter has a ±2% accuracy rating.

In a sedation unit in which a minimum O_2 flow of 2.5 L/min is delivered, the N_2O control knob may be turned up as high as the administrator desires, but the flow of N_2O gas will not exceed 5.5 L/min. This provides a 31% O_2 concentration (2.5 L/min per 8.0 L/min). If, however, the flow of O_2 is

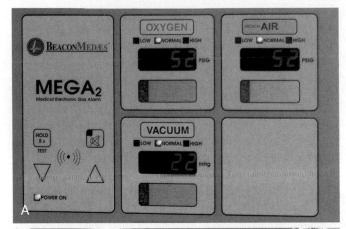

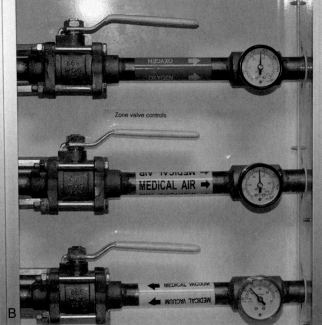

Figure 14.38 A, Alarm system for central system. Alarm is activated when O_2 or N_2O pressures are low or high and when reserve tanks are in use. **B,** Central medical gas valve shutoff.

increased above the minimum flow rate, the volume flow of N_2O may also be increased.

Oxygen Fail Safe

In either the portable or central systems, the O_2 cylinder will become depleted before the cylinder of N_2O. Approximately 2.5 O_2 cylinders will be used for each N_2O cylinder of comparable size. It is obvious that a potentially dangerous situation exists because if the O_2 cylinder becomes depleted during a procedure, the patient could conceivably receive 100% N_2O.

The O_2 fail-safe system is designed to prevent this from happening by automatically terminating the flow of N_2O whenever the delivery pressure of O_2 falls below a predetermined level. For example, both N_2O and O_2 are delivered to the patient at a pressure of approximately 50 psig. When the pressure in the O_2–compressed-gas cylinder nears zero (but

is not quite at zero), the delivery pressure of O_2 through the reducing valve can no longer be maintained at 50 psig. As this pressure falls (e.g., to 40 psig), the O_2 fail-safe mechanism is activated and the flow of N_2O gas (from a cylinder that may be almost full) is terminated. The patient at no time receives 100% N_2O. Several other safety devices are activated once the O_2 fail safe is brought into use. These are discussed in the following paragraphs.

Emergency Air Inlet

Located on top of the bag-tee outlet, the emergency air inlet is maintained in a closed position as long as O_2 or N_2O-O_2 is delivered through the sedation unit. When the flow of gas ceases, as in the preceding example in which the O_2 fail safe is activated, the emergency air inlet valve opens, permitting the patient to continue to breathe comfortably, although the gas inhaled now is atmospheric air. Should the termination of gas flow through the machine fail to be noticed by the administrator and assistant, the patient will gradually become less and less sedated or may mention an increasing resistance to inhalation.

Alarm

An alarm may be attached to the O_2 fail-safe system that is audible when this system is activated. This will prevent a situation in which the administrator, so involved in the dental procedure at hand, fails to notice the shutting off of the gas flows on the unit. In central systems, an alarm system is placed in an area (e.g., the reception desk) where personnel are frequently located (Fig. 14.38, *A*).

Oxygen Flush Button

The O_2 flush button permits the rapid delivery of high flows of O_2 to the patient. With the older pneumatic mixers, the N_2O had to be manually turned off to be able to deliver 100% O_2. With the newer electronic devices, 100% O_2 delivery is ensured by the unit automatically stopping the N_2O delivery when the O_2 flush button is pressed. All of this can be accomplished without user intervention. This automation of pure O_2 delivery is a distinct advantage during emergency situations. The button is ideally located on the front of the sedation unit in easy view (see Fig. 14.4). Most O_2 flush buttons permit the delivery of at least 35 L/min of O_2. This is intended for use in emergency situations. This one feature alone is reason enough to purchase an inhalation sedation unit. Positive-pressure O_2 can also be delivered with this system.

Reservoir Bag

The reservoir bag may be considered a safety feature because it may be used to assist or control respiration in emergency situations (see Figs. 14.19 and 14.22). All inhalation sedation units should have a reservoir bag.

Color Coding

Although simple, color coding is an important safety feature of all inhalation sedation units. All parts of the unit that carry or operate O_2 are colored green in the United States (white internationally), whereas tubes, knobs, and other parts handling N_2O are colored light blue (blue internationally).

Lock

Locks may be included in the inhalation sedation unit and on protective caps found on the larger cylinders. As discussed in Chapter 17, abuse of N_2O is not uncommon. Although persons in the dental profession are prime candidates for abuse of this technique, there are instances in which nondental persons have gained access to dental systems. The use of a lock on the cylinders makes it less likely that this situation will develop.

Quick Connect for Positive-Pressure Oxygen

All inhalation sedation units have a quick-connect attachment for positive-pressure O_2 located on the head. If it is not present, the units must be adaptable to this device.

AVAILABLE INHALATION SEDATION UNITS

Many inhalation sedation units are currently available for use in the dental or medical office. The underlying mechanism in all is quite similar; however, there are significant differences in appearance. Some units have a wooden veneer, whereas

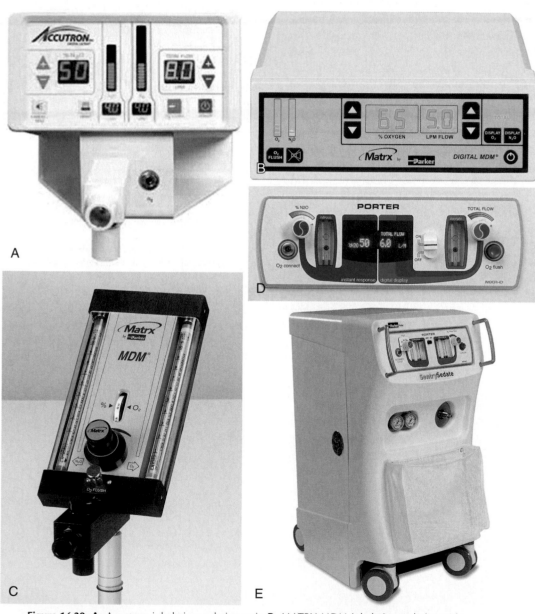

Figure 14.39 A, Accutron inhalation sedation unit. **B,** MATRX MDM inhalation sedation unit. **C,** Porter inhalation sedation unit. **D,** Porter Sentry inhalation sedation unit. **E,** Porter Sentry Sedate. (A, © 2017 Accutron, Inc., a subsidiary of Crosstex International, Inc. B-E, Courtesy Porter Instrument, Parker Hannifin Corporation.)

others are made of molded plastic; some are quite large, and others are more compact. Several machines are advertised with unique features relating to safety, appearance, or operation. Several examples of inhalation sedation units are illustrated in Fig. 14.39, A–D.

One factor that I believe must be present regarding the inhalation sedation unit is that the unit should have received an acceptable rating from the ADA's Council on Scientific Affairs.[16] The ADA has adopted an acceptance program for inhalation sedation units that permits the dentist to better evaluate those units considered for purchase. The ADA's Council on Scientific Affairs has developed Guidelines for Nitrous Oxide-Oxygen Conscious Sedation Systems (2002) that suggest what types of testing these devices should be able to meet. One important addition in these guidelines are requirements that are aimed at making it difficult, if not impossible, to administer less than 20% O_2 to the patient. To receive a satisfactory classification, the manufacturer must submit its devices to the Council on Scientific Affairs for evaluation. The council publishes a listing of acceptable devices in the *Journal of the American Dental Association,* the *Dentist's Desk Reference,*[19] and on the ADA website (www.ada.org). All of the devices listed have been accepted by the Council on Scientific Affairs of the ADA. The decision as to the most appropriate unit for your dental or medical office should be made after careful consideration of your needs and available space.

Effective in September 1994, the ADA discontinued the acceptance program for N_2O-O_2 scavenging devices after rescinding the then-current ADA guidelines used in evaluation of N_2O scavenging systems.[20]

REFERENCES

1. McCarthy FM, Shuken RA: Appraisal of the demand flow anesthetic machine and review of the literature. *J Oral Surg* 27(8):624–626, 1969.
2. Gauert WB, Husted RF: Differences in metered and measured oxygen concentrations during nitrous oxide analgesia. *Anesth Analg* 47(4):441–445, 1968.
3. Allen GD: *Dental anesthesia and analgesia,* ed 2, Baltimore, 1979, Williams & Wilkins.
4. Department of Transportation, Office of Federal Regulations, National Archives Administration: Code of federal regulations, title 49, section 178, Washington, DC, October 1, 2015.
5. Follmer KE: Anesthetic gas fires are preventable. *Anesth Prog* 19(2):38–39, 1972.
6. Hogg CF: Pin-indexing failures. *Anesthesiology* 38(1):85–87, 1973.
7. Steward DJ, Sloan IA: Additional pin-indexing failures. *Anesthesiology* 39(3):355, 1973.
8. Sawhney KK, Yoon YK: Erroneous labeling of a nitrous oxide cylinder. *Anesthesiology* 59:260, 1983.
9. Davis PD, Kenny GNC: *Basic physics and measurement in anesthesia,* ed 5, Oxford, 2003, Butterworth-Heinemann.
10. Dorsch JA, Dorsch SE: *Understanding anesthesia equipment,* ed 5, Philadelphia, 2008, Lippincott, Williams & Wilkins.
11. Eisenkraft JB: The anesthesia machine and workstation. In Ehrenwerth J, Eisenkraft JB, Berry JM, editors: *Anesthesia equipment: principles and applications,* Philadelphia, 2013, Saunders.
12. Compressed Gas Association: *Compressed gas cylinder valve outlet and inlet connections* (vol 1). ed 13, New York, 2013, The Association.
13. Compressed Gas Association: *Diameter-index safety system,* ed 6, New York, 2013, The Association.
14. Bowie E, Huffman LM: *The anesthesia machine: essentials for understanding,* Madison, 1985, Ohmeda, BOC Health Care.
15. ASTM F1850-00: Standard Specification for Particular Requirements for Anesthesia Workstations and Their Components, ASTM International, West Conshohocken, PA, 2005, www.astm.org. (Accessed 7 December 2015).
16. ADA Council on Scientific Affairs, ADA Council on Dental Practice: Nitrous oxide in the dental office. *J Am Dent Assoc* 128(3):364–365, 1997.
17. Council on Scientific Affairs: Acceptance program guidelines: nitrous oxide-oxygen conscious sedation systems, Chicago, 2000, American Dental Association.
18. National Fire Protection Association: NFPA99: Health Care Facilities Code, Quincy, 2015, The Association, www.nfpa.org/codes-and-standards. (Accessed 7 December 2015).
19. *Dentist's desk reference: materials, instruments and equipment,* Chicago, 1983, American Dental Association.
20. Fan PL: Letter to manufacturers of nitrous oxide scavenging systems and other interested parties, Sep 1, 1994. In *ADA guidelines for nitrous oxide scavenging systems,* Chicago, 1994, American Dental Association.

chapter 15

Inhalation Sedation: Techniques of Administration

CHAPTER OUTLINE

GENERAL DESCRIPTION
ADMINISTRATION
    Pretreatment Visit and Instructions
    Day of Appointment
    Subsequent Appointments
COMPARISON OF TECHNIQUES OF
ADMINISTRATION
    Constant Liter Flow Technique
    Constant O_2 Flow Technique

NORMAL DISTRIBUTION CURVE
TITRATION AND TIME
SIGNS AND SYMPTOMS OF
OVERSEDATION
    Clinical Indicators of Oversedation

The administration of nitrous oxide-oxygen (N_2O-O_2) for pharmacosedation is a very easy and straightforward procedure. It requires an approved sedation unit, a trained administrator, and a patient desiring sedation. Proper training conveys confidence to the patient and, as a result, an expectation of a successful outcome. Training, as defined by the American Dental Association guidelines, requires instruction in pain and anxiety control consisting of 14 hours of course content, including a clinical component during which competency in inhalation sedation technique is achieved.[1] Even though N_2O-O_2 is considered a very safe drug, a number of unpleasant and potentially dangerous complications can still develop. Therefore the person responsible for the administration of N_2O-O_2 must be aware of these potential problems, know how to prevent them from occurring, and know how to recognize and manage them.

Some operators insist on turning on a sedation unit to a fixed percentage of N_2O. This fixed percentage is either arbitrary or the one that was used at a previous appointment. This concept clearly violates the principle of titration, which allows for the correct amount (percentage) of N_2O-O_2 for the desired level of sedation. Titration, an important concept in the administration of any drug to a patient, is the primary guiding principle, along with monitoring the patient for depth of sedation. Titration for each appointment is necessary both to compensate for individual variation in patient response to N_2O and because patients may respond differently at each

appointment and may not require the same level of sedation for different procedures. The ability to quickly increase or decrease the flow of N_2O permits every patient to achieve the level of sedation that he or she and the administrator are seeking. It allows for comfortable sedation for those who are difficult to sedate and those who are easily affected by the gas.

The techniques described emphasize titration as the guiding principle to successful N_2O-O_2 administration for both the patient and the administrator. This will result in fewer adverse side effects (e.g., nausea, vomiting, or poor behavioral reactions) and an overall normal pleasant experience.

GENERAL DESCRIPTION

The technique of inhalation sedation for the cooperative adult patient (an apprehensive patient who willingly accepts the nasal hood) is as follows. Management of the more difficult patient, such as the child or adult with a disability or the pediatric patient, is described in Chapters 35 and 38.

1. A flow rate (liter per minute) of 100% oxygen (O_2) is established, and the nasal hood is placed on the patient's nose. The patient is instructed to self-adjust the hood as needed for comfort.
2. The appropriate flow rate is established while the patient is breathing 100% O_2. The bag is neither expanding nor shrinking in size, but remains uniform during breathing.

3. The percentage of N_2O is started, approximately 20% initially. The N_2O percentage is increased in approximately 10% increments every 60 seconds.

4. When the patient states that he or she feels pleasant and more relaxed, the ideal level of clinical sedation has been achieved. (*Note:* The "ideal" level of sedation being sought will vary from patient to patient and from doctor to doctor.)

5. Once the ideal level of sedation is achieved, local anesthetic may be administered (if necessary) and the planned dental/surgical procedure completed.

6. N_2O flow is terminated, and the patient is administered 100% O_2 at a flow rate equivalent to the established rate for this patient. This may be started earlier than the absolute completion of the procedure to ensure a more expedient recovery. O_2 is administered for minimally 3 to 5 minutes, or longer if clinical signs of sedation persist.

7. The patient may leave the dental office unescorted if he or she is, in the dentist's estimation, completely recovered from sedation.

The approach to the N_2O-O_2 sedation technique is divided into three phases: the induction phase (steps 1 to 4), the injection and treatment phase (step 5), and the recovery phase (steps 6 and 7).

ADMINISTRATION

The following description of the administration of N_2O-O_2 applies to the adult patient (teenager included) who willingly accepts the nasal hood, is able to breathe through the nose, and is able to sit in the dental chair without involuntary muscular movements interfering with the procedure. The technique of administration will differ slightly for a patient who has never before received N_2O-O_2. At appropriate points in the technique, these differences are explained.

Pretreatment Visit and Instructions

A patient who has a deep fear or phobia of dentistry may not be a candidate for N_2O-O_2 administration. N_2O-O_2 may or may not be effective in patients with severe fear and/or phobias. Whether the patient has a deep fear or phobia is best determined through an appointment for discussion and possible demonstration of the use of N_2O-O_2. Because fear of the unknown often leads to phobias, an appointment to discuss N_2O-O_2 procedures in advance can help identify potential candidates for its use. The ideal time to introduce an apprehensive patient to inhalation sedation for the first time is not at an appointment at which actual dental or surgical treatment is scheduled. A further increase in anxiety can occur if the dentist or hygienist attempts to use N_2O-O_2 without having previously described the technique. Even the first sight of the nasal hood might remind the patient of unpleasant experiences that have occurred in the past, such as nausea and vomiting after general anesthesia or a sense of suffocation produced by the nasal hood.

In the ideal situation, the dentist, recognizing the patient's need for N_2O-O_2 sedation (e.g., anxiety, medically compromised,

gagging), will discuss with the patient the reasons for selecting this technique and the benefits to be gained from its use, both for the dentist and for the patient. This appointment can be used for a "demonstration" of the N_2O-O_2 equipment and to allow the patient the opportunity to ask questions about the upcoming procedure. It is remarkable how this familiarization can help relieve fear and promote a positive interaction between the clinician and the patient.

It is unusual to find an adult patient who has not heard of or been given N_2O-O_2. *Laughing gas,* or so-called *sweet air,* is a common term to the lay public. Some may have had a previous unpleasant experience with it. It is important for these patients to know that they are not obligated to experience it again, but it may be worthwhile to explain that they could have been easily overdosed (they were not titrated) and that you are confident you can provide a better experience. In any event, this time spent with the patient without the concern of an actual procedure is often all that is needed to get the partnership with the patient that you are seeking. These patients can be, and often are, your best practice ambassadors.

In discussing with the patient what he or she can expect from the experience, it is crucial to present honesty and clarity in the preoperative and the operative appointment. Do not tell the patient what he or she will or will not feel during this experience because each patient may respond differently. Instead of informing the patient that "you will feel tingling in your fingers or toes," use a more open-ended statement, such as "you should feel more relaxed and at ease." Some patients who do not experience the suggested signs, such as tingling, will think that the N_2O-O_2 is not working for them or that something is wrong. It is better to be more vague and general in describing the clinical signs and symptoms of sedation. In a patient who, for religious, medical, or other personal reasons, does not use or like the effects of alcohol, comparing the actions of N_2O with those of alcohol or other drugs will make the patient less willing to try and accept it. For the sake of these patients and the patient who has had a personal negative experience with substance abuse, the comparison of N_2O and alcohol should be avoided.

At the conclusion of this initial visit, preoperative medications, such as prophylactic antibiotics, antianxiety drugs, or sleeping medication, may be prescribed. Oral antianxiety drugs are useful in the patient who becomes increasingly fearful as the dental appointment nears. Oral drugs help reduce these fears. However, care should be taken, especially in children, when giving concomitant sedation agents because synergistic effects with subsequent possibly dangerous levels of sedation may occur. Once in the dental office, the patient may then receive N_2O-O_2 for any additional sedation required during the dental treatment. Postoperative instructions can be given and financial matters handled before the patient is released.

Patients may have a light meal a few hours before an appointment for N_2O-O_2 administration. A heavy meal, particularly with children, should be avoided because this can often lead to nausea and vomiting. Conversely a patient who has had nothing to eat can also become nauseous.

Day of Appointment
Monitoring During Inhalation Sedation
The following is the recommended monitoring for inhalation sedation procedures:
1. Baseline vital signs, preoperatively
2. Verbal communication with patient
3. Vital signs recorded periodically during the procedure
4. Postoperative vital signs

Other monitors, such as the pretracheal stethoscope and the electrocardiogram (ECG), are considered optional in both the adult and pediatric patient whenever inhalation sedation is used as a sole technique. Pulse oximetry, although not mandatory or required, is relatively inexpensive and an excellent way to ensure that the patient is, in fact, adequately O_2 saturated. This is the surest way to confirm that all N_2O-O_2 equipment and anatomic systems are functioning properly. In all instances, the administrator of N_2O-O_2 must monitor the patient as per the requirements of the appropriate state or provincial dental regulatory body.

Preparation of the Equipment
Experts in the use of N_2O-O_2 met in 1995 at the request of the American Dental Association to consider the then-current use of N_2O-O_2 in the dental office.[2] One outgrowth of that meeting was the development of guidelines for equipment inspection and use. They are as follows.

On the day of the scheduled appointment, the dental assistant prepares the sedation unit by opening one O_2 and one N_2O cylinder. Compressed gas cylinders are opened by turning the knob on the top of the cylinder in a counterclockwise direction. Start by turning the knob only slightly, just barely opening the cylinder, permitting the pressure gauge to rise slowly. Once the pressure reaches its maximum level, the knob may be turned freely until fully open. The purpose of slowly opening the cylinder is to minimize any increase in internal temperature within the reducing valve as gas under high pressure rushes from the cylinder into the reducing valve.

After the cylinders have been prepared, the nasal hood is checked to be certain that it is clean, and other equipment (tubes and reservoir bag) is checked for leaks.

Preparation of the Patient
1. *Request that the patient visit the restroom and void if necessary before the start of the sedative procedure.*

> **COMMENT:** Patients receiving N_2O-O_2 sedation do not urinate any more frequently than other persons; however, more urine is produced when a person is in the supine position than when standing. In addition, the patient who has to urinate while receiving N_2O-O_2 must first be unsedated (given 100% O_2), permitted to visit the restroom, and then resedated, a process requiring approximately 10 minutes. This time may be saved by requesting the patient to void, if necessary, before treatment commences.

2. *Review the medical history questionnaire and record preoperative vital signs before the start of the N_2O-O_2.*

> **COMMENT:** Vital signs to be recorded include blood pressure, heart rate and rhythm, and respiratory rate. Vital signs may be recorded by the dentist, the dental hygienist, the dental assistant, or a nurse.

3. *If the patient wears contact lenses, the lenses should be removed before the start of inhalation sedation.*

> **COMMENT:** Gas leaks from the mask around the bridge of the nose may produce drying of the eyes with potential irritation of the patient.

Technique of Administration
1. *Position patient in comfortable, reclined position in dental chair.*

> **COMMENT:** The preferred position (Fig. 15.1) is first a consideration of patient comfort. The partially reclined position may be used, if necessary, for the patient's

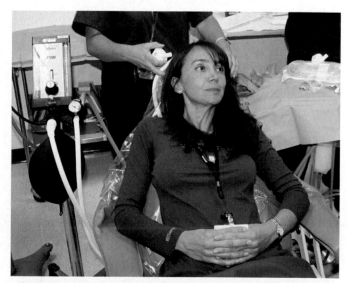

Figure 15.1 Patient is positioned in a comfortable, reclined position.

comfort or the convenience of the dentist during the procedure. The upright position is not recommended unless essential for the procedure, such as when taking impressions or radiographs.

2. *Position the inhalation sedation unit.*

COMMENT: This procedure applies only to the use of the portable inhalation sedation unit (Fig. 15.2), as opposed to the fixed, central systems commonly found in dental offices. The N$_2$O-O$_2$ unit should always be placed behind the patient, out of his or her line of sight. A positive placebo response will occur in some patients receiving N$_2$O-O$_2$, but if the patient can see the unit and watch as the administrator adjusts the controls, this response can be negated.

3. *Start the flow of O$_2$ at 6 L/min, place the nasal hood over the patient's nose, and remind the patient to breathe through the nose.*

COMMENT: Placing the nasal hood on the patient (Fig. 15.3) after starting the flow of O$_2$ will prevent the patient from feeling suffocated when breathing through the nose if the O$_2$ flow is not begun before placement of the nasal hood.

Although it may appear ridiculous to remind a patient to breathe through the nose once the nasal hood has been positioned, this is a very important part of the procedure. Many persons will continue to breathe through their mouths unless they are specifically reminded not to do so, and this contaminates the environment with exhaled N$_2$O.

4. *Secure the nasal hood.*

COMMENT: The nasal hood usually has two hoses coming from the N$_2$O-O$_2$ unit. These are placed around the sides of the dental chair, and the nasal hood is secured by adjusting the slip ring behind the headrest (Fig. 15.4). The patient is asked to hold the nasal hood in a comfortable position as this is done. Care must be taken in adjusting the nasal hood because one of the tubes is often pulled more than the other, making the nasal hood tilt to one side.

If the nasal hood has only one hose, it is placed over the patient's forehead and secured.

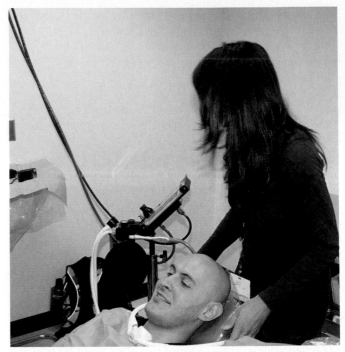

Figure 15.2 Inhalation sedation unit is best placed behind the patient, out of line of sight.

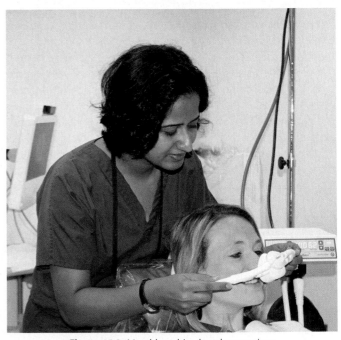

Figure 15.3 Nasal hood is placed on patient.

The nasal hood should not be too tight or too loose. The patient should have some lateral and up-and-down movement of the head. The *patient* serves as the final check as to whether the nasal hood is secure.

Leaks develop on occasion around an ill-fitting mask. Nasal hoods are available in a variety of sizes. The size is checked before the start of the procedure. The nasal hood used should fit the patient's nose. An overly small

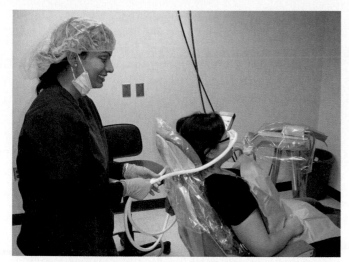

Figure 15.4 Nasal hood is secured by adjusting slip ring behind back of chair.

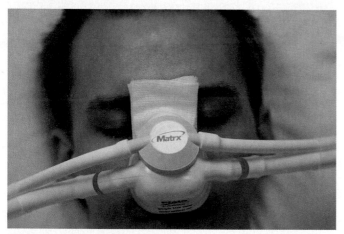

Figure 15.5 Folded 2 × 2-inch gauze on bridge of nose prevents leaks.

or overly large mask will leak. Leaks may also develop with masks of the appropriate size. Most often, these leaks occur around the bridge of the nose, with the patient complaining of "air" exhaled into his or her eyes. Permitting the patient to adjust the nasal hood is often all that is needed to correct this situation. If this simple solution is ineffective, the hood is removed, a folded 2-inch square gauze pad is placed over the bridge of the nose, and the nasal hood is replaced. This usually seals the leak (Fig. 15.5).

When a scavenging nasal hood (recommended) is used, the exhalation tubes must be connected to the vacuum system. It is important to adjust the vacuum so that the patient is able to exhale and inhale comfortably.[2] If the vacuum is too weak, the patient may experience difficulty in breathing out, and if the vacuum is too forceful, the patient may not receive any N_2O-O_2 because the gases are rapidly sucked from the nasal hood into the overly efficient vacuum system.

5. *Determine proper flow rate for the patient.*

COMMENT: This is one of the most important steps in the successful use of N_2O-O_2 sedation. The patient must be able to breathe comfortably at this point, before the start of N_2O flow, to be comfortable throughout the procedure.

At the onset of the procedure, a 6-L/min flow of 100% O_2 is initiated for the adult (3 or 4 L/min for smaller pediatric patients), the nasal hood is placed on the patient, and the patient instructed to breathe only through the nose. In most adult patients (and virtually all children), this minute volume will be more than adequate for the patient to breathe comfortably. Breathing comfortably implies that the patient is able to take a normal breath and feel as though the volume of "air" is adequate, as opposed to the patient who states that the machine is not delivering enough "air," causing him or her difficulty in breathing. I have never seen the opposite situation, in which the patient states that there is too much "air" delivered.

It is impossible to predict which patient will require a minute volume greater than 6 L/min. Larger patients may be quite comfortable at 6 L/min, whereas petite patients may require higher flow rates. Persons who participate in endurance sports, such as marathon running, swimming, and bicycle racing, are more likely to require larger minute volumes. In addition, persons with chronic obstructive pulmonary disease (COPD), heart failure (HF), or partial nasal obstruction may also require larger volumes.

The patient is asked, "Can you breathe normally?" or "Are you comfortable?" If the answer is Yes, the flow rate is left at 6 L/min; if the patient requests a greater volume, the O_2 flow rate is increased to 7 L/min and allowed to remain there for a minute, and the same question is asked. This process is repeated until the patient becomes comfortable. The appearance of the reservoir bag is a reliable indicator of appropriate flow rate (see later).

It is not uncommon for a patient to require a higher flow rate at the beginning of N_2O-O_2 sedation. This is especially so for the patient receiving N_2O-O_2 sedation for the first time. Placing the nasal hood on the patient's nose may pose a subconscious threat, and the individual may overcompensate by breathing more deeply and/or rapidly until satisfied that he or she will not suffocate. This same phenomenon is seen in early training of SCUBA (Self-Contained Underwater Breathing Apparatus) divers. After the N_2O-O_2 provides sedation at this elevated flow rate, the dentist might return the flow rate to the original 6 L/min (without telling the patient). In almost all cases, the patient will be unable to detect the change.

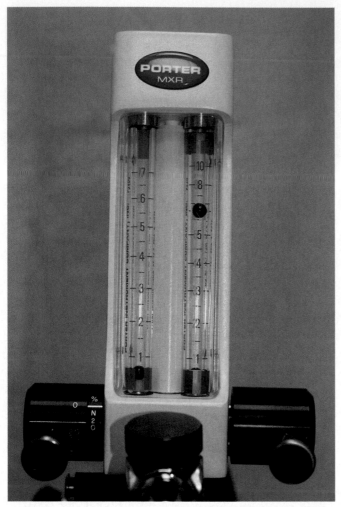

Figure 15.6 Establishing minimum O_2 flow before the start of titration.

The reservoir bag that remains partially inflated (deflated) (Fig. 15.7, *A*), deflating and inflating partially with each breath, usually indicates that the minute volume is adequate (the bag remains partially inflated throughout the procedure) and that the seal of the nasal hood is tight (inflates and deflates with each breath).

A bag that remains totally deflated (Fig. 15.7, *B*) may indicate one of the following:

- The minute volume of gas is inadequate; in this situation, the patient will usually complain of not receiving enough "air."
- The nasal hood has relatively large leaks; in this case the patient will have no difficulty breathing because any lack of gas from the N_2O-O_2 unit is compensated for by ambient air entering through the leaks. The patient may also say, "Air is blowing into my eyes every time I breathe."
- The vacuum on the scavenging system is too high, forcing gases directly out of the nasal hood into the vacuum system. The patient will usually complain of not receiving enough "air."

A bag that is overly inflated (Fig. 15.7, *C*), looking like a balloon about to burst, may indicate one of the following:

- The minute volume is too great for the patient. Although an unlikely occurrence, the patient might complain about an inability to breathe against the rapid flow of air into the nasal hood.
- The hoses leading from the sedation unit have become kinked (occluded). In this case the patient will complain about an inability to breathe comfortably through the nasal hood.

Of these two situations involving an overly inflated bag, the second—occluded tubes—is the more likely to occur.

7. *Begin titration of N_2O.*

Establishing the minimal flow rate is important because if it is assumed that the patient can tolerate 6 L/min comfortably but actually cannot, then this individual will probably never become comfortably sedated with N_2O-O_2 during the procedure. This step is always carried out with the patient receiving 100% O_2 (Fig. 15.6).

6. *Observe the reservoir bag.*

COMMENT: The appearance of the reservoir bag indicates the respiratory depth and rate. The reservoir bag on the sedation unit will provide an indication of the seal on the nasal hood in addition to allowing a determination of the adequacy of the minute volume of gas delivered to the patient. However, the patient is always the most reliable indicator of the signs and symptoms of inhalation sedation, including the seal of the hood and the adequacy of minute volume.

COMMENT: Once an adequate minute volume of gas flow for the patient has been determined, the administration of N_2O may begin. Two methods of administering N_2O to the patient are presented, both of which are quite acceptable. In the first, the total liter flow of gases (N_2O and O_2) per minute is kept constant throughout the procedure (**the constant liter flow technique**). In the second method, the liter flow of O_2 remains constant (**the constant O_2 flow technique**), and the volume of N_2O is adjusted. Advantages and disadvantages of both techniques are discussed. These techniques are used with inhalation sedation units that possess separate control knobs for the N_2O and the O_2 flows. On inhalation sedation units with a mixing dial, the operator needs only to adjust the dial to the desired concentration of N_2O or O_2. These units operate by keeping the total volume of gas flow constant throughout the procedure (constant liter flow technique).

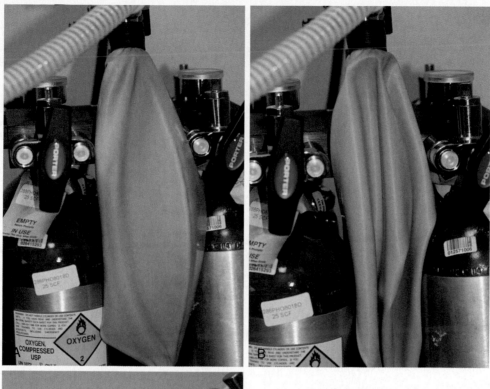

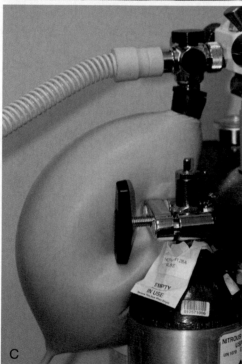

Figure 15.7 A, Partially inflated reservoir bag usually indicates adequate seal and minute volume.
B, Deflated reservoir bag usually indicates either a leak around the nasal hood or a deficient minute
volume. **C,** Distended reservoir bag indicates either an overly large minute volume or occluded
breathing tubes.

In all situations, regardless of the type of unit or the technique used, the initial percentage of N$_2$O should be approximately 20%. With the mixing dial units, the administrator needs merely to adjust the percentage dial to either 20% N$_2$O or 80% O$_2$. Flows of the individual gases are automatically adjusted. If a 6-L/min O$_2$ flow is adequate for the patient, when the dial is adjusted to 20% N$_2$O, the N$_2$O flowmeter will read 1.2 L/min and the O$_2$ flowmeter will decrease from 6 to 4.8 L/min.

When operating a unit with individual control knobs for N$_2$O and O$_2$ and using the *constant liter flow* technique, the administrator increases the N$_2$O flow to 1 L/min and then decreases the O$_2$ flow rate to 5 L/min (Fig. 15.8). This produces an N$_2$O percentage of 16.6% (1 L/min N$_2$O /6 L/min total gas flow). In the *constant O$_2$ flow* technique, the O$_2$ flow is left at its initial rate (6 L/min in this case) and the N$_2$O flow is increased to 1 L/min. The N$_2$O concentration is 14.3% (Fig. 15.9).

In my experience, many persons learning to use N$_2$O-O$_2$ inhalation sedation have difficulty determining the concentrations of the gases delivered. One of the most common misconceptions is that the liter flow of the N$_2$O is equal to the percentage of the gas delivered. For example, a 2-L/min flow of N$_2$O actually does not equal 20%. The only situation in which this would be the case is when the total gas flow (O$_2$ + N$_2$O) is 10 L/min. The percentage of a gas delivered through the N$_2$O-O$_2$ unit can readily be determined by dividing the liter flow per minute of the gas by the total volume of both gases delivered:

$$\text{Percentage N}_2\text{O} = \frac{\text{L/min N}_2\text{O}}{\text{L/min O}_2 + \text{L/min N}_2\text{O}}$$

$$\text{Percentage O}_2 = \frac{\text{L/min O}_2}{\text{L/min O}_2 + \text{L/min N}_2\text{O}}$$

Table 15.1 provides an easy method of determining the percentage of N$_2$O delivered at common flow rates.

8. *Observe the patient.*

COMMENT: The patient breathes this concentration of N$_2$O for approximately 60 to 90 seconds. During this time, the administrator should observe the patient, looking for

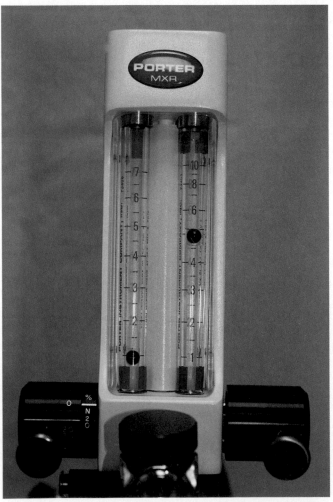

Figure 15.8 Constant liter flow technique: O$_2$ flow decreases 1 L/min to 5 L/min, N$_2$O flow increases 1 L/min to 1 L/min, and N$_2$O percentage equals 16.6%.

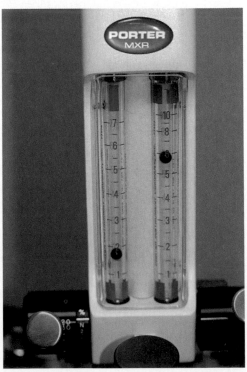

Figure 15.9 Constant O$_2$ flow technique: O$_2$ flow remains constant at 6 L/min, N$_2$O flow is raised 1 L/min, and N$_2$O percentage equals 14.3%.

| Table 15.1 | N₂O Percentage Chart | | | | | | | | | |

L/MIN O₂	L/min N₂O									
	1	2	3	4	5	6	7	8	9	10
10	9	17	23	29	33	38	41	44	47	50
9	10	18	25	31	36	40	44	47	50	53
8	11	20	27	33	38	43	47	50	53	56
7	13	22	30	36	42	46	50	53	56	59
6	14	25	33	40	45	50	54	57	60	63
5	17	19	38	44	50	55	58	62	64	67
4	20	33	43	50	56	60	64	67	69	71
3	25	40	50	57	63	67	70	73	75	77
2	33	50	60	67	71	75	78	80	82	83
1	50	67	75	80	83	86	88	89	90	91

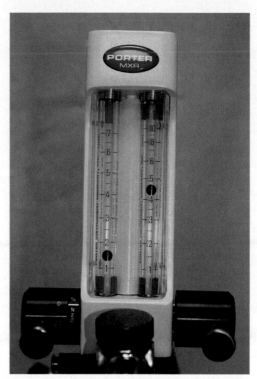

Figure 15.10 Constant liter flow technique; subsequent changes in gas flow every 60 to 90 seconds are a 0.5-L/min O₂ decrease and 0.5-L/min N₂O increase.

signs and symptoms of sedation. At the end of the 60- to 90-second period, the patient is asked, "What are you feeling?" It is important to ask open-ended questions that require the patient to respond with more than a simple Yes or No. "What are you feeling?" requires the patient to answer in sentences, stating "I feel no different from before," or "I feel a little lightheaded." The question, "Do you feel good?" brings responses of only Yes or No.

The typical patient receiving approximately 20% N₂O will have little or no effect after 1 to 2 minutes. In this case the titration of the N₂O continues.

Two points that may appear minor must be mentioned:

1. *During the titration of N₂O to a patient, the administrator or assistant must remain by the patient at all times, in visual, physical, or verbal contact.* Otherwise, the patient may think that he or she has been left alone during the procedure and may panic, remove the nasal hood, and become agitated. Visual, physical, or verbal contact with the patient prevents this.

2. *The patient's legs should be uncrossed during sedation.* The significance of this lies in the fact that once sedated, the patient rarely moves at all. Should the legs be crossed for prolonged periods, circulation of blood to the periphery may be compromised and paresthesia may develop. As blood flow returns, the feeling of hyperesthesia (e.g., "pins and needles") will be quite uncomfortable.

9. *Continue titration of N₂O.*

COMMENT: If the initial concentration of N₂O proves inadequate, the level of N₂O is increased. Following the initial level of 20% N₂O, all subsequent increases will be smaller, approximately 10%.

With the *mixing dial units*, the administrator simply turns the percentage dial to 30% N₂O (or 70% O₂). The machine will automatically adjust the individual gas flows.

In the *constant liter flow technique*, all subsequent increases in N₂O and decreases in O₂ will be 0.5-L/min changes. Thus with a 6-L/min flow, the N₂O is increased to 1.5 L/min and the O₂ is decreased to 4.5 L/min, giving a concentration of 33% N₂O (Fig. 15.10).

With the *constant O₂ flow technique*, the O₂ remains at 6 L/min and the N₂O is increased to 2 L/min, an N₂O concentration of 28.6% (Fig. 15.11).

10. *Observe the patient.*

COMMENT: Questioning the patient after 60 to 90 seconds at approximately 30% N₂O is more likely to provide positive responses about the clinical effects of N₂O. Table 15.2 lists the usual sequence of signs and symptoms of N₂O-O₂ inhalation sedation. Following are the more common signs and symptoms:

• *Lightheadedness:* The first clinical evidence of the effect of N₂O is usually the feeling of lightheadedness. Many patients, having never received N₂O, may describe this as dizziness, which they may find uncomfortable. The administrator should immediately tell the patient that this feeling is normal but transient and will pass as the concentration of N$_2$O is increased. The feeling of lightheadedness develops at a level that is clinically inadequate for the management of most patients.

- *Tingling (paresthesia) sensation of arms, legs, or oral cavity:* After the sensation of lightheadedness, the typical patient will describe a sensation of tingling in the arms, legs, or oral cavity. This symptom also develops at a level that is still inadequate to permit the ideal management of the fearful patient. However, advantage may be taken of the paresthesia that develops. Dental procedures involving soft tissues (i.e., scaling, curettage) can usually be completed without the use of local anesthesia and with minimal, if any, discomfort. The patient receiving N$_2$O-O$_2$ may state that the "pain" is still felt but that it no longer hurts. In other words, the nature of the discomfort has been altered from a sharp, knifelike pain to a duller, much more tolerable one. Similar to opioids (e.g., narcotics), nitrous oxide "separates pain from suffering."[3-5]

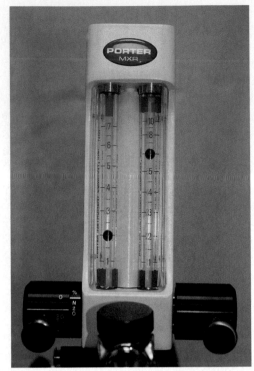

Figure 15.11 In constant O$_2$ flow technique, subsequent changes in gas flow are a 1-L/min increase in N$_2$O every 60 to 90 seconds.

Advantage may also be taken of the paresthesia developing in the patient's arms during venipuncture and intravenous sedation. N$_2$O -induced paresthesia will make venipuncture more tolerable for the patient fearful of injections.

Another area of medicine in which peripheral paresthesia is of value is in surgery of the foot. Injections of local anesthetic or steroids into the sole of the foot are extremely painful. The use of N$_2$O-O$_2$ sedation and the ensuing anesthesia will make this procedure significantly more tolerable.

- *Feeling of warmth, floating, or heaviness:* The next symptoms that develop usually indicate entry into a level of sedation

Table 15.2	Signs and Symptoms of N$_2$O-O$_2$ Sedation	
PHASE	**SYMPTOMS**	**SIGNS**
1. Early to ideal sedation	Lightheadedness (dizziness) Tingling of hands and feet Wave of warmth Feeling of vibration throughout body Numbness of hands and feet Numbness of soft tissues of oral cavity Feeling of euphoria Feeling of lightness or heaviness of extremities Analgesia	Blood pressure and heart rate elevated slightly early in procedure, then return to baseline values Respirations are normal, smooth Peripheral vasodilation Flushing of extremities, face Decreased muscle tone as anxiety decreases (arms and legs relax)
2. Heavier sedation/slight oversedation	Hearing, especially of distant sounds, becomes more acute Visual images become confused (patterns on ceiling begin to move) Sleepiness Sweating increases Laughing, crying Dreaming Nausea	Increased movement Increased heart rate, blood pressure Increased rate of respiration Increased sweating Possibly lacrimation
3. Oversedation	Nausea	Vomiting Loss of consciousness (unlikely with at least 20% O$_2$)

at which the patient is either at or near the ideal for treatment. The ideal sedation level was described as a stage at which the patient is relaxed and comfortable and at which the administrator is also relaxed and able to treat the patient without compromising the quality of dental care delivered. This ideal level varies from dentist to dentist according to the patient's needs, the training and experience of the dentist and the staff, and the desires of the dentist.

The clinical sensations of heaviness, warmth, and floating usually indicate that the patient is approaching the desired level. Warmth develops first in most cases, with the patient stating that he or she feels warmer. Observation will show the patient to be more flushed, a finding most noticeable on the patient's forehead, where perspiration may be observed. The patient's hands and arms may also feel warmer. A few patients may begin to perspire heavily, a situation that may be uncomfortable. If this occurs, the percentage of N_2O should be lowered by approximately 5% (a 0.5-L/min decrease in N_2O and a 0.5-L/min increase in O_2) to attempt to decrease perspiration without significantly altering the sedative action of the N_2O. A feeling of heaviness or floating may also be noted. The patient may state that his or her arms and legs feel either quite heavy (so heavy that they cannot be moved) or extremely light (so light that they float).

Because clinical signs and symptoms may vary considerably from patient to patient, I rarely describe these symptoms in detail to patients before the procedure. I have found it useful to be purposefully vague, describing the effects of N_2O-O_2 sedation in general terms. Patients are told only that they will feel more relaxed and comfortable. When patients have been told specifically that they will experience lightheadedness, tingling, numbness, warmth, and heaviness, it has sometimes been observed that they become upset if any of these symptoms fail to develop, as indeed may be the case.

The administrator always observes the patient throughout the sedative technique. Watching the apprehensive patient begin to experience the effects of N_2O-O_2 is of great benefit in determining the proper level of sedation. As mentioned, a patient who has never before received N_2O-O_2 sedation will prove a little more difficult to sedate than one who has. Patients who have previously achieved ideal sedation (have "been there") can simply tell the administrator when they are "there" again. The patient for whom N_2O-O_2 is used for the first time finds it somewhat more difficult to gauge the proper level of sedation.

Careful observation of the patient aids in determining this. The appearance of apprehensive patients is described in Chapter 4. They do not appear comfortable when seated in the dental chair. Hands may firmly clench the armrest in the so-called *"white-knuckle" syndrome* (Fig. 15.12, *A*), and their legs may seem quite stiff. As sedation develops, the patient's arms and legs relax, and he or she eventually achieves a "sedated look" (Fig. 15.12, *B*).

The verbal response of the patient will also change as the effect of N_2O increases. Early in the procedure, the patient may state that he or she feels relaxed; however, this may be said in a very rapid, unrelaxed

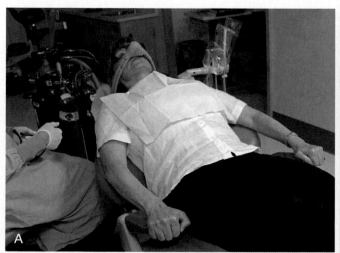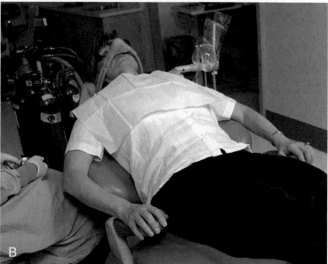

Figure 15.12 A, White-knuckle syndrome exhibited by apprehensive patient at start of procedure. **B,** Relaxation of hands is commonly observed when patient becomes sedated. (From Darby ML, Walsh MM: *Dental hygiene: theory and practice,* ed 3, St Louis, Saunders, 2010.)

manner. In fact, the patient does feel somewhat relaxed (compared with the feeling on first entering the dental office). However, should the administrator mistake this level of relaxation for the ideal sedative state and attempt to treat the patient, the result would likely prove to be less than adequate. As sedation increases, the patient's responses slow down, with an increasing lag time observed between questions and the patient's response to them. It appears almost as though the patient experiences difficulty in phrasing replies. The patient's state is now more near the ideal.

The state produced by N_2O-O_2 should not be compared with that of alcohol unless the patient volunteers the comparison spontaneously. To compare the effects of N_2O-O_2 with alcohol to patients who do not consume alcohol for religious, medical, or other personal reasons will probably make them less likely to want to try the technique.

11. *Begin dental treatment.*

> **COMMENT:** The patient appears quite relaxed at this point. Titration has continued, with approximately 10% increases in the level of N_2O until the signs and symptoms associated with adequate sedation have been noted. Despite this, the only way of determining with absolute accuracy whether the proper sedative level has been achieved is to begin the planned treatment and observe the patient's response.

If the planned treatment proceeds without any overt signs of discomfort from the patient, it can be assumed that sedation is successful. However, once the procedure begins, it is not unusual for the patient to make movements, especially when potentially traumatic procedures, such as the administration of local anesthetics, are carried out. If the movements are significant or disruptive, the procedure should be halted and the level of sedation increased by approximately 5% N_2O. This apparent lack of adequate sedation can easily be explained when it is realized that the signs and symptoms of ideal sedation observed earlier were produced while N_2O-O_2 was administered to a patient who was merely sitting in the dental chair. Placing a local anesthetic syringe into a fearful patient's mouth raises his or her anxiety level considerably, potentially to a point beyond which the concentration of N_2O-O_2 inhaled can effectively manage the patient's fears. Halting the procedure and increasing the percentage of N_2O slightly (5%) usually eliminates this problem.

Once pain control (via local anesthetic) has been obtained, the procedure usually continues with little difficulty. However, the patient may experience periods when the level of sedation may lessen and conversely when the level becomes too intense. N_2O, because of its analgesic and sedative qualities, is excellent in combination with local anesthetic to achieve cooperation for most patients in a dental or surgical environment.

One of the prime benefits of inhalation sedation with N_2O-O_2 is the ability to tailor the sedation to the needs of the patient. The administrator and assistant must continually observe the patient for any indication of changes in level of sedation. The level of sedation may become too light when a particularly traumatic part of the procedure is started. For example, the patient may be relaxed until the handpiece is placed in the mouth and turned on. In some patients, the sound of the handpiece is quite anxiety provoking. At this point, the patient may tell the administrator that the effect of the N_2O is gone, as though the machine were turned off. As before, the dental procedure should be temporarily halted, the percentage of N_2O increased by approximately 5% (or more, if needed), the patient resedated, and the procedure resumed.

A sedative level that has been particularly effective during therapy may become too intense when the procedure is finished (e.g., a lull in dental treatment while the assistant prepares a material for the doctor) and the patient's anxiety level lessens. The percentage of N_2O inhaled by the patient is too great for the now-diminished anxiety level, and the patient becomes overly sedated (e.g., less responsive). Management of this situation simply requires a decrease of the N_2O flow by approximately 5%. Within 30 to 60 seconds, the patient will become less sedated.

12. *Observe the patient and inhalation sedation unit during the procedure.*

> **COMMENT:** Throughout the procedure, the patient and the inhalation sedation unit must be observed by the dentist, hygienist, or assistant. The level of sedation sought with N_2O-O_2 is such that communication between the administrator or assistant and the patient is readily achieved. The patient should be able to respond to any requests or questions posed. Lack of response to any command should indicate to the staff that dental treatment be terminated immediately and the patient evaluated. In most cases a decrease in the N_2O by 5% to 10% quickly brings about a response from the patient. The assistant or dentist should also observe the N_2O-O_2 unit periodically to reconfirm that the gases are indeed still flowing. All units have fail-safe devices designed to prevent the inadvertent administration of 100% N_2O, and these devices are usually quite effective. However, very rare situations have occurred

in which these devices have failed and patients have received 100% N_2O, often with catastrophic consequences.[6,7] Visual observation of the N_2O-O_2 unit will prevent this from occurring.

13. *Terminate the flow of N_2O.*

> **COMMENT:** At the completion of treatment or of that portion of it requiring sedation, the N_2O flow will be terminated. In all instances, the O_2 will be returned to the original flow rate determined at the start of the procedure. (This will not be necessary, of course, in the constant O_2 flow technique.) The patient is permitted to breathe 100% O_2 for not less than 3 to 5 minutes. Longer periods may be necessary should the patient exhibit any clinical signs or symptoms of sedation at the end of this period. There is no formula for determining the length of time to breathe 100% O_2, but for most patients, the longer the N_2O-O_2 sedation procedure is, the greater the length of time is required to reverse the sedative effects.

N_2O is not titrated "out of the patient" at the end of the procedure the way it must be done at the induction of sedation. The O_2 flow is increased to its original L/min level and the N_2O flow turned to 0 L/min (0%). It is suggested that the reservoir bag not be emptied of any residual gas when the N_2O flow is terminated; the thought is that the reservoir bag contains some N_2O that will contaminate the atmosphere.

The proper time to terminate the flow of N_2O varies from patient to patient. For example, in the extremely fearful patient whose anxieties relate to all aspects of dental or surgical treatment, it is advisable to continue the N_2O flow until the entire procedure is completed. However, in the more typical patient, whose apprehensions about dentistry are more specific, such as the administration of local anesthesia or the sound or feel of the handpiece, it is possible to terminate the N_2O flow after the traumatic element of treatment is completed but before the end of the entire procedure. There are several benefits to the early termination of the N_2O flow, especially when the duration of treatment has been prolonged.

When the N_2O flow is terminated before the end of a long procedure (in excess of 1 hour), discharge of the patient from the office is hastened. Rather than waiting until completion of the procedure to remove the N_2O and start the 100% O_2 flow, the dentist elects to administer 100% O_2 after completing the preparation of the teeth but before placing the restorations. The dentist or assistant will increase the O_2 flow to its original value and turn off the N_2O. This can be done without the patient's awareness, if possible. The reason for this apparent subterfuge is that when asked how they feel, many patients, unaware that the N_2O has been turned off and that they have been breathing 100% O_2 for many minutes, will state that they are still as relaxed as they were before N_2O was terminated. There is a 15% to 20% positive placebo response for most drugs,[8] and if approached carefully, this response may be used to advantage in many N_2O-O_2 patients. In the event that the placebo response does not occur in a patient, the patient will simply state that the effect of the N_2O is no longer felt, to which the dentist will reply that it has been turned off because the procedure is almost completed.

For the more apprehensive patient or for shorter procedures, N_2O-O_2 may be administered for the entire treatment. On completion, the same procedure of returning the O_2 flow to its original levels and of turning off the N_2O is carried out. The patient inhales 100% O_2 for not less than 3 to 5 minutes.

14. *Discharge the patient.*

> **COMMENT:** Determination of recovery from the effects of inhalation sedation is quite important because in most cases the patients will be dismissed from the office and be allowed to resume their normal activities without any prohibitions. For this reason, the dentist must be absolutely certain that recovery is complete before considering discharge of the patient. Not all patients receiving inhalation sedation with N_2O-O_2 will recover adequately enough to permit their discharge from the office without an escort.

Because it is common practice to permit most patients to leave the office unescorted after inhalation sedation and to operate a motor vehicle or other potentially dangerous machinery, valid objective criteria must be used to determine the degree of recovery. Several factors are used in evaluating the recovery process: response of the patient to questioning, vital signs, and a test for motor coordination.

The response of the patient to questioning is the primary determinant of recovery from sedation. However, because this is a purely subjective response, other, more valid (from a medicolegal standpoint), objective criteria should also be used. The patient has, at this point in the procedure, received 100% O_2 for at least 3 to 5 minutes. This is adequate to bring about an almost total reversal of symptoms in most patients. Longer periods may be necessary in some patients, particularly

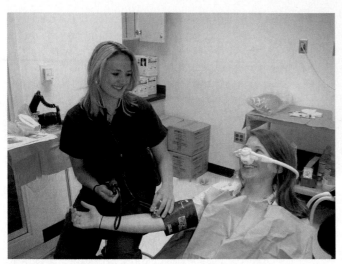

Figure 15.13 Vital signs are valuable adjuncts in the evaluation of recovery from sedation.

those who received N_2O-O_2 for a longer duration. The reason for insisting on a minimum of 3 to 5 minutes of 100% O_2 at the end of the procedure is to decrease the possibility of diffusion hypoxia. Diffusion hypoxia can occur when the N_2O exits through the lungs at a much faster rate than the nitrogen (N_2) that replaces it, thereby diluting and reducing the O_2 supply and blood saturation. Diffusion hypoxia is discussed further in Chapter 18.

The position of the patient is altered from the supine or semisupine (during dental treatment) to a more upright one as recovery continues. The nasal hood remains in position at this time. The patient is asked what he or she is feeling. Any reply other than "I feel perfectly normal" or "I feel the way I did when I arrived in the office" indicates the need for additional O_2. The nasal hood, providing O_2, should be left on the patient for an additional 2 to 3 minutes, and the question then repeated. The patient should not be discharged while any signs or symptoms of sedation remain. In those cases in which N_2O-O_2 was used in combination with other sedation techniques (oral, rectal, intranasal, intramuscular, or intravenous), the patient must have a responsible adult in attendance to escort him or her from the office.

Vital signs are valuable adjuncts in the evaluation of recovery from sedation (Fig. 15.13). They are objective parameters that indicate the state of function of the patient's cardiorespiratory system. Vital signs to be measured and recorded on the sedation record include blood pressure, heart rate and rhythm, and respiratory rate. It must be understood that vital signs recorded after the procedure will not be exactly the same as those recorded preoperatively or even those obtained at the patient's preliminary visit to the office. Fluctuation

in either direction is normal. Parameters that may be useful in determining the degree of recovery following sedation are the following:

- Blood pressure: ±20 mm Hg/10 mm Hg from baseline
- Heart rate and rhythm: ±15 beats/min from baseline; same rhythm as baseline
- Respirations: ±3 breaths/min from baseline

Variations in vital signs beyond these parameters are normal, or they may indicate a residual effect of the drugs. There may be no correlation between the changed vital signs and the use of inhalation sedation. Significant alteration in one or more of the vital signs should be evaluated before the patient is discharged.

Another modified neurologic test such as touching the tip of the nose with the index finger can indicate recovery. A most valuable criterion in determining recovery from inhalation sedation will be an evaluation of the patient's motor coordination called the *Trieger test*. This test is an objective measurement of the patient's ability to perform fine motor movements. The test was originally introduced in 1941 as the Bender Gestalt test and was used as an adjunct in the diagnosis and psychotherapy of organic brain damage in children.[9] In 1967 Dr. Norman Trieger modified the original test by selecting one figure and replacing its solid lines with dots (Figs. 15.14 and 15.15). The adaptation of this test for measuring recovery from anesthesia and sedation is based on the fact that fatigue and central nervous system (CNS)-depressant drugs exaggerate psychomotor dysfunction.[10] Disturbance in motor coordination is determined by successive trials on the test by the same individual.

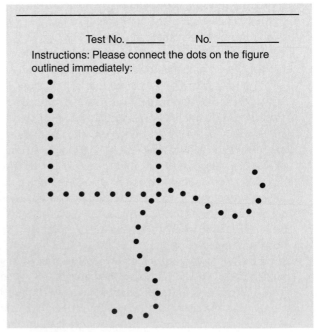

Figure 15.14 Trieger test for motor coordination.

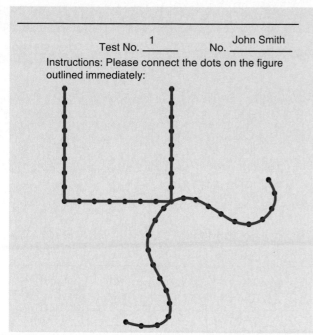

Test No. _____ 1 _____   No. _____ John Smith _____

Instructions: Please connect the dots on the figure outlined immediately:

Figure 15.15 Baseline Trieger test. All dots are connected and quality of lines is good.

The patient is requested to complete the test preoperatively. This test provides a baseline with which subsequent tests are compared. The test is supported on a firm surface (e.g., clipboard), and the patient is asked to carefully connect all of the dots. Scoring of the test is based on the number of dots that are missed completely. Two other factors that may be evaluated are (1) the time required for the patient to complete the test (e.g., 10 seconds) and (2) the general quality of the lines (i.e., straight, wavy, or erratic).

After the administration of 100% O_2 and the patient's subjective response that he or she feels normal, the postsedation Trieger test is administered. The patient is returned to the same position he or she was in for the preoperative test and is reminded to carefully complete the test by connecting all the dots; the results are then evaluated. The patient may miss more or fewer dots than preoperatively; however, the numbers should be close. Seven missed dots after sedation with five dots missed preoperatively is not significant, provided the time and quality of the lines are approximately the same as they were earlier.

Use of the Trieger test with patients *during* their sedation procedure is interesting. The degree of motor dysfunction evident at this time is often quite significant. In Trieger's original study, return to the baseline level occurred within 2 to 4 minutes after the termination of the N_2O.[11] If the postsedation Trieger test demonstrates a residual effect of N_2O, the patient should recover for several more minutes and then retake the Trieger test.

When it has been determined to the administrator's satisfaction that the patient has fully recovered from the effects of the N_2O-O_2, the nasal hood is removed and the patient is returned to the upright position and permitted to stand. At this point, it is important for a member of the office staff (e.g., assistant) to stand in front of the patient so that if the patient becomes dizzy or his or her legs feel weak on standing (possible postural [orthostatic] hypotension), the staff member can provide support and return the patient to the chair, preventing possible injury. This is not more likely to occur with the use of N_2O-O_2 than with other sedation techniques or when no sedation is used. It is merely good practice to be prepared for this potentially dangerous situation that can develop in any patient following prolonged recumbency (the time required varies from patient to patient) or in patients receiving certain drugs, especially antihypertensives.

It is not unusual for a patient to feel normal while seated in the dental chair and then lightheaded upon first standing. If this happens, the patient should be placed back in the chair, O_2 administered for several more minutes, and the patient then allowed to try to stand again. The patient should never be permitted to leave the office if any signs or symptoms of sedation remain. Although virtually all patients will recover fully in a few minutes, some individuals will require a significantly longer period. This patient and others with similar symptoms should neither be discharged from the office unescorted nor permitted to drive a car or return to work where mental alertness is required. Provisions must be made for a companion to escort the patient home. Although this negates a major advantage in the use of inhalation sedation, strict adherence to this provision will prevent potential injury to the patient and potential liability to the dentist.

In some situations, it may be prudent to insist on an escort for all patients receiving inhalation sedation. Standard operating procedure in the U.S. Navy for inhalation sedation includes the requirement of a responsible adult for the patient.

Most patients recover completely following inhalation of 100% O_2 for at least 3 to 5 minutes. If the dentist is satisfied that this is the case, the patient may be permitted to leave the office unescorted. This is the only technique of sedation in which this may be considered.

The patient's ability to operate a motor vehicle after receiving inhalation sedation has been studied.[12] Several parameters were evaluated, including steering errors, speeding errors, and braking reaction time (Table 15.3). Subjects were evaluated before, during, and after the administration of N_2O-O_2. In all categories, subjects demonstrated a deterioration of ability during the inhalation of N_2O-O_2 similar to that produced by

Table 15.3	Recovery From Nitrous Oxide		
	PRESEDATION	**SEDATION**	**POSTSEDATION**
Speeding errors	4.33 ± 2.15	3.75 ± 2.05	2.58 ± 1.31
Max possible = 11			
Mean + s/d			
Steering errors	9.73 ± 2.87	11.09 ± 3.33	9.09 ± 2.43
Max = 16			
Braking errors	24.25 ± 4.47	30.42 ± 2.16	23.42 ± 5.50
Max = 35			
Signaling errors	7.17 ± 1.85	10.42 ± 4.46	4.92 ± 1.93
Max = 19			
Mean braking time (sec)	0.486	0.578	0.474
(range)	(0.442–0.608)	(0.448–0.986)	(0.412–0.604)

Data from Jastak JT, Orendorff D: *Anesth Prog* 22:113, 1975.

alcohol. Following the administration of O_2 and then room air, all measured parameters had returned to baseline values or exceeded them. It was concluded that the typical patient may safely operate a motor vehicle following recovery from N_2O-O_2 inhalation sedation.

Postoperative instructions relevant to the dental or surgical procedure are given in written form to the patient. The patient is then dismissed from the office.

15. *Record data concerning the sedation procedure.*

COMMENT: The assistant should record in the patient's chart that inhalation sedation was used (Fig. 15.16). A sample entry in the chart follows.

The patient received _____% N_2O- _____% O_2 at a total liter flow of _____ L/min. The procedure lasted approximately _____ minutes. At the termination of the procedure, the patient received 100% O_2 for _____ minutes at a flow of _____ L/min. The patient tolerated the procedure well and was dismissed from the office in good condition.

Vital Signs	*Baseline*	*After Procedure*
Blood pressure	112/76	118/78 (mm Hg)
Heart rate	88	82 (beats/min)
Respirations	18	16 (breaths/min)

In addition, any postoperative instructions should be indicated on the chart. A rubber stamp or preglued labels may be prepared with this information and included in the patient's chart and the blanks filled in after the procedure.

Date:_____ Patient: _____ Age: ____

ASA classification: I   II   III   IV

Med consult needed: Yes/No   Operative procedure: _____

Procedural data:

	PREOPERATIVE	POSTOPERATIVE
BP:	_____	_____
Pulse/quality:	_____	_____
Respiration:	_____	_____

N_2O Start time: _____ N_2O Finish time: _____

Titrated % of N_2O: _____   Postoperative O_2: _____
  (for documentation purposes   (in minutes)
  only)

Comments:

Clinician signature: _____

Figure 15.16 Example of clinical record for conscious sedation. (From Clark MS, Brunick AL: *Handbook of nitrous oxide and oxygen sedation*, St Louis, 2008, Mosby.)

16. *Cleanse the equipment.*

COMMENT: The "rubber goods" of the inhalation sedation unit are in contact with the patient's skin and exhaled breath and will naturally become contaminated with foreign material, bacteria, and viral agents. Serious respiratory infections have resulted from the use of contaminated anesthesia machines in operating rooms.[13–15] Nasal hoods for inhalation sedation have also been demonstrated to be contaminated with multiple human pathogens capable of transmission from one patient to another.[16] In a study by Yagiela, Hunt, and Hunt,[17] 100% of nasal hoods used for 10-minute sedative procedures were inoculated with bacteria.

Cleansing of nasal hoods is mandatory. Simple washing of the nasal hood with soap and water has been shown merely to decrease the number of bacterial and viral contaminants.[18] Other techniques have been used, including using alcohol, glutaraldehyde, and iodophor; autoclaving; and microwaving.[15,18–20] All of these techniques have disadvantages when used on nasal masks.

Under the Spaulding classification of inanimate surfaces, nasal hoods are considered semicritical in terms of infection risk.[21] Items in this group come into contact with intact mucous membranes and are therefore resistant to infection by common bacterial spores.[15]

The following is the current recommended procedure for sterilization of nasal hoods.[15,17] After each use, the nasal hood is washed with soap and warm water and then immersed in glutaraldehyde solution for 10 minutes. It is then rinsed thoroughly with tap water to remove the disinfectant solution. At the end of each week, all tubing, reservoir bags, and nasal hoods are stored in glutaraldehyde for 10 hours to achieve complete sterilization. After this 10-hour period, the equipment is rinsed in warm tap water for 1 hour.

Subsequent Appointments

Once a patient has successfully received inhalation sedation, it is highly likely that the use of N_2O-O_2 will be desired for future treatment. At subsequent visits, the same technique should be used. The experience and information gathered from the initial N_2O-O_2 experience will facilitate any such future procedures. The rate at which the sedation at these subsequent appointments is induced should not be increased. Increasing the speed of induction often leads to increased patient discomfort. Patients should be better able to tell the administrator when they are "there" (at ideal sedation), having been "there" before. The ultimate goal, however, is to have patient acceptance of dental treatment fearlessly without the need for N_2O-O_2.

It is important to note that the concentration of N_2O required for ideal sedation may vary somewhat from visit to visit. Ideally, this percentage will decrease over time as a patient's level of comfort with treatment increases; however, other nondental or medical factors will come into play. Factors such as the patient's social life, working life, altered physical condition, and time of day may decrease or increase the percentage of N_2O required by the patient. Normally, variation from visit to visit is slight (35% today, 40% or 30% at the next visit). Only

rarely will significant differences be noted over short periods (e.g., 35% to 65%). To use the same concentration of N_2O at each visit or not to titrate as a means of "saving time" (see the following discussion) is to increase the risk of discomfort to the patient.

COMPARISON OF TECHNIQUES OF ADMINISTRATION

Both the constant liter flow and the constant O_2 flow technique may be used in the delivery of N_2O-O_2. There is little clinical difference between these techniques. The few differences that do exist are presented. The selection of the technique to be used clinically is made at the discretion of the administrator.

Constant Liter Flow Technique
Summary of Technique
1. Establish O_2 flow rate.
2. Increase N_2O to 1 L/min, and decrease O_2 by 1 L/min.
3. Subsequently increase N_2O at 0.5 L/min and decrease O_2 at 0.5 L/min, maintaining the same total flow rate during the procedure.

Advantages
1. Smaller volumes of gases used
2. Less costly
3. Decrease in exhaled N_2O contamination

Disadvantage
Percentage increments of N_2O are fixed; thus it is easier to oversedate the patient.

Examples of Technique
Most inhalation sedation units are incapable of delivering less than a 2.5- or 3-L/min flow of O_2. In this case the O_2 flow rate will not fall below 2.5 or 3 L/min even as the N_2O rate continues to be increased at its usual 1-L/min increment. Thus this becomes equivalent to the constant O_2 flow technique:

6.0-L/Min Flow		
N_2O L/Min	**O_2 L/Min**	**Percentage of N_2O**
0	6.0	0
1.0	5.0	16
1.5	4.5	25
2.0	4.0	33
2.5	3.5	41
3.0	3.0	50
3.5	2.5	58
4.0	2.5*	61
4.5	2.5*	64

Unable to deliver less than 2.5 L/min.

7.0-L/Min Flow		
N₂O L/Min	O₂ L/Min	Percentage of N₂O
0	7.0	0
1.0	6.0	14
1.5	5.5	21
2.0	5.0	28
2.5	4.5	35
3.0	4.0	42
3.5	3.5	50
4.0	3.0	58
4.5	2.5	65
5.0	2.5*	67
5.5	2.5*	69

Unable to deliver less than 2.5 L/min.

Constant O₂ Flow Technique
Summary of Technique
1. Establish O₂ flow rate.
2. Increase N₂O flow rate to 1 L/min and leave O₂ constant.
3. Subsequently increase N₂O in increments of 1 L/min.
4. O₂ flow rate remains constant throughout procedure.

Advantages
1. Slightly easier to use; requires adjustment of one dial
2. Larger volumes of gases used; thus little difficulty in breathing adequately
3. Percentage increments of N₂O decrease as the percentage of N₂O increases (see charts), minimizing risk of inadvertent oversedation

Disadvantages
1. Larger volumes of gases used; thus more costly to administer
2. Larger volumes of N₂O used; thus potentially greater contamination of environment with N₂O

Examples of Technique

6.0-L/Min O₂		
N₂O L/Min	O₂ L/Min	Percentage of N₂O
0	6.0	0
1.0	6.0	14
2.0	6.0	26
3.0	6.0	33
4.0	6.0	40
5.0	6.0	45
6.0	6.0	50
7.0	6.0	54

7.0-L/Min O₂		
N₂O L/Min	O₂ L/Min	Percentage of N₂O
0	7.0	0
1.0	7.0	12
2.0	7.0	22
3.0	7.0	30
4.0	7.0	36
5.0	7.0	41
6.0	7.0	46
7.0	7.0	50

NORMAL DISTRIBUTION CURVE

As has been stressed throughout this book, patients vary in their response to drugs. However, if the percentage of N₂O required to achieve ideal sedation is summarized for many hundreds or thousands of patients, then a normal distribution curve may be formulated.

The following information is a compilation of more than 6000 N₂O-O₂ inhalation sedations administered at the University of Southern California School of Dentistry from 1973 through September 2006.[22] Statistics were obtained at sea level. At higher altitudes (e.g., 1584 meters [5200 feet] in Denver or 2194 meters [7200 feet] in Mexico City), greater percentages of N₂O will be required to achieve comparable sedation levels. An increase of approximately 5% is necessary at Denver's altitude.

Normal Distribution Curve for Adults Successfully Sedated With N₂O-O₂	
Percentage of Patients	Percentage of N₂O Achieving Ideal Sedation
10	<1
15	1
20	4
25	7
30	22
35	24
40	24
45	10
50	4
55	1
60	2
65	<1
70	<1

When the patients are divided into larger groups, it can be seen that 70% of patients who achieve ideal sedation with inhalation sedation did so at an N_2O percentage between 30% and 40%. Approximately 12% required concentrations of N_2O below 30%, whereas 18% required N_2O concentrations in excess of 40% to achieve the same level of sedation.

This chart includes only patients who reached ideal sedation with N_2O-O_2. Not included are the approximately 3% of patients receiving N_2O-O_2 who did not achieve clinically adequate sedation levels. For whatever reason (e.g., too fearful, required more than 70% N_2O, mouth breathing, claustrophobia), the technique failed to achieve its goals. This is to be expected with inhalation sedation as well as with every other technique of sedation.

TITRATION AND TIME

One of the major problems that develops over time in the typical dental practice where inhalation sedation is used is that the dentist stops titrating.[23] Fixed concentrations are delivered to all patients, with the percentage of N_2O approximately 40% or 50%. This technique of not titrating N_2O cannot be recommended for routine use and is reviewed in Chapters 16 and 18. The rationale presented for not titrating N_2O is that titration takes too long to be done properly and that in the typical dental office, such time is not available. Table 15.4 demonstrates that when titrated according to the schedule presented in this chapter (every 60 to 90 seconds), the typical patient requiring approximately 30% to 40% N_2O will be sedated within 3 to 6 minutes.

The 3 to 6 minutes required for sedation to be achieved is compensated for by the fact that, once relaxed, the patient will move little, if at all, during the remainder of the procedure. This is in stark contrast to a fearful, unsedated patient who moves constantly, making treatment more difficult and stressful for both the staff and the patient. Achieving effective pain control is considerably more difficult (and potentially dangerous) as the patient moves during local anesthetic administration. Once treatment begins, the patient will often ask to have it stopped so that he or she may do any number of things that prevent the dentist from completing treatment (e.g., drinking water, going to the restroom). The few minutes required to achieve ideal sedation with inhalation sedation are well worth the effort and time invested.

SIGNS AND SYMPTOMS OF OVERSEDATION

If titration is adhered to, it is unlikely that the patient will become uncomfortable or oversedated. However, it is possible that at various times during treatment, the depth of sedation will become greater without the N_2O percentage having been altered. This occurs most often when a part of the treatment is completed and there is a lull (a lack of stimulation of the patient) while additional equipment or materials are prepared for use. During tooth preparation, for example, a constant stimulus is provided by the sound and vibration of the handpiece. The patient is receiving a concentration of N_2O adequate to produce a calming effect at this time. However, when the preparation is completed and the restorative material is being prepared and inserted, little or no stimulation of the patient occurs. This same percentage of N_2O will produce a deepening of the sedation at this time.

Following are some clinical indicators of oversedation.[24] Management of this situation is simply to decrease the level of N_2O by approximately 5% to 10%. There is no need to use the O_2 flush or to terminate the flow of N_2O. Within 30 seconds of decreasing the N_2O flow (approximately 0.5 to 1 L/min), the patient will be more responsive.

Clinical Indicators of Oversedation
The Patient Persistently Closes the Mouth
Patients receiving N_2O-O_2 sedation should be capable of keeping their mouths open without use of mouth props during the entire procedure. The administrator will tell patients at the start of the sedation that they are to breathe through their nose but are to keep their mouth open. If the patient needs constant reminders to keep the mouth open during dental treatment, the N_2O flow is decreased by 0.5 L/min.

Mouth props (with dental floss tied through them) may be used, but are not recommended for the inexperienced N_2O-O_2 administrator because they take away one of the earliest signs of oversedation. With clinical experience, other clinical clues of oversedation are recognizable to the dentist and assistant, and mouth props may again be recommended.

Most medical procedures in which N_2O-O_2 is used occur away from the mouth. The need for maintaining the mouth in an open position is, of course, nonexistent. In these cases,

Table 15.4	Titration Times According to Percentage of N_2O Required for Sedation					
	Constant Liter Flow			Constant O_2 Flow		
TIME (MIN)	N_2O (L/MIN)	O_2 (L/MIN)	PERCENTAGE OF N_2O	N_2O (L/MIN)	O_2 (L/MIN)	PERCENTAGE OF N_2O
0	0	6.0	0	0	6.0	0
1.0–1.5	1.0	5.0	16	1.0	6.0	16
2.0–3.0	1.5	4.5	25	2.0	6.0	25
3.0–4.5	2.0	4.0	33	3.0	6.0	33
4.0–6.0	2.5	3.5	41	4.0	6.0	40

the physician loses an important guide to early detection of oversedation. The physician or surgical nurse must become more aware of the "other" aspects of patient monitoring.

The Patient Spontaneously Begins Mouth Breathing

Patients receiving N_2O-O_2 have been told by the administrator to breathe only through the nose. A possible sign of oversedation is a spontaneous reversion to mouth breathing, especially in adults (children are more likely to do this in the absence of oversedation). The first time this occurs, the patient is simply reminded to breathe through the nose; however, after several recurrences, the N_2O flow is decreased by 0.5 L/min.

Mouth breathing is easy for the dentist, hygienist, and dental assistant to detect. Mouth mirrors become fogged, and the exhalation of air through the mouth can be felt. Use of a rubber dam effectively eliminates the potential for mouth breathing.

For physicians and other health professionals working at a distance from the mouth, the occurrence of mouth breathing will be rarer than in dentistry. Patients should be told at the start of the procedure to breathe solely through their nose and not to open their mouth.

The Patient Complains of Nausea and Effects of Sedation Felt as Too Intense or Uncomfortable

When a patient says that he or she is uncomfortable, the administrator should immediately decrease the flow of N_2O. Most patients tolerate a degree of discomfort in silence, so at any mention of discomfort, the N_2O flow should be decreased by 0.5 L/min.

If this plea is ignored by the administrator or if the patient does not volunteer the information, it is not unusual for the patient to suddenly and without warning remove the nasal hood. As patients begin to lose control (become oversedated), they respond by attempting to remove the cause of this feeling—the nasal hood. Listening to and watching the patient carefully can prevent these unpleasant situations from arising.

The Patient Fails to Respond Rationally or Gives Sluggish Responses

The sedated patient becomes distracted from the office environment. To a degree this is desirable; however, when a patient no longer responds to verbal command, the level of sedation should be decreased.

It is not uncommon for a patient to respond more slowly than usual to spoken commands during N_2O-O_2 sedation. However, when the command must be repeated more than twice, decrease the flow of N_2O by 0.5 L/min. The patient receiving N_2O-O_2 moderate sedation should be able to respond rationally and relatively quickly to commands.

The Patient Begins to Lose Control

As mentioned, a level of sedation will develop at which the patient feels as though he or she is losing control. In the absence of the patient volunteering this information to the administrator, a sudden jerking movement by the patient will be noticed and the patient may remove the nasal hood. The N_2O flow should be decreased slightly with the O_2 increased the same amount, and within 30 seconds, the patient will recover. When questioned about their experience, patients will say, "I felt as though I was falling into a bottomless, black hole." This is similar to the feeling that many persons experience when lying down to sleep when quite tired. Commonly the person will suddenly jerk his or her body upward. This is in response to the feeling of falling into the bottomless hole—an attempt to grab hold of something.

The Patient Speaks Incoherently or Dreams

Speaking incoherently indicates that the level of sedation is too great. The patient is probably dreaming, and the speaking is a part of the dream. In any case, it becomes impossible for dental therapy to be continued at this time. The N_2O flow should be decreased by 0.5 L/min and the patient carefully tended to.

The Patient Becomes Uncooperative

One of the goals of sedation is for the patient to become more cooperative. As with any technique of sedation, this goal will not always be obtainable. In this case the patient, as sedation progresses, becomes more outgoing and verbal and may even be somewhat physical (moving about in the chair more than before). Decreasing the level of N_2O by 0.5 L/min may decrease this effect yet still provide adequate sedation for the planned treatment to continue.

This effect on patients may be seen with any CNS depressant, including N_2O, but it is especially common with alcohol. Many persons become more "outgoing" and "friendly" after several drinks as their blood alcohol level increases. Alcohol produces a generalized depression of the cerebral cortex, decreasing inhibitions and allowing the individual to act in an out-of-the-ordinary manner. Unlike the effect of alcohol, this effect of N_2O may be readily reversed by decreasing the flow of N_2O.

The Patient Laughs, Cries, or Becomes Giddy

N_2O is commonly known as *laughing gas* because of the propensity of many persons receiving it to begin uncontrollable laughter. Its administration can also lead to uncontrolled crying.

N_2O does not make a person happy or sad. It merely decreases the inhibitions of the patient and increases the intensity of emotions. For example, a person in a very good, happy mood will feel even better when N_2O is administered. This person will be more likely to enjoy the sedative experience and to start laughing should humorous thoughts come to mind. Conversely the patient coming to the appointment in a poor mood will be more apt to release these feelings when N_2O-O_2 is administered. Without N_2O-O_2 the person would not cry, but does so quite readily once the N_2O is administered.

In either case, laughing or crying, the continuation of dental treatment becomes impossible. The concentration of N$_2$O must therefore be decreased to a more appropriate level.

The Patient Has Uncoordinated Movements

When a patient receiving N$_2$O-O$_2$ makes uncoordinated movements, the concentration of N$_2$O must be decreased. For example, consider a 20-year-old woman receiving 40% N$_2$O for dental treatment because of her fears of dentistry. She was well sedated, but occasionally during the procedure she suddenly, without warning, lifted her legs upward as high as she could and then let them drop back onto the chair. After reducing the N$_2$O flow by 0.5 L/min, the patient was asked about this reaction. She stated that she was unaware of lifting her legs but that she did remember that her legs had become extremely light and began to float upward by themselves. She then would "catch them" and bring them back down. Such uncoordinated movement is potentially injurious. Immediate reduction of the N$_2$O flow by 0.5 L/min remedied this situation.

In each of the situations presented, the patient has entered into a level of sedation that is just slightly beyond that which is deemed ideal. Management is not dramatic; the simple reduction of N$_2$O flow by approximately 5% to 10% corrects the situation. It is very rare indeed when the flow of N$_2$O must quickly be terminated. N$_2$O-O$_2$ has the unique ability to quickly allow for physiologic change by increasing or decreasing the concentration.

REFERENCES

1. House of Delegates, American Dental Association: *Guidelines for teaching pain control and sedation to dentists and dental students*, Chicago, 2016, American Dental Association.
2. American Dental Association Council on Scientific Affairs: Nitrous oxide in the dental office. *J Am Dent Assoc* 128(3):364–365, 1997.
3. Gillman MA: Possible mechanisms of action of nitrous oxide at the opioid receptor. *Med Hypotheses* 15(2):109–114, 1984.
4. Quock RM, Curtis BA, Reynolds BJ, Mueller JL: Dose-dependent antagonism and potentiation of nitrous oxide antinociception by naloxone in mice. *J Pharmacol Exp Ther* 267(1):117–122, 1993.
5. Gillman MA, Lichtigfeld FJ: Clinical role and mechanisms of action of analgesic nitrous oxide. *Int J Neurosci* 93(1–2):55–62, 1998.
6. Donaldson M, Donaldson D, Quarnstrom FC: Nitrous oxide-oxygen administration: when safety features no longer are safe. *J Am Dent Assoc* 143(2):134–143, 2012.
7. Tracy Press: Dentist scrutinized after child's death. October 30, 2015. Tracy, California.
8. Geers AL, Miller FG: Understanding and translating the knowledge about placebo effects: the contribution of psychology. *Curr Opin Psychiatry* 27(5):326–331, 2014.
9. Trieger N, Newman MG, Miller JG: An objective measure of recovery. *Anesth Prog* 16(1):4–7, 1969.
10. Trieger NT, Laskota WI, Jacobs AW, et al: Nitrous oxide: a study of physiological and psychological effects. *J Am Dent Assoc* 82(1):142–150, 1971.
11. Newman MG, Trieger NT, Millar JC: Measuring recovery from anesthesia: a simple test. *Anesth Analg* 48(1):136–140, 1969.
12. Jastak JT, Orendorff D: Recovery from nitrous oxide sedation. *Anesth Prog* 22(4):113–116, 1975.
13. Joseph JM: Disease transmission by inefficiently sanitized anesthetizing apparatus. *JAMA* 149:1196, 1952.
14. Olds JW, Kisch AL, Eberle BJ, Wilson JN: *Pseudomonas aeruginosa* respiratory tract infection acquired from a contaminated anesthesia machine. *Am Rev Respir Dis* 105(4):628–632, 1974.
15. Jastak JT, Donaldson D: Nitrous oxide. In Dionne RA, Phero JC, editors: *Management of pain and anxiety in dental practice*, New York, 1991, Elsevier.
16. Hunt LM, Yagiela JA: Bacterial contamination and transmission by nitrous oxide sedation apparatus. *Oral Surg Oral Med Oral Pathol* 44(3):367–373, 1977.
17. Yagiela JA, Hunt LM, Hunt DE: Disinfection of nitrous oxide inhalation equipment. *J Am Dent Assoc* 98(2):191–195, 1979.
18. Christensen RP, Robison RA, Robinson DF, et al: Antimicrobial activity of environmental surface disinfectants in the absence and presence of bioburden. *J Am Dent Assoc* 119(4):493–505, 1989.
19. Rohrer MD, Bulard RA: Microwave sterilization. *J Am Dent Assoc* 110(2):194–198, 1985.
20. Young SK, Graves DC, Rohrer MD, Bulard RA: Microwave sterilization of nitrous oxide nasal hoods contaminated with virus. *Oral Surg Oral Med Oral Pathol* 60(6):581–585, 1985.
21. Favero MS: Chemical disinfection of medical and surgical materials. In Block SS, editor: *Disinfection, sterilization and preservation*, ed 3, Philadelphia, 1985, Lea & Febiger.
22. School of Dentistry, University of Southern California: Statistics from section of anesthesia & medicine, Los Angeles, 2006, unpublished.
23. Clark M, Brunick A: *Handbook of nitrous oxide and oxygen sedation*, ed 4, St Louis, 2015, Mosby.
24. Bennett CR: *Conscious sedation in dental practice*, ed 2, St Louis, 1978, Mosby.

chapter 16

Inhalation Sedation: Complications

Complications associated with the administration of nitrous oxide and oxygen are rare.[1] However, there is no technique of sedation that does not have a potential for complications. The most common cause is inadequate or incomplete training of the doctor and staff. Combining N_2O-O_2 with one or more other sedative agents can cause oversedation if the N_2O is not titrated. The technique of N_2O-O_2 is forgiving in that most issues that arise can be quickly corrected by proper technique. Most complications of inhalation sedation are associated with the following:

1. Inadequate or incomplete sedation
2. Poor patient experience
3. Equipment performance

INADEQUATE OR INCOMPLETE SEDATION

Inadequate or incomplete sedation usually involves poor patient selection for the use of N_2O-O_2 sedation. An example would be the *authoritarian type of personality*, who when faced with the prospect of loss of control or the sense of this loss becomes uncomfortable. The patient, not wanting to lose control, will consciously or subconsciously "fight" the effects of the agent (N_2O). Unfortunately, other similar sedative procedures produce the same effects, and the success rate of most will be poor in the authoritarian type of patient unless more potent agents are used.

Patients who are *emotionally or psychologically unstable* may not fare well with N_2O-O_2. Patients who use *mind-altering drugs* may also have residual conflicting or counterproductive effects from N_2O administration. These patients, particularly if chronic abusers, may be "resistant" to the effects of N_2O and/or expect or require a level of potency that is beyond the capacity of N_2O in therapeutic percentages. *Hyporesponders,* representing approximately 15% of the population, may not respond to the highest levels of N_2O that can possibly be given (70% concentration). N_2O-O_2 may not be adequate for the *severely fearful* patients. Choose your patient carefully and be mindful that N_2O-O_2 works best in conjunction with local anesthetic.[2]

POOR PATIENT EXPERIENCE

The second classification of potential complications—poor patient experience—can be best managed by prevention. Prevention is most easily and best accomplished by titration of the N_2O during administration. Titration allows for enough N_2O to be given to achieve the desired clinical effect for a given patient for a particular procedure. Most patients who have complications are oversedated. Physical signs and symptoms such as excessive perspiration, nausea and vomiting, hallucinations, and increased agitation rather than sedation are all clear signs and symptoms of oversedation. If a patient demonstrates any of these signs, the N_2O concentration should be decreased by 0.5 to 1.0 lpm, and in approximately 30 to

60 seconds, a reversal of these adverse reactions will be evident and the patient's status returned to their previous level of sedation. It is truly impressive to observe how quickly a patient will return to a level of cooperation and acceptance of treatment after this minimal decrease in N_2O concentration. It is important to keep the oxygen (O_2) flow unchanged. The built-in features of modern inhalation sedation units prevent a concentration of more than 70% N_2O from occurring. This safety feature helps reduce the possibility of oversedation and possible hypoxia.

The primary reason to administer N_2O-O_2 is to provide a pleasant experience for the patient by altering his or her mood. Anything less is unacceptable. Some patients can have an inexplicable idiosyncratic reaction to any drug, but this is extremely rare with N_2O, and there are no true absolute contraindications, only relative contraindications. Contraindications to the administration of N_2O-O_2 are discussed in Chapter 12.

EQUIPMENT PERFORMANCE

The last classification of potential complications is equipment performance. This has become extremely rare as a result of the intense scrutiny placed on manufacturers by numerous professional agencies and the extreme desire by the manufacturers to provide a safe and excellent product. The manufacturers have succeeded in producing a safe machine with backup systems that ensure that adequate levels of O_2 are present to maintain operation. Even with a failure in the O_2 supply, the machine still allows the patient to receive room air without impediment. The possibility for machine or equipment failure usually revolves around purposeful alteration of the equipment as sold or the use of outdated equipment. The rubber parts of the sedation machine can tear, leak, or malfunction and should therefore be frequently inspected per the American Dental Association's protocol.[3] The chance of equipment failure in today's environment is extremely small. Equipment failure can best be prevented by routine examination and inspection of the inhalation sedation unit.

COMPLICATIONS

Complications, as mentioned, rarely occur. When a complication does arise, it is commonly the result of a higher concentration of N_2O than is required by the patient (lack of titration) and long duration of use (greater than 1 hour).

Nausea and Vomiting

The incidence of nausea and vomiting (N&V) with the administration of N_2O-O_2 inhalation sedation is extremely low.[4] The most common cause of N&V during dental treatment is the inadvertent swallowing of blood. When related to the sedation technique N&V most often occur as a result of hypoxia or oversedation. Historically, N_2O was administered without the addition of supplemental O_2. The "technique" was to create an intentionally anoxic (cyanotic) patient and then work as

rapidly as possible until the patient recovered. Some did not recover; others awoke very nauseated and vomiting. This history has in some areas persisted to the erroneous conclusion that N_2O-O_2 was the cause of the N&V.[2] It has been shown through years of clinical experience that N&V occur in fewer than 0.5% of patients.[5] When N&V does occur, it is usually associated with the following causes.

Presence of Food in the Stomach

Heavy meals preceding an inhalation sedation administration can easily cause N&V, particularly in pediatric patients. The converse can also be true. Patients treated on an empty stomach may also be more susceptible to N&V. I ask patients to have a high-carbohydrate meal 4 to 6 hours before the appointment. This prevents starvation and yet allows for stomach contents to be minimized.

Oversedation

A reliable and consistent sign of oversedation is a response from the patient that he or she feels bad or "sick to the stomach," usually preceded by sweating and pallor. No matter the percentage of N_2O concentration, the patient is oversedated. The N_2O flow should be discontinued (allowing the patient to breathe 100% O_2), and the patient will quickly recover (30 to 60 seconds).

The "Roller Coaster Ride"

Administration of N_2O-O_2 allows the best possible degree of titration of any drug route. However, this great advantage can become a disadvantage by increasing, decreasing, increasing, and decreasing the N_2O-O_2 flow, causing a so-called "roller coaster ride." This may increase the risk of N&V. Titration for all patients is encouraged, but wide swings in the concentration of N_2O can have a deleterious effect on the patient. Levels of sedation may also fluctuate considerably if the patient is allowed to maintain a conversation and breathe through his or her mouth.

Length of Sedation

The longer the patient has N_2O-O_2 sedation, the greater is the incidence of N&V. Although this is not nearly as problematic as high concentrations and oversedation, length of sedation should be monitored. There is no absolute maximum time limit for N_2O-O_2 procedures though prudence dictates that a shorter duration is better than longer.

Prior History of Nausea and Vomiting

Some people are more prone to N&V than others. Although this is most likely related to their psychological profile, it is nonetheless a factor of predisposition. Serious consideration should be given to whether these patients should receive an antiemetic. This is especially true for children.[6] Antiemetics can be delivered orally or rectally to help prevent nausea in patients (Table 16.1). Ondansetron (Zofran) has become a favored drug to manage N&V.

Table 16.1	Antiemetics	
GENERIC NAME	PROPRIETARY NAME	ADULT ORAL DOSE (MG)
Dimenhydrinate*	Dramamine	50–100
Cyclizine*†	Marezine	50
Meclizine*†	Bonine	25–50
Hyoscine, scopalamine	—	0.6–1
Hydroxyzine†	Vistaril	25–100
Diphenidol†	Vontrol	25–50
Trimethobenzamide	Tigan	100–300
Prochlorperazine	Compazine	5–10
Promethazine	Phenergan	12.5–25
Ondansetron	Zofran	8
Dolasetron	Anzemet	100
Metoclopramide	Reglan	10

*Nonprescription.
†Should be used with caution; can be teratogenic in pregnancy.

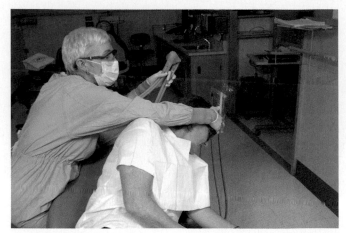

Figure 16.1 If vomiting occurs, turn the patient's head and body to the side away from the operator. (Courtesy Dr. Mark Dellinges.)

Patient Positioning

Patient positioning should promote comfort. If a patient is moving a lot in the chair, encourage them to get comfortable because this, to a minor degree, is thought to contribute to N&V.

Management of Nausea and Vomiting

Historically, before the development of fail-safe machines that ensure delivery of supplemental O_2, hypoxia or anoxia would commonly result in N&V. As a result, the administration of N_2O-O_2 was associated with N&V. With the advent of the fail-safe machine in 1976, the incidence of vomiting diminished significantly. In the clinical experience with inhalation sedation at the University of Southern California, the incidence of vomiting was found to be 0.3% of the 6500 patient experiences reviewed.[5] The most dangerous circumstance (although this is extremely unlikely to occur), in my opinion, is for a patient to become unconscious while receiving N_2O-O_2 and have a secondary sequela of silent regurgitation with aspiration of vomitus into the trachea. This life-threatening situation would most likely occur only with an unmonitored patient receiving a high level of N_2O. The greater the depth of sedation, the more likely is the incidence of nausea and vomiting. Parkhouse et al[7] demonstrated that the incidence of nausea rose with increasing concentration of N_2O. The duration of sedation was also of importance, but not as great as that of depth of sedation.

Management of nausea. The goal of sedation is to make a patient's dental experience more comfortable. If at any time a patient appears to be uncomfortable or actually complains of being uncomfortable, the administrator of the sedation should recognize and manage this. As the doctor is working intently

in the oral cavity, quite often it is the dental assistant who first notices this discomfort. The patient, whose arms have been draped on the arm rest of the dental chair in a relaxed manner may move them onto their abdomen and begin to rub or press. Facially the patient may appear to be in distress. The dental assistant should immediately indicate this (nonverbally) to the doctor, who will ask the patient, "Are you still comfortable?" (do not ask "Are you nauseous?"). A nauseous patient will reply they are not comfortable, and the administrator should decrease the flow of N_2O by 0.5 to 1.0 lpm. The nausea should resolve within a minute or two. If not, continue to decrease the flow of N_2O by 0.5 to 1.0 lpm every minute until relief occurs. The incidence of nausea—as low as it is—is much more common than that of vomiting.

Management of vomiting. Patients who are about to vomit usually have a period of impending awareness of the event: hypersalivation, diaphoresis (sweating), and nausea. If the patient expresses this awareness, the following should be carried out:

1. The clinician should turn off the N_2O flow and have the patient continue breathing 100% O_2.
2. If vomiting begins, remove the nasal hood or other delivery apparatus from the patient's face.
3. Remove the rubber dam, if present, and any other dental equipment from the oral cavity.
4. Turn the patient's head and body to the side away from the side on which the person treating the patient is stationed (Fig. 16.1). This permits the vomitus to pool in the cheek instead of flowing back into the patient's pharynx, where airway obstruction may occur. A kidney or emesis basin and high-volume suction tip may be used to assist in removing the vomitus (Fig. 16.2). A dry 4" × 4" piece of gauze can also quickly aid in removing vomitus.
5. Following the incident, replace the nasal hood on the patient's nose so that he or she may be permitted to breathe 100% O_2 for at least 3 to 5 minutes. The patient may be somewhat

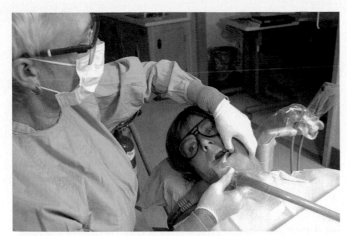

Figure 16.2 Vomitus is removed with suction or finger. The patient should receive 100% O_2. (Courtesy Dr. Mark Dellinges.)

reluctant to have the nasal hood placed back on for fear of becoming sick again. Explain to the patient that he or she will breathe only 100% O_2 and that the reason for doing so is to minimize the chance of becoming sick again.

If the patient does not wish to continue with N_2O-O_2 during treatment, it is best to adhere to these wishes. However, the door should not be closed on the future use of this valuable form of sedation. It should be stressed to the patient that vomiting is a very unusual occurrence and that it is unlikely to occur again. If necessary, antiemetics may be prescribed preoperatively for this patient (see Table 16.1).

Tooth Pain Associated With Sinus Pressure

N_2O displaces air from the maxillary sinus, thereby increasing pressure within the sinus cavities.[8] This increase in sinus pressure can cause a patient to experience "aching" in maxillary teeth and is usually associated with prolonged use (>1 hour) of N_2O-O_2. Because the anterior, middle, and posterior superior alveolar nerves pass through the sinus membrane, the increased pressure within the sinus cavity on the nerve(s) can lead to the feeling of a toothache. This increased pressure can, on rare occasion, lead to earache as pressure increases within the inner ear cavity.[9]

Vertigo

Prolonged exposure of the vestibulocochlear complex to N_2O can result in vertigo.[9] This complication can cause increased tension on the tympanic membrane. This tension can result in an alteration in hearing acuity, and the patient may complain of this alteration in hearing.

Bowel Discomfort

As in other closed spaces (e.g., sinus, inner ear), airspaces in the gut can be displaced by N_2O. This nonrigid potential space can have an enlargement to the extent that discomfort and flatulence occur as a result of high concentration and prolonged use of N_2O.[10]

Claustrophobia

Claustrophobia is a disorder that is shared by many patients. The nasal hood and/or face mask of the sedation unit can precipitate a claustrophobic response in severely claustrophobic individuals. Patients will often pinpoint the mask coming into contact with their face as the most unpleasant part of a general anesthesia experience in the hospital. Allowing a patient with this concern to adjust the nasal hood to their liking can help improve the experience. Claustrophobia is a real fear that requires understanding on the part of the health care provider. In extreme instances of claustrophobia, inhalation sedation may be contraindicated.

Contact Lens Wearers

Large numbers of patients wear contact lenses today. People usually think of them as a part of their normal anatomy. The nasal mask, if not snugly in place over the nose, will potentially allow the dry gas to affect the lens and cause irritation to the eye. Patients should be requested to remove their contact lenses before receiving inhalation sedation.

Anatomic Obstruction

Anatomic variations, such as enlarged tonsils and/or adenoids, can present a significant obstacle to the adequate administration of N_2O-O_2. A deviated nasal septum can also potentially decrease the ease of gas flow through the entirety of the airway. It is worth exploring these possible anatomic considerations with patients to anticipate possible interference.

Understanding of the Language

The continual change in demographics in the United States and the increase in cultural diversity have presented a potential complicating factor because of the increasing difficulty in verbal communication. Although simple instructions may seem to be clear and well understood, the dentist must try to anticipate the need for additional resources for the communication of more detailed instruction.

Esoteric Potential Complications

Pulmonary conditions such as chronic obstructive pulmonary disease (COPD), emphysema, cystic fibrosis, decompression illness ("bends"), or pneumothorax are all pathophysiologic circumstances that can be initiated or exacerbated by the administration of N_2O. These "complications" can certainly be real, but practically they are not recorded in the literature to be significant. The astute clinician should understand that the N_2O dynamics should apply to the clinical situation.

MANAGING COMPLICATIONS

As mentioned, most complications are preventable through the use of titration and an awareness that high concentrations and, to a lesser degree, prolonged administration can precipitate these events. Monitoring allows observation of the patient to assess his or her level of sedation and allows general assessment of the physiognomy. A preoperative evaluation of baseline vital signs is important. The use of a pulse oximeter while administering N_2O-O_2 has no parallel for detection of O_2 perfusion at the cellular level. A pulse oximeter reading will usually be at 100% O_2 saturation concentration throughout the administration of N_2O-O_2. Pulse oximeters are inexpensive and, although not mandated or necessary, provide an added level of confidence to the clinician. Periodic recording of vital signs, most importantly postoperative vital signs, is highly recommended. A postoperative vital signs record is essential before the patient is discharged.

In conclusion, N_2O-O_2 as a technique for sedation is very useful and safe.[11] As with all medications and procedures, we should be prepared to treat the unexpected. The complications that can and do present are easily managed or possibly prevented by the trained practitioner and staff.

REFERENCES

1. Hulland SA, Freilich MM, Sandor GKB: Nitrous oxide-oxygen or oral midazolam for pediatric outpatient sedation. *Oral Surg Oral Med Oral Pathol Oral Radiol Endod* 93(6):643–646, 2002.
2. Langa H: *Relative analgesia in dental practice: inhalation analgesia with nitrous oxide*, Philadelphia, 1968, WB Saunders.
3. American Dental Association: ADA campaign urges twice yearly checks on the status of dental equipment, supplies, ADA News, March 19, 2012.
4. Fernandez-Guisasola J, Gomez-Arnau JI, Cabrera Y, del Valle SG: Association between nitrous oxide and the incidence of postoperative nausea and vomiting in adults: a systematic review and meta-analysis. *Anaesthesia* 65(4):379–387, 2010.
5. School of Dentistry, University of Southern California: Statistics from section of anesthesia & medicine, Los Angeles, 2006. unpublished.
6. Houck WR, Ripa LW: Vomiting frequency in children administered nitrous oxide-oxygen in analgesic doses. *J Dent Child* 38:404, 1971.
7. Parkhouse J, Henrie JR, Duncan GM, Rome HP: Nitrous oxide analgesia in relation to mental performance. *J Pharmacol Exp Ther* 128:44–54, 1960.
8. Farber NE, Stuth EAE, Stucke AG, Pagel PS: Inhaled anesthetics: pulmonary pharmacology. In *Miller's anesthesia*, ed 8, Philadelphia, 2015, Saunders, pp 670–705.
9. Taylor E, Feinstein R, White PF, Soper N: Anesthesia for laparoscopic cholecystectomy: is nitrous oxide contraindicated? *Anesthesiology* 76(4):541–543, 1992.
10. Longnecker DE, Miller FL: Pharmacology of inhalational anesthetics. In Longnecker DE, Tinker JH, Morgan G, Jr, editors: *Principles and practice of anesthesiology*, ed 2, St Louis, 1998, Mosby.
11. Clark M, Brunick A: *Handbook of nitrous oxide and oxygen sedation*, ed 4, St Louis, 2008, Mosby.

chapter 17

Contemporary Issues Surrounding Nitrous Oxide

CHAPTER OUTLINE

Nitrous oxide–oxygen inhalation sedation (N_2O-O_2) remains popular in clinical use in medical, dental, nursing, and paraprofessional offices. The advantage of stress reduction in the apprehensive and/or medically compromised patient is responsible for this popularity. The aging population that in years past would not have come to the dental office because of systemic illness is now capable of undergoing extensive treatment because of advances in medical technology. These new patients not only are increasing in numbers, but also have the affluence to pay for treatment and comfort.

The evolution of sedation should include advances in supportive medications and therapies in addition to the heightened awareness of the public to the possibility of increased therapeutic service with sedation; these factors have helped thrust N_2O-O_2 to the forefront. Professional education became more formalized and took a significant step forward approximately 45 years ago when the Council on Dental Education of the American Dental Association accepted standards for educational programs for inhalation sedation.[1]

Along with the increased use of N_2O-O_2 has come a greater concern for the safety of personnel who are in contact with it for the greatest length of time—the dentist and dental office staff. The following three categories are addressed in this regard:
1. Potential biohazards from long-term exposure to trace anesthetic gas
2. Recreational abuse of N_2O
3. Sexual phenomenon and N_2O

POTENTIAL BIOHAZARDS FROM LONG-TERM EXPOSURE TO TRACE ANESTHETIC GAS

Throughout the history and evolution of N_2O, it was widely recognized to exert an influence on the general physiognomy of humans. What was not understood was the concept of addiction. From Horace Wells to Sigmund Freud, we see through the pages of history the great scientists and many unknowns who have succumbed to experimentation, usually without thought of chemical consequence.

As times have passed, the fact that chemicals have biologic effects and are even capable of causing death has come to be recognized. Health agencies around the world have been organized to protect the public from hazardous products circulating in society.

N_2O is found naturally in the atmosphere in extremely minute quantities. It is quickly reversible in action, but is it totally harmless?

Little was known of the possible effects of inhalation of minute amounts of anesthetic vapors until the late 1960s.

Before then little was done to eliminate anesthetic vapors delivered into the ambient air from anesthesia machines. In 1967 Vaisman[2] published the results of a survey of Russian anesthesiologists in which it was demonstrated that they suffered a higher incidence of irritability, headache, fatigue, nausea, pruritus, spontaneous abortion, and fetal malformation than non–operating room personnel. This was the first report that inhalation gases may exert a negative influence on human physiology. Subsequent retrospective studies followed that seemed to confirm Vaisman's result.[3-5] It must be emphasized that in these studies, N_2O was but one of many gases under investigation. Because it is the most commonly used inhalation anesthetic, N_2O is found in all samples of air taken from operating theaters. It is used in conjunction with O_2 and other, more potent inhalation anesthetics such as halothane, enflurane, sevoflurane, and isoflurane. Therefore it has been impossible to separate the effects of any one of these gases from the others. In other words, the findings presented here are potentially produced by any one of the anesthetic gases found in the operating theater. Because of the special nature of dental practice, in which virtually the only inhalation anesthetic used is N_2O, the findings of these operating theater studies were not applicable to the dental profession.

In the United States Cohen et al[6,7] published articles in the 1970s dealing with anesthetic health hazards in the dental setting. One article contained a study that surveyed more than 50,000 dentists and dental assistants who were exposed to trace anesthetics. The results suggested that long-time exposure to anesthetic gases could be associated with an increase in general health problems and with disease of the reproductive system in particular. This study was retrospective in nature, and it only fueled concern regarding the safety of N_2O in the dental office. Unfortunately, this "study" did not contain any measured data on these trace gases that were involved in any of the environs reported.

In 1974 Bruce, Bach, and Arbit[8] "investigated the possibility of N_2O affecting perceptual cognition and psychomotor skills of personnel exposed to varying concentrations of the gas." They reported that just hours of exposure to as little as 50 ppm could result in audiovisual impairment. Despite multiple attempts to duplicate their results, all efforts failed. However, the National Institute for Occupational Safety and Health (NIOSH) and the Occupational Safety & Health Administration (OSHA) became interested in these studies and established 50 ppm to be the maximum exposure limit for personnel in the dental setting. It was determined that 25 ppm was achievable in the operating room, and therefore this became the standard in that setting.[9] Multiple attempts to reproduce the research results of Bruce, Bach, and Arbit[8] have failed. Interestingly, these researchers have retracted their conclusions, indicating that the results were not based on biologic factors.[10]

The results of this "research," as one would expect, caused a concern and subsequent decline in the use of N_2O-O_2. Indeed, there was alarm in the manufacturing and equipment industry for N_2O-O_2 that bordered on a crisis. In 1995 Clark conducted a worldwide literature search on the topic of biohazards associated with N_2O-O_2 use.[11] Of the 850 citations reviewed, only 23 met the predetermined criteria for scientific merit. The conclusion drawn from this literature review was that there was no scientific basis for the previously established threshold levels for the hospital operating room or the dental setting. This research became the impetus for a meeting of interested parties representing dentistry, government, and manufacturing. A result of the September 1995 meeting, sponsored by the American Dental Association's Council on Scientific Affairs and Council on Dental Practice, was the formal position statement that a maximum N_2O exposure limit in parts per million has not been determined.[12]

The specific biologic issue is the inactivation of methionine synthase. This enzyme is linked to vitamin B12 metabolism. Vitamin B12 is necessary for DNA production and subsequent cellular reproduction. N_2O does affect methionine synthase and does, in high concentration and under long exposure (24 hours or greater), have an effect on reproduction.[13] However, to date there is no evidence that a direct causal relationship exists between reproductive health and scavenged low levels of N_2O.[14,15] Sweeney et al[16] were the first to link reproductive problems in humans with long-term N_2O exposure. They used a sensitive test—the deoxyuridine suppression test—to accurately determine the first signs of this biologic effect in humans. Sweeney et al found that long-term exposure levels of 1800 ppm of N_2O did not exert any detectable biologic effect in humans. They suggest that a level of 400 ppm is a reasonable exposure level that is both attainable and significantly below the biologic threshold. The NIOSH has set the exposure limit for operating theaters within the United States at 25 ppm, with dental offices set at 50 ppm.[9] The Health and Safety Executive in the United Kingdom (HSE UK) Occupational Exposure Limits set a figure of 100 ppm as a time-weighted average for 8 hours.[17] Other countries' exposure limits range from 25 ppm to 100 ppm with short-term peaks up to 500 ppm (Table 17.1).

Table 17.1	Occupational Exposure Limits From a Sampling of Countries	
COUNTRY	**EXPOSURE LIMIT (ppm)**
Australia	25
United Kingdom	100
Canada (Ontario)	25
Sweden	100
France	25
Denmark	25
Germany	100
United States	25 (NIOSH)
	50 (ACGIH)

From Clark MS, Brunick AL: Handbook of nitrous oxide and oxygen sedation, ed 4, St Louis, 2014, Mosby.

An additional specific biologic issue surrounding N_2O includes the fact that N_2O in very high nontherapeutic doses can cause leukopenia and reduction in megaloblastic erythropoiesis resembling pernicious anemia. Neurologic disorders associated with long-term N_2O exposure appear as myeloneuropathy.[18–22] Symptoms, such as sensory and proprioception impairment, may be permanent, but are usually temporary with a slow recovery.

Scavenging

Today, it is below the standard of care to not utilize a scavenging nasal hood[12] (see Figs. 14.31 and 14.36). They are inexpensive, disposable, and readily available. The scavenging nasal hood is a double mask—an inner mask contained within a slightly larger outer mask. Each mask has two tubes entering into it so that the entire apparatus has four tubes, two on either side of the nasal hood. The inner mask receives a fresh supply of N_2O-O_2 from the inhalation sedation unit and delivers gas to the nose of the patient through two tubes that are slightly larger in diameter than the other two tubes. The outer, slightly larger, mask connects to the two slightly smaller tubes that connect with the vacuum system. A small vacuum is created in the space between the inner and outer masks. On exhalation through the nose, all exhaled gases are vented into the outer nasal hood and then, via the vacuum, are carried away from the patient and the treatment area (Fig. 17.1).

The Silhouette scavenging nasal hood (see Figs. 14.32 and 14.37) is considerably smaller in size than other scavenging nasal hoods, is transparent, contains no metal, and provides ease of access during dental treatment.

An additional benefit of the scavenging nasal hood is that peripheral leakage of gases resulting from improper fit of the mask is prevented because the outer nasal hood is attached to the vacuum system and will remove any such gases before they reach the ambient air.[23] The optimum and recommended vacuum flow rate is 45 L/min. At this rate, leakage of N_2O-O_2 into the room is prevented even when the mask is removed from the patient and a gas flow of 4 L of each N_2O and O_2 is delivered through the nasal hood.[24] It is important to remember that the vacuum should not be so strong as to prevent adequate ventilation of the lungs with N_2O-O_2 to achieve sedation. Allowing the patient to adjust the mask will invariably create a snugger fit and seal of the nasal hood periphery than the administrator would be able to achieve alone.

The ventilation system in the operatory can be extremely effective as a scavenging tool. A strategically placed, well-designed venting system can not only minimize trace N_2O levels in one operatory, but can expedite separation of gas from one area of a building to another. This tremendous source of scavenging is often overlooked and underused. It can also be relatively inexpensive.

Air sweeps are simply oscillating fans that can be placed in such a way as to "sweep" the trace N_2O from a specific area. The air sweep is probably most useful in interrupting the transfer of exhaled gas from the patient to operator. The 12-inch area

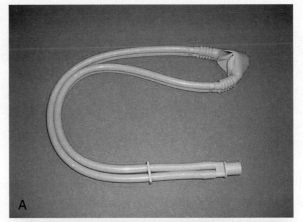

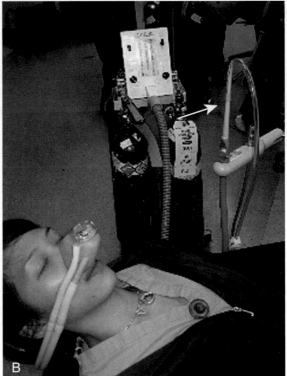

Figure 17.1 A, Scavenging nasal hood and tubing. **B,** Attached to vacuum system (arrow), exhaled gases are vented away from the operating area.

between the patients mouth and the operators face, sometimes called the *breathing zone,* contains high concentrations of gas that may be directed toward the venting system (Table 17.2).

The number-one cause of N_2O contamination in the office is from the patient talking (Box 17.1). The clinician should recognize this and attempt to modify the situation to make verbal interaction with the patient as brief and concise as possible. This is best done by simply explaining to the patient that N_2O-O_2 is most effective when breathed through the nose. The use of rubber dam is a highly effective means of decreasing trace N_2O exposure. Remember that all vocal discourse, laughing, and so forth create a direct source of N_2O into the treatment area.[25]

Table 17.2	Levels of N₂O (Ppm) in Breathing Zones When Using Conventional Nasal Hood With Expiratory Valve		
CATEGORIES	DENTIST	ASSISTANT	ROOM AVERAGE
General dentist's office	775 ± 63	440 ± 52	310 ± 37
Pediatric dentist's office	940 ± 92	112 ± 23	280 ± 52
Oral surgeon's office	1000 ± 130	1600 ± 250	310 ± 47

Box 17.1	Potential Sources of Nitrous Oxide

1. *Normal gas flow*
   Exhaling valve
   Around perimeter of nasal hood
2. *Patient*
   During the procedure—mouth breathing, talking, laughing
   After the procedure—30 L N₂O exhaled within 3 to 5 min
3. *Inhalation sedation unit*
   High-pressure system
   Worn wall connectors
   Loose high-pressure hose connections
   Deformed compression fittings
   Low-pressure system
   Loose, defective, or missing gaskets and seals
   Worn or defective bags and breathing tubes
   Loosely assembled slip joints and threaded connections
   Loose flowmeters
4. *Air conditioning*

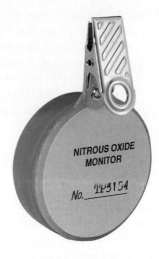

Figure 17.2 Time-weighted nitrous oxide vapor monitor. (Courtesy NevinLabs. Chicago, Illinois.)

Monitoring of Trace Nitrous Oxide
Infrared N₂O Analyzer

The most accurate and effective method of determining N₂O levels in ambient air is through an infrared (IR) N₂O analyzer.[27] IR light is absorbed at different wavelengths by different gases. The advantage of IR spectrophotometry is the ability to detect minute levels of gases, such as N₂O, in ambient air at levels of as low as 1 ppm. The IR analyzer takes surrounding air samples into a nozzlelike opening and transfers them to a sampling cell. Differences in N₂O concentrations in the sampled air result in proportional changes in the quantity of IR energy that is transmitted through the sampling cell, sensed by the detector, and then amplified and displayed on the monitor. This occurs almost instantaneously. The IR analyzer can be used to detect many different gases in addition to N₂O and can detect gases from the previously mentioned 1 ppm to an upper limit of 2000 ppm. The machine is extremely accurate to within one-half of a percentage point. IR analyzers are very expensive, but can

be rented from a gas service company. The supplier of your compressed gases will have the resource for contacts to allow you to rent an IR spectrophotometer for N₂O analysis.

Time-Weighted Monitoring

TWM devices are commonly used in medical and dental offices.[28] The devices detect the amount of N₂O absorption over a given period. A dosimeter badge is worn by anyone (usually staff) who desires to know the amount of N₂O he or she has been exposed to in a particular setting. The dosimeters are sent back to the company laboratory with the history of exposure time to N₂O. The laboratory returns a time-weighted value of exposure. Although they are not nearly as accurate as IR, they serve a useful purpose (Fig. 17.2).

The American Dental Association published in its March 1997 journal recommendations for responsible maintenance and monitoring of N₂O and its equipment (Box 17.2).[12]

In conclusion, we hope always to challenge ourselves to deliver the very best care to our patients. We are guided by our conscience and our knowledge. To date, no direct evidence of any causal relationship between long-term, low-level exposure to N₂O and potential biologic effects exist.

RECREATIONAL ABUSE OF NITROUS OXIDE

N₂O causes euphoria and, therefore, as Sir Humphrey Davy discovered in 1798, has a potential for abuse.[29,30] It is usually not as addictive as some drugs,[31] but nonetheless it can be a "steppingstone" to other drugs and can cause incapacitation of the affected person. Dr. Gardner Colton traveled the world displaying the "exhilarating" effect of N₂O. These same pleasant effects are used to abate fear in our practices. N₂O should be given the same respect that is given to all drugs.[31,32] When chronically abused, N₂O can have serious health consequences.[33]

Box 17.2	Recommendations for Responsible Maintenance and Monitoring of Nitrous Oxide and Equipment

1. The dental office should have a properly installed N_2O delivery system. This includes appropriate scavenging equipment with a readily visible and accurate flowmeter (or equivalent measuring device), a vacuum pump with the capacity for up to 45 L of air per minute per workstation, and a variety of sizes of masks to ensure proper fit for individual patients.
2. The vacuum exhaust and ventilation exhaust should be vented to the outside (e.g., through the vacuum system) and not close to fresh-air intake vents.
3. The general ventilation should provide good room air mixing.
4. Each time the N_2O machine is first turned on, and every time a gas cylinder is changed, the pressure connections should be tested for leaks. High-pressure line connections should be tested for leaks on a quarterly basis. A soap solution may be used to test for leaks. Alternatively a portable IR spectrophotometer can be used to diagnose an insidious leak.
5. Before their first daily use, all N_2O equipment (reservoir bag, tubing, mask, connectors) should be inspected for worn parts, cracks, holes, or tears (Fig. 17.3). Replace as necessary.
6. The mask may then be connected to the tubing and the vacuum pump turned on. All appropriate flow rates (i.e., up to 45 L/min or per manufacturer's recommendations) should be verified.
7. A properly sized mask should be selected and placed on the patient. A good, comfortable fit should be ensured. The reservoir (breathing) bag should not be overinflated or underinflated while the patient is breathing O_2 (before administering N_2O).
8. The patient should be encouraged to minimize talking and mouth breathing while the mask is in place.
9. During administration, the reservoir bag should be periodically inspected for changes in tidal volume and the vacuum flow rate verified.
10. On completion of administration, 100% O_2 should be delivered to the patient for 5 min before the mask is removed. In this way, both the patient and the system will be purged of residual N_2O. Do not use an O_2 flush.
11. Periodic (semiannual interval is suggested) personal sampling of dental personnel, with emphasis on chairside personnel exposed to N_2O, should be conducted (e.g., use of diffusive sampler [dosimeters] or IR spectrophotometer).

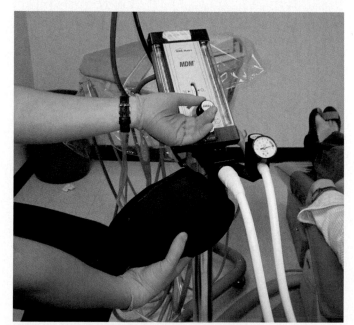

Figure 17.3 The reservoir bag may be checked for leaks by overinflating the bag, occluding conducting tubes, and squeezing the bag. If the bag deflates, a leak is present in the system.

Agents that can produce euphoria when inhaled are readily available. This includes such products as solvents, model glue, nail polish remover, or typewriter correction fluid, to name a few. These products are sold commercially to everyone. It is particularly unfortunate that children and adolescents have a higher incidence of abuse than even older adolescents and young adults. It also appears that these inhalation products are attractive because they are cheap and easily attained. N_2O is legally available in small cylinders called *whippets* (Fig. 17.4). These are used in the manufacturing of whipping cream; N_2O is the propellant gas in whipped cream cylinders (Fig. 17.5). When these cylinders are used properly, whipping cream fluffed up by N_2O emerges; if they are held improperly, 100% N_2O escapes. A quick glance at a can of whipping cream on the grocer's shelf reveals N_2O as an ingredient. Often these whippets can be purchased at music concerts or, at one time in the recent past, in areas of repute for good times, such as Bourbon Street in New Orleans. The pharmacokinetics of N_2O do not allow for screening detection as with other drugs. This does not imply that there is no physiologic effect on the user.

Typical abusers of N_2O are usually older and commonly from middle- to upper-class society. If they have an inhalation sedation unit available, it has probably been altered in

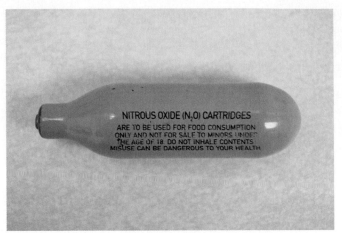

Figure 17.4 Nitrous oxide whippet. (From Clark MS, Brunick AL: *Handbook of nitrous oxide and oxygen sedation*, ed 4, St Louis, 2014, Mosby.)

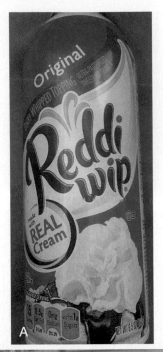

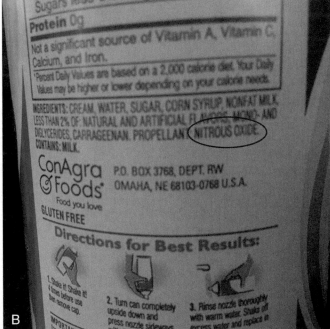

Figure 17.5 Whipped cream container uses N_2O as its whipping gas.

an attempt to deliver a higher concentration of gas. A dentist living in Colorado placed a blanket over his head to increase the concentration. He became asphyxiated because of this and the fact that he altered the sedation machine to deliver 100% N_2O. He could not be revived. Chronic inhalation (abuse) of N_2O may lead to various neuropathies.[30,33] This is particularly disconcerting if the loss of tactile sensation is associated with interference with one's occupation (e.g., dentist).[32,33] The N_2O-induced neuropathy is generally reversible, but can be permanent.

N_2O is used for mood alteration, sedation, and analgesia. It is the weakest of all general anesthetic agents. In certain circumstances (e.g., <21% O_2), it has the potential to cause unconsciousness. Today, most states and provinces have programs that are part of the licensing board to help practitioners effectively treat addictive and self-abusive drug issues. All drug addiction requires just "a little bit more" to maintain or reach that desired "high." It is the principle of addiction and always, if not aborted, leads to death.[34,35] The stakes are high when a decision is made by anyone to abuse a substance. Finally, as we should have learned from Horace Wells, whose life took a tragic turn because of abuse, "Let's make original mistakes."

SEXUAL PHENOMENON AND NITROUS OXIDE AND OTHER SEDATION TECHNIQUES

The goal being sought by administering sedation is to distract the fearful patient and take their mind off of what is being done by the dentist (e.g., drilling, cutting). Fearful patients are overly alert and overly aware of what is being done to them while in the dental chair. They overreact to any and all stimuli, be they painful (nociceptive) or (usually) nonpainful (e.g., blowing air in their mouth), making it difficult for the dentist to treat them effectively and safely.

All drugs administered for sedation, by all routes, including N_2O, are classified as central nervous system (CNS) depressants. Our goal is to take the fearful patient's mind away from what is happening to them in the dental chair to some other, less threatening place. Under the influence of this CNS-depressant drug the patient relaxes, allowing the doctor to carry out the required dental treatment safely and efficiently.

By depressing the patient's brain (CNS) the drug (e.g., N_2O) alters their state of consciousness, making them less aware of their surroundings. At the same time, by depressing the CNS all sedative drugs also depress the patient's inhibitions, making it easier for them to "'let out"' whatever it is they are feeling at that time, thus the common term *"laughing gas"* for nitrous oxide. N_2O does *not* make you happy. If you *are* happy when the drug is administered, you become happier and are more likely to express it outwardly and laugh (you are less inhibited). Likewise, if a person is in a foul mood when administered a sedative drug—including N_2O—we could call N_2O *'crying gas,'* as their sorry feelings would be more likely to be expressed.

These outward expressions of mood are seen in all patients, with all sedation techniques, including inhalation sedation.

When sedative drugs are administered in higher doses, the level of CNS depression increases and patients may dream. Though less common, dreaming can also occur with the "usual" dose of a CNS-depressant drug. Dreaming can be "good" (dreaming of happy times in the past, of relaxing on a beach, of skiing), where the patient lies back in the dental chair with a smile on their face, or "bad" ("nightmares"), where the patient suddenly grabs the nasal hood (nosepiece) and sits up in the dental chair telling the doctor, "I don't like this stuff. It's too intense" (specifically with N_2O-O_2 sedation).

Dreams can also be of a sexual nature.

History

Sir Humphrey Davy (1778–1829) in his book *Researches, Chemical and Philosophical; Chiefly Concerning Nitrous Oxide* (1798), described experiencing "voluptuous sensations" while inhaling nitrous oxide[36] (see Chapter 11).

Reports of sexual hallucinations while receiving anesthetic drugs (of all sorts and by all routes of administration) have occurred ever since they were first used in the early 1840s.[37] The first reported case of alleged sexual abuse during anesthesia occurred in Paris, France, in 1847. This was less than 1 year after the first public demonstration of ether anesthesia in Boston, Massachusetts, on October 16, 1846. A Parisian dentist was accused of using ether to assist in sexually assaulting two girls.[38]

Less than 2 years later, physicians were debating whether sexual dreaming could be a side effect of anesthesia. In January 1849 a discussion of "Chloroform in Midwifery" occurred during a meeting of the Westminster Medical Society in England.[37,39] One of the physicians, Dr. G. T. Gream (Obstetrician, Queen Charlotte's Lying-In Hospital, London, England), enumerated several reasons why he did not think that chloroform was appropriate for obstetric use, and in so doing, he "alluded to several cases in which women had, under the influence of chloroform, made use of obscene and disgusting language. This latter fact alone he considered sufficient to prevent the use of chloroform in English women."[37,39]

What is readily apparent from these accounts is that within 3 or 4 years of its introduction, inhalation analgesia and anesthesia were well recognized to cause sexual dreams or ideations. The refined sensibilities and decorum of certain English physicians might be contravened by the use of these drugs.[37,38]

Concern about sexual dreaming with anesthesia also occurred in the United States, where in 1854 a Philadelphia dentist, Dr. Stephen T. Beale, was accused of sexually assaulting a young woman while administering ether for a dental extraction.[37,38] Writing about this case, the *Boston Medical and Surgical Journal* stated, "It is our decided opinion, that the evidence of even a partially etherized person should not be received as valid, without corroboration. We believe that such persons *are totally incapable of making a correct statement of what transpires during the time they are under the influence of the ether* ... [italics original]."[37,40]

Dr. Moreton Stille, a physician prominent in the realm of American medical jurisprudence, discussed the topic of altered sensations during the use of chloroform and ether.[41,42] Stille detailed the reports of dreams and hallucinations during analgesia and anesthesia that other physicians had published. Most of these dreams were of happy times or pleasant places, but occasionally dreams were unpleasant. He recognized that they could contain sexual ideations.[37] One example is of a female rendered insensible by ether who, after some unintelligible phrases, related some most circumstantial details of her private life. This involuntary confidence, which might have been followed by serious consequences had it taken place anywhere but in a hospital, was discovered afterward to have been perfectly true.[41]

An additional published case occurred in Montreal, Quebec, in 1858, where a dentist was accused of attempted rape while using chloroform during a dental procedure.[43] The husband of another patient testified that his wife also thought she had been assaulted by the dentist, but the husband was present for the entire procedure and no assault had occurred. Yet the court found the dentist "guilty of an attempt to commit rape, with recommendation to mercy."[43] Therefore, by the late 1850s, the concept that ether and chloroform could produce sexually related dreams and ideations was well known in Europe, Britain, and the United States.[37]

Stille also listed six points about "etherization" (ether or chloroform), two of which are significant to this discussion: (1) that the memory of what has passed during the state of etherization is either of events wholly unreal or of real occurrences perverted from their actual nature, and (2) that there is reason to believe that the impression left by the dreams occasioned by ether may remain permanently fixed in the memory with all the vividness of real events.[37,41]

More recent studies confirmed many other studies that dreaming of various scenes is a frequent event during anesthesia, occurring in as many as 22% of patients if questioned immediately after anesthesia emergence.[44,45] The dreaming patients tended to be younger and healthier,[44,45] and dreaming was thought to occur during anesthesia recovery.[45] This period of anesthesia recovery could be equated with the level of "minimal" to "moderate" sedation employed in the outpatient dental office setting. In most of these studies, women more commonly had dreams compared with men, and the reported dreams that were related to sex were infrequent.[44,45] These studies seem to confirm the observations of the physicians and dentists of the mid-1800s, although the anesthetics are completely different.

All but one historical report has involved women patients receiving treatment from male physicians or dentists. This same phenomenon has been observed, though less commonly, in men using current anesthetics and sedatives.[46–48] The sex of the physician, dentist, or nurse does not protect him or her against allegations of malfeasance.[46,47] Just as in these cases of women, men may have dreams about their female anesthetist,[49] recovery room nurse,[46] dentist, and dental hygienist.

Present Day

Situations continue to be reported in which a male doctor has been accused by a female patient of sexual assault during their receipt of dental care under sedation.[50,51] Though some accusations followed the administration of intravenous sedation,[52,53] the overwhelming majority followed the use of N_2O-O_2 inhalation sedation. A significant number of these accusations led to formal complaints being lodged with law enforcement agencies, frequently leading to criminal charges of sexual assault being lodged against the dentist.[54–56] Most have involved formal hearings before state dental boards with a consideration of loss of professional licensure. The possibility of being accused of sexual improprieties, when in fact the patient may have been dreaming, presents a serious problem for the administrator of inhalation sedation as well as all other sedation techniques.

Nitrous Oxide-Oxygen Inhalation Sedation and Dreaming

When N_2O-O_2 inhalation sedation is administered by titration technique, the patient receives progressively larger concentrations of N_2O (at increments of 1 minute) until the desired level of sedation is achieved. This process of titration usually requires a 5- or 6-minute period of time to achieve this desired level. On the normal distribution curve ("bell-shaped curve") the "average" patient will require between 35% and 45% N_2O. Some require higher N_2O concentrations and others less. The titration technique permits the dentist to provide each patient with his or her "ideal" level of N_2O.

With the built-in "fail-safe" devices, a contemporary N_2O-O_2 delivery system cannot deliver more than 70% N_2O and no less than 30% O_2. Because atmospheric air contains ~21% O_2, it becomes impossible to administer to the patient less than "normal" levels of oxygen during their sedation procedure.

If the titration technique is employed, it becomes highly unlikely that an overly deep level of sedation will occur, minimizing the occurrence of complications such as nausea and vomiting and dreaming.

However, all too many dentists, in an effort to "save time," do not titrate N_2O. They administer a fixed concentration of the agent to all of their patients. Most often these doctors administer a concentration of 40% N_2O (60% O_2) or 50% N_2O (50% O_2). Though in no way dangerous (the patient is still receiving >21% O_2), this technique does increase the risk of oversedation in those patients who, in fact, require a lesser

N_2O concentration than that being delivered to them. For example, a patient requiring only 25% N_2O who receives 40% or 50% N_2O has a greater likelihood of experiencing the previously mentioned complications, including dreaming.

Dreaming need not be sexual in nature. As mentioned earlier, when patients enter into a too-deep level of sedation, they become more dissociated with reality. They remain conscious but oblivious to what is happening around and to them. Their response to verbal commands—such as "open your mouth"—is sluggish or nonexistent. The explanation for this is akin to what happens when a person is sleeping deeply and "dreams" that they hear a telephone ringing. After a number of "rings" they slowly awaken to the fact that their bedside telephone is really ringing. But during their "dream" of lying on a beach in Hawai'i they couldn't comprehend *why* a telephone would be ringing. Back to our dental patient receiving too much N_2O: "Why, when lying on that very same beach, would someone be asking me to 'open your mouth'?"

Management of this scenario is for the doctor to decrease the flow of N_2O while increasing the flow of O_2, thereby lessening the level of sedation and returning the patient back to the desired level.

As for dreams with sexual content, the incidence appears to be quite rare, although it is likely to be considerably greater than reported, as reporting of sexual dreams is embarrassing for most people.

In a 1975 paper reviewing 1331 sedation cases, 3 cases of sexual dreaming and hallucinations were uncovered (0.00225% incidence).[57] Rosenberg found an increased incidence of dreaming from 2% to 29% when the percentage of N_2O was increased from 40% to 80%, respectively, in young, healthy females. Other responses observed in this study included paranoid auditory and visual hallucinations, panic, anger, and emotionally kaleidoscopic dreams.[58]

Dr. Jed Allen, in his textbook on dental sedation, wrote in 1979: "A female chaperone is essential in an office where nitrous oxide-oxygen is administered, owing to the propensity of females under nitrous oxide-oxygen to have sexual abreactions."[59]

In a 1988 anonymous survey of 50 female dental hygiene students (average age 20 years) at the University of Southern California School of Dentistry, 18% expressed a feeling of "sexual arousal" or "increased sexuality" while receiving N_2O-O_2 sedation.[60]

In a second survey (1988) of dental students (average age 22 years) receiving N_2O-O_2 sedation during their preclinical training, 10% of both male and female students (N = 88) reported feelings of increased sexuality or arousal.[61] There was no difference in the occurrence of sexual arousal in persons describing themselves as sexually active from those classifying themselves as not sexually active.

Commonalities in Reported Cases of Alleged Sexual Misconduct on Sedated Patients

Having been in the position of reviewing too many cases of alleged sexual misconduct on dental patients receiving sedation—primarily inhalation sedation—many similarities appear:

1. All complaints were from young female patients (e.g., teenage to early 30s) and involved male dentists.
2. No patient discussed her experience with the doctor after recovery from the sedation.
3. Many of the women commented later on how shocked or stunned they were that this might have occurred.
4. Several patients mentioned that they were unable to think clearly until the next day.
5. Formal complaints to either a law enforcement agency or a state dental board did not occur until either family members or friends were told of the experience and advice was sought as to how to proceed. Several more recent cases (allegations) were brought many years (e.g., 20 to 30 years) after the alleged occurrence, when the now-adult patient went through psychotherapy.[54]
6. No patient gave any indication of distress during treatment, but most mentioned spontaneously that they were frightened by the experience, explaining their not accusing the doctor at that very moment.
7. At the time of the perceived occurrence, the male doctor was alone in the treatment room with the female patient. In only two cases was a dental assistant or any other person present in the treatment room with the doctor and patient. This appears to be the key factor that allowed these cases to be seriously considered by law enforcement authorities.
8. Concentrations of N_2O in excess of 50% were administered in every situation in which allegations of sexual misconduct were involved.

As it does in skin, N_2O-O_2 also alters tactile sensation throughout the body. Consider a dental patient in the supine position during dental treatment and sedation. The dentist is treating mandibular teeth. He or she would be seated at an 8:00 position at the dental chair facing the patient. As the doctor brings his or her hand around to administer a local anesthetic injection or begin to drill on a tooth, their forearm and elbow will usually be in contact with, and applying pressure on, the patient's chest. It is quite difficult for a dentist to accomplish dental treatment in the lower jaw without coming into physical contact with portions of the patient's chest, abdomen or, in smaller patients, upper pelvic region.

An unsedated dental patient would not consider this pressure or sensation to be a sexual assault. It is quite obviously the dentist coming into incidental contact with the body as he or she "assaults" the mouth with the drill or syringe. However, when a patient's mind has been depressed by N_2O-O_2 (or other sedative drugs), they are not aware of what the doctor is doing in their mouth, but they may be aware of this "pressure" on their chest (breasts of a female patient). Because their sensation is altered, this may be interpreted by the patient as sexually arousing. But they are dreaming at the time and are unable to connect what is happening dentally with their "real" sexual dream.

Patients experiencing a sexual dream do believe it is really happening. Sleeping dogs aside one's bed will bark, pant, and move their paws as they dream of chasing a rabbit. When a human experiences a nightmarish dream, they awaken bathed in sweat, with a rapid heart rate, and breathing rapidly. During a sexual dream the person is physically (sexually) aroused, not realizing it is a dream until they awake.

Dreams are real to the person having them. Therefore a complainant in a N_2O-O_2 sexual assault matter will give evidence that she honestly believes to be truthful, even though in reality it may have been a result of a hallucination or dream. It is difficult or almost impossible for the patient to distinguish between "fact and fiction" in these circumstances while their brain is under the influence of N_2O.

Unfortunately, some physicians, surgeons, and dentists use CNS-depressant drugs to sexually assault their patients.[62–64] Their defense simply is that the drug the patient received for sedation could have caused a sexual hallucination to occur, and hence the sexual assault was not real and did not actually occur. This makes it very difficult for the difference between a dream and actual reality to be shown in court.

Recommendations

The allegation of sexual impropriety against a health professional is devastating in its potential impact on the livelihood of that person, whether the allegation is subsequently proved or disproved. Loss of dental license and/or incarceration may result. As with all situations involving potential risk, it is best to attempt to avoid their occurrence. To do so in this one area is easily accomplished. If put into practice, the following recommendations related to the administration of N_2O-O_2 inhalation sedation will essentially eliminate the possibility of such allegations:

1. **Never sedate any patient, with any technique of sedation, without an assistant present in the room.** Require the assistant to remain in the room throughout the entire sedation procedure.
2. **Do not routinely administer N_2O in concentrations greater than 50%. Always titrate N_2O-O_2.** For the concerned doctor who employs sedation frequently, the installation of a closed-circuit television (CCTV) monitoring system would effectively disprove such allegations.[65] Signage indicating that CCTV is in use must be posted.

It is extremely likely that the incidence of sexually oriented dreams or hallucinations during inhalation sedation is higher than is imagined, but in the typical dental office environment, with both a chairside assistant and a busy office setting, potential complaints by a patient are probably obviated by the relative unlikelihood of the experience having occurred (e.g., "It must have been a dream!"). In addition, patients seem to be somewhat reticent to report such phenomena, although the frequency of such accusations appears to be increasing.

As Dr. Dudley W. Buxton (member of the Royal College of Physicians and member of the Royal College of Surgeons of England; 1855–1931) stated more than 120 years ago, "[N]o administrator of an anesthetic is safe from having such a charge preferred against him, and if he and his supposed victim are alone, it is simply a case of word against word."[66] This admonition continues to be prudent for those who administer anesthetics or intravenous sedatives and for all postanesthesia care unit personnel: It is mandatory to have a third party in the immediate vicinity.

REFERENCES

1. American Dental Association: Council on Dental Education guidelines for teaching the comprehensive control of pain and anxiety in dentistry. *J Dent Educ* 36:62, 1972.
2. Vaisman A: Work in surgical theatres and its influence on the health of anesthesiologists. *Eksp Khir Anestheziol* 3:44, 1967.
3. Askrog V, Harvald B: Teratogen effect of inhalation anesthetics. *Nord Med* 83(16):498–500, 1970.
4. Lencz L, Nemes C: Morbidity of Hungarian anesthesiologists in relation to occupational hazard. In Corbett TH, ed: anesthetics as a cause of abortion. *Fertil Steril* 23:866, 1972.
5. Bruce D, Eide KA, Linde HM, Eckenhoff JE: Causes of death among anesthesiologists: a 20 year survey. *Anesthesiology* 35(3):565–569, 1968.
6. Cohen EN, Brown BW, Jr, Bruce DL, et al: A survey of anesthetic health hazards among dentists. *J Am Dent Assoc* 90(6):1291–1296, 1975.
7. Cohen EN, Gift HC, Brown BW, Jr, et al: Occupational disease in dentistry and chronic exposure to trace anesthetic gases. *J Am Dent Assoc* 101(1):21–31, 1980.
8. Bruce DL, Bach MJ, Arbit J: Trace anesthetic effects on perceptual, cognitive, and motor skills. *Anesthesiology* 40(5):453–458, 1974.
9. Bruce DL, Bach MJ: *Trace effects of anesthetic gases on behavioural performance of operating room personnel.* HEW pub no (NIOSH) 76-169, Cincinnati, 1976, U.S. Department of Health, Education, and Welfare.
10. Yagiela JA: Health hazards and nitrous oxide: a time for reappraisal. *Anesth Prog* 38(1):1–11, 1991.
11. Clark M, Brunick A: Potential biohazards for health personnel associated with chronic exposure to N₂O. In Clark M, Brunick A, editors: *Handbook of nitrous oxide and oxygen sedation,* ed 4, St Louis, 2015, Mosby, pp 188–202.
12. ADA Council on Scientific Affairs: ADA Council on Dental Practice: nitrous oxide in the dental office. *J Am Dent Assoc* 128(3):364–365, 1997.
13. Fujinagra M, Baden JM, Mazze RI: Susceptible period of nitrous oxide teratogenicity in Sprague-Dawley rats. *Teratology* 40(5):439–444, 1989.
14. Rowland AS, Baird DD, Weinberg CR, et al: Reduced fertility among women employed as dental assistants exposed to high levels of nitrous oxide. *N Engl J Med* 327(14):993–997, 1992.
15. Eger EI, II: Fetal injury and abortion associated with occupational exposure to inhaled anesthetics. *AANA J* 59(4):309–312, 1991.
16. Sweeney B, Bingham RM, Amos RJ, et al: Toxicity of bone marrow in dentists exposed to nitrous oxide. *BMJ* 291(6495):567–569, 1985.
17. Dookun R, Lyne JP, Robb ND: Nitrous oxide: past, present, and future. *SAAD Dig* 14(1-2):13–35, 1997.
18. Layzer RB, Fishman RA, Schafer JA: Neuropathy following abuse of nitrous oxide. *Neurology* 28(5):504–506, 1978.
19. Lassen HC, Henriksen E, Neukirch R, Kristensen HS: Treatment of tetanus, severe bone marrow depression after prolonged nitrous oxide anesthesia. *Lancet* 270(6922):527–530, 1956.
20. Stacy CB, DiRocci A, Gould RJ: Methionine in the treatment of nitrous oxide-induced neuropathy and myeloneuropathy. *J Neurol* 239(7):401–403, 1992.
21. Weimann J: Toxicity of nitrous oxide. *Best Pract Res Clin Anaesthesiol* 17(1):47–61, 2003.
22. Myles PS, Leslie K, Silbert B, et al: A review of the risks and benefits of nitrous oxide in current anesthetic practice. *Anaesth Intensive Care* 32(2):165–172, 2004.
23. Certosimo F, Walton M, Hartzell D, Farris J: Clinical evaluation of the efficacy of three nitrous oxide scavenging units during dental treatment. *Gen Dent* 50(5):430–435, 2002.
24. Chessor E, Verhoeven M, Hon CY, Teschke K: Evaluation of modified scavenging system to reduce occupational exposure to nitrous oxide in labor and delivery rooms. *J Occup Environ Hyg* 2(6):314–322, 2005.
25. Allen WA: Nitrous oxide in the surgery; pollution and scavenging. *Br Dent J* 159(7):222–230, 1985.
26. Nitrous oxide gas monitor, Medigas 3010. *Dent Econ* 90(9):120, 2000.
27. Lane GA: Measurement of anesthetic pollution in oral surgery offices. *J Oral Surg* 36(6):444–446, 1978.
28. Landauer RS, Jr. Co, Division of Tech Ops, Products and Services Division, Landauer, Glenwood Science Park, Glenwood, Ill 40425.
29. Gillman MA: Nitrous oxide abuse in perspective. *Clin Neuropharmacol* 15(4):297–306, 1992.
30. Malamed SF, Orr DL, II, Hershfield S, et al: The recreational abuse of nitrous oxide by health professionals. *J Calif Dent Assoc* 8:38, 1980.
31. Gillman MA: Nitrous oxide: an opioid addictive agent. Review of the evidence. *Am J Med* 81(1):97–102, 1986.
32. Aston R: Drug abuse: its relationship to dental practice. *Dent Clin North Am* 28(3):595–610, 1984.
33. Layzer RB, Fishman RA, Schafer JA: Neuropathy following abuse of nitrous oxide. *Neurology* 28(5):504–506, 1978.
34. Wagner SA, Clark MA, Wesche DL, et al: Asphyxial deaths from recreational use of nitrous oxide. *J Forensic Sci* 37(4):1008–1015, 1992.
35. Suruda AJ, McGlothlin JD: Fatal abuse of nitrous oxide in the workplace. *J Occup Med* 32(8):682–684, 1990.
36. Davy H: Researches, chemical and philosophical; chiefly concerning nitrous oxide. In Fullmer JZ, editor: *Sir Humphry Davy's published works,* Cambridge, MA, 1969, Harvard University Press, p 1800.
37. Strickland RA, Butterworth JF, IV: Sexual dreaming during anesthesia: early case histories (1849–1888) of the phenomenon. *Anesthesiology* 106(6):1232–1236, 2007.
38. Hartshorne E: Remarks on the case of a dentist convicted of violating a patient while under the influence of ether inhalation. *Med Examiner* 10:706–730, 1854.
39. Westminster Medical Society: Chloroform in midwifery. *Lancet* 53:99–100, 1849.
40. Sentence of Dr. Beale, the dentist. *Boston Med Surg J* 51:384–385, 1854.
41. Stille M: The psychical effects of ether inhalation. *Med Examiner* 10:730–739, 1854.
42. Wharton F, Stille M: *A treatise on medical jurisprudence,* Philadelphia, 1855, Kay & Brother, pp 337–342.
43. Alleged criminal assault by a dentist. *Boston Med Surg J* 59:287, 1858.
44. Leslie K, Myles PS, Forbes A, et al: Dreaming during anaesthesia in patients at high risk of awareness. *Anaesthesia* 60:239–244, 2005.

45. Leslie K, Skrzypek H, Paech MJ, Kurowski I: Dreaming during anesthesia and anesthetic depth in elective surgery patients. *Anesthesiology* 106:33–42, 2007.

46. Playford RJ: Allegation of sexual assault following midazolam sedation in a man. *Anaesthesia* 47(9):818, 1992.

47. Balasubramaniam B, Park GR: Sexual hallucinations during and after sedation and anaesthesia. *Anaesthesia* 58:549–553, 2003.

48. Hansen-Flaschen J, Adler BS: Allegations of sexual abuse in an intensive care unit. *Crit Care Med* 27(2):437–440, 1999.

49. Thomson KD, Knight AB: Hallucinations after propofol. *Anaesthesia* 43(2):170–171, 1988.

50. Jastak JT, Malamed SF: Nitrous oxide and sexual phenomena. *J Am Dent Assoc* 101(1):38–40, 1980.

51. Lambert C: Sexual phenomena, hypnosis, and nitrous oxide sedation. *J Am Dent Assoc* 105(6):990–991, 1982.

52. Dundee JW: Fantasies during sedation with intravenous midazolam or diazepam. *Med Leg J* 58(Pt 1):29–34, 1990.

53. Weller MPI: Midazolam and sexual fantasies. *Plast Reconstr Surg* 92(7):1368–1370, 1993.

54. Gardiner S: Dentist Rodger Garry Leighton guilty of indecent assaults on young girls. *Sydney Morning Herald*. November 11, 2015, http://www.smh.com.au/nsw/dentist-rodger-garry-leighton-guilty-of-indecent-assaults-on-young-girls-20151111-gkwc2t.html. (Accessed 14 January, 2016).

55. Mencarini M: Former dentist convicted of sexual assault to get new trial. *Detroit Free Press*. September 3, 2015. http://www.freep.com/story/news/local/michigan/2015/09/03/dentist-sexual-assault-wendell-racette/71665506/. (Accessed 14 January, 2016).

56. Marzulli J: Dentist wanted for sexually assaulting patient under anesthesia arrested at Kennedy Airport. *New York Daily News*. January 12, 2016. http://www.nydailynews.com/news/crime/cops-nab-dentist-kennedy-sexual-assault-patient-article-1.2493651. (Accessed 14 January, 2016).

57. Jastak JT, Paravecchio R: An analysis of 1331 sedations using inhalation, intravenous or other techniques. *J Am Dent Assoc* 91(6):1242–1249, 1975.

58. Rosenberg P: The effect of N_2O-oxygen inhalation on subjective experiences of healthy young adults. *Ann Chir Gynaecol Fenn* 63(6):500–504, 1974.

59. Allen GD: *Dental anesthesia and analgesia (local and general)*, ed 2, Baltimore, 1979, Williams & Wilkins, p 180.

60. Malamed SF, Serxner K, Weidenfeld AM: The incidence of sexual phenomena in females receiving nitrous oxide and oxygen inhalation sedation. *J Am Analgesia Soc* 22(2):9–10, 1988.

61. Malamed SF: Current concerns, chronic exposure, recreational abuse, and sexual phenomena. In Malamed SF, editor: *Sedation: a guide to patient management*, ed 3, St Louis, 1995, CV Mosby, Inc., pp 291–292.

62. Canadian doctor sexually assaulted 21 sedate women, *USA Today*. February 26, 2014. www.usatoday.com. (Accessed 20 January, 2016).

63. In the Matter of the Disciplinary Action Against the Dentist License of Joseph H. Wang. No. C6-87-1337. Court of Appeals of Minnesota. December 29, 1987.

64. In the Matter of the Disciplinary Action Against the Dentist License of Joseph H. Wang. No. C6-87-1337. Supreme Court of Minnesota. June 9, 1989.

65. The law and ethics of recording in dental surgeries, *DDU J*. March 2014. www.theddu.com/guidance-and-advice/journals/march-2014/the-law-and-ethics-of-recording-in-dental-surgeries. (Accessed 20 January, 2016).

66. Buxton DW: *Anaesthetics: their uses and administration*, Philadelphia, 1888, P. Blakiston, Son, pp 149–151.

chapter 18

Practical Considerations

CHAPTER OUTLINE

$\mathcal{P}$revious chapters of this section, the technique of administration, complications, and current concerns associated with inhalation sedation have been discussed. In this chapter, a number of additional factors are discussed in an attempt to reflect on and evaluate other factors that are important in the completeness of the overall training of the administrator of nitrous oxide–oxygen (N_2O-O_2). Many of these questions do not usually arise until the clinician has been using inhalation sedation for a while. It should be remembered that realistically, complications of N_2O-O_2 sedation are indeed rare, and N_2O is a very safe agent for use in the health sciences.

DETERMINATION OF PROPER TITRATION AT SUBSEQUENT VISITS

One of the most important factors to consider when using inhalation sedation is that the gases have a very rapid onset of action. Because of this rapid onset, it becomes possible for patients to be titrated to a precise level of sedation. The ability to titrate with inhalation sedation is of considerable importance because it is quite possible that a patient may require different concentrations of N_2O-O_2 to achieve the same level of sedation at subsequent visits. The absence of titration leads to increased patient reports of negative reactions (e.g., nausea, "it's too intense!") to N_2O-O_2, and clinicians begin to shy away from its use. Titration is the only means for the administrator to satisfactorily determine the appropriate level of sedation. Factors

that may influence the concentration of N_2O-O_2 necessary for adequate sedation include the patient's level of anxiety, expected level of pain, age, and presence of other sedatives or CNS depressants.

Procedural Anxiety

As the patient's anxiety decreases and the bulk of discomfort associated with the procedure is complete, the percentage of N_2O necessary to achieve a given level of sedation will correspondingly decrease, with all other variables remaining equal. With proper patient management by both the administering clinician and ancillary staff, a fearful patient should become less apprehensive about subsequent procedures—"It wasn't that bad!" If the patient is titrated carefully to his or her "ideal sedation level," it will likely be observed that the patient requires somewhat lower N_2O concentrations as he or she becomes progressively less anxious over time.

Although this is true for most patients and for most forms of procedural treatment, it is also possible that a patient who has been responding quite well at 30% N_2O will have an inadequate clinical effect from that concentration when a different type of procedure is undertaken. For example, this patient may respond well at 30% N_2O for restorative treatment; however, when undergoing periodontal surgery, the patient may require 45% N_2O. This is explained by the increased level of anxiety produced in this patient by the prospect of a surgical procedure in contrast with the more benign (in this patient's mind) restorative treatment.

Baseline Level of Stress

A significant influence on the level of N_2O required for sedation is the patient's baseline level of stress. The patient's state of mind has a significant bearing on the manner in which central nervous system (CNS)–depressant drugs act. A patient may arrive at the facility on a day when things have just not gone well. If this patient has any degree of procedural anxiety, it becomes obvious that our sedation technique has a formidable task ahead. Contrast this with the same patient who arrives at the facility having had a simply wonderful day. The concentration of N_2O required to sedate this patient will probably be lower than that required in the first situation.

It is impossible, and indeed foolhardy, to discount the influence of outside stresses on the patient. All practicing clinicians have encountered remarkably different behavior patterns from the same patient at different visits. The process of titrating N_2O will help compensate for the effects of these outside influences.

As discussed in Chapter 4, it is recommended that the anxious patient and the medically compromised patient be scheduled for their procedure earlier in the day. At this time, presumably following a period of restful sleep, the medically compromised patient is rested and better able to tolerate any additional stresses imposed by the procedure. The fearful patient ought to be treated early in the day for the simple reason that the patient will want to get "it" over with as soon as possible. The procedural appointment might well be the most unpleasant part of this patient's day. An appointment scheduled late in the day allows the patient more time to worry and for their level of anxiety to increase. Scheduled later in the day, this patient might require significantly greater levels of N_2O to achieve sedation than would have been necessary if he or she had been treated earlier in the morning.

Level of Fatigue

The level of baseline fatigue has an effect on the patient's pain reaction threshold and therefore on the response to $N_2O\text{-}O_2$ sedation. Patients who are tired and unable to sleep the night before the appointment because of procedural fear overreact to most stimuli. With their "nerves on edge," they interpret usually nonpainful stimuli as painful. $N_2O\text{-}O_2$ inhalation sedation may still prove to be effective; however, the patient may require greater concentrations of N_2O.

When a patient appears to be apprehensive about an upcoming treatment, it is prudent for a clinician to address this fact and consider prescribing a sedative-hypnotic for the patient 1 hour before bedtime the evening before the scheduled treatment (e.g., triazolam). A well-rested patient may require lower concentrations of N_2O to achieve comparable levels of sedation than the overtired patient.

When the three factors mentioned are considered, it becomes obvious that the same person may respond to $N_2O\text{-}O_2$ in an entirely different manner at subsequent appointments. When titration is not used, it is entirely possible that the level of N_2O used at prior visits will produce the same level of sedation, decreased levels of sedation, or overly deep sedation of the same patient. The use of titration at each and every appointment minimizes the significance of these factors.

POOR PATIENT EVALUATION

Patient evaluation relates to the administrator observing the many signs and symptoms that the patient will be exhibiting during the procedure. One of the most important safety features of all pharmacosedative techniques is that the patient remains conscious and is able to respond to verbal and physical stimuli. To ignore a patient's input during the important induction phase of sedation is foolhardy. The sedation should be to a level at which the patient feels comfortable. Information imparted by the patient is quite important in the overall assessment of his or her well-being. The patient should be used as a vital component of the overall monitoring of conscious (minimal or moderate) sedation.

PATIENT UNATTENDED DURING SEDATION

Occasions may develop during the treatment of a particular patient when the clinician will be called away for a few moments to attend to some other business. When a patient is undergoing $N_2O\text{-}O_2$ sedation, the patient must *never* be left unattended by the clinician administering the $N_2O\text{-}O_2$.

When $N_2O\text{-}O_2$ is administered, a constant flow of gases is delivered to the patient. Procedural stimulation serves to lighten the level of sedation. When procedural stimulus stops but the N_2O level is left constant, the depth of sedation will increase. The lack of treatment stimulation is the primary reason for this occurrence. This normally does not result in any serious difficulty when someone is present in the treatment room and monitoring the patient. In the absence of a trained person to monitor the patient and to promptly recognize and manage the situation, significant complications are possible.

Should it become essential for the clinician to leave a patient receiving $N_2O\text{-}O_2$ for even a few short minutes, a well-trained assistant should be available to remain with the patient in the treatment area. In addition, because of the lack of procedural-induced stimulation of this patient, the level of N_2O should be decreased by approximately 10% whenever there is a pause in treatment for more than a few minutes. In the absence of an N_2O credentialed person to monitor the patient, the clinician must terminate the flow of N_2O, reestablish a flow of 100% O_2, and return the patient to the presedative state before leaving the treatment area. Although this second option is more cumbersome, it should be followed whenever there is no other person available to monitor the patient.

As mentioned in Chapter 17, there is yet another, more important reason for the N_2O clinician to have a second person available during sedative procedures—that of minimizing the possibility of being accused (perhaps falsely) of sexual improprieties. A second person must always be present in the treatment area whenever a patient receives N_2O-O_2 or any other pharmacosedative drug.

IMPROPER RECOVERY PROCEDURES

Too many clinicians will terminate the flow of N_2O and simply remove the nasal hood, permitting the patient to breathe atmospheric air rather than 100% O_2. As is noted in the following situation, such practice leads to an increased incidence of postinhalation sedation complications. Many clinicians who do administer 100% O_2 to their patients following N_2O-O_2 sedation do so for a fixed period of time (e.g., 2 minutes), regardless of the length of the inhalation sedation that preceded it. As was discussed in earlier chapters on pharmacology and technique of administration, a minimum period of from 3 to 5 minutes of 100% O_2 is required for the majority of the N_2O to be eliminated from the patient's body After 3 to 5 minutes, the degree of recovery is assessed and, if necessary, the patient continues to receive 100% O_2 for an additional period.

Means of assessing recovery ought to be employed routinely whenever inhalation sedation is used if the patient is to be permitted to leave the facility alone to drive a vehicle or return to work.

Two means of assessment of recovery from sedation are recommended: (1) monitoring of vital signs and (2) a brief neurologic assessment. These have been discussed earlier in this section. Vital signs, especially blood pressure, heart rate, and respiratory rate, are monitored at a patient's first visit to the dental office to establish baseline vital signs. Neurologic assessment after N_2O administration is done to ensure a complete return to presedation cognitive ability and confirm the presence of steady gate with ambulation. The postoperative assessments are compared with both the preoperative and baseline values; if they are reasonably close to these readings, it may be assumed that the medications administered to the patient are no longer exerting a depressant action on the cardiorespiratory system. Proper oxygenation at the end of inhalation sedation and proper assessment of recovery before discharge will prevent virtually all of the uncomfortable side effects and potential problems associated with N_2O-O_2 sedation.

POSTSEDATION NAUSEA, HEADACHE, AND LETHARGY

After N_2O-O_2 sedation, the patient, feeling symptom free and having completed appropriate recovery tests, may be discharged from the facility. In most instances, the patient will continue to feel normal, with no evidence of any side effects from the N_2O. A few patients will experience a postsedation feeling of being "hung over"; this effect may deter these few patients from future inhalation sedation appointments. Among the signs and symptoms of this postsedation hangover effect are nausea, headache, and lethargy.

In most cases, this effect does not develop within the first few minutes after the termination of the sedative procedure. Most patients will have returned to their home or business when the symptoms develop. Management is symptomatic. In most cases, tincture of time is the recommended treatment.

It is also possible for a patient to have received O_2 for the recommended 3 to 5 minutes or even longer and still encounter these same effects postoperatively. The normal distribution curve provides evidence that some persons still respond to the very low levels of N_2O found in their blood after at least 3 to 5 minutes (or longer) of 100% O_2. It is usually not possible for the clinician to prevent this occurrence the first time that the patient receives N_2O, but on subsequent visits, the patient, having informed the clinician of this unpleasant experience, will be administered 100% O_2 for a longer period. Although this increased period of oxygenation may prove adequate to prevent a recurrence of the signs and symptoms, it is entirely possible that even careful attention to the patient's recovery will fail to produce the desired result in extremely sensitive patients.

The term *diffusion hypoxia* is often mentioned in regard to this situation.[1] As discussed in Chapter 15, N_2O is rapidly removed from a patient's blood after the cessation of the N_2O gas flow. If the patient breathes atmospheric air rather than 100% O_2 at this time, the alveoli become filled with a mixture of nitrogen (N_2), O_2, carbon dioxide (CO_2), water vapor, and N_2O. Some N_2O will be reabsorbed into the circulatory system of the patient, and the O_2 present in the alveoli will be diluted to approximately 10% during the first few minutes following termination of the N_2O flow. These factors produce the signs and symptoms described. It appears that this effect is more commonly noted in cigarette smokers.[2]

One of these symptoms, lethargy, may not be caused completely by the mechanisms just described. A feeling of "not quite being back to normal" does occur in some patients who have received N_2O-O_2. When asked to describe this feeling, the patient usually describes a feeling similar to that experienced when first arising from a pleasant sleep. The patient, although not tired, is not quite fully awake, feeling perhaps 90% normal. After a few moments of activity, the patient is fully functional. This type of postsedation response is not uncommon and will develop immediately after treatment. If this occurs, the patient should be permitted to move about for a few moments. If this added movement does not return the patient to the presedative state, he or she should be placed back into the chair and given 100% O_2 until alert.

WHO ADMINISTERS NITROUS OXIDE?

The following points are mentioned because of the legalities of inhalation sedation administration within the dental or medical facility. It is not at all uncommon within the practice of dentistry for the dental assistant to be the person to administer

N_2O-O_2 to the patient. In some states, it is permissible for a dental assistant, under the direct supervision of the dentist (the dentist is physically present in the room at all times), to adjust the flow of gases delivered to the patient. In this situation, the dentist would tell the dental assistant to "raise the N_2O 1 L/min" or "decrease the O_2 by one half of a liter per minute." The dentist controls the sedative process; the assistant is an extension of the dentist in this case.

However, in other dental offices, it is common practice for the dental assistant to administer the N_2O-O_2 without the dentist physically present in the treatment area. In this situation, it is considered by the parties involved to be acceptable because the dental assistant remains with the patient. In other cases, the dentist is the one to place the nasal hood on the patient; however, the dentist will then leave the room, permitting the assistant to complete the sedative procedure alone with the patient.

Because of the legalities involved in the delegation of expanded functions to auxiliaries, such liberties as described cannot be condoned unless (1) such delegation of duty is specifically permitted under the state or provincial dental practice act and (2) the auxiliary permitted to administer the inhalation sedation has received thorough training in all aspects of N_2O-O_2 sedation, including the recognition and management of side effects and complications. For this reason, dentists using N_2O-O_2 sedation must be aware of their state's or province's dental practice act and its provisions in this area.

A similar situation involves the use of N_2O-O_2 inhalation sedation by the dental hygienist. Although 32 states permit a certified registered dental hygienist to administer N_2O-O_2 to patients, in all cases, the dental practice act specifies that a dentist must be physically present in the dental office.[3] The certified registered dental hygienist is not permitted to administer inhalation sedation to patients when the dentist is not present within the office. Unfortunately, such desirable practices do not always develop, and in many instances, N_2O-O_2 is administered to the patient without the presence of the dentist in the office. From a purely medical-legal perspective, it must be stated that this practice cannot be condoned. It is, at this time, the dentist's ultimate responsibility should anything undesirable result from the administration of inhalation sedation.[4] Although the well-trained dental hygienist is fully capable of recognizing and managing such situations, the dentist should always be immediately available to direct the patient's management and to render such additional assistance as is deemed necessary under the specific circumstances of the situation.

In dentistry, the dentist should always be present in the office when inhalation sedation is administered by the certified registered dental hygienist, and the dentist must always be physically present in the treatment area, directing the administration of N_2O-O_2 by the dental assistant if this is permitted in the state or province. As dental practice acts continue to be revised, it is recommended that the dentist, hygienist, and assistant regularly keep abreast of such changes as might affect their practices.

Registered nurse–administered N_2O programs also take similar considerations as noted earlier. Although the well-trained registered nurse is fully capable of recognizing and managing potential complications, a licensed independent practitioner should be available to offer additional support if needed. The state board of nursing in which the registered nurse is currently practicing regulates the scope of practice for the registered nurse along with institutional policy and procedures. Advisory position statements published by the various licensing agencies vary from state to state and may or may not offer a clear interpretation of the nurse practice act associated with N_2O administration by the registered nurse. One example of clear support related to registered nurse–administered N_2O is the Arizona State Board of Nursing, which published specific recommendations and guidelines surrounding nurse-administered N_2O sedation.[5] It is recommended that registered nurses and employers regularly keep abreast of practice changes by their licensing agency because changes could affect current practices. States that do not issue position statements often take a position that empowers nurses to determine their own scope of practice as established by the nurse practice act of that state.[6] When the registered nurse determines N_2O-O_2 sedation is in his or her scope of practice, administration of N_2O must be administered in accordance with institutional policy and procedures and administered in accordance with a licensed health care provider's written order.

EQUIPMENT

It is important that all members of the dental or medical team are knowledgeable and comfortable around the N_2O-O_2 sedation unit. This is essential for patient comfort and reassurance. Old and outdated equipment should be replaced with modern equipment. Updated and safe equipment will allow the practitioner to maximize skills and take full advantage of one of the most time-tested positive adjuncts in our armamentarium for the reduction of patient anxiety.

REFERENCES

1. Papageorge MB, Noonan LW, Jr, Rosenberg M: Diffusion hypoxia: another view. *Anesth Pain Control Dent* 2(3):143–149, 1993.
2. Burrows B, Knudson RL, Cline MG, Lebowitz MD: Quantitative relationships between cigarette smoking and ventilatory function. *Am Rev Respir Dis* 115(2):195–205, 1977.
3. American Dental Hygienists' Association: *States where dental hygienists can administer nitrous oxide*, Chicago, Sept 2015, American Dental Hygienists' Association. Available at: www.adha.org. (Accessed 21 January 2016).
4. Clark M, Brunick A: *Handbook of nitrous oxide and oxygen sedation*, ed 4, St Louis, 2015, Mosby.
5. Scope of practice position statement: nitrous oxide. Available at www.azbn.gov. (Accessed 21 January 2016).
6. Determining your RN scope of practice. Available at www.dora.state.co.us. (Accessed 21 January 2016).

chapter 19

Teaching Inhalation Sedation: History and Present Guidelines

CHAPTER OUTLINE

The history of inhalation sedation and its use are well documented. Inhalation sedation with nitrous oxide (N_2O) and oxygen (O_2) has withstood the test of time as the safest of all sedation techniques used in the history of medicine and dentistry. The story of N_2O began with its discovery by Sir Joseph Priestley and the experimentation and subsequent documentation of some of the effects by Sir Humphrey Davy. The involvement of Gardner Colton and even Samuel Colt, inventor of the popular revolver – the Colt-45 – as entrepreneur showmen added color, entertainment, and most importantly, clinical experience to the use of N_2O. Horace Wells, a dentist and acknowledged discoverer of anesthesia, ushered into the medical field the tremendous possibility for pain control. However, this initial discovery did not burst onto the scene; in fact, it was almost overlooked, but ended up changing human history forever.

Reading the history of N_2O can give one a special appreciation for Gardner Quincy Colton. His unselfishness in teaching Horace Wells how to manufacture N_2O led to its discovery. His documentation of more than 170,000 cases of N_2O administration without mortality gave testimony to his clinical skill and dedication to the advancement of pain control.

As has been mentioned throughout this section, inhalation sedation with N_2O-O_2 is the safest of all sedation techniques currently available. Factors responsible for this include the nature of the gases used, the manner in which they are administered (with no less than 30% O_2), the addition of fail-safe devices to inhalation sedation units, and the upgrading of education in the use of inhalation sedation. This last factor is discussed in this chapter, for although great strides have been taken in improving the educational process in teaching inhalation sedation, there remain many persons who seek an easy way out, looking for shortcuts to make the technique even simpler to learn. To maintain the safety of inhalation sedation, high standards for education must be ensured and gradually increased as our knowledge of the technique continues to grow.

As mentioned in Chapter 11, one reason for the failure of inhalation sedation to maintain its popularity among the dental profession in the 1930s and 1940s was the absence of educational programs. Dental schools did not include the use of N_2O-O_2 in their curricula, and continuing education programs were essentially nonexistent at that time. Drs. Harry Langa and Harry M. Seldin were instrumental in providing education with some uniformity and baseline criteria for didactic and clinical training of dental students.

In an effort to provide a uniform level of education in the teaching of different techniques of anesthesia and sedation within the dental school curriculum, three groups—the American Dental Society of Anesthesiology (ADSA), the American Dental Association (ADA), and the American Association of Dental Schools (AADS; now American Dental Education Association [ADEA])—sponsored four workshops on pain control in 1964, 1965, 1971, and 1977. From these conferences emerged the *Guidelines for Teaching the Comprehensive Control of Pain and Anxiety in Dentistry*.[1,2] The guidelines provide outlines for a curriculum in pain control at three levels: (1) the undergraduate dental student (doctoral student), (2) graduate dental student (postdoctoral student), and (3) in a continuing education program. These guidelines were approved by the ADA's Council on Dental Education in May 1971.[2] In 1977 part III of the guidelines, relating to continuing education programs, was revised. The revised guidelines were approved by the House of Delegates of the ADA in 1978.[3] Part I of the guidelines underwent revision in 1979,[4] with the entire document revised again in 1989,[5] 1992,[6] 2007,[7] and 2012.[8] A more recent revision to the guidelines occurred in 2016, and portions relating to the administration of inhalation sedation are presented following the 2016 educational guidelines.[9]

2016 GUIDELINES – GENERAL PRINCIPLES OF MINIMAL SEDATION

Education Courses

Education may be offered at different levels (competency, update, survey courses, and advanced education programs). A description of these different levels follows:

1. **Competency Courses** are designed to meet the needs of dentists who wish to become competent in the safe and effective administration of local anesthesia, minimal and moderate sedation. They consist of lectures, demonstrations, and sufficient clinical participation to assure the faculty that the dentist understands the procedures taught and can safely and effectively apply them so that mastery of the subject is achieved. Faculty must assess and document the dentist's competency upon successful completion of such training. To maintain competency, periodic update courses must be completed.
2. **Update Courses** are designed for persons with previous training. They are intended to provide a review of the subject and an introduction to recent advances in the field. They should be designed didactically and clinically to meet the specific needs of the participants. Participants must have completed previous competency training (equivalent, at a minimum, to the competency course described in this document) and have current experience to be eligible for enrollment in an update course.
3. **Survey Courses** are designed to provide general information about subjects related to pain control and sedation. Such courses should be didactic and not clinical in nature, since they are not intended to develop clinical competency.
4. **Advanced Education Courses** are a component of an advanced dental education program, accredited by the Commission on Dental Accreditation in accord with the Accreditation Standards for advanced dental education programs. These courses are designed to prepare the graduate dentist or postdoctoral student in the most comprehensive manner to be competent in the safe and effective administration of minimal, moderate, and deep sedation and general anesthesia.

Teaching Administration of Minimal Sedation

The faculty responsible for curriculum in minimal sedation techniques must be familiar with the ADA Policy Statement: Guidelines for the Use of Sedation and General Anesthesia by Dentists, and the Commission on Dental Accreditation's Accreditation Standards for dental education programs.

These Guidelines present a basic overview of the recommendations for teaching minimal sedation. These include courses in nitrous oxide/oxygen sedation, enteral sedation, and combined inhalation/enteral techniques.

General Objectives

Upon completion of a competency course in minimal sedation, the dentist must be able to:

1. Describe the adult anatomy and physiology of the respiratory, cardiovascular, and central nervous systems as they relate to the above techniques.
2. Describe the pharmacological effects of drugs.
3. Describe the methods of obtaining a medical history and conduct an appropriate physical examination.
4. Apply these methods clinically in order to obtain an accurate evaluation.
5. Use this information clinically for ASA classification risk assessment and pre-procedure fasting instructions.
6. Choose the most appropriate technique for the individual patient.
7. Use appropriate physiologic monitoring equipment.
8. Describe the physiologic responses that are consistent with minimal sedation.
9. Understand the sedation/general anesthesia continuum.
10. Demonstrate the ability to diagnose and treat emergencies related to the next deeper level of anesthesia than intended.

INHALATION SEDATION (NITROUS OXIDE-OXYGEN)

Inhalation Sedation Course Objectives

Upon completion of a competency course in inhalation sedation techniques, the dentist must be able to:

1. Describe the basic components of inhalation sedation equipment.
2. Discuss the function of each of these components.

3. List and discuss the advantages and disadvantages of inhalation sedation.
4. List and discuss the indications and contraindications of inhalation sedation.
5. List the complications associated with inhalation sedation.
6. Discuss the prevention, recognition, and management of these complications.
7. Administer inhalation sedation to patients in a clinical setting in a safe and effective manner.
8. Discuss the abuse potential, occupational hazards, and other untoward effects of inhalation agents.

Inhalation Sedation Course Content

1. Historical, philosophic, and psychological aspects of anxiety and pain control
2. Patient evaluation and selection through review of medical history taking, physical diagnosis, and psychological considerations
3. Definitions and descriptions of physiologic and psychological aspects of anxiety and pain
4. Description of the stages of drug-induced central nervous system depression through all levels of consciousness and unconsciousness, with special emphasis on the distinction between the conscious and the unconscious state
5. Review of adult respiratory and circulatory physiology and related anatomy
6. Pharmacology of agents used in inhalation sedation, including drug interactions and incompatibilities
7. Indications and contraindications for use of inhalation sedation
8. Review of dental procedures possible under inhalation sedation
9. Patient monitoring using observation and monitoring equipment (i.e., pulse oximetry), with particular attention to vital signs and reflexes related to the pharmacology of N_2O
10. Importance of maintaining proper records with accurate chart entries recording medical history, physical examination, vital signs, drugs and doses administered, and patient response
11. Prevention, recognition, and management of complications and life-threatening situations
12. Administration of local anesthesia in conjunction with inhalation sedation techniques
13. Description, maintenance and use of inhalation sedation equipment
14. Introduction to potential health hazards of trace anesthetics and proposed techniques for limiting occupational exposure
15. Discussion of abuse potential

Inhalation Sedation Course Duration

While length of a course is only one of the many factors to be considered in determining the quality of an educational program, the course should be a minimum of 14 hours plus management of clinical dental cases, during which clinical competency in inhalation sedation technique is achieved. The inhalation sedation course most often is completed as a part of the predoctoral dental education program. However, the course may be completed in a postdoctoral continuing education competency course.

Participant Evaluation and Documentation of Inhalation Sedation Instruction

Competency courses in inhalation sedation techniques must afford participants with sufficient clinical experience to enable them to achieve competency. This experience must be provided under the supervision of qualified faculty and must be evaluated. The course director must certify the competency of participants upon satisfactory completion of training. Records of the didactic instruction and clinical experience, including the number of patients treated by each participant must be maintained and available.

Faculty

The course should be directed by a dentist or physician qualified by experience and training. This individual should possess an active permit or license to administer moderate sedation in at least one state, have had at least 3 years of experience, including the individual's formal postdoctoral training in anxiety and pain control. In addition, the participation of highly qualified individuals in related fields, such as anesthesiologists, pharmacologists, internists, cardiologists, and psychologists, should be encouraged.

A participant-faculty ratio of not more than ten-to-one when inhalation sedation is being used allows for adequate supervision during the clinical phase of instruction; a one-to-one ratio is recommended during the early state of participation.

The faculty should provide a mechanism whereby the participant can evaluate the performance of those individuals who present the course material.

Facilities

Competency courses must be presented where adequate facilities are available for proper patient care, including drugs and equipment for the management of emergencies.

2016 GUIDELINES FOR THE USE OF SEDATION AND GENERAL ANESTHESIA BY DENTISTS[10]

I. *Introduction* – The administration of local anesthesia, sedation, and general anesthesia is an integral part of dental practice. The American Dental Association is committed to the safe and effective use of these modalities by appropriately educated and trained dentists. The purpose of these guidelines is to assist dentists in the delivery of safe and effective sedation and anesthesia.

Dentists must comply with their state laws, rules, and/or regulations when providing sedation and anesthesia and will only be subject to Section III. Educational Requirements as required by those state laws, rules, and/or regulations.

Level of sedation is entirely independent of the route of administration. Moderate and deep sedation or general anesthesia may be achieved via any route of administration, and thus an appropriately consistent level of training must be established.

For children, the American Dental Association supports the use of the American Academy of Pediatrics/American Academy of Pediatric Dentistry Guidelines for Monitoring and Management of Pediatric Patients During and After Sedation for Diagnostic and Therapeutic Procedures.

II. *Definitions.* Methods of Anxiety and Pain Control

Minimal sedation (previously known as anxiolysis) is a minimally depressed level of consciousness, produced by a pharmacological method, that retains the patient's ability to independently and continuously maintain an airway and respond normally to tactile stimulation and verbal command. Although cognitive function and coordination may be modestly impaired, ventilatory and cardiovascular functions are unaffected.[1]

Patients whose only response is reflex withdrawal from repeated painful stimuli would not be considered to be in a state of minimal sedation.

The following definitions apply to administration of minimal sedation:

Maximum recommended dose (MRD) – maximum FDA-recommended dose of a drug, as printed in FDA-approved labeling for unmonitored home use.

Dosing for minimal sedation via the enteral route – minimal sedation may be achieved by the administration of a drug, either singly or in divided doses, by the enteral route to achieve the desired clinical effect, not to exceed the maximum recommended dose (MRD).

The administration of enteral drugs exceeding the maximum recommended dose during a single appointment is considered to be moderate sedation, and the moderate sedation guidelines apply.

Nitrous oxide/oxygen when used in combination with sedative agent(s) may produce minimal, moderate, deep sedation, or general anesthesia.

If more than one enteral drug is administered to achieve the desired sedation effect, with or without the concomitant use of nitrous oxide, the guidelines for moderate sedation must apply.

Note: In accord with this particular definition, the drug(s) and/or techniques used should carry a margin of safety wide enough never to render unintended loss of consciousness. The use of the MRD to guide dosing for minimal sedation is intended to create this margin of safety.

IV. ***Clinical Guidelines* – A. Minimal Sedation**

1. Patient History and Evaluation

Patients considered for minimal sedation must be suitably evaluated prior to the start of any sedative procedure. In healthy or medically stable individuals (ASA I, II)

this should consist of a review of their current medical history and medication use. In addition, patients with significant medical considerations (ASA III, IV) may require consultation with their primary care physician or consulting medical specialist.

2. Preoperative Evaluation and Preparation
   - The patient, parent, legal guardian, or caregiver must be advised regarding the procedure associated with the delivery of any sedative agents, and informed consent for the proposed sedation must be obtained.
   - Determination of adequate oxygen supply and equipment necessary to deliver oxygen under positive pressure must be completed.
   - An appropriate focused physical evaluation should be performed.
   - Baseline vital signs including body weight, height, blood pressure, pulse rate, and respiration rate must be obtained unless invalidated by the nature of the patient, procedure, or equipment. Body temperature should be measured when clinically indicated.
   - Preoperative dietary restrictions must be considered based on the sedative technique prescribed.
   - Preoperative verbal and written instructions must be given to the patient, parent, escort, legal guardian, or caregiver.

3. Personnel and Equipment Requirements
   Personnel:
   - At least one additional person trained in Basic Life Support for Healthcare Providers must be present in addition to the dentist.

   Equipment:
   - A positive-pressure oxygen delivery system suitable for the patient being treated must be immediately available.
   - Documentation of compliance with manufacturers' recommended maintenance of monitors, anesthesia delivery systems, and other anesthesia-related equipment should be maintained. A pre-procedural check of equipment for each administration of sedation must be performed.
   - When inhalation equipment is used, it must have a fail-safe system that is appropriately checked and calibrated. The equipment must also have either (1) a functioning device that prohibits the delivery of less than 30% oxygen or (2) an appropriately calibrated and functioning in-line oxygen analyzer with audible alarm.
   - An appropriate scavenging system must be available if gases other than oxygen or air are used.

4. Monitoring and Documentation
   Monitoring: A dentist, or at the dentist's direction, an appropriately trained individual, must remain in the operatory during active dental treatment to monitor the patient continuously until the patient meets the criteria for discharge to the recovery area. The

appropriately trained individual must be familiar with monitoring techniques and equipment. Monitoring must include:

Consciousness:

- Level of sedation (e.g., responsiveness to verbal commands) must be continually assessed.

Oxygenation:

- Oxygen saturation by pulse oximetry may be clinically useful and should be considered.

Ventilation:

- The dentist and/or appropriately trained individual must observe chest excursions.
- The dentist and/or appropriately trained individual must verify respirations.

Circulation:

- Blood pressure and heart rate should be evaluated preoperatively, postoperatively, and intraoperatively as necessary (unless the patient is unable to tolerate such monitoring).

Documentation: An appropriate sedative record must be maintained, including the names of all drugs administered, time administered, and route of administration, including local anesthetics, dosages, and monitored physiological parameters.

5. Recovery and Discharge

- Oxygen and suction equipment must be immediately available if a separate recovery area is utilized.
- The qualified dentist or appropriately trained clinical staff must monitor the patient during recovery until the patient is ready for discharge by the dentist.
- The qualified dentist must determine and document that levels of consciousness, oxygenation, ventilation, and circulation are satisfactory prior to discharge.
- Postoperative verbal and written instructions must be given to the patient, parent, escort, legal guardian, or caregiver.

6. Emergency Management

- If a patient enters a deeper level of sedation than the dentist is qualified to provide, the dentist must stop the dental procedure until the patient returns to the intended level of sedation.
- The qualified dentist is responsible for the sedative management, adequacy of the facility and staff, diagnosis, and treatment of emergencies related to the administration of minimal sedation and providing the equipment and protocols for patient rescue.

REFERENCES

1. Guidelines for postgraduate and continuing education in pain and anxiety control. *Anesth Prog* 20:167, 1973.
2. American Dental Association, Council on Dental Education: Guidelines for teaching the comprehensive control of pain and anxiety in dentistry. *J Dent Educ* 36(1):62–67, 1972.
3. American Dental Society of Anesthesiology: Guidelines for the teaching of pain and anxiety control and management of related complications in a continuing education program, part III. *Anesth Prog* 26:51, 1979.
4. AADS Special Report: Curricular guidelines for comprehensive control of pain and anxiety in dentistry. *J Dent Educ* 44(5):279–286, 1980.
5. American Dental Association, Council on Dental Education: Guidelines for teaching the comprehensive control of pain and anxiety in dentistry. *J Dent Educ* 53(5-6):305–310, 1989.
6. American Dental Association, Council on Dental Education: Guidelines for teaching the comprehensive control of pain and anxiety in dentistry, Chicago, 1992, The Association.
7. American Dental Association, Council on Dental Education: Guidelines for teaching pain control and sedation in dentists and dental students, Oct. 2007 ADA House of Delegates. Chicago, 2007, The Association.
8. American Dental Association, Council on Dental Education: Guidelines for the use of sedation and general anesthesia by dentists, Oct. 2007 ADA House of Delegates. Chicago, 2012, The Association.
9. American Dental Association, Council on Dental Education: Guidelines for teaching pain control and sedation in dentists and dental students, Oct. 2016 ADA House of Delegates. Chicago, 2016, The Association.
10. American Dental Association, Council on Dental Education: Guidelines for the use of sedation and general anesthesia by dentists. Oct. 2016 ADA House of Delegates. Chicago, 2016, The Association.

Section V

INTRAVENOUS SEDATION

The intravenous (IV) route of sedation is the subject of Section V. Drugs administered directly into the cardiovascular system produce clinical actions significantly more rapidly than drugs administered via other routes (e.g., oral, intranasal, or intramuscular). Rapid onset of action is both of benefit and of potential danger. It is beneficial because it permits the doctor to effectively titrate the drug to a desired clinical effect; it is potentially dangerous because the actions of intravenously administered drugs develop more rapidly and because their actions are more pronounced than those of drugs administered via other routes with slower onset and less complete absorption. It is therefore of the utmost importance that every person using the IV route of drug administration or contemplating its use receive thorough training in the procedures involved in its safe and effective use.

The chapters that follow provide the basic didactic material for an intensive course in IV moderate sedation. They consist of two parts: The first, a discussion of venipuncture, includes the anatomy for venipuncture, the armamentarium for the continuous IV infusion, and the technique of venous cannulation (venipuncture). The second portion of the IV sedation didactic program is the discussion of drugs and specific techniques of IV sedation, including the clinical pharmacology of intravenously administered drugs, the techniques of administering these agents, and the complications associated with the use of this route of drug administration.

Chapter 29 may prove to be the most important chapter in this section. This chapter is titled "Guidelines for Teaching," and it outlines the fundamentals of training required for this very valuable technique. It is my belief that IV sedation is an important part of the dentist's armamentarium in the management of pain, fear, and anxiety; however, because of the nature of this technique (e.g., its rapid onset of action, more profound effects of drugs), the dentist using it must undergo a degree of training that is beyond that required for employment of many of the techniques already discussed in Sections III and IV.

All 50 states in the United States[1] and six provinces in Canada[2-4] have enacted legislation requiring a dentist to possess a special permit to use the IV route for sedation. Minimum educational requirements have been established by these states and provinces and by various organizations, including the American Dental Association,[5-7] American Dental Society of Anesthesiology,[8] American Academy of Pediatric Dentistry,[9] American Academy of Periodontology,[10,11] and the American Association of Oral and Maxillofacial Surgeons.[12] Specific guidelines are presented in Chapter 29. It is strongly recommended that all dentists either currently using or contemplating the use of the IV route for moderate sedation read this section carefully. Courses not meeting the requirements presented in this chapter are not considered adequate to properly prepare the dentist and the office staff to use IV moderate sedation.

Like Section IV on inhalation sedation, this section is presented in chapters that are shorter than those in other parts. Its purpose is to better enable the reader to locate the specific material that is of importance to him or her.

The IV route of drug administration is extremely valuable. It is only through proper education of those dentists wishing to use the technique that IV moderate sedation can remain a safe procedure. The reader must always keep in mind that this section was designed to be used in conjunction with an intensive course in IV moderate sedation, a course containing both didactic and clinical components. Use of IV moderate sedation after having simply read this section is foolhardy and should not be considered.

REFERENCES

1. American Dental Association: *Department of State Government Affairs*, Chicago, 2009, The Association. http://www.ada.org/~/media/ADA/Advocacy/Files/anesthesia_sedation_permit.ashx. (Accessed February 1, 2017).
2. College of Dental Surgeons of British Columbia. Standards and Guidelines. Minimal and moderate sedation services in dentistry (Non-hospital facilities). 2014. https://www.cdsbc.org/CDSBCPublicLibrary/Minimal-Moderate-Sedation-Standards.pdf. (Accessed February 1, 2017).
3. Alberta Dental Association + College. Standard of practice: Use of sedation in non-hospital dental practice. https://www.cdsbc.org/CDSBCPublicLibrary/Minimal-Moderate-Sedation-Standards.pdf. (Accessed February 1, 2017).
4. Royal College of Dental Surgeons of Ontario. Sedation and Anesthesia. http://www.rcdso.org/members/sedationandanesthesia. (Accessed February 1, 2017).
5. American Dental Association: *Guidelines for the use of sedation and general anesthesia by dentists*. As adopted by the October 2007 ADA House of Delegates, Chicago, 2007, American Dental Association.
6. American Dental Association: *Guidelines for teaching pain control and sedation to dentists and dental students*. As adopted by the October 2007 ADA House of Delegates, Chicago, 2007, American Dental Association.
7. American Dental Association, Council on Dental Education: *Guidelines for the use of sedation and general anesthesia by dentists*. Oct 2007 ADA House of Delegates, Chicago, 2012, The Association.
8. Rosenberg MB, Campbell RL: Guidelines for intraoperative monitoring of dental patients undergoing conscious sedation, deep sedation, and general anesthesia. *Oral Surg* 71(1):2–8, 1991.
9. American Academy of Pediatric Dentists (AAPD): Guideline for monitoring and management of pediatric patients before, during, and after sedation for diagnostic and therapeutic procedures: Update (2016), Developed through a collaborative effort between the American Academy of Pediatrics and the AAPD. Available at http://www.aapd.org/media/Policies_Guidelines/G_Sedation1.pdf. (Accessed February 1, 2017).
10. American Academy of Periodontology (AAP): Guidelines: in-office use of conscious sedation in periodontics. Available at www.perio.org/resources-products/posppr3-1.html. (Accessed January 27, 2016).
11. Committee on Anesthesia. American Academy of Periodontology: American Academy of Periodontology Statement on the Use of Moderate Sedation by Periodontists. *J Periodontol* 84(4):435, 2013.
12. American Association of Oral and Maxillofacial Surgeons (AAOMS): Parameters of care: clinical practice guidelines for oral and maxillofacial surgery (AAOMS ParCare 2012). Anesthesia in outpatient facilities. http://www.aaoms.org/images/uploads/pdfs/parcare_anesthesia.pdf. (Accessed February 1, 2017).

chapter 20

Intravenous Sedation: Historical Perspective

CHAPTER OUTLINE

The historical development of intravenous (IV) anesthesia and sedation is reviewed in this chapter. Although the impact made by the development of the IV route of drug administration was not quite as dramatic as was that of inhalation anesthesia (see Chapter 11), the ability to administer medications directly into the cardiovascular system proved to be a boon to the medical and dental professions.

THE EARLY DAYS

As was true with inhalation anesthetics, it seems as though some of the techniques and drugs had been available for many years before the thought occurred to put them to any therapeutic use. Indeed, with the IV route, it was not until well after the development of inhalation anesthesia that the administration of drugs directly into the cardiovascular system of a human being occurred.

William Harvey (1578–1657) (Fig. 20.1) provided much of the groundwork for the future of IV medication with the publication of the results of experiments on the circulation of blood. Harvey stated that there was a continuous circulation of blood within a closed system.[1] Before Harvey's findings, a multitude of theories relating to the flow of blood in the human body abounded. Most of these suggested that blood flowed to tissues within the body in an open system. Harvey was born in England and received his medical training at Oxford University. Following graduation he went to Padua, Italy, then the leading medical center in the world, where he began to formalize his theories on the circulation of blood. Andrea Cesalpino (1519–1603) was an important predecessor of Harvey. Cesalpino was the first person to use the word *circulation* in reference to blood and its travels throughout the body.[2] Cesalpino was also first to propose that capillaries connect

arteries and veins, meaning that there is no free flow of blood into the tissues of the body as had been assumed for many years. The one major drawback to Cesalpino's theory was his proposal that there were direct connections between major arteries and veins.

On returning to England in 1602, Harvey entered into private medical practice and prospered. He became the court physician for King James I and for King Charles I. Despite his busy practice, Harvey continued to experiment; most of his research involved the circulation of blood. As early as 1615, Harvey spoke of the circulation of blood within a closed system; however, it was not until 1628 that he published one of the most important textbooks in the history of medicine and biology: *Exercitatio Anatomica de Motu Cordis et Sanguinis in Animalibus (On the Movement of the Heart and Blood in Animals)*[1] (Fig. 20.2).

Harvey demonstrated for the first time that because of the presence of valves within the heart and veins, blood flow within the circulatory system was unidirectional. In addition, he discussed capillaries, microscopic vessels that connect smaller arteries and smaller veins, thus providing a closed circulatory system. Despite his description of capillaries, Harvey was never able to see them; it was not until after his death that Marcello Malpighi (1628–1694) first saw capillaries through the microscope.

Harvey's book produced great controversy because it attempted to disprove theories relating to blood flow that had been held for many years. Controversy over Harvey's book raged for approximately 20 years after its publication. Today, Harvey's work is considered the seventeenth century's most significant achievement in physiology and medicine.

As a logical extension of Harvey's work, the first IV administration of a drug occurred in the same century (1657). Sir

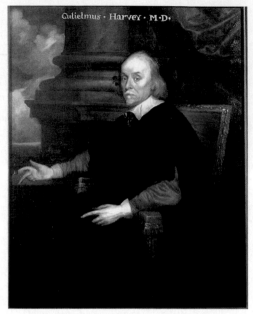

Figure 20.1 William Harvey (1579–1657).

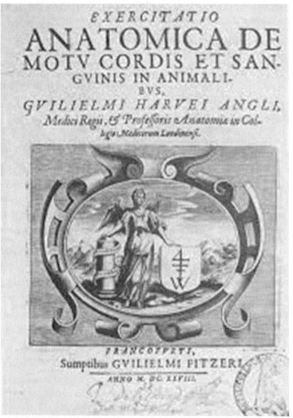

Figure 20.2 William Harvey's *Exercitatio Anatomica de Motu Cordis et Sanguinis in Animalibus* – 1628. (Reprinted with permission from Wellcome Library, London.)

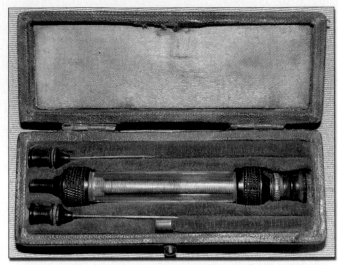

Figure 20.3 Anel syringe – 1839. (Courtesy Museum of Drugs.)

Christopher Wren and Robert Boyle administered tincture of opium intravenously into a dog by using a sharpened quill to which a bladder had been attached.[3] Eight years later, Richard Lower successfully transfused blood from one animal to another.

THE 1800S

The late 1700s and early 1800s saw the development of anesthesiology, with the advent of ether, chloroform, and nitrous oxide-oxygen (N_2O-O_2). This history is chronicled in Chapter 11.

In 1839 in New York, Isaac E. Taylor and James Augustus Washington administered a solution of morphine in an Anel syringe[4] (Fig. 20.3). The Anel syringe had originally been designed for entry into the lacrimal duct and had a finely elongated tapering nozzle instead of a sharp point. Taylor and Washington had to make a skin incision with a knife to deposit the morphine under the skin of the patient. This was not an IV injection, but more than likely subcutaneous. By 1842, modifications in syringes had occurred that eliminated the necessity to make a separate skin incision. The Jayne syringe was similar to the earlier Anel syringe; however, a sharp point had replaced the tapered nozzle, permitting a direct puncture of the skin. Charles Gabriel Pravaz (of Lyon, France) was the first to design a syringe with a separate needle. His syringe, manufactured from glass, was introduced in 1853. The Anel, Jayne, and Pravaz syringes were used primarily to deposit morphine along or near the path of a nerve in cases of neuralgia.

Professor W. W. Green,[5] from the University of Maine School of Medicine, published in 1868 in the *American Journal of Dental Sciences* a paper entitled "The Hypodermic Use of Morphia during Anesthesia."[5] Green advocated the subcutaneous administration of 0.5 to 1 grain of morphine while the patient was receiving ether anesthesia. Green's reasons for his recommendation included the probability of pain, prevention of

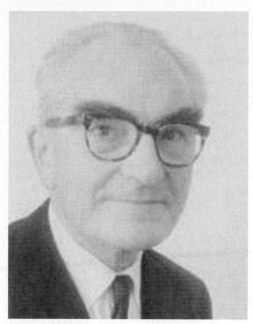

Figure 20.4 Dr. Stanley Drummond-Jackson. (Courtesy Society for the Advancement of Anaesthesia in Dentistry.)

shock, a shortening of the anesthetic's influence, and the prevention of delirium and nausea.

Pierre-Cyprien Oré of Bordeaux, France was the first person to administer a drug intravenously when he administered chloral hydrate to animals to achieve general anesthesia in 1872.[6] Two years later he administered chloral hydrate general anesthesia to a human being.

THE 1900S

Further development of the IV route was somewhat slow. The major developments in anesthesia during the late 1800s occurred in local anesthesia and in the refinement of the techniques of inhalation anesthesia. However, in 1903, Emil Fisher and J. von Mering synthesized the first barbiturate barbitone (Veronal).[7] For his part in the development of this important drug, Fisher received the Nobel Prize in Chemistry in 1902.

In 1929 sodium amobarbital (Amytal) was administered intravenously by L. G. Zerfas.[8] This represented the first IV administration of a rapidly acting barbiturate. However, amobarbital was not administered by Zerfas for the purpose of producing anesthesia. Rather, amobarbital was used primarily as an anticonvulsant. Its function as an anesthetic was limited to those patients in whom inhalation anesthetics could not be administered. A year later in 1930 pentobarbital (Nembutal) was synthesized.

In 1935 John S. Lundy, at the Mayo Clinic in Rochester, Minnesota, introduced sodium thiopental (Pentothal).[9] This rapid-acting, short-duration IV anesthetic eventually became the most popular drug in the United States for the induction of general anesthesia via the IV route.

At approximately the same time in England, Stanley L. Drummond-Jackson pioneered the use of IV barbiturate anesthesia for both oral surgery and conservative dental procedures[10] (Fig. 20.4). The agent employed by Drummond-Jackson was methohexital, known as Brevital in the United States and Brietal in Europe.

Studying at the Mayo Clinic with Lundy was Adrian Hubbell. Hubbell, along with two others, B. S. Wyckoff and O. K. Bullard, was a pioneer in the administration of IV general anesthesia for ambulatory oral surgical patients.[11] In addition, Hubbell was the first person in North America to use IV general anesthesia without premedication as a sole agent for ambulatory patients having oral operations in a dental office. In 1933 Victor Goldman[12] published the first English-language article dealing with the subject of IV anesthesia for dental surgery.

Thus far we have discussed the evolution of IV general anesthesia. As also occurred with the use of N_2O general anesthesia in the early to mid-1900s, an evolutionary process was taking place. With the advent of better, more effective local anesthetics for pain control, the requirement of anesthesia and analgesia from IV medications was diminishing.

In 1945 Niels Bjorn Jorgensen became probably the first person to use the IV route to provide what Jorgensen himself termed *intravenous premedication*.[13] Jorgensen refined the technique of administering IV barbiturates and combined pentobarbital administration with an opioid (meperidine) and an anticholinergic (scopolamine). This technique was first used in 1945 at the Loma Linda University School of Medicine. In 1955 this technique for producing IV sedation was first taught to the third-year dental students at the Loma Linda School of Dentistry, where it has been taught to all succeeding classes.

This technique gradually became known as the *"Loma Linda technique"* and is now known as the *"Jorgensen technique,"* after Niels Bjorn Jorgensen, its founder and the father of IV sedation in dentistry.[14]

In 1965 A. Davidau[15] in Paris, France, first used diazepam (Valium) as a sedative agent in dentistry. Shortly thereafter, D. M. G. Main[16] reported on his first case of diazepam sedation in dentistry. Main used diazepam as an adjunctive agent in the Jorgensen technique.

R. O'Neil and P. J. Verrill[17,18] used diazepam as the sole sedative agent for patients undergoing oral surgical procedures. The Verrill sign, considered by some an indicator of the proper level of sedation and others of a slightly oversedated state, came from these studies. Diazepam became the most commonly employed IV sedative agent within dentistry. With the introduction of the benzodiazepines, the Jorgensen technique, the original IV sedative technique, has become a historical afterthought. In 1986 midazolam, a water-soluble benzodiazepine, was introduced into clinical practice in the United States following its earlier introduction elsewhere in the world. Although similar in many respects to diazepam, midazolam has a number of distinct advantages and has become the most popular IV sedative drug in both medicine and dentistry, eclipsing diazepam.[19]

Another major change in IV sedation has been the increased attention placed on patient monitoring during sedation and general anesthesia. Noninvasive forms of monitoring have become available that help increase patient safety during IV moderate sedation and general anesthesia.[20,21] Examples of these devices include the pulse oximeter and end-tidal carbon dioxide monitor. Their use is described in Chapters 5 and 31.

REFERENCES

1. Harvey W: *Exercitatio anatomica de motu cordis et sanguinis in animalibus, 1628,* (Leake CD, transl), Springfield, IL, 1931, Charles C Thomas.
2. Lee JA, Atkinson RS: *A synopsis of anesthesia,* ed 5, Baltimore, 1964, Williams & Wilkins.
3. Bankoff G: *The conquest of pain: the story of anesthesia,* London, 1946, MacDonald.
4. Archer WH: *A manual of dental anesthesia,* Philadelphia, 1952, WB Saunders.
5. Green WW: Hypodermic use of morphia during anaesthesia. *Am J Dent Sci* (3rd ser) 2:207, 1868.
6. Sykes WS: *Essays on the first hundred years of anaesthesia,* Edinburgh, 1960, E & S Livingstone.
7. Driscoll EJ: Dental anesthesiology: its history and continuing evolution. *Anesth Prog* 25(5):143–152, 1978.
8. Zerfas LG: Induction of anesthesia in man by intravenous injection of sodium iso-amyl-ethyl barbiturate. *Proc Soc Exp Biol Med* 26:399, 1929.
9. Lundy JS: Intravenous anesthesia: preliminary report of use of two new thiobarbiturates. *Proc Staff Meetings Mayo Clin* 10:536, 1935.
10. Drummond Jackson SL: Epival anesthesia in dentistry. *Dent Cosmos* 77:130, 1935.
11. Hubbell AO, Adams RC: Intravenous anesthesia for dental surgery with sodium ethyl (1-methylbutyl) thiobarbituric acid. *J Am Dent Assoc* 27:1186, 1940.
12. Goldman V: "Evipan" in dentistry. *Dent Mag Oral Top* 50:1153, 1953.
13. Jorgensen NB, Leffingwell FE: Premedication in dentistry. *J South Calif Dent Assoc* 21:1, 1953.
14. Jorgensen NB, Hayden J, Jr: *Sedation, local and general anesthesia in dentistry,* ed 2, Philadelphia, 1972, Lea & Febiger.
15. Davidau A: New methods in anaesthesiology and their use in dentistry: treatment of difficult patients and execution of complex procedures. *Rev Assoc Med Israelites* (France) 16:663, 1967.
16. Brown PRH, Main DMG, Lawson JM: Diazepam in dentistry, report on 108 cases. *Br Dent J* 125(11):498–501, 1968.
17. O'Neil R, Verrill PJ: Intravenous diazepam in minor oral surgery. *Br J Oral Surg* 7(1):12–14, 1969.
18. O'Neil R, Verrill PJ, Aellig WH, Laurence DR: Intravenous diazepam in minor oral surgery. *Br Dent J* 128(1):15–18, 1970.
19. Trieger N: Intravenous sedation in dentistry and oral surgery. *Int Anesth Clin* 27(2):83–91, 1989.
20. Eichhorn JH, Cooper JB, Cullen DJ, et al: Standards for patient monitoring during anesthesia at Harvard Medical School. *JAMA* 256(8):1017–1020, 1986.
21. Holzman RS, Cullen DJ, Eichhorn JH, Philip JH: Guidelines for sedation by non-anesthesiologists during diagnostic and therapeutic procedures. The risk management committee of the department of anesthesia of Harvard Medical School. *J Clin Anesth* 6(4):265–275, 1994.

chapter 21

Intravenous Moderate Sedation: Rationale

CHAPTER OUTLINE

General anesthesia has a long history in dentistry, starting with Drs. Horace Wells and William T. G. Morton in the mid-1800s. Intravenous (IV) sedation is a relatively new technique in dentistry. It is only in the past 55 to 60 years that IV moderate sedation has gained a foothold. Until the late 1960s, the IV route was used almost exclusively by oral and maxillofacial surgeons, primarily because their postdoctoral training placed great emphasis on the IV route of drug administration. Until recently, most dental schools in the United States did not include training in IV drug administration in their curricula, and today only a few courses are available wherein the postgraduate dentist can receive such training. The past 40 years, however, have seen the implementation of predoctoral courses in IV moderate sedation by a small, but still growing, number of U.S. dental schools. Because of this and the present availability of a handful of excellent postgraduate programs in IV moderate sedation and the availability of 3-year residencies in general anesthesia for dentists, the number of dentists using IV moderate sedation has grown. It is impossible to even guess at the number of dentists (excluding oral and maxillofacial surgeons) employing the IV route today; however, for the patient requiring this mode of treatment, it has become considerably easier to locate a dentist who administers IV moderate sedation for nonsurgical procedures.

A factor that deterred many dentists from the use of IV moderate sedation was the high cost of professional liability insurance. The 1980s saw a dramatic increase in the cost of liability insurance in many areas of life in the United States,

not only in the health professions. However, the fact was that the cost of liability insurance for a dentist using IV conscious sedation (as it was then termed) was, in many states, prohibitively high. This became a major consideration in a dentist's decision whether to use this valuable technique of patient management. As the mid-1990s arrived, the cost of liability insurance leveled off and in certain circumstances (e.g., a periodontist using IV moderate sedation in the state of California) actually decreased. As more complete risk assessment surveys were completed, the cost of liability insurance for dentists using IV moderate sedation continued along this promising pathway.

ADVANTAGES

1. The onset of action of intravenously administered drugs is arguably the most rapid of all techniques discussed in this book. Hand–heart–brain circulation time is approximately 20 to 25 seconds. Although some individual variation exists in this and in the onset of action for different drugs, overall, the IV route of drug administration permits the most rapid onset of action (or at least almost as rapid an onset as inhalation drugs).

2. Because of the rapid onset of action of most intravenously administered drugs, the drug dosage can be tailored to meet the specific needs of the patient. The guesswork associated with determining proper dosage of an orally, intranasally, or intramuscularly administered drug is eliminated when the IV route is used. This concept of

individualizing drug dosages is termed *titration* and represents one of the most important safety features associated with IV drug administration.

3. Because of the rapid onset of action of most IV drugs, the dentist is able to provide the patient with a suitable level of sedation. The level of sedation must never, of course, exceed that level to which the dentist has been trained. Minimal, moderate, and deep levels of sedation can all be achieved via the IV route, and the dentist must always remain cognizant of his or her limitations, as based on prior experience and training.

4. The recovery period for most intravenously administered drugs is significantly shorter than that seen for the same drug administered via the oral, rectal, intranasal (IN), or intramuscular (IM) routes. Recovery from intravenously administered drugs will, however, be considerably longer and less complete than that following nitrous oxide-oxygen (N_2O-O_2) inhalation sedation. An escort, a responsible adult—a person who has a vested interest in the health and safety of the patient—is required for dismissal of the patient following the IV sedation procedure.

5. In the continuous IV infusion technique recommended in this book, a patent vein is maintained throughout the procedure. This facilitates reinjection of any additional central nervous system (CNS)–depressant drug (although this is rarely necessary). However, the major significance of maintaining a patent vein is that through it a portal exists for the administration of any rescue (emergency) drugs that may be required in the unlikely event an emergency arises during IV therapy.

6. The side effects of nausea and vomiting are extremely uncommon when drugs are administered intravenously as recommended.

7. Effective control of salivary secretions is possible through the IV administration of anticholinergics. This will be of benefit to the dentist during various types of dental therapy, such as the taking of impressions.

8. The gag reflex is diminished. Patients receiving IV moderate sedation rarely experience difficulty with gagging. This action is similar to that occurring with N_2O-O_2 inhalation sedation. If the only requirement in a patient is to minimize the gag reflex, inhalation sedation is preferred over IV moderate sedation. Only in the event that inhalation sedation fails to diminish the hyperactive gag reflex should IV moderate sedation be employed solely for this purpose.

9. Many of the drugs administered intravenously for sedation effectively diminish motor disturbances (e.g., seizure activity and cerebral palsy), making this route advantageous for the seizure-prone patient.

10. The ability to readily gain IV access (venipuncture) may prove to be important in any emergency situation. Although antidotal drug therapy is not recommended as the initial step in the effective management of emergency situations, the ability to establish an IV line provides immediate access to the cardiovascular system should it become necessary

to administer drugs to the victim. Through the use of IV moderate sedation on a regular basis, the dentist is better able to maintain proficiency in the technique of venipuncture.

DISADVANTAGES

1. Venipuncture is necessary. Although most adult patients tolerate venipuncture with little or no difficulty, some patients are psychologically unable to "handle" needles anywhere in their body. Children may be particularly difficult to manage via this route because veins are proportionally smaller in smaller patients, making venipuncture itself more difficult. Younger children requiring IV moderate sedation will usually pose severe management problems (the "precooperative" patient) or be physically unable to control themselves. Not all patients, even adults, have veins that are easy to visualize and gain access to with a needle. Probably the most significant challenge facing the dentist learning IV moderate sedation is to develop a degree of proficiency at venipuncture. Venipuncture is a learned skill, one that becomes easier to perform as experience is gained.

2. Complications may arise at the venipuncture site. As discussed in Chapter 27, a variety of minor and some major complications can develop at the venipuncture site. These include hematoma, phlebitis, and intraarterial injection of a drug.

3. Monitoring of the patient receiving IV moderate sedation must be more intensive than that required in most other moderate sedation techniques. Because intravenously administered drugs act rapidly, the entire dental team must be trained to assess the physical and mental status of the patient throughout the procedure. The greater the depth of sedation (deep > moderate > minimal), the greater is the need for increased patient monitoring.

4. Recovery from intravenously administered drugs is not complete at the end of the dental treatment. All patients receiving any intravenously administered CNS depressant must be escorted from the dental office by a responsible adult companion.

5. Although the depth of sedation provided by intravenously administered drugs can be increased rapidly (by administration of additional drug), the converse is not true. Many intravenously administered drugs cannot be reversed by specific drug antagonists. Although antagonists do exist for several drug groups, specifically opioids, benzodiazepines, and anticholinergics, they are not recommended for routine administration.[3-5] Should a patient become overly sedated (deep instead of moderate; moderate instead of minimal), the initial, and most effective, management in all situations is the maintenance of basic life support: assess the patient's airway, assist or support ventilation, and provide for the effective circulation of oxygenated blood. Following these steps (P-C-A-B [basic life support]), consideration may be given to antidotal drug therapy.

Box 21.1	Advantages and Disadvantages of Intravenous Sedation
Advantages	**Disadvantages**
1. Rapid onset of action	1. Venipuncture is necessary
2. Titration is possible	2. Venipuncture complications may occur
3. Highly effective	3. More intensive monitoring required
4. Recovery shorter than other techniques (IM, IN, oral)	4. Recovery not complete—escort needed
5. Patent vein is safety factor	5. Some IV drugs cannot be reversed
6. Nausea and vomiting are uncommon	
7. Control of salivary secretions possible	
8. Gag reflex diminished	
9. Motor disturbances (epilepsy, cerebral palsy) diminished	
10. Ability to perform IV is benefit in serious emergency situations	

Box 21.1 summarizes the advantages and disadvantages of the IV route of drug administration.

CONTRAINDICATIONS

1. Unless a doctor has received specific training in the administration of CNS-depressant drugs to patients younger than 16 years, IV moderate sedation is relatively contraindicated in this group. In the continuing dental education programs in IV sedation that this author has been involved with, we have changed the lower age limit for IV moderate sedation to patients 16 years and older.[1,2] The major reason for this recommendation is that in younger patients there is a greater-than-usual incidence of overresponsiveness to the "usual" dosages of CNS depressants. In other words, many of these patients require smaller dosages of a drug to achieve a desired clinical level of sedation. This ought not to be a problem because the doctor administering the drug should always titrate slowly; however, extreme caution must be exercised whenever the younger patient receives CNS depressants via any route. Because of the rapid onset of action of intravenously administered drugs, this route should be reserved for use by the individual specifically trained or experienced in managing these patients (e.g., pediatric dentist).

2. Older patients (by definition, those 65 years of age and older) also demonstrate a greater "sensitivity" to drugs, including CNS depressants. The same precautions should be instituted (e.g., slow titration).

3. Pregnancy represents a relative contraindication to the administration of IV moderate sedation because most CNS depressants cross the placenta into the fetus. With some drugs, there is an increased risk of birth defects in the developing fetus. The subject of sedation and pregnancy is more fully discussed in Chapter 4.

4. A history of significant hepatic dysfunction contraindicates (either relatively or absolutely) the use of IV moderate sedation. Most intravenously administered drugs undergo biotransformation in the liver into pharmacologically inactive (and in some cases, active) products. The presence of significant hepatic dysfunction (American Society of Anesthesiologists [ASA] 3 or 4) may alter the rate at which these drugs undergo metabolism. This may lead to a prolonged period of higher blood levels of the drug and may lead to a prolongation of the clinical actions of the drug and/or a more profound effect from the same dose. Many patients with significant hepatic dysfunction (e.g., ASA 4 or 5 cirrhosis, hepatitis) are not ambulatory; however, when presented with a history of liver disease, the dentist should pursue an in-depth dialog history and consider medical consultation should any doubt remain as to the patient's physical status.

5. Thyroid dysfunction is a relative contraindication to the use of IV moderate sedation. Patients who are clinically *hypothyroid* are particularly sensitive to CNS depressants, such as sedative-hypnotics, antianxiety agents, and opioid analgesics. Patients exhibiting clinical signs and symptoms of hypothyroidism should probably not be administered IV moderate sedation. Box 21.2 lists clinical signs and symptoms of hypothyroidism. This represents a relative (not an absolute) contraindication, because if other sedative techniques (e.g., inhalation sedation) prove inadequate, lighter levels of IV moderate sedation may be provided. Titration should be carried out even more slowly than is usually recommended. Patients who are hypothyroid but are currently treated with thyroid medications (e.g., levothyroxine [Synthroid]) can safely receive IV moderate sedation. Patients who are clinically *hyperthyroid* (signs and symptoms present) are likely to prove extremely difficult to sedate. In addition, drugs such as the anticholinergics atropine and scopolamine ought not to be administered to the clinically hyperthyroid patient. Both drugs possess vagolytic properties, increasing the heart rate. Because hyperthyroid individuals may already have a significant elevation in their heart rate, further increases might prove deleterious to the patient's well-being by increasing the workload of the heart and also the risk of possible myocardial ischemia and decreased cardiac output.

	Signs and Symptoms of
Box 21.2	**Hypothyroidism and**
	Hyperthyroidism

Hypothyroidism	Hyperthyroidism
Weakness	Nervousness
Dry skin	Increased sweating
Lethargy	Hypersensitivity to heat
Slow speech	Palpitation
Sensation of cold	Fatigue
Gain in weight	Eye signs (exophthalmos)
Cold skin	Increased appetite
Thick tongue	Tachycardia
Edema of face	Goiter
Pallor of skin	Tremor
Memory impairment	Weight loss
Decreased sweating	Weakness
Loss of hair	

Patients with a hyperthyroid history but who, through surgery, radiation, or drug therapy, are presently euthyroid (normal thyroid function) may receive IV moderate sedation with minimal to no increase in risk.

6. Adrenal insufficiency represents a relative contraindication to the use of IV moderate sedation. Patients receiving chronic corticosteroid therapy or patients with Addison disease may be less able physiologically to handle the stresses associated with dental care than are patients with normal adrenal cortices. Although these patients require careful management (see stress-reduction protocol, Chapter 4), deeper levels of sedation are not recommended. IV moderate sedation may be used; however, only light-to-moderate sedation levels are suggested.

7. Patients receiving either monoamine oxidase inhibitors (MAOIs) or tricyclic antidepressants (TCAs) should be evaluated carefully before the administration of any CNS depressant. These drugs are used in the management of depression. Before administration of any other drug that is able to alter mental function (e.g., CNS depressants), medical consultation with the patient's psychiatrist or physician is recommended. Opioid agonists and barbiturates are synergistic with these two groups of drugs.

8. IV moderate sedation is not contraindicated in patients with a history of psychiatric disorders; however, it is strongly recommended that medical consultation be obtained before CNS-depressant drugs are given.

9. Patients who are extremely obese (morbid obesity, body mass index [BMI] >40) have a variety of potential problems.[1,2] Because of the excessive amounts of skin and superficial fat, venipuncture may prove to be extremely difficult. Of greater importance is the fact that in markedly obese persons, there is usually a concomitant decrease in cardiovascular and pulmonary reserve. Other forms of sedation, especially inhalation sedation, should be considered first, with IV moderate sedation considered only when other techniques prove ineffectual.

10. One of the most significant contraindications to the use of IV moderate sedation in the dental office is a dearth of visible superficial veins. All IV procedures in a dental office environment will be of an elective nature. It seems patently unfair for an already phobic patient to have to endure multiple unsuccessful venipuncture attempts so that we can give them a drug to help them relax. As is discussed in Chapter 24, the preliminary IV visit is used to determine whether the patient is an acceptable candidate for the proposed IV procedure. One of the objectives of this visit is to confirm the presence of superficial veins.

11. When using IV moderate sedation, the dentist must specifically question the patient regarding any history with each of the drugs considered for the procedure. Allergic responses and "hyperresponders" may be uncovered before the offending drug is administered. In addition, each drug has specific contraindications to its use. The drug package insert or Chapter 25 of this book should be reviewed for this important information. These contraindications include opioids (specifically meperidine)—asthma; and anticholinergics—glaucoma, prostatic hypertrophy.

INDICATIONS

The major indications for the administration of IV moderate sedation are essentially those of other sedative techniques. However, there are a number of indications for IV moderate sedation that are unique to this technique. These include the control of salivary secretions and the production of amnesia.

IV moderate sedation is not a technique that should be used as readily as is inhalation sedation. Before employing IV techniques, the doctor should carefully consider other techniques, especially inhalation sedation. IV moderate sedation should be considered for use only in situations in which there exists a specific indication.

Anxiety

As with inhalation sedation and the other sedation techniques discussed in this book, the primary indication for use of sedation is the presence of fear and anxiety. Unlike inhalation sedation, however, the use of the IV route should be reserved for those patients in whom other techniques have proved inadequate or for patients in whom prior history or the doctor's experience indicates that the IV route is the method most likely to succeed.

In most instances, the IV route should be reserved for patients exhibiting pronounced levels of apprehension and fear of the dental situation. Inhalation sedation can often effectively manage the patient with a lesser degree of fear and anxiety. However, there will be occasions when IV moderate sedation is required even for these patients.

Amnesia

A unique advantage of IV drug administration is the ability of some drugs to provide a degree of amnesia (lack of recall). Whether amnesia develops or does not develop after IV drug administration depends on several items. Some drugs are much more likely to provide amnesia than others. Diazepam, midazolam, lorazepam, and scopolamine are examples of drugs that have a greater degree of amnesia associated with their administration; meperidine and other opioids are less likely to provide an amnestic effect.

The depth of CNS depression (sedation) has, to some degree, an effect on whether amnesia develops and on the duration of the amnestic period. In general, given the same patient and the same drug (e.g., midazolam), more profound levels of sedation provide a greater likelihood of amnesia. This factor is the reason for my considering amnesia to be "the icing on the cake" during a sedation procedure. The prime goal of sedation is to relax the patient. In many cases, this result can be obtained with the patient only lightly sedated. The patient may tolerate the procedure quite well, but at its conclusion, may not be amnesic. In this situation, the sedation procedure must be considered a success. The primary goal—that of managing the difficult patient more easily and effectively—was accomplished. Should there also be a lack of recall of events that occurred during the procedure, so much the better. It is wiser to provide a patient comfortable dental treatment with total recall (no amnesia) at a lighter level of sedation than it is to provide comfortable dental treatment with total lack of recall at a deeper level of sedation. With loss of consciousness, lack of recall (amnesia) is virtually 100%, yet is associated with increased risk to the patient.

As with all other factors relating to drug response, there is a significant degree of individual variation in the occurrence of amnesia. Some patients will be amnesic following seemingly very light levels of sedation, whereas others may demonstrate no apparent amnesia with deeper levels of sedation. Such response is consistent with normal variation in response to drug administration.

Medically Compromised Patients

The IV route of sedation is indicated in the management of persons who are medically compromised and unable to tolerate stress in a normal manner. Although inhalation sedation is the preferred technique in most of these patients, light levels of IV moderate sedation may also be used in many of these situations.

ASA 2 or 3 Cardiovascular-Risk Patients. Examples of cardiovascular situations in which the IV route may be considered include angina pectoris, previous myocardial infarction, certain dysrhythmias, heart failure, and high blood pressure. The preferred route of sedation for all of these disorders is inhalation sedation with N_2O-O_2. In each of these cardiovascular disorders, the clinical status of the patient will deteriorate should the level of O_2 in the myocardium or in the blood become inadequate to meet the demands of the heart. With N_2O-O_2 sedation, the occurrence of such situations is minimized. Whenever IV moderate sedation is used in the management of the ASA 3 patient, there are two recommendations:
1. Employ light-to-moderate levels of sedation.
2. Administer 3 L/min of O_2 via a nasal cannula or 6 L/min via a nasal hood throughout the sedative procedure.

Previous Cerebrovascular Accident

The patient who has suffered a cerebrovascular accident (CVA, stroke, "brain attack") falls into the ASA 2, 3, or 4 category. The ASA status of the patient is determined by the duration of time since the CVA and by the presence or absence of residual signs and symptoms of CNS dysfunction.

As with the cardiovascular-risk patient, the CVA patient may require sedation during dental treatment. Although N_2O-O_2 is the preferred technique because of the increased percentage of O_2 administered, IV moderate sedation can be used if these same recommendations (as listed earlier for cardiovascular-risk patients) concerning depth of sedation (light to moderate only) and the administration of O_2 are observed.

Epilepsy

Epileptic patients are acceptable candidates for IV moderate sedation. In most cases, the seizure activity of the patient is controlled through daily administration of anticonvulsant (antiepileptic) drugs (many of which, coincidentally, are used intravenously as sedatives). Such patients will be able to tolerate almost any technique of sedation with little or no difficulty. It is in the patient whose seizure activity has not been controlled effectively that the IV route may prove particularly beneficial. Stress is a factor that acts to precipitate acute seizure activity; therefore use of the stress-reduction protocol is recommended. Although inhalation sedation may prove effective, the use of intravenously administered benzodiazepines, particularly midazolam or diazepam, is recommended. These drugs are effective anticonvulsants and can be administered intravenously should a protracted seizure (e.g., status epilepticus) develop. Their use as IV sedatives will greatly diminish (although not entirely eliminate) the likelihood of a seizure occurring during treatment. Consultation with the patient's physician is recommended before use of IV moderate sedation in these epileptic patients. The use of O_2 via nasal cannula or nasal hood is strongly recommended in epileptic patients because any degree of hypoxia may precipitate a seizure. Light-to-moderate levels of sedation may be safely employed in these patients.

Other Medically Compromised Patients. The IV route may also be used for many other medically compromised patients. ASA 4 patients should not receive IV moderate sedation within the dental office; such treatment is relegated to the operating room or the hospital dental clinic, where medical consultation and a more controlled treatment environment can be provided. ASA 2 and 3 patients are usually acceptable candidates for sedation. Whether or not the IV route is appropriate can be determined through consultation with the patient's physician, if felt necessary. The administration of supplemental O_2 throughout the IV procedure is recommended for all ASA 2, 3, and 4 patients.

Control of Secretions

Occasions arise during dental treatment when it is beneficial to decrease the volume of salivary secretions. The major indication for this will be impression taking following the preparation of teeth for full coverage. A dry mouth may also prove to be beneficial during restorative dentistry and surgical procedures. Anticholinergics can be administered orally, intramuscularly, and intravenously, with the IV route providing the most reliable and effective results. Agents such as atropine, scopolamine, and glycopyrrolate may be administered intravenously, either alone or in conjunction with other CNS depressants.

Analgesia

Although far from the ideal method of pain control in dentistry, intravenously administered opioid analgesics assist in obtaining clinically adequate pain control. Local anesthetics remain the ideal drugs for eliminating pain during dental treatment; however, though rare, occasions do arise where these drugs do not provide entirely adequate relief of discomfort. In such situations, the administration of CNS depressants, such as N_2O-O_2 or opioid analgesics, elevates the pain reaction threshold of the patient, thereby decreasing, or at least modifying, the patient's response to noxious stimulation.

The use of intravenously administered drugs as the sole means of achieving pain control is ineffective in the absence of general anesthesia. General anesthesia should not be considered unless the doctor has completed a residency in anesthesiology (see Section VI).

Diminished Gag Reflex

Some dental patients have a significant problem with gagging whenever instruments or fingers are placed in the posterior part of their oral cavity. Whatever the underlying reason for this response, it becomes difficult, if not impossible, for the dentist to treat these patients successfully. Several sedation techniques possess the added benefit of diminishing the gag reflex. Most notable among these is IV moderate sedation, followed closely by inhalation sedation with N_2O-O_2.

In most instances, the use of inhalation sedation is recommended to control a hyperactive gag reflex. To obtain a few intraoral radiographs or an impression takes but a few minutes, and because IV sedative techniques are too long acting for these procedures, inhalation sedation is recommended. If a patient has difficulty whenever anything is placed in his or her mouth (e.g., handpiece, explorer) and treatment is to last for an hour or more, the use of IV moderate sedation becomes a more reasonable option.

Indications for the use of intravenously administered drugs are quite numerous. Although the obvious indication is fear and apprehension, the dentist should be aware that many other indications for the use of IV moderate sedation do exist.

REFERENCES

1. Continuing Dental Education, Herman Ostrow School of Dentistry of U.S.C., Intravenous sedation syllabus – 2014. Herman Ostrow School of Dentistry of U.S.C.
2. Oregon Academy of General Dentistry – Oregon Health Sciences University. Intravenous sedation syllabus – 2017. Oregon Academy of General Dentistry – Oregon Health Sciences University.
3. Brogden RN, Goa ZL: Flumazenil. A reappraisal of its pharmacological properties and therapeutic efficacy as a benzodiazepine antagonist. *Drugs* 42(6):1061–1089, 1991.
4. The Flumazenil in Intravenous Conscious Sedation With Diazepam Multicenter Study Group II: Reversal of central benzodiazepine effects by flumazenil after intravenous conscious sedation with diazepam and opioids: report of a double-blind multicenter study. *Clin Ther* 14(6):910–923, 1992.
5. Magruder MR, Delaney RD, DiFazio CA: Reversal of narcotic-induced respiratory depression with nalbuphine hydrochloride. *Anesth Rev* 9:34, 1982.

chapter 22

Armamentarium

INTRAVENOUS DRUG ADMINISTRATION

The equipment required for venipuncture and for intravenous (IV) drug administration is discussed in this chapter. IV drugs may be administered in several ways, including the following:

1. Direct IV drug administration; patency of the vein not maintained
2. Needle maintained in the vein without a continuous infusion; patency maintained by periodic flushing
3. Continuous IV infusion; patency maintained by a continuous infusion of solution

Direct Intravenous Administration

In direct IV administration, a tourniquet is placed on the patient's arm, engorging the veins; the injection site is prepared; and the needle of the syringe containing the drug(s) is placed into the lumen of the vein, in effect doing the venipuncture with the drug-containing syringe. After ensuring that the needle tip lies within the lumen of the vein (aspiration of blood back into the syringe), the dentist or assistant removes the tourniquet, and the drug is slowly administered into the vein. Following drug administration, the needle is removed from the vein, pressure is applied to the site to stop the bleeding, and the planned treatment begins. No access to the vein is maintained during the procedure (Fig. 22.1).

Needle Maintained in the Vein Without Continuous Infusion

When the needle is maintained in the vein without an infusion, the tourniquet is placed, the veins are engorged, and the tissues are prepared in the usual manner. A winged infusion set or a hollow metal needle is used for venipuncture. Following successful venipuncture, the tourniquet is removed, and the syringe (without a needle attached) is connected to the needle that has been left in the vein and taped into place. After the drug is titrated to effect, the syringe is detached from the needle, and a second syringe containing a solution such as sterile water for injection is attached to the needle. The dental procedure is begun, with the dentist or assistant periodically flushing the needle with 1 mL of solution to keep the vein patent (Fig. 22.2).

Continuous Intravenous Infusion

With a continuous IV infusion, an indwelling needle or catheter is attached to a length of tubing that in turn is connected to a bag of IV infusion fluid. The same venipuncture procedure is carried out that was described for the first two techniques. Following removal of the tourniquet, the flow of IV solution is started, and the needle or catheter is secured. The IV drugs are administered through an injection port on the tubing, and the drug syringe is then removed. The rate of the IV infusion is adjusted to maintain a slow flow that will prevent needle

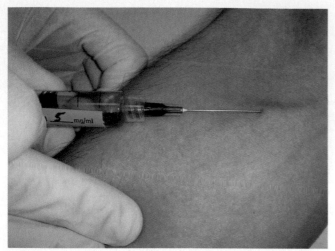

Figure 22.1 Direct IV drug administration. Blood is aspirated into syringe before injection to determine that needle is still within lumen of vein.

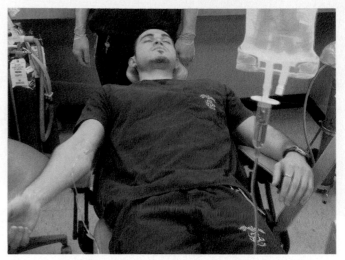

Figure 22.3 Continuous IV infusion.

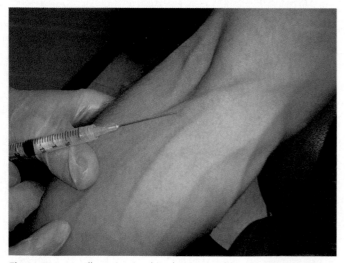

Figure 22.2 Needle maintained in the vein without continuous infusion.

occlusion during the dental procedure, which is then begun (Fig. 22.3).

ADVANTAGES AND DISADVANTAGES OF VARIOUS METHODS

The first technique, direct IV administration, in which the syringe is removed from the vein after drug administration, cannot be recommended for routine use in IV sedation. The only reasons for considering use of this technique, in my opinion, are:
1. Emergency situations in which IV drug administration is required and time or the lack of equipment does not permit establishment of an IV infusion

2. Situations in which the needle needs to be maintained in the vein for only a very brief period (as in drawing of blood for laboratory analysis)

Why do I believe this technique should not be used? As is evident in later chapters and during training in IV sedation, the most exacting part of learning to use IV sedation is becoming technically proficient at venipuncture. Although not a hard technique to master, venipuncture can be difficult on some occasions in even the most experienced of hands. Why, then, if placing a needle into the vein is the most difficult task in IV sedation, should the needle be removed from the patient's vein after a successful venipuncture? Adherents of the needle-removal technique claim that the patient is bothered by the needle remaining in the vein and that the presence of the needle in the vein throughout the procedure reminds the patient of a hospital. However, once the needle is placed into a vein and the sedative drug titrated to effect, the patient has little, if any, awareness of its presence, whether it is in for 1 minute or several hours. In response to the belief about the hospital setting, I can only state that the presence of a needle within the vein throughout the procedure is routine in hospital practice simply because it increases safety. Patients will accept as normal most practices within the dental office. A valid argument in favor of the needle-removal technique is that removal of the needle from the vein makes it difficult for additional drugs to be administered following the initial titration, minimizing the chance of a drug overdose.

Removal of the needle from the vein is illogical because, on occasion, additional IV sedative drugs may be required later in the procedure or a reversal agent may be needed later during the treatment period. Drugs, such as flumazenil, naloxone, or physostigmine, may (rarely) be required during or at the end of the IV sedation procedure. In both of these situations, a venipuncture would need to be redone. Because venipuncture is the only part of the IV sedation procedure that might be considered difficult, is it not logical to leave the needle in situ during the entire procedure? In addition, should a situation arise in which the patient's blood pressure decrease significantly, superficial veins will become more difficult to visualize and cannulate.

The second technique, in which the needle remains in the vein throughout the procedure and its patency maintained by periodic flushing with some solution, is an improvement on the previous technique. The only drawback to this technique is that periodic flushing of the needle is required to prevent clotting of the lumen from occurring. During a busy dental procedure, it is not uncommon for the dentist and the assistant to become deeply engrossed in the oral cavity and to neglect to flush the needle, in which case the lumen of the needle becomes clotted with blood and a vein must be recannulated.

Continuous IV infusion is the most highly recommended technique in all situations in which a patent vein is to be maintained for a period of time exceeding but a few minutes. In this technique, patency of the needle and vein are maintained by the constant infusion of IV solution from the bag into the needle and the patient's vein. The only drawback to this procedure is the possibility that (1) the infusate might become contaminated (an extremely unlikely occurrence) and (2) the drip rate might be too rapid, causing the bag of solution to be emptied during the procedure.

Readministration of sedative or administration of emergency drugs is easily carried out by simply inserting the syringe needle into the injection site on the IV tubing. The ease of maintaining a patent vein and the increased safety afforded the patient by the continuous IV infusion are the primary reasons for considering this technique as the ideal for IV drug administration. The equipment and techniques discussed in this section relate to continuous IV infusion.

INTRAVENOUS INFUSION SOLUTION
Choice of Solution
A number of fluids are available for IV therapy. Although the type of solution chosen is of potential significance in the hospitalized patient receiving prolonged IV therapy, for a short-duration IV procedure (less than 1 hour to several hours' duration) on a relatively healthy patient (American Society of Anesthesiologists [ASA] 1 or 2), the choice of infusate becomes academic. Solutions available for IV administration include the following:

Solution	Abbreviation
Lactated Ringer's	LR
Sterile water for injection	SW
5% dextrose in water	D_5W
Sodium chloride injection	¼ NS

Although other infusion solutions are available, these represent the most commonly used solutions.

In the ambulatory ASA 1, 2, or 3 patient considered a candidate for IV moderate sedation on an outpatient basis, there will be no contraindication to the use of any of these solutions. The question of whether a patient with insulin-dependent diabetes mellitus (type 1, or IDDM) should receive 5% dextrose in water often arises—will this solution elevate the patient's blood sugar level?

The answer is that a 5% dextrose and water solution is not contraindicated in the diabetic patient. First, the concentration of dextrose (5%) is not great enough to produce significant changes in the blood sugar level of this patient.[1] Second, as stressed in Chapter 26, the patient receiving IV moderate sedation is required to fast (be NPO) for 6 hours before the planned procedure. The patient arrives at the dental office with a decreased blood sugar level, perhaps not quite hypoglycemic but definitely not hyperglycemic. The addition of approximately 250 to 500 mL of 5% dextrose and water will produce a slight elevation in blood sugar level, a desirable effect at this time. It must be remembered that when a person with diabetes becomes clinically hypoglycemic, treatment of choice is the administration of 50% dextrose, a solution 10 times that which is infused during IV sedation.

Volume of Solution
All IV infusion solutions (fluids) are packaged in plastic bags (Fig. 22.4).

IV fluids are available in a variety of sizes. Most commonly used sizes include 1000, 500, and 250 mL. The 1000-mL (1-L [liter]) size is common in the hospital setting when a patient is receiving long-term IV therapy. The patient usually receives 3 L of IV fluid daily. Under general anesthesia, during which time the patient must be kept hydrated throughout the surgery, 1-L bags are also commonly used. Use of the 1-L bag for dental outpatient procedures is not the most highly recommended, although there is no significant reason why it could not be used. However, for the typical IV procedure in the dental office, the 1-L bag is simply too large. For example, during a 1-hour procedure, the typical patient may receive 250 to 500 mL of infusion fluid. At the conclusion of the procedure, the infusion bag represents one of the three items in the IV armamentarium that must be discarded. It is a single-use item and must never be reused despite the fact that, in this example, approximately 500 to 750 mL of infusate remains unused.

The 250-mL or 500-mL bags of IV fluid represent the most nearly ideal sizes for the typical 1- to 4-hour dental IV moderate sedation procedure. With proper management of the flow rate (as discussed in Chapter 26), a 250-mL or 500-mL bag can easily last for 3 to 4 hours.

The solution found within the IV bag is sterile. However, problems with contaminated fluids have developed in the past.[2] Care must be exercised by the user of such fluids to try to ensure their continued sterility. Administration of contaminated

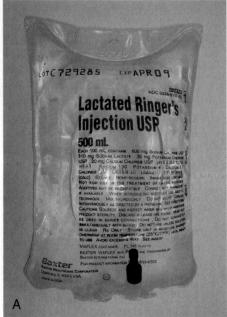

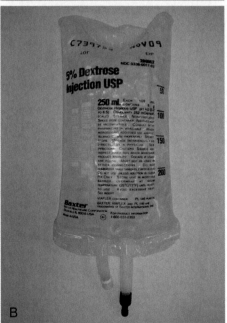

Figure 22.4 IV infusion solution of lactated Ringer's (LR) **(A)** 5% dextrose in water (D5W) **(B)**.

3. Once the seal on the bag of infusate has been opened, the fluid cannot be stored for any length of time without the possibility of contamination. If a bag of fluid is prepared for an IV procedure and the appointment is canceled, the bag could still be used if another procedure is scheduled for that same day. However, the bag should be discarded if it would not be used for a day or more. Bags of IV fluid do not contain preservatives or bacteriostatic agents; therefore they represent excellent culture media for bacterial growth.

4. *If there is ever any doubt as to the sterility of an unopened bag of IV infusion fluid, it should not be used.* However, the bag should not be discarded. On the contrary, the bag should be returned to the manufacturer for assay. The manufacturer will be very concerned about the possibility of a contaminated IV solution being used clinically.

The following checklist summarizes precautions for IV infusion solution:

1. Is the IV fluid clear?
2. Has the expiration date of the IV solution passed?
3. If an IV bag is open, has it been stored for more than a few hours?
4. Is there any doubt regarding its sterility? (Never use a bag of IV fluid when any doubt exists as to its sterility.)

INTRAVENOUS ADMINISTRATION SET

Delivery of the IV infusion from the bag to the patient requires tubing. IV administration sets, or IV tubing, as they are commonly known, have several components in common (Fig. 22.5).

The *piercing pin* is that part of the IV set that is inserted into the bag of IV fluid. It is a rigid plastic piece that must be kept sterile before its insertion into the bag of solution.

Located immediately below the piercing pin is the *drip chamber.* The drip chamber is an enlarged, flexible, clear plastic chamber into which fluid from the bag (infusate) will drip. The drip chamber has two functions: to prevent air from entering into the IV tubing and to permit regulation of the solution's flow rate.

The drip chamber should be filled approximately halfway with IV fluid to prevent air bubbles from entering into the IV tubing. Although isolated air bubbles within the tubing are of little consequence (see Chapter 27), the naive patient may be quite disturbed to see any bubble of air enter into his or her body. An unfilled drip chamber or one just barely filled with solution will allow air bubbles to enter the tubing as each drop of solution falls from the bag into the drip chamber.

Conversely, overfilling of the drip chamber prevents the dentist from assessing the flow rate of the IV fluid. Although this factor is not as critical in the ambulatory dental or surgical patient as it is in the hospitalized patient, the flow rate does require adjustment at various times during the IV procedure (see Chapter 26). In addition, in two groups of patients—the

fluids directly into the cardiovascular system of the patient can produce bacteremia or septicemia and has led to deaths and significant morbidity.[3]

The following should be checked before using a bag of solution:

1. *All IV infusion fluids are clear.* A solution that has any coloration to it or any particulate matter floating within it should never be used.
2. In addition to the name of the solution, the bag will have an expiration date. *IV infusion should never be used after its expiration date has passed* (see Fig. 22.4).

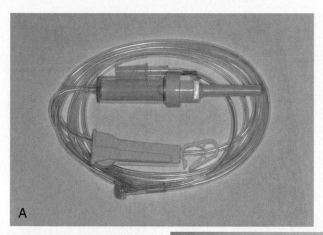

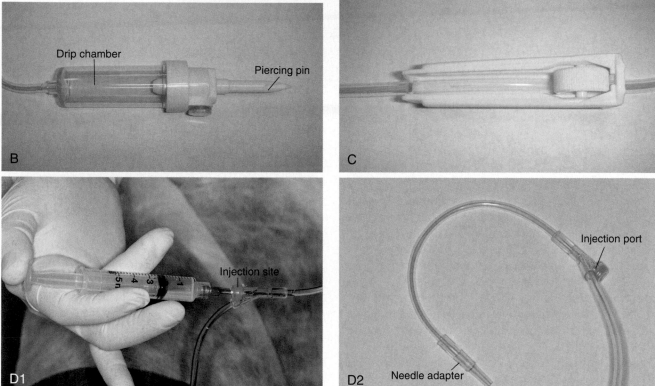

Figure 22.5 A, IV administration set. **B,** Piercing pin and drip chamber. **C,** Rate adjustment knob. **D,** Injection site and needle adapter.

smaller child and the patient with more advanced heart failure (ASA 3 or 4)—overhydration is a complication to be avoided. The ability to determine the precise rate of flow is of importance in these situations.

When the typical adult IV infusion set is used, 10 drops equal 1 mL of solution. Therefore for a 250-mL bag of IV solution to last for 2 hours (120 minutes), we can adjust the flow rate to 20 drops per minute (2 mL/min; 120 min = 240 mL). Some adult IV infusion sets are 15 drops per mL. The number of drops per milliliter will be found on the bag of solution.

Pediatric infusion sets provide a finer adjustment such that 60 drops equal 1 mL of solution (Fig. 22.6). Use of the pediatric

infusion is recommended in the smaller child and in the adult with more advanced heart failure (ASA 3, 4), neither of whom is a recommended candidate for IV moderate sedation.

Extending from the drip chamber is a variable length of plastic tubing, commonly 78 inches long, to which the IV needle will be attached. Along the length of this tubing are found several items (see Fig. 22.5):
- Rate adjustment knob
- Injection port or syringe port
- Rubber bulb (not present on all infusion sets)
- Adapter for needle or syringe

The *rate adjustment knob* permits regulation of the rate of flow of the IV fluid into the drip chamber. By rolling the round

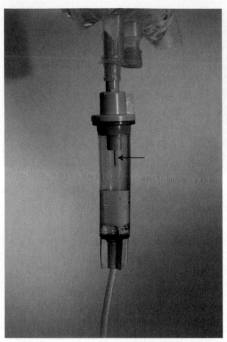

Figure 22.6 Pediatric infusion set. Note small pin within drip chamber (*arrow*).

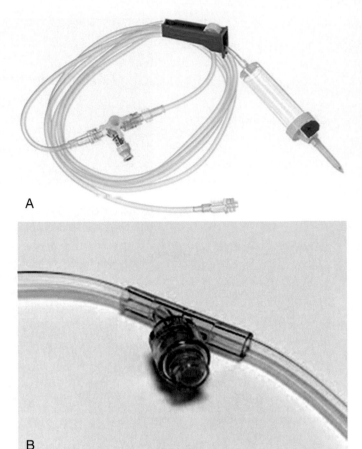

Figure 22.7 **A,** Needleless infusion set. **B,** Syringe attachment site.

controller, the IV tubing is either compressed or opened, slowing or accelerating the rate of flow of the IV fluid.

The *injection port* is usually a rubber diaphragm that fits over a hard plastic spur off of the main IV tubing. The needle of the syringe containing the drug to be injected is inserted into this port, and the drug is injected into the flowing infusion. The rubber diaphragm should not be removed from the plastic before injection.

Because of the potential danger of needle-stick injury, infusion sets are available in which the syringe connects to the injection port through a Luer-Lok connection, so-called "*needleless systems*" (Fig. 22.7).

On some IV sets near the distal end of the IV tubing just above where the needle adapter is found is a rubber bulb. This bulb is larger than the plastic tubing and serves as a means of checking if the needle or catheter tip lies within the lumen of a vein. The bulb need only be squeezed and released. If the needle or catheter tip lies within the lumen of a vein, a flash of blood appears in the tubing just above the entry point of the needle into the patient's skin. A second possible use of the rubber bulb is to serve as an alternative site for injection of a drug. The syringe needle is inserted into the bulb (with care not to perforate the other side of the tubing, sticking one's own finger), and the drug is injected into the IV fluid. Multiple punctures of the rubber bulb, however, can lead to leakage. The injection port is the recommended site for drug administration on the IV tubing.

At the very end of the IV tubing is the *needle adapter.* A variety of shapes and sizes of needles may be used for venipuncture. In addition, there are a multitude of manufacturers of each needle. To ensure that needles and tubing from different manufacturers can be used interchangeably, a standard female Luer connector is used. Any needle in the following discussion easily attaches onto standard IV tubing.

Under no circumstances should reuse of the IV infusion tubing ever be considered because the tubing will always become contaminated with the patient's blood at its most distal end. This blood may be quite visible as it surges back into the tubing when the needle tip enters into the lumen of the vein during venipuncture, or it may be quite dilute and perhaps not visible to the eye. Reuse of the IV tubing runs an unacceptably high risk of transmission of potentially very serious diseases. Do not do it!

NEEDLES

To deposit a drug beneath the skin, as in the case of intramuscular or subcutaneous injection, or directly into a blood vessel, as in the case of IV administration, a needle must be used. Needles are usually referred to by gauge and type.

Gauge

Gauge usually refers to the outside diameter of the needle. However, in discussions of the hypodermic needle, standard gauge numbers have come to be associated with the size of the lumen. Therefore the gauge number of a needle may refer to the internal diameter (ID) or the outside diameter (OD) of the needle lumen. Needles used for venipuncture generally range from 14 gauge to approximately 24 gauge. The lower (smaller) the gauge number, the larger the size of the lumen. Therefore a 16-gauge needle has a larger lumen than a 24-gauge needle.

The term *gauge* is often quite confusing. The term derives from the number of pieces of wire (in this case needles) that can be placed into a 1-mm circle. Therefore only 16 needles of 16 gauge will fit into the same space occupied by 23 needles of 23 gauge. Table 22.1 lists commonly used needle gauges and their major functions.

Types

Several types of needles are available for venipuncture; all have their adherents, their advantages, and their disadvantages. The following are the three most commonly employed needles (Fig. 22.8):

1. Hollow metal needle
2. Winged needle (scalp vein needle)
3. Indwelling catheter

The *hollow metal needle* is the prototypical needle (i.e., the traditional IV needle). This needle represents the basic design from which other needles in the following discussions have been modified. Fig. 22.9 illustrates the components of the hollow metal needle.

The needle is inserted directly into the vein and then attached via its hub to the IV tubing or directly to the syringe containing the drug to be administered. Since the development of the scalp vein needle and the indwelling catheter, use of the hollow metal needle for venipuncture has become limited to emergency situations in which other needles are not readily available or situations in which blood is to be drawn from a patient for laboratory analysis.

The hollow metal needle may be used to review the anatomy of the IV needle. At one end of the needle is a sharp tip. A triple bevel slopes backward from this tip and ends at the heel of the shaft. The shaft runs from this point to the hub. The length of the shaft varies, but is commonly between ⅝ inch and 1.2 inches in length. The hub is an enlarged metal or plastic portion that permits the needle to be attached to the IV tubing or a syringe.

The *winged needle* is a popular needle for IV moderate sedation procedures in the ambulatory patient within both dentistry and medicine. Some regard the winged needle as the device of choice for venipuncture of superficial veins in patients of all ages. The primary advantage over other types of needles is its ease of manipulation.

The winged needle (Fig. 22.10) consists of a sharp stainless steel needle, one or two flexible winglike projections mounted to the shaft of the needle, a variable length of flexible tubing, and a female Luer adapter that connects with any standard IV administration set.

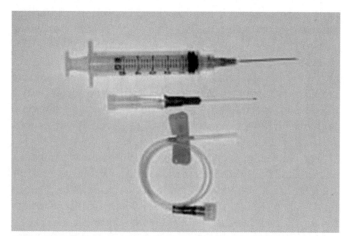

Figure 22.8 Hollow metal needle (*top* [attached to syringe]), indwelling catheter (*middle*), and winged needle (*bottom*) are available for IV drug administration.

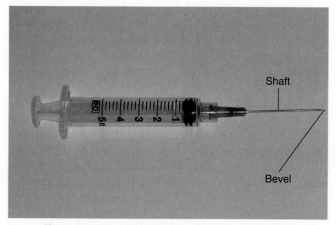

Figure 22.9 Components of the hollow metal needle.

Table 22.1	Needle Gauge and Function
GAUGE	FUNCTION
14	Phlebotomy Administration of blood
16	Phlebotomy Surgical procedures in which blood is likely to be required
18	Common during general anesthesia in which blood administration is unlikely
20, 21	Intramuscular drug administration Occasionally, IV during short procedure on ASA 1 or 2 patients IV sedation in dentistry
23	IV sedation in dentistry
25, 27	Intraoral local anesthetic administration
30	Intraoral local anesthetic administration Acupuncture

ASA, American Society of Anesthesiologists; *IV,* intravenous.

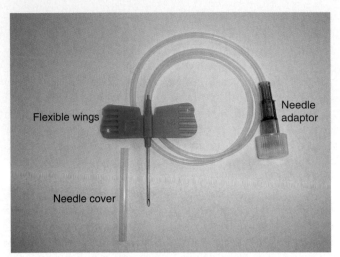

Figure 22.10 Components of the winged needle.

The wings allow the user to hold the needle more firmly, permitting greater ability to manipulate the needle and to gain greater "feel" during the procedure. In addition, following successful venipuncture, the wings may be taped down to better secure the needle within the vein. The winged needle has several synonyms: *winged infusion set, Butterfly needle, and scalp vein needle.*

Butterfly is a proprietary name for the winged infusion set. However, like other proprietary names, such as Ping Pong and Linoleum, common usage has turned the proprietary name into the most commonly used name of the device. The term *Butterfly needle* is very commonly used and is acceptable, although technically not correct.

The winged infusion set evolved from what was termed the *scalp vein needle.* Superficial veins in most neonates and infants are quite small and frequently difficult to cannulate. Often the physician had to surgically expose a vein (called a *venous cutdown*) to manually insert a catheter. The scalp vein needle evolved because among the most prominent veins found in the neonate or infant are those on the scalp (Fig. 22.11). The scalp vein needle is shorter, thereby minimizing the problem of needle perforation of the back wall of the vein, which can lead to either an infiltration or a hematoma.

Though available in a variety of gauges, the 21- and 23-gauge winged infusion sets are most used in dentistry, with the 21-gauge needle preferred because it will permit a greater volume of solution to flow through it per minute than the 23-gauge needle (13 to 3 mL/min).[4]

A potential problem with both the hollow metal needle and the winged infusion set is their rigidity. Should they be placed into a vein in a mobile area, such as the wrist or antecubital fossa, special precautions must be observed to prevent the patient from moving that area, or the needle, lying within the lumen of the vein, will perforate its posterior wall, producing a hematoma, requiring recannulation into a vein at a different site. Common terminology states that "we have lost the vein."

To minimize this risk, the flexible indwelling catheter was devised. Several types of *indwelling catheter* are available, among them the catheter–overneedle unit and the catheter–inside-needle unit. Within dentistry, the catheter–overneedle is recommended. "Safety catheters" have been developed that minimize risk of needle-stick injury. Following successful venipuncture, the metal needle retracts into a protective plastic sheath, preventing inadvertent needle-stick injury (Fig. 22.12). Materials used for the plastic catheter include polyvinyl chloride (PVC), Silastic, and Teflon. Modern catheters are radiopaque so that they may easily be visualized on x-ray examination.

The indwelling catheter, called the *catheter–overneedle,* when first designed, consisted of a metal hub to which a plastic catheter was attached. The catheter was physically connected to the separate metal hub by means of a piece of plastic. The safety of this design was called into question because the link between the catheter and the hub may not be secure and the catheter could come loose and migrate through the patient's veins. Such occurrences did occur, leading to the development of the modern indwelling catheter in which the catheter is of one-piece design (Fig. 22.13).[5] The catheter migration problem is essentially nonexistent with the catheter–overneedle unit. (Small pieces of catheter may still be severed and can migrate within the venous circulation if the metal needle [introducer] is reinserted into the catheter while it is still within the vein, a procedure that cannot be condoned—and is discussed fully in Chapter 24.)[6,7]

Regardless of the particular design of the indwelling catheter, its basic format is the same. A metal needle (called the *introducer* because it is used to "introduce" the catheter into the vein), ranging in gauge from 14 to 23, has a very tight-fitting plastic catheter placed over it. The catheter's length is just slightly less than that of the metal needle so that several millimeters of the introducer extend beyond the catheter (see Fig. 22.13, *A*).

Following successful venipuncture with the introducer (blood visibly returns into the needle), the catheter is advanced into the vein, the introducer removed, the IV infusion set attached, and the catheter secured. The actual technique of venipuncture using the indwelling catheter is presented in Chapter 24.

The indwelling catheter is recommended for use within the operating room and in most general anesthetic procedures. It has also become the preferred needle for IV moderate sedation. In situations in which maintenance of a patent vein is essential, indwelling catheters are recommended. The reason indwelling catheters are not universally taught as the primary venipuncture needle for most ambulatory procedures is that the winged infusion set is somewhat easier for a beginner to master. With some experience using the winged infusion set, the student has little or no difficulty moving to the indwelling catheter. Because the most "difficult" part of the IV moderate sedation technique is venous cannulation, use of the indwelling catheter has become preferred.

The IV infusion, the administration set, and the needle are all single-use, disposable items.

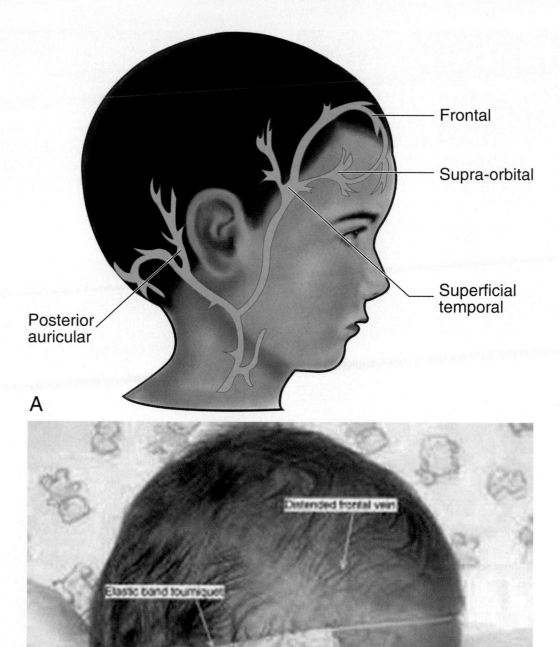

Figure 22.11 Scalp vein needle. **A,** Neonatal venous anatomy. **B,** A rubber band and is used as tourniquet when accessing scalp veins

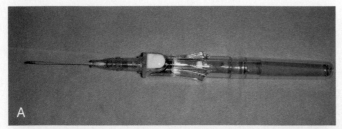

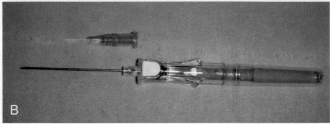

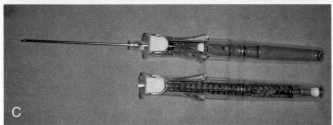

Figure 22.12 Components of the indwelling catheter. **A,** Intact unit. **B,** Catheter *(top)*; metal needle *(bottom)*. **C,** Catheter with "safe" needle retracted *(bottom)*.

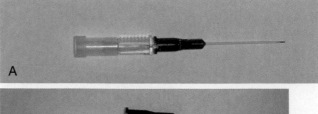

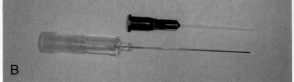

Figure 22.13 A, Intact IV catheter–overneedle. **B,** Components of catheter–overneedle.

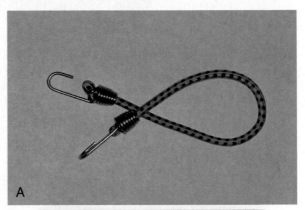

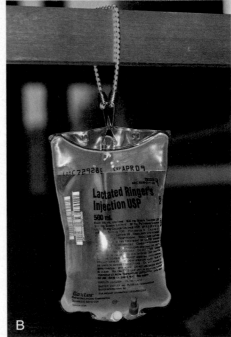

Figure 22.14 A, B, Bungee cord.

OTHER ITEMS

A number of additional items are of importance during venipuncture. An *IV stand* is used to elevate the bag of IV solution. As is discussed in Chapter 24, the height of the bag of IV solution above the patient's heart will, in part, determine the rate of flow of the solution.

IV poles mounted on a portable stand are commonly used within the operating room. Such devices are usually too cumbersome for use within the dental environment, there simply not being enough room for the dentist, one or two assistants, and the IV pole. In addition, portable IV stands are somewhat expensive, whereas the following device is inexpensive but functional.

To conserve precious floor space, the bag of IV fluid may be hung from the ceiling. A bolt and hook, as used for hanging plants, with several links of chain hung from the ceiling to the side of the patient's head, function quite well as an IV stand. An alternative is to use a small bungee cord wrapped around the light standard on the dental chair (Fig. 22.14).

A *tourniquet* is used to prevent the return of venous blood from the periphery to the heart while allowing for the unimpeded flow of arterial blood into the limb, thereby engorging the veins and making them more visible and easier to cannulate. A number of items may be used as tourniquets (Fig. 22.15):
1. Thin rubber tubing (e.g., Penrose drain)
2. Velcro tourniquet
3. Blood pressure cuff (sphygmomanometer)

Adhesive tape is needed to secure the needle to the patient's arm. An inexpensive tape, such as transparent adhesive tape, is usually adequate. Tegaderm has become quite popular because it combines ease of application and a secure fit with visibility (Fig. 22.16). Patients allergic to the adhesive used on tape will require the use of hypoallergenic tape. Always ask the patient about allergy to adhesive before the start of the IV procedure.

To cleanse the skin before venipuncture and to dry the tissue, *sterile 2 × 2-inch gauze wipes* are needed.

Prepackaged *alcohol wipes*, or simply a 2 × 2-inch gauze pad moistened with isopropyl alcohol (Fig. 22.17), are needed to cleanse the skin before venipuncture. Alcohol can also be used to cleanse the rubber covering of the injection site on the IV tubing and the rubber stopper on multiple-dose vials of drugs.

An *armboard* or immobilizer is required when venous cannulation is accomplished in either the wrist or antecubital fossa with a rigid needle (winged set or straight metal needle). The device is used to immobilize a portion of the arm, preventing it from being flexed by the patient, potentially dislodging the metal needle from the vein (Fig. 22.18). An immobilizer is not necessary when a flexible catheter has been inserted.

An *elbow immobilizer* consists of two rigid metal pieces connected at either end by two adjustable plastic straps. In the center is a Velcro strap that is used to fasten the immobilizer in position. The elbow immobilizer is available in both adult and pediatric sizes, is easy to work with, does an excellent job of immobilizing the antecubital fossa, and is not very expensive. This device is not as effective in immobilizing the wrist.

Adhesive bandages are used at the end of the procedure to protect the site of venipuncture.

The items previously described are the essentials for venipuncture and IV moderate sedation. Several other items should always be available not only for IV moderate sedation, but also in every dental office.

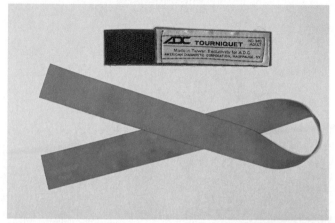

Figure 22.15 Tourniquets: Velcro tourniquet (*top*) and rubber tubing (*bottom*).

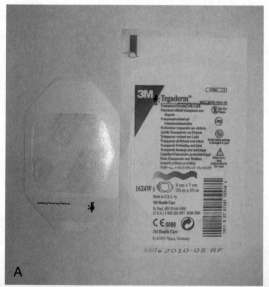

Figure 22.16 Tegaderm. **A,** Intact. **B,** In use.

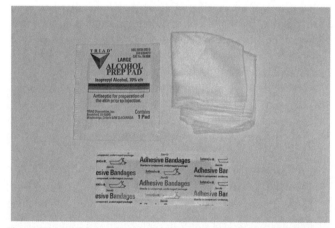

Figure 22.17 Additional items for venipuncture: alcohol, sterile gauze, and bandages.

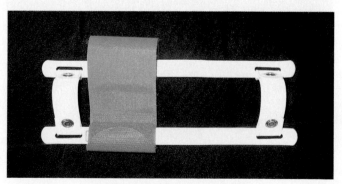

Figure 22.18 Elbow immobilizer.

A *sphygmomanometer* and *stethoscope* are required for monitoring of the patient's blood pressure before, during, and after the sedative procedure. In addition, the stethoscope may be used to auscultate both the heart and lungs at any time before or during the procedure.

The blood pressure cuff (sphygmomanometer) may be used as a tourniquet during venipuncture by simply inflating it to a pressure above the patient's diastolic blood pressure but below their systolic blood pressure (e.g., to approximately 100 mm Hg when the patient's blood pressure is 120/80 mm Hg).

Patients must be monitored throughout the IV sedation procedure. A variety of *monitoring devices* are available, ranging from the inexpensive (pretracheal stethoscope) to the more costly (end-tidal carbon dioxide [CO_2] monitor). The use of these monitors and recommendations for monitoring during the various levels of sedation and general anesthesia are discussed in Chapters 5 and 26.

Oxygen (O_2) should be available in all dental offices whether or not IV moderate sedation is used. Although its primary use is in the management of emergency situations, the routine administration of O_2 through a nasal cannula or nasal hood (Fig. 22.19) to patients receiving IV sedation is recommended (see Chapter 26).

An *emergency drug kit* and *emergency equipment* must also be available in all dental offices. The emergency kit in the dental office in which IV moderate sedation is used contains several drugs that are not considered mandatory in the typical dental office emergency drug kit (Fig. 22.20):

1. Opioid antagonist: naloxone
2. Benzodiazepine antagonist: flumazenil
3. Antiemergence delirium: physostigmine
4. Vasodilator: procaine 1% or 2% or phentolamine mesylate

These items and their uses are discussed in Chapter 27; the emergency drug kit and equipment are reviewed in Chapter 33.

A handheld near-infrared (NIR) *vein finder* should be considered for inclusion in the armamentarium for IV moderate sedation (Fig. 22.21). Chiao et al demonstrated a significantly increased rate of successful venipuncture compared with

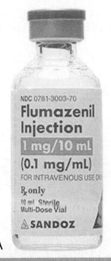

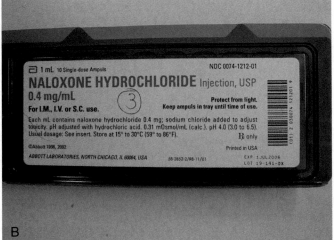

Figure 22.20 A, Flumazenil. **B,** Naloxone

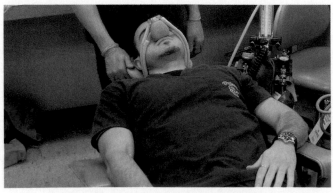

Figure 22.19 Patient receives O_2 during IV sedation.

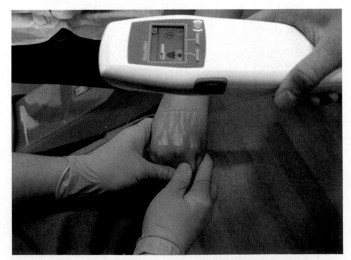

Figure 22.21 Near infrared vein finder aids in locating veins. (Photo courtesy of Dr. Kenneth Lee, SOLIS Surgical Arts, Tarzana, CA.)

conventional venipuncture technique in obese, African American, and Asian subjects,[8] though other clinical trials demonstrated no increase in cannulation success.[9,10] It has been our experience that persons who perform venipuncture daily all enthusiastically recommend inclusion of an NIR vein finder in their armamentarium.

REFERENCES

1. Moltra VK, Meiler SE: The diabetic surgical patient. *Curr Opinion Anaesthesiol* 19(3):339–345, 2006.
2. Moore KL, Kainer MA, Badrawi NA, et al: Neonatal sepsis in Egypt associated with bacterial contamination of glucose-containing intravenous fluids. *Pediatr Infect Dis J* 24(7):590–594, 2005.
3. Garrett DO, McDonald LC, Wanderley A, et al: An outbreak of neonatal deaths in Brazil associated with contaminated intravenous fluids. *J Infect Dis* 186(1):81–86, 2002.
4. Trieger NT: *Pain control*, ed 2, St Louis, 1994, Mosby.
5. Galdun JP, Paris PM, Weiss LD, Heller MB: Central embolization of needle fragments: a complication of intravenous drug abuse. *Am J Emerg Med* 5(5):379–382, 1987.
6. Hart BL, Newell JD, II, Davis M: Pulmonary needle embolism from intravenous drug abuse. *Can Assoc Radiol J* 40(6):326–327, 1989.
7. Angelos MG, Sheets CA, Zych PR: Needle emboli to lung following intravenous drug abuse. *J Emerg Med* 4(5):391–396, 1986.
8. Chiao FB, Resta-Flarer F, Lesser J, et al: Vein visualization: patient characteristic factors and efficacy of a new infrared vein finder technology. *Br J Anaesth* 110(6):966–971, 2013.
9. deGraff JC, Cuper NJ, van Dijk A, et al: Evaluating NIR vascular imaging to support intravenous cannulation in awake children difficult to cannulate: a randomized clinical trial. *Pediatr Anesth* 24(11):1174–1179, 2014.
10. Aulagnier J, Hoc C, Mathieu E, et al: Efficacy of Accuvein to facilitate peripheral intravenous placement in adults presenting to an emergency department: a randomized clinical trial. *Academ Emerg Med* 21(8):858–863, 2014.

chapter 23

Anatomy for Venipuncture

enipuncture is a technique separate and distinct from intravenous (IV) sedation. All health care professionals should become proficient with this route of drug administration, whether IV sedation is practiced or not, because the ability to establish an IV line may prove to be important in emergency situations.

Venipuncture is not a difficult technique to learn. Indeed, Malamed demonstrated that the initial attempt at venipuncture by untrained dental students had a greater than 90% success rate.[1] However, proficiency requires practice. Once learned, knowledge of the technique remains with the dentist forever; yet because it is an acquired skill, if not used regularly, the level of the dentist's ability will diminish.

In theory, venipuncture may be attempted in any superficial vein of a size sufficient to accommodate the needle. Fig. 23.1 illustrates the major superficial veins in the human body. In practice, however, elective venipuncture is usually confined to one of the patient's extremities. Either an arm or leg may be used. The usual preference is the arm, with the leg used when arm veins are inadequate or in emergency situations in which the arm may be unavailable or unsuitable for use.

IV sedation in the dental setting in an ambulatory patient is almost always an elective procedure. Selection of a venipuncture site will therefore usually be limited to one of the arms. Use of the leg for venipuncture is usually reserved for the infant or child, in whom arm veins are smaller and less superficial than in the adult, or the adult with a disability, in whom a venipuncture site in the foot may be more easily secured than one on the arm.

In this chapter, the anatomy of the circulation to the arm is described in detail. Both the venous circulation and the arterial circulation are discussed, because it is necessary to be aware of those sites where anatomically important structures, such as arteries and nerves, lie in close proximity to veins. Knowing where not to attempt a venipuncture is valuable knowledge.

ARTERIES OF THE UPPER LIMB

Blood to the right upper limb leaves the aortic arch through the short, wide brachiocephalic (innominate) trunk, which divides into the right common carotid and right subclavian arteries, the latter delivering arterial blood to the upper limb. On the left side, the subclavian artery is a direct branch of the arch of the aorta. From this point onward, the arteries of the two sides are symmetric.[2]

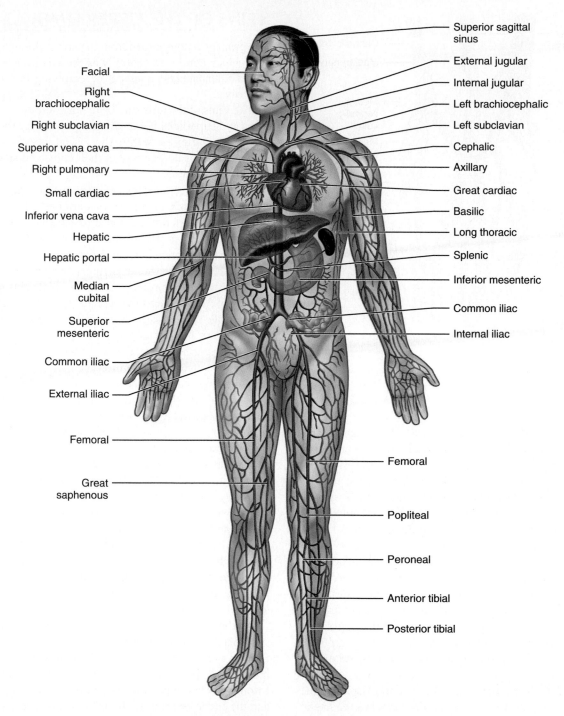

Figure 23.1 Principal veins of the human body.

At the outer border of the first rib, the *subclavian artery* turns laterally to enter into the axilla. At this point, it is termed the *axillary artery.* The axillary artery leaves the axilla at the lower border of the teres major muscle to enter the arm or brachium as the *brachial artery.* Approximately 1 inch below the antecubital fossa, the brachial artery bifurcates into the *radial* and *ulnar arteries* (Fig. 23.2), which travel distally in the forearm and terminate in the palm as an *arterial arch.* The

ulnar artery forms the *superficial palmar arch,* which travels to the level of the web of the thumb, where it is completed by a small branch arising from the radial artery, the superficial palmar branch. The radial artery crosses the bottom of the so-called *snuffbox* (the hollow at the base of the thumb), reaching the dorsum of the hand and then entering the palm. There it forms the *deep palmar arch,* which is completed by a small branch from the ulnar artery, the deep palmar branch.

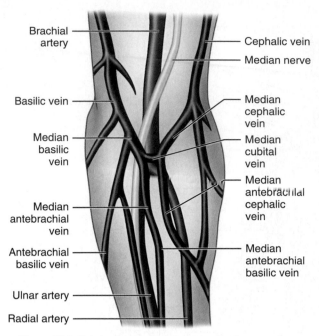

Figure 23.2 Relative location of major arteries in upper arm.

The location of these arteries has great clinical significance. Within the antecubital fossa, the brachial artery is commonly found beneath the median basilic vein, usually the most prominent vein in the antecubital fossa. The brachial artery is located just medial of the midline in the antecubital fossa and is the primary reason that the medial aspect of the antecubital fossa is low on my list of preferred venipuncture sites for the neophyte phlebotomist.

Approximately 2.5 cm (1 inch) below the antecubital fossa, the radial and ulnar arteries arise from the brachial artery. The radial artery lies on the lateral aspect of the ventral surface of the forearm, the ulnar on its medial aspect. Although it is not superficial at its origin, approximately 5% of the population does possess a recurrent radial artery, which is located on the lateral side of the antecubital fossa and is relatively superficial.

The radial artery continues down the ventral aspect of the forearm, not lying near the surface until it reaches the lateral aspect of the wrist, at the base of the snuffbox. At this point, on the ventral surface of the wrist, the radial artery is quite superficial. It is at this point that the radial pulse and arterial blood for blood gas analysis may be obtained. Care must be exercised whenever venipuncture is contemplated in this region. Fortunately, venous anatomy does not readily lend itself to venipuncture at this site.

The ulnar artery descends through the forearm, lying more deeply within the tissues than does the radial. It lies on the medial aspect of the forearm, but at no point does it become superficial enough to be palpable.

VEINS OF THE UPPER LIMB

The primary venous return from the arm is through the *axillary vein,* which continues centrally as the *subclavian* and *brachiocephalic (innominate) veins* before emptying into the *superior vena cava.*

The veins of the arm may be divided into two groups: deep veins and superficial veins. The deep veins, for the most part, accompany arteries within the fascial sleeve, whereas the superficial veins lie for most of their course outside the fascial sleeve.

Deep veins, except for the axillary veins, are arranged in pairs, one on either side of the various arteries. The axillary vein, which is a direct continuation of the basilic vein, crosses the axilla and becomes the subclavian vein at the outer border of the first rib. Its branches correspond to those of the axillary artery, except for the thoracoacromial, which joins the cephalic vein. The axillary vein receives the brachial veins in the lower portion of the axilla and the cephalic vein in the upper portion of the axilla. These deep veins will not be of significance in venipuncture.

The *superficial veins* of the upper limb are the veins selected for most elective venipuncture. Their anatomy is discussed in the following sections (see Fig. 23.1).

Blood to the digits is drained through an anastomosis of *palmar* and *dorsal digital veins.* From the palmar aspect of the hand, most blood flows to the dorsum of the hand, especially through the *intercapitular veins* that lie between the heads of the metacarpal bones (aka knuckles) and around the margins of these heads. Blood from the digits and palm therefore drains primarily into the *dorsal venous network* on the back of the hand. Two major veins arise from this dorsal venous network. The *cephalic vein* arises from the radial aspect of this network, and the *basilic vein* arises from the ulnar side. These veins ascend the forearm, the cephalic on the lateral aspect, the basilic medially. Within the forearm, the *median vein of the forearm* arises and ascends the forearm on its medial aspect.

At the antecubital fossa, a number of veins, somewhat superficial, are usually visible. From lateral to medial are the *cephalic vein,* the *median cephalic,* the *median vein,* the *median basilic,* and the *basilic.* The cephalic vein continues upward through the clavipectoral fascia to drain into the *axillary vein,* and the *basilic vein* runs to the axilla, where it continues directly as the axillary vein.

ANATOMY

Clinically the arm provides the phlebotomist with four distinct areas for venipuncture. At the upper part of the arm is found the antecubital fossa, which is discussed as two separate areas: (1) the medial aspect of the antecubital fossa and (2) the lateral aspect of the antecubital fossa. In our descent down the arm, the ventral aspect of the forearm is next, followed by the dorsum of the wrist and the dorsum of the hand. Each of

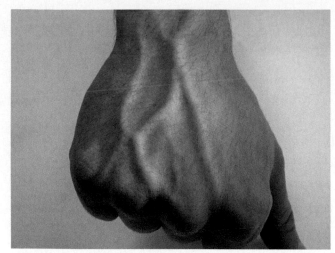

Figure 23.3 Superficial veins of dorsum of hand and wrist.

these potential venipuncture sites presents its own advantages and disadvantages.

Dorsum of the Hand

The dorsum of the hand is the preferred site for venipuncture of anesthesiologists (Fig. 23.3). It has several distinct advantages over other sites and few disadvantages. It is one of my two preferred sites.

Anatomically, it is extremely rare to find arteries on the dorsal aspect of the hand; most arteries are located on its palmar aspect. In addition, most blood returning to the heart is routed into the veins that form the dorsal venous network, a group of superficial veins. The location of most of the veins on the dorsum of the hand and of most arteries in the palm obviates the obstructive pressures that occur on the dorsum when a fist is formed, thereby maintaining intact the arterial blood supply into the hand during a "fight or flight" situation. This pattern is similar to the dorsal venous arch of the foot, which is distant from the pressure applied to the sole when a person stands.

The veins within the dorsal venous network have the obvious advantage of being quite superficial. Ease of accessibility is important when elective venipuncture is considered. A second advantage of the dorsum of the hand is the anatomic safety of the region. Rarely (but not never) will an artery be found on the dorsal aspect of the hand.

There are two disadvantages to the dorsal veins of the hand. First, these veins are smaller than veins found more proximally. Second, because these veins are superficial, they tend to be mobile.

As to the first disadvantage, it is common practice within anesthesia to start an IV infusion on the dorsum of the hand using a needle not smaller than 18 gauge. Quite frequently a 16-gauge needle is used in this area. In virtually all children and adults, the dorsum of the hand can readily accommodate these large-gauge needles. In dentistry, a 20- or a 22-gauge

needle may be used for venipuncture, needles easily accommodated by the lumen of these smaller veins.

The mobility of veins on the dorsum of the hand can, in some cases, make successful venipuncture more difficult to accomplish. Fortunately, several techniques are available for immobilizing veins during venipuncture:
1. Holding the hand in a fist during venipuncture
2. Pulling the skin of the dorsum toward the knuckles during venipuncture
3. Use of the inverted Y configuration, if present

These immobilization techniques are discussed more fully in Chapter 24.

It is sometimes said that venipuncture on the dorsum of the hand is more painful for the patient than at other sites. I personally have found that venipuncture in the dorsum is neither more nor less comfortable than at any other site on the arm. The most important factor determining comfort or discomfort is the technical prowess of the person attempting the venipuncture. With experience usually comes increasing technical ability and greater comfort for the patient.

Wrist

The dorsal venous network continues proximally, draining subcutaneously along the margins of the hand and wrist into two major veins (see Fig. 23.3). In most persons, the veins of the wrist are not so uniform that they can be assigned names. However, on the lateral (radial) aspect of the wrist in the snuffbox is found the so-called *intern's or resident's vein*. This vein becomes the cephalic vein as it ascends the forearm. Although usually visible, this vein has the disadvantage of being quite mobile and located in an area that is difficult to immobilize.

Another vein, which ultimately becomes the basilic vein, is commonly found on the ulnar aspect of the dorsum of the wrist. It, too, is located in an area where mobility is great and immobilization difficult. Another vein may be found toward the middle of the dorsal aspect of the wrist. Of the three veins, this last represents the most logical choice for venipuncture in this region. It is both superficial and mobile, but immobilization may usually be achieved through the techniques discussed previously.

The ventral aspect of the wrist is not as desirable an area for elective venipuncture. Though several veins are usually visible, they possess several undesirable characteristics: They are not as large as those on the dorsum of the wrist; the anatomy of the region leaves much to be desired—relatively superficial arteries, nerves, and tendons make the region both more sensitive and more risky for attempted venipuncture; and the wrist must be immobilized if a rigid metal needle is to be used. The ventral aspect of the wrist is more difficult to immobilize than the dorsum.

In summary, the dorsum of the wrist is greatly preferred to its ventral aspect. However, significant disadvantages to use of the wrist for venipuncture exist, including vein mobility and the need to immobilize the wrist during the entire IV

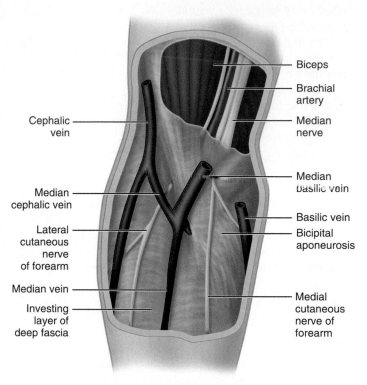

Cephalic vein

Median cephalic vein

Lateral cutaneous nerve of forearm

Median vein

Investing layer of deep fascia

Biceps

Brachial artery

Median nerve

Median basilic vein

Basilic vein

Bicipital aponeurosis

Medial cutaneous nerve of forearm

Figure 23.4 Veins of the ventral forearm and antecubital fossa.

procedure should a rigid metal needle be used. Immobilization of the wrist is not necessary when an indwelling catheter is used.

Forearm

The forearm represents one of the preferred sites for venipuncture on the upper limb (Fig. 23.4). The basilic and cephalic veins are the major veins of the forearm, with the basilic coursing up the medial (ulnar) aspect of the arm and the cephalic on its lateral or radial aspect. The basilic and cephalic veins are not as superficial as the veins found in the dorsum of the hand and the wrist; however, they are usually visible and often palpable, especially following application of the tourniquet.

A third vein, the median vein of the forearm, travels subcutaneously along the midline of the ventral surface. It lies somewhat deep at the distal end of the forearm, becoming more superficial just below the antecubital fossa.

The dorsal aspect of the forearm may also be considered for venipuncture. However, because of a lack of obvious veins and the presence of hair, this site is not of primary importance.

Advantages of the veins of the forearm include the following:

1. The veins are larger than those found in the wrist and dorsum of the hand.
2. Veins, because they are not superficial, do not roll during venipuncture attempts.

3. There is no need to immobilize either the wrist or the antecubital fossa when the forearm is used for venipuncture with a rigid metal needle. (This increases patient comfort during the IV procedure.)
4. Anatomically the superficial ventral (and dorsal) aspects of the forearm are devoid of any major arteries or nerves that might lie close to the usual venipuncture sites.

A disadvantage of the ventral aspect of the forearm is the lack of superficiality of the veins, making successful venipuncture more difficult to accomplish in some patients.

Antecubital Fossa

The antecubital fossa, or elbow joint, has for many years been one of the most popular sites for venipuncture. The usual pattern of veins in this region is illustrated in Figs. 23.1 and 23.2.

The cephalic and basilic veins traverse the lateral and medial aspects of the antecubital fossa, respectively. They represent relatively large targets for venipuncture. However, in some persons, they may be located so far laterally or medially that venipuncture becomes technically more difficult to carry out successfully, and in patients in whom venipuncture is successful, stabilization of the rigid needle or flexible catheter is difficult.

The median vein of the forearm usually becomes somewhat more superficial as it approaches the antecubital fossa. It lies almost directly in the midline of the forearm. Just below the border of the antecubital fossa, the median vein bifurcates.

In most persons, the median vein divides into two major branches: the median cephalic and the median basilic veins. The median cephalic, as its name implies, runs laterally to join with the cephalic vein, and the median basilic runs medially, joining with the basilic vein.

In this, the most common pattern, the largest of the veins in the antecubital fossa is the median basilic vein. This is so because a deep vein connects with the median basilic vein in this area. Indeed, the median basilic vein is usually the first choice of phlebotomists. The median cephalic vein is also large, though not as large as the median basilic vein. The cephalic and basilic veins are also large, but because of their location (lateral and medial, respectively), they are more difficult to enter and to stabilize the needle in.

Although many of the veins of the antecubital fossa appear large and therefore present as inviting targets for venipuncture, there is a potential problem when venipuncture is carried out (by the neophyte) on the medial aspect of the antecubital fossa. The problem lies in the anatomy of this region.

As is evident in a cross-sectional diagram of the antecubital fossa (Fig. 23.5), important structures are located directly below the medial aspect of the fossa. Centrally the biceps tendon passes deeply down to the upper end of the radius. Medial to this lies the bicipital aponeurosis. On the aponeurosis lies the large median basilic vein with the median cutaneous nerve of the forearm on its medial side. This vein is somewhat mobile

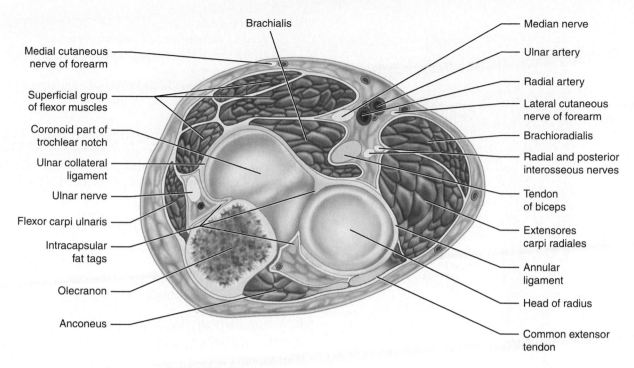

Figure 23.5 Cross-section of antecubital fossa (ventral area on top).

(although not as mobile as the dorsal wrist veins) and may slip away from the needle tip during venipuncture if not immobilized adequately. Should the vessel be nicked, a large hematoma will develop. During immobilization, the vein may be flattened, making venipuncture more difficult.

Of far greater importance, however, is the fact that immediately below the bicipital aponeurosis and the median basilic vein lie the median nerve and the brachial artery or its branches, the radial and ulnar arteries. It is not impossible for a novice to miss the median basilic vein and to enter into the brachial artery or to injure the median nerve.

No such potential problem exists on the lateral aspect of the antecubital fossa. The median cephalic vein, although smaller in size than the median basilic, is relatively immobile and can readily accommodate a 20-gauge needle. The lateral cutaneous nerve of the forearm lies nearby, but no important structures lie deep to the fascia. The radial nerve is lateral to the biceps tendon, but it lies in an intramuscular groove deep on the bone, well out of harm's way.

Advantages of the antecubital fossa as a venipuncture site include the following:
1. Veins are larger than other sites on the arm.
2. Veins are not mobile or are not as mobile as those on the wrist and dorsum of the hand.
3. The lateral aspect of the antecubital fossa is anatomically safe.

Disadvantages of the antecubital fossa for venipuncture are as follows:
1. Veins are not as superficial as in other sites, making venipuncture more difficult in some patients.

2. Anatomically the medial aspect of the fossa has significant anatomy that should be avoided.
3. The antecubital fossa must be immobilized throughout the procedure when a rigid metal needle is used for venipuncture.

It is recommended that the lateral aspect of the antecubital fossa be used preferentially, especially by the less experienced phlebotomist. As technical prowess increases, the medial aspect may also be used.

Foot

On rare occasion, it may be impractical or impossible to use the arm for venipuncture. Within the dental setting in an elective procedure on an American Society of Anesthesiologists (ASA) 1 or 2 patient, it might be advisable to forgo the IV route in favor of another technique of sedation (e.g., intramuscular [IM], intranasal [IN]). However, in pediatric dentistry, where superficial veins of the arm may be small and difficult to locate and cannulate, the foot may be considered as an IV route as more of a necessity than as an elective procedure. In addition, many younger children are not willing to sit quietly in the chair while venipuncture is performed on the arm. This is especially so in pediatric patients who require IV sedation for their management. A child can relatively easily move their arm or grab at it with the opposite hand, dislodging the needle or catheter. In this situation, the foot may prove a more appropriate site for venipuncture.

The superficial veins of the foot are illustrated in Fig. 23.6. Anatomically the dorsum of the foot and the medial and lateral aspects of the ankle offer safe sites for venipuncture.

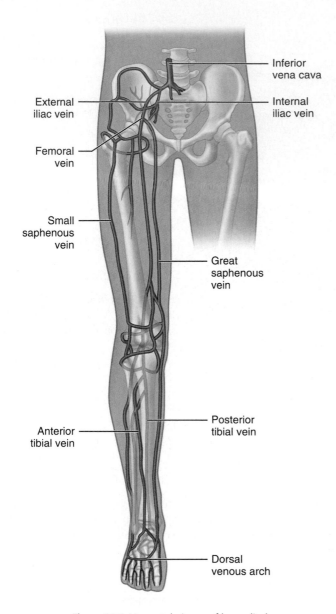

Figure 23.6 Venous drainage of lower limb.

In addition, the dorsal veins of the foot are usually quite superficial.

The dorsum of the foot contains a dorsal venous network similar to that found on the dorsum of the hand. As these veins progress toward the ankle, they drain into two major superficial vessels. Located immediately above the medial malleolus is the great saphenous vein, the largest superficial vein in the ankle or foot. On the opposite side, just below the lateral malleolus, is found the small saphenous vein.

Advantages of the foot or ankle for venipuncture include the following:
1. Superficial vessels
2. Relatively large vessels

3. Anatomically safe
4. No need to immobilize the venipuncture site
    Disadvantages of the foot and ankle as a venipuncture site include the following:
1. Accessibility is more limited than with the upper limb.
2. Veins roll when contacted by the needle.

SELECTION OF VENIPUNCTURE SITE

Several factors should be considered when determining the ideal site for venipuncture.[3] These are discussed in the following sections.

Condition of the Superficial Veins

Veins may appear tortuous, straight, hardened by age, scarred from previous use or abuse, sore, or inflamed from recent venipuncture. The preferred vein is one that is unused, easily visible, and relatively straight.

Relationship of the Vein to Other Anatomic Structures

Potential venipuncture sites in which other anatomic structures of importance, such as nerves and arteries, might be contacted or damaged should be avoided, if possible. In the arm, the primary area where this is of significance is the medial aspect of the antecubital fossa.

Duration of the Venipuncture

During prolonged IV infusion (more than 2 hours), a site that permits the patient the greatest freedom of movement is important. Thus a vein traversing a joint, such as the antecubital fossa or wrist, is not ideal for prolonged IV therapy because the joint will require immobilization if a rigid metal needle is used. Venipuncture on the dorsum of the hand or the ventral forearm will be better tolerated in this situation. Patients have complained during 2- to 4-hour IV sedation cases that their elbow has become quite stiff or sore because of the necessity for immobilization. For shorter durations (less than 2 hours) this should not be a factor.

Clinical Status of the Patient

Injury or disease involving one of the limbs may preclude the use of that area for venipuncture. Prior recent venipuncture in the selected site should lead the dentist to search for another potential site.

A history of phlebitis in the patient should forewarn the dentist to either reconsider the use of the IV route or to search for the largest vein possible in the selected limb. Patients who have undergone major surgical reconstruction (e.g., following breast cancer) in the upper limb or axilla may have deficits in venous drainage from that arm.

Age (Size) of the Patient

In neonates, who are unlikely to be patients in a dental office, scalp veins are preferred because of their accessibility and to simplify the problem of restraint of the infant. In seriously ill newborn infants, the umbilical vein may be used during the first 24 to 48 hours of life.

Smaller children, because their limbs are "pudgier," may have superficial veins of the upper limb that are quite difficult to visualize. The foot may prove a more acceptable site for venipuncture. Once again, these patients are not recommended as candidates for elective IV moderate sedation.

In very obese adult patients, veins may prove difficult or impossible to locate. A careful search of both arms and, if necessary, the feet will usually be fruitful in locating one or more veins. If the planned dental procedure is elective, the absence of superficial veins should be considered a contraindication to the use of IV sedation. Should it be essential to establish an IV line, hospitalization of the patient, with subsequent surgical cutdown to cannulate a vein, may be the most prudent course of action.

Type of Intravenous Procedure

The chemical nature of the drugs administered, the size of the vein to be cannulated, and the size of the needle are important because they all may produce irritation of the inner wall of the vein, a situation increasing the risk of phlebitis.

In general, the larger the vein is in relation to the size of the needle or catheter, the less likelihood there is that irritation and phlebitis will develop. This is because the drugs and infusion solution will undergo more rapid dilution in the blood where the caliber of the vein exceeds the outside diameter of the needle or cannula. Mechanical irritation by the needle or cannula against the endothelial wall of the vein is another cause of phlebitis. Cannulation of larger veins is a means of decreasing risk of venous irritation and subsequent phlebitis.

Two drugs discussed in this section are capable of producing significant venous irritation. These drugs, diazepam (frequently used) and pentobarbital (not recommended, rarely used), are used intravenously as sedatives in dentistry and medicine. Methods of minimizing the risk of phlebitis when these drugs are administered are discussed in Chapter 26. These drugs should be administered slowly into a rapidly running IV infusion. In addition, the use of larger veins will minimize, but not eliminate, the risk of developing venous irritation.

RECOMMENDED SITES FOR VENIPUNCTURE

Five potential sites for venipuncture in the upper limb have been reviewed in this chapter. They are, in my order of preference (Fig. 23.7), as follows:
1. Dorsum of hand
2. Ventral forearm
3. Lateral antecubital fossa

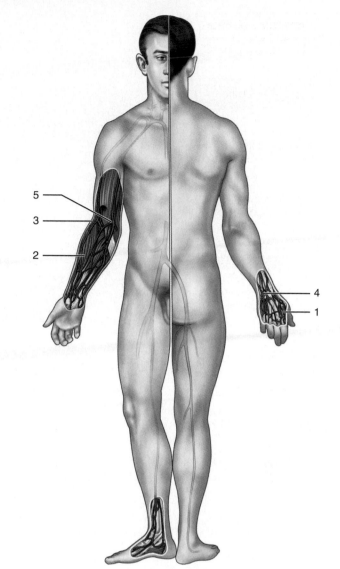

Figure 23.7 Sites of venipuncture in order of preference: *1*, dorsum of hand; *2*, ventral forearm; *3*, lateral antecubital fossa; *4*, dorsal wrist; and *5*, medial antecubital fossa. (Adapted from Abbott Laboratories: *Venipuncture and venous circulation*, Chicago, 1971, Abbott Laboratories.)

4. Dorsal wrist
5. Medial antecubital fossa

The *dorsum of the hand* remains the most preferred site because its veins are superficial and because of the anatomic safety of the site. However, the dorsum is not always an appropriate site for drugs that may produce venous irritation (e.g., diazepam). A close second on my list is the *ventral forearm*. This site is preferred for longer-duration procedures and when the dorsum of the hand is not available. The absence of a need for immobilization of a joint, anatomic safety, and larger veins make this site suitable for most venipuncture procedures. A third preferred site, the *lateral antecubital fossa*, is chosen for its larger veins and anatomic safety.

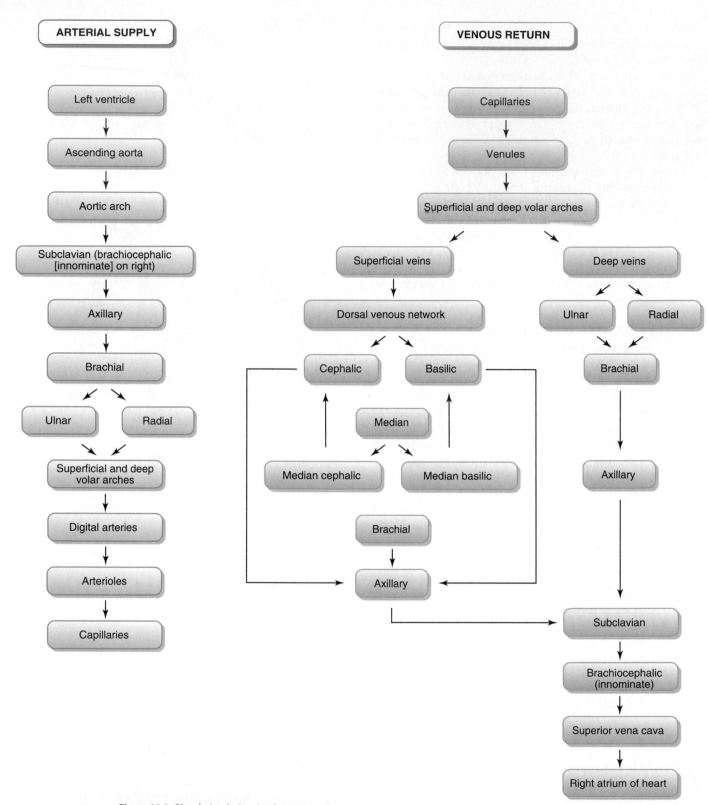

Figure 23.8 Blood circulation in the upper extremity. Blood leaves the left ventricle; traverses arteries, arterioles, capillaries, venules, and veins; and returns to the right atrium via the superior vena cava.

Table 23.1	Comparison of Venipuncture Sites			
ORDER OF PREFERENCE	SITE	PROXIMITY TO IMPORTANT ANATOMY	SIGNIFICANT "ROLL" OR MOVEMENT OF VEIN	JOINT IMMOBILIZATION (METAL NEEDLE ONLY)
1	Dorsum of hand	No	Yes	No
2	Ventral forearm	No	No	No
3	Lateral antecubital fossa	No	No	Yes
4	Dorsal wrist	No	Yes	Yes
5	Medial antecubital fossa	Yes	No	Yes

Running far behind these first three sites are the *dorsal wrist,* with its superficial veins, and last, the *medial antecubital fossa,* with its larger veins but with its significant anatomy just below the surface. These last three sites also require immobilization of a joint if rigid metal needles are used, but not with flexible catheters.

Table 23.1 summarizes some of the important features of the five venipuncture sites on the upper limb. Fig. 23.8 summarizes blood flow through the arm.

REFERENCES

1. Malamed SF: Unpublished data, 1993.
2. Grant JCB: *An atlas of anatomy,* Baltimore, 1962, Williams & Wilkins.
3. Abbott Laboratories: *Venipuncture and venous cannulation,* Chicago, 1971, Abbott Laboratories.

chapter 24

Venipuncture Technique

The preparation of the equipment for a continuous intravenous (IV) infusion and venipuncture technique is described in this chapter.

PREPARATION OF EQUIPMENT

1. The armamentarium discussed in Chapter 22 is laid out and removed from its packaging.
2. The flow-regulating clamp or screw on the IV infusion set is turned to the closed position so that no fluid will run through the tubing when it is inserted into the bag of IV fluid.
3. If a winged infusion set is used, it is removed from its box and attached to the end of the IV tubing. The protective sheath covering the needle is left on. If an indwelling catheter is used, it is not attached to the IV tubing.
4. The cap or cover is removed from the entry port on the bag of IV infusion fluid (blue in Fig. 24.1).
5. The protective covering over the piercing pin on the IV tubing is removed carefully so as not to contaminate the pin.
6. The IV infusion bag is held securely in one hand while the piercing pin is firmly pushed through the entry port into the IV solution.
7. The bag of IV fluid is inverted and suspended from the IV pole.
8. The drip chamber on the IV tubing should be filled approximately halfway with IV fluid. If it is not, the

chamber can be squeezed and released to draw additional fluid into it (Fig. 24.2). If the chamber is overfilled to the extent that it is impossible to visualize individual drops of solution as they exit the IV bag, the bag and drip chamber are inverted and the drip chamber squeezed to force fluid back into the IV bag (Fig. 24.3). Care should be taken to prevent the entry of air bubbles into the IV tubing at this time.

9. The flow-regulating clamp or screw is slowly opened, allowing fluid to run through the entire length of the IV tubing (and the attached needle if winged infusion set is used), removing all the air bubbles, if possible, from the tubing. On occasion, it will be impossible to remove every bubble from the tubing. Although there is little significance to a few air bubbles entering the patient's cardiovascular system, it is best to attempt to eliminate them. The highly unlikely problem of air embolism is discussed in Chapter 27.
10. The flow-regulating screw is closed to stop the flow of fluid. The IV infusion is now ready for use.

Additional equipment required for venipuncture includes the following:

- Tourniquet
- Adhesive tape to secure the site
- Alcohol wipe
- Dry sterile gauze squares
- Armboard: wrist or elbow immobilizer (optional with flexible catheter)

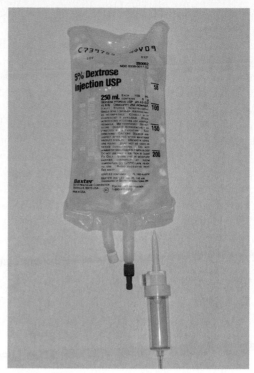

Figure 24.1 Protective caps are removed from the infusion solution *(blue)* and the piercing pin.

- Bandage
- Sphygmomanometer
- Stethoscope
- Monitoring devices
- Oxygen (O$_2$) and emergency kit
- Near infrared vein finder (optional)

PREPARATION FOR VENIPUNCTURE

The patient is asked to visit the restroom, if necessary, before the start of the venipuncture. Once the IV has been started and central nervous system (CNS)–depressant drugs administered, it will be more difficult for the patient, even assisted by office staff, to accomplish a visit to the restroom.

The patient is seated comfortably in the dental chair. A semireclined-to-supine position is recommended as physiologically superior to the upright position for maintenance of cerebral blood flow and adequate respiration.

Preoperative vital signs are recorded on the patient's sedation record sheet (Fig. 24.4 and see Fig. 5.19 *top*). Included should be the blood pressure, heart rate and rhythm, respiratory rate, and O$_2$ saturation. The patient's baseline vital signs have been recorded at a prior visit to the dental office.

The blood pressure cuff (sphygmomanometer) is placed on the left arm and left in place throughout the IV procedure. The right arm should be used if the dentist is left-handed.

The patient's arms (without the tourniquet in place) are scanned for obvious veins. Often veins will be made readily

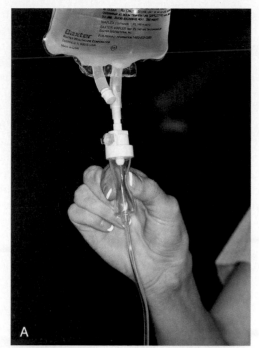

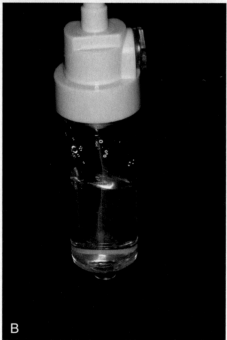

Figure 24.2 A, B, The drip chamber should be approximately half-filled with solution.

visible if the arm is permitted to hang down below the level of the patient's heart for a few minutes as this augments venous distention. One of the goals of the preoperative visit is to determine whether the patient has suitable veins for the IV procedure.

On occasion, a patient who had very visible, superficial veins at the preoperative visit will appear in the office on treatment day with no obvious veins. This is explained by the presence of a greater degree of anxiety with attendant higher levels of circulating catecholamines (producing peripheral vasoconstriction). When veins are not readily apparent, the patient should be asked at what site on the arm he has previously had blood drawn successfully. Sometimes a patient will boast that "they had to try four times before they found a vein" or that "three people had to try before they succeeded." This should alert the dentist that a difficult venipuncture may be in the offing. However, such a statement by the patient may also be used to the dentist's advantage. If, by using "special care," the dentist is able to successfully complete the venipuncture on the first or second attempt, the patient will be more confident in that dentist's overall

ability. Several methods of distending veins are available and are discussed later.

If the Trieger test for evaluation of recovery is to be used (see Chapter 5), the baseline Trieger test is now completed by the patient. Any other monitoring devices, such as the pulse oximeter, capnograph, pretracheal stethoscope, or electrocardioscope, are now placed on the patient.

Because of the possibility of accidental inoculation of health professionals with viral and other organisms found in some patients' blood, universal precautions are essential in situations involving potential contact with blood. All persons working with the venipuncture should wear masks, glasses, and gloves. Gloves must be worn throughout the procedure, from the point of preparation until the IV is removed, the bleeding stops, and a bandage is in place.

Caution
Gloves should always be worn by all personnel while preparing for and performing venipuncture.

A tourniquet is placed on the limb (arm or leg) selected for venipuncture. On the arm, the tourniquet is placed superior to the antecubital fossa. The commonly used soft rubber tubing (e.g., Penrose drain) is applied in a slipknot (Fig. 24.5). The tourniquet should be sufficiently tight to prevent venous drainage from the arm without obstructing arterial flow into the arm. A radial pulse should still be palpable with the tourniquet in place.

When a blood pressure cuff is used as a tourniquet, the pressure in the cuff is raised and maintained at a point between the patient's systolic and diastolic pressures (e.g., ~120 mm Hg if the blood pressure is 140/90 mm Hg). This produces venous distention in the same manner as the tourniquet.

The patient is then asked to repeatedly open and close his or her hand into a fist. Muscular activity forces more blood into the veins, allowing additional arterial blood to enter into the limb, further distending the veins. Once the veins have

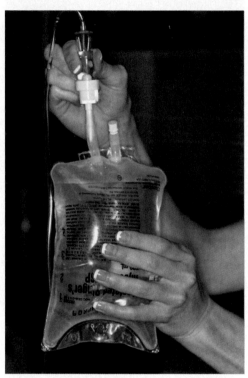

Figure 24.3 If the drip chamber is overfilled, the bag is inverted, and the chamber squeezed to remove solution.

SEDATION RECORD

Date	14 March 2016		Pre-op vitals	BP 136/76	HR 82	SpO₂ 99	RR 14

Name	John Smith	Age 45	Gender M F	Weight 185 Lbs	Height 71"	BMI 25.8	Mallampati 1	ASA 1

Medical History	WNL	NPO Status Solids 10 Hours Clear liquids 4 Hours	NIBP L R Pulse oximeter
		Procedures	Precord ECG EtCO₂
Medications	simvastatin 20 mg po aspirin 81 mg	Multiple restoratons, SRP	
		Operator K. Lee Assistants B. Chanpong	
Drug Allergies	NKDA		IV 20G 22G 24G
		Start Finish Premed	R L
		ANES 1055	Site
		SURG	

TIME	1100									
Oxygen (L/min)										
Nitrous Oxide (L/min)										

Figure 24.4 Baseline evaluation and preoperative vital signs are entered prior to the start of the procedure.

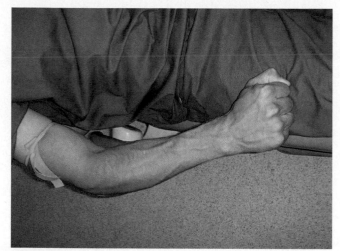

Figure 24.5 A tourniquet is applied, using a slipknot, above the antecubital fossa. Opening and closing of the hand further aids venous distention.

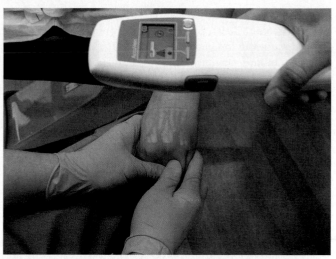

Figure 24.6 Near infrared (NIR) vein finder aids in locating veins. Photo courtesy of Dr. Kenneth Lee, SOLIS Surgical Arts, Tarzana, CA.

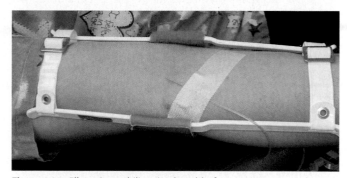

Figure 24.7 Elbow immobilizer is placed before venipuncture when a rigid needle is used.

been distended, the patient is asked to keep the fist clenched until venipuncture has been successfully completed.

At this point, most persons will have one or more readily visible veins; however, some others may not have visible or even palpable veins. Several methods are available to increase venous distention.

1. *Light slapping* or *rubbing of the skin* over the vessel will aid in venodilation.
2. Heat dilates blood vessels. Direct application of heat to the area is also a great aid.
   a. A *warm, moist towel* may be applied for several minutes to the entire region proximal and distal to the proposed venipuncture site.
   b. It has been suggested that an *electric hair dryer* can be used as a quick method to produce vasodilation at almost any site.
   c. Near infrared vein locators have been introduced to help in detection of difficult-to-find veins (Fig. 24.6).
3. Another means of producing vasodilation is to use nitrous oxide-oxygen (N_2O-O_2) sedation, which produces the following beneficial effects during venipuncture:
   a. Peripheral vasodilation
   b. A degree of analgesia, making the venipuncture less traumatic
   c. Relaxation of the apprehensive patient

When N_2O-O_2 is used as an aid during venipuncture, the patient should be sedated as described in Chapter 15 (titrated) and returned to a nonsedated state before the administration of any IV drugs.

Once the vein chosen for cannulation has been adequately distended, the site must be prepared. Physical restraints are seldom required in adults because most patients rarely object strenuously to venipuncture (although they may not "like it"). When a vein in the antecubital fossa or wrist is selected, an elbow or wrist immobilizer should be placed before the start of the venipuncture if a rigid metal needle is to be used (Fig.

24.7). An immobilizer is unnecessary if a flexible catheter is to be inserted.

Some experts recommend that any solution used to cleanse the injection site be warmed to body temperature. Because the arm is warm, it is more sensitive to cold so that the blood vessel may contract (i.e., disappear or "collapse") almost immediately on exposure to a cold or rapidly evaporating solution, such as alcohol.

When needles larger than 20 gauge (18, 16, or 14 gauge) are used, venipuncture can be rendered virtually painless by simply raising a wheal in the skin over the vein by injecting 0.2 to 0.3 mL of a 1% lidocaine hydrochloride solution without epinephrine. A 25-gauge needle should be used. However, use of needles of 20 gauge or smaller (e.g., 22 gauge) for venipuncture is not associated with excessive discomfort, so the preceding technique is not necessary. Indeed, the injection of lidocaine itself produces a stinging sensation. Lidocaine buffered with sodium bicarbonate to a pH of about 7.6 can be used to obviate the discomfort of "traditional" lidocaine, with a pH of 3.5.[1]

For the truly needle-phobic patient, the use of EMLA should be considered. EMLA, eutectic mixture of local anesthetics, is an anesthetic ointment consisting of base forms of prilocaine and lidocaine.[2,3] It is applied to the proposed venipuncture site 1 hour before the procedure and covered with an occlusive bandage. In most instances, it is recommended that two sites, one on either arm, be treated with EMLA.

Patients who are fearful about both the dental and the IV procedure should have received preoperative oral sedative drugs approximately 1 hour before the planned start of the procedure. Sedation with N_2O-O_2 should also be considered at this time.

The venipuncture site must now be cleansed. In many hospitals, it is common to prepare the venipuncture site using both a defatting agent and an antibacterial agent. Commonly available preparations are benzalkonium chloride tincture and 70% alcohol solution and 99% isopropyl alcohol and Betadine (povidone–iodine). Povidone–iodine solution is preferred to tincture of iodine because it is considerably less irritating and equally effective; on the other hand, tincture of iodine acts more rapidly. In most short-term IV situations, the traditional isopropyl alcohol wipe is still used and is considered the minimal preparation recommended at the IV site. The site is thoroughly cleansed with the alcohol wipe and permitted to air-dry, or a sterile, dry gauze wipe may be used to dry the area before venipuncture.

INDWELLING CATHETER

The indwelling catheter represents the current "state of the art" for venous cannulation in dental and medical procedures. The IV infusion is prepared for use as described previously. The catheter is not attached to the IV tubing.

The vein is selected, distended, and prepared for venipuncture in the usual manner. The indwelling catheter is held at a 30° angle to the skin with its bevel facing up either lateral to or directly atop the vein, depending on the site of venipuncture (Fig. 24.8, A).[4,5] The skin is pulled in the direction opposite to which the needle ("introducer") is advanced to facilitate passage through the skin (Fig. 24.13, B). Resistance is lost once the skin is penetrated; the angle of the needle is decreased and the needle is directed toward the vein. On entry of the needle into the vein, blood is seen in the plastic chamber (Fig. 24.8, B). The introducer is now angled parallel to the course of the vein and advanced several millimeters further into the lumen of the vessel.

The hub of the metal needle (introducer) is held firmly in one hand by the operator while fingers of the other hand securely grasp the plastic hub of the catheter. The entire length of the plastic catheter is slowly and gently advanced into the vein (Fig. 24.9). It is important that *the catheter not be forced if any resistance is encountered.* It is equally important that only the catheter itself, not the metal introducer, be advanced into the vein and also that the metal introducer not be withdrawn from the catheter until the catheter has been fully advanced.

Following complete insertion of the catheter, the tourniquet is removed, decreasing venous pressure. An assistant holds the needle adapter end of the IV tubing while the doctor

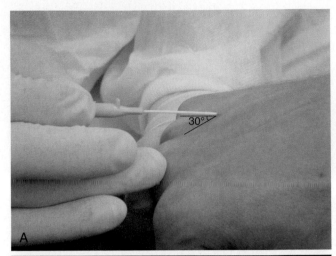

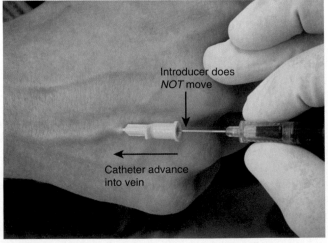

Figure 24.8 A, The needle is inserted into vein at 30° angle **(B)** until blood return is observed in plastic window *(arrow).*

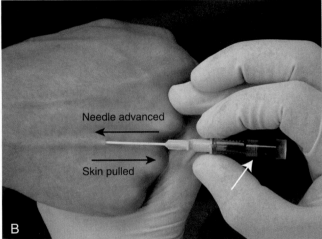

Figure 24.9 The entire length of the plastic catheter is slowly and gently advanced into the vein.

removes the metal introducer needle from the indwelling catheter. The needle adapter of the IV tubing is expeditiously connected to the catheter hub and the IV flow started. The needle adapter and catheter must not be let go of at this time because they have yet to be secured. Once the introducer needle is removed from the catheter, blood will flow back into the catheter and onto the patient or floor if the catheter is not quickly attached to the IV tubing. The importance of removing the tourniquet before this step is obvious because what amounts to a mere oozing of blood out of the catheter without the tourniquet would quickly become a river of blood if the tourniquet were left in place. Even in experienced hands, this step can become untidy. To minimize this possibility, the following procedure is suggested:

1. Release the tourniquet.
2. Press your fingertip onto the skin directly above the tip of the plastic catheter within the vein. This will occlude the catheter, preventing any blood loss (Fig. 24.10).
3. Place a dry gauze wipe beneath the end of the catheter. This will absorb any small volume of blood that might be lost between removal of the introducer and connecting of the IV tubing.
4. Securely attach the needle adapter and the catheter.

If step 2 is done properly, this entire process can be completed at a leisurely pace, without loss of any blood.

The IV drip is now started and the catheter and tubing secured. Although several taping techniques are available (the reader is referred to previous editions of this text for their description),[6] we have turned to the use of a single large clear adhesive square (Tegaderm), which provides a secure site and is transparent and "neat" (Fig. 24.11).

Because the flexible catheter lies within the vein, neither armboard nor elbow immobilizer is necessary. The patient is now ready for the administration of the IV medications.

WINGED INFUSION SET

The winged infusion set, or butterfly needle, is somewhat easier for the neophyte sedationist or phlebotomist to learn with than is the indwelling catheter. One simple step, puncturing of the vein wall, is all that is required for this needle to be successful. However, because a rigid sharp metal needle remains inside of the vein throughout the procedure, it is also easier for the vein wall to be damaged accidentally by slight movements by the patient. Use of a joint immobilizer is necessary if venipuncture is accomplished in the wrist, antecubital fossa, or, in some instances, the dorsum of the hand.

Basic Technique—Winged Infusion Set

The plastic wings of the needle are held by the thumb and middle finger, with the index finger squeezed between the wings (Fig. 24.12).[7] This permits the operator the greatest control over the needle. Holding the needle with a finger beneath the needle interferes with the venipuncture. The protective sheath over the needle is removed. Care must be taken from this point on to not contaminate the needle by touching it to any object. Should this occur, the needle is immediately replaced with a new, sterile one. Air in the tubing of the new needle must be removed by running the IV infusion solution through the needle.

Basic venipuncture technique with the winged infusion set is the same as that described previously for the indwelling catheter. It is described in detail later in this chapter. Once the blood return is noted, the needle is advanced several millimeters further into the vein and the "wings" of the needle laid flat against the skin and secured (taped down). The tourniquet is removed and IV fluid administered.

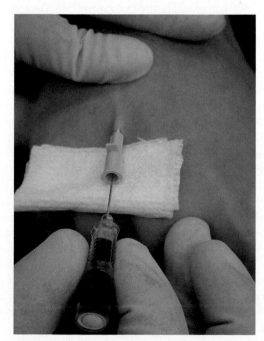

Figure 24.10 Fingertip placed on skin at tip of catheter to prevent leakage of blood when introducer is removed.

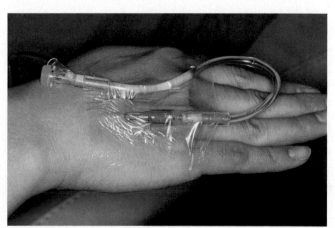

Figure 24.11 Transparent adhesive provides stability and visibility at venipuncture site (Tegaderm).

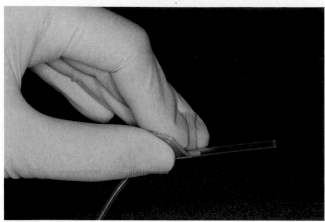

Figure 24.12 The index finger is placed between the wings of the needle, and the wings are folded over by thumb and middle fingers. This provides the dentist with increased control and tactile sensation during venipuncture.

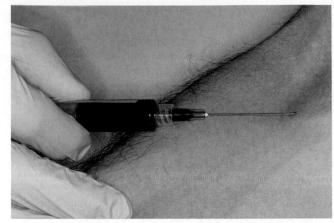

Figure 24.13 Barbotage. Blood pulled into syringe to dilute drug.

HOLLOW METAL NEEDLE

Although not recommended for use in routine IV drug administration, the hollow metal needle may be used for venipuncture in emergency situations or in procedures, such as the drawing of blood samples for laboratory analysis, when only short-term cannulation is required. The hollow metal needle will almost always be attached to a syringe, which contains a drug to be injected or into which blood is to be drawn.

Basic Technique—Hollow Metal Needle

The basic technique of venipuncture is the same as that described earlier for the winged infusion set. However, once the metal needle enters the vein, great care must be taken as the needle is advanced, because it is often difficult to obtain the correct needle angulation within the vein with a syringe attached (syringes are available that have an eccentrically placed needle, making venipuncture somewhat easier). The tourniquet is removed and the syringe held securely in place.

Before the administration of the drug, an aspiration test must be performed to confirm that the needle tip remains within the vessel's lumen. With one hand holding the syringe in position, the other hand gently pulls the plunger of the syringe until a backflow of blood is observed. This technique (drawing of blood into the syringe) is called *barbotage* (Fig. 24.13). The drug is then administered.

VENIPUNCTURE TECHNIQUE

Dorsum of Hand

The patient's hand is kept in a clenched fist until venipuncture is completed. The patient's fist is supported by the dentist's left hand, with the thumb of the dentist's left hand placed below the patient's knuckles pulling the skin of the dorsum of the hand over the knuckles toward the dentist (Fig. 24.14).

These two procedures minimize mobility of the vein during venipuncture. Should this be ineffective, the patient should bend his or her fist down, further immobilizing the vein. Care is needed with these techniques because in some patients the vein may actually collapse (the vein disappears) when attempts are made to immobilize it.

The site of needle entry into the skin on the dorsum of the hand is usually lateral to the vein and approximately 1 cm (0.4 inch) below the desired point of entry of the needle into the vein (Fig. 24.15). This takes into account the mobility of these veins. Should the needle be placed directly atop the vein, the vein will invariably roll out from under the needle as pressure is applied with the needle.

The optimum angle of entry of the needle through the skin is 30° (Fig. 24.16). An angle greater than 30° will increase the risk of the needle traveling through the vein, whereas angles less than 30° are associated with increased discomfort during passage of the needle through the skin. *The bevel of the needle will always be facing up* (see Fig. 24.16). The tip of the needle is placed gently against the skin at the site of entry, with the needle directed parallel to the course of the vein. With the skin of the dorsum still pulled over the knuckles, the tip of the needle penetrates skin lateral to the vein. Resistance is noted as the needle passes through the skin. Once through the skin, resistance markedly decreases. At this point, the angle of the needle is decreased (to avoid going "too deep") so that the needle shaft is held parallel to the skin. Veins on the dorsum of the hand are quite superficial, and if directed deeper, the needle may miss the vein entirely, going under it. The direction of the needle is also altered at this time. The needle should be directed toward the spot on the vein where the needle tip is to penetrate the vein wall. The angle of entry into the vein should be gentle so that the needle meets with the vein about 5 to 10 mm above the point of entry into the skin (this may be likened to a car merging onto a highway).

The needle is slowly advanced toward the vein. There should be little resistance and no discomfort to the patient at this time. As the needle tip comes into contact with the vein wall on the dorsum of the hand, the doctor may observe the vein

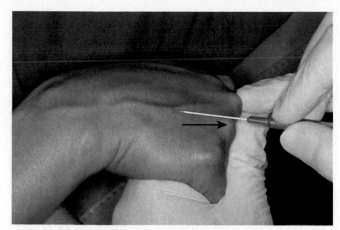

Figure 24.14 The dentist supports the patient's hand and pulls the skin of the hand over the knuckle (*arrow*).

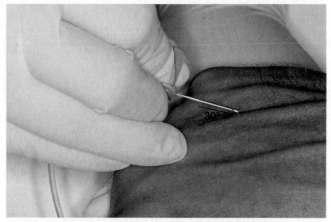

Figure 24.16 Optimum angle of needle entry is 30° with bevel facing up.

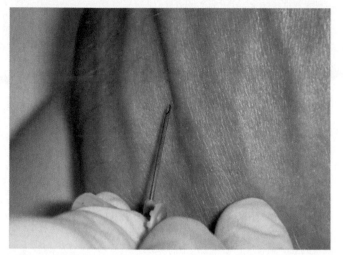

Figure 24.15 Entry point of the needle is just lateral to the vein.

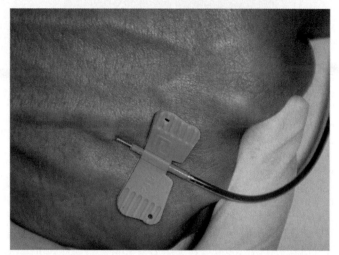

Figure 24.17 Return of blood into IV tubing signifies successful venipuncture.

move as the needle tip pushes it. This is common and is desirable. The needle tip has yet to enter into the lumen of the vein, but the tip has come in contact with the vein wall. As the needle continues to move in the same direction, the vein may continue to be pushed along with the needle. Because the vein cannot move indefinitely within the confines of the skin, it will soon appear to "pop," returning to its original position on the hand. (This is similar to increasing pressure applied to the outside of an inflated balloon until the balloon finally pops.) As this occurs, the needle tip enters into the lumen, and resistance is lost. On occasion, the patient may be aware of this (painless) "popping" feeling.

A backflow of blood into the tubing is the one sure sign of successful venipuncture (Fig. 24.17). The needle is redirected so that it lies parallel to the direction of the vein and advanced very carefully several more millimeters into the lumen of the vessel. This minimizes the risk of a needle that is tenuously placed within a vein becoming dislodged as it is secured or if the patient accidentally moves his or her hand.

Care must be taken as the metal needle is advanced so that its sharp tip does not puncture or tear the inferior wall of the

vessel. To prevent this, the needle tip is angled so that it is held slightly upward within the lumen of the vein as the needle is advanced. The shaft of the needle must be placed only a few millimeters into the lumen of the vein. Attempts to advance the entire length of the needle into the vessel may result in loss of the vein through inadvertent laceration or puncture of the wall ("blowing the vein") and formation of a hematoma.

Winged infusion set: Once the needle tip has entered the vein, the plastic wings of the butterfly needle are placed against the patient's skin and held in position by the doctor while the assistant performs several important tasks. The doctor's primary job at this time is to maintain the needle within the vein.

The assistant releases the tourniquet on the patient's arm. Blood is seen to leave the IV tubing, returning into the blood vessel.

Next the assistant starts the IV drip by opening the flow screw or knob on the tubing, and drops of IV solution should be noticed in the drip chamber. The IV drip is opened immediately to prevent clotting of blood within the needle or tubing. The next task is to secure the catheter or needle within the vein with tape using the method previously described.

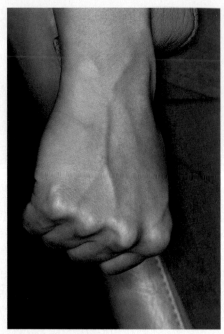

Figure 24.18 Inverted Y formed by merging of two veins is ideal configuration for venipuncture.

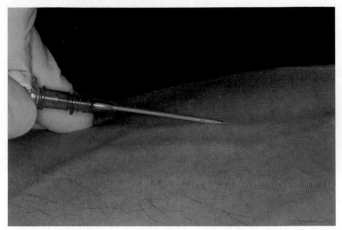

Figure 24.19 Angle of penetration of skin is 30°. Skin is retracted by the fingers of the other hand.

The most pressing problem in establishing an IV infusion on the dorsum of the hand is the mobility of the veins; any method of immobilization is appreciated. Three means of so doing have been described (clenched fist, bending hand, and thumb pulling skin over knuckles). A fourth, a naturally occurring anatomic configuration of veins, may also be used to advantage. This configuration involves the formation of an inverted Y from the merging of two smaller veins to form a larger one. Often this configuration is located just above the knuckles as two digital veins converge (Fig. 24.18). Basic venipuncture technique is essentially identical to that just described; the primary difference is that entry of the needle into the vein occurs at the point of confluence of these three vessels. If the needle is inserted between the two digital veins and aimed for the point at which they meet, the veins are prevented from rolling away from the needle.

The needle enters into the skin about 5 mm below the convergence of the veins and is directed toward that spot. Pressure is exerted on the needle, which then enters the lumen of the vein; the needle or catheter is advanced and then secured as previously described. The inverted Y is a highly recommended site for venipuncture on the dorsum of the hand.

Rigid needle: Following successful venipuncture on the dorsum of the hand with a rigid needle, immobilization of the wrist should be considered if the needle's tip is located in its proximity.

Dorsum of Wrist

The technique of venipuncture on the dorsum of the wrist is identical to that just described for the dorsum of the hand. It is extremely rare to find the inverted Y configuration on the wrist; however, where it is present, its use is recommended.

The use of an immobilizing device is necessary if a rigid needle is used in this site.

Ventral Forearm

The ventral aspect of the forearm is a recommended site for venipuncture. Because veins at this site are not as superficial as those of the dorsum of the hand and wrist, they tend to be less mobile. As a result of this decreased mobility, there is a slight variation in the venipuncture technique on the ventral forearm.

On the ventral forearm, the needle is placed directly atop the vein to be entered rather than on its side. Held at the same 30° angle, the needle is directed into the skin and then directly into the vein. Once blood returns into the tubing, signifying successful entry into the vein, the angle of the needle is decreased so that it is held almost parallel to the skin and slowly advanced several millimeters into the vein.

During venipuncture, the thumb of the opposite hand of the dentist should be placed on the skin several inches below (distal [peripheral] to) the planned entry site, pulling skin at the site in a direction opposite to that of the needle (Fig. 24.19). This facilitates entry of the needle through the skin. All other components of venipuncture at this site are identical to the basic procedure previously described. Immobilization is not required when the forearm is used for venipuncture.

Antecubital Fossa

The technique of venipuncture at either the medial or lateral antecubital fossa is identical to that of the ventral forearm, with the important exception that the antecubital fossa must be immobilized if a rigid metal needle is used. Immobilization is not needed with the flexible indwelling catheter. If required, it is suggested that immobilization of the joint occur before venipuncture rather than after, when any accidental movement by the patient might dislodge the needle.

On occasion, veins in the antecubital fossa will be superficial. In this case it is possible that the vein will roll out from under the needle as venipuncture progresses. Should this occur, the attempt is continued using the technique described for the dorsum of the hand, with the needle entering from the side of the vein.

Before discussing termination of an IV infusion, several comments are warranted concerning the technique of venipuncture.

1. Experienced phlebotomists commonly spend more time locating a suitable vein than actually performing the venipuncture. Time spent in distending veins is time well spent because the likelihood of successfully entering a larger-diameter vein is greater than that of entering a small vein.

2. If the tourniquet is placed on the arm or leg for an extended time, the skin will become mottled, then purple, and will feel cool. The patient will likely complain of discomfort as a period of hyperesthesia develops. Should this occur, the tourniquet is removed, restoring circulation to the tissues. After 2 to 3 minutes, the tourniquet may be reapplied and the procedure restarted. Venipuncture should not take long to accomplish. Each of the steps described is performed sequentially. As experience and technical ability are acquired, the speed with which venipuncture is successfully completed will increase.

3. If the needle gets "lost" within the tissues during venipuncture (e.g., the needle should be in the vein, but it is not), do not use the needle as a probe in an attempt to locate the vein. Using the needle as a probe simply traumatizes the tissues, increasing patient discomfort and greatly increasing the risk of accidentally puncturing the vein and producing a hematoma. The following sequence is recommended in this situation (Fig. 24.20):

   a. Locate the tip of the needle by lifting the needle tip up and looking for the imprint it makes under the skin.

   b. If the tip is located under and beyond the vein, the vein will appear to be lifted up by the needle. Withdraw the needle slightly so that the tip is pulled back to the other side of the vein. Elevate the tip of the needle and readvance it toward the vein.

   c. If the needle tip has advanced over and beyond the vein, the outline of the needle will be apparent, not the vein.

Withdraw the needle slightly so that the tip is pulled back to the original side of the vein. Readvance the needle with the tip pointed more parallel to the vein than in the previous attempt.

TERMINATING THE INTRAVENOUS INFUSION

At the conclusion of the IV procedure, the catheter or needle must be removed before the patient is discharged from the office. Criteria for terminating the IV infusion are discussed in Chapter 26. It is assumed here that all criteria have been satisfactorily met by the patient.

1. If an IV infusion is used, the flow is stopped by tightening the rate-control screw or knob.

2. The needle or catheter is held gently in position while the adhesive tape is carefully removed from the skin.

3. A sterile gauze square is placed over the site of the catheter or needle entry into the skin. No pressure is exerted because pressure on the skin if a rigid metal needle is still within the vein will be uncomfortable for the patient and might injure the vein as the needle is withdrawn. This is not a factor with a flexible catheter.

4. The catheter or needle is carefully removed from the vein. The assistant should cap or discard the needle immediately so that no one is accidentally stuck with the contaminated needle.

5. As soon as the catheter or needle is withdrawn from the skin, firm, direct finger pressure is applied onto the gauze square over the site of penetration of the skin. Pressure is maintained for at least 3 to 5 minutes. Failure to do so may result in leakage of blood and formation of a hematoma.

6. When the antecubital fossa is used for venipuncture, a common mistake is to place a gauze square on the site and have the patient bend his or her elbow (Fig. 24.21), assuming

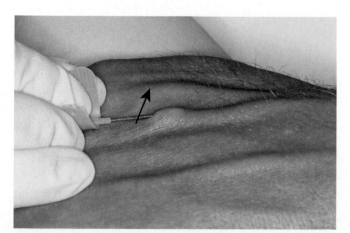

Figure 24.20 Locate needle tip by LIFTING tip upward and looking for imprint. If needle has gone BELOW vein, the vein will appear to be lifted up. If needle has gone OVER the vein, the outline of the needle will be apparent.

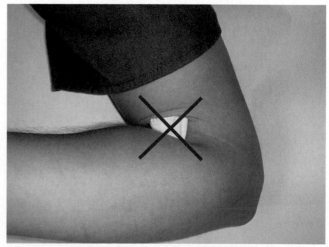

Figure 24.21 Placing gauze over the injection site and bending the elbow does not provide adequate pressure and often results in hematoma formation.

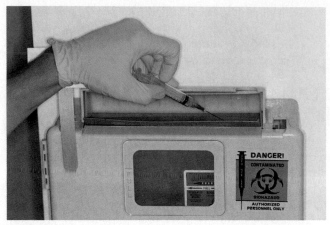

Figure 24.22 An appropriate sharps disposal should be available for used needles.

that this provides pressure adequate to stop the bleeding. Bending of the elbow does not provide adequate pressure and commonly results in hematoma formation. Regardless of the location of the venipuncture, it is important that firm, direct pressure with a gloved hand be applied for at least 3 to 5 minutes.

7. After 3 to 5 minutes a bandage is placed over the puncture site.

8. The needle is destroyed (Fig. 24.22), and the IV needle, tubing, and bag are discarded in appropriate receptacles.

REFERENCES

1. Fetzer SJ: Reducing the pain of venipuncture. *J Perianesth Nurs* 14(2):95–101, 1999.
2. Celik G, Ozbek O, Yilmaz M, et al: Vapocoolant spray vs. lidocaine/prilocaine cream for reducing the pain of venipuncture in hemodialysis patients: a randomized, placebo-controlled, crossover study. *Int J Med Sci* 8(7):623–627, 2011.
3. Travenol Laboratories: Quik-Cath, product information sheet, Deerfield, IL, 1978, Travenol Laboratories.
4. Abbott Laboratories: Venipuncture and venous cannulation, Chicago, 1971, Abbott Laboratories.
5. Malamed SF: Venipuncture technique. In *Sedation: a guide to patient management*, ed 4, St Louis, 2003, CV Mosby, p 325.
6. Abbott Laboratories: I.V. tips #6: how to use the butterfly infusion set, Chicago, 1972, Abbott Laboratories.
7. Scarfone RJ, Jasani M: Pain of local anesthetics: rate of administration and buffering. *Ann Emerg Med* 31(1):36–40, 1998.

chapter 25

Pharmacology

CHAPTER OUTLINE

A variety of drugs are available for intravenous (IV) sedation. These include a number of categories, primarily sedative-hypnotics, opioids, and anticholinergics. Drugs commonly used in IV moderate sedation are listed in Box 25.1. Also listed in Box 25.1 are several drugs (indicated by ‡) that are not recommended for IV use by dentists who have not completed a 3-year residency in anesthesiology. These drugs are discussed briefly so that the dentist may more fully understand the rationale for their not being recommended. Other drugs, such as the barbiturates, which at one time were *the* drugs of choice

in IV sedation, have fallen from favor as newer, safer, and more effective drugs have been introduced. Discussion of the barbiturates has been minimized. For a more in-depth discussion of these drugs, the reader is directed to previous editions of this textbook.

BENZODIAZEPINES

The benzodiazepines have become the most commonly used IV sedative drugs in both dentistry and medicine. Four

<table>
<tr><td>Box 25.1</td><td>Drugs Available for Intravenous Moderate Sedation</td></tr>
</table>

Sedative-Hypnotics and Antianxiety Drugs
Benzodiazepines
Diazepam
Midazolam
Lorazepam*
Flunitrazepam†

Histamine Blockers
Promethazine

Opioid Agonists
Meperidine
Morphine
Fentanyl
Sufentanil
Alfentanil
Remifentanil*

Opioid Antagonist
Naloxone

Anticholinergics
Atropine
Scopolamine
Glycopyrrolate

Antidotal Drugs
Flumazenil
Naloxone
Nalbuphine
Physostigmine
Procaine

Others
Ketamine‡
Propofol‡

Not recommended for use in IV moderate sedation.
†*Not available for clinical use in the United States (March 2017).*
‡*Not recommended for use in IV moderate sedation without general anesthesia training.*

benzodiazepines are discussed (Table 25.1); three of them are presently available in the United States, whereas one (flunitrazepam) is available in Central and South America.[1]

Diazepam

Diazepam was synthesized in 1959 by Sternbach and Reeder. The drug became available as Valium (Hoffmann-La Roche) in 1963 and shortly thereafter became the most prescribed oral drug in the Western world.[2] Diazepam is also available in a parenteral preparation for intramuscular (IM) (see Chapter 10) and IV use. Diazepam was originally approved by the Food and Drug Administration (FDA) in November 1963.

IV administration of diazepam appears to have begun with the work of Davidau in Paris in 1965.[3] This was followed shortly thereafter by a report by Main[4] in 1967, who used diazepam as an adjunct to the Jorgensen technique. In 1968 Brown reported on 40 cases in which diazepam was used alone, with the drug administered until the patient felt sleepy.[5]

In 1969 O'Neill and Verrill[6] reported on the use of IV diazepam for sedation in minor oral surgical procedures, with good-to-excellent results in 51 of 52 patients treated. In 1970 O'Neill et al reported on 55 patients undergoing dental surgical procedures lasting between 20 and 45 minutes. IV diazepam provided successful sedation and cooperation in 49 patients; 4 others moved and spoke occasionally but were able to be treated, and 2 patients required additional IV medications (methohexital) for treatment to be completed successfully.[7]

The dosage used in these patients was that required to produce marked ptosis (drooping of the upper eyelid; Fig. 25.1). Halfway ptosis of the upper eyelid is now recognized as the Verrill sign.[8] The practice of administering diazepam until the appearance of the Verrill sign produces a level of

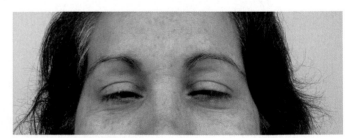

Figure 25.1 Verrill sign: eyelids at "half-staff."

	Benzodiazepines for Intravenous Moderate Sedation			
Table 25.1				
Generic Name	**Proprietary Name**	**Usual Concentration (mg/mL)**	**Duration of Action (min)**	**Average Sedation Dose (mg)**
Diazepam	Valium*	5	45	10–12
Lorazepam	Ativan	2	6–8 hr	2–4
Midazolam	Versed,* Dormicum, Hypnovel	1	45	2.5–7.5

*The proprietary names Valium and Versed are no longer in use in the United States. Valium was discontinued in 2014, Versed in 2003.

sedation (central nervous system [CNS] depression) that is considered by many to be more profound than is usually necessary and is therefore not recommended for routine use.[9]

Peter Foreman,[10] in New Zealand, used diazepam in combination with atropine and incremental doses of methohexital. Although successful, he stated that the addition of even small amounts of methohexital greatly increased the risk of overdose. In a subsequent study, Foreman used diazepam alone for a variety of dental treatments, finding that although the degree of amnesia produced by diazepam varied significantly from patient to patient, virtually all patients agreed that dental treatment had been at least tolerable rather than an ordeal. He found that IV diazepam had made it possible to treat those patients who may not have received proper treatment in the past because of fear. Foreman stated, "Diazepam has become the drug of choice for the trained general dental practitioner, as well as for the introduction of dental students to intravenous sedation."[11]

With the introduction of midazolam into clinical practice, the use of IV moderate sedation with diazepam has decreased. However, as discussed in Chapter 26, there are still occasions to consider diazepam as a first-line agent for IV moderate sedation or as a supplement to IV midazolam.

Chemistry

Diazepam is a member of the 1,4-benzodiazepine group of compounds. The chemical formula for diazepam is 7-chloro-1,3-dihydro-1-methyl-5-phenyl-2H-1,4-benzodiazepin-2-one. It is a pale yellow-white crystalline powder with virtually no odor. It is considerably soluble in chloroform and acetone, moderately soluble in ethanol and ether, and poorly soluble in water.[12]

General Pharmacology

It is believed that emotions are largely controlled by the limbic system (i.e., the portion of the brain composed of the amygdala, hippocampus, and septal areas).[13] The midbrain reticular formation, hypothalamus, and thalamus are also involved with the experience or transmission of emotions.

In very small doses, diazepam appears to act on the hippocampus, whereas other areas of the brain remain unaffected and the patient remains alert.[14] Following oral administration of diazepam, this action of the drug would be appropriate; however, when diazepam is administered intravenously, a more intense effect is desirable. Administered to the point at which sedation and ataxia (loss of muscular coordination) occur, a more generalized depression of the CNS is observed.

Research suggests that the anxiolytic properties of benzodiazepines are mediated by increased inhibitory nerve transmission.[15] γ-Aminobutyric acid (GABA) is an important inhibitory neurotransmitter in the brain. Glycine (aminoacetic acid), the simplest nonessential amino acid, may be the major inhibitory transmitter of the spinal cord. The anticonvulsant and sedative properties of benzodiazepines may result from a direct agonist effect on stereospecific benzodiazepine receptors, which in turn facilitate the inhibitory action of GABA on its own postsynaptic receptors.

Fate of Intravenous Diazepam

Following IV administration, diazepam reaches a peak blood level in approximately 1 to 2 minutes. The onset of clinical activity is therefore quite rapid.[16] Blood levels of approximately 1.0 µg/mL may be achieved after an IV dose of 10 to 20 mg of diazepam.[17] Clinically, this would equate with a deeper level of moderate sedation (not deep sedation) and a period of anterograde amnesia.

As mentioned in Chapters 7 and 10, diazepam has a plasma half-life of approximately 30+ hours.[18] A commonly held misconception is that a drug with a long half-life will possess a long duration of action, whereas one with a shorter half-life will have a shorter duration of action. This is untrue, and diazepam is an excellent example of this. The β-half-life is an indicator of the rate at which a drug undergoes biotransformation (in the liver for diazepam), whereas the factor most responsible for a drug's duration of action is its degree of receptor-site (protein) binding.

Over a period of approximately 45 minutes following titration of an appropriate sedative dose of diazepam, the patient will remain sedated and anxiety free (anxiolytic). In many patients, the following distinct phases of sedation can be observed, each lasting approximately 15 minutes.

Phase 1: 0 to 15 minutes. During phase 1 of IV moderate sedation with diazepam, the cerebral blood level of diazepam is at its peak, and the patient is sedated to his or her maximal degree. The patient remains responsive to verbal and physical stimulation, but response is slowed, speech slurred, and the patient may have difficulty enunciating words. The patient may not appear to be aware of the presence of the dentist or the assistant during this phase. Anterograde amnesia, if it is to occur, usually includes procedures carried out at this time.

Phase 2: 16 to 30 minutes. The level of sedation is somewhat lessened (the patient becomes somewhat more aware of his or her surroundings than in phase 1 because the cerebral blood level of diazepam begins to decrease as the drug undergoes redistribution [α-half-life] to those organs and parts of the body that are less vessel rich than the brain). However, he or she is definitely still sedated. Patient response to stimulation (both verbal and physical) is increasingly more rapid, the slowing of responses in phase 1 having diminished or disappeared. Patients can usually recall events occurring during this phase, although in isolated cases, amnesia may occur in this phase as well.

Phase 3: 31 to 45 minutes. During this period, the typical patient will state that he or she feels "normal" again; in other words, the feeling of sedation has dissipated. It may be tempting to administer additional diazepam to the patient; however, this is normally not necessary. Although no longer feeling sedated, the patient is also no longer apprehensive. The now-decreasing cerebral blood level of diazepam is no longer adequate to maintain the earlier depth of sedation, but it is sufficient to provide an anxiolytic state (similar to the desired actions of oral diazepam; minimal sedation). With treatment nearing completion and the patient free of pain (as a result of the administration of local anesthesia), there is usually no need for the readministration of diazepam at this time.

Phase 4: 46 to 60 minutes. At this time after receiving diazepam, almost all patients will feel and look recovered. This is not a result of the β-half-life of the drug (30+ hours), but because of redistribution: α-half-life. The blood level of diazepam at 60 minutes after IV administration of 20 mg is 0.25 μg/mL.[17] The patient is not recovered at this time. Under no circumstances should the dentist ever believe that this patient is capable of operating a car or leaving the dental or surgical office unescorted.

As redistribution of diazepam continues during this first hour after IV administration, the level of the drug increases in several storage sites, including fat, the walls of the intestines, and the gallbladder. Diazepam stored in fat will usually remain there because diazepam is quite lipid soluble and the blood supply of fat is quite poor.

A clinically significant phenomenon can arise at this point, a result of the diazepam stored in the gallbladder and intestinal walls. Known as the *rebound effect* or *second-peak effect,* it involves a recurrence of symptoms of sedation and drowsiness approximately 1 hour after the first meal taken after the patient leaves the treatment site.[19] In most cases, this will occur about 4 to 6 hours following the drug's administration (start of the procedure). After a meal, particularly one rich in lipids, the gallbladder constricts, releasing its contents of bile and unmetabolized diazepam into the small intestine, where over the next hour or so diazepam is reabsorbed back into the cardiovascular system. In some patients, the diazepam blood level may reach a point at which clinical signs and symptoms of sedation recur: The patient feels quite tired and will want to lie down for a few minutes. It becomes absolutely essential therefore that the patient receiving diazepam and his or her escort be advised of this possibility before their discharge from the dental office. The rebound effect is less likely to be observed in a patient whose gallbladder has been removed.

Because diazepam is extremely lipophilic, it cannot be excreted through the kidneys and therefore must undergo biotransformation in the liver.

Biotransformation

Diazepam is biotransformed by one of two pathways. In the first, the diazepam molecule undergoes demethylation to desmethyldiazepam, which possesses anxiolytic, but not sedative, effects. Desmethyldiazepam is too lipophilic to permit its excretion by the kidney. Desmethyldiazepam has a half-life of 96 hours and eventually undergoes hydroxylation to oxazepam, another pharmacologically active drug.[20]

The second pathway involves the hydroxylation of the diazepam molecule to 3-hydroxydiazepam, yet another pharmacologically active metabolite also known as *temazepam.* Temazepam undergoes demethylation into oxazepam.

Oxazepam is still another water-insoluble anxiolytic benzodiazepine. It is used as an anxiolytic agent by the oral route of administration. The pharmacology of oxazepam (Serax) is discussed in Chapter 7. The half-life of oxazepam ranges between 3 and 21 hours. It is rapidly biotransformed into its major metabolite, oxazepam glucuronide.

Effects of Age and Disease

It is often stated that drug dosages should be decreased in very young (e.g., under 6 years) and older patients (over 65 years) in addition to patients with significant liver disease. The pharmacokinetics of diazepam have been well studied in these groups of patients.[21-24] The following is presented as a summary of that research.

In patients 2 years and older, diazepam is handled as in the adult. The only significant clinical advice is to adjust the dose of the drug appropriately. With titration via the IV route, clinical results are usually achieved at smaller doses than in adults (assuming a cooperative patient—not a very likely situation).

In elderly patients, the dose of diazepam by the IV (or any other) route should be decreased for several reasons. The rate at which the diazepam undergoes biotransformation is decreased in older patients. In addition, when administered orally, the drug is absorbed in the gastrointestinal tract somewhat more slowly. However, the most important reason for the apparent increased sensitivity of older patients to diazepam (and other drugs) is related primarily to protein binding. Older patients exhibit decreased protein binding of drugs.[21] This means that there will be more of the free, unbound drug available within the blood to cross the blood–brain barrier and produce CNS depression. Diazepam is offered as an example: In the younger patient, diazepam is approximately 98.5% protein bound.[22] Therefore the clinical effects of diazepam are produced by only 1.5% of the dosage administered, the non–protein-bound diazepam. In the older patient in whom protein binding is decreased, diazepam may be 97% protein bound, still a significant figure, but one permitting 3% (or twice as much) non–protein-bound diazepam to be available to produce CNS depression. It becomes obvious that when administered the same dose of the drug, the clinical actions on the older patient will be exaggerated. The dosages of diazepam by the oral and IM routes must be decreased in older patients. With IV administration, titration will provide effective sedation at what will likely be a smaller dose of the drug than is usually given.

Skeletal Muscle Relaxation

Diazepam and other benzodiazepines produce skeletal muscle relaxation. Research has demonstrated that the muscle-relaxant properties of benzodiazepines are caused by central rather than peripheral effects.[25] Monosynaptic reflexes, such as the knee jerk, are essentially unaffected by even large doses of diazepam, whereas polysynaptic reflexes are depressed by rather small doses.

Anticonvulsant Activity

Benzodiazepines, as CNS depressants, possess anticonvulsant properties. Diazepam, midazolam, chlordiazepoxide, and nitrazepam (and other benzodiazepines) have the ability to antagonize the convulsive effects of local anesthetic overdose produced by lidocaine, mepivacaine, bupivacaine, cocaine, and procaine.

In one study, the seizure threshold for lidocaine-induced tonic-clonic seizure activity was 8.5 mg/kg.[26] When IM diazepam was administered 60 minutes before treatment in a dose of 0.25 to 0.5 mg/kg, the seizure threshold was elevated to 16.8 mg/kg of lidocaine.[27]

In the management of generalized tonic-clonic seizures, the benzodiazepines have not supplanted phenytoin and phenobarbital as oral maintenance anticonvulsants; however, IV midazolam and diazepam are drugs of choice in the management of status epilepticus and acute seizure activity.[28,29] Once the seizure has been controlled, maintenance therapy with other anticonvulsants is initiated.

Cardiovascular System

Hemodynamic studies show that diazepam produces little effect on the cardiovascular system of healthy human subjects.[30] IV diazepam, in a dose of 0.3 mg/kg, produces no clinically significant changes in either blood pressure or cardiac output.

Diazepam was compared with thiopental (at the time [1991] *the* IV induction agent of choice) as a preanesthetic induction agent in the cardiovascularly compromised patient (American Society of Anesthesiologists [ASA] 3 and 4).[31] Administered intravenously in a dose of 0.2 mg/kg, less than 1% of the patients studied experienced a reduction of cardiac output of more than 15%, and none had a mean blood pressure reduction of more than 15%. In contrast, on receiving 2 mg/kg of thiopental, 85% of the patients exhibited more than a 15% reduction in cardiac output, whereas 68% demonstrated more than a 15% reduction in blood pressure. Adverse hemodynamic effects attributable to the benzodiazepines are rare in humans, even in patients with significant cardiac or pulmonary disease.[32]

Respiratory System

All sedative-hypnotics, including the benzodiazepines, are potential respiratory depressants. When these drugs are studied in patients without pulmonary disease, respiratory depression produced by intravenously administered benzodiazepines is barely detectable.[33] In addition, and quite significantly, the benzodiazepines do not potentiate the respiratory-depressant actions of opioids.[34]

Hepatic Disease

Agitation and combativeness are occasionally encountered in patients with liver disease. Murray-Lyon et al, in a study of patients with severe parenchymal liver disease, administered diazepam intravenously.[35] Adequate sedation was achieved in all patients with no deterioration of their clinical status.

Diazepam, administered with care, is an appropriate sedative for patients with impaired liver function.

Pain

In general, studies have failed to demonstrate specific analgesic properties of the benzodiazepines; however, large doses of benzodiazepines (e.g., "deep sedation") will impair motor response to painful stimulation.[36] These studies show that benzodiazepines are much more capable of attenuating the emotional response to pain than of altering the actual sensation of pain.

Other studies have demonstrated that diazepam may possess some slight analgesic properties.[37] These findings do not, however, alter the fact that in clinical situations in which pain control is a factor during dental treatment, local anesthetics must still be administered in the usual manner.

Amnesia

Intravenously administered diazepam produces *anterograde amnesia* (i.e., a lack of recall occurring from the time of injection onward).[38] Retrograde amnesia, a lack of recall of events occurring before drug administration, is quite rare. Amnesia after diazepam IM administration is uncommon and is essentially nonexistent after oral administration.

After IV diazepam administration, the duration of the amnesic period is approximately 10 minutes, with considerable variation noted. During this time, patients respond normally to stimulation, but at a later time (immediately postoperatively or 24 hours later), they are unable to recall the event.

In my experience with IV diazepam sedation, amnesia developed in approximately 75% of patients in whom diazepam had been titrated to a clinically adequate level of moderate sedation. The length of amnesia has varied, but it has been limited in most persons to the first 10 to 15 minutes after diazepam administration. In a very few patients, the amnesic effect has lasted through the entire appointment.

The importance of the amnesic phase is that traumatic procedures may be completed with the patient responding normally to them; however, at the end of the procedure, the patient will have no recall of what took place. The most common procedure during this period is the administration of local anesthetic. The patient may respond to the initial administration of the local anesthetic (although administration of local anesthetic should be performed as atraumatically as possible at all times). At the end of the dental or surgical procedure, patients often question their dentist to find out how their lips or tongue became "numb" or "frozen" without a "shot" or "how the drug injected in their arm (diazepam/midazolam) kept them from 'feeling' the procedure." Unfortunately, the amnesic period does not encompass the time period preceding the administration of the benzodiazepine (retrograde amnesia); therefore the patient will almost always recall the venipuncture attempt or attempts.

Although amnesia is usually a welcome benefit of IV moderate sedation, the absence of amnesia does not imply that the procedure was a failure. The primary goal of sedation is relaxation of the patient so that the treatment can be completed in a more ideal manner. The presence or absence of amnesia does not alter this fact. Lack of recall should be considered the "icing on the cake."

Contraindications

Injectable diazepam is contraindicated in patients with the following: known allergy to diazepam or other benzodiazepines and acute narrow-angle glaucoma and open-angle glaucoma, unless the patient is receiving appropriate therapy. True allergy (e.g., itching, hives, rash, bronchospasm) to benzodiazepines, though possible, is an extremely rare occurrence. Other contraindications include alcohol intoxication, CNS depression, and age less than 6 months.

Cautions include psychosis, impaired pulmonary function, impaired renal function, impaired liver function, and advanced patient age.

Warnings

Probably the most significant side effect of intravenously administered diazepam is the occurrence of venous thrombosis, phlebitis, local irritation, or swelling. Although these complications are rare with the administration of IV diazepam as recommended in Chapter 26, a manufacturer of diazepam recommends the following as a means to minimize this possibility[39]:

1. The solution should be injected slowly, taking at least 1 minute for each milliliter (5 mg).
2. Small veins, such as those on the dorsum of the hand or wrist, should not be used.
3. Extreme care should be taken to prevent intraarterial administration or extravasation.
4. Diazepam should not be mixed or diluted with other solutions or drugs in a syringe or infusion flask.
5. If it is not feasible to administer diazepam directly intravenously, it may be injected slowly through the infusion tubing as close as possible to the vein insertion.

Other warnings include the following:

1. Extreme care must be exercised when diazepam is administered to elderly or debilitated patients and to those with limited pulmonary reserve because of the possibility of apnea or cardiac arrest or both.
2. Concomitant use of barbiturates, alcohol, or other CNS depressants increases depression with increased risk of apnea.
3. When diazepam is administered with an opioid analgesic, the dose of the opioid should be reduced by at least one third and should be administered in small increments.

The administration of IV diazepam as recommended in Chapter 26 takes into account these warnings. Titration will prevent accidental overdose in the preceding situations.

Use in Pregnancy

Any drug that crosses the blood–brain barrier also crosses the placenta, entering into the fetus. An increased risk of congenital malformation associated with the administration of benzodiazepines during the first trimester of pregnancy has been suggested in several studies.[40] Because the administration of these drugs in dentistry is rarely a matter of urgency, their use at this time cannot be recommended. The possibility that a woman of childbearing potential may be pregnant at the time diazepam is used should always be considered.

Pediatric Use

Children 2 years and older handle diazepam as adults do. The major consideration is dosage. If diazepam is administered intravenously, titration will provide the proper safeguard to prevent overdose.

The administration of IV diazepam alone to younger children in the dental setting has not always provided ideal sedation. Difficulties exist in establishing venipuncture in any of these patients. Even more significant, however, is the child's response to the feeling of being sedated (IV moderate sedation). Whereas the adult will become more relaxed and cooperative as the effect of the diazepam increases, many younger children will appear to "fight" the effect, becoming increasingly agitated and uncomfortable. Some may call this a "paradoxical reaction" to the drug. It is my belief that the child is simply responding to the altered sensations he or she is experiencing (in his or her head). Because the child is unaccustomed to this feeling, he or she moves around so as to "get away" from it. IV diazepam when used as a sole agent in younger children does not provide a consistently adequate level of sedation.

Precautions

When diazepam is combined with other psychotropic agents, careful consideration must be given to possible potentiation of the drug effect.[39] Categories such as the phenothiazines, opioids, barbiturates, monoamine oxidase inhibitors (MAOIs), and other antidepressants are included.

Because metabolites of diazepam are excreted in the kidneys, the administration of diazepam in patients with compromised renal function should be undertaken with care. Lower dosages may be required for elderly or debilitated patients. Titration!

Patients receiving diazepam intravenously must be cautioned against engaging in hazardous occupations requiring complete mental alertness, such as operating machinery or driving a motor vehicle. Patients should also be advised against the use of alcoholic beverages after the administration of IV diazepam. In general, it is my policy to recommend that patients neither drive their car nor consume alcohol for the remainder of the treatment day at least and the next day if recovery at that time is not complete.

Adverse Reactions

The most frequently reported adverse reaction to intravenously administered diazepam is phlebitis at the site of injection. This is discussed in Chapter 27. Other, less frequent adverse reactions include the following:

- Hyperactivity

- Confusion
- Nausea (extremely rare)
- Changes in libido
- Hiccups (not uncommon; more annoying than anything)
- Decreased salivation (a benefit in dental treatment)

Paradoxical reactions such as acute hyperexcited states, anxiety, hallucinations, increased muscle spasticity, rage, and stimulation are also seen. The general term for this phenomenon is *emergence delirium*. It is seen more frequently with scopolamine administration and is discussed thoroughly in Chapter 27.

Dosage

The following directions regarding recommended dosage are taken from the diazepam package insert.[39]

Dosage should be individualized for maximal beneficial effect. The usual recommended dose in older children and adults ranges from 2 to 20 mg IV, depending on the indication and its severity. Lower doses, usually 2 to 5 mg, should be used for elderly or debilitated patients.

The dose of intravenously administered diazepam will always be determined by titrating the drug slowly (1 mL per minute) into a rapidly running IV infusion. In this manner, each patient will receive only the dose appropriate for sedation, and overdose should not occur.

Availability

Diazepam (generic): 5 mg/mL in 2-mL ampules, 10-mL multiple-dose vials, and 2-mL preloaded syringe.[39] Injectable diazepam consists of the following ingredients:

- 40% propylene glycol
- 10% ethyl alcohol
- 5% sodium benzoate and benzoic acid as buffers
- 1.5% benzyl alcohol as preservative

Diazepam is classified as a Drug Enforcement Administration (DEA) Schedule IV drug. Propylene glycol and ethyl alcohol are included because diazepam is lipid soluble and relatively water insoluble; it therefore requires a nonaqueous-solvent system. Many of the complications and side effects attributed to diazepam, especially phlebitis, are in fact produced by the propylene glycol, which is closely related to ethylene glycol, a major component of antifreeze.[41]

The IV administration of diazepam can produce a sensation of burning in some patients. This is caused not by the diazepam, but by the propylene glycol vehicle. It is recommended that the patient be advised of this possibility as the drug is administered. The dentist will tell the patient, "There may be a feeling of warmth as the drug is administered. This is entirely normal and will pass within a few minutes." As the drug is carried in venous blood away from the injection site, this sensation fades. Its occurrence may be minimized by opening the IV infusion to a rapid rate before injecting the diazepam. Some persons recommend the administration of 1 mL of 1% lidocaine or procaine into the IV line immediately before the administration of diazepam. The analgesic properties of lidocaine and procaine

prevent the burning sensation from occurring. In my experience with diazepam, slow injection of diazepam into a rapidly running infusion prevents this sensation from arising. IV lidocaine administration is not necessary.

The search for a water-soluble benzodiazepine with clinical properties similar to diazepam but without its potential for venous irritation led to the development of midazolam. Diazepam was, until recently, the most commonly used IV sedative within dentistry. When used as recommended, it is safe and extremely effective in the management of severe apprehension and fear of the dental or surgical situation. IV diazepam is recognized as one of the two "basic" IV moderate sedation techniques in dentistry.

Diazepam
The medical history of patients to receive diazepam should be checked for the following: • Allergy or hypersensitivity to benzodiazepines • Glaucoma (untreated) • Phlebitis, thrombophlebitis

Diazepam	
Proprietary name:	Generic only in USA
Classification:	Benzodiazepine
Availability:	5 mg/mL
Average sedative dose (IV):	10–12 mg
Maximum single dose:	20 mg
Maximum total dose:	30 mg

Diazepam	
Pregnancy category	D
Lactation	Possibly unsafe
Metabolism	Liver extensively; active metabolites
Excretion	Urine, half-life 30–60 hr
DEA schedule	IV

Midazolam

Midazolam is a 1,4-benzodiazepine compound that is similar in most pharmacologic aspects to diazepam. It possesses several attributes, however, that make it more attractive than diazepam in certain clinical situations.

Synthesized in 1975 by Walser and Fryer at Hoffmann-La Roche Laboratories, midazolam was available in many parts of the world in the early 1980s and was released for use in the United States in 1986. Midazolam first received FDA approval in December 1985. The chemical formula is

8-chloro-5(2′-fluorophenyl)-1-methyl-4H-imidazo (1,5-α)(1,4) benzodiazepine maleate. It is a colorless crystal in an aqueous solution. Each milliliter of the injectable solution contains either 1 or 5 mg midazolam maleate buffered to a pH of 3.3.[42] The acidic pH maintains the benzodiazepine ring in an open configuration, which is required for its water solubility (the diazepam ring is closed, and it is insoluble in water). Once in the body, the physiologic pH (7.4) acts to close the ring, providing the chemical structure of the drug that is required for its clinical efficacy.

Its water solubility differentiates midazolam from other parenteral benzodiazepines—diazepam, lorazepam, and chlordiazepoxide. The need for potentially irritating solvents, such as propylene glycol, is eliminated with midazolam. The water solubility of midazolam is produced by the substitution of imidazole at the 1,2 position of the 1,4-benzodiazepine ring structure and is aided because midazolam is the salt of an acid. This water solubility is responsible for the positive findings of a lack of burning sensation on injection and the absence of phlebitic sequelae at the injection site.

Pharmacokinetics and Biotransformation

Midazolam undergoes metabolism in the liver by hydroxylation into three major metabolites.[43] Whereas the major metabolites of diazepam are pharmacologically active anxiolytics, the major metabolites of midazolam have no pharmacologic activity. In addition, because of its lack of active metabolites and shorter half-life, a rebound effect is not evidenced with midazolam.

The α-half-life (distribution and redistribution) of midazolam has been recorded as 4 to 18 minutes. The β-half-life (metabolism and excretion) is 1.7 to 2.4 hours. By contrast, diazepam's β-half-life is 31.3 hours.[44] The shorter half-lives of midazolam make the drug more suitable for ambulatory sedation procedures: a relatively short duration of action combined with a relatively rapid inactivation and excretion of the drug.

Midazolam is 94% protein bound, with the binding occurring primarily in serum albumin. Midazolam possesses a relatively rapid onset of action, with the induction of general anesthesia having ranged from 55 to 143 seconds.[45]

Amnesia

Midazolam, like the other parenteral benzodiazepines, has the ability to produce anterograde amnesia. Conner et al demonstrated the incidence of amnesia in patients receiving IV midazolam (Table 25.2).[46]

The results shown in Table 25.2 indicate that midazolam is superior to other benzodiazepines or IV drug combinations in providing anterograde amnesia. In one study, 71% of the patients did not recall being in the recovery room.[46] Other studies have not demonstrated these same remarkable results, but in all cases, the degree of anterograde amnesia provided by midazolam was at least equal to that produced by diazepam.[47] Retrograde amnesia is not produced by midazolam.

Table 25.2	Incidence of Amnesia in Patients Receiving Intravenous Midazolam	
TIME AFTER INJECTION (min)	**AMNESIC PATIENTS (%)**	
2	96	
30	87.5*	
32	69	
43	57	

*Data from Fragen RJ, Caldwell NJ: Awakening characteristics following anesthesia induction with midazolam for short surgical procedures, *Arzneimittelforschung* 31(12a):2261-2263, 1981.

Since the introduction of midazolam for clinical use in the United States, I have seen the dramatic effects of midazolam-induced amnesia; most are beneficial, but some are potentially dangerous. For the typical 1-hour IV moderate sedation procedure in dental or outpatient surgical practice (e.g., colonoscopies), most patients have little recall of most or all of the procedure, and for most patients, this is quite acceptable and positive. One case, however, must be mentioned as a caution.

A young, healthy (ASA I) woman received IV midazolam and local anesthesia for the removal of three third molars. Following the 20-minute procedure, the patient appeared alert and was quite responsive to questions. Gauze packs (2" × 2") had been placed at the sites of extraction, and the patient had been told to bite down hard on the gauze and not to swallow. She responded verbally that she would do as directed. Within 2 minutes, the patient was complaining of a lump in her throat. Observation of the mouth indicated that all gauze packs had disappeared—the patient had swallowed them. Fortunately, they were located in the upper part of the esophagus and were of no great consequence. However, when questioned, the patient had absolutely no recall either of receiving the instructions given her by the dentist or of swallowing the gauze pads.[48]

It becomes imperative, therefore, for the patient to be observed much more carefully during the in-office recovery period, that special precautions be taken to prevent such events from recurring (e.g., 4" × 4" gauze packs with dental floss attached be used, not 2" × 2"), and that postoperative instructions (verbal and written) be given to both the patient and his or her escort. The benzodiazepine antagonist flumazenil has been shown to decrease the duration of midazolam's amnesic period.[49]

Duration of Clinical Activity

Because of its short α-half-life, the duration of clinical sedation noted with midazolam is somewhat shorter than that of diazepam. Its duration of action is therefore quite compatible with the typical 1-hour dental or surgical procedure.

Midazolam differs in another manner from diazepam. It appears that midazolam is much more effective than diazepam when amnesia is a desired result of the drug's administration.

However, when sedation is of higher priority, diazepam is a more effective agent. These are personal observations (anecdotes) that have not received the careful scientific study (evidence-based medicine) required to make a categorical statement.

Cardiorespiratory Activity

Midazolam, as is typical of benzodiazepines, has minimal effect in usual doses on the cardiovascular and respiratory dynamics of the ASA 1 or 2 patient. IV doses of 0.15 mg/kg of midazolam in healthy persons have produced statistically significant, but clinically insignificant, decreases in arterial blood pressure and increases in heart rate.[50] However, other researchers noted no untoward cardiovascular response with similar doses.[51] Gath et al[52] recommend midazolam as an induction agent for patients with ischemic heart disease because of its rapid onset of action and minimal effects on the cardiovascular system.

Diazepam and midazolam both produce the same effects on the respiratory system. Doses of 0.3 mg/kg of diazepam and 0.15 mg/kg of midazolam produced comparable depression of respiratory response to carbon dioxide (CO_2) in healthy volunteers.[50] It was concluded that midazolam and diazepam injected intravenously in equipotent doses depress respiration significantly and similarly. The results of the study indicate that this is mediated by direct depression of central respiratory drive rather than caused by a simultaneous depression of the muscles of respiration, although this possibility cannot be excluded. In the doses administered, equivalent to 21 mg of diazepam and 10 mg of midazolam for the typical 70-kg adult male, such a response might be expected. Since publication of this study in 1980, it has been demonstrated that equipotent doses of midazolam are approximately one fourth of the diazepam dose.[53]

In all cases, the cardiovascular and respiratory depression noted with midazolam were typical for parenteral benzodiazepines and significantly less than those observed following equipotent doses of barbiturates (thiopental, pentobarbital). No cardiac dysrhythmias were provoked by midazolam administration.

In November 1987, Roche Laboratories, the manufacturer of midazolam, sent a warning to physicians about the use of midazolam in moderate sedation.[54] It stated that the administration of midazolam had been associated with respiratory depression and respiratory arrest. Guidelines for the safe administration of this agent were offered (see "Dosage and Administration"). These guidelines emphasized the need for the slow titration of midazolam to all patients, especially the medically compromised.

Side Effects

The most frequently noted complaint after midazolam administration is dizziness. In the study by Conner et al,[46] 46% of patients mentioned experiencing dizziness. Despite this, 92% stated that they enjoyed the feeling produced by midazolam, and 100% said that they would accept the drug again if they required another operation.

Dosage and Administration

When midazolam was introduced, initial reports implied that midazolam was 1.5 times as potent as diazepam. Subsequent clinical experience with midazolam has shown it to be approximately four times as potent as diazepam.[53] The mean effective dose for 50% of subjects (MED50) for the induction of general anesthesia is 0.2 mg/kg, although significant patient variation exists.[55] Clinically adequate IV moderate sedation with midazolam should always be achieved by slow titration. In its 1987 letter, Roche recommended "an initial intravenous dose for conscious sedation as little as 1 mg, but not exceeding 2.5 mg for a normal, healthy adult."[54] Lower doses are necessary for older (over 60 years) or debilitated patients and for patients receiving concomitant opioids or other CNS depressants. The initial dose and all subsequent doses should never be given as a bolus; administer over at least 2 minutes and allow an additional 2 or more minutes to fully evaluate the sedative effect. The use of the 1 mg/mL or dilution of the 5 mg/mL formulation is recommended to facilitate slower injection.[54]

The following is the most recent (February 2016) recommendation[56] for the IV administration of midazolam to adult patients[56]: "Titrate slowly to achieve the desired effect. The usual dosage range is between 1–5 mg IV given over a 2-minute period, immediately before the procedure. Initially, do not exceed 2.5 mg (or 1.5 mg for elderly, debilitated, or those receiving other CNS depressants). If an adequate response is not achieved after 2-minutes, titrate upward in small increments. A total dose of 5 mg is generally sufficient for normal healthy adults and 3.5 mg for geriatric or debilitated patients. Premedication with an opiate agonist may potentiate the response to midazolam, reduce the midazolam dose by 30–50%."[56]

Doses of midazolam administered to normal, healthy (ASA 1) adult patients at the University of Southern California School of Dentistry and Oregon Health Sciences University IV moderate sedation continuing dental education programs have ranged from as little as 2 to 10 mg for an initial titrating dose. As with all drugs, there is significant patient variation in response to dosage.

Availability

Midazolam: 1 and 5 mg/mL in 2- and 10-mL vials (Hypnovel, Dormicum [Roche Laboratories] in the United Kingdom and other parts of the world). Midazolam is classified as a DEA Schedule IV drug. The proprietary name, Versed, was discontinued in the United States on July 28, 2003.[56,57]

As with other CNS depressants, the dosage of midazolam must be decreased when other CNS depressants are administered concomitantly. In addition, following IV moderate sedation, the patient must be escorted from the dental office in the company of a responsible adult and advised not to have any alcohol and not to engage in any hazardous occupation requiring complete mental alertness, such as operating machinery or driving a motor vehicle, for approximately 24 hours.

Midazolam

The medical history of patients receiving midazolam should be checked for the following:
- Allergy or hypersensitivity to benzodiazepines
- Acute pulmonary insufficiency
- Respiratory depression

Midazolam

Proprietary name:	Generics (USA)
	Hypnovel, Dormicum (UK)
Classification:	benzodiazepine
Availability:	1 mg/mL, 5 mg/mL
Average sedative dose (IV):	2.5–7.5 mg
Maximum single dose:	6–8 mg
Maximum total dose:	10 mg

Midazolam

Pregnancy category	D
Lactation	S (Safety conditional)
Metabolism	Liver
Excretion	Urine (<1% unchanged); half-life 2.5 hr
DEA schedule	IV

Lorazepam

Lorazepam is a benzodiazepine with sedative and antianxiety effects. It may be administered either intramuscularly or intravenously. Chemically, it is 7-chloro-5-(o-chlorophenyl)-1,3-dihydro-3-hydroxy-2H-1,4-benzodiazepin-2-one. Lorazepam, like diazepam, is virtually insoluble in water. Although available for IV use, lorazepam is seldom used in the outpatient ambulatory patient because of the relative inability to titrate the drug and its prolonged duration of action.[58] Lorazepam was approved by the FDA in September 1977.

Lorazepam differs from most IV drugs in that its onset of clinical action is quite slow. After IV administration, lorazepam produces little or no clinical effect for about 5 minutes, with its maximum effect noted approximately 20 minutes after administration. "Average" dosages of lorazepam must be administered, a situation that takes away one of the most important safety features of the IV route of drug administration—the ability to titrate.

From personal experience with IV lorazepam, I have found that it is rather easy to oversedate the patient. Administration of 1 or 2 mg of lorazepam usually provides adequate sedation, but because of the bell-shaped curve, some patients become overly sedated at this same dose.

The duration of clinical action of lorazepam is too long for most dental procedures. The usual duration of sedative effects of lorazepam is 6 to 8 hours; however, some degree of unsteadiness and sensitivity to the CNS-depressant effects of other drugs (e.g., opioid analgesics prescribed for postsurgical pain control) may persist for as long as 24 hours. I recall a patient who contacted me 36 hours after receiving 2 mg of lorazepam intravenously and asked me when the effect of the drug would go away.

The introduction of flumazenil offers a means of reversing the sedative effects of lorazepam at the conclusion of the procedure. However, the clinical actions of flumazenil, especially after IV administration, are shorter than the clinical actions of lorazepam, leading to a possible (probable?) recurrence of sedation after the patient is discharged from the office, a potentially dangerous situation. As discussed in the section on flumazenil, antidotal drugs, and complications (see Chapter 27), consideration should be given for IM flumazenil administration whenever IV flumazenil is used.

The amnesic properties of lorazepam are impressive and include both anterograde and a degree of retrograde amnesia. Lack of recall is maximal approximately 15 to 20 minutes after IV administration and may include events occurring throughout the treatment day. This feeling of "losing a day" may not be very comfortable for the ambulatory patient. Lorazepam is more highly recommended for use in the hospitalized, monitored patient as a preoperative IM or IV drug than in the ambulatory outpatient.

Warnings and Precautions

Patients receiving lorazepam must be warned against operating a motor vehicle or machinery or engaging in hazardous occupations for 24 to 48 hours after its administration. Dosages of lorazepam should be decreased in patients older than 50 years to minimize the risk of oversedation.[59]

The use of scopolamine with lorazepam is not recommended because there is no beneficial effect to be gained; however, additive CNS depression, hallucination, and irrational behavior may be more likely to occur.

Patients must be advised that getting out of bed unassisted may result in falling and injury if undertaken within 8 hours of receiving parenteral lorazepam. Alcohol should not be consumed for at least 24 to 48 hours after lorazepam injection. Other warnings and precautions for lorazepam are similar to those for diazepam and other benzodiazepines.

Pediatric Use

Data are insufficient to support the use of lorazepam in patients younger than 18 years. Its administration in outpatient pediatric dentistry appears unwarranted, especially in light of its prolonged clinical action.

Adverse Reactions

The most frequently noted adverse reactions to lorazepam are caused by a direct extension of its CNS-depressant properties and include the following[60]:

1. *Excessive sleepiness* that interfered with regional nerve block developed in 6% of patients studied. Patients older than 50 years had a significantly greater incidence of excessive sleepiness than did younger patients.
2. Restlessness, confusion, depression, and delirium occurred in 1.3% of patients.
3. Visual and self-limiting hallucinations developed in 1% of patients.

Because of its lack of water solubility, lorazepam may produce a burning sensation at the site of IV administration similar to that of diazepam. This occurred in 1.6% of patients receiving the drug. At 24 hours after injection, 0.5% still complained of discomfort. Patients should be advised that there may be slight warmth felt at the injection site as the drug is administered and that this is entirely normal and will pass within a few minutes. Slow injection of lorazepam into a rapidly running IV infusion minimizes this reaction.

Dosage

The following directions regarding recommended dosage are taken from the lorazepam package insert[61]:

For the primary purpose of sedation and relief of anxiety, usual recommended initial IV dose of lorazepam is 2 mg total, or 0.044 mg/kg (0.02 mg/lb), whichever is smaller. This dose will suffice for sedating most adults and should not ordinarily be exceeded in patients older than 50 years.[61]

Administration

Lorazepam should be diluted immediately before IV administration with an equal volume of a compatible solution. When properly diluted, lorazepam may be administered directly into a vein or into the tubing of an existing IV infusion. The rate of injection of lorazepam should not exceed 2.0 mg/min. Lorazepam may be diluted with the following[61]:

- Sterile water for injection
- Sodium chloride injection
- 5% dextrose injection

Availability

Ativan (Wyeth): 2 and 4 mg/mL in 10-mL vials and 1-mL preloaded syringes.

Lorazepam is not highly recommended for use in outpatient sedation because of its prolonged clinical action, its extreme amnesic properties, and primarily the lack of ability of the administrator to titrate the drug to clinical effect. Lorazepam is classified as a Schedule IV drug. It is an excellent IV sedative for nonambulatory hospitalized patients for whom close post-treatment monitoring is available for extended periods.[60]

Lorazepam
The medical history of patients receiving lorazepam should be checked for the following: • Allergy or hypersensitivity to benzodiazepines

Lorazepam	
Proprietary name:	Ativan
Classification:	Benzodiazepine
Availability:	2 and 4 mg/mL
Average sedative dose (IV):	2 mg
Maximum single dose:	2 mg
Maximum total dose:	4 mg

Lorazepam	
Pregnancy category	D
Lactation	Possibly unsafe
Metabolism	Liver
Excretion	Urine, half-life 14 hr
DEA schedule	IV

Flunitrazepam

Flunitrazepam is a water-soluble benzodiazepine derivative that is chemically and pharmacologically related to diazepam and other drugs of this group. The chemical formula for flunitrazepam is 5-(o-fluorophenyl)-1,3-dihydro-1-methyl-7-nitro-2H-1,4-benzodiazepin-2-one. The sedative, antianxiety, amnesic, and muscle-relaxing properties of flunitrazepam are similar to those of diazepam except that its sedative and sleep-inducing properties are more pronounced and longer lasting than those of diazepam.[62] Foreman[63] reported flunitrazepam to be approximately 15 times as potent as diazepam and suggested that the drug be diluted before administration to ensure precise titration.

Flunitrazepam is available in a 1-mL ampule containing 2 mg. The manufacturer suggests diluting the drug with 1 mL of sterile water for injection before use, providing a solution of 1 mg/mL.[64] Foreman, however, suggests that further dilution is warranted, recommending the dilution of 2 mg (1 mL) of flunitrazepam in 9 mL of sterile water, providing a solution of 0.2 mg/mL.[63]

Flunitrazepam is known on the street as "roofies." It is sometimes snorted to offset cocaine withdrawal. It has also acquired the title "the date-rape drug" because of its ability to induce anterograde amnesia, preventing the victim from recalling specific events while under the influence of the drug.[64,65]

Following IV administration for the induction of general anesthesia, flunitrazepam produces its clinical effects within

1 to 3 minutes, and the peak effect is noted in 5 minutes. The duration of clinical action ranged from 10 to 60 minutes, with significant variation with dosage (1 to 6 mg). The α-half-lives and β-half-lives of flunitrazepam are 19 and 34 hours.

Side Effects and Complications

The side effects and complications associated with flunitrazepam administration are similar to those of other benzodiazepines. As with most benzodiazepines, flunitrazepam is remarkably free of respiratory- or cardiovascular-depressant effects. The most frequently reported side effects associated with flunitrazepam administration are diaphoresis, ataxia, erythema, blurred vision, hypersalivation, dry mouth, weakness, hypothermia, hypoventilation, and prolonged drowsiness.[66] The dosage of flunitrazepam should be decreased in elderly and debilitated patients. The use of alcohol and driving should be prohibited for 24 hours after the administration of flunitrazepam.

Flunitrazepam Sedation in Dentistry

Foreman reported on 10 patients who received IV flunitrazepam moderate sedation.[63] The dosages ranged from 1.4 to 2 mg. Treatment conditions ranged from good to excellent in 8 of the 10 patients. No patient recalled receiving a local anesthetic during treatment (though they all did receive local anesthetics), nor did they recall any of the dental treatment. They did remember being escorted to the recovery area and driven home after discharge from the office.

The duration of sedation produced by flunitrazepam is somewhat longer than that produced by diazepam. This would contraindicate its use in shorter procedures (those lasting less than 1 hour), but would be an indication for its administration in longer procedures. Recovery from sedation was less complete than that seen with diazepam, even at 24 hours. In cases in which a more rapid patient recovery is important, flunitrazepam may not be the desired drug for IV moderate sedation.

Availability

Rohypnol (Roche Laboratories): 2 mg in 1-mL ampules. Flunitrazepam is not available in the United States (February 2017). It is available in both oral and parenteral preparations in Central and South America.[64]

Chlordiazepoxide

Chlordiazepoxide, the first benzodiazepine, was approved by the FDA in 1960. The parenteral formulation of chlordiazepoxide has been discontinued in the United States.[67]

SUMMARY

The benzodiazepines represent the most nearly ideal drugs for IV moderate sedation in the ambulatory patient. Pharmacologically, they normally demonstrate little significant effect on the cardiovascular and respiratory systems when administered in recommended doses via recommended techniques (e.g., titration). Midazolam and diazepam are the drugs of choice for IV moderate sedation procedures with a duration of 60 minutes or less. Midazolam possesses a number of advantages, most important of which are its amnesic qualities, lack of irritation to blood vessels, and the lack of a rebound, or second-peak, effect. Flunitrazepam is recommended for administration where procedures in excess of 1 hour are contemplated, whereas lorazepam should be reserved, in most instances, for nonambulatory, well-monitored patients undergoing longer procedures.

BARBITURATES

The barbiturates served as an important group of sedative drugs in dentistry for almost 50 years. Niels B. Jorgensen, the father of IV sedation in dentistry, included a barbiturate in his technique of IV premedication, known worldwide as the *Jorgensen technique.*[68]

Although several barbiturates are available for IV administration (Table 25.3), only one, pentobarbital, was used to any significant degree—as a component of the Jorgensen technique.

With the introduction of the benzodiazepines, initially diazepam and now midazolam, the need for and use of barbiturates decreased to the point where, today, they are rarely, if ever, indicated for use in moderate sedation. One can argue effectively that their negative attributes (e.g., respiratory depression at therapeutic sedation levels, hangover, excitation [increased talkativeness during sedation], circulatory depression, and laryngospasm) outweighed their benefit (sedation).[69]

Table 25.3	Barbiturates for Intravenous Administration			
GENERIC NAME	PROPRIETARY NAME	USUAL CONCENTRATION (mg/mL)	DURATION OF ACTION	AVERAGE SEDATIVE DOSE (mg)
Pentobarbital	Nembutal	50	2–4 hr	125–175
Secobarbital	Seconal	50	2–4 hr	100–150
Methohexital	Brevital (U.S.)	10	5–7 min	*
	Brietal (U.K.)			
Thiopental	Pentothal	25	—	*
Thiamylal	Surital	25	—	*

*Not recommended for IV moderate sedation without anesthesiology training.

The summary section on barbiturates from the fourth edition of this text follows.

SUMMARY

Although a number of barbiturates are available for IV administration, there are important reasons for some not being recommended for use in IV moderate sedation. The potent respiratory depressant properties of the barbiturates, combined with the steep dose-response curves of methohexital, thiopental, and thiamylal, are reason enough to recommend against their use by any doctor not extensively trained in general anesthesia and in the management of the airway of the unconscious patient. It is simply too easy to get into trouble (e.g., inadvertent loss of consciousness and airway obstruction) with these drugs. There are, however, two barbiturates—pentobarbital and secobarbital—that are recommended for use as IV sedatives. Although pharmacologically similar, pentobarbital is the more commonly used. Possessing a relatively flat dose-response curve, pentobarbital is an excellent drug for sedative procedures requiring 2 to 4 hours.

Those wishing a detailed description of the barbiturates, specifically pentobarbital (Nembutal), secobarbital (Seconal), methohexital (Brevital, Brietal), sodium thiopental (Pentothal), and thiamylal (Surital) are referred to the previous edition of this textbook.[70]

HISTAMINE BLOCKERS (ANTIHISTAMINICS)

Promethazine, classified as a histamine blocker, is, on rare occasion, employed for IV moderate sedation. The basic pharmacology of histamine blockers has been discussed in Chapters 7 and 10. In this section, only those aspects of promethazine's pharmacology relevant to IV administration are reviewed.

Promethazine

Promethazine is a phenothiazine derivative used primarily in pediatric dentistry as a sedative-hypnotic administered either orally or intramuscularly for the production of moderate-to-deep sedation. Promethazine may also be administered intravenously either as a sole agent or in combination with an opioid. Promethazine was approved by the FDA in 1951.

The clinical duration of action of promethazine following IV administration is approximately 1 to 2 hours. Clinical recovery of the patient at this time is somewhat greater than that observed after pentobarbital administration; however, it is significantly less than that seen with diazepam or midazolam. Promethazine is indicated for sedation procedures of approximately 1 hour to 2 or more hours.

The most significant adverse reaction to the administration of promethazine is the occurrence of extrapyramidal reactions. Clinical signs and symptoms of extrapyramidal reactions and their management are discussed in Chapter 7.

Dosage

The usual dose of promethazine required for moderate sedation after IV administration is approximately 25 to 35 mg. This drug should be administered in a concentration of 25 mg/mL.[71]

Availability

Generic only. The proprietary name Phenergan has been discontinued. 25 mg/mL in 1-mL ampules and 10-mL vials. It is also available in a 50-mg/mL concentration that is recommended for IM use only. Promethazine is not a scheduled drug.

Promethazine	
Pregnancy category	C
Lactation	Possibly unsafe
Metabolism	Liver
Excretion	Feces and urine; half-life 7–14 hr
DEA schedule	Not controlled; prescription required

SUMMARY

Though rarely employed, promethazine is an effective IV sedative. Its primary indication is for IV procedures requiring more than 1 to 2 or more hours to complete, though the benzodiazepines, midazolam and diazepam, can easily be retitrated and used for these very same procedures.

PROPOFOL

Propofol (2,6-diisopropylphenol) is an IV nonbarbiturate anesthetic that is chemically unrelated to other IV anesthetics. Propofol is used to induce general anesthesia that can be maintained by continuous infusion or with inhalation anesthetics. Propofol induces general anesthesia as quickly as thiopental, but emergence from anesthesia is 10 times more rapid than with thiopental and is associated with minimal postoperative confusion. Propofol has no analgesic activity and causes sedation at a lower dosage than that needed for anesthesia. Unlike many other general anesthetics, propofol possesses antiemetic activity. Propofol (Diprivan) received FDA approval in October 1989.[72] Propofol formulated in a lipid vehicle supports the growth of microorganisms. There have been worldwide reports of extrinsic microbial contamination of propofol leading to outbreaks of serious postoperative nosocomial infections. The antimicrobial agent ethylenediaminetetraacetic acid (EDTA) has been added to the propofol formulation. In vitro studies confirmed that EDTA added to propofol retards microbial growth. Data on the incidence of nosocomial infections before and after the introduction of propofol with EDTA indicates that there have been no further cluster outbreaks and individual nosocomial infections appear to have been reduced.[73]

Pharmacodynamics

Central Nervous System

Propofol decreases cerebral metabolism, blood flow, and intracranial pressure.[74,75] However, when larger doses are administered, marked lowering of systemic arterial pressures can significantly diminish cerebral perfusion.[76]

Respiratory System

Propofol, like most other IV CNS depressants, possesses respiratory-depressant properties. Propofol depresses respiration similarly to the barbiturates in normal patients (ASA 1), but to a greater degree than the benzodiazepines.[77]

Cardiovascular System

Propofol's cardiovascular-depressant effects are more profound than those of thiopental.[78] Both a direct myocardial depression and decreased systemic vascular resistance have been implicated in producing profound hypotension following large bolus doses of propofol.[78,79] Age also affects cardiovascular response to propofol, and caution is mandatory when propofol is administered to elderly patients.[80]

Miscellaneous Effects

Propofol may have antiemetic effects. Studies have demonstrated an extremely low incidence of emetic sequelae after outpatient anesthesia with propofol.[81] Propofol has a distribution half-life of 2 to 4 minutes and an elimination half-life of 3 to 12 hours (due to its slow release from fat stores).[72,77]

Like most IV anesthetics, propofol is eliminated via hepatic metabolism followed by renal excretion of the more water-soluble metabolites. There is some evidence that an extrahepatic route of elimination, such as the lungs, contributes to the clearance of propofol.[72,77] Propofol is rapidly and extensively metabolized to inactive, water-soluble sulfate and glucuronic acid conjugates that are eliminated by the kidney.[82] No changes in propofol's pharmacokinetics have been reported to date in the presence of hepatic or renal disease.

Clinical Use

IV administration of propofol results in a rapid onset of action (approximately 40 seconds, depending on dose, rate of administration, and presence of premedication) that is comparable with that of barbiturate induction agents.[83,84] Recovery from propofol's sedative-hypnotic effects is equally rapid, approximately 3 to 5 minutes following an IV bolus of 2 to 2.5 mg/kg.[72,85] The duration of propofol's central depressant effects increases in a dose-dependent fashion.[86] In contrast to the barbiturates, there appears to be less residual postoperative sedation, fatigue ("hangover"), and cognitive and psychomotor impairment with propofol.[87]

Propofol received considerable interest in the area of moderate sedation in hospital settings such as the operating theater and intensive care units and may offer advantages over other sedative-hypnotics because of its short duration of effect, rapid recovery, and minimal side effects.[88-90] A carefully titrated subhypnotic dose of propofol (0.5 to 1 mg/kg followed by 3 to 4.5 mg/kg/hr) produces excellent sedation with minimal respiratory depression and a short recovery period.[91]

The use of propofol for IV moderate sedation by non-general anesthesia–trained dentists is **not** recommended.

Warnings

Propofol is contraindicated for use in patients 16 years of age and under because safety and effectiveness have not been established.[72,92] Propofol administration is contraindicated in patients with a known hypersensitivity to the drug or its components.

Patients receiving propofol should be continuously monitored by persons not involved in the conduct of the surgical or diagnostic procedure; oxygen supplementation should be immediately available and provided where clinically indicated, and oxygen saturation should be monitored in all patients.[72,92]

Adverse Reactions

The most common adverse reactions, which occurred in more than 3% of patients receiving propofol, included hypotension, nausea, headache, and injection site pain or hotness.

Dosage and Administration

Drug dosages should always be individualized. The following are general dosage guidelines.[72,92]

Induction of General Anesthesia

Adults: 2 to 2.5 mg/kg or approximately 40 mg every 10 seconds until induction. Elderly, debilitated patients: 1 to 1.5 mg/kg or approximately 20 mg every 10 seconds until induction. Variable-rate infusion: titrated until the desired clinical effect is obtained.

Maintenance of Anesthesia

Adults: most patients require 100 to 200 μg/kg/min, or 6 to 12 mg/kg/hr. Elderly, debilitated, and ASA 3 or 4 patients: most require 50 to 100 μg/kg/min, or 3 to 6 mg/kg/hr. With an intermittent bolus of propofol, a dose of 25 to 50 mg as needed is suggested. Variable-rate infusion: titrated to desired clinical effect.[72]

Sedation

Dosage and rate should be individualized. A slow infusion or slow injection is preferred to rapid bolus administration. Most require an infusion of 100 to 150 μg/kg/min (6 to 9 mg/kg/hr) or a slow injection of 0.5 mg/kg over 3 to 5 minutes.

Most elderly, debilitated, and ASA 3 or 4 patients require doses similar to healthy adults, but they must be given as a slow infusion or slow injection and not as a rapid bolus. Bolus and rate should be titrated to clinical effect. A variable-rate infusion technique is preferred over an intermittent bolus technique. Most patients require an infusion of 25 to 75 μg/ kg/min (1.5 to 4.5 mg/kg/hr) or incremental bolus doses of 10 or 20 mg.

Elderly, debilitated, and ASA 3 or 4 patients require a 20% reduction of the adult dose. A rapid (single or repeated) bolus dose should not be used.

Propofol has been shown to be compatible with the following IV fluids when administered into a running IV catheter:

- 5% dextrose injection
- Lactated Ringer's injection
- Lactated Ringer's and 5% dextrose injection
- 5% dextrose and 0.45% sodium chloride injection
- 5% dextrose and 0.2% sodium chloride injection

Strict aseptic technique must always be maintained during handling because propofol is a single-use parenteral preparation and contains no antimicrobial preservative. The vehicle is capable of supporting rapid growth of microorganisms. Failure to follow recommended handling procedures may result in microbial contamination causing fever, infection or sepsis, or other adverse consequences that could lead to life-threatening illness. Propofol should be prepared for use just before administration. Administration should be completed within 6 hours after opening the ampules or vials.

Availability

Propofol (Diprivan; APP Pharmaceuticals) is available in ready-to-use 20-mL ampules and 50-mL infusion vials containing 10 mg/mL of propofol. Propofol is not a scheduled drug, but does require a prescription.

Propofol	
Pregnancy category	B
Lactation	Probably safe
Metabolism	Liver
Excretion	Kidney; half-life 3–12 hr >70% of elimination occurs during distribution phases with half-lives of 2–4 min and 30–64 min
DEA schedule	Not controlled; requires prescription

The administration of propofol for IV moderate sedation by nongeneral anesthesia–trained dentists is *not* recommended.

The administration of propofol for moderate sedation cannot be recommended for any dentist or physician who has not completed a dental or medical residency in anesthesiology.

OPIOID ANALGESICS

Opioids are administered primarily for their analgesic properties. They are excellent drugs for the management of moderate-to-severe pain.[93] Although they affect many systems throughout the body, their primary therapeutic actions derive from their effects on the CNS. Opioids are able to produce analgesia, drowsiness, changes in mood, and mental clouding. Of significance is that analgesia is produced without the loss of consciousness. The use of these drugs by the oral and IM routes is discussed in Chapters 7 and 10, with relevant pharmacology reviewed in Chapter 10. In this section, the use of these drugs in IV moderate sedation is discussed.

Opioid analgesics may be divided into the following categories: (1) opioid agonists, (2) opioid agonist-antagonists, and (3) opioid antagonists. *Opioid agonists* are those drugs that interact with an opioid receptor producing a physiologic change. An *opioid antagonist* is a drug that occupies a receptor site with no resultant pharmacologic effect. Opioids of the third group, *opioid agonist-antagonists*, possess properties of opioids of both of the preceding groups. With the appearance in the 1960s of drugs such as pentazocine, which had both agonist and antagonist properties, it became necessary to formulate a concept of multiple opioid receptors in the CNS.

In 1976 Martin[94] proposed a theory of multiple receptors rather than a single target for opiate agonists. Three separate opioid receptors, mu (μ), kappa (κ), and sigma (σ), were defined. A fourth, delta (δ), has since been identified. Table 10.3 lists the opioid receptors and agonist and antagonist drugs for each. Box 25.2 lists the various physiologic responses attributed to the various opioid receptors.[95,96]

Propofol	
The medical history of patients receiving propofol should be checked for the following:	
• Allergy or known hypersensitivity to propofol or its components	
• Nursing women	

Propofol	
Proprietary name:	Diprivan
Classification:	IV anesthetic/sedative-hypnotic
Availability:	10 mg/mL
Average sedative dose (IV):	An infusion of 100–150 μg/ kg/min (6–9 mg/kg/hr) or a slow injection of 0.5 mg/kg over 3–5 min
Maximum single dose:	Remains to be determined
Maximum total dose:	Remains to be determined

Box 25.2	Opioid Receptor Activation and Physiologic Effects

μ Receptor
Euphoria
Supraspinal analgesia
Indifference to stimuli
Respiratory depression
Depressed flexor reflexes
Locomotion
Hypothermia
Muscular rigidity
Dependence

κ Receptor
Sedation
Spinal analgesia
Miosis
Limited respiratory depression
Catalepsy

σ Receptor
Dysphoria
Hallucinations
Catatonia
Mydriasis
Tachycardia
Respiratory stimulation
Vasomotor stimulation

δ Receptor
Sedation
Euphoria

From Pallasch TJ, Gill CJ: Butorphanol and nalbuphine: a pharmacologic comparison, Oral Surg Oral Med Oral Pathol 59(1):15-20, 1985.

OPIOID AGONISTS

A number of opioid agonists—meperidine, morphine, fentanyl, alfentanil, sufentanil, and remifentanil—are available for use intravenously during sedation (moderate or deep) in dentistry.

Meperidine

Meperidine was, for many years, the most commonly used IV opioid in dentistry. (It has since been superseded by fentanyl.) The basic pharmacology of meperidine is discussed in Chapter 10. After IV administration, meperidine exhibits clinical actions in 2 to 4 minutes. Its duration of action is approximately 30 to 45 minutes, with considerable variation noted between patients and with administration of larger doses.

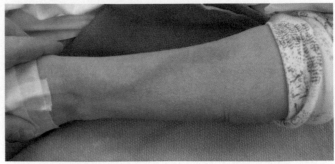

Figure 25.2 "Tracking" of vein following IV meperidine administration.

Meperidine has atropine-like properties, having been initially synthesized in the 1930s as an anticholinergic.[97] Patients receiving meperidine may demonstrate decreased salivary secretions and an increased heart rate because of its vagolytic properties. In the doses recommended later, these responses are usually nominal. Meperidine was approved by the FDA and marketed in 1942.[98]

Meperidine may also produce localized histamine release, resulting in the phenomenon of "tracking" at the site of meperidine administration (Fig. 25.2). The skin overlying the vein into which meperidine is injected will appear red, and the patient may mention that itching is present. As meperidine is carried by veins centrally up the patient's arm toward the heart, the reddening may continue to follow (tracking) the path of the vein. It is important to remember that this is a normal response to meperidine administration, not an allergic reaction. Meperidine-induced histamine release will be localized to the path of the vein, whereas an allergic response would be more generalized over the entire region. Management of meperidine-induced histamine release is simply to allow it to dissipate spontaneously, which occurs over the next 10 to 15 minutes. Because of the possibility of histamine release, the administration of meperidine is contraindicated in asthmatics (histamine produces bronchospasm).[98]

Dosage

When meperidine is administered intravenously during moderate sedation, the recommended maximum dose is 50 mg. In our IV moderate sedation programs we recommend an absolute maximum meperidine dose of 100 mg.[99,100] At this dose, the typical patient response is an increase in his or her pain reaction threshold (analgesia) without any significant change in the depth of sedation. Opioids may be administered either before or after the sedative-hypnotic drug (the primary drug used to produce sedation). At a maximum dose of 50 to 100 mg, meperidine produces virtually no cardiovascular or respiratory depression in the typical patient.[101] Meperidine should be administered in a concentration not exceeding 10 mg/mL. When the 50-mg/mL concentration is used, 1 mL of meperidine is placed into a 5-mL syringe, and 4 mL of diluent (e.g., 5% dextrose and water) is added. The resulting solution contains 50 mg of meperidine in 5 mL of fluid, or 10 mg/mL.

Availability

Demerol (Sanofi-Aventis) (Pethidine in the United Kingdom): 10 mg/mL in 1-mL ampules, 25 mg/mL in 0.5- and 1-mL ampules, 50 mg/mL in 0.5- and 1-mL ampules and 30-mL vials, 75 mg/mL in 1- and 1.5-mL ampules, and 100 mg/mL in 1- and 2-mL ampules and 20- and 30-mL vials. Meperidine is classified as a Schedule II drug (DEA).

It has been our clinical experience that the 50-mg/mL dosage form of meperidine is the most convenient to work with. More concentrated solutions are potentially dangerous because it is too easy for a mistake in calculation to lead to the administration of an overly large dose. The 10- and 25-mg/mL dosage forms are also appropriate; however, with the 10-mg/mL form, larger volumes of solution will be used.

Single-use 1-mL ampules are recommended instead of multidose vials unless meperidine is used on a regular basis. The 20- or 30-mL vial may become contaminated if permitted to remain unused for a considerable time. Because meperidine (and other opioid analgesics) is a Schedule II drug, precise records must be kept of the drug's administration. One-mL ampules simplify this task considerably.

Morphine

Morphine sulfate represents the classic opioid agonist. Morphine was in use for many years before its approval by the newly formed FDA in 1939. It is useful, but rarely used for IV moderate sedation in outpatient situations because of its long duration of action (1.5 to 2 hours).[102] The pharmacology of morphine is discussed in Chapter 10.

Dosage

When it is administered for IV moderate sedation in dentistry, the maximum dose of morphine should not exceed 8 mg. The drug is diluted to a concentration of 1 mg/mL before use. Little change in the depth of sedation will normally occur at this dose level, yet the patient's pain reaction threshold will be elevated.

Availability

Morphine sulfate: 2, 4, 8, 10, and 15 mg/mL. Morphine sulfate is classified as a Schedule II drug.[102] The use of morphine sulfate should be restricted to dental procedures requiring more than 2 hours.

Meperidine

The medical history of patients receiving meperidine should be checked for the following:
- Allergy or known hypersensitivity to opioid analgesics
- Asthma
- MAOIs taken within 14 days
- COPD and decreased respiratory reserve

Morphine

The medical history of patients receiving morphine should be checked for the following:
- Allergy or known hypersensitivity to opioid analgesics
- Asthma
- MAOIs taken within 14 days
- COPD and decreased respiratory reserve

Meperidine

Proprietary name:	Demerol
Classification:	Opioid agonist
Availability:	10, 25, 50, 75, and 100 mg/mL
Average sedative dose (IV):	37.5–50 mg
Maximum single dose:	50 mg
Maximum total dose:	100 mg

Morphine

Proprietary name:	Morphine
Classification:	Opioid agonist
Availability:	2, 4, 8, 10, and 15 mg/mL
Average sedative dose (IV):	5–6 min
Maximum single dose:	8 mg
Maximum total dose:	8 mg

Meperidine

Pregnancy category	C
Lactation	Probably safe
Metabolism	Liver, mostly; active metabolite
Excretion	Urine; half-life 2.5–4 hr
DEA schedule	II

Morphine

Pregnancy category	C
Lactation	Probably safe
Metabolism	Liver; GI tract
Excretion	Urine 85% (9%–12% unchanged); bile/feces 7%–10%; half-life 2–4 hr
DEA schedule	II

Hydromorphone

Hydromorphone is a hydrogenated ketone, semisynthetic analog of morphine. Hydromorphone has a more rapid onset of analgesia than morphine, but its duration of action is somewhat shorter, thereby limiting its use in patients with chronic pain. Hydromorphone binds to various opioid receptors, producing analgesia and sedation (opioid agonist). Opiates do not alter the pain threshold of afferent nerve endings to noxious stimuli, nor do they affect the conductance of impulses along peripheral nerves. Analgesia is mediated through changes in the perception of pain at the spinal cord and higher levels in the CNS. There is no ceiling effect of analgesia for opiates. The emotional response to pain is also altered. Opioids 'separate pain from suffering.' In the dental environment where local anesthetics are the primary drugs administered to manage pain, this is of little concern. Hydromorphone was initially marketed before 1962.[103]

Hydromorphone is administered via the oral, rectal, subcutaneous, IM, and IV routes. Hydromorphone metabolites are primarily excreted in the urine; only a small amount of the hydromorphone dose is excreted unchanged in the urine. The half-life of immediate-release hydromorphone is 2 to 3 hours with a duration of analgesia of 3 to 4 hours.[104] Following intravenous administration, analgesia normally develops within 5 to 10 minutes. The primary indication for administration of hydromorphone is the management of moderate-to-severe pain.

Coda et al administered three different doses (10, 20, and 40 µg/kg) of hydromorphone and placebo, via IV bolus, to 10 healthy volunteers to determine the effect on experimental pain.[105] During each session subjects underwent repeated electrical tooth pulp stimulation at intensities sufficient to elicit a rating of "strong pain" before drug administration. Although the peak effect was poorly defined, the onset of analgesia was rapid, within 5 minutes, and maximum analgesic effect was seen between 10 and 20 minutes after maximum plasma hydromorphone concentration. However, within sessions they found a poor relationship between hydromorphone plasma concentration and its clinical effect. Compared with pain report data from other human studies done in their laboratory, hydromorphone has a shorter time to peak effect compared with morphine, and overall, hydromorphone hydrochloride is approximately five times as potent as morphine sulfate on a milligram basis.[105]

Dosage

When it is administered for IV moderate sedation in dentistry, the maximum dose of hydromorphone should not exceed 1 mg. The drug is diluted to a concentration of 0.2 mg/mL before use. Little change in the depth of sedation will normally occur at this dose level, yet the patient's pain reaction threshold will be elevated.

Availability

Hydromorphone: 1, 2, 4, and 10 mg/mL. Hydromorphone is classified as a Schedule II drug.[103] The use of Dilaudid should be restricted to dental procedures requiring more than 2 hours.

Hydromorphone	
The medical history of patients receiving hydromorphone should be checked for the following: • Allergy or known hypersensitivity to opioid analgesics • Asthma • COPD and decreased respiratory reserve	

Hydromorphone	
Proprietary name:	Dilaudid, Exalgo, Palladone
Classification:	Opioid agonist
Availability:	1, 2, 4, and 10 mg/mL
Average sedative dose (IV):	0.2–0.5 mg
Maximum single dose:	1 mg
Maximum total dose:	1 mg

Hydromorphone	
Pregnancy category	C, but trimester specific
Lactation	Probably safe
Metabolism	Primarily liver
Excretion	Urine primarily; bile. half-life (IV) 2.3 hr
DEA schedule	II

Fentanyl

Fentanyl is a rapid-onset, short-acting opioid agonist that is approximately 100 times more potent than morphine (0.1 mg of fentanyl is equianalgesic to 10 mg of morphine).[106] It was originally synthesized and introduced as one of the components of the drug combination known as Innovar. The FDA approved fentanyl for IV administration in February 1968.[107]

Fentanyl has replaced meperidine as the most used opioid analgesic in IV moderate sedation.

Following IV administration of fentanyl, peak analgesia occurs within minutes and lasts for 30 to 60 minutes after a single dose; duration is directly dose related. Respiratory depressant effects persist longer than analgesic actions, and residual fentanyl from one dose can potentiate the effect of subsequent doses. Serum concentrations appear to fall rapidly, within 5 minutes, from a peak level after IV dosage, but residual drug can be detected for at least 6 hours.[107,108]

Respiratory depression is a side effect of all opioid agonists, with the respiratory-depressant effect of fentanyl lasting longer than its analgesic properties. This potential must always be considered before discharge of an apparently "recovered" patient from the office in the custody of a person who is not trained to recognize respiratory depression or to manage it (e.g., a parent or other non–medical professional guardian).

As with other opioid agonists, fentanyl decreases the respiratory rate. This action of fentanyl is rarely observed for more than 30 minutes after the drug's administration. After IV administration of a single dose of fentanyl, peak respiratory depression is noted 5 to 15 minutes later.[109] Depression of breathing (decreased sensitivity to CO_2 stimulation) has been demonstrated for up to 4 hours in healthy volunteers.

Indications

Fentanyl is indicated for use as the following:

- As an analgesic in short anesthetic procedures and in the recovery room
- As an analgesic to supplement general or regional anesthesia
- In combination with a neuroleptic as a premedication for the induction of anesthesia and as an adjunct in the maintenance of general and regional anesthesia

Contraindications

Fentanyl is contraindicated for use in patients with known allergy or intolerance to it.

Warnings

Fentanyl may cause muscular rigidity, especially involving the muscles of respiration (thoracic and abdominal).[110] This action appears to be related to rate of injection, occurring more frequently following rapid administration. This can usually be prevented by the slow IV administration of the drug.

Should muscular rigidity develop, management consists of assisted or controlled ventilation or, if necessary, the administration of a neuromuscular-blocking agent, such as succinylcholine. This latter step must never be considered unless the dentist or physician has been trained to administer skeletal muscle relaxants and is intimate with the technique of controlled ventilation. Patients who have received MAOIs within the past 14 days should not receive fentanyl or any other opioid agonist because of the potential for severe and unpredictable potentiation of the opioid effect.[111]

The safety of fentanyl in patients younger than 2 years has not been established; therefore it cannot be recommended for use in dental outpatient sedation in this population. Fentanyl should not be administered to pregnant patients unless the benefits of its administration clearly outweigh the potential hazards of opioid administration.[107,112]

Precautions

Fentanyl should be administered with caution to patients with chronic obstructive pulmonary disease (COPD) and to patients with decreased respiratory reserve (ASA 3, 4, and 5). In these patients, opioids may decrease respiratory drive to an even greater degree than usual. Significant liver and renal dysfunction also represent relative contraindications to fentanyl administration.

Adverse Reactions

The most frequently noted adverse reactions to fentanyl administration include respiratory depression, apnea, muscular rigidity, and bradycardia. If untreated, these may progress to respiratory arrest, circulatory depression, or cardiac arrest. Other adverse reactions include hypotension, dizziness, blurred vision, nausea and vomiting, laryngospasm, and diaphoresis.[107,112]

Dosage

Fentanyl is administered in conjunction with other antianxiety or sedative-hypnotic medications for sedation. The recommended dose of fentanyl is therefore predicated on the fact that the patient has already received, or is going to receive, one or more other CNS depressants. The maximum dose of fentanyl recommended for use in outpatient sedative procedures is 0.05 to 0.06 mg (1.0 to 1.2 mL). This dose is equivalent to approximately 8 mg morphine and about 50 mg of meperidine. Fentanyl should always be diluted from its initial concentration of 0.05 mg/mL by adding 4 mL of diluent (e.g., 5% dextrose and sterile water) to produce a final concentration of 0.01 mg/mL.

Availability

The proprietary name Sublimaze (Akorn, Inc.) has been discontinued in the United States. Fentanyl is available as 0.05 mg/mL (50 μg/mL) in 2-, 5-, 10-, and 20-mL ampules.

Fentanyl is classified as a Schedule II drug.

Fentanyl
The medical history of patients receiving fentanyl should be checked for the following: • Allergy or known hypersensitivity to opioid analgesics • MAOIs taken within 14 days • COPD and decreased respiratory reserve

Fentanyl	
Proprietary name:	Generic
Classification:	Opioid agonist
Availability:	0.05 mg/mL (50 μg/mL)
Average sedative dose (IV):	0.05–0.06 mg (50–60 μg)
Maximum single dose:	0.08 mg (80 μg)
Maximum total dose:	0.1 mg (100 μg)

Fentanyl	
Pregnancy category	C
Lactation	Safe
Metabolism	Liver
Excretion	Urine (10%–25% unchanged); half-life 3.7 hr
DEA schedule	II

Alfentanil, Sufentanil, and Remifentanil

Three analogs of fentanyl—alfentanil, sufentanil, and remifentanil—are in clinical use in the United States. The FDA approved sufentanil in 1984,[113] alfentanil in 1986,[114] and remifentanil in 1996.[115] Clinical actions of these drugs are similar to those of fentanyl, but there are some significant differences. Although the onset of clinical action of alfentanil is very rapid, occurring within 1 minute after injection, its duration is very short (11 minutes at twice its MED50).[116] The elimination half-life of alfentanil is 97 ± 22 minutes in adults, whereas in geriatric patients and persons with liver dysfunction, clearance rates are slower.[117-119] Alfentanil is a tetrazole derivative of fentanyl with many pharmacologic actions similar to those of fentanyl and sufentanil; however, alfentanil has a quicker onset of action than fentanyl and a shorter duration of action than either fentanyl or sufentanil.[120] In addition, alfentanil has a shorter half-life and may produce less respiratory depression than either fentanyl or sufentanil.

The use of alfentanil and sufentanil in general anesthesia has been evaluated in depth[121,122]; they are quite well accepted, especially for short surgical procedures. Alfentanil has received considerable attention in dentistry and other outpatient surgical procedures.[123-127] It is frequently administered in conjunction with propofol.[128] Both alfentanil and sufentanil are opioid agonists and as such should be managed with the same care as other members of this group.

Remifentanil is an opioid agonist for use during general anesthesia and monitored anesthesia care.[115,129-132] Remifentanil is a member of the phenylpiperidine class of opiate agonists. It has a rapid onset and peak effect and an ultrashort duration of action. The effects subside within 5 to 10 minutes after discontinuation of therapy. New steady-state concentrations occur within 5 to 10 minutes after changes in infusion rates. Remifentanil is useful in attenuating the hemodynamic response to intubation and helps maintain cardiovascular stability during anesthesia. Remifentanil alone does not provide reliable amnestic effects or adequate anesthetic depth for general surgery; the concurrent use of inhaled anesthetics and/or hypnotics is required. The respiratory-depressant effects of remifentanil must be taken into consideration when given to critically ill patients. Remifentanil has analgesic effects and may be used in pain management of intensive care and postoperative patients; however, the injection is rarely given for extended periods.

Only personnel specifically trained in the use of IV and general anesthetics should administer remifentanil. Remifentanil differs from other β-receptor agonists in that it is metabolized by esterases located in the systemic circulation; other agents are hepatically metabolized.

Availability

Alfenta (Akorn, Inc.): 500 µg/mL (alfentanil as hydrochloride) per milliliter in 2-, 5-, 10-, and 20-mL ampules. Sufentanil (generic): 50 µg (sufentanil as citrate) per milliliter in 1-, 2-, and 5-mL ampules. Ultiva (Bioniche Pharma): (remifentanil) 1-mg/3-mL vial, 2-mg/5-mL vial, and 5-mg/10 mL vial. Alfentanil, sufentanil, and remifentanil are classified as Schedule II drugs.

OPIOID AGONIST-ANTAGONISTS

Because of the potentially significant side effects associated with administration of opioid agonists, considerable research was conducted to find a potent analgesic that possesses the efficacy of morphine but lacks its respiratory-depressant actions, its drug dependence, and abuse liability.

In the 1960s success was attained with the introduction of pentazocine, the first drug with both opioid agonist and opioid antagonist properties to be marketed (1967).[133] In succeeding years, some of the initial fervor for pentazocine waned as significant side effects were reported.[134,135] Pentazocine is rarely employed during IV moderate sedation. Two other drugs in this same category—nalbuphine and butorphanol—were developed and are used in IV moderate sedation for both dental and medical outpatient procedures.[136,137] The three drugs classified as opioid agonist-antagonists are pentazocine, nalbuphine, and butorphanol.

Pentazocine

The chemical formula for pentazocine is 1,2,3,4,5,6-hexahydro-6,11-dimethyl-3-(3-methyl-2-butenyl)-2,6-methano-3-benzazocin-8-ol lactate. Pentazocine was introduced in 1967 as a nonnarcotic opioid in both oral and parenteral formulations.[133] Pentazocine injection was originally FDA approved in 1967.[138] Only the IV form of pentazocine is currently available.[138]

A dose of 30 mg of pentazocine is equivalent to approximately 10 mg of morphine or 75 mg of meperidine. Administered intravenously, pentazocine's onset of action is 1 to 2 minutes, with a duration of approximately 1 hour, although the patient may still exhibit alterations in consciousness for a number of hours following discharge from the office.

Pentazocine has opioid antagonist effects and sedative properties. Administered to patients receiving morphine-type opioids, pentazocine weakly antagonizes the analgesic, cardiovascular, respiratory, and CNS-depressant effects produced by these agents.[139] The sedative effect of a 30-mg IV dose of pentazocine is equivalent to that of approximately 10 mg of IV diazepam.[140] Pentazocine does not provide the same degree of amnesia as does diazepam.

Pentazocine is indicated for use in the management of moderate-to-severe pain and is also used as a preoperative or preanesthetic medication and as a supplement during general anesthesia (administered intravenously). Pentazocine initially gained some popularity within dentistry as an alternative to the opioid agonists.[141] However, with the introduction of butorphanol, nalbuphine, alfentanil, and sufentanil, the dental use of pentazocine has markedly decreased.

Contraindications

Pentazocine is contraindicated for use in patients with a documented allergy to it, COPD, and during pregnancy.[138]

Warnings

Despite early claims to the contrary, experience with pentazocine has demonstrated that both psychological and physical dependence can develop.[142] Abrupt discontinuance of pentazocine has produced a clinical syndrome consisting of abdominal cramps, elevated temperature, rhinorrhea, restlessness, anxiety, and lacrimation.[143]

Pentazocine should be administered to the pregnant patient only in situations in which the benefits of administration clearly outweigh its potential hazards. For routine outpatient sedation in the dental setting, there is rarely an indication for pentazocine administration in pregnant patients.

Another significant untoward effect of pentazocine is the occurrence of acute neuropsychiatric manifestations, such as visual hallucinations, disorientation, confusion, mental depression, disturbing dreams, and dysphoria.[144] These responses usually resolve spontaneously within a few hours. The responsible mechanism is as yet unknown. Administration of naloxone may end in recovery. Management of reactions that do occur is symptomatic, with vital signs monitored and recorded regularly during the reaction, although stimulation of the δ receptor will produce these same responses. Readministration of pentazocine to this same patient at future dates should be avoided, if possible, to minimize the possibility of recurrence.

The administration of pentazocine to patients younger than 12 years is not recommended because of a lack of clinical data. The drug package insert for pentazocine recommends that ambulatory patients receiving parenteral pentazocine be cautioned not to operate machinery, drive cars, or unnecessarily expose themselves to hazards.[145]

Precautions

Patients with asthma, COPD, or other conditions associated with decreased respiratory reserve should be given pentazocine with caution, if at all. Patients with extensive liver disease appear to exhibit a greater number of adverse side effects from the usual clinical dose, a response indicating a decreased rate of metabolism of the drug by the liver. The plasma half-life of pentazocine is approximately 2 hours.

Pentazocine should be administered with caution to patients with seizure disorders. Seizures have developed after administration of pentazocine, although a direct cause-and-effect relationship has never been established.[146]

Adverse Reactions

Pentazocine exhibits the same adverse reactions as the opioid agonists previously discussed, including nausea and vomiting, xerostomia, diarrhea, constipation, blurred vision, euphoria, dysphoria, respiratory and cardiovascular depression, and allergic reactions. In addition, pentazocine produces the neuropsychiatric reactions noted.

Dosage

Pentazocine is commonly administered in conjunction with an antianxiety or sedative-hypnotic agent for moderate sedation. It is therefore usually administered after the patient has received one or more drugs. The maximum recommended dose of pentazocine in IV moderate sedation is 30 mg. When titrated slowly, the usual dose required (in combination with other drugs) for sedation is approximately 20 mg.

Availability

Talwin (Winthrop): 30 mg/mL in 1-mL, 1.5-mL, and 2-mL ampules and in 10-mL vials. Each mL contains pentazocine lactate equivalent to 30 mg base and 2 mg acetone sodium bisulfite, 1.5 mg sodium chloride, and 1 mg methylparaben as preservative, in water for injection. Pentazocine is classified as a Schedule IV drug.

Nalbuphine

Nalbuphine, 17-(cyclobutylmethyl)-4,5α-epoxymorphinan-3,6α,14-triol hydrochloride, was synthesized in 1965 and approved by the FDA in 1979.[147] It is not a controlled substance. The chemical incorporates the molecular features of the opioid agonist oxymorphone hydrochloride (Numorphan) with that of the opioid antagonist naloxone hydrochloride (Narcan).[147]

Pharmacology

Nalbuphine has an analgesic potency approximately 0.8 to 0.9 times that of morphine. In clinical practice, nalbuphine is considered equianalgesic to morphine when administered in equal doses (e.g., 10 mg of nalbuphine is equal to 10 mg of morphine).[148]

After IV administration, nalbuphine's onset of action is 2 to 3 minutes. Its duration of action is slightly longer than that of morphine (approximately 3 to 6 hours). A 10-mg dose of nalbuphine is equivalent to approximately 50 to 75 mg of meperidine.[149]

Studies of the effectiveness of nalbuphine as a preoperative sedative agent are lacking, and there are few studies evaluating IV nalbuphine in dental procedures.[150-153] This author used nalbuphine several hundred times in IV moderate sedation on dental outpatients, most often with acceptable results.

Nalbuphine possesses opioid antagonist effects at the μ-opioid receptor. Nalbuphine is 10 times as effective as pentazocine as an opioid antagonist and one fourth as potent as nalorphine in morphine-dependent subjects.[147] Quite interesting, and potentially significant, is that nalbuphine may be used as an opioid antagonist in place of naloxone. Gal et al[154] substituted nalbuphine (0.1 mg/kg) for naloxone to reverse respiratory depression produced by oxymorphone or hydromorphone. They noted a dramatic reversal of respiratory depression and a restoration of normal ventilation within 5 minutes. Of greater importance is that nalbuphine provided substantial analgesia *after* reversal of the opioid-induced respiratory depression, which extended well into the postoperative period. These differential μ- (opioid antagonism) and κ- (agonist analgesia) receptor actions of nalbuphine may be of value in preventing the adverse cardiovascular stimulation observed in some patients suffering from surgical pain when naloxone is administered to reverse opioid-induced CNS depression; unfortunately, however, naloxone also acts to reverse the analgesia produced by the opioid.[155]

Pharmacokinetics

Following IV administration, the analgesic effects of nalbuphine appear in 2 to 3 minutes. The analgesic effects of the drug persist for approximately 3 to 6 hours. The plasma half-life of nalbuphine is 5 hours. The drug undergoes metabolism in the liver; oral doses of nalbuphine undergo a significant hepatic first-pass effect, and only 20% of an orally administered dose is biologically available.[156]

Nalbuphine is physically compatible with most aqueous drugs and can thus be combined in the same syringe. Nalbuphine cannot, however, be combined with diazepam because a milky white precipitate forms.

Adverse Effects

When nalbuphine is used solely as an analgesic, the most frequently noted adverse effect is sedation, which is reported in 36% of patients.[157] This "side effect" is used to advantage in IV moderate sedation procedures. Other common adverse responses (occurring in more than 3% of patients) include the following:

Sweaty, clammy feeling	9%
Nausea and vomiting	6%
Dizziness, vertigo	5%
Dry mouth	4%
Headache	3%

Psychotomimetic effects occurred only rarely and included depression, confusion, dysphoria, euphoria, feelings of unreality, feelings of hostility, and hallucinations. The incidence of these is significantly less than that seen with pentazocine.[157]

The potentially most serious adverse effect associated with nalbuphine administration is respiratory depression. When the pure opioid agonists (morphine, meperidine, and fentanyl) are administered, both the rate and depth of respiration are depressed in a dose-related manner until apnea occurs. For outpatient ambulatory procedures, the potential for respiratory depression is the factor most significantly limiting the use of opioid agonists. Nalbuphine possesses ceiling effects for respiratory depression, whereas its analgesic effects may become more pronounced with increasing doses. Gal et al demonstrated a plateau effect for both respiratory depression and analgesia for nalbuphine in doses up to 0.6 mg/kg.[158] In other studies, it was demonstrated that the normal dose of nalbuphine (7 to 10 mg/70 kg) produced the same degree of respiratory depression as an equivalent dose of morphine; however, nalbuphine-induced respiratory depression peaked at 30 mg/70 kg (equivalent to 20 mg/70 kg morphine) and remained the same even at nalbuphine doses of 3 mg/kg (210 mg/70 kg), whereas morphine-induced depression continued to increase in a dose-related manner.[159,160] Larger doses of nalbuphine do not extend the duration of respiratory depression beyond the usual 3 hours. Nalbuphine therefore possesses a ceiling effect on both the degree and the duration of respiratory depression. This is in contrast to butorphanol, which has a ceiling effect only on the degree of respiratory depression, not its duration.[161]

When administered to medically compromised patients, especially the cardiovascular-risk patient, nalbuphine produces a slight decrease in cardiac workload, a potentially beneficial effect. Romagnoli and Keats considered nalbuphine an ideal drug for patients with heart disease because it was devoid of hemodynamic effects except those associated with the relief of pain and anxiety.[162] Lefevre et al compared clinically equivalent doses of fentanyl with nalbuphine for "IV analgesia" in medically compromised patients (ASA 3 or 4).[163] Respiratory rates and SpO_2 were significantly lower ($p > .05$) for the patients receiving fentanyl.

One of the potential benefits of the opioid agonist-antagonist analgesics is a limited or absent drug dependence and abuse liability (e.g., psychic dependence, physical dependence, tolerance) as a result of their opioid antagonist actions compared with complete μ-receptor agonists such as morphine.[164]

Overdose

Overdose of nalbuphine is exceptionally rare but possible. Signs and symptoms of overdose include CNS depression and respiratory depression, both of which are managed with basic life support and completely reversed with the IV administration of naloxone.

Contraindications

In the dental outpatient environment nalbuphine is contraindicated for use in patients who are allergic or hypersensitive to it. The drug package insert should be consulted for additional contraindications.[147,165]

Warnings

Because nalbuphine produces CNS depression, patients receiving this drug must be cautioned against the performance of potentially dangerous tasks, such as driving a car and operating machinery.[147,165] Nalbuphine is not recommended for administration to patients younger than 18 years because of a lack of clinical experience in patients in this age group. Pregnant patients should not receive nalbuphine unless the advantages of its administration clearly outweigh its potential disadvantages.

Nalbuphine may exhibit additive effects with other CNS depressants administered concurrently. The dosage of one or both of the drugs should be reduced. This should not pose a significant problem with IV administration if the drugs are titrated to effect.

Precautions

Nalbuphine should be administered with caution, at reduced dosages, to patients with impaired respiratory drive, including asthma and COPD (ASA 3, 4, and 5). Because nalbuphine is metabolized in the liver and excreted through the kidneys, it is possible that patients with impaired hepatic or renal function may overrespond to usual dosages. Dosages should be reduced in these patients. Titration minimizes this risk.

Dosage

When administered intravenously, nalbuphine should be titrated to clinical effect. The maximum dose of nalbuphine recommended for IV moderate sedation is 10 mg. This represents both the maximum single and total doses. Onset of action after IV administration is 2 to 3 minutes, with a duration of analgesic effect of 3 to 6 hours. The average IV dose of nalbuphine is approximately 7 to 8 mg.

When nalbuphine is administered after diazepam or midazolam, the depth of sedation is rarely increased. However, recovery from sedation is somewhat less complete than that observed when diazepam or midazolam is administered alone.

Because of the doses recommended here (10 mg maximum), the beneficial effects of nalbuphine's ceiling level for respiratory depression (30 mg) will not be observed. It is only at dosages considerably greater than these that the ceiling effect on respiratory depression is noted. In doses up to 10 mg of nalbuphine, the degree of respiratory depression should not be profound, but will be equivalent to that induced by 10 mg of morphine or 50 to 75 mg of meperidine.

Availability

The proprietary name, Nubain, has been discontinued in the United States. The generic form of nalbuphine is available as 10 mg/mL and 20 mg/mL.

Nalbuphine is not a scheduled drug.

Nalbuphine	
Proprietary name:	Generic
Classification:	Opioid agonist-antagonist
Availability:	10 mg/mL; 20 mg/mL
Average sedative dose (IV):	7–8 min
Maximum single dose:	10 mg
Maximum total dose:	10 mg

Nalbuphine	
Pregnancy category	B
Lactation	Safety unknown
Metabolism	Liver
Excretion	Urine; bile and feces; half-life 5 hr
DEA schedule	May be over-the-counter (OTC), OTC with restrictions; Rx, or Schedule II–IV. Status determined by state laws.

Butorphanol

Butorphanol was synthesized in 1971 by Monkovic, approved by the FDA, and introduced in the United States in 1978.[166] Butorphanol is a synthetic agonist-antagonist analgesic similar in pharmacology to nalbuphine. The chemical formula of butorphanol is *levo-N*-cyclobutylmethyl-6,10α,β-dihydroxy-1,2,3,9,10,10α-hexahydro-(4H)-10,4α-iminoethanophenanthrene tartrate. Though not a controlled substance, in June 1997 the DEA recommended that butorphanol be classified as a controlled substance.[166]

Pharmacology

When butorphanol is compared with morphine for analgesia, 2 mg of butorphanol (administered intramuscularly) is approximately as effective as 10 mg of morphine, 80 mg of meperidine, and 40 mg of pentazocine. Data indicate that butorphanol is approximately 3.5 to 7 times as potent as morphine, 15 to 20 times more potent than pentazocine, and 30 to 40 times more potent than meperidine on a weight basis.[167]

Pharmacokinetics

After IV administration, butorphanol's analgesic actions are noted within minutes. Maximum blood levels occur in 5 minutes and thereafter decline in a biphasic manner. The α-half-life of rapid elimination (distribution) is approximately 0.1 hour, and the β-half-life (metabolism and excretion) is 2.15 to 3.5 hours. Duration of analgesic properties is 3 to 4 hours.[168]

Butorphanol undergoes extensive metabolism in the liver before excretion through the kidneys. Less than 5% of a

Nalbuphine	
The medical history of patients receiving nalbuphine should be checked for the following:	

The medical history of patients receiving nalbuphine should be checked for the following:
- Known or suspected opioid dependence
- Allergy or known hypersensitivity to nalbuphine
- Pregnancy or childbearing potential
- Asthma, COPD, or other types of decreased respiratory drive

dose is excreted unchanged in the urine. The major route of elimination of butorphanol and its metabolites is through the kidney (75%), with biliary excretion accounting for 15% of the dose. It is 80% bound to human serum protein and distributed extensively to tissues. Butorphanol is highly lipid soluble and concentrates in adipose tissue and excretory organs. Accumulation may occur with repeated doses of the drug.[169]

Effect on Respiration

Butorphanol has properties similar to those of pentazocine and nalbuphine with respect to respiratory depression and opioid antagonist properties.[168] As an antagonist, butorphanol is 30 times as potent as pentazocine, but only one-fortieth as potent as naloxone. In a study by Nagashima et al, 2- and 4-mg IV doses of butorphanol were compared with 10- and 20-mg doses of morphine.[170] Respiratory depression produced by 4 mg of butorphanol was found to be statistically and clinically equivalent to that produced by 2 mg of butorphanol or 10 mg of morphine. This and other studies have demonstrated that butorphanol does not produce a dose-related effect on respiration in contrast to that observed with opioid agonists, such as morphine and meperidine.

Increasing doses of butorphanol did, however, produce a longer duration of respiratory depression, although the degree of depression did not increase.[171] Butorphanol possesses a ceiling effect only on the degree of respiratory depression, but not for its duration, whereas nalbuphine possesses a ceiling effect on both the depth and duration of respiratory depression. As with other opioid agonists and opioid agonist-antagonists, these respiratory-depressant properties of butorphanol are reversible with naloxone.

Cardiovascular Effects

Unlike nalbuphine, butorphanol does possess cardiovascular effects similar to, but less intense than, those of pentazocine. The administration of butorphanol as part of an IV sedation regimen to cardiovascular-risk patients (ASA 3 and 4) is not recommended. These include increased pulmonary artery pressure, increased pulmonary wedge pressure, increased left ventricular end-diastolic pressure, increased systemic arterial pressure, and increased pulmonary vascular resistance. Both the cardiac index and cardiac workload are increased with butorphanol.[172]

Butorphanol and pentazocine administration should be restricted in patients with acute myocardial infarction, coronary insufficiency or ventricular dysfunction, and high blood pressure (ASA 4 and 5). Butorphanol, like nalbuphine, is an agonist-antagonist analgesic with a low physical-dependence liability, which distinguishes it from traditional potent opioid agonists.

When butorphanol is administered in large doses, the incidence of unpleasant psychotomimetic effects is increased. This factor may serve to limit the abuse potential of butorphanol.

Side Effects

Side effects reported after butorphanol administration are similar to those for other parenteral analgesics. The most frequently reported side effect was sedation (37%), a side effect that is used to advantage during IV moderate sedation. Other common side effects were as follows[166,173]:

Floating, pleasant feelings	7%
Nausea	7%
Clamminess, sweating	5%
Headache	2%
Vertigo	2%
Dizziness	2%
Lethargy	2%

Overdose

Overdose of butorphanol is extremely unlikely; however, it is a clinical possibility. Signs and symptoms relate to exaggerated CNS and respiratory depression. Management consists of basic life support, with consideration for airway patency and ventilation, followed by the administration of naloxone or another opioid antagonist.

Warnings

Because of its opioid antagonist properties, the use of butorphanol is not recommended in patients known to be physically dependent on opioids. Administration in such patients may induce an acute abstinence syndrome (withdrawal).[166,173] Because of the increased workload of the heart occurring with butorphanol administration, this drug is not recommended in patients with ventricular dysfunction or coronary insufficiency.

Precautions

Because butorphanol produces some respiratory depression, it should be administered with caution to patients with preexisting respiratory depression, such as patients receiving other CNS depressants; patients with asthma, COPD, or other types of decreased respiratory reserve; or patients with high blood pressure (ASA 3, 4, or 5).

Patients with hepatic or renal dysfunction may overrespond to usual doses of butorphanol. If it is administered to these patients, the dosage should be adjusted to account for this response. With IV administration, slow titration will minimize this potential response.

Use of butorphanol in patients younger than 18 years or in pregnant patients is not recommended because of a lack of clinical experience to demonstrate its safety in these groups. Ambulatory patients receiving butorphanol must, of course, be cautioned against possible hazardous situations, such as driving a car or operating machinery.[166,173]

Dosage

This author had only limited experience with the use of butorphanol in IV moderate sedation (approximately 115 cases).

However, it has been my impression that butorphanol may effectively be substituted for the traditional opioid agonists with no decrease in effectiveness and with the possible addition of decreased risk of respiratory depression. The doses recommended for IV use should preclude significant respiratory depression, regardless of the pharmacologic properties of butorphanol.

After IV administration of 1 to 2 mg, onset of analgesic and sedative actions is quite rapid (1 to 2 minutes). Administered after diazepam or midazolam, titrated butorphanol usually will not deepen the sedative level of the patient; for this reason the maximum recommended dose (2 mg) is usually given. Recovery from diazepam-butorphanol or midazolam-butorphanol sedation is not as complete clinically as from diazepam or midazolam sedation alone.

Availability

The proprietary name, Stadol, has been discontinued in the United States. Butorphanol generic is supplied as 1 mg/mL in 1-mg/mL and 2 mg/mL.

Butorphanol

The medical history of patients receiving butorphanol should be checked for the following:
- Allergy or known hypersensitivity to butorphanol
- Known or suspected opioid dependence
- Asthma, COPD, or other types of decreased respiratory drive
- High blood pressure
- Cardiovascular disease

Butorphanol

Proprietary name:	Generic
Classification:	Opioid agonist-antagonist
Availability:	1 and 2 mg/mL
Average sedative dose (IV):	1.5 mg
Maximum single dose:	2 mg
Maximum total dose:	2 mg

Butorphanol

Pregnancy category	C
Lactation	Probably safe
Metabolism	Liver, extensively
Excretion	Urine 70%–80%; feces 15%; half-life 4.7 hr; 6.6 hr >65 yr)
DEA schedule	IV

SUMMARY

The mixed opioid agonist-antagonists offer several advantages over pure opioid agonists, such as meperidine, fentanyl, and morphine. Although respiratory depression is a significant consideration in opioid agonist administration, this risk has been reduced (although not eliminated) with the opioid agonist-antagonists. Respiratory problems may still develop with administration of these agents, but appear to be less frequent.

Pentazocine has been available for more than 30 years. It is rarely used intravenously for sedation because of the significant incidence of negative psychotomimetic effects. In addition, it is known today that physical dependence on pentazocine does occur.[138,174]

Butorphanol, a more recent addition to the armamentarium, appears to have fewer significant adverse effects than pentazocine. However, it produces an increase in cardiovascular workload, which mitigates against its use in cardiovascular-risk patients.[166,172]

Nalbuphine appears to have all the advantages of butorphanol; however, it does not increase cardiovascular workload and is an excellent opioid antagonist.[147,165] One additional benefit of butorphanol and nalbuphine is that they are non-scheduled drugs, requiring no special forms or paperwork for their purchase or administration. Pentazocine is a Schedule IV drug, whereas the opioid agonists are Schedule II drugs.

Note: Throughout this discussion of the opioid agonists and opioid agonist-antagonists, it has been mentioned in the "Warnings" and "Precautions" sections that the use of these agents in patients with significant liver or renal dysfunction, or both, and in patients with significant pulmonary disease (COPD) is contraindicated. Please bear in mind that the use of IV moderate sedation was earlier recommended for patients who have been categorized as ASA physical status classifications 1 and 2, with only a selected few ASA 3 patients considered acceptable. The patients mentioned in the "Warnings" and "Precautions" sections are considered, at best, ASA 3 and are usually ASA 4. Adherence to basic tenets of patient selection for IV moderate sedation will minimize the number of problems that may develop in these patients.

OPIOID ANTAGONISTS

The only drug presently available that possesses pure opioid antagonist properties is naloxone. The pharmacology and clinical importance of this drug are reviewed in the section on antidotal drugs.

ANTICHOLINERGICS

Anticholinergics, also known as *belladonna alkaloids* and *cholinergic blocking agents,* are important to the practice of anesthesia and are valuable adjuncts to intravenously administered sedatives. Indications for the use of anticholinergics in the practice of anesthesia and IV moderate sedation include the following:

(1) as preoperative medication to reduce salivary secretions, (2) to treat vagally induced bradycardia, and (3) to reverse muscle paralysis (in general anesthesia) when administered with neostigmine. Three anticholinergics—atropine, scopolamine, and glycopyrrolate—are discussed. These drugs are popular during IV moderate sedation in dentistry, administered primarily for their antisalivary actions. Atropine was formally approved by the FDA in 1938,[175] scopolamine in 1939,[176] but they had been used clinically for many years before that. Glycopyrrolate was approved by the FDA in 1961.[177]

Pharmacology

The belladonna alkaloids are widely distributed in nature. Atropine, chemically a racemic mixture of *levo*- and *dextro*-hyoscyamine (only the *levo* form is pharmacologically active), is found in the following botanicals:

- *Atropa belladonna,* known as the deadly nightshade
- *Datura stramonium,* Jamestown weed, Jimson weed, stinkweed, thorn apple, and devil's apple

Scopolamine, chemically *levo*-hyoscine, is found in the following:

- *Hyoscyamus niger,* black henbane
- *Scopolia carniolica*

Glycopyrrolate, a synthetic anticholinergic, was introduced in 1961. It is a quaternary ammonium compound with the chemical name 1-methyl-3-pyrrolidyl-phenyl-cyclopentane-glycolate methobromide.

Mechanism of Action

The anticholinergics act as competitive antagonists to acetylcholine (Ach) at the postganglionic receptor located at the neuroeffector junction of the parasympathetic nervous system. Although the actions of these drugs are essentially similar, the degree to which the individual drug possesses a certain property may differ. For example, scopolamine has a greater effect on salivary glands than does atropine, but atropine has a greater effect on the heart and bronchial musculature. In clinical doses, atropine does not produce CNS depression; however, scopolamine does and is therefore frequently used as a component in preoperative sedation.

Central Nervous System

Atropine produces a stimulation of the medulla and higher cerebral centers. In clinical doses of 0.5 to 1.0 mg, this effect is noted as a mild vagal stimulation in which both the rate and depth of breathing are increased.[178] This effect is a result of bronchiolar dilation and increased physiologic dead space. Atropine is not effective in reversing significant respiratory depression.

Scopolamine in therapeutic doses produces a degree of CNS depression, clinically noted as drowsiness, euphoria, amnesia, fatigue, and dreamless sleep. Unfortunately, in some patients, the same clinical dose may produce excitement, restlessness, hallucinations, and delirium and is more likely to occur in the presence of pain.[176]

Glycopyrrolate, a quaternary ammonium compound, does not cross the blood–brain barrier. It also does not produce the CNS actions noted for atropine and scopolamine.

In cases in which sedation is a desirable effect, the administration of scopolamine is preferred to either atropine or glycopyrrolate. Scopolamine provides 5 to 15 times the sedative effects of the other two drugs.[178]

Amnesia may be a desirable action of an anticholinergic drug. Of the three, only scopolamine produces this effect. Although amnesia may occur after scopolamine administration, it is not as consistent a finding as it is with midazolam or diazepam. When present, however, amnesia tends to be prolonged, often persisting for 2 to 4 hours. Although anterograde amnesia—lack of recall of events occurring after administration of scopolamine—is most common, retrograde amnesia, the lack of recall of events occurring before administration of the drug, may also occur.[179]

Eye

Anticholinergics block the responses of the sphincter muscle of the iris and the ciliary muscle of the lens to cholinergic stimulation. They therefore produce mydriasis (dilation of the pupil) and cycloplegia (paralysis of accommodation). Administered in therapeutic doses, atropine (0.4 to 0.6 mg) produces little ocular effect. However, scopolamine in therapeutic doses produces significant mydriasis and cycloplegia.

Administered parenterally, the anticholinergics have little effect on intraocular pressure except in patients with acute narrow-angle glaucoma, in whom dangerously high intraocular pressures may develop. This occurs when the iris, which is crowded back into the angle of the anterior chamber of the eye, interferes with drainage of the aqueous humor.[180] In the more commonly seen wide-angle glaucoma, such an increase in intraocular pressure seldom occurs, and the anticholinergics may be used with little increase in risk to the patient. The administration of anticholinergics is contraindicated for patients who wear contact lenses.

Respiratory Tract

The anticholinergic drugs decrease secretions of the nose, mouth, pharynx, and bronchi, thereby drying the mucous membranes of the respiratory tract. This, of course, represents one of the indications for administration of these drugs as preanesthetic medications. Clinically the antisialagogic actions of 0.4 mg of atropine are equal to those of a dose of 0.2 mg of glycopyrrolate.

Bronchial smooth muscle is also dilated after administration of anticholinergic drugs; atropine is considerably more potent in this regard than either scopolamine or glycopyrrolate. Atropine, scopolamine, and glycopyrrolate decrease the incidence of laryngospasm during general anesthesia. This is because of the decrease in respiratory tract secretions that might precipitate reflex laryngospasm, which is produced by contraction of laryngeal skeletal muscle.

Cardiovascular Actions

The principal effect of the anticholinergics on the heart is an alteration in rate. Clinical doses of 0.4 to 0.6 mg of atropine produce a decrease in heart rate of 4 to 8 beats/min. This effect is not seen if the drug is administered rapidly intravenously. Larger doses produce a tachycardia by blocking the effects of the vagus nerve at the sinoatrial (SA) pacemaker. The rate may rise as much as 35 to 40 beats above the resting rate (in a study with young men receiving 2 mg of atropine intramuscularly).[181] This action of the anticholinergics is most notable in young healthy adults in whom vagal tone is great. In very young patients and geriatric patients, atropine may fail to accelerate the heart rate.

Scopolamine in small doses (0.1 to 0.2 mg) produces even more profound cardiac slowing than atropine. With larger doses, the resultant tachycardia is equal to that of atropine, but shorter lived. The heart rate will return to baseline or perhaps result in bradycardia.

Glycopyrrolate produces less tachycardia than either atropine or scopolamine and thus is indicated for use in patients in whom atropine- or scopolamine-induced tachycardia is not desirable. Conversely, in situations in which significant bradycardia has developed, the administration of glycopyrrolate will not provide the desired increase in heart rate. Atropine or scopolamine is necessary at this time.

Gastrointestinal Tract

Therapeutic doses of anticholinergics do not greatly affect gastric secretion. Doses in excess of 1 mg (atropine) must be administered to alter gastric secretion significantly. The anticholinergics have little effect on the secretion of pancreatic juice, bile, or succus entericus.

On the other hand, anticholinergics have profound actions on gastrointestinal motility. In both healthy patients and in those with gastrointestinal disease, therapeutic doses inhibit the motor activity of much of the small and large intestine. Motility is reduced along with muscle tone, in addition to the amplitude and frequency of peristaltic activity. This is termed the *antispasmodic effect of the anticholinergics.*[182]

Secretory Glands

The actions of the anticholinergics on respiratory and digestive tract secretions have been discussed. Even small doses inhibit the activity of sweat glands. The skin becomes hot and dry. If sweating is depressed, body temperature may rise, a finding usually noted only after toxic doses. The lacrimal glands are also inhibited by the anticholinergics, but to a smaller extent than other secretory glands. The secretion of milk is not significantly affected.

Biotransformation

The anticholinergics are rapidly removed from the blood and distributed throughout the body. Atropine is approximately 50% protein bound in the blood. Approximately 13% to 50% of a dose of atropine is found unchanged in the urine. The liver is the primary organ of biotransformation. A small amount of the drug is found in the feces, and an even smaller amount is found in expired air.[183] Less than 1% of a dose of scopolamine is recovered unchanged in the urine.

Atropine

In clinical doses (0.5 to 1 mg), atropine produces stimulation of the medulla and higher cerebral centers, resulting in a mild central vagal stimulation and moderate respiratory stimulation. Its primary IV use is for the reduction of salivary and bronchial secretions.[184]

Contraindications to the administration of atropine include glaucoma, adhesions (synechiae) between the iris and the lens of the eye, and asthma.[175,185] The effects of atropine on the developing fetus are not known with any degree of certainty; therefore, the use of atropine during pregnancy should be reserved for those cases in which its effects are truly important. This effectively rules out its use in most dental situations.

Adverse Reactions

Although systemic tolerance to drug effects varies greatly (the normal distribution curve), Table 25.4 lists the "normal" response to increasing doses of atropine.

Table 25.4	Normal Response to Increasing Doses of Atropine
DOSE (mg)	**EFFECT**
0.5	Slight dryness of nose and mouth
	Bradycardia
1.0	Greater dryness of nose and mouth, with thirst
	Slowing, then acceleration, of the heart
	Mydriasis
2.0	Very dry mouth
	Tachycardia with palpitation
	Mydriasis
	Slight blurring of near vision
	Flushed, dry skin
5.0	Increase in the preceding symptoms plus the following:
	Disturbance of speech
	Difficulty in swallowing
	Headache
	Hot, dry skin
	Restlessness with asthenia (lack of energy)
10.0	The preceding symptoms to an extreme degree plus the *following*:
	Ataxia
	Excitement
	Disorientation
	Hallucinations
	Delirium
	Coma

Table 25.5	Atropine Doses for Children	
Weight		
KG	LB	DOSE (mg)
3–7	7–16	0.1
8–11	17–24	0.15
12–18	25–40	0.2
19–29	41–65	0.3
30–41	66–90	0.4
>41	>90	0.4–0.6

Intoxication to atropine has been described as follows: "Dry as a bone, red as a beet, and mad as a hatter."[186] Fortunately, atropine intoxication is rarely fatal if rapidly diagnosed and antidotal therapy instituted. Physostigmine, 1 to 5 mL of a dilution of 1 mg of physostigmine in 5 mL (0.2 mg/mL) administered intravenously, is the drug of choice in the management of this reaction. The dose may be repeated every 5 minutes if necessary for a total dose of 2 mg in children and 6 mg in adults.[187]

Dosage

The usual adult dose of atropine is 0.4 to 0.6 mg. Recommended doses for children are found in Table 25.5.

Availability

Atropine sulfate: 0.05 and 0.1 mg/mL. Atropine is not a scheduled drug.

Atropine Sulfate

The medical history of patients receiving atropine sulfate should be checked for the following:
- Glaucoma
- Prostate disease
- Asthma
- Adhesions between iris and lens of eye
- Myasthenia gravis
- Contact lenses

Atropine Sulfate

Classification:	Anticholinergic
Availability:	0.3–1.3 mg/mL
Average therapeutic dose:	0.4–0.6 min
Maximum single dose:	0.4–0.6 mg
Maximum total dose:	0.4–0.6 mg

Atropine Sulfate

Pregnancy category	C
Lactation	Probably safe
Metabolism	Liver
Excretion	Urine primarily (13%–50% unchanged); half-life 2–3 hr
DEA schedule	Not controlled, prescription required

Scopolamine Hydrobromide

Scopolamine hydrobromide differs in several significant ways from atropine. Scopolamine can produce a degree of CNS depression, whereas atropine does not. Scopolamine is a frequently used constituent of preanesthetic medication. In this regard, scopolamine provides the following beneficial effects:
- Decreases in salivary and bronchial secretions
- Some sedative effect (minor)
- Anterograde amnesia

The latter two effects are unique to scopolamine and form the basis for its use in anesthesia practice.[188] Unfortunately, scopolamine is also more apt to produce the phenomenon known as *emergence delirium* than either atropine or glycopyrrolate.[176] Because this reaction, which involves vivid dreaming, nightmares, and hallucinations, develops most often in very young and elderly patients, the use of scopolamine in patients younger than 6 years and older than 65 years is discouraged.[176,189]

Dosage

The usual adult therapeutic dose is 0.32 to 0.65 mg. Recommended doses for children are found in Table 25.6.[190]

Availability

Scopolamine hydrobromide (Hope Pharmaceuticals): 0.4 mg/mL.

Scopolamine is not a scheduled drug.

Scopolamine Hydrobromide

The medical history of patients receiving scopolamine hydrobromide should be checked for the following:
- Glaucoma
- Adhesions between iris and lens
- Asthma
- Prostatic disease
- Myasthenia gravis
- Contact lenses

Table 25.6	Scopolamine Hydrobromide Doses for Children
AGE	**DOSE (mg)**
6 mo to 3 yr	0.1–0.15
3–6 yr	0.15–0.2
6–12 yr	0.2–0.3

Scopolamine Hydrobromide	
Classification:	Anticholinergic
Availability:	0.3–0.6 mg/mL
Average therapeutic dose:	0.3 mg
Maximum single dose:	0.3 mg
Maximum total dose:	0.3 mg

Scopolamine Hydrobromide	
Pregnancy category	C
Lactation	Caution in nursing
Metabolism	Liver extensively
Excretion	Urine (<5% unchanged); half-life 8 hr
DEA schedule	Not controlled, prescription required

Glycopyrrolate

Glycopyrrolate is a quaternary ammonium compound. As such it does not cross lipid membranes such as the blood–brain barrier; this is in contrast to both atropine and scopolamine. Glycopyrrolate is less likely to produce unwanted CNS depression or delirium-type reactions.

After IV administration, the onset of clinical action develops within 1 minute. Glycopyrrolate has a duration of action of vagal blocking effects for 2 to 3 hours and antisialagogue effects for up to 7 hours.[191] This latter effect may be undesirable in the ambulatory patient.

Warnings

Ambulatory patients receiving glycopyrrolate must be advised not to perform hazardous work, operate machinery, or drive a motor vehicle because the drug may produce drowsiness or blurred vision.[177,192] In the presence of a high environmental temperature, heat prostration (heat stroke and fever caused by decreased sweating) can occur with the use of glycopyrrolate.

Precautions

Glycopyrrolate should be used with caution in patients with tachycardia because the drug may cause a further increase in the heart rate.[192] In addition, patients with ischemic heart disease, coronary artery disease, heart failure, dysrhythmias, hypertension, or hyperthyroidism should be evaluated carefully before administration of glycopyrrolate.

Although glycopyrrolate has been shown to be nonteratogenic in animal studies, its effect on the human fetus is unknown; therefore the use of glycopyrrolate in pregnancy is not recommended and should be reserved for those cases in whom it is truly required.

Dosage

The usual therapeutic dose of glycopyrrolate in adults is 0.1 mg (0.5 mL) as needed and may be repeated every 2 to 3 minutes. In children, the IV dose of glycopyrrolate is 0.02 mg (0.1 mL) per pound of body weight, not to exceed a dose of 0.1 mg (0.5 mL) in a single dose. As with the adult, this dose may be repeated every 2 to 3 minutes as needed.

Availability

Robinul (West-Ward Pharmaceutical Corp): 0.2 mg/mL.
Glycopyrrolate is not a scheduled drug.

Glycopyrrolate
The medical history of patients receiving glycopyrrolate should be checked for the following:
• Allergy to glycopyrrolate
• Glaucoma
• Prostatic disease
• Asthma
• Myasthenia gravis
• Ischemic heart disease
• Contact lenses

Glycopyrrolate	
Proprietary name:	Robinul
Classification:	Anticholinergic
Availability:	0.2 mg/mL
Average therapeutic dose:	0.1 mg
Maximum single dose:	0.1 mg
Maximum total dose:	0.2 mg

Glycopyrrolate	
Pregnancy category	B
Lactation	Safety unknown
Metabolism	Unknown
Excretion	Urine 85% (>80% unchanged), bile (>80% unchanged); half-life 0.83 hr
DEA schedule	Not controlled, prescription required

SUMMARY

The anticholinergics serve primarily as adjunctive drugs during IV sedation in outpatients. The selection of the appropriate anticholinergic will be based on the indication for its use; for example:

- Longer procedures (more than 2 to 3 hours): glycopyrrolate
- Amnesia: scopolamine
- Sedation: scopolamine
- Decreased cardiovascular action: glycopyrrolate
- Short procedure, no amnesia, no sedation: atropine

Anticholinergics may be administered in combination with any of the drugs discussed in this section, with the notable exception of lorazepam (Ativan). The use of scopolamine is not recommended in conjunction with lorazepam because of the intense amnesic effect and the increased possibility of emergence delirium produced by this combination.[193]

KETAMINE

Ketamine hydrochloride is a cyclohexane derivative closely related chemically and pharmacologically to phencyclidine, a veterinary anesthetic and drug of abuse (known as *angel dust*). It is a sedative hypnotic used to provide anesthesia for short diagnostic and surgical procedures, as an induction agent, as an adjunct to supplement low-potency anesthetics such as nitrous oxide, and as a supplement to local and regional anesthesia.[194]

Anesthesia produced by ketamine has been termed *dissociative anesthesia*.[195] It is a state in which the patient appears awake, has his or her eyes open, and is capable of (involuntary) muscular movement, but appears to be unaware of or dissociated from the environment. Another term for the state induced by ketamine is *cataleptic anesthesia*. Profound analgesia and amnesia are associated with ketamine administration. Ketamine received FDA approval in 1970.[194]

Ketamine is similar in structure, mechanism of action, and activity to phencyclidine (PCP), but ketamine is much less potent and has a shorter duration of action. Ketamine has been associated with substance abuse and illicit use. Reportedly, ketamine has been used to facilitate rape (i.e., acquaintance or date rape) because the drug can be easily administered in beverages to unknowing victims. Slang terms for ketamine include K, Special K, Keets, Green, Jet, Super Acid, and Super C.[196] Ketamine is also widely used in veterinary medicine.

The dissociative state produced by ketamine is an excitatory state, completely dissimilar from that seen after administration of traditional general anesthetics, such as isoflurane, sevoflurane, propofol, and fentanyl. Ketamine has a sympathomimetic activity resulting in tachycardia, hypertension, increased myocardial and cerebral oxygen consumption, increased cerebral blood flow, and increased intracranial and intraocular pressure. Ketamine is a potent bronchodilator and can be used to treat refractory bronchospasm. Clinical effects observed following ketamine administration include increased blood pressure, increased muscle tone (may resemble catatonia), opening of eyes (usually accompanied by nystagmus), increased myocardial oxygen consumption, and minimal respiratory depression. Ketamine has no effects on pharyngeal or laryngeal reflexes; thus the patient's airway remains intact.[194] When used in dental procedures, it is important to place an oropharyngeal pack to prevent contamination of the pharynx and/or larynx with debris.

In the operating room, IV ketamine is used for short procedures, such as dilatation and curettage (D&C), surgical procedures on the skin, or dental procedures, such as extraction or restorative dentistry in pediatric patients. Another use of ketamine is in patients in whom numerous surgical procedures will be required, such as burn victims requiring multiple débridements and skin grafts over a brief period.

The onset of action of ketamine after IV administration is rapid (less than 1 minute), with a duration of clinical effect of approximately 10 minutes.[197] The usual IV induction dose of ketamine is 1 to 4.5 mg/kg (approximately 0.5 to 2 mg/lb) administered over 1 minute. More rapid administration results in respiratory depression and an exaggerated pressor response. The duration of anesthesia may be extended with readministration of ketamine in doses of 0.5 mg/kg. Recovery from ketamine anesthesia is prolonged when larger doses of ketamine are administered. An even more effective method of prolonging ketamine anesthesia is by administering local anesthesia for pain control and nitrogen-oxide-oxygen (N_2O-O_2) for additional CNS depression. Administration of these drugs along with ketamine reduces the dose of ketamine required, speeds recovery, and minimizes adverse recovery room phenomena (hallucinations).

Recovery from ketamine-induced anesthesia is prolonged and often associated with vivid dreams, hallucinations, and delirium.[198] These emergence reactions are significantly more common in adults than in children and may last from minutes to hours. Flashbacks—recurrence of these experiences—have occurred months after the administration of ketamine. This is somewhat similar to flashbacks occurring after administration of LSD. Sussman reported that 24% of patients older than 16 years reported emergence reactions, whereas only 8% of those younger than 16 years had the same response.[199] Patients older than 65 years have decreased incidence of adverse emergence phenomena. The incidence of recovery phenomena may be minimized if the patient is permitted to remain undisturbed in a quiet, darkened recovery area.[200] IM administration of ketamine is associated with a decreased incidence of these reactions.

Ketamine is commonly used in the younger patient as an induction agent (via IM administration), after which an IV infusion is started and the patient maintained with IV ketamine or other IV or inhalation agents as needed. Ketamine is also used as an anesthetic agent for diagnostic procedures, for minor operations of shorter duration, and for patients undergoing multiple procedures under a general anesthetic.

Having considerable experience with ketamine anesthesia with both inpatients and outpatients, I adamantly believe that ketamine use should be limited to those doctors who have completed a residency in anesthesiology, have experience with ketamine (because it is so different from "traditional" general anesthetics), and have adequate recovery room facilities and monitoring available in the office.

> **The administration of ketamine for IV moderate sedation by non-general anesthesia trained dentists is *not* recommended.**

ANTIDOTAL DRUGS

In concluding this section on the pharmacology of drugs recommended for IV moderate sedation, several others demand attention. These drugs are used but rarely; however, like an umbrella on a cloudy day, their ready availability is important. This group is called antidotal drugs because their use is reserved for reversing adverse effects of drugs that have been previously administered. The following categories of drugs are included:

- Opioid antagonist
- Benzodiazepine antagonist
- Agent for reversal of emergence delirium
- Vasodilator for extravascular or intraarterial drug administration

Each of these categories should be represented in the emergency kit of any doctor administering parenteral sedation by the subcutaneous (SC), IM, or IV routes or IV general anesthesia.

Opioid Antagonists

The most significant side effect of opioid analgesics is respiratory depression. This, more than anything else, limits their use in outpatient dentistry. Less-than-adequate monitoring of respiratory efforts in the sedated patient has led to significant morbidity and death.[201] Management of respiratory depression is reviewed in Chapter 27 and potentially includes the administration of an opioid antagonist. IV administration of an opioid antagonist rapidly reverses the respiratory-depressant effects of the opioid agonist.

The first opioid antagonist, nalorphine, became available in 1951, followed a year later by levallorphan. Both of these drugs reverse the analgesic effects of opioids and their respiratory-depressant properties. Administered to an opioid-dependent individual, these drugs induce acute abstinence syndrome (withdrawal). When administered in the absence of opioid-induced respiratory depression, both nalorphine and levallorphan are capable of producing respiratory depression and of enhancing respiratory depression produced by barbiturates.[202]

In the late 1960s, naloxone was introduced and has replaced both levallorphan and nalorphine as the drug of choice in reversing opioid-induced respiratory depression. It is the only opioid antagonist currently available that is free of opioid agonist effects.[203] Naloxone was approved by the FDA in 1971.

Auto-injector and nasal spray formulations of naloxone are now available, specific for use in opioid overdose outside of a medical setting[204-206]

Naloxone

Naloxone is a semisynthetic congener of the opioid analgesic oxymorphone from which it differs by the replacement of the methyl group on the nitrogen (N_2) atom by an allyl group.[203] Naloxone hydrochloride is soluble in water and dilute acids and strong alkali. It is only slightly soluble in alcohol and practically insoluble in ether and chloroform.

Naloxone hydrochloride is a pure opioid antagonist. It does not possess any "agonistic" or opioid-type properties. Naloxone does not produce respiratory depression, unlike levallorphan and nalorphine, nor does it produce psychotomimetic effects or miosis. When administered in the absence of opioids, naloxone exhibits essentially no pharmacologic activity. Administered to a patient who is physically dependent on opioids, naloxone induces withdrawal symptoms. Naloxone in and of itself does not produce tolerance or lead to physical or psychological dependence.

Following IV administration of naloxone, improvement in respiration may be observed in 1 to 2 minutes. The duration of naloxone's effect is relatively short after IV use (about 30 minutes). The duration of respiratory depression produced by the opioid varies considerably with different opioids. It is therefore possible for naloxone to successfully reverse opioid-induced respiratory depression, only to have respiratory depression recur later after the clinical activity of naloxone has regressed. For this reason, it has become common practice to administer an IM dose of naloxone following the IV dose. Onset of action following IM administration of naloxone is 2 to 5 minutes. Onset may be delayed in hypotensive patients.[204] The IM dose provides a longer duration of clinical action. After the administration of naloxone, the patient should not be discharged from the office for 2 hours so that any recurrence of respiratory depression may be recognized and managed by readministration of naloxone, if necessary.

Naloxone is indicated for use in opioid depression, including respiratory depression, induced by any of the natural or synthetic opioids, propoxyphene, and the opioid agonist-antagonists pentazocine, nalbuphine, and butorphanol.

Contraindications

Naloxone is contraindicated for use in patients who are allergic or hypersensitive to it.

Warnings. Naloxone must be administered with extreme care to persons with known or suspected physical dependence on opioids. The abrupt and complete reversal of opioid agonist effects may precipitate an acute abstinence syndrome. After naloxone reversal of opioid-induced respiratory depression, the patient must be kept under surveillance in the event that repeated doses of naloxone might be needed. Respiratory depression produced by nonopioids (e.g., benzodiazepines, barbiturates) is not reversed by naloxone.

Precautions. In the event of opioid-induced respiratory depression, naloxone is neither the most important nor the first step in patient management. Of greater importance is patency of the airway and adequate ventilation. All persons administering parenteral opioid analgesics must be capable of maintaining the airway of the unconscious patient and of assisting or controlling the ventilation of the patient.

Adverse reactions. Administered to patients in the absence of opioids, naloxone is essentially free of any side effects. In the presence of opioids, abrupt reversal of opioid depression may produce the following:
- Nausea and vomiting
- Sweating
- Tachycardia
- Increased blood pressure
- Tremulousness

In the presence of pain, reversal of opioid depression by large doses (greater than 0.4 mg) of naloxone may also significantly reverse analgesia, resulting in extreme discomfort and excitement. It has been reported in cardiac-risk patients that rapid reversal of opioid-induced respiratory depression by large doses of naloxone has produced tachycardia and dramatic elevations in blood pressure, resulting in left ventricular failure and pulmonary edema.[207]

Dosage

Naloxone may be administered subcutaneously, intramuscularly, or intravenously. As mentioned, the onset of action after IV administration is 1 to 2 minutes. After IM or SC administration, approximately 10 minutes may be required for onset of action. Duration of action is 30 minutes after IV administration and 1 to 4 hours following IM or SC administration. The potency of naloxone will be greater after IV administration.[208]

For the adult: Initially, titrated at 0.1 to 0.2 mg IV at 2- to 3-minute intervals until the desired response is obtained.[204,208] Naloxone is diluted to a concentration of 0.1 mg/mL. This is accomplished by taking 1 mL of the 0.4-mg/mL concentration and adding 3 mL of diluent (e.g., 5% dextrose and water). Every 2 to 3 minutes, 0.1 to 0.2 mg should be injected slowly intravenously while the patient is observed for adequate reversal of respiratory depression: increased ventilation effort and increased alertness without significant pain or discomfort.

Additional doses of naloxone may be required in some patients, depending on the type and dose of opioid administered and the patient's response to naloxone. If repeated administration of naloxone is necessary, it is recommended that the IM route be given serious consideration because the duration of action of naloxone will be prolonged by this route of administration.

In children 5 years or older or weighing more than 20 kg: initially, 0.005 to 0.01 mg IV at 2- to 3-minute intervals until the desired degree of reversal is obtained.[209] The dose may be administered intramuscularly or subcutaneously if systemic perfusion is adequate. If, for some reason, naloxone must be administered subcutaneously or intramuscularly, the adult dose is 0.4 mg and the pediatric dose is 0.01 mg/kg. The onset of action is slower; however, the duration of action will be significantly longer than noted after IV administration.

Availability

Narcan (brand discontinued in the United States; available as generic): adults and children, 0.4 mg/mL.

Naloxone is not a scheduled drug.

Naloxone
The medical history of patients receiving naloxone should be checked for the following: • Allergy or known hypersensitivity to naloxone • Opioid dependence

Naloxone	
Proprietary name:	Generic
Classification:	Opioid antagonist
Availability:	0 0.4 mg/mL
Average reversal dose (IV):	0.4 mg (adult)
Maximum single dose:	0.4 mg (adult)
Maximum total dose:	1.2 mg (adult)* *Lack of improvement after two or three doses usually indicates that respiratory depression is not produced by opioids.

Naloxone	
Pregnancy category	B
Lactation	Safety unknown
Metabolism	Liver
Excretion	Urine (half-life 64 min)
DEA schedule	May be over-the-counter (OTC), OTC with restrictions, Rx, or Schedule II–V; status determined by state laws

SUMMARY

The availability of drugs capable of reversing significant undesirable effects of opioids is quite important. However, it is significantly more important to remember that the occasion to use these drugs will almost never develop if IV sedatives and opioids are administered in a reasonable manner (e.g., titrated to clinical effect). The maximum doses of opioids recommended in this and in succeeding chapters will not produce respiratory depression in any but the most debilitated or acutely hyperresponsive patients. However, maximum doses rarely must be administered. Adequate clinical effects are usually obtained with doses below these maximums. The secret to success and safety with opioids, as with all drugs, is slow titration of the drug to the desired effect.

In more than 40 years of teaching IV moderate ("conscious") sedation on the doctoral, postdoctoral, and continuing education levels, I have never treated a patient who required an opioid antagonist for reversal of opioid-induced respiratory depression. Having the drug readily available is absolutely essential if opioids of any type are administered by any route. Routine opioid reversal, recommended by some, is unnecessary and may in some cases increase patient risk (as in cases in which postoperative pain is present, overstressing the cardiovascular system).

Benzodiazepine Antagonist

Although the benzodiazepines have been described as the most nearly ideal drugs for anxiety control and sedation, there are still adverse drug reactions (ADRs) associated with their administration. Emergence delirium, excessive duration of sedation, and possible respiratory depression are but a few of these ADRs. Though rare, their occurrence can wreak havoc on a procedure. Flumazenil, a specific benzodiazepine antagonist, was introduced into clinical practice in the late 1980s and in the United States in 1992. Flumazenil was approved by the FDA in December 1991.[210]

Flumazenil, administered intravenously after the IV administration of midazolam, diazepam, and other benzodiazepines, produces a rapid reversal of sedation and improved ability to comprehend and obey commands.[211] Flumazenil will also antagonize the sedative actions of zolpidem (Ambien) and eszopiclone (Lunesta).[210] Administered intravenously, the drug rapidly enters the brain with an onset of action of 1 to 2 minutes. Peak concentrations are dose proportional and occur 1 to 3 minutes after its administration. Flumazenil also reduces the duration of anterograde amnesia produced with midazolam: 91 minutes (with flumazenil) compared with 121 minutes (no flumazenil).[212,213] When administered in a geriatric population (72 ± 9 years) following midazolam sedation, patients required less recovery time from sedation and demonstrated increased alertness and a decreased amnesic effect. Two patients became somewhat anxious following flumazenil administration.[213]

Whereas flumazenil reverses benzodiazepine-induced sedation, it has no proven effectiveness in the treatment of hypoventilation induced by benzodiazepines.

Adults: Initially, 0.2 mg IV. The dose may be repeated after 45 seconds if the desired level of consciousness is not achieved, and subsequently at 1-minute intervals, until a maximum of four doses have been administered (1 mg total over 5-minute period). If resedation occurs, repeat the regimen at 20-minute intervals, up to a maximum of 3 mg/hour.[214]

Adolescents and children: Initially, 0.01 mg/kg IV (max: 0.2 mg) administered over 15 seconds. The dose may be repeated after 45 seconds if the desired level of consciousness is not achieved, and subsequently at 1-minute intervals (maximum of four additional times) up to a maximum cumulative dose of 0.05 mg/kg or 1 mg, whichever is lower.[214] Safety and efficacy of flumazenil administration in pediatric patients experiencing resedation have not been established.[214]

Flumazenil is used clinically as a means of terminating oversedation or overdose associated with the benzodiazepines. The "routine" administration of flumazenil at the termination of every IV benzodiazepine procedure is unnecessary and not recommended.

Dosage

Initial IV dose of 0.2 mg (2 mL) and subsequently at 1-minute intervals, until a maximum of four doses have been administered (1 mg total over 5-minute period).[214]

Availability

Romazicon (Genentech) is supplied in 5-mL multiple-use vials containing 0.1 mg/mL flumazenil.

Flumazenil
The medical history of patients receiving flumazenil should be checked for the following: • Allergy or known hypersensitivity to flumazenil or benzodiazepines • Patients who have been given benzodiazepines for control of a life-threatening condition, such as status epilepticus, or control of intracranial pressure

Flumazenil	
Proprietary name:	Romazicon
Classification:	Benzodiazepine antagonist
Availability:	0.1 mg/mL
Average reversal dose (IV):	0.2 mg
Maximum single dose:	0.2 mg every 45 seconds
Maximum total dose:	1.0 mg

Flumazenil	
Pregnancy category	C
Lactation	Safety unknown
Metabolism	Liver extensively
Excretion	Urine (90–95%) <1% unchanged; feces 5–10%; half-life 54 min
DEA schedule	Not controlled, requires prescription (Rx)

Reversal of Emergence Delirium

Several of the drugs previously discussed in this chapter have the disturbing ability to produce what is known as *emergence delirium.*[215] During recovery from clinical sedation with a benzodiazepine or scopolamine (the drugs used in dentistry most likely to produce emergence delirium), the patient appears to lose contact with reality. There may be increased muscular activity, and the patient may speak, but is unintelligible. A variety of clinical responses may be noted; however, in all of them, it is apparent that the patient is not returning to his or her "normal" state of consciousness. Until the mid-1970s, management of emergence delirium consisted of monitoring the patient and symptomatic treatment. Antidotal therapy was not available.

Physostigmine

Physostigmine is a reversible anticholinesterase similar in action to neostigmine, with the important difference that neostigmine, a quaternary compound, does not cross the blood–brain barrier, whereas physostigmine, a tertiary ammonium compound, readily crosses it. Physostigmine was synthesized in 1935 and accepted by the FDA as a pre-1938 drug.[216]

Actions

Physostigmine is extracted from the seeds of *Physostigma venenosum* (Calabar bean). It is a reversible anticholinesterase that increases the concentration of ACh at cholinergic transmission sites. The action of ACh is normally quite transient because of its rapid hydrolysis by the enzyme anticholinesterase. Physostigmine inhibits this action of anticholinesterase and thereby prolongs and intensifies the actions of ACh.[217]

Because it is a tertiary ammonium compound, physostigmine crosses the blood–brain barrier to reverse the central toxic effects of anticholinergia and emergence delirium: anxiety, delirium, disorientation, hallucinations, hyperactivity, and seizures. Physostigmine is rapidly metabolized (60 to 120 minutes).

Contraindications

Physostigmine should not be administered to patients with asthma, diabetes, cardiovascular disease, or mechanical obstruction of the gastrointestinal or genitourinary tracts.[216,218]

Warnings

Physostigmine may produce excessive salivation, emesis, urination, and defecation. These are unlikely to develop if the drug is administered intravenously at a rate of 1 mg/min. More rapid administration can produce the preceding signs and symptoms as well as bradycardia; hypersalivation, leading to respiration difficulties; and possibly convulsions.

Precautions

Atropine sulfate should always be available whenever physostigmine is administered because it is an antagonist and antidote for physostigmine.

Dosage

Adults: 0.5 to 2 mg IM or slow IV (not to exceed 1 mg/min IV). May repeat every 10 to 30 minutes as needed. For overdoses of drugs that cause toxic anticholinergic effects, the manufacturer recommends a dose of 2 mg IM or slow IV; repeat if life-threatening signs, such as dysrhythmia, convulsions, or coma, occur. For postanesthesia care, the manufacturer recommends a dose of 0.5 to 1 mg IM or slow IV; may repeat every 10 to 30 minutes as needed.[218] Peak effects are seen in approximately 5 minutes when given IV. Cholinesterase hydrolyzes physostigmine, making its duration of action approximately 1 to 2 hours when given IV.[216]

Children

0.02 mg/kg (range 0.01 to 0.03 mg/kg) IM or slow IV (not to exceed 0.5 mg/min IV); may repeat at 5- to 10-minute intervals as needed until a total dose of 2 mg is reached or an adverse cholinergic reaction occurs.[218] Reserve use for life-threatening situations only.

Availability

The proprietary name, Antilirium, is no longer available in the United States. Physostigmine is available as 1.0 mg/mL.

Physostigmine is not a scheduled drug.

Physostigmine

The medical history of patients receiving physostigmine should be checked for the following:
- Asthma
- Diabetes mellitus
- Cardiovascular disease
- Mechanical obstruction of gastrointestinal or genitourinary tract

---

Physostigmine

Proprietary name:	Generic
Classification:	Reversible anticholinesterase
Availability:	1 mg/mL
Average therapeutic dose (IV):	0.5–2.0 mg
Maximum single dose:	2 mg
Maximum total dose:	4 mg

Physostigmine

Pregnancy category	C
Lactation	Safety unknown
Metabolism	Hydrolysis
Excretion	Urine minimally; half-life 15–40 min
DEA schedule	Not controlled; prescription required

SUMMARY

Although emergence delirium is an uncommon complication of sedation procedures, it does occur. It is most often seen following administration of scopolamine to a patient who is under 6 years old or older than 65 years old. Management of emergence delirium is based primarily on symptomatic treatment. Physostigmine administration hastens the reversal of signs and symptoms.

It is important to note that agitation and excessive movement during or after sedation may also be a sign of hypoxia. The patency of the patient's airway and oxygenation of the lungs must always be considered before administration of a drug for what is presumed to be emergence delirium.

Vasodilator for Extravascular or Intraarterial Drug Administration
Procaine

Procaine, the last of the antidotal drugs recommended for the emergency kit of the doctor administering parenteral sedation or general anesthesia, is a local anesthetic with significant vasodilating properties. The following are indications for use of this drug:

- Extravascular administration of an irritating chemical
- Intraarterial administration of a drug

In both cases, the major problem is that of compromised circulation to either a localized area of tissue (extravascular injection) or a limb (intraarterial). Proper management requires the immediate restoration of blood flow.

A property of all injectable local anesthetics (with the notable exception of cocaine) is vasodilation. Of the available injectable local anesthetics, procaine (Novocain) possesses the most vasodilating effects. This property makes procaine less effective as a local anesthetic (without addition of a vasopressor), but makes it eminently suitable for reversal of blood vessel spasm.

Procaine should be used in a 1% concentration without vasopressor. More detailed discussion of management of these problems is found in Chapter 27.

Dosage

For management of extravascular drug administration, 1 to 5 mL of 1% procaine is administered as described in Chapter 27. For intraarterial administration, 1 to 2 mL of 1% procaine is usually sufficient.

Availability

The proprietary name, Novocain, is not available in the United States. Generic procaine is available as 1% procaine in 2-mL and 6-mL ampules and 30-mL vials.

Procaine	
Proprietary name:	Generic
Classification:	Local anesthetic
Availability:	1% (10 mg/mL)
Average reversal dose (IV):	1–5 mL
Maximum single dose:	1–5 mL
Maximum total dose:	5 mL

Procaine	
Pregnancy category	C
Lactation	Safety unknown
Metabolism	Plasma cholinesterase
Excretion	Urine (<2% unchanged); half-life 40 sec
DEA schedule	Not controlled; prescription required

Procaine
The medical history of patients receiving procaine should be checked for the following: • Allergy or known hypersensitivity to ester type of local anesthetics   • Familial history of atypical plasma cholinesterase

REFERENCES

1. ClinicalKey. Flunitrazepam drug monograph. www.clinicalkey.com. June 30, 2002. (Accessed 16 February 2016).
2. Giovannitti JA, Trapp LD: Adult sedation: oral, rectal, IM, IV. In Dionne RA, Phero JC, editors: *Management of pain and anxiety in dental practice*, New York, 1991, Elsevier.
3. Davidau A: Premedication for problem patients or for long-lasting treatments. *Rev Stomatol Chir Maxillofac* 67(10):589–595, 1966.
4. Main DMG: The use of diazepam in dental anaesthesia. In Knight PF, Burgess CG, editors: *Diazepam in anaesthesia*, Bristol, 1968, John Wright.
5. Brown PRH, Main DMG, Wood N: Intravenous sedation in dentistry: a study of 55 cases using pentazocine and diazepam. *Br Dent J* 139(2):59–60, 1975.
6. O'Neill R, Verrill P: Intravenous diazepam in minor surgery. *Br J Oral Surg* 7(1):12–14, 1969.
7. O'Neill R, Verrill PF, Aellig WH, Laurence DR: Intravenous diazepam in minor oral surgery. Further studies. *Br Dent J* 128(1):15–18, 1970.
8. Trieger N: Intravenous sedation in dentistry and oral surgery. *Int Anesthesiol Clin* 27(2):83–91, 1989.
9. Trieger N: Intravenous sedation. In Trieger N, editor: *Pain control*, ed 2, St Louis, 1974, Mosby., pp 98–122.
10. Foreman PA: Diazepam in dentistry: clinical observations based on the treatment of 167 patients in general dental practice. *Anesth Prog* 15(9):253–259, 1968.
11. Foreman PA: Intravenous diazepam in general dental practice. *NZ Dent J* 65(302):243–253, 1969.
12. Danneberg P, Weber KH: Chemical structure and biological activity of the diazepines. *Br J Clin Pharmacol* 16(Suppl 2):231S–244S, 1983.
13. Joseph R: The limbic system: emotion, laterality and unconscious mind. *Psychoanal Rev* 79(3):405–456, 1991.
14. Medina JH, Novas ML, DeRoberts E: Chronic RO 15-1788 treatment increases the number of benzodiazepine receptors in rat cerebral cortex and hippocampus. *Eur J Pharmacol* 90(1):125–128, 1983.

15. Haefely W: The biological basis of benzodiazepine actions. *J Psychoactive Drugs* 15(1):19–39, 1983.

16. Jack ML, Colburn WA, Spirt NM, et al: A pharmacokinetic/ pharmacodynamic/receptor binding model to predict the onset and duration of pharmacological activity of the benzodiazepines. *Prog Neuropsychopharmacol Biol Psychiatry* 7(4-6):629–635, 1983.

17. Ghoneim MM, Mewaldt SP, Hinrichs JV: Behavioral effects of oral versus intravenous administration of diazepam. *Pharmacol Biochem Behav* 21(2):231–236, 1984.

18. Colburn WA, Gibson M: Composite pharmacokinetic profiling. *J Pharm Sci* 73(11):1667–1669, 1984.

19. Baird ES, Hailey DM: Delayed recovery from a sedative: correlation of the plasma levels of diazepam with clinical effects after oral and intravenous administration. *Br J Anaesth* 144(8):803–808, 1972.

20. Vree TB, Hekster CA, vander Kleijn E: Significance of apparent half-lives of a metabolite with a higher elimination rate than its parent drug. *Drug Intell Clin Pharm* 16(2):126–131, 1982.

21. Salzman C, Shader RI, Greenblatt DJ, Harmatz JS: Long v. short half-life benzodiazepines in the elderly. Kinetics and clinical effects of diazepam and oxazepam. *Arch Gen Psychiatr* 40(3):293–297, 1983.

22. Greenblatt DJ, Divoll M, Abernethy DR, et al: Benzodiazepine kinetics: implications for therapeutics and pharmacogeriatrics. *Drug Metab Rev* 14(2):251–292, 1983.

23. Pacifici GM, Cuoci L, Placidi GF, et al: Elimination of kinetics of desmethyldiazepam in two young and two elderly subjects. *Eur J Drug Metab Pharmacokinet* 7(1):69–72, 1982.

24. Pomara N, Stanley B, Block R, et al: Adverse effects of single therapeutic doses of diazepam on performance in normal geriatric subjects: relationship to plasma concentrations. *Psychopharmacology (Berl)* 84(3):342–346, 1984.

25. Zbinden G, Randall LO: Pharmacology of benzodiazepines: laboratory and clinical correlations. *Adv Pharmacol* 5:213–291, 1967.

26. Ausinch B, Malagodi MH, Munson ES: Diazepam in the prophylaxis of lignocaine seizures. *Br J Anaesth* 48(4):309–313, 1976.

27. de Jong RH: Clinical physiology of local anesthetic action. In Cousins MJ, Bridenbaugh PO, editors: *Neural blockade*, ed 2, Philadelphia, 1988, Lippincott.

28. Ramsay RE: Treatment of status epilepticus. *Epilepsia* 34(Suppl 1):S71–S81, 1993.

29. Yamanouchi H: Treatment of status epilepticus. *Nippon Rinsho* 72(5):895–901, 2014.

30. Darmansjah I, Muchtar A: Dose-response variation among different populations. *Clin Pharmacol Ther* 52(2):449–452, 1992.

31. Luo A, Huang Y, Liu Y, et al: Midazolam as a main anesthesia induction agent: a comparison with thiopental and diazepam. *Chin Med Sci J* 6(3):172–174, 1991.

32. Jacka MJ, Johnson GD, Milne B: Diazepam's effect on systemic vascular resistance during cardiopulmonary bypass is not caused by its vehicle (alcohol-propylene glycol). *J Cardiothorac Vasc Anesth* 7(1):28–29, 1993.

33. Taburet AM, Tollier C, Richard C: The effect of respiratory disorders on clinical pharmacokinetic variables. *Clin Pharmacokinet* 19(6):462–490, 1990.

34. Paakkari P, Paakkari I, Landes P, et al: Respiratory m-opioid and benzodiazepine interactions in the unrestrained rat. *Neuropharmacology* 32(4):323–329, 1993.

35. Murray-Lyon IM, Young J, Parkes JD, et al: Clinical and electroencephalographic assessment of diazepam in liver disease. *Br Med J* 4(5782):265–266, 1971.

36. DeFeudis FV: GABA-ergic analgesia: a naloxone-insensitive system. *Pharmacol Res Commun* 14(3):383–389, 1982.

37. Sawynok J: GABAergic mechanisms of analgesia: an update. *Pharmacol Biochem Behav* 26(2):463–474, 1987.

38. Unrug-Neervoort A, van Luijtelaar G, Coenen A: Cognition and vigilance: differential effects of diazepam and buspirone on memory and psychomotor performance. *Neuropsychobiology* 26(3):146–150, 1992.

39. Roche Laboratories: *Valium. Drug package insert*, Nutley, NJ, 1990, Roche Laboratories.

40. Bergman U, Rosa FW, Baum C, et al: Effects of exposure to benzodiazepines during fetal life. *Lancet* 340(8821):694–696, 1992.

41. Doenicke A, Lorenz W, Hoernecke R, et al: Histamine release after injection of benzodiazepines and of etomidate. A problem associated with the solvent propylene glycol. *Ann Fr Anesth Reanim* 12(2):166–168, 1993.

42. Amrein R, Hetzel W: Pharmacology of drugs frequently used in ICU's: midazolam and flumazenil. *Intensive Care Med* 17:S1–S10, 1991.

43. Fraser AD, Bryan W, Isner AF: Urinary screening for midazolam and its major metabolites with the Abbott ADx and TDx analyzers and the EMIT d.a.u. benzodiazepine assay with confirmation by GC/MS. *J Anal Toxicol* 15(1):8–12, 1991.

44. Jones RD, Chan K, Rouolson CJ, et al: Pharmacokinetics of flumazenil and midazolam. *Br J Anaesth* 70(3):286–292, 1993.

45. Ouellette RG: Midazolam: an induction agent for general anesthesia. *Nurse Anesth* 2(3):134–137, 1991.

46. Conner JT, Katz RL, Pagano RR, Graham CW: RO 21-3981 for intravenous surgical premedication and induction of anesthesia. *Anesth Analg* 57(1):1–5, 1978.

47. Hennessy MJ, Kirkby KC, Montgomery IM: Comparison of the amnesic effects of midazolam and diazepam. *Psychopharmacology (Berl)* 103(4):545–550, 1991.

48. Malamed SF, Nikchevich D, Jr, Block J: Anterograde amnesia as a possible postoperative complication of midazolam as an agent for intravenous conscious sedation. *Anesth Prog* 35(4):160–162, 1988.

49. Longmire AW, Seger DL: Topics in clinical pharmacology: flumazenil, a benzodiazepine antagonist. *Am J Med Sci* 306(1):49–52, 1993.

50. Forster A, Gardaz JP, Suter PM, Gemperle M: Respiratory depression by midazolam and diazepam. *Anesthesiology* 53(6):494–497, 1980.

51. Brown CR, Sarnquist FH, Canup CA, Pedley TA: Clinical, electroencephalographic, and pharmacokinetic studies of a water-soluble benzodiazepine, midazolam maleate. *Anesthesiology* 50(5):467–470, 1979.

52. Gath I, Weidenfeld J, Collins GI, Hadad H: Electrophysiological aspects of benzodiazepine antagonists, Ro 15-1788 and Ro 15-3505. *Br J Clin Pharmacol* 18(4):541–547, 1984.

53. Zakko SF, Seifert HA, Gross JB: A comparison of midazolam and diazepam for conscious sedation during colonoscopy in a prospective double-blind study. *Gastrointest Endosc* 49(6):684–689, 1999.

54. Roche Laboratories: Important new information on the administration of Versed (midazolam hydrochloride/Roche) injection for conscious sedation, Letter, Nov 1987.

55. Jones RD, Lawson AD, Andrew LJ, et al: Antagonism of the hypnotic effect of midazolam in children: a randomized, double-blind study of placebo and flumazenil administered after midazolam-induced anaesthesia. *Br J Anaesth* 66(6):660–666, 1991.

56. ClinicalKey. Midazolam drug monograph. February 1, 2016. www.clinicalkey.com (Accessed 20 February 2016).

57. Epocrates. Midazolam. www.epocrates.com. (Accessed 13 March 2016).

58. Saano V, Hansen PP, Paronen P: Interactions and comparative effects of zopiclone, diazepam and lorazepam on psychomotor performance and on elimination pharmacokinetics in healthy volunteers. *Pharmacol Toxicol* 70(2):135–139, 1992.

59. ClinicalKey. Lorazepam drug monograph. January 26, 2016. www.clinicalkey.com (Accessed 21 February 2016).

60. Eldor J: High dose flunitrazepam anesthesia. *Med Hypotheses* 38(4):352–354, 1992.

61. Wyeth-Ayerst Laboratories: *Ativan. Drug package insert,* Philadelphia, PA, 2005, Wyeth-Ayerst Laboratories.

62. Young C, Knudsen N, Hilton A, Reves JG: Sedation in the intensive care unit. *Crit Care Med* 28(3):854–866, 2000.

63. Foreman PA: Flunitrazepam in outpatient dentistry. *Anesth Prog* 29(2):50–54, 1982.

64. ClinicalKey. Flunitrazepam drug monograph. July 1, 2002. www.clinicalkey.com (Accessed 21 February 2016).

65. Druid H, Holmgren P, Ahlner J: Flunitrazepam: an evaluation of use, abuse and toxicity. *Forensic Sci Int* 122(2-3):136–141, 2001.

66. Dixon RA, Bennett NR, Harrison MJ, et al: I.V. flunitrazepam and i.v. diazepam in conservative dentistry: a cross-over trial. *Br J Anaesth* 52(5):517–526, 1980.

67. ClinicalKey. Chlordiazepoxide drug monograph. February 1, 2016. www.clinicalkey.com (Accessed 21 February 2016).

68. Jorgensen NB: Local anesthesia and intravenous premedication. *Anesth Prog* 13(6):168–169, 1966.

69. Becker DE, Bennett CR: Intravenous and intramuscular sedation. In Dionne RA, Phero JC, Becker DE, editors: *Management of pain and anxiety in the dental office,* Philadelphia, 2002, WB Saunders.

70. Malamed SF: Pharmacology. In Malamed SF, editor: *Sedation: a guide to patient management,* ed 4, St Louis, 2000, CV Mosby, pp 340–346.

71. ClinicalKey. Promethazine drug monograph. December 21, 2015. www.clinicalkey.com (Accessed 22 February 2016).

72. ClinicalKey. Propofol drug monograph. September 18, 2015. www.clinicalkey.com (Accessed 22 February 2016).

73. Jansson JR, Fukada T, Ozaki M, Kimura S: Propofol EDTA and reduced incidence of infection. *Anaesth Intensive Care* 34(3):362–368, 2006.

74. Vandesteene A, Trempont V, Engelman E, et al: Effect of propofol on cerebral blood flow and metabolism in man. *Anaesthesia* 43(Suppl):42–43, 1988.

75. Van Hemelrijck J, Fitch W, Mattheussen M, et al: Effect of propofol on the cerebral circulation and autoregulation in the baboon. *Anesth Analg* 71(1):49–54, 1990.

76. Van Hemelrijck J, Van Aken H, Plets C, et al: The effects of propofol on intracranial pressure and cerebral perfusion pressure in patients with brain tumors. *Acta Anaesthesiol Belg* 40(2):95–100, 1989.

77. Hemelrijck JV, Gonzales JM, White PF: Pharmacology of intravenous anesthetic agents. In Rogers MC, Tinker JH, Covino BG, et al, editors: *Principles and practice of anesthesiology,* St Louis, 1993, Mosby.

78. Grounds RM, Twigley AJ, Carli F, et al: The haemodynamic effects of intravenous induction, comparison of the effects of thiopentone and propofol. *Anaesthesia* 40(8):735–740, 1985.

79. Patrick MR, Blair IJ, Feneck RO, Sebel PS: A comparison of the hemodynamic effects of propofol (Diprivan) and thiopentone in patients with coronary artery disease. *Postgrad Med J* 61(Suppl 3):23–27, 1985.

80. Dundee JW, Robinson FP, McCollum JS, Patterson CC: Sensitivity to propofol in the elderly. *Anaesthesia* 41(5):482–485, 1986.

81. McCollum JSC, Milligan KR, Dundee JW: The antiemetic action of propofol. *Anaesthesia* 43(3):239–240, 1988.

82. Shafer SL: Advances in propofol pharmacokinetics and pharmacodynamics. *J Clin Anesth* 5(6 Suppl 1):14S–21S, 1993.

83. Rogers KM, Dewar KM, McCubbin TD, Spence AA: Preliminary experience with ICI 35868 as an IV induction agent: comparison with althesin. *Br J Anaesth* 52(8):807–810, 1980.

84. Rutter DV, Morgan M, Lumley J, Owen R: ICI 35868 (Diprivan): a new intravenous induction agent. *Anaesthesia* 35(12):1188–1192, 1980.

85. Weightman WM, Zacharias M: Comparison of propofol and thiopentone anaesthesia (with special reference to recovery characteristics). *Anaesth Intensive Care* 15(4):389–393, 1987.

86. Kay B, Stephenson DF: Dose-response relationship for disoprofol (IC 135868; Diprivan). *Anaesthesia* 36(9):863–867, 1981.

87. MacKenzie N, Grant IS: Comparison of the new emulsion formulation of propofol with methohexitone and thiopentone for induction of anaesthesia in day cases. *Br J Anaesth* 57(8):725–731, 1985.

88. MacKenzie N, Grant S: Comparison of propofol with methohexitone in the provision of anesthesia for surgery under regional blockade. *Br J Anaesth* 57(12):1167–1172, 1985.

89. MacKenzie N, Grant IS: Propofol for intravenous sedation. *Anaesthesia* 42(1):3–6, 1987.

90. Grounds RM, Lalor JM, Lumley J, et al: Propofol infusion for sedation in the intensive care unit. *Br Med J (Clin Res Ed)* 294(6569):397–400, 1987.

91. White PF, Negus JB: Sedative infusions during local or intravenous regional anesthesia: a comparison of propofol and midazolam. *J Clin Anesth* 3(1):32–39, 1991.

92. Stuart Pharmaceuticals: *Diprivan. Drug package insert,* Wilmington, Del, 1992, Stuart Pharmaceuticals.

93. Stanley TH: Opiate anaesthesia. *Anaesth Intensive Care* 15(1):38–59, 1987.

94. Martin WR: Naloxone. *Ann Intern Med* 85(6):765–768, 1976.

95. Phillips WJ: Central nervous system pain receptors. In Faust RJ, editor: *Anesthesiology review,* New York, 1991, Churchill Livingstone.

96. Shields SE: Pharmacokinetics of epidural narcotics. In Faust RJ, editor: *Anesthesiology review,* New York, 1991, Churchill Livingstone.

97. Pallasch TJ: *Clinical drug therapy in dental practice,* Philadelphia, 1973, Lea & Febiger.

98. ClinicalKey. Meperidine drug monograph. November 19, 2015. www.clinicalkey.com (Accessed 23 February 2016).

99. Malamed SFM, Reed KR: *Intravenous moderate sedation syllabus,* Los Angeles, CA, 2014, Herman Ostrow School of Dentistry of U.S.C.

100. Reed KR, Malamed SFM: *Intravenous moderate sedation syllabus,* Portland, OR, 2016, Oregon Academy of General Dentistry, Oregon Health Sciences University.

101. Rosow C: Pharmacology of opioid analgetic agents. In Longnecker DE, Tinker JH, Morgen G, Jr, editors: *Principles and practice of anesthesiology,* ed 2, St Louis, 1998, Mosby.

102. ClinicalKey. Morphine drug monograph. January 11, 2016. www.clinicalkey.com (Accessed 23 February 2016).

103. ClinicalKey. Hydromorphone drug monograph. August 17, 2015. www.clinicalkey.com (Accessed 23 February 2016).

104. *Dilaudid (hydromorphone) oral liquid and tablet package insert*, Stamford, CT, 2013, Purdue Pharma L.P.

105. Coda B, Tanaka A, Jacobson RC, et al: Hydromorphone analgesia after intravenous bolus administration. *Pain* 71(1):41–48, 1997.

106. Wedell D, Hersh EV: A review of the opioid analgesics fentanyl, alfentanil, and sufentanil. *Compendium* 12(3):184–187, 1991.

107. ClinicalKey. Fentanyl drug monograph. January 22, 2016. www.clinicalkey.com (Accessed 1 March 2016).

108. Gracely RH, Dubner R, McGrath PA: Fentanyl reduces the intensity of painful tooth pulp sensations: controlling for detection of active drugs. *Anesth Analg* 61(9):751–755, 1982.

109. Shook JE, Watkins WD, Camporesi EM: Differential roles of opioid receptors in respiration, respiratory disease, and opiate-induced respiratory depression. *Am Rev Respir Dis* 142(4):895–909, 1990.

110. Rosenberg M: Muscle rigidity with fentanyl: a case report. *Anesth Prog* 24(2):50–52, 1977.

111. Mackenzie JE, Frank LW: Influence of pretreatment with a monoamine oxidase inhibitor (phenelzine) on the effects of buprenorphine and pethidine in the conscious rabbit. *Br J Anaesth* 60(2):216–221, 1988.

112. Janssen: Sublimaze injection. *Drug package insert*, August 12, 2014 JANSSEN-CILAG Pty Ltd, Macquarie Park NSW 2113 Australia.

113. ClinicalKey. Sufentanil drug monograph. February 24, 2016. www.clinicalkey.com (Accessed 4 March 2016).

114. ClinicalKey. Alfentanil drug monograph. February 26, 2016. www.clinicalkey.com (Accessed 4 March 2016).

115. ClinicalKey. Remifentanil drug monograph. June 9, 2015. www.clinicalkey.com (Accessed 4 March 2016).

116. Janssens F, Torremans J, Janssen PA: Synthetic 1,4-disubstituted-1,4-dihydro-5H-tetrazol-5-one derivatives of fentanyl: alfentanil (R 39209), a potent, extremely short-acting narcotic analgesic. *J Med Chem* 29(11):2290–2297, 1986.

117. Meistelman C, Saint-Maurice C, Lepaul M, et al: A comparison of alfentanil pharmacokinetics in children and adults. *Anesthesiology* 66(1):13–16, 1987.

118. Helmers JH, Noordiun H, van Leeuwen L: Alfentanil used in the aged: a clinical comparison with its use in young patients. *Eur J Anaesthesiol* 2(4):347–352, 1985.

119. Shafer A, Sung ML, White PF: Pharmacokinetics and pharmacodynamics of alfentanil infusions during general anesthesia. *Anesth Analg* 65(10):1021–1028, 1986.

120. Reitz JA: Alfentanil in anesthesia and analgesia. *Drug Intell Clin Pharm* 20(4):336–341, 1986.

121. Fone KC, Wilson H: The effects of alfentanil and selected narcotic analgesics on the rate of action potential discharge of medullary respiratory neurones in anesthetized rats. *Br J Pharmacol* 89(1):67–76, 1986.

122. Bagshaw ON, Singh P, Aitkenhead AR: Alfentanil in day-case anaesthesia. Assessment of a single dose on the quality of anaesthesia and recovery. *Anaesthesia* 48(6):476–481, 1993.

123. Ghosh YK, Beamer J, Ahluwalia HS: A new technique of alfentanil-induced conscious sedation for oculoplastic surgery. *Orbit* 30(2):70–71, 2011.

124. McHardy FE, Fortier J, Chung F, et al: A comparison of midazolam, alfentanil and propofol for sedation in outpatient intraocular surgery. *Can J Anaesth* 47(3):211–214, 2000.

125. Phitayakorn P, Melnick BM, Vuicinie AF: Comparison of continuous sufentanil and fentanyl infusions for outpatient anaesthesia. *Can J Anaesth* 34(3 Pt 1):242–245, 1987.

126. Davis PJ, Chopyk JB, Nazif M, Cook DR: Continuous alfentanil infusion in pediatric patients undergoing general anesthesia for complete oral restoration. *J Clin Anesth* 3(2):125–130, 1991.

127. Edgin WA, Ford ML, Mansfield MJ: Alfentanil for general anesthesia in oral and maxillofacial surgery. *Oral Maxillofac Surg* 47(10):1039–1042, 1989.

128. Bostek CC, Fiducia DA, Klotz RW, Herman N: Total intravenous anesthesia with a continuous propofol-alfentanil infusion. *CRNA* 3(3):124–131, 1992.

129. Burkle H, Dunbar S, Van Aken H: Remifentanil: a novel, short-acting, m-opioid. *Anesth Analg* 83(3):646–651, 1996.

130. Glass PS: Remifentanil: a new opioid. *J Clin Anesth* 7(7):558–563, 1995.

131. Beers R, Camporesi E: Remifentanil update: clinical science and utility. *CNS Drugs* 18(15):1085–1104, 2004.

132. Kapila A, Glass PS, Jacobs JR, et al: Measured context-sensitive half-times of remifentanil and alfentanil. *Anesthesiology* 83(5):968–975, 1995.

133. Goldstein G: Pentazocine. *Drug Alcohol Depend* 14(3-4):313–323, 1985.

134. Burstein AH, Fullerton T: Oculogyric crisis possibly related to pentazocine. *Ann Pharmacother* 27(7-8):874–876, 1993.

135. Wilkinson DJ: Opioid agonist/antagonists in general anaesthesia. *Br J Hosp Med* 38(2):130–133, 1987.

136. Pallasch TJ, Gill CJ: Butorphanol and nalbuphine: a pharmacologic comparison. *Oral Surg* 59(1):15–20, 1985.

137. Zallen RD, Cobetto GA, Bohmfalk C, Steffan K: Butorphanol/diazepam compared to meperidine/diazepam for sedation in oral and maxillofacial surgery: a double-blind evaluation. *Oral Surg* 64(4):395–401, 1987.

138. ClinicalKey. Pentazocine drug monograph. May 12, 2015. www.clinicalkey.com (Accessed 4 March 2016).

139. Woolverton WL, Schuster CR: Behavioral and pharmacological aspects of opioid dependence: mixed agonist/antagonists. *Pharmacol Rev* 35(1):33–52, 1983.

140. Donadoni R, Rolly G, Devulder J, Verdonck R: Double-blind comparison between nalbuphine and pentazocine in the control of postoperative pain after orthopedic surgery. *Acta Anaesthesiol Belg* 39(4):251–256, 1988.

141. Davidson-Lamb R: Nalbuphine hydrochloride (Nubain) versus pentazocine for analgesia during dental operations. A double blind, randomized trial. *SAAD Dig* 6(4):76–81, 1985.

142. Baum C, Hus JP, Nelson RC: The impact of the addition of naloxone on the use and abuse of pentazocine. *Public Health Rep* 102(4):426–429, 1987.

143. Kewitz H: Rare but serious risks associated with non-narcotic analgesics: clinical experience. *Med Toxicol* 1(Suppl 1):86–92, 1986.

144. Jago RH, Restall J, Stonham J: The effect of naloxone on pentazocine induced hallucinations. *J Roy Army Med Corps* 130(1):64–65, 1984.

145. Hospira: *Pentazocine hydrochloride. Drug package insert*, Lake Forest, IL, 2009, Hospira.

146. Roytblat L, Bear R, Gesztes T: Seizures after pentazocine overdose. *Isr J Med Sci* 22(5):385–386, 1986.

147. ClinicalKey. Nalbuphine drug monograph. February 24, 2016. www.clinicalkey.com (Accessed 8 March 2016).

148. Miller RR: Evaluation of nalbuphine hydrochloride. *Am J Hosp Pharm* 37(7):942–959, 1980.

149. Lefevre B, Freysz M, Lepine J, et al: Comparison of nalbuphine and fentanyl as intravenous analgesics for medically compromised patients undergoing oral surgery. *Anesth Prog* 39(1-2):13–18, 1993.

150. Parsons JD: The use of nalbuphine (Nubain) and midazolam in sedation for dentistry. *SAAD Dig* 6(6):125–131, 1986.

151. Hunter PL: Use of nalbuphine for analgesia in combination with methohexital sodium. *Anesth Prog* 36(4-5):150–168, 1989.

152. Dolan EA, Murray WJ, Ruddy MP: Double-blind comparison of nalbuphine and meperidine in combination with diazepam for intravenous conscious sedation in oral surgery outpatients. *Oral Surg* 66(5):536–539, 1988.

153. Milnes AR, Maupome G, Cannon J: Intravenous sedation in pediatric dentistry using midazolam, nalbuphine and droperidol. *Pediatr Dent* 22(2):113–119, 2000.

154. Gal TJ, DiFazio CA, Moscicki J: Analgesic and respiratory depressant activity of nalbuphine: a comparison with morphine. *Anesthesiology* 57(5):367–374, 1982.

155. Pallasch TJ, Gill CJ: Naloxone-associated morbidity and mortality. *Oral Surg* 52(6):602–603, 1981.

156. Schmidt WK, Tam SW, Shotzberger GS, et al: Nalbuphine. *Drug Alcohol Depend* 14(3-4):339–362, 1985.

157. Hameroff SR: Opiate receptor pharmacology: mixed agonist/antagonist narcotics. *Contemp Anesth Pract* 7:27–43, 1983.

158. Gal TJ, DiFazio CA, Moscicki J: Analgesic and respiratory depressant activity of nalbuphine: a comparison with morphine. *Anesthesiology* 57(5):367–374, 1982.

159. Errick JK, Heel RC: Nalbuphine: a preliminary review of its pharmacological properties and therapeutic efficacy. *Drugs* 26(3):191–211, 1983.

160. Crul JF, Smets MJ, van Egmond J: The efficacy and safety of nalbuphine (Nubain) in balanced anesthesia. A double blind comparison with fentanyl in gynecological and urological surgery. *Acta Anaesthesiol Belg* 41(3):261–267, 1990.

161. Bowdle TA: Clinical pharmacology of antagonists of narcotic-induced respiratory depression. A brief review. *Acute Care* 12(Suppl 1):70–76, 1988.

162. Romagnoli A, Keats AS: Ceiling effect for respiratory depression by nalbuphine. *Clin Pharmacol Ther* 27(4):478–485, 1980.

163. Lefevre B, Freysz M, Lepine J, et al: Comparison of nalbuphine and fentanyl as intravenous analgesics for medically compromised patients undergoing oral surgery. *Anesth Prog* 39(1-2):13–18, 1993.

164. Preston KL, Jasinski DR: Abuse liability studies of opioid agonist-antagonists in humans. *Drug Alcohol Depend* 28(1):49–82, 1991.

165. Hospira: *Nalbuphine. Drug package insert*, Lake Forest, IL, 2007, Hospira.

166. ClinicalKey. Butorphanol drug monograph. August 31, 2015. www.clinicalkey.com (Accessed 8 March 2016).

167. Bowdle TA: Clinical pharmacology of antagonists of narcotic-induced respiratory depression. *Acute Care* 12(Suppl 1):70–76, 1988.

168. Vogelsang J, Hayes SR: Butorphanol tartrate (Stadol): a review. *J Post Anesth Nurs* 6(2):129–135, 1991.

169. Vandam LD: Butorphanol. *N Engl J Med* 302(7):381–384, 1980.

170. Nagashima H, Karamanian A, Malovany R, et al: Respiratory and circulatory effects of intravenous butorphanol and morphine. *Clin Pharmacol Ther* 19(6):738–745, 1976.

171. Roscow CE: Butorphanol in perspective. *Acute Care* 12(Suppl 1):2–7, 1988.

172. O'Hair KC, Dodd KT, Phillips YY, Beattie RJ: Cardiopulmonary effects of nalbuphine hydrochloride and butorphanol tartrate in sheep. *Lab Anim Sci* 38(1):58–61, 1988.

173. Hospira: *Butorphanol tartrate. Drug package insert*, Lake Forest, IL, 2004, Hospira.

174. From RP: Substance dependence and abuse by anesthesia care providers. In Rogers MC, Tinker JH, Covino CG, et al, editors: *Principles and practice of anesthesiology*, St Louis, 1993, Mosby.

175. ClinicalKey. Atropine drug monograph. February 3, 2016. www.clinicalkey.com (Accessed 8 March 2016).

176. ClinicalKey. Scopolamine drug monograph. January 27, 2016. www.clinicalkey.com (Accessed 8 March 2016).

177. ClinicalKey. Glycopyrrolate drug monograph. January 27, 2016. www.clinicalkey.com (Accessed 8 March 2016).

178. Finder RL, Bennett CR: Use of scopolamine for dental anesthesia and analgesia techniques. *J Oral Maxillofac Surg* 42(12):802–804, 1984.

179. Izquierdo I: Mechanism of action of scopolamine as an amnestic. *Trends Pharmacol Sci* 10(5):175–177, 1988.

180. Fassi A, Rosenberg M: Atropine, scopolamine and glycopyrrolate. *Anesth Prog* 26(6):155–159, 1979.

181. Das G: Therapeutic review: cardiac effects of atropine in man: an update. *Int J Clin Pharmacol Ther Toxicol* 27(10):473–477, 1989.

182. Noronha-Blob L, Lowe VC, Peterson JS, Hanson RC: The anticholinergic activity of agents indicated for urinary incontinence is an important property for effective control of bladder dysfunction. *J Pharmacol Exp Ther* 251(2):586–593, 1989.

183. Kanto J, Klotz U: Pharmacokinetic implications for the clinical use of atropine, scopolamine and glycopyrrolate. *Acta Anaesth Scand* 32(2):69–78, 1988.

184. Bryant DH: Anti-cholinergic drugs and their use in asthma. *Prog Clin Biol Res* 263:379–391, 1988.

185. Hospira: *Atropine. Drug package insert*, Lake Forest, IL, 2015, Hospira.

186. Ramjan KA, Williams AJ, Isbister GK, Elliott EJ: 'Red as a beet and blind as a bat' Anticholinergic delirium in adolescents: lessons for the paediatrician. *J Paediatr Child Health* 43(11):779–780, 2007.

187. Repreht J: The central muscarinic transmission during anaesthesia and recovery: the central anticholinergic syndrome. *Anaesth Reanim* 16(4):250–258, 1991.

188. Nuotto E: Psychomotor, physiological and cognitive effects of scopolamine and ephedrine in healthy man. *Eur J Clin Pharmacol* 24(5):603–609, 1983.

189. Schneck HJ, Rupreht J: Central anticholinergic syndrome (CAS) in anesthesia and intensive care. *Acta Anaesthesiol Belg* 40(3):219–228, 1989.

190. Helfaer MA, Rock P: Formulary: guide to physiologic assessment and pharmacologic dosing in common anesthetic practice. In Rogers MC, Tinker JH, Covino CG, et al, editors: *Principles and practice of anesthesiology*, St Louis, 1993, Mosby.

191. el Hakim M: Cardiac dysrhythmias during dental surgery, comparison of hyoscine, glycopyrrolate and placebo medication. *Anaesth Reanim* 16(6):393–398, 1991.

192. West-ward Pharmaceutical Corp: Robinul Injectable. *Drug package insert*, Eatontown, NJ, November 2011.

193. Preston GC, Ward CE, Broks P, et al: Effects of lorazepam on memory, attention and sedation in man: antagonism by Ro 15-1788. *Psychopharmacology (Berl)* 97(2):222–227, 1989.

194. ClinicalKey. Ketamine drug monograph. March 2, 2016. www.clinicalkey.com (Accessed 9 March 2016).

195. Reich DL, Silvay G: Ketamine: an update on the first twenty-five years of clinical experience. *Can J Anaesth* 36(2):186–197, 1989.

196. Smith KM: Drugs used in acquaintance rape. *J Am Pharm Assoc (Wash)* 39(4):519–525, 1999.

197. Haas DA, Harper DG: Ketamine: a review of its pharmacologic properties and use in ambulatory anesthesia. *Anesth Prog* 39(3):61–68, 1992.

198. Becsey L, Malamed SF, Radnay P, Foldes FF: Reduction of the psychotomimetic and circulatory side effects of ketamine by droperidol. *Anesthesiology* 37(5):536–542, 1972.

199. Sussman DR: A comparative evaluation of ketamine anesthesia in children and adults. *Anesthesiology* 40(5):459–464, 1974.

200. White PF, Way WL, Trevor AJ: Ketamine: its pharmacology and therapeutic uses. *Anesthesiology* 56(2):119–136, 1982.

201. Goodson JM, Moore P: Life-threatening reactions following pedodontic sedation: an assessment of narcotic, local anesthetic and antiemetic drug interaction. *J Am Dent Assoc* 107(2):239–245, 1983.

202. Lasagna L, Beecher HK: The analgesic effectiveness of nalorphine and nalorphine-morphine combinations in man. *J Pharmacol Exp Ther* 112(3):356–363, 1954.

203. Sharts-Engel NC: Naloxone review and pediatric dosage update. *Am J Maternal Child Nurs* 16(3):182, 1991.

204. ClinicalKey. Naloxone drug monograph. December 4, 2015. www.clinicalkey.com (Accessed 9 March 2016).

205. *Evzio (naloxone hydrochloride injection) package insert*, Richmond, VA, 2014, Kaleo, Inc.

206. *Narcan (naloxone hydrochloride) nasal spray package insert*, Radner, PA, 2015, Adapt Pharma, Inc.

207. Wride SR, Smith RE, Courtney PG: A fatal case of pulmonary edema in a healthy young male following naloxone administration. *Anaesth Intens Care* 17(3):374–377, 1989.

208. Hospira: *Narcan hydrochloride. Drug package insert*, Lake Forest, IL, 2007, Hospira, Inc.

209. ECC Committee, Subcommittees and Task Forces of the American Heart Association: 2010 American Heart Association Guidelines for Cardiopulmonary Resuscitation and Emergency Cardiovascular Care. Part 14: Pediatric Advanced Life Support. *Circulation* 122:s876–s908, 2010.

210. ClinicalKey. Flumazenil drug monograph. February 5, 2016. www.clinicalkey.com (Accessed 9 March 2016).

211. Rodrigo MR, Rosenquist JB: The effect of Ro 15-1788 (Anexate) on conscious sedation produced with midazolam. *Anaesth Intensive Care* 15(2):185–192, 1987.

212. Wolff J, Carl P, Clausen TG, Mikkelsen BO: Ro 15-1778 for postoperative recovery: a randomized clinical trial in patients undergoing minor surgical procedures under midazolam anaesthesia. *Anaesthesia* 41(10):1001–1006, 1986.

213. Ricou B, Forster A, Bruckner A, et al: Clinical evaluation of a specific benzodiazepine antagonist (Ro 15-1788): studies in elderly patients after regional anaesthesia under benzodiazepine sedation. *Br J Anaesth* 58(9):1–11, 1986.

214. *Flumazenil (Romazicon) package insert*, Nutley, NJ, 2007, Roche Pharmaceuticals.

215. Olympio MA: Postanesthetic emergence delirium: historical perspective. *J Clin Anesth* 3(1):60–63, 1991.

216. ClinicalKey. Physostigmine drug monograph. July 2, 2014. www.clinicalkey.com (Accessed 9 March 2016).

217. Lauven PM, Stoeckel H: Flumazenil (Ro 15-1788) and physostigmine. *Resuscitation* 16(Suppl):S41–S48, 1988.

218. Akorn, Inc.: *Physostigmine salicylate injection. Drug package insert*, Lake Forest, IL, 2008, Akorn, Inc.

chapter 26

Intravenous Moderate Sedation: Techniques of Administration

CHAPTER OUTLINE

Techniques of intravenous (IV) moderate sedation are discussed in this chapter employing the drugs presented in Chapter 25. In this sixth edition, several techniques of IV sedation, including the classic Jorgensen and Foreman techniques, have been deemphasized, having been supplanted by techniques involving benzodiazepines that are discussed later. The reader seeking in-depth description of these two classic techniques, and others, is referred to the fourth edition of this text.[1]

MONITORING DURING INTRAVENOUS SEDATION

Whenever drugs are administered parenterally, it is of paramount importance that the patient be monitored closely. Guidelines for monitoring during moderate sedation have been developed.[2-7] Every dentist must adhere to those regulations regarding monitoring that have been established by the dental governing body in the state or province in which they are licensed to practice.

The following represents this author's recommendation for monitoring during IV moderate sedation:
1. Baseline vital signs are recorded at preliminary appointment.
   a. Blood pressure
   b. Heart rate and rhythm
   c. Respiratory rate (may include oxygen saturation and end-tidal CO_2 levels)
   d. Height and weight (BMI)
   e. Temperature (optional)
2. Preoperative vital signs are recorded on the day of treatment before the start of the procedure.
3. Immediately following IV drug administration, vital signs are recorded.
4. Periodically during the procedure (commonly interpreted as every 5 minutes), vital signs should be recorded.
5. Postoperatively, vital signs are recorded.
6. Following recovery and immediately before patient discharge from the office, a final set of vital signs is recorded.

The following monitoring devices are available:
1. Precordial or pretracheal stethoscope
2. Pulse oximeter
3. End-tidal carbon dioxide (CO_2) monitor (capnography)
4. Electrocardiograph (ECG)

> **Monitoring is done CONTINUOUSLY.**
> **Recording is done PERIODICALLY.**

The pretracheal stethoscope is recommended for use during IV moderate sedation procedures. The pulse oximeter is a standard monitoring device used during IV moderate sedation. Functioning as a continuous monitor of arterial oxygen (O_2) saturation and heart rate, the pulse oximeter represents the standard of care for monitoring during parenteral sedation. Recent graduates from U.S. dental schools who employ IV moderate sedation would not even consider starting an IV sedation case in the absence of an oximeter.[8] End-tidal CO_2 monitors (capnographs) are now mandatory during general anesthesia and IV deep sedation and are more gradually being required for IV moderate sedation.[9,10] The ECG is less essential during parenteral sedation procedures than are techniques for monitoring the respiratory system. The ECG, though desirable, should, in this author's opinion, be considered an optional monitor for IV moderate sedation. Regulatory bodies in a number of states have mandated the use of an ECG during IV moderate sedation.

The most important system to be monitored during IV moderate sedation is the central nervous system (CNS). This is accomplished through direct verbal contact with, and the response of, the patient. Based on the definition of moderate sedation, patients are able to respond appropriately to verbal or physical stimulation throughout parenteral moderate sedation procedures.

Box 26.1   Intravenous Moderate Sedation Techniques

Basic Techniques
Benzodiazepine

Modifications of Basic Techniques
Benzodiazepine with anticholinergic

Advanced Techniques
Benzodiazepine with opioid
Opioid with benzodiazepine

Others (Historical)
Jorgensen technique
Diazepam with methohexital (Foreman technique)
Berns technique
Shane technique

Monitors and monitoring recommendations for all modalities of sedation are discussed in detail in Chapter 5.

Classification of Intravenous Drugs

Antianxiety/Sedative-Hypnotic Drugs
Diazepam
Midazolam

Opioid-Type Analgesics
Meperidine
Morphine
Hydromorphone
Fentanyl
Alfentanil
Sufentanil
Remifentanil
Nalbuphine
Butorphanol

Anticholinergics
Atropine
Glycopyrrolate

BASIC INTRAVENOUS MODERATE SEDATION TECHNIQUES

These sedation techniques form the backbone of IV moderate sedation. Knowledge of these techniques will enable the trained dentist to meet the needs of a dental or surgical procedure of any duration, achieving satisfactory sedation for virtually all patients requiring IV moderate sedation (Box 26.1).

The *Jorgensen technique* is, arguably, the original IV moderate sedation technique.[11] Despite efforts at modifying (e.g., improving) it, the original Jorgensen technique was used successfully for many years, providing excellent sedation with few reports of any significant complications. The primary indication for the Jorgensen technique was a dental procedure requiring 2 or more hours to complete. Since the introduction of the benzodiazepines diazepam and midazolam, and because of the inability to reverse the clinical actions of the barbiturate, pentobarbital, use of the Jorgensen technique has dramatically decreased. For an in-depth discussion of the Jorgensen technique, the reader is referred to earlier editions of this textbook.[1]

IV moderate sedation using a benzodiazepine has replaced the Jorgensen technique as the most popular technique in dentistry.[12] IV benzodiazepine sedation meets the needs of contemporary dental practice (i.e., sedation for approximately 1 hour). Midazolam, introduced in the United States in 1985, has supplanted diazepam to become the most used IV technique in the area of 1-hour IV moderate sedation.[12]

With the availability of these drugs, virtually all patients requiring IV moderate sedation will be successfully managed, regardless of the length of the procedure.

Midazolam or Diazepam?

Patients who are receiving benzodiazepines orally for prolonged periods may exhibit a tolerance to the IV administration of diazepam or midazolam. Robb and Hargrave[13] reported three cases of patients who required doses of 47 and 50 mg midazolam, 26 mg midazolam, and 30 and 34 mg midazolam for IV moderate sedation. Discontinuance of the oral benzodiazepine produced a return to more normal response.

Given one titrating dose, the duration of midazolam-induced sedation is slightly shorter than that of diazepam. Clinical experience has demonstrated that recovery is as complete as with diazepam. Some patients may exhibit a degree of residual sedation up to 60 minutes after drug administration, though this is rare. It also appears, subjectively, that the depth of sedation provided by midazolam is not as intense as that noted with diazepam; however, the degree and length of midazolam-induced anterograde amnesia are considerably greater than that produced by diazepam.

The decision as to which benzodiazepine to use must take into account several factors, including the following:

1. Possibility of phlebitis (venous inflammation) – diazepam relatively contraindicated; midazolam preferred.
2. Requirement for sedation – diazepam slightly greater level of sedation, though not significantly better than midazolam.
3. Requirement for amnesia – midazolam clearly superior to diazepam.

Intravenous Benzodiazepine (Midazolam or Diazepam)
Preliminary Appointment

When either midazolam or diazepam is considered for use, specific questions must be asked of the patient regarding any prior exposure to the drug(s) and how they reacted to them. Specific contraindications to their use must be addressed. For midazolam and diazepam, these include the following:

1. Allergy or hypersensitivity to benzodiazepines
2. Glaucoma (untreated)
3. History of phlebitis or thrombophlebitis (contraindication to diazepam)
4. Acute pulmonary insufficiency (contraindication to midazolam)
5. Preexisting respiratory depression

Patients classified as American Society of Anesthesiologists (ASA) 1 and 2 are candidates for IV moderate sedation. ASA 3 patients might be considered, but only on a case-by-case basis.

Before the day of treatment, the following items concerning the patient's suitability for IV moderate sedation are evaluated by the dentist and staff.

Degree of Apprehension

Which route of sedation (oral, intramuscular [IM], inhalation, IV) is most appropriate for this patient? If the IV route is selected, which technique is most appropriate for this patient?

Informed Consent

If the IV route is selected, informed consent must be provided to the patient, describing the IV procedure, its alternatives (e.g., IM, general anesthesia), and the most likely complications associated with its use. The patient signs the consent form, which is then added to the patient's dental record. A specific informed consent for IV sedation should be signed before each IV procedure when multiple IV sedation visits are planned.[14]

Medical History

The medical history questionnaire, dialog history, and vital signs are reviewed, seeking the presence of contraindications, either relative or absolute, to the use of the drugs considered.

Nature and Length of Dental Procedure Contemplated

The degree of trauma associated with the planned procedure must be considered in evaluating a potential sedative technique. In addition, the length of the procedure is a consideration. Selection of appropriate drugs can tailor the length of sedation to almost any duration.

Presence of Superficial Veins

The presence of suitable superficial veins is a primary requisite for elective IV procedures. Lack of "good" (visible) veins is an acceptable reason for avoiding the IV route and selecting an alternative route of drug administration.

Recording of Baseline Vital Signs

Baseline vital signs are obtained at this visit if they have not been previously recorded.

Preoperative Instructions

The following is an example of preoperative instructions for IV moderate sedation:

1. Arrangements must be made for a responsible adult to drive the patient home after the IV moderate sedation appointment. The patient cannot be discharged from the dental office unescorted.

COMMENT: A "responsible adult" may be defined as "a person who has a vested interest in the health and safety of the patient." When the patient arrives for treatment, the name, address, and telephone number of his or her escort should be obtained immediately. If treatment is planned to last up to 1 hour, the escort is requested to accompany the patient to the office and remain during the procedure. For procedures lasting more than 2 hours, the escort is still requested to accompany the patient to the office. However, the dentist may elect to permit the escort to leave the office for the duration of the procedure and to return before the procedure is scheduled to end. In either case, it is extremely important to have seen or at least spoken to the patient's escort before the start of the procedure. It is my policy to cancel the planned procedure whenever a suitable escort is not available at the start of treatment.

When oral sedation is prescribed preoperatively to be taken at home, an escort must drive the patient to the office.

2. The patient should be NPO (nil per os) for approximately 6 hours before the procedure.

> **COMMENT:** The goal of NPO is to provide an empty stomach and gastric fluids with a higher pH in the highly unlikely event that the patient should become nauseous and vomit during or following the IV procedure. There is less likelihood of aspiration of solid or particulate matter if food is not present in the stomach. Patients may be permitted to ingest clear liquids, such as water or apple juice, along with any medications they may be required to take (e.g., antihypertensives). If the scheduled appointment is before noon, the patient is told not to eat anything that morning. For an afternoon IV sedation, the patient is advised to avoid anything by mouth after 8 am. A light, carbohydrate-rich breakfast consisting of dry cereal and juice may be taken before 8 am that morning. Medications may be taken normally, with water.

Standard anesthesia NPO protocol before sedation or general anesthesia follows the 2 – 4 – 6 rule. No clear liquids within 2 hours of the start of the procedure; no breast milk within 4 hours; and no infant formula, nonhuman milk, or light meal within 6 hours[15] (Table 26.1).

3. The patient is advised to wear loose-fitting garments.

> **COMMENT:** This will minimize any possibly excessive respiratory depression caused by mechanical means. The upper garment worn by the patient should be of short-sleeved length or have no sleeves so that access may readily be gained to both arms.

Many dentists using IV moderate or deep sedation or general anesthesia have the patient change into a surgical shirt (or "scrubs"). Loose fitting and short sleeved, a scrub top allows the anesthesia team immediate and unimpeded access to the patient's chest and upper body throughout the procedure.

4. The patient should plan to arrive at the office approximately 15 minutes before the scheduled appointment.

5. Should the patient develop a cold, flu, sore throat, or any other illness, the appointment will be canceled and rescheduled at a time when the patient is more physically fit. The patient should call if any of these symptoms develop.

Table 26.1	NPO Recommendations
INGESTED MATERIAL	**MINIMUM FASTING PERIOD, H**
Clear liquids: water, fruit juices without pulp, carbonated beverages, clear tea, black coffee	2
Breast milk	4
Infant formula	6
Nonhuman milk: because nonhuman milk is similar to solids in gastric emptying time, the amount ingested must be considered when determining an appropriate fasting period	6
Light meal: a light meal typically consists of toast and clear liquids. Meals that include fried or fatty foods or meat may prolong gastric emptying time; both the amount and type of foods ingested must be considered when determining an appropriate fasting period	6

> **COMMENT:** Research has demonstrated that morbidity and mortality following anesthesia in patients with upper respiratory infections (URIs) are significantly greater in the time following the patient's apparent "recovery" from the URI.[16] Most of this morbidity is related to respiratory disease.

6. The medications, if any, to be taken before arrival in the office for treatment are prescribed, and the names of drugs, dosages, and instructions are given.

7. If an oral antianxiety drug is to be administered in the dental office, the patient should be requested to appear 1 hour before the scheduled start of the dental procedure.

8. The time, date, and place of appointment are given to the patient.

Day of Treatment

The day of the scheduled dental treatment arrives, and the dental-phobic patient is in the waiting room. Knowing that the patient is fearful of the upcoming procedures, the dentist will not wish to prolong his or her wait any longer than necessary because the patient's anxiety and fears will increase during this time.

An exception to this will be the patient receiving oral sedation before IV sedation. Oral sedative drugs ought not be taken by the patient at home. Rather they should be administered to the patient by a member of the dental office staff (e.g., dentist) in the office on the day of the scheduled sedation. The patient should be scheduled to arrive in the office approximately 1 hour before the scheduled start of the IV procedure, the oral sedative administered, and the patient asked to remain in the reception area.

During this time, the assistant will prepare the IV infusion and drugs for use (see Chapter 24). Once all is ready, the patient is asked to visit restroom to void (the patient *MUST* be accompanied to the restroom if they have previously received oral sedation), if necessary, following which the patient is taken to the treatment room and seated in a semiupright (comfortable) position. The availability of the patient's escort must be determined at this time.

Once the patient is seated in the dental chair, monitors are placed, and preoperative vital signs monitored and recorded on the anesthesia record sheet (Fig. 26.1). Ideally the blood pressure cuff is placed on the arm opposite the working side of the dentist, remaining in place throughout the procedure. If used, the pretracheal stethoscope and ECG electrodes are applied along with the pulse oximeter and/or end-tidal CO_2 monitor. A nasal cannula or nasal hood is positioned, and a 3- to 6-L/min flow of O_2 is administered throughout the IV procedure.

Because of an increased risk of phlebitis following diazepam administration, it is suggested that, when possible, smaller veins, such as those on the dorsum of the hand or wrist, be avoided when venipuncture is performed.[17,18] This is not necessary with midazolam. Because midazolam is water soluble, phlebitis is uncommon, and venipuncture may be established at any available site, including the dorsum of the hand and wrist. Venipuncture is completed, and the IV infusion is established and secured (see Chapter 24).

Midazolam – as Sole IV Drug

Midazolam may now be administered to the patient. The midazolam has previously been readied for use by the dental assistant. This is now reviewed.

Midazolam is commonly administered intravenously in a concentration of 1 mg/mL. When the 5-mg/mL formulation of midazolam is used, 1 mL of the drug is placed into a 5-mL syringe and 4 mL of IV fluid (e.g., D5W or 0.9% sodium chloride) added. This provides a final concentration of 1 mg/mL midazolam. The syringe is recapped and labeled "midazolam 1 mg/mL." Syringes containing drugs should always be labeled, even when only one drug is to be administered.

Drug Administration – Midazolam

The patient is placed in a supine position before drug administration. It is good practice to open up the IV infusion so that the rate of flow is rapid during the administration of any drug. This further dilutes the drug, minimizing any local irritation that might develop when the drug comes into contact with the vein wall.

Immediately before beginning drug administration, the assistant or dentist should make one final check to confirm that the IV infusion is still patent. By squeezing the flash bulb of the tubing or holding the bag of IV solution below the level of the patient's heart, a return of blood into the tubing should be noted, a sign of a still-patent IV line (Fig. 26.2).

A test dose of 0.2 mL (each small delineation on the 3-mL or 5-mL syringe is 0.2 mL) of midazolam is administered to determine whether any unusual response (e.g., hypersensitivity, allergy) is to develop (Fig. 26.3).

After waiting about 20 seconds, titration of midazolam starts. The recommended rate of injection of midazolam is 1 mL/min, the equivalent of 1 mg of midazolam per minute.

The dentist should start by administering 0.5 mL slowly and continuously over 30 seconds. Because of the great individual variation in drug response, the dentist must always titrate carefully to the desired level of sedation for each patient. Midazolam titration should continue at a rate of 1 mL/min until this ideal level of sedation is achieved.

When first learning to use IV moderate sedation, a dentist's natural tendency will be to cease titration of midazolam at the very first sign of any change in the patient's level of consciousness. Because of the uncertainty of the dentist, many patients may be undersedated. As clinical experience is gained, the dentist will develop a "feel" for the proper level of moderate sedation.

The following are clinical signs and symptoms associated with the desired level of moderate sedation:

- The patient will appear to become more relaxed in the dental chair in contrast to his or her earlier, more visibly tense demeanor. The patient may stretch out, uncross his or her legs, and relax his or her grip on the arm of the chair.
- The patient's response to questions will be somewhat slower than it was earlier, and the patient may appear to have some difficulty in putting thoughts together into words.
- The patient may appear to be having difficulty keeping his or her eyelids open (as occurs when we are tired and begin to doze off). This is not to be considered the primary criterion for proper sedation. Halfway ptosis of the upper eyelid, the Verrill sign (Fig. 26.4), usually occurs when the patient is somewhat overly sedated.[17,18]

When midazolam is administered at the recommended rate, the typical (normoresponding) patient in the middle of the "bell-shaped" curve requiring approximately 4 to 8 mg of midazolam will be sedated within 4 to 8 minutes of the start of drug administration. Once the desired level of sedation is reached, the rate of the IV infusion is slowed. Whenever a drug is not being administered, the infusion rate is adjusted to approximately 1 drop every 5 to 10 seconds. The purpose is to maintain patency of the needle (by preventing a blood clot from forming in the needle) during the procedure. This slow drip rate is commonly abbreviated as t.k.o. (to keep open).

Immediately after the administration of midazolam, vital signs and the drug dose (in milligrams) are recorded on the anesthesia record. Vital signs should be recorded immediately after any subsequent IV drug administration and at 5- to 10-minute intervals throughout the procedure. All drugs administered during IV moderate sedation, including local anesthetics, must be recorded on the anesthesia record in milligrams (mg) of drug (e.g., 36 mg lidocaine), not volume (e.g., 1.8 mL)

Dosage – Midazolam

The average dose of midazolam required for clinically adequate IV moderate sedation is between 4 and 8 mg (based on more

Date	29 MARCH 2016		Pre-op Vitals	BP 118/68	HR· 54	SpO₂ 99	RR 16

Name Stanley Smith

Age 67	Gender M Ⓜ F	Weight 195 lbs.	Height 6'0"	BMI 26.4	Mallampati 1	ASA 1

Medical History ↑ cholesterol

Medications Simvastatin 20 mg

Drug Allergies NkDA

NPO
Solids 8 Hours 6 Clear Liquids 6 Hours
Procedure(s): Multiple restorations
Operator: SFM   Assistants: KLR

NIBP Ⓛ R
Pulse Oximeter ✔
Precordial ✔
ECG ✔
EtCO₂

	Start	Finish	Premedication	IV 20G 22G
ANES	0910		NONE	R L
SURG				Site

TIME	9⁻	15	30	45	10⁻	15	30	45	11⁻						Used	Wasted
Oxygen (LPM)		5⁻														
Nitrous Oxide (LPM)																
Midazolam (mg)																
Diazepam (mg)																
Fentanyl (mcg)																
Meperidine (mg)																
Hydromorphone (mg)																
Sufentanil (mcg)																
Ketorolac (mg)																
NS (mL)																---
2% lidocaine 1:100K epi (mg)																---
4% articaine 1:100K epi (mg)																---
Response to Verbal Stimuli																
SpO₂		99														
Respiratory Rate		16														
EtCO₂ Present																
ECG Pattern		NSR														

Discharged to:

BP

HR

SpO₂

RR

☐ Awake

☐ Alert

☐ Ambulatory

	9⁻	15	30	45	10⁻	15	30	45	11⁻

150

100

50

Comments

Operator Signature: _____   Faculty Signature: _____

Figure 26.1 Patient information and preoperative vital signs are recorded and entered onto the patient's chart.

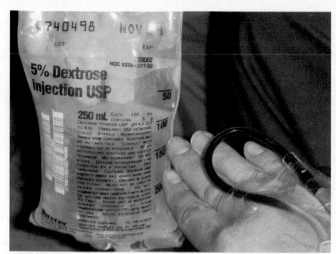

Figure 26.2 Holding bag of IV solution below the level of the vein should produce a return of blood into the tubing, a sign of a still-patent IV.

than 2500 midazolam sedation procedures). The range of these doses is of far greater importance because it illustrates the tremendous individual variability in response to midazolam (and all drugs). In my experience with midazolam as a sole agent for sedation, clinically adequate sedation has been achieved with as little as 0.5 mg (0.5 mL) in some patients, whereas others have received in excess of 10 mg and have not even come close to the desired level of sedation.

The following is suggested as a means of determining the maximum dose of midazolam for a given patient:

Midazolam is titrated at a rate of 1 mg (1 mL) per minute until "ideal" sedation is achieved. The average dose of diazepam required to produce this clinical effect is 4 to 8 mg. Once this effect is achieved, titration ceases, the IV infusion is slowed to t.k.o., and the operative phase of treatment is begun (see later discussion).

If, however, a midazolam dose of 8 mg has been administered with the patient demonstrating some, but not close to ideal, clinical sedation, additional midazolam may be titrated up to a total of 10 mg. On the other hand, if the patient has received 8 mg of midazolam but exhibits virtually *no signs or symptoms* of sedation, it is suggested that the administration of midazolam cease. Experience with benzodiazepines has demonstrated that when no evidence of sedation occurs with an 8-mg dose of midazolam, its continued administration will probably not prove beneficial to the patient, but may increase the risk of occurrence of several dose-related complications. My recommendation to the neophyte at IV moderate sedation is that when a dose of 8 mg midazolam fails to produce any signs or symptoms of clinical sedation, the administration of midazolam is terminated, and the planned dental or surgical procedure is attempted without the administration of additional IV drugs.

The dentist experienced in IV moderate sedation and/or general anesthesia has several additional options available at this time, but in the hands of the dentist without anesthesiology

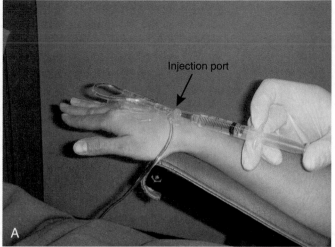

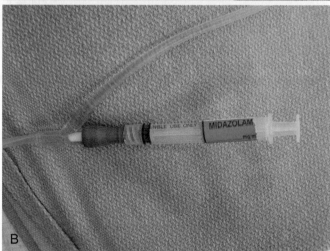

Figure 26.3 A, Needle inserted into injection port *(arrow).* **B,** Needleless syringe system.

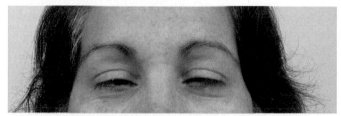

Figure 26.4 Halfway ptosis of the upper eyelid is often seen when a benzodiazepine (e.g., midazolam, diazepam) is employed as an IV sedative.

training, the most prudent course of action at this time is to cease IV drug administration and begin the planned procedure. Midazolam is an excellent amnestic drug, and I am no longer surprised by the number of patients who, lacking any obvious signs or symptoms of sedation, do extremely well and have a significant degree of amnesia at the end of the procedure. Should this attempt to treat fail, the patient should be dismissed (following adequate recovery) and rescheduled for a different IV moderate sedation technique at a later date.

Midazolam	
Average sedative dose	4–8 mg
Sedative dose range	2–10 mg
Maximum dose, no sedation	8 mg
Maximum dose, some sedation	10 mg

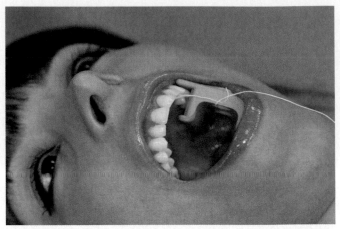

Figure 26.5 Rubber bite block with string (dental floss) tied to it.

Intraoperative Period – Midazolam

Local anesthetic is administered to the patient exactly as it would be if the patient was not sedated. This includes the use of topical anesthetic and all of the other steps involved in the atraumatic administration of local anesthesia.[19] The patient may react to any pain associated with the local anesthetic injection, but this usually is nothing more than a slight moan, grimace, or minor movement. Adequate time should be allowed for the local anesthetic to take effect before starting the planned dental procedure.

During the first 1 to 5 minutes following IV midazolam titration, the level of sedation (CNS depression) is greatest. Although overresponse to the drug can occur, the patient who has overresponded to midazolam will be somewhat sluggish in response to verbal commands, such as "open your mouth." For this reason, the use of a mouth prop should be considered, at least at the outset of the IV moderate sedation procedure. Within 5 to 10 minutes, the depth of midazolam sedation has usually lessened so that the patient's mouth can be voluntarily kept open. A rubber bite block with a piece of string (dental floss) tied around it or a ratchet type of (Molt) mouth prop may be used at this time (Fig. 26.5).

Lack of response to verbal command or, more significantly, a lack of response to a painful stimulus (i.e., local anesthetic injection) may indicate that the patient is overly sedated. Lack of response to sensory stimulation is always reason for the dentist to stop treatment and reevaluate the patient's level of CNS depression and airway and ventilatory status (e.g., to "rescue" the patient from unintended entry into the next level of sedation [deep]).[20]

Following local anesthetic administration, a rubber dam should be applied, if necessary, for the planned procedure. The rubber dam serves two important functions during IV moderate sedation:

1. It aids in maintaining the mouth in an open position (it may be used in place of the mouth prop).
2. It minimizes the risk of tracheal aspiration by preventing extraneous material from falling into the posterior part of the mouth, throat, and pharynx.

Dental treatment begins at this time. Because of the 45- to 60-minute duration of sedation provided by IV midazolam, the dental treatment should be planned to fit into this time period. Midazolam produces a period of anterograde amnesia in most patients, lasting for most of the duration of the dental procedure (if not longer).[20] Potentially painful or traumatic procedures completed during this time will likely not be remembered by the patient later, though they will still respond to the stimulus in a somewhat normal manner when they occur.

Planned properly, as the sedative effect begins to noticeably wane (about 30 minutes after drug administration), relatively innocuous procedures are being performed, such as completing restorations, suturing, or adjusting occlusion. In addition, having received local anesthesia earlier, the patient will be pain free at this time and able to tolerate these procedures without complaint. In most patients, actual treatment time, with one initial titrating dose of midazolam, can usually be extended well beyond 1 hour because of the lack of pain and the relative innocuousness of the procedures carried out at the end of the treatment period.

It is uncommon for a patient to require a second dose of midazolam if the duration of the planned procedure was appropriate (about 1 hour). As discussed in Chapter 25, midazolam sedation may be divided into several phases: stage 1 (minutes 1 to 10): good sedation plus amnesia; stage 2 (minutes 11 to 30): "OK" sedation plus amnesia; stage 3 (minutes 31 to 45): sedation wanes (patient more alert), amnesia still present; and stage 4 (minutes 46 to 60): clinical recovery of patient, amnesia may still be present. With entry into the third phase, the patient may opine that he or she feels "normal" once again, and the dentist might be tempted to administer additional midazolam. However, by this time, treatment should be nearing completion, the procedure performed is usually atraumatic, the patient has effective pain management (local anesthesia), and although the patient feels normal, he or she is still anxiety free, if not visibly sedated. Readministration of midazolam is rarely necessary in this typical 1-hour IV moderate sedation procedure.

Occasionally, readministration of midazolam might become necessary to permit successful completion of the procedure. For example, a patient is scheduled for restorative procedures planned for about 1 hour. All goes well, but one of the teeth unexpectedly requires endodontic treatment. The patient becomes increasingly aware of the surroundings approximately 45 minutes into the procedure and has become somewhat apprehensive again. The treating dentist has two options: first, to temporarily fill the canal, dismiss the patient, and reschedule for another IV visit; or second, to titrate additional midazolam and continue with endodontic care at the same visit. Retitration of midazolam or diazepam will be discussed later in this chapter.

Posttreatment Period – Midazolam

Following completion of the planned treatment, the IV infusion is discontinued if, in the opinion of the dentist, there is no further need for drug administration. By this time, the patient should be responding relatively normally with no adverse or bizarre signs or symptoms noted (e.g., emergence delirium). The technique for termination of the IV infusion is discussed in Chapter 24. Nasal O_2 can also be terminated at this time.

Recovery Criteria – Midazolam

The patient is never to be discharged alone from the office after IV moderate sedation, regardless of the patient's apparent state of recovery or the degree to which the patient protests. Criteria for discharge from the office include the vital signs and the physical reaction of the patient.

The patient's vital signs should approximate those of baseline level (taken at the preliminary visit). If blood pressure appears significantly depressed (more than 30 mm Hg below baseline) and/or clinical signs and symptoms of sedation remain, the patient must be permitted additional time to recover while continuing to receive supplemental O_2.

The most important criterion for discharge is the patient's response, which is highly subjective. Under no circumstance can a patient ever be permitted to leave the office feeling poorly or unable to walk without assistance. In a few cases, the patient may feel dizzy, mildly nauseous, or weak. In such cases, the patient should be permitted to rest until he or she feels better (thus the importance of a recovery area in the office supervised by a trained assistant). A sedated patient should never be left unattended in any room for any length of time; the dentist or a trained member of the staff is physically present at all times, if at all possible.

When it is believed that the patient has recovered sufficiently to be discharged, all monitoring devices are removed and the patient is permitted to stand. A member of the dental team, the dentist or assistant, should position himself or herself in front of the patient so that if the patient's legs are a little weak, that person can support the patient, preventing a fall and potential injury.

The chair is adjusted from semisupine to an almost 90-degree position. This is done slowly, preferably in several steps, to allow the patient's cardiovascular system to readapt to the increasing effect of gravity, thereby preventing postural hypotension, dizziness, and, possibly, syncope.

The patient turns and sits with his or her legs touching the floor before standing. If the patient is able to accomplish this without difficulty (following midazolam or diazepam IV moderate sedation, there is rarely difficulty in standing after 45 minutes), the patient is requested to take a few steps toward the dentist or assistant. If all is well, the patient is reseated in the dental chair and their escort brought in.

The foremost criterion in permitting patients to be discharged from the office is their ability to take care of themselves should they, for any reason, be left alone during the remainder of the day. They should be able to stand and walk without assistance. If such is not the case, the patient is permitted additional time to recover.

When midazolam or diazepam is used for IV moderate sedation, clinical recovery usually appears to be quite complete at 45 to 60 minutes.

Once recovery is deemed adequate for discharge, the patient is returned to the dental chair and their responsible adult escort brought in. In the presence of both persons, postoperative instructions are presented verbally and in writing. It is potentially possible with midazolam (less likely with diazepam) for the patient to still be amnesic at this time in the procedure, thus the necessity of the escort and written instructions. Instructions given to the patient should be recorded on the anesthesia record and a copy included in the patient's dental chart.

Usual postsedation instructions are presented in Box 26.2. Additional instructions should be included if mandated by the dental treatment. This might include restrictions on diet or the need for ice or heat application. Once again, these are presented verbally to both the patient and his or her escort, given to the patient in writing, and recorded on the patient's chart.

The companion accompanies the patient from the office. A member of the office staff should remain with the patient until he or she is seated safely in the car with the seat belt secured (in a passenger's seat, not the driver's seat).

The anesthesia record sheet and the patient's treatment chart are completed, disposable IV equipment (needle, tubing, syringes, and infusion solution) discarded properly, and any unused drug discarded (and the discard recorded). A note in the chart and anesthesia record sheet is made: "x mg midazolam discarded." Recording of the disposition of all drugs, especially the Schedule II opioid agonists, is a very important part of the IV procedure.

Fig. 26.6 illustrates a typical anesthesia record at the conclusion of the IV moderate sedation procedure. The following (sample) entry is made in the patient's dental chart when the anesthesia record sheet is included in the chart:

Date. Patient received intravenous moderate sedation. Anesthesia record enclosed. Dental treatment: extraction 27, 30, 31; MOD 15, etc., signature or initials of dentist.

When an anesthesia record is not available (every effort should be taken to avoid this because its absence is somewhat difficult to explain), the following chart entry is suggested:

IV started with a 21-gauge indwelling catheter in the left ventral forearm. The patient received 7 mg midazolam in one titrating dose. Duration of IV procedure = 45 minutes, the patient receiving 5 L/min 100% O_2 via nasal hood throughout the procedure. A total of 180 mL of 0.9 normal saline was administered. Monitoring included continuous pulse oximetry and BP q 5 min. The patient tolerated the procedure well and was discharged in good condition from

Box 26.2	Postsedation Instructions

1. Go home and rest for the remainder of the day.
2. Do not perform any strenuous activity. You should remain in the company of a responsible adult until you are fully alert.
3. Do not attempt to eat a heavy meal immediately. If you are hungry, a light diet (liquids and toast) will be more than adequate.
4. A feeling of nausea may occasionally develop after sedation. The following may help you feel better: (a) lying down for a while and/or (b) a glass of cola beverage or ginger ale.
5. Do not drive a motor vehicle or perform any hazardous tasks for the remainder of the day.
6. Do not take any alcoholic beverages or any medications for the remainder of the day unless you have contacted me first.
7. The following medication(s) have been ordered for you by the dentist. Take them only as directed.
8. If you have any unusual problems, you may call (office telephone number).

the office in the custody of Mary Smith at 12:05 PM. Postoperative instructions were given verbally and in writing to both the patient and companion.

Although this may appear to be voluminous and perhaps excessive, especially considering the nature of the usual treatment entry in dental records, this type of recordkeeping is absolutely essential whenever sedative procedures are employed. There should be no doubt at a later date as to exactly what transpired during the sedative procedure.

One more important task remains on the day of the IV moderate sedation: each and every patient who receives IV (or other parenteral sedation technique [IM, intranasal (IN)]) sedation should be contacted by telephone by the dentist in the late afternoon if the IV was in the morning or early that evening following an afternoon IV procedure. This is one of the most important actions a health care provider can perform for his or her patient. It demonstrates to the patient the dentist's sincerity and concern and is a means of circumventing potential posttreatment problems (e.g., the development of pain or

bleeding) before they become significant. Note of this conversation is entered in the patient's chart.

Diazepam – as Sole IV Drug

Diazepam may now be administered to the patient. The diazepam has previously been readied for use by the dental assistant. This is now reviewed.

Diazepam is available in a 10-mL vial at a concentration of 5 mg/mL. The assistant takes a sterile, disposable 3- or 5-mL syringe and after wiping the rubber diaphragm of the vial with isopropyl alcohol (and waiting 1 minute for the alcohol to dry) injects 3 mL of air into the vial of diazepam and withdraws an equal volume of the yellowish diazepam solution. The syringe is recapped, labeled "diazepam 5 mg/mL," and put aside for later use. Syringes containing drugs must always be labeled, even when only one drug is used. Diazepam is not, and cannot, be diluted.

Drug Administration – Diazepam

The patient is placed in a supine position before drug administration. It is good practice to open up the IV infusion so that the rate of flow is rapid during the administration of any drug. This further dilutes the drug, minimizing any local irritation that might develop when the drug comes into contact with the vein wall.

Immediately before beginning drug administration, the assistant or dentist should make one final check to confirm that the IV is still patent. By squeezing the flash bulb of the tubing or holding the bag of IV solution below the level of the patient's heart, a return of blood into the tubing, a sign of a patent IV line, should be noted (see Fig. 26.2).

Diazepam, an oily, viscous liquid, has the ability to cause a burning sensation in some patients as it is administered, with the sensation lasting until the diazepam is flushed from the injection site. A rapidly running IV drip minimizes this sensation. In addition, it is advisable to tell the patient that he or she may experience a brief period of warmth when the drug is injected, that this is normal, and that it will subside quickly.

A test dose of 0.2 mL (each small delineation on the 3-mL or 5-mL syringe is 0.2 mL) diazepam is administered to determine whether any unusual response (e.g., hypersensitivity, allergy) will develop (see Fig. 26.3).

After waiting about 20 seconds, titration of diazepam starts. The recommended rate of injection of diazepam is 1 mL/min, the equivalent of 5 mg of diazepam per minute.

The dentist should start by administering 0.5 mL slowly and continuously over 30 seconds. Because of the great

	BASELINE	PREOPERATIVE	POST-IV DRUG ADMINISTRATION	POSTOPERATIVE
Blood pressure (mm Hg)	124/68	132/74	128/70	124/72
Heart rate (beats/min)	66	78	74	74
Respiratory rate (breaths/min)	16	18	14	16
O_2 saturation (%)	97	97	98	98
Dentist's signature: _____				

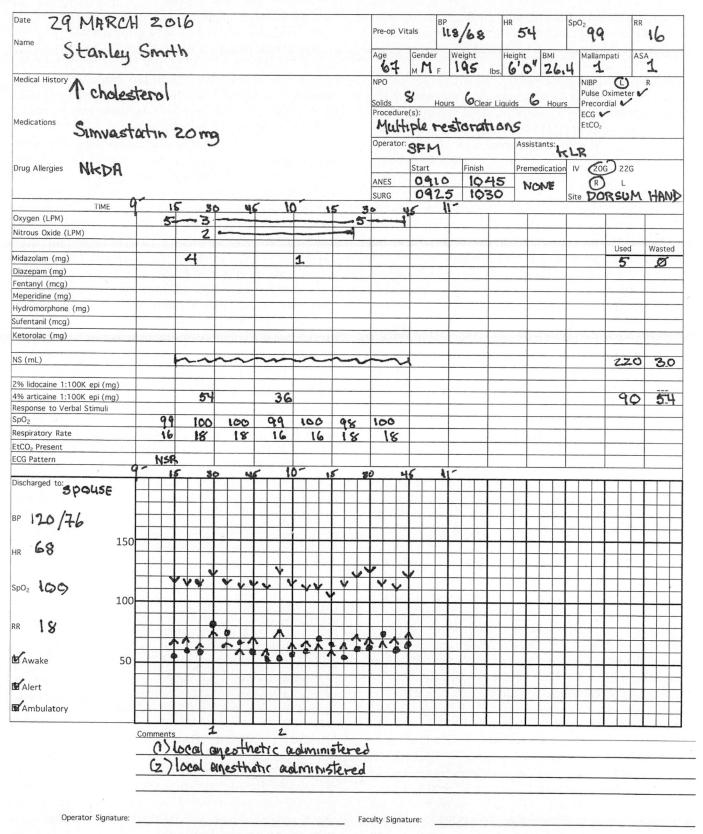

Date: 29 MARCH 2016

Name: Stanley Smith

Medical History: ↑ cholesterol

Medications: Simvastatin 20 mg

Drug Allergies: NKDA

Pre-op Vitals — BP: 118/68 HR: 54 SpO₂: 99 RR: 16

Age: 67 Gender: M (M) F Weight: 195 lbs. Height: 6'0" BMI: 26.4 Mallampati: 1 ASA: 1

NPO — Solids: 8 Hours 6 Clear Liquids 6 Hours

NIBP: (L) R Pulse Oximeter ✓ Precordial ✓ ECG ✓ EtCO₂

Procedure(s): Multiple restorations

Operator: SFM   Assistants: KLR

	Start	Finish	Premedication	IV (20G) 22G
ANES	0910	1045	NONE	(R) L
SURG	0925	1030		Site DORSUM HAND

TIME	9⁻	15	30	45	10⁻	15	30	45	11⁻						Used	Wasted
Oxygen (LPM)		5→3					5→									
Nitrous Oxide (LPM)			2				→									
Midazolam (mg)		4			1										5	Ø
Diazepam (mg)																
Fentanyl (mcg)																
Meperidine (mg)																
Hydromorphone (mg)																
Sufentanil (mcg)																
Ketorolac (mg)																
NS (mL)															220	30
2% lidocaine 1:100K epi (mg)																
4% articaine 1:100K epi (mg)		54		36											90	54
Response to Verbal Stimuli																
SpO₂	99	100	100	99	100	98	100									
Respiratory Rate	16	18	18	16	16	18	18									
EtCO₂ Present																
ECG Pattern	NSR															

Discharged to: SPOUSE

BP 120/76
HR 68
SpO₂ 100
RR 18

☑ Awake
☑ Alert
☑ Ambulatory

TIME	9⁻	15	30	45	10⁻	15	30	45	11⁻

150

100

50

Comments: 1   2

(1) local anesthetic administered
(2) local anesthetic administered

Operator Signature: _____   Faculty Signature: _____

Figure 26.6 Completed sedation record for an IV diazepam procedure.

individual variation in drug response, the dentist must always titrate carefully to the desired level of sedation for each patient. Diazepam should continue to be titrated at a rate of 1 mL/min until this ideal level of sedation is achieved.

When first learning to use IV moderate sedation, a dentist's natural tendency will be to cease titration of diazepam at the very first sign of a change in the patient's level of consciousness. Because of the uncertainty of the dentist, many patients may be undersedated. As clinical experience is gained, the dentist will develop a "feel" for the proper level of moderate sedation.

The following are clinical signs and symptoms associated with the desired level of moderate sedation:

- The patient will appear to become more relaxed in the dental chair in contrast to his or her earlier, more visibly tense demeanor. The patient may stretch out, uncross his or her legs, and relax his or her grip on the arm of the chair.
- The patient's response to questions will be somewhat slower than it was earlier, and the patient may appear to have some difficulty in putting thoughts together into words.
- The patient may have difficulty keeping the eyelids open (as happens when one is tired and falling asleep). This is not to be considered the primary criterion for proper sedation. Halfway ptosis of the upper eyelid, the Verrill sign (see Fig. 26.4), usually occurs when the patient is somewhat too heavily sedated.[18,21]

When diazepam is administered at the recommended rate, the typical patient (middle of the "bell-shaped" curve), requiring approximately 10 to 12 mg of diazepam, should be sedated within 2 to 3 minutes of the start of drug administration. Once the desired level of sedation is reached, the rate of the IV infusion is slowed. Whenever a drug is not being administered, the infusion rate is adjusted to approximately 1 drop every 5 to 10 seconds. The purpose is to maintain patency of the needle (by preventing a blood clot from forming in the needle) during the procedure. This slow drip rate is commonly abbreviated as t.k.o.

Immediately after the administration of diazepam, vital signs and the drug dose (in milligrams) are recorded on the anesthesia record. Vital signs should be recorded immediately after any subsequent IV drug administration and at 5- to 10-minute intervals throughout the procedure. All drugs administered during IV moderate sedation, including local anesthetics, must be recorded on the anesthesia record in milligrams (mg) of drug (e.g., 8 mg diazepam), not volume (e.g., 1.6 mL)

Dosage – Diazepam

The average dose of diazepam required for clinically adequate IV moderate sedation is between 10 and 12 mg (based on more than 3750 cases). The range of these doses is of far greater importance because it illustrates the tremendous individual variability in response to diazepam (and all drugs). In my experience with diazepam as a sole agent for sedation, clinically adequate sedation has been achieved with as little as 2.5 mg (0.5 mL) in some patients, whereas others have received in excess of 30 mg and have not even approached the desired level of sedation.

The following is suggested as a means of determining the appropriate dose of diazepam for a given patient:

Diazepam is titrated at a rate of 5 mg (1 mL) per minute until the ideal sedation level for that patient is achieved. The average dose of diazepam required to produce this clinical effect is 10 to 12 mg. Once this is achieved, titration ceases, the IV infusion is slowed to t.k.o., and the operative phase of treatment is begun (see later discussion).

However, if a diazepam dose of 20 mg has been administered with the patient demonstrating some, but not close to ideal, clinical sedation, additional diazepam may be titrated up to a total of 30 mg. If, on the other hand, the patient has received 20 mg of diazepam but exhibits virtually no *signs or symptoms* of sedation, it is suggested that the administration of diazepam cease. Experience with diazepam has demonstrated that when no evidence of sedation occurs with a 20-mg dose, the addition of another 10 or 20 mg probably will not prove beneficial to the patient, but may increase the risk of occurrence of several dose-related complications. My recommendation to the neophyte at IV moderate sedation is that when a dose of 20 mg of diazepam fails to produce any signs or symptoms of clinical sedation, the administration of diazepam is terminated, and the planned dental or surgical procedure attempted without the administration of additional IV drugs.

The dentist experienced in IV moderate sedation and/or general anesthesia has several additional options available at this time, but in the hands of the dentist without anesthesiology training, the most prudent course of action at this time is to cease IV drug administration and begin the planned procedure. I am no longer surprised by the number of patients who, lacking any obvious signs or symptoms of sedation, do extremely well and have a significant degree of amnesia at the end of the procedure. Should this attempt to treat fail, the patient should be dismissed (following adequate recovery) and rescheduled for a different IV moderate sedation technique at a later date.

Diazepam	
Average sedative dose	10–12 mg
Sedative dose range	2.5 to >30 mg
Maximum dose, no sedation	20 mg
Maximum dose, some sedation	30 mg

Intraoperative Period – Diazepam

Local anesthetic is administered to the patient exactly as it would be if the patient was not sedated. This includes the use of topical anesthetic and all of the other steps involved in atraumatic administration of local anesthesia.[19] The patient may react to any pain associated with the local anesthetic injection, but this usually is nothing more than a slight moan, grimace, or minor movement. Adequate time must be allowed for the local anesthetic to take effect before starting the planned procedure.

During the first 1 to 5 minutes following IV diazepam titration, the level of sedation (CNS depression) is greatest. Although overresponse to the drug can occur, the patient who has overresponded to diazepam will be somewhat sluggish in response to verbal commands, such as "open your mouth." For this reason, the use of a mouth prop should be considered, at least at the outset of the IV diazepam procedure. Within 5 to 10 minutes, the depth of sedation has usually lessened so that the patient's mouth can be voluntarily kept open. A rubber bite block with a piece of string (dental floss) tied around it or a ratchet type of (Molt) mouth prop may be used at this time (see Fig. 26.5).

Lack of response to verbal command or, more significantly, a lack of response to a painful stimulus (i.e., local anesthetic injection) may indicate that the patient is overly sedated. Lack of response to sensory stimulation is always an indication for the dentist to stop treatment and evaluate the patient's level of CNS depression and airway and ventilatory status.

Following local anesthetic administration, a rubber dam should be applied, if necessary, for the planned procedure. The rubber dam serves two important functions during IV moderate sedation:

1. It aids in maintaining the mouth in an open position (it may be used in place of the mouth prop).
2. It prevents extraneous material from falling into the posterior part of the mouth, throat, and pharynx.

Dental treatment begins at this time. Because of the 45- to 60-minute duration of sedation provided by IV diazepam, treatment should be planned to fit into this time period.[21] Diazepam produces a period of anterograde amnesia in approximately 75% of patients, lasting approximately 10 minutes.[22] It is recommended that potentially painful or traumatic procedures be completed at the start of the treatment, if possible, to take advantage of this amnesic period.

In this manner, as the sedative effect begins to wane (about 30 minutes after drug administration), relatively innocuous procedures are being performed, such as completing restorations, suturing, or adjusting occlusion. In addition, having received local anesthesia earlier, the patient should remain pain free at this time and able to tolerate these procedures without complaint. In most patients, actual treatment time, with one initial titrating dose of diazepam, can usually be extended well beyond 1 hour because of the lack of pain and the relative innocuousness of the procedures carried out at the end of the treatment period.

It is uncommon for a patient to require a second dose of diazepam if the duration of the planned procedure was appropriate (about 1 hour). As discussed in Chapter 25, diazepam sedation may be divided into several phases: stage 1 (minutes 1 to 5): decreased awareness, good sedation, amnesia; stage 2 (minutes 6 to 30): "good" sedation, no amnesia; stage 3 (minutes 31 to 45): sedation wanes, no amnesia; stage 4 (minutes 46 to 60): anxiolysis, no amnesia; and stage 5 (60 minutes and beyond): clinical recovery. With entry into the third or fourth phase, the patient may mention that he or she feels "normal" once again, and the dentist might be tempted to administer additional diazepam. However, by this time, treatment should be nearing completion; the procedure being performed is usually atraumatic, the patient has effective pain management (local anesthesia), and although the patient feels "normal," he or she is still anxiety free, if not visibly sedated. Thus readministration of diazepam is rarely necessary in the typical 1-hour IV moderate sedation procedure.

Occasionally, readministration of diazepam might be necessary to permit successful completion of the procedure. For example, a patient is scheduled for restorative procedures with IV diazepam. All goes well, but one of the teeth unexpectedly requires endodontic treatment. The patient becomes increasingly aware of the surroundings approximately 40 minutes into the procedure and has become somewhat apprehensive again. The treating dentist has two options: first, to temporarily fill the canal, dismiss the patient, and reschedule for another IV visit or second, titrate additional diazepam and continue with dental care at the same visit. Retitration of diazepam or midazolam will be discussed later in this chapter.

Posttreatment Period – Diazepam

Following completion of the planned dental procedure, the IV infusion is discontinued if, in the opinion of the dentist, there is no further need for drug administration. By this time, the patient should be responding normally with no adverse or bizarre signs or symptoms noted (e.g., emergence delirium). The technique for termination of the IV infusion is discussed in Chapter 24. Nasal O_2 can also be terminated at this time.

Recovery Criteria

The patient is never to be discharged alone from the office after IV moderate sedation, regardless of the patient's apparent state of recovery or the degree to which the patient protests. Criteria for discharge from the office include the vital signs and the reaction of the patient.

The patient's vital signs should approximate those of baseline level (taken at the preliminary visit). If blood pressure appears significantly depressed (more than 30 mm Hg below baseline) and/or clinical signs and symptoms of sedation remain, the patient must be permitted additional time to recover while continuing to receive supplemental O_2.

The most important criterion for discharge is the patient's physical response, which is highly subjective. Under no circumstances can a patient ever be permitted to leave the office feeling poorly or unable to walk without assistance. In a few cases, the patient may feel dizzy, mildly nauseous, or weak. In such cases, the patient should be permitted to rest until he or she feels better (thus the importance of a recovery area in the office, supervised by a trained assistant). A sedated patient should never be left unattended in any room for any length of time; the dentist or a trained member of the staff is physically present at all times, if at all possible.

When it is believed that the patient has recovered sufficiently to be discharged, all monitoring devices are removed and the patient is permitted to stand. A member of the dental team, the dentist or assistant, should position himself or herself in front of the patient so that if the patient's legs are a little weak, that person can support the patient, preventing a fall and potential injury.

The chair is adjusted from semisupine to an almost 90-degree position. This is done slowly, preferably in several steps, to allow the patient's cardiovascular system to readapt to the increasing effect of gravity, thereby preventing postural hypotension, dizziness, and, possibly, syncope.

The patient turns and sits with his or her legs touching the floor before standing. If the patient is able to accomplish this without difficulty (following midazolam or diazepam IV moderate sedation, there is rarely difficulty in standing after 45 minutes), the patient is requested to take a few steps toward the dentist or assistant. If all is well, the patient is reseated in the dental chair and their escort brought in.

The foremost criterion in permitting patients to be discharged from the office is their ability to take care of themselves should they, for any reason, be left alone during the remainder of the day. They should be able to stand and walk without assistance. If such is not the case, the patient is permitted additional time to recover.

When diazepam is used for IV moderate sedation, clinical recovery usually appears to be quite complete at 45 to 60 minutes.

Once recovery is deemed adequate for discharge, the patient is returned to the dental chair and his or her responsible adult escort brought in. In the presence of both persons, postoperative instructions are presented verbally and in writing. It is potentially possible, although quite unlikely with diazepam, that the patient may still be amnesic at this time in the procedure, thus the necessity for the escort and written instructions. Instructions given to the patient should be recorded on the anesthesia record and a copy included in the patient's dental chart.

Usual postsedation instructions are presented in Box 26.2. Additional postoperative instructions should be included if mandated by the dental treatment. This might include restrictions on diet or the need for ice or heat application. Once again, these are presented verbally to both the patient and the escort, given to the patient in writing, and recorded on the patient's chart.

The companion accompanies the patient from the office. A member of the office staff must remain with the patient until the patient is seated safely in the car with the seat belt secured (in a passenger's seat, not the driver's seat).

The anesthesia record sheet and the patient's treatment chart are completed, disposable IV equipment (needle, tubing, syringes, and infusion solution) safely discarded, and any unused drug discarded and recorded. A note in the chart and anesthesia record sheet is made: "x mg diazepam discarded." Recording of the disposition of all drugs, especially the Schedule II opioid agonists, is a very important part of the IV procedure.

Fig. 26.6 illustrates a typical anesthesia record at the conclusion of the IV moderate sedation procedure. The following entry is made in the patient's dental chart when the anesthesia record sheet is included in the chart:

Date. Patient received intravenous moderate sedation. Anesthesia record enclosed. Dental treatment: extraction 27, 30, 31; MOD 15, etc., signature or initials of dentist.

When an anesthesia record is not available (every effort should be taken to avoid this because this is somewhat difficult to defend legally), the following chart entry is suggested:

IV started with a 21-gauge indwelling catheter in the left ventral forearm. The patient received 13 mg diazepam in one titrated dose. Duration of IV procedure = 45 minutes, the patient receiving 5 L/min 100% O$_2$ via nasal hood throughout the procedure. A total of 180 mL of 0.9 normal saline was administered. Monitoring included continuous pulse oximetry and BP q 5 min. The patient tolerated the procedure well and was discharged from the office in the custody of Mary Smith at 12:05 pm. Postoperative instructions were given verbally and in writing to both the patient and companion.

Although this may appear to be voluminous and perhaps excessive, especially considering the nature of the usual entry in dental records, this type of recordkeeping is absolutely essential whenever sedative drugs are employed. There should be no doubt at a later date as to exactly what transpired during the sedative procedure.

One more important task remains on the day of the IV moderate sedation procedure: each and every patient who receives IV (or other parenteral sedation technique [IM, IN]) sedation should be contacted by telephone by the dentist in the late afternoon if the IV was in the morning or early that evening if the IV was in the afternoon. This is one of the most important actions a health care provider can perform for his or her patient. It demonstrates to the patient the dentist's sincerity and concern and is a means of circumventing potential problems (e.g., the development of pain or bleeding) before they become significant. Note of this conversation is entered in the patient's chart.

Retitration of Midazolam or Diazepam

The administration of a single titrating dose of either midazolam or diazepam for sedation provides approximately 45 to 60 minutes of sedation. When combined with adequate local anesthesia, treatment time usually exceeds 1 hour. There are occasions, however, when treatment requires approximately 2 hours or more to complete.

In situations where the dental procedure is planned to exceed 1 hour or where a planned 1-hour procedure is unexpectedly prolonged, the duration of sedation may be extended by additional titrating doses of either midazolam or diazepam.

Should the decision be made to retitrate and continue treatment, the rate of flow of the IV drip is increased and additional midazolam or diazepam titrated at a rate of 1 mL/min (1 mg/min midazolam; 5 mg/min diazepam) until the patient becomes sedated once again or until a total dose (including the initial titration) of 10 mg midazolam or 30 mg diazepam has been administered. Following retitration, the IV drip rate is again slowed to t.k.o. and the dental treatment is recommenced.

Retitration with midazolam or diazepam will almost always require a smaller dose than that required for the initial titration. For example, if 6 mg of midazolam was required initially, a midazolam dose of 2 or 3 mg might produce the same clinical level of sedation on retitration. For reasons that are explained in Chapter 27, the total combined dose of midazolam administered at one appointment should, if possible, be kept to not more than 10 mg, whereas that of diazepam to not more than 30 mg. When midazolam or diazepam is readministered, vital signs are once again recorded on the anesthesia record sheet

SUMMARY

Basic techniques of IV moderate sedation have been presented. It is my belief that the benzodiazepines form the backbone of the dentist's IV sedation armamentarium. When these techniques are used as described, serious complications will not arise. Retrospective studies on the Jorgensen technique and IV midazolam and/or diazepam have demonstrated beyond doubt that these procedures are sound, safe, and effective.[12,23,24]

Availability of these procedures enables the dentist to pick an appropriate IV technique based on the time allotted for treatment:

- Up to 1 hour: Diazepam or midazolam
- From 1 to 2 hours: Midazolam or diazepam (retitrated)
- More than 2 hours: Dental procedures requiring 2 or more hours to complete utilizing IV moderate sedation are discouraged. The incidence of complications and adverse events increases with increased duration of the procedure.

In addition, the following applies to IV drug administration:

- Titrate the drugs slowly.
- Remain within the dosage limits recommended for each technique.
- Failures (the inability to provide adequate sedation within the dosage recommended), although rare, do occur and are to be expected. When this happens, no other drug should be administered to the patient. This includes, for the relatively inexperienced operator, nitrous oxide-oxygen (N_2O-O_2). An attempt is made to treat the patient as best as possible. If this proves to be futile, the procedure is terminated and rescheduled for another time, at which a different technique of sedation will be used. The administration of additional drug or of a different drug to the patient can increase the risk of problems (e.g., unconsciousness, airway obstruction), especially in the hands of the less experienced dentist. Finding out the hard way that this is true is discouraged.

MODIFICATIONS OF BASIC TECHNIQUES

Anticholinergic + Benzodiazepine

In this section, a modification of basic technique is described: the addition of an anticholinergic to midazolam or diazepam.

Selection of a suitable anticholinergic is based on the needs of the patient and the desired duration of its action. Where a slight degree of sedation and amnesia is desired, scopolamine (0.3 mg) is recommended. Its use is appropriate in a procedure of any duration. If the patient is younger than 6 years or older than 65 years, scopolamine is not recommended because of an increased risk of emergence delirium.

Atropine (0.4 mg) is used when a drying effect is desired without amnesia or additional sedation and the duration of the procedure is less than 2 hours. Glycopyrrolate (0.2 mg) is recommended for procedures in excess of 2 hours when a drying effect is required. Table 26.2 summarizes the properties of anticholinergics.

Technique

Anticholinergics should be administered in a separate syringe. The patient receives diazepam or midazolam as discussed previously, and the anticholinergic is then administered. The anticholinergic drug is slowly injected over 1 minute.

The use of diazepam and scopolamine (0.3 mg) may provide a longer duration of amnesia in some patients than will either drug alone. Rather than the amnesic period lasting approximately 10 minutes, it may extend over greater lengths of time. This is not the case when midazolam is administered because the duration of amnesia associated with midazolam is considerably longer than that produced by scopolamine.

One of the disadvantages of employing anticholinergics is that some patients will complain that the drying effect is bothersome, both during the procedure and in some cases after the procedure on returning home. Although drugs are available to reverse anticholinergics (the reversible cholinesterase inhibitors neostigmine and physostigmine), their routine use is not recommended because of possible undesirable side effects.

Opioid + Benzodiazepine

In this section, the addition of an opioid analgesic, either fentanyl, meperidine, or hydromorphone, to midazolam or diazepam is discussed.

When used for a well-defined purpose, the combination of a benzodiazepine and an opioid is quite rational.

Table 26.2	Indications for Anticholinergics			
	SALIVARY SECRETIONS	AMNESIA	SEDATION	DURATION (HR)
Atropine	+	−	−	<2
Glycopyrrolate	+	−	−	>2
Scopolamine	+	+	+	<2

Use of techniques described in this section should be limited to dentists meeting one or both of the following requirements:

1. Dentists who have successfully completed training in general anesthesia techniques and in the management of the airway of an unconscious patient
2. Dentists with considerable experience in the basic techniques of IV moderate sedation (e.g., single benzodiazepine)

Because these techniques involve administration of two or more CNS depressants, there is an increased likelihood of additive drug effects, especially in the medically compromised or elderly populations. Clinically this would produce either an increased depth of sedation possibly beyond that which is desirable and/or transient periods of apnea, both of which require the dentist to immediately terminate dental treatment and evaluate the patient's status (e.g., 'rescue' the patient).

When the listed drugs are administered as suggested (dosage, rate of injection, and monitoring), clinical problems are unlikely to develop. Deviation from these guidelines will increase the potential for adverse side effects.

Rationale for Advanced Techniques

Why discuss the addition of a second drug to the basic IV moderate sedation technique? Two reasons are presented.

First, maximum, safe, and effective doses of each of the basic drugs have been presented. If no clinical effect has developed at that dose, further administration of the same drug is unlikely to provide acceptable sedation until extremely large doses are given. It was suggested in the discussion of basic techniques that the inexperienced (IV sedation) dentist not administer additional IV drugs, attempt to complete the dental procedure—if possible—or attempt a different IV technique at a subsequent appointment.

The dentist who meets one or both of the aforementioned criteria listed may, however, elect to administer a second CNS depressant to this patient—if permitted to do so by the dentist's state or provincial dental regulatory body. Opioids are an excellent choice, with small doses usually providing the additional sedation required for the patient to accept dental treatment and remain comfortable.

Second, a degree of analgesia is provided by the opioid during potentially painful procedures. When used in this regard, a larger dose of opioid is desirable.

The sequence in which the benzodiazepine and opioid are administered depends on the reason for the opioid's inclusion in the technique.

Requirement: Sedation

In the situation in which midazolam or diazepam has been administered to its maximum recommended dose yet the patient remains unsedated, careful administration of an opioid will likely aid in providing the desired sedation. The opioid is slowly titrated (at a rate of 1 mL per minute), with the dentist and assistant carefully observing the patient for signs of increasing sedation. Titration of the opioid ceases when the desired sedation level is reached or the maximum recommended dose of 50 micrograms

(μg) of fentanyl, 50 mg meperidine, or 1 mg hydromorphone is administered. The end point of depth of sedation achieved in this manner should be no greater than that "ideal" level observed with the basic techniques described earlier.

In this first technique, in which the primary requirement is sedation, the patient will have received a larger dose of the antianxiety drug and a smaller dose of the opioid analgesic (e.g., midazolam 8 mg and fentanyl 30 μg; diazepam 20 mg and meperidine 25 mg, or 10 mg midazolam and 0.4 mg hydromorphone).

Requirement: Analgesia

When the planned dental procedure involves a significant potential for pain (either perioperative or postoperative), such as oral surgery or endodontic or periodontal surgery, the benefits of an opioid analgesic may be desirable. The primary technique of pain control during dental treatment will always be local anesthesia. The addition of IV opioids will help the patient during the procedure should the local anesthetic effect begin to lessen. The nature of the discomfort experienced by the patient will be altered—opioids separate pain from suffering.

When used for this purpose, the analgesic drug is administered first and titrated until one of two things occurs: (1) clinically adequate sedation develops or (2) the maximum recommended opioid dose has been administered. In most situations, the slow administration of the opioid does not produce significant sedation, so the maximum recommended dose is usually administered; however, the opioid must always be titrated slowly to prevent a hyperresponding patient from overreacting. Following opioid administration, if additional sedation is desired, either midazolam or diazepam may be slowly titrated.

It is obvious that when this technique is used, the patient will receive a larger dose of the opioid analgesic and a smaller dose of the antianxiety or sedative-hypnotic drug (e.g., meperidine 50 mg and diazepam 7 mg; fentanyl 50 μg and midazolam 4 mg; and 0.8 mg hydromorphone and 6 mg midazolam).

Some patients are quite sensitive to the CNS-depressant actions of opioids and will become adequately sedated at a dose below the maximum recommended for that drug. Should this occur, titration of the opioid is stopped when the desired sedative level is reached, and neither midazolam nor diazepam is administered, and the planned treatment started. The maximum doses and the recommended dilutions of the opioids are presented in Table 26.3.

Techniques

Midazolam or Diazepam With Opioid

When either midazolam or diazepam is the primary drug for sedation, the most appropriate opioids to use are meperidine and fentanyl. Duration of sedation will usually not be increased; however, it is possible that clinical recovery at 60 minutes will not be as complete as that seen when midazolam or diazepam is administered alone. Administration of longer-acting opioids (hydromorphone, morphine) will only delay recovery.

Midazolam or Diazepam With Opioid Plus Anticholinergic

Addition of an anticholinergic is based on the criteria previously discussed. The use of glycopyrrolate is not recommended because of its prolonged duration of action compared with midazolam or diazepam.

Opioid Followed by Benzodiazepine

In reversing the order of drug administration, we are seeking a greater analgesic effect from our drugs. The management of anxiety is not the primary reason for the IV procedure.

Selection of the opioid should be based on the anticipated duration of the procedure, as discussed. Anticholinergics may be administered if desired. Table 26.4 illustrates the different doses of sedative and opioid drugs required when administered alone or in combination. These results are taken from more than 35 years of IV (conscious) moderate sedation continuing education courses.

When any of these advanced IV techniques are used, the drugs must always be titrated slowly (1 mL/min) unless otherwise recommended. The patient is observed for signs of increasing sedation so that oversedation does not occur.

Do not combine the opioid in the same syringe as the benzodiazepine. The administrator loses control over drug action when this is done.

Table 26.3	Opioids: Doses and Dilutions		
	AVAILABILITY (MG/ML)	MAXIMUM DOSE (MG)	DILUTION FOR USE (MG/ML)
Meperidine	50	50	10
Morphine	10	8	1
Fentanyl	0.05 (50 µg/mL)	0.08	0.01
Hydromorphone	1	1.0	0.2
Pentazocine	30	30	10
Nalbuphine	10	10	2
Butorphanol	2	2	0.4

Table 26.4	Average Drug Doses From 2153 Cases		
DRUG 1	DOSE (MG)	DRUG 2	DOSE (MG)
Diazepam	12.5	—	—
Diazepam	19.1	Meperidine	35.1
Meperidine	48.2	Diazepam	8.4
Midazolam	4.8	—	—
Midazolam	7.5	Meperidine	38.0
Meperidine	46.7	Midazolam	3.6
Promethazine	41.2	—	—
Promethazine	48.6	Meperidine	31.1
Meperidine	45.2	Promethazine	21.4

OTHER TECHNIQUES—A BRIEF REVIEW

Other IV moderate sedation techniques are available. Most of these techniques are, today, primarily of historical interest rather than clinically relevant. These techniques kindled interest within dentistry in IV sedation and led inexorably to the benzodiazepine technique used today.

The depth of sedation provided with some of these techniques is considered deep sedation compared with the moderate sedation techniques described in the previous sections of this chapter. The point at which deep sedation ends and general anesthesia (the loss of consciousness) begins is a gray area to be avoided by all but the most well-trained individuals.[20] Indeed, most state dental boards and legislative bodies have determined that deep sedation, to all intents and purposes, is general anesthesia and must be treated in the same manner.

These techniques are mentioned for historical accuracy and to make our discussion more inclusive. Doctors Niels Bjorn Jorgensen, Sylvan Shane, Joel Berns, and Peter Foreman were pioneers in the administration of IV drugs in dentistry.

The Jorgensen Technique—An Overview

The Jorgensen technique is a combination of three drugs administered intravenously providing 2 or more hours of moderate sedation. Niels Bjorn Jorgensen first used this technique, which he called *intravenous premedication,* in 1945 at the Loma Linda University School of Medicine.[25] Jorgensen introduced the technique because of his dissatisfaction with the vagaries of oral and IM routes of sedation. IV drug administration permitted a more precise and reliable level of sedation than was possible with any of the other techniques then available.

The Jorgensen technique has been used successfully at the Loma Linda University School of Dentistry since 1965. Originally designed for use during oral surgical procedures, its appropriateness in all branches of dentistry has been reaffirmed many times. The technique became known as the *Loma Linda technique* because of Jorgensen's affiliation with that school and is now known as the Jorgensen technique, after the man considered by many to be the father of IV sedation in dentistry.

Three drugs are administered in the Jorgensen technique:
1. Pentobarbital, a barbiturate
2. Meperidine, an opioid agonist
3. Scopolamine, an anticholinergic

Everett and Allen,[26] discussing the physiologic effects of the Jorgensen technique, demonstrated that minimal physiologic alteration is produced, although three of their subjects did develop nausea. This latter effect was most likely caused by the opioid. In my experience with the Jorgensen technique, nausea and vomiting are extremely rare and are rarely significant complications.

Function of the Individual Drugs

Pentobarbital

Pentobarbital is the drug that produces the desired depth of sedation associated with the Jorgensen technique. Pentobarbital is also the drug that provides the 2- to 4-hour duration of action associated with the Jorgensen technique. Pentobarbital, a generalized CNS depressant, also has the disquieting effect of making patients more likely to overreact to stimulation (barbiturates produce disinhibition). This is a negative action of the drug and is one reason for inclusion of the opioid in the technique.

Meperidine

Meperidine is an opioid agonist and, as such, has a number of potentially adverse side effects, including respiratory depression, postural hypotension, nausea, and vomiting. Its functions in the Jorgensen technique are threefold:

1. To provide some additional sedation
2. To provide some analgesia, counterbalancing the negative actions of the barbiturate
3. To provide some euphoria

In the dosage of meperidine used in the Jorgensen technique (not greater than 25 mg), the major effect of meperidine is its analgesic action. Patients who have received pentobarbital alone commonly overreact to painful or traumatic stimulation; however, with the addition of up to 25 mg of meperidine, this response is moderated, with most patients responding to stimulation "normally."

Scopolamine

Scopolamine is an anticholinergic with several functions in the Jorgensen technique:

1. Scopolamine provides anterograde amnesia in some patients.
2. It inhibits salivary secretions, thus providing a drier operating field.
3. It produces a degree of CNS depression, although this is rarely, if at all, clinically significant.

Scopolamine may also produce emergence delirium, which is why it is contraindicated in patients younger than 6 years and those older than 65 years.

Diazepam With Methohexital (Foreman Technique)

The combination of diazepam with methohexital, an ultrashort-acting barbiturate, was used with success by many persons, foremost among them Peter Foreman of New Zealand.[27-30] After initially titrating diazepam to baseline sedation (see diazepam technique discussion), a small bolus of 5 to 10 mg of methohexital is administered in anticipation of unpleasant procedures. This includes the administration of local anesthetics or surgery on osseous structures. The 5- to 10-mg increments of methohexital provide a deepening of sedation (into deep sedation) that lasts from 5 to 7 minutes.

Foreman found this technique to be valuable in dental procedures requiring 30 to 90 minutes for completion. In his experience, the usual dose of drugs administered in a procedure lasting more than 1 hour is diazepam 10 to 20 mg and methohexital 50 to 100 mg (in 5- to 10-mg increments). Amnesia is greatly enhanced by addition of the methohexital.

Care must be taken to administer only small increments of methohexital with this technique because larger doses will produce deep sedation bordering on unconsciousness, with attendant depression of protective reflexes, skeletal muscle relaxation, difficulty in maintaining a patent airway, and possible laryngospasm.

The Berns Technique

Joel Berns[31] describes a technique involving the administration of three drugs: a barbiturate, secobarbital; the opioid, meperidine; and another barbiturate, methohexital. Secobarbital is administered first and slowly titrated to baseline sedation (the dose range is from 25 to 75 mg) followed by 25 to 50 mg meperidine. Local anesthesia is administered and the procedure started. Methohexital in increments of 10 to 20 mg is administered just before any traumatic procedure, which may include administration of local anesthesia or extractions.

This technique is similar to the Foreman technique previously described, with the barbiturate, secobarbital, replacing diazepam. The same benefits and potential problems exist in this procedure. An additional consideration is the absence of any pharmacologic antagonist for the barbiturates, whereas flumazenil is available to reverse any unwanted actions of the benzodiazepines.

The Shane Technique

Sylvan Shane[32,33] from Maryland developed a technique, first described in 1966, that he called *intravenous amnesia*. The technique consists of two components: (1) a verbal component that precedes drug administration; and (2) a drug component that involves the IV administration of alphaprodine (an opioid), hydroxyzine (sedative/histamine blocker), atropine, and methohexital and local anesthesia for pain control.

The verbal component is extremely important in the Shane technique. Before drug administration, the patient is told the following:

1. You will be asleep during the procedure.
2. Before falling asleep, you will feel the calming effects of the medications.
3. "Pentothal" is being administered.
4. No pain will be felt during the procedure.
5. When the procedure is complete, you will express disbelief and insist that you were never asleep. (This must be said to the patient before the patient says it to the dentist.)
6. You will know when the procedure is over because your lips, tongue, and teeth will feel numb. When you feel the numbness, you will know that "something must have happened," and this numbness confirms that the procedure is over.
7. (The patient is then exposed to the sound of the drill, air blower, and amalgam condenser.) You will hear these sounds, and they also mean that the procedure is over. These instruments are used to polish, carve, and smooth the fillings,

Table 26.5	Shane Technique Drug Schedule		
	Dose (mg)*		
Drug	**Age 2–6 Yr**	**Age 7–18 Yr**	**Adult**
Alphaprodine	6	7–18 (same as age in yr)	18–24
Hydroxyzine	25	25–50	50
Atropine	0.3	0.4	0.6

*Normal saline is added to dilute the mixture as needed to a total of 5 mL in the syringe.

and this is done during the hour required for you to awaken sufficiently to get up out of the chair.

8. (Gauze is placed over the patient's eyes [taped in place].) The gauze will be over your eyes when you awaken to keep the polishing dust out of your eyes.

9. (The patient's later response to all of the above is anticipated.) You will swear that you were never asleep, yet the treatment will be completed, and you will feel as though only a minute has passed.

The drugs are then administered as listed in Table 26.5. Shane recommended combining alphaprodine, hydroxyzine, and atropine in one syringe and the methohexital in a second syringe.

Following the administration of the drugs in the first syringe to clinical effect, 1 to 2 mL (10 to 20 mg) of methohexital is administered. Local anesthesia of the entire oral cavity (as needed) is obtained. On completion of local anesthetic administration, the patient is told to close his or her mouth, and nothing is said or done for the next 2 minutes.

The dentist then tells the patient that the treatment is completed, all the fillings are done, and the patient may now go home. Of course, the dentist has not even started treatment yet. Patients normally respond to this by saying, "You're fooling me" or "You're kidding."

The dentist counters this by reminding the patient that the mouth is numb and that he or she was told previously that when awakened, he or she would be numb. The patient will then lie back in the chair and begin sleeping.

At this point, the dentist states, "I am going to be polishing your fillings or trimming your bony spicules from the extraction sites." The actual dental procedure starts.

Shane et al[34,35] term the verbal component of the procedure the *Therapeutic Lie*. Shane reported on at least 15,000 sedations without fatality.

The level of CNS depression noted during the Shane technique is deep sedation. The dentist using this technique must be well trained (and in the United States must have a general anesthesia "permit" from their state's regulatory agency) in the management of patients at this level of CNS depression. Factors that severely limited use of the Shane technique were the recommendation by the manufacturer of hydroxyzine that the drug not be administered intravenously and the removal of alphaprodine from clinical use in the United States.

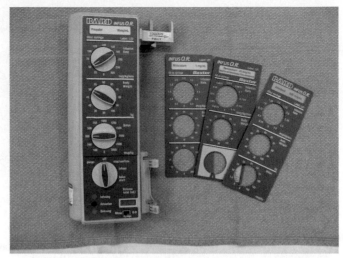

Figure 26.7 Drug infusion pump.

Propofol

Propofol has been used for IV sedation in a number of medical specialties, including ophthalmology,[36] radiology,[37] gynecology,[38,39] gastroenterology,[40] neurosurgery,[41] intensive care medicine,[42,43] and pediatric surgery[44] in addition to dentistry.[45–47] Among propofol's advantages are a very rapid onset of action and an extremely rapid recovery following termination of administration. Following propofol sedation patients are ready for discharge (are "street ready") in a considerably shorter period than following the IV benzodiazepines, diazepam and midazolam.[48]

Not the least of the disadvantages of propofol administration is its potential to produce levels of CNS and respiratory depression that may be beyond the training of the IV moderate sedation dentist.

When propofol is administered intravenously, many patients mention a "burning sensation" at the site of injection.[49] This may be prevented or minimized by the initial administration (IV) of 1 mL of lidocaine (1%) or any other IV drug (midazolam, diazepam, or meperidine).

Because of the short duration of action of propofol, microcomputer-based syringe pumps have been developed that enable a continuous controlled dose of drug to be administered (Fig. 26.7). This enables the dentist to maintain a therapeutic blood level of propofol for prolonged periods. Drugs administered via infusion pumps are administered on a dose/weight/time basis (e.g., μg/kg/min).

Oei-Lim et al[47] found that a syringe-infusion pump set at an initial rate of 3 mg/kg/hr induced moderate sedation in approximately 11.6 minutes in severely apprehensive patients and/or those with mental or physical disabilities. The infusion rate was then adjusted to accommodate for variations in the level of sedation during the dental procedure (average duration of treatment = 55 minutes). The mean infusion rate was 3.6 mg/kg/hr. Sedation was successful in 17 of 19 patients. Cohen et al[50] used an initial bolus dose of 0.5 mg/kg, followed by an infusion of 4 mg/kg/hr to provide deep sedation for ambulatory oral surgery.

Propofol may also be administered as a bolus by syringe without an infusion pump. Propofol must be administered

	Table 26.6	**Summary of Intravenous Drug Doses, Duration, Amnesia**				
DRUG	**CONCENTRATION USED (MG/ML)**	**AVERAGE DOSE (MG)**	**MAXIMUM DOSE (MG)***	**MAXIMUM DOSE (MG)†**	**DURATION**	**AMNESIA ‡INDUCED**
Sedatives						
Diazepam	5	10–12	20	30	45 min	Yes
Midazolam	1	2.5–7.5	8	10	45 min	Yes
Promethazine	10	25–35	50	75	1–2 hr	Somewhat
Opioids						
Meperidine	10	37.5	50	50	<1 hr	No
Morphine	1	5–6	8	8	1.5–2.5 hr	No
Fentanyl	0.01	0.05–0.06	0.08	0.08	30–45 min	No
Hydromorphone	0.2	0.2–0.5	1	1	2 hr	No
Pentazocine	10	20	30	30	1 hr	No
Nalbuphine	2	7–8	2	2	1.5–2 hr	No
Butorphanol	0.4	1.5	2	2	1.5–2 hr	No
Anticholinergics						
Atropine	0.4	0.4–0.6	0.4–0.6	0.4–0.6	3–4 hr	No
Scopolamine	0.3	0.3	0.3	0.3	3–4 hr	Yes
Glycopyrrolate	0.1	0.1	0.1	0.2	7 hr	No

*Maximum dose at one titration.
†Maximum total dose at appointment.
‡Amnesic effect when used in maximum dose recommended.

frequently by this method to maintain the patient in a sedated state.

> **It is my recommendation that propofol not be used by dentists trained solely in IV moderate sedation.**

SUMMARY

Several techniques of IV moderate sedation were presented in this chapter. As a rule, there is no necessity for any one dentist to have all of these techniques available for use in his or her dental practice.

The most rational means of employing these techniques is to start initially with the basic techniques. To learn them well will require at least 50 to 100 cases with each technique.

The only means of obtaining the knowledge and training in the safe and effective use of IV moderate sedation techniques is through dental school, postgraduate residency programs, and continuing education courses. The safe administration of IV moderate sedation cannot be learned by reading a textbook.

Strict adherence to the recommendations presented for each of the drugs and techniques, without exception, no matter how tempting alterations might appear, is essential. If these simple rules are followed, problems do not often occur. A summary of recommended drugs, dosages, and durations is presented in Table 26.6.

REFERENCES

1. Malamed SF: Intravenous sedation: techniques of administration. In *Sedation: a guide to patient management*, Malamed SF. 4th ed, St Louis, 2002, CV Mosby, pp 387–398.
2. Rosenberg MB, Campbell RL: Guidelines for intraoperative monitoring of dental patients undergoing conscious sedation, deep sedation, and general anesthesia. *Oral Surg* 71(1):2–8, 1991.
3. Council on Dental Education, American Dental Association: Guidelines for the use of sedation and general anesthesia by dentists, Adopted by the ADA House of Delegates, Oct 2016 Chicago, 2016, The Association.
4. Council on Dental Education, American Dental Association: Guidelines for teaching pain control and sedation to dentists and dental students, Adopted by the ADA House of Delegates, Oct 2016 Chicago, 2016, The Association.
5. American Academy of Periodontology: Guidelines: In-Office use of conscious sedation in periodontics. *J Periodontol* 72:968–975, 2001. Available at: www.perio.org/resources-products/posppr3-1.html.
6. American Association of Oral and Maxillofacial Surgeons, Committee on Anesthesia: *Office anesthesia evaluation manual*, ed 4, Rosemont, IL, 1991, The Association.
7. American Academy of Pediatrics, American Academy of Pediatric Dentistry, Cote CJ, Wilson S, Work Group on Sedation: Guidelines for monitoring and management of pediatric patients during and after sedation for diagnostic and therapeutic procedures: an update. *Paediatr Anaesth* 18(1):9–10, 2008.
8. Malamed SF: Survey of doctors using IV conscious sedation, unpublished data, 2007.

9. Sims PG, Kates CH, Moyer DJ, et al: Anesthesia in outpatient facilities. *J Oral Maxillofac Surg* 70(11 Suppl 3):e31–e49, 2012.

10. Dental Practice Act. 2015 Legislative session. Oregon Administrative Rules, Chapter 818-026-0060. Moderate sedation permit, State of Oregon Board of Dentistry. 2015, pages 126-128.

11. Jorgensen NB, Hayden J, Jr: *Premedication, local and general anesthesia in dentistry*, Philadelphia, 1967, Lea & Febiger.

12. Dionne RA, Yagiela JA, Moore PA, et al: Comparing efficacy and safety of four intravenous sedation regimens in dental outpatients. *J Am Dent Assoc* 132(6):740–751, 2001.

13. Robb ND, Hargrave SA: Tolerance to intravenous midazolam as a result of oral benzodiazepine therapy: a potential problem for the provision of conscious sedation in dentistry. *J Anesth Pain Control Dent* 2(2):94–97, 1993.

14. Legal Medicine Perspectives, Starozyntk vs. Reich, Superior Ct. of NJ, Case #A-4706-03T1, Sep/Oct 2005, pp 75-76.

15. American Society of Anesthesiologists (ASA): Practice guidelines for preoperative fasting and the use of pharmacological agents to reduce the risk of pulmonary aspiration: application to healthy patients undergoing elective procedures. An updated report by the American Society of Anesthesiologists Committee on Standards and Practice Parameters. *Anesthesiology* 114(3):495–511, 2011.

16. Tait AR, Knight PR: The effects of general anesthesia on upper respiratory tract infection in children. *Anesthesiology* 67(6):930–935, 1987.

17. ClinicalKey. Midazolam drug monograph. February 1, 2016. www.clinicalkey.com Accessed February 20, 2016.

18. O'Neill R, Verrill PJ, Aellig WH, Laurence DR: Intravenous diazepam in minor oral surgery. *Br Dent J* 128(1):15–18, 1970.

19. Malamed SF, Sykes P, Kubota Y, et al: Local anesthesia: a review. *J Anesth Pain Control Dent* 1(1):11–24, 1992.

20. American Society of Anesthesiologists: American Society of Anesthesiologists Task Force on Sedation and Analgesia by Non-Anesthesiologists: Practice guidelines for sedation and analgesia by non-anesthesiologists. *Anesthesiology* 96(4):1004–1017, 2002.

21. ClinicalKey. Diazepam drug monograph. March 11, 2016. www.clinicalkey.com Accessed March 23, 2016.

22. O'Boyle CA: Benzodiazepine-induced amnesia and anaesthetic practice: a review. *Psychopharmacol Ser* 6:146–165, 1988.

23. Shepherd SR, Sims TN, Johnson BW, Hershman JM: Assessment of stress during periodontal surgery with intravenous sedation and with local anesthesia only. *J Periodontol* 59(3):147–154, 1988.

24. Daniel SR, Fry HR, Savard EG: Intravenous "conscious" sedation in periodontal surgery: a selective review and report of 1,708 cases. *J West Soc Periodontol/Periodont Abstr* 32(4):133–146, 1984.

25. Jorgensen NB, Leffingwell FE: Premedication in dentistry. *J Philipp Dent Assoc* 20(3):21–28, 1967.

26. Everett GB, Allen GD: Simultaneous evaluation of cardiorespiratory and analgesic effects of intravenous analgesia using pentobarbital, meperidine, and scopolamine with local analgesia. *J Am Dent Assoc* 83(1):155–158, 1971.

27. Foreman PA: Pharmacosedation: intravenous route. In McCarthy EM, editor: *Emergencies in dental practice*, ed 3, Philadelphia, 1979, WB Saunders.

28. Foreman PA: Control of the anxiety/pain complex in dentistry: intravenous psychosedation with techniques using diazepam. *Oral Surg* 37(3):337–349, 1974.

29. Foreman PA: Intravenous diazepam in general dental practice. *NZ Dent J* 65(302):243–253, 1969.

30. Foreman PA, Neels R, Willetts PW: Diazepam in dentistry, Clinical observations based on treatment of 167 patients in general dental practice. *Anesth Prog* 15(9):253–259, 1968.

31. Berns JM: "Twilight sedation": a substitute for lengthy office intravenous anesthesia. *J Conn Dent Assoc* 37:4, 1963.

32. Shane SM: Intravenous amnesia to obliterate fear, anxiety and pain in ambulatory dental patients. *J Md Dent Assoc* 9(2):94–98, 1966.

33. Shane SM: Intravenous amnesia for total dentistry in one sitting. *J Oral Surg* 24(1):27–32, 1966.

34. Shane SM, Carrel R, Vandenberge J: Intravenous amnesia: an appraisal after seven years and 10,500 administrations. *Anesth Prog* 21(2):36–46, 1974.

35. Shane SM: Intravenous amnesia for total dentistry in one sitting: an appraisal after 15,000 administrations, Fifth Annual Continuing Education Seminar in Practical Considerations in IV and IM Dental Sedation, Miami Beach, Fla, 1979.

36. Kost M, Emerson D: Propofol-fentanyl versus midazolam-fentanyl: a comparative study of local sedation techniques for cataract surgery. *CRNA* 3(1):7–15, 1992.

37. Bloomfield EL, Masaryk TJ, Caplin A, et al: Intravenous sedation for MR imaging of the brain and spine in children: pentobarbital versus propofol. *Radiology* 186(1):93–97, 1993.

38. Sherry E: Admixture of propofol and alfentanil: use for intravenous sedation and analgesia during transvaginal oocyte retrieval. *Anaesthesia* 47(6):477–479, 1992.

39. Silverman DG: New anesthetic approaches to gynecologic surgery. *Curr Opin Obstet Gynecol* 3(3):375–378, 1991.

40. Chin NM, Tai HY, Chin MK: Intravenous sedation for upper gastrointestinal endoscopy: midazolam versus propofol. *Singapore Med J* 33(5):478–480, 1992.

41. Silbergeld DL, Mueller WM, Colley PS, et al: Use of propofol (Diprivan) for awake craniotomies: technical note. *Surg Neurol* 38(4):271–272, 1992.

42. Niccolai I, Barontini L, Paolini P, et al: Long-term sedation with propofol in ICU: hemocoagulation problems. *Minerva Anestesiol* 58(6):375–379, 1992.

43. Ewart MC, Yau KW, Morgan M: 2% propofol for sedation in the intensive care unit: a feasibility study. *Anaesthesia* 47(2):146–148, 1992.

44. Bifarini G, Spaccatini A, Ciammitti B, et al: Sedation with continuously infused propofol in caudal block for elective pediatric surgery. *Minerva Anestesiol* 58(4):181–184, 1992.

45. Oei-Lim VL, Kalkman CJ, Bouvy-Berends EC, et al: A comparison of the effects of propofol and nitrous oxide on the electroencephalogram in epileptic patients during conscious sedation for dental procedures. *Anesth Analg* 75(5):708–714, 1992.

46. Rudkin GE, Osborne GA, Curtis NJ: Intra-operative patient-controlled sedation. *Anaesthesia* 46(2):90–92, 1991.

47. Oei-Lim LB, Vermeulen-Cranch DM, Bouvy-Berends EC: Conscious sedation with propofol in dentistry. *Br Dent J* 170(9):340–342, 1991.

48. Dembo JB, Kirkwood CA, Marsh RA: A comparison of propofol (Diprivan) and methohexital for outpatient oral surgery. Proceedings of the 40th annual meeting of the American Society of Anesthesiology, Toronto, Ontario, 1993.

49. Cillo JE, Jr: Propofol anesthesia for outpatient oral and maxillofacial surgery. *Oral Surg Oral Med Oral Pathol Oral Radiol Endo* 87(5):530–538, 1999.

50. Cohen M, Eisig S, Kraut RA: Infusion pump for deep conscious sedation with propofol and methohexital. Proceedings of the 40th annual meeting of the American Society of Anesthesiology, Toronto, Ontario, 1993.

chapter 27

Intravenous Sedation: Complications

CHAPTER OUTLINE

VENIPUNCTURE COMPLICATIONS
Nonrunning Intravenous Infusion
Venospasm
Hematoma
Infiltration
Localized Venous Complications
Air Embolism
Overhydration
LOCAL COMPLICATIONS OF DRUG ADMINISTRATION
Extravascular Drug Administration
Intraarterial Injection
Local Venous Complications

COMPLICATIONS
Nausea and Vomiting
Localized Allergy
Respiratory Depression and Respiratory Obstruction
Emergence Delirium
Laryngospasm
SPECIFIC DRUG COMPLICATIONS
Benzodiazepines
Promethazine
Opioids
Scopolamine

A number of complications may occur when the intravenous (IV) route of drug administration is used. Fortunately, most are relatively benign and easily managed. Others, however, are more significant and can lead to serious morbidity or death.

The complications associated with IV drug administration are divided into four groups: (1) those associated with venipuncture, (2) localized complications related to drug administration, (3) general drug-related problems, and (4) drug-specific complications. These are outlined in Box 27.1.

VENIPUNCTURE COMPLICATIONS

Nonrunning Intravenous Infusion

One of the most common and vexing complications of venipuncture and IV drug administration is the nonrunning or very slowly running IV infusion. Once venipuncture has been successfully completed (e.g., blood returning into the tubing), the tourniquet is removed and the IV drip started. During drug administration, the drip rate should be increased; at other times, the rate should be slowed. The causes of a nonrunning or slowly running IV infusion follow.

IV Infusion Bag Too Close to the Heart Level

Gravity forces the IV infusate from the bag down into the patient. The greater the difference in height between the bag and the patient's heart is, the more rapid the flow of solution can be. A simple experiment demonstrates this: The IV bag is held high above the patient's heart level, and the rate of flow is checked. With the rate-adjusting knob opened fully, the drip should be rapid. As the bag is gradually lowered toward the level of the patient's heart, the rate of flow of the drip decreases until, when held at the patient's heart level, the flow ceases entirely. When the bag is lowered below the level of the patient's heart, blood returns into the tubing (Fig. 27.1).

This is a situation that might arise when the dental chair is placed low to the floor at the start of a procedure and is elevated at a later time. Increasing the distance between the bag of IV infusion solution and the patient's heart will correct the situation.

Bevel of Needle Against Wall of Vein

It was recommended that the bevel of the needle be facing upward during venipuncture to allow entry through the skin

Box 27.1	Complications Associated With IV Drug Administration

Venipuncture Complications
- Nonrunning IV infusion
- Venospasm
- Hematoma
- Infiltration
- Local venous complications
- Air embolism
- Overhydration

Local Complications of Drug Administration
- Extravascular drug administration
- Intraarterial injection
- Local venous complications

General Drug-Related Complications
- Nausea and vomiting
- Localized allergy
- Respiratory depression
- Emergence delirium
- Laryngospasm

Specific Drug Complications
Benzodiazepines
- Local venous complications
- Emergence delirium
- Recurrence of amnesia
- Oversedation

Promethazine
- Oversedation
- Extrapyramidal reactions

Opioids
- Nausea and vomiting
- Respiratory depression
- Rigid chest

Scopolamine
- Emergence delirium

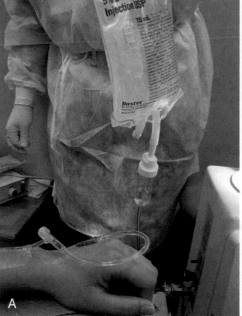

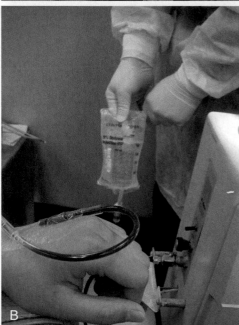

Figure 27.1 A, Bag of IV solution held above level of patient's heart (vein) allows fluid to run into patient. **B,** Lowering bag of IV solution below level of patient's heart (vein) allows blood to return into tubing from patient.

to be as atraumatic as possible. Following entry into the skin, the needle is advanced into the vein, with blood returning into the tubing a sign of a successful venipuncture. At this point, the tourniquet is removed and the infusion started. If the IV drip rate that is flowing rapidly until the scalp vein or metal needle is taped into position is noted to slow considerably, it is quite possible that in taping the needle into position, the bevel of the needle was lifted and now lies against the wall of the vein. This will restrict or prevent the flow of fluid from the IV drip into the patient.

To determine whether this is the cause of a slow or nonrunning drip, the needle is carefully untaped and the wings of the butterfly needle gently lifted. This lowers the bevel of the needle off the wall of the vein. If the drip rate increases, the protective cap from the scalp vein needle (Fig. 27.2) or a 2 × 2-inch gauze square is carefully placed under the wings of the needle and the needle retaped.

This is unlikely to occur when an indwelling catheter is used for venipuncture because there is no bevel on the catheter.

However, when a catheter is positioned in either the dorsum of the hand or antecubital fossa, it is possible for the tip of the catheter to lie in a bend in the vein, creating a slow flow of IV solution. Determine this by straightening the patient's wrist or elbow and looking for an increase in the rate of flow of the IV drip. This may be minimized by preventing the patient from bending the joint through the use of an elbow immobilizer or wrist board.

Tourniquet Not Removed

An embarrassing but not uncommon cause of a nonrunning IV drip following successful venipuncture may simply be that the tourniquet has been left on the patient because it has become hidden from view by a sleeve of a garment that has inched down. Following the return of blood into the IV tubing, the dentist or assistant opens up the control knob to start the IV drip. It is noted that the drip is not flowing and that blood does not leave the IV tubing as normally occurs. It is usually noted that more blood appears to be entering into the IV tubing (as it is forced from the vein into the tubing) (Fig. 27.3). Once excessive blood is noticed in the tubing, simple removal of the tourniquet will alleviate this embarrassing situation.

Infiltration

Following successful entry into the vein, the metal needle somehow becomes dislodged while being secured. The dentist or assistant, unaware of this, opens the rate knob, but little or no solution flows. If no solution is flowing, the three causes of nonrunning IVs previously discussed should be considered. If the drip rate is extremely slow and cannot be increased, one should first look at the site where the needle tip is located beneath the patient's skin. If the needle tip has left the vein and fluid is still flowing, a small colorless swelling will develop at this site. This is termed an *infiltration* (see discussion later).

In all cases in which an IV drip that was previously running well has either slowed or stopped entirely, the needle should not be removed from the vein until it has been determined definitively that the needle tip is no longer within the vein. The following procedure is recommended to determine the cause of the slow or nonrunning IV drip:

1. Open the drip rate knob.
2. Elevate the IV bag. Does flow rate increase?
3. Place the IV bag below heart level. Does blood return?
4. Check the IV site. Is tissue swelling present? Does the skin at the needle site feel cooler than surrounding tissues? (See "Infiltration" section.)
5. Elevate the wings of the butterfly needle or straighten the patient's arm or wrist as appropriate with a catheter. Does flow improve?
6. If infiltration has occurred, the IV drip is stopped and the needle or catheter removed with the venipuncture reattempted at another site.

This is unlikely to occur when an indwelling catheter has been used for venipuncture.

Venospasm

Venospasm is a protective mechanism in which the vein wall reacts to stimulation from the needle by going into spasm. As the needle approaches, the vein appears to disappear or "collapse." Venospasm is occasionally accompanied by a burning sensation in the immediate area. This burning sensation ends without any specific treatment as the spasm resolves. Venospasm may occur before or after entry of the needle into the vein, securing of the catheter or needle, or starting of the IV drip.

Prevention

Venospasm cannot always be prevented.

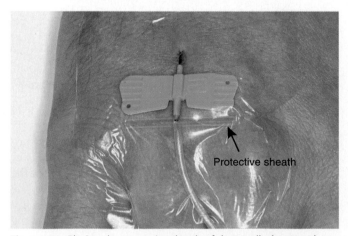

Figure 27.2 Placing the protective sheath of the needle (or gauze) beneath the wings of the needle (*arrow*) increases the rate of IV infusion if the bevel is pressing against the vein wall.

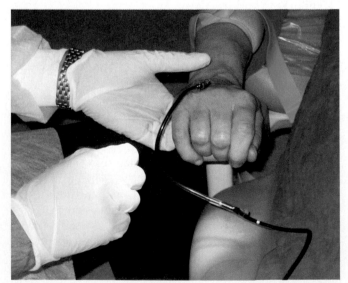

Figure 27.3 Tourniquet left in place forces blood to flow from patient into IV tubing.

Recognition

Venospasm is identified by the disappearance of a previously visible vein during attempted venipuncture. A burning sensation may or may not accompany venospasm.

Management

The needle should not be removed from the site because the vein has not been entered or damaged. The needle is pulled back slightly (1 to 2 mm), and heat applied to the site in an attempt to dilate the vessel. If and when the vein reappears, the venipuncture attempt is continued.

A sensation of burning during venipuncture and IV drug administration is associated with several other complications and with one cause that is not a complication—the IV administration of diazepam. Intravenous administration of diazepam is occasionally associated with the sensation of warmth or burning; however, this sensation travels up the patient's arm (centrally) as the drug travels through the veins. Intraarterial (IA) injection of a drug will produce a burning sensation or pain traveling down (peripherally) the arm toward the fingers. Extravascular injection of a drug produces a burning sensation at the site of injection that remains at the site of administration. The injection of meperidine may cause the release of histamine and a burning or itching sensation along the path of the vein. Venospasm occurs more frequently in apprehensive patients, presumably as a result of their higher levels of circulating catecholamines (predisposing them to peripheral vasoconstriction).

Hematoma

Hematoma is the most common complication associated with venipuncture. It represents the extravasation of blood into interstitial spaces surrounding a blood vessel. The presence of blood in this space leads to localized swelling and discoloration.

When venipuncture is successful, the needle itself acts as an obturator, sealing the hole in the vein wall made during entry of the needle. In some patients, particularly older patients in whom blood vessel walls have lessened elasticity, leakage of blood around the needle may occur during the IV procedure even though the needle tip still lies within the lumen of the vein.

Hematoma may occur at two distinct times during the IV procedure. First, it may develop during attempted venipuncture if the vessel wall is damaged (Fig. 27.4). This is not always preventable. The second cause of hematoma is usually preventable. In this situation, the IV procedure has been completed and the catheter or needle removed from the vein. Improper application of pressure or inadequate duration of pressure at the venipuncture site can result in a hematoma.

Prevention

It is not always possible to prevent hematoma *during* venipuncture, although careful adherence to recommended

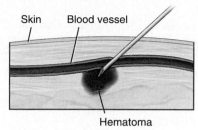

Figure 27.4 Hematoma occurs when blood extravasates from blood vessel into surrounding tissues.

technique minimizes its likelihood. Hematoma developing *after* the procedure may be prevented by application of firm pressure for a minimum of 5 to 6 minutes. The commonly used technique of placing gauze over the venipuncture site in the antecubital fossa and having the patient flex his or her arm (illustrated in Fig. 24.21) does not always provide pressure adequate to prevent hematoma.

Recognition

Hematoma is a painless, bluish discoloration, frequently with swelling, noted under the skin at the site of needle puncture. It develops during attempted venipuncture or at the conclusion of the IV procedure on removal of the catheter or needle.

Management

When hematoma develops during attempted venipuncture, swelling increases rapidly because the tourniquet is still on the patient's arm (significantly increasing the pressure of blood within the vein). Immediate management consists of the following:

1. Remove the tourniquet (to decrease venous blood pressure).
2. Remove the needle from the site.
3. Apply firm pressure with sterile gauze for 5 to 6 minutes.
4. If the site is tender, ice may be applied in the first few postoperative hours. Ice acts as a vasoconstrictor and as an analgesic. Do not use heat because heat is a vasodilator.

When hematoma develops following removal of the IV catheter or needle, immediate management consists solely of direct pressure with gauze followed by the application of ice to the area.

Subsequent management of either form of hematoma can best be described as "tincture of time." It will require approximately 10 to 14 days for the subcutaneous blood to be resorbed by the body. Nothing can be done to speed this process. Should the patient experience discomfort or soreness (more likely if the hematoma is located in a joint [wrist, antecubital fossa]), he or she can be advised to use moist heat on the area for 20 minutes every hour. Heat should not be used within the first 4 hours after the onset of the hematoma because it acts as a vasodilator and might induce further bleeding.

Infiltration

Infiltration is similar to a hematoma in that a fluid is deposited into the tissues surrounding the blood vessel. A hematoma is the infiltration of blood outside of a blood vessel. Extravascular injection of a drug is the infiltration of drug outside of the blood vessel. Infiltration is defined as a painless, colorless swelling that develops at the site of the needle (cannula) tip when the IV infusion is started.

In this situation, we are discussing the deposition of the IV infusate (e.g., 0.9% normal saline, lactated Ringer's, D5&W) into the tissues surrounding the blood vessel. The infiltration discussed here differs from hematoma in that the swelling that develops does not occur until the IV drip is turned on, whereas the hematoma occurs as soon as the vein wall is damaged.

In the continuous IV infusion technique, when infiltration does occur, it only consists of a solution that does not produce any degree of tissue irritation or damage. In contrast, in IV techniques in which the drug is injected directly into a blood vessel, it is much more likely that the drug will produce tissue damage (e.g., diazepam) and/or a delayed onset of sedation if deposited outside the blood vessel.

Prevention

Infiltration can be prevented by careful venipuncture technique and by not starting the IV drip or injecting drugs until it has been confirmed that the needle tip or catheter still lies within the lumen of the vein. Checking for this is quite easy. The rubber flash bulb (if present) on the IV tubing may be squeezed, with blood returning into the tubing when the pressure is released, or the IV bag may be held below the level of the patient's heart (see Fig. 27.1B).

Cause

Movement of the metal needle either while it is being secured or through movement of the patient's arm during the sedation procedure may cause the rigid metal needle to perforate the vein wall, producing an infiltration or hematoma. Common causes of a needle becoming dislodged are (1) attempting to thread (insert) a rigid metal needle too far into the vein and (2) carelessness during taping of the needle. Infiltration is much less likely to occur when a plastic catheter is used for venipuncture.

Recognition

Infiltration is a painless, colorless swelling that occurs around the tip of the needle when the IV drip is started. The tissue around the needle tip is raised, and the skin at this site feels cooler than skin at a distance from this site. This is because the infusate is at room temperature (22°C/72°F), not body temperature.

Management

The IV infusion is stopped immediately and the needle or catheter removed. Sterile gauze is placed at the site and pressure applied for 5 to 6 minutes. Pressure will stop any bleeding and also spread out any fluid within the tissue. The fluid will be resorbed into the cardiovascular system. Little or no residual soreness will be noted.

Localized Venous Complications

Localized venous complications can develop after IV sedation procedures. Many factors are responsible for their development, and there are a number of different clinical expressions that venous complications can take. Trauma to the vein wall produced by the needle or cannula is a possible cause of this problem. In the dental outpatient environment, the most likely cause of venous complications is chemical irritation of the vein wall produced by the drug administered, usually diazepam. Localized venous complications are discussed later in this chapter (see "Local Complications of Drug Administration").

Air Embolism

Air embolism is a possible, although extremely unlikely, complication of IV sedation. It is best prevented by using a technique that is free of air: eliminating air bubbles from syringes and from the IV tubing before the procedure and periodically observing the IV infusion bag to prevent it from emptying.

In the highly likely event that one or more small bubbles of air enter into the venous circulation, they will be absorbed by the blood quite rapidly with no clinical sequelae. It is not always possible for all air bubbles to be removed from the IV tubing or syringes, and it is quite probable that small bubbles may enter into the venous circulation of the patient. The patient, noticing the air bubble moving slowly down the IV tubing toward his or her arm, may become quite anxious, believing (from television or movies) that as little as one bubble of air is lethal. Fortunately, this is not so. A rule of thumb in a hospital environment is that a patient can tolerate up to 1 mL/kg of body weight of air in the peripheral venous circulation without adverse effect.[1]

The typical IV administration set can hold approximately 15 to 27 mL of fluid.[2] Because 10 drops of solution (or air) equals 1 mL (adult infusion set), the chances of introducing large volumes of air into the patient's circulation are extraordinarily low. A 50-kg (110-lb) patient can tolerate 50 mL of air. This is equivalent to 500 to 750 drops of air from an adult IV administration set (10 or 15 drops/mL).

In small children, air embolism is a more significant problem because their smaller bodies cannot tolerate large volumes of air in the cardiovascular system. A 13-kg (30-lb) child is at greater risk of this complication than is a larger patient. The pediatric infusion set delivers smaller drops – 60 drops per mL – allowing for a finer degree of control over IV fluid delivery.

Management

Should air embolism occur, management is based on the attempt to prevent this air from entering into the cerebral and pulmonary circulations. This is accomplished by positioning the patient in the dental chair lying on his or her left side (preventing entry into the pulmonary circulation) and in a head-down position (preventing entry into the cerebral circulation).

Overhydration

Overhydration of the patient is another not very common problem associated with IV procedures in the dental office. The two most likely candidates for overhydration, however, are children and patients with heart failure (American Society of Anesthesiologists [ASA] 3, 4). Signs of overhydration include pulmonary edema, respiratory distress, and an increase in heart rate and blood pressure. These are also the signs and symptoms occasionally noted in a patient with acute pulmonary edema.

A rule of thumb for replacement of fluid in a patient is that the initial dose of IV solution administered is equal to 1.5 times the number of hours a patient has gone without food times the patient's weight in kilograms.[3] This is the volume of fluid in milliliters required to replace the fluid deficit created by the patient's taking nothing by mouth (NPO) before the procedure. If a patient has been NPO for 6 hours before coming to the office, the initial volume of IV solution administered is nine times the patient's body weight in kilograms. The maintenance dose of IV solution is 3 mL/kg. The problem of underhydration (dehydration) is not significant in the usual outpatient environment.

When IV drugs are administered to pediatric patients, it is recommended that a pediatric infusion set be used. This set, which permits 60 drops/mL instead of the usual 10 or 15, allows for the more precise administration of fluids to the younger, smaller patient or to the adult with more serious heart failure (ASA 3, 4). In most instances, these two groups of patients are not candidates for elective IV moderate sedation in the outpatient dental setting.

LOCAL COMPLICATIONS OF DRUG ADMINISTRATION

Extravascular Drug Administration

When a drug is injected into subcutaneous tissues instead of the blood vessel, three problems may develop:
1. Pain
2. Delayed absorption of the drug
3. Tissue damage

Pain associated with extravascular drug administration occurs at the site of the needle tip under the skin and tends to remain localized to that area. This distinguishes extravascular injection from IA and IV injections, where a burning sensation radiates either peripherally or centrally. The patient will complain of discomfort as the drug is injected in all three situations.

A potentially greater problem (depending on the drug and the dose administered) is delayed absorption of the drug into the cardiovascular system, especially if larger volumes have been deposited into the tissues. In essence, the drug has been administered subcutaneously instead of intravenously. Uptake of a subcutaneously administered drug is slow, with an onset of clinical activity (e.g., sedation) occurring anywhere from about 10 to 30 minutes later.

A third problem that might arise is damage to the tissues into which the drug has been deposited. Some drugs used intravenously are potentially irritating to tissues, primarily diazepam. The initial response of the tissues is arteriolar and capillary constriction, which decreases the blood supply to the area. If vascular constriction is prolonged or if the chemical is irritating enough, necrosis and sloughing of tissue may occur.

Causes

There are two causes of extravascular drug administration. The first is the needle or cannula slipping out of the vein. This usually leads to an immediate formation of a hematoma that is quickly recognized. No drug has usually been injected at this time. The second cause is the needle entering the vein and then being pushed through the other side as the dentist attempts to advance it farther into the vein. Blood will have returned into the tubing as the needle entered the vein originally, thereby giving the (false) impression that the needle or catheter tip remains in the vein. However, with removal of the tourniquet, it is unlikely that the blood will leave the tubing, as normally occurs, because the tip of the needle no longer lies in the vein but in subcutaneous tissue. On very rare occasions, the blood will leave the IV tubing and reenter the patient, allowing the IV infusion to run even though the needle tip is no longer in the vein. This will occur when the bag of IV solution is quite high above the patient's heart or if the patient's skin and underlying soft tissues are not "firm," allowing gravity to force the solution into the tissues. The latter is seen more often in older, frailer patients.

Use of a continuous IV drip technique really minimizes the possibility of extravascular injection of the drug because an infiltration of infusate produces an immediate swelling of the tissue at the tip of the needle. Second, before administration of any drug, it is recommended that patency of the vein be reconfirmed by squeezing the flash bulb or holding the IV bag below the level of the patient's heart. Despite these precautions, a subtle movement of a patient's wrist or elbow just after this check but just before drug administration can produce this complication when a rigid metal needle is used for venipuncture and IV maintenance. Use of an indwelling catheter minimizes this risk. The administration of a 0.2-mL test dose of a drug is a means of detecting this complication before a larger, potentially more damaging bolus of drug is deposited.

Recognition

As the irritating drug, especially diazepam, is injected extravascularly, the patient will complain of an intense pain occurring at the site of the needle tip that does not migrate up or down their arm. In addition, as an increasing volume of drug is injected, the tissue at the site of the needle tip will become raised as the solution is forced into the subcutaneous tissues. If the chemical is irritating, the skin overlying the raised tissue will become ischemic as blood vessels in the area constrict in response to the irritation. A second possible reaction is for the tissues to become erythematous as a result of inflammation.

Management

The two major problems to be managed are (1) possible delayed absorption of the drug and its effect on the patient and (2) potential damage to the tissues at the site of deposition. Management initially consists of removing the needle and applying pressure at the site of injection to stop the bleeding and to disperse the solution deposited under the skin. If less than 1 or 2 mL of drug has been deposited extravascularly, these steps are all that are required for effective management.

In the highly unlikely situation that larger volumes of drug have been deposited extravascularly and the overlying tissue is raised and ischemic, two problems must be addressed: (1) tissue damage and (2) delayed-onset sedation. Pressure alone may not be adequate to disperse the solution, and additional drug management may be required. The drug of choice is 1% procaine, a local anesthetic with profound vasodilating properties. Several milliliters of procaine can be infiltrated into the affected tissues using a single puncture point and a "fan-type" injection. This increases the rate of drug absorption and eliminates any discomfort that may be present.

The possible delayed onset of sedation produced by the slow absorption of the drug must be managed symptomatically, with basic life support procedures ("rescue")—maintaining the circulation, airway, and ventilation—implemented as needed. When diazepam is the drug injected extravascularly, a mild increase in the level of sedation might be noted about 30 to 40 minutes later. This should not lead to a significant alteration in the observed level of consciousness.

In the conscious patient receiving drugs via an IV infusion, it is unlikely that a large volume of drug will be administered extravascularly. If the drug is titrated at the recommended rate of 1 mL/min, it becomes obvious well within a minute that the needle is not in the vein. Drug administration is immediately stopped and IV patency rechecked.

Intraarterial Injection

The most significant of the localized complications of IV drug administration is IA injection of the drug. There are numerous reasons why this serious complication occurs only infrequently. However, when it does occur, immediate and vigorous therapy is indicated to prevent tissue damage, gangrene, and possible loss of the limb.[4-8] Drugs injected into an artery produce irritation of the muscular arterial wall as the drug is carried peripherally. As the diameter of the artery decreases, the drug is increasingly in contact with the artery wall. The immediate response of the artery to this chemical insult is spasm. Arterial spasm, especially if it occurs in one of the larger arteries of the upper limb, as is likely in this situation, will compromise the circulation to all or a large portion of the tissue distal to the injection site.

Prevention

Prevention is the most important feature in this discussion of IA injection. Fortunately, it is rather difficult to accidentally enter into an artery and even more difficult to accidentally administer a drug intraarterially. Many signs and symptoms occur that alert the dentist and assistant to the fact that the needle does not lie within a vein.

1. The vessel should be palpated before venipuncture is attempted. *Arteries conduct a pulse that can be palpated before the tourniquet is placed on the patient's arm.* Once a tourniquet is in place, the artery may not pulsate and the vessel may be mistaken for a vein. This is especially likely to happen on the medial aspect of the antecubital fossa, where the brachial artery is somewhat superficial.
2. As the needle approaches the arterial wall, the vessel will begin to spasm. Arterial spasm is much more intense than venospasm and is associated with a more intense burning sensation. For this reason alone, it is usually very difficult to accidentally (and on many occasions even purposefully) enter into an artery.
3. If the needle does enter the artery (or any vessel, for that matter), a return of blood into the IV tubing will be noted. With the tourniquet still in place, the return of blood will be similar to that seen in venipuncture; however, the color of the blood differs: Arterial blood (oxygenated) is a brighter cherry red, whereas venous blood (decreased O_2 concentration) is a darker maroon.
4. On removal of the tourniquet, a significant difference is noted. On release of the tourniquet, blood pressure within the vein decreases to about 4 to 6 mm Hg (in the arm), and blood leaves the IV tubing returning into the patient. Following removal of the tourniquet, arterial blood pressure will increase (e.g., 120/80 mm Hg) with the bright red arterial blood remaining in the IV tubing and, perhaps, exhibiting a pulsatile flow with every contraction of the heart.

To this point, no damage has been done to the patient or to the artery (except for the needle puncture). If the IA puncture is noted at this time, the needle is carefully removed and firm pressure exerted over the site for at least 10 minutes.

However, if a drug is injected into the artery, additional problems may develop rapidly.

Recognition

A number of signs and symptoms are associated with IA injection of a drug:

1. The patient complains of a severe pain that radiates peripherally from the site of injection of the drug toward the hand and fingers.
2. The radial pulse should be checked. Absence of the radial pulse indicates that arterial spasm is severe and that immediate management is essential. Presence of the radial pulse, though it may be weak, indicates that at least some arterial blood is entering into the hand and fingers. A problem may exist, but it is not as acute.

3. The skin color of the affected hand should be compared with that of the opposite hand. Lack of blood flow into the affected limb produces a loss of normal skin color. A paler color or a mottled appearance may be noted initially.

4. Both limbs should be felt to determine temperature. The flow of blood into the hand provides warmth. When blood flow to the limb is compromised, that limb becomes cooler than the opposite limb with normal blood flow.

The major cause of injury from IA injection is chemical endarteritis that results in thrombosis and ischemia. Crystals of the drug precipitate as a result of the change in pH, leading to further occlusion of vessels. Results of this range from small areas of gangrene to the loss of fingers or a limb (Fig. 27.5).[6]

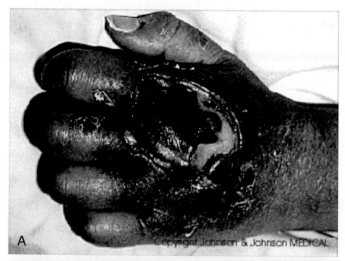

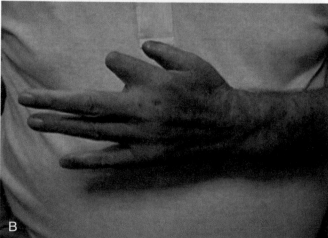

Figure 27.5 A and **B,** Left forearm of a healthy 20-year-old male after promethazine was unintentionally infused into his radial artery. Both images show the appearance during a "washout" procedure after fasciotomies and debridement were performed for skin necrosis. (From Sen S, Chini EN, Brown MJ: Complications after unintentional intraarterial injection of drugs: risks, outcomes, and management strategies, *Mayo Clin Proc* 80:783–795, 2005.)

Management

Management of IA injection is best achieved by the following steps:

1. *Leave the needle in place.* Do not remove the IA needle that has been accidentally placed. It provides an avenue for the administration of the drug used in management of this situation.

2. *Administer procaine.* Slowly inject 1% procaine, to a volume of between 2 and 10 mL, into the artery. Procaine serves four functions at this time: (1) anesthetic, to decrease pain; (2) vasodilator, to break the arterial spasm, reinitiating blood flow; (3) pH about 5, counterbalance for drugs with alkaline pH (e.g., pentobarbital); and (4) diluent, decreasing the concentration of the previously administered IA drug. Procaine frequently breaks the arterial spasm, which is noted by a return of color and warmth to the limb and a return of a pulse wave equal in strength to that of the opposite limb.

3. *Hospitalize the patient.* All patients who have had accidental IA drug administration should be seen in the emergency department of a hospital where a vascular surgeon or anesthesiologist will be consulted. The dentist should accompany the patient to the hospital so that the treating physicians can be advised of the drug(s) administered intraarterially and the treatment rendered. Additional treatment may also be deemed necessary. Such treatment may consist of a sympathetic nerve block, such as a stellate ganglion block or brachial plexus block. When indicated, general anesthesia or surgical endarterectomy may be required. Heparinization may be used, if needed, to prevent further thrombosis. If treatment fails to reestablish effective blood flow to the limb, amputation of gangrenous parts may be required. Hyperbaric oxygen (O₂) is often used to force oxygen into the tissues when arterial spasm is not readily broken by the aforementioned procedures.[9] Other treatment may include administration of urokinase and heparin.[10]

The IA injection of a drug is a serious complication that should not occur if basic concepts of venipuncture and IV drug administration, recommended in earlier chapters of this section, are followed. In the unlikely situation that IA drug administration does occur, management as described is recommended, followed by accurate recordkeeping and contacting one's insurance carrier immediately.

IA Drug Injection
Prevention
Palpate vessel before placement of the tourniquet.
Avoid anatomically at-risk sites (e.g., median antecubital fossa), if possible (at least as a neophyte phlebotomist).
Recognition
Intense pain during venipuncture attempt
Bright cherry red blood

Pulsatile flow of blood in IV tubing when tourniquet
  is released
Intense pain radiating down arm toward fingers as
  drug is injected
Loss of color in limb
Loss of warmth in limb
Weakening or loss of radial pulse in limb

Local Venous Complications

Following a successful IV sedation procedure, the patient is discharged home. The patient may feel fine through the next day only to find, 2 days after the procedure, that the area in which the needle and drug were placed is swollen, red, hot, and painful.

The general category of local venous complications is used here because of the multiple names given to the situation discussed.

Phlebitis is an inflammation of a vein: "phlebo" means vein; "itis" means inflammation.

Thrombophlebitis is a condition in which inflammation of the vein wall has preceded the formation of a thrombus (blood clot).

Phlebothrombosis is the presence of a clot within a vein, unassociated with inflammation of the wall of the vein (Fig. 27.6).

Gelfman, Driscoll, and colleagues[11–13] reported on several prospective and retrospective studies of the problem of local venous complications. Criteria that they established for identification of these entities were the following:

- Thrombophlebitis: pain, induration, and a delay in onset of these symptoms
- Phlebothrombosis: a condition of venous thrombosis without inflammation; occurs much more immediately, and pain is not a prominent feature

It appears that the primary problem developing after IV sedation is thrombophlebitis. Clinical features of thrombophlebitis include the following:

- Edema
- Inflammation
- Tenderness
- Delayed onset: 24 to 48 hours, but may develop up to a week after venous insult

Causes of thrombophlebitis include anything that produces either mechanical or chemical irritation of a vein. Among the factors involved in the development of thrombophlebitis are those listed in Box 27.2.

IV solutions, infusions, or drugs that have pH values at either end of the spectrum (basic or acidic) are associated with a greater incidence of venous complications. Some drugs injected intravenously have vehicles, such as propylene glycol and alcohol, that are irritating to vein walls. Diazepam is an example of a drug containing such a vehicle (propylene glycol).[14] It was mentioned earlier in this section that some patients experience pain on IV administration of diazepam. Gelfman and Driscoll[12] reported that in patients experiencing such discomfort on injection, the incidence of phlebothrombosis, but not thrombophlebitis, was increased.

The duration of the IV infusion is not as great a concern in outpatient sedation as it is with a hospitalized patient, where an IV infusion may be maintained for days at a time. It is common practice within hospitals for an IV team to change the site of the IV infusion every few days, thereby minimizing the risk of developing local venous complications.

Improper technique, use of dull needles (highly unlikely with disposable needles), and improper fixation of the needle or catheter are mechanical causes of irritation. A needle or catheter that is not well secured will continually irritate the walls of the vein.

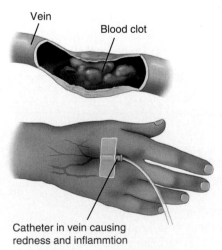

Figure 27.6 Thrombophlebitis.

Box 27.2	Factors Involved in the Development of Thrombophlebitis

pH of the infusion liquid
Components of the infusate
pH of the drug(s)
Duration of the IV infusion
Mechanical factors:
- Bevel and dullness of needle
- Technique of venipuncture
- Improper fixation of needle or catheter
- Size of needle in relation to vein lumen
- Type of needle (metal vs. plastic catheter)
- Presence of infection or disease
- Age and sex of the patient
- Site of venipuncture

Placement of a very large needle or catheter within the lumen of a smaller vein will potentially produce greater irritation with an increased risk of thrombophlebitis. As recommended in this section, the 21-gauge needle or catheter will not impinge on the walls of any vein in the upper limb.

The site of venipuncture is also a factor. Venipuncture of the femoral or saphenous vein of the leg is associated with a higher incidence of thrombophlebitis and thromboembolism. There are significantly fewer complications with superficial veins of the arm and the dorsum of the hand. Within the upper limb, there are differences in the incidence of thrombophlebitis. Nordell et al[15] reported five cases of thrombophlebitis in 52 patients. Table 27.1 is a summary of sites of venipuncture and incidence of thrombophlebitis.[15]

Other studies have demonstrated similar statistics. Chambiras found a twofold greater incidence of venous complications in the hand than in the antecubital fossa.[16]

Prevention

It is not always possible to prevent local venous irritation when one of the factors responsible for its development is mechanical irritation produced by the venipuncture or the needle. Fortunately the superficial veins of the upper limb are less likely to suffer serious postinjection complications than are the veins of the leg. Prevention is based on the following:

- Using sharp, sterile needles
- Following atraumatic, sterile venipuncture technique
- Securing the needle firmly in position
- Injecting IV drugs slowly into a rapidly running infusion
- Diluting IV drugs, when possible

When dilution is not possible (e.g., with diazepam or propofol), use of larger veins (antecubital fossa and forearm) is recommended.

Recognition

The patient is usually asymptomatic for 1 or more days following the IV procedure. The inflammatory process requires approximately 24 to 48 hours to fully develop, at which time the patient usually contacts the dental office complaining of soreness, (possibly) swelling, redness of the area, and (possibly) warmth.

Management

Management of any localized venous complication requires that the patient return to the dental office for evaluation. The dentist should examine the patient to determine the nature and extent of the situation. All findings are recorded in the patient's chart, and the patient is examined regularly until the situation resolves. The key to successful management is patient cooperation and satisfaction.

Management of thrombophlebitis includes the following:

1. Activity in the limb should be limited through the use, if possible, of a sling.
2. The affected limb should be elevated when possible.
3. Moist heat should be applied for 20 minutes three to four times a day.
4. Should thrombophlebitis occur in a joint (elbow or wrist), immobilization is more difficult, but should still be attempted. Constant movement of the affected area leads, in some patients, to increased discomfort. Management of pain consists of the administration of nonsteroidal antiinflammatory analgesics (NSAIDs), such as aspirin or ibuprofen, every 4 to 6 hours as needed for pain.
5. Anticoagulants and antibiotics are not part of the usual therapy and will not be required unless the situation worsens. By this time, however, it is likely that the patient will have been referred to a physician (ideally a vascular surgeon) for definitive management.

In the usual course of events, the acute phase of thrombophlebitis, involving tenderness, swelling, and discomfort, resolves within a few days, leading to a chronic phase in which the discomfort is gone but the vein remains hard and knotty.[13] This may occur at the site of the venipuncture or anywhere along the path of this vein and its tributaries. The extent of these lumps and bumps subsides over time. Treatment of choice during this phase is tincture of time.

The patient is seen in the office on a less and less frequent basis as the situation resolves. Records are maintained of the findings at each visit. In most cases, full resolution is noted within 3 to 4 weeks, although cases have been reported in which patients have suffered lingering tenderness for more than 3 years (wrist vein).

In the unlikely event that fever or malaise develops, consultation with a vascular surgeon (the person most likely to be familiar with the management of this complication) is recommended. In any situation in which a patient is referred for medical (or dental) consultation, it is recommended that the referring dentist speak with the physician (discussing management of the case) before the patient is seen. Another clinical indication for referral to a physician is patient dissatisfaction. If the patient expresses doubt over the dentist's handling of

Table 27.1	Site of Venipuncture and Incidence of Thrombophlebitis		
SITE	NO. OF VENIPUNCTURES	NO. OF CASES OF THROMBOPHLEBITIS	INCIDENCE OF THROMBOPHLEBITIS (%)
Hand, wrist	26	3	11.5
Forearm	15	2	13.33
Antecubital fossa	11	0	0
From Nordell K, Mogensen L, Nyquist O, Ornius E: Thrombophlebitis following intravenous lidocaine infusion, *Acta Med Scand* 192(4):263–265, 1972.			

the problem (after all, this is, in their mind, no longer a dental problem), immediate consultation with an appropriate physician is recommended.

Management of phlebothrombosis, a small, painless nodule located at the site of venipuncture, is essentially the same as that described for thrombophlebitis:

1. Immobilization of the affected limb
2. Moist heat applied to the area for 20 minutes three to four times a day
3. Tincture of time

Virtually all cases of local venous complications resolve within a short period without residual effects.

COMPLICATIONS

In this section, systemic reactions brought about through the administration of IV drugs are discussed.

Nausea and Vomiting

The incidence of nausea and vomiting associated with IV moderate sedation is quite low. However, the potential does exist for some of the drugs administered to produce this problem. Of the drugs recommended for use via the IV route, opioids are most likely to induce nausea and vomiting. Promethazine and scopolamine, which possess antiemetic properties, are among those drugs least likely to produce nausea and vomiting.

Causes of Nausea and Vomiting

1. Swallowing blood
2. Opioid administration
3. Hypoxia

The potential problem is not the development of nausea, but in the act of vomiting, especially in the patient with central nervous system (CNS) depression (i.e., the sedated patient). The patient who vomits while lying supine in a dental chair faces the possibility of aspirating vomitus into his or her respiratory tract (trachea, bronchi, lungs) and suffocating on the vomitus or developing a pneumonitis. The fact that a patient has received a CNS-depressant drug only increases this risk because their protective reflexes may be somewhat depressed.

As mentioned, it is the general category of opioids in which the incidence of vomiting is greatest. The production of nausea and vomiting related to opioid use is dose related. The larger the dose of the opioid is, the higher the incidence of nausea and vomiting. With the dosages recommended in Chapters 25 and 26, the incidence of vomiting has proven to be virtually zero. When I first began the clinical use of nalbuphine, it was used in doses greater than those currently recommended. Of the first 10 patients receiving nalbuphine, 5 either became nauseous or vomited later that same day. Decreasing the dosage of the drug eliminated this problem while maintaining the drug's clinical effectiveness.

The incidence of vomiting following opioid administration is greater in ambulatory patients than in hospitalized, nonambulatory patients.[17] Patients receiving very large doses of opioids during general anesthesia do not have as high an incidence of postoperative vomiting, whereas patients undergoing ambulatory surgery and receiving significantly lower doses of opioids have a greater incidence of vomiting. This increased rate of vomiting is related to the more frequent changes of body position that occur in the ambulatory patient. Unfortunately, this is a fact of life with which we must live. Happily, however, when opioid dosages are kept within the limits recommended herein, the incidence of this complication is extremely low.

Management of Nausea

Should nausea develop while the patient is still in the dental office, he or she can be returned to the dental chair and O_2 administered. This alone usually leads to recovery. Hypoxia is a frequent cause of nausea. Since recommending that O_2 be administered routinely during IV sedation, we have seen the virtual disappearance of nausea in our patient population. If nausea develops after discharge of the patient from the office, postoperative instructions suggest that the patient lie down for a while and drink a cola beverage or ginger ale, if available, as this may settle their stomach and prevent vomiting.

An antiemetic may be administered intravenously or intramuscularly if the patient is still in the dental office when nausea develops. Ondansetron (Zofran) is recommended, 4 mg administered IV 10 to 15 minutes before the end of the case.[18]

Ondansetron[18]	
Proprietary name:	Zofran
Classification:	Antiemetic
Availability:	Oral – 4-mg and 8-mg tablets; 4-mg/5-mL injectable
Recommended antiemetic dose:	8 mg PO q8h prn; 4 mg IV or IM

Management of Vomiting

Should nausea progress to vomiting when the patient is at home, the most important thing for the patient to remember is that he or she should not be lying supine because the possibility of aspiration of vomitus is greater in this position. This is one of the reasons for strict adherence to the discharge criteria recommendation that the patient be able to manage himself or herself at home before discharge from the office.

If vomiting occurs during dental treatment (a situation that has occurred only once in more than 6000 cases at the University of Southern California), the airway must immediately be cleared of all dental equipment. The patient's head should be turned to the side (away from the operator) so that the vomitus pools on one side of the mouth, leaving a patent airway. Suction is then applied so that the remaining vomitus may be removed.

Localized Allergy

It is not uncommon for a patient receiving IV drugs to mention that the skin at the site of injection itches. There may be a localized or diffuse reddening of the tissues. Several possibilities exist as to the cause of this reaction.

Most opioids, but primarily meperidine, induce the localized release of histamine. As the drug enters and travels up the vein toward the heart, a red line tracing the course of the vein may be noted (see Fig. 25.2). The patient may mention that his or her arm itches. Histamine release is a normal pharmacologic property of meperidine and does not represent allergy. Within 5 to 10 minutes, this response resolves by itself. Treatment is usually not required. If the itching is intense, IV administration of a histamine blocker, such as diphenhydramine, should be considered.

Less frequently, it will be observed that the skin around the site of the needle is diffusely erythematous with raised areas noted. The word "blotchy" may appropriately be used to describe its appearance. The site may "burn" or be quite itchy. The reaction is localized to the immediate area, but is not as localized to the path of the blood vessels, as is the meperidine-induced histamine reaction. The most frequently observed cause of this type of localized allergic response is the adhesive on the tape used to secure the needle or catheter.[19] A significant number of persons are allergic to the adhesive used on tape. The erythematous reaction will appear to be located under and around the tape. Management of this situation dictates the IV administration of the histamine blocker diphenhydramine. The use of hypoallergenic tape should prevent recurrence of this reaction.

If the allergic response appears to be more directly related to drug administration, treatment must be more vigorous and more immediate. The chemical mediators of allergy that are released from mast cells into the venous circulation in response to antigenic challenge will be traveling toward the heart and may soon involve the skin and respiratory and cardiovascular systems. Management of this potentially life-threatening reaction (anaphylaxis) involves placing a tourniquet high on the patient's arm as soon as the reaction is noted. This may prevent or at least slow the development of a generalized reaction. If the reaction is still limited to the limb, parenteral administration of a histamine blocker is recommended; however, once the reaction becomes more generalized, 0.3 mg of a 1:1000 epinephrine solution is administered intramuscularly or subcutaneously,[20] followed by activation of emergency medical service (EMS) and the IV (or intramuscular [IM]) administration of a histamine blocker.[21] The IV administration of epinephrine 1:1000 is never indicated. Epinephrine used intravenously is always administered as a 1:10,000 concentration, not 1:1,000.

Prevention of allergic reactions is greatly preferred to their management. Prevention is based on a careful pretreatment discussion of the patient's prior allergic history and response to any of the drugs administered. The patient should be questioned about any previous reactions to adhesives. In addition, the 0.2-mL test dose recommended for all drugs will aid in determining whether allergy is present. Although the administration of a dose as small as 0.2 mL of an allergen can, in some cases, induce anaphylactic reactions, in most circumstances, the observed reaction may be less severe, and management can proceed as previously described.

Epinephrine[20]	
Proprietary name:	Adrenalin, EpiPen
Classification:	Endogenous catecholamine
Availability:	0.3 mg (prefilled autoinjector)
Dose (SC/IM):	0.3 mg SC/IM

Diphenhydramine HCL[21]	
Proprietary name:	Benadryl
Classification:	H$_1$ antagonist (histamine blocker; antihistamine)
Availability:	50 mg/mL
Average dose (IV):	50 mg (>30 kg); 25 mg up to 30 kg

Respiratory Depression and Respiratory Obstruction

Morbidity and mortality associated with IV moderate sedation have frequently been related to the development of unrecognized respiratory depression, leading to respiratory arrest, cardiac dysrhythmias, and cardiac arrest. *All* of the sedative drugs discussed in this book are respiratory depressants (although to varying degrees at therapeutic doses). All are capable, in some doses and in some patients, of producing respiratory arrest. Respiratory depression is a more significant problem with certain drug groups, such as opioid agonists and barbiturates (one of the reasons why barbiturate use is no longer recommended).

Respiratory obstruction occurs as a result of the relaxing of the skeletal muscle of the tongue leading to soft tissue obstruction, either partial (e.g., "snoring") or complete (no "sound"). It is more often noted following benzodiazepine administration.

Respiratory depression following drug administration is dose related. Smaller doses of the drug produce little or no respiratory depression in the "average patient" (middle of the bell-shaped curve); however, increasing the drug dose increases its CNS-depressant effects and ultimately leads to respiratory depression.

Respiratory depression may occur following extremely low doses of any drug if the patient lies on the hyperresponding slope of the normal distribution curve. Unfortunately, little can be done before drug administration to determine this fact other than questioning the patient about his or her prior response to drugs, such as analgesics and anxiolytics (e.g., oral diazepam). A response from a patient who mentions becoming extremely drowsy after one 2-mg diazepam tablet should alert the dentist to the possibility of hyperresponsiveness to benzodiazepines. The 0.2-mL IV test dose, followed by a wait of 30 seconds before administering any additional drug, is another means of discovering a patient's hypersensitivity to a drug. One other means of accounting for variations in patient response to drugs is titration. Whenever possible, drugs should always be titrated to clinical effect. When titrated, oversedation and respiratory depression following IV drug administration should not occur or will do so only infrequently. The drug doses recommended in Chapters 25 and 26 will provide effective sedation with little or no respiratory depression in the typical normoresponding patient.

The two drug categories most likely to produce respiratory depression are opioid analgesics and barbiturates, though benzodiazepines, more likely to produce respiratory obstruction, may also produce respiratory depression in the hyperresponsive patient. Opioid-induced respiratory depression is characterized by a decrease in the rate of breathing. The adult respiratory rate, normally between 14 and 18 breaths/min, may decrease to 5 or 6 deeper breaths/min. Barbiturate-induced respiratory depression was one of the primary factors leading to the decreased use of these drugs today.

Recognition

Use of the pulse oximeter permits the early detection of desaturation of the blood, an early sign of respiratory depression. A subtle progression of decline in O_2 saturation readings from the high 90s to the mid-90s should lead the dentist to pause treatment and assess the patient's airway and respiratory status. The pulse oximeter alarm for low O_2 saturation is usually set at 90. Respiratory obstruction is noted through both a drop in O_2 saturation readings and sound. Partial airway obstruction produced by the relaxed tongue muscles is associated with the sound of snoring.

Management

The initial steps in management of respiratory depression or obstruction are universal, regardless of the cause of the problem. Following are the steps of basic life support:
- *Position:* If not already supine (most patients receiving IV moderate sedation *will* already be in the supine position during treatment), the patient is immediately placed into the supine position. The patient's feet are elevated slightly (10 to 15 degrees) to aid the return of venous blood to the heart.
- *Circulation:* The carotid pulse is palpated to determine the functional status of the cardiovascular system. If respiratory depression is recognized early, the carotid pulse will still be strong and regular. A pulse oximeter's rhythmic beeping should reassure the dentist that the patient's heart is beating.
- *Airway:* Probably the most important step in managing an airway problem, be it respiratory obstruction or depression, is ensuring airway patency. This is accomplished through the head tilt–chin lift maneuver (Fig. 27.7). Proper

performance of this step lifts the tongue off of the hypopharynx, providing for a patent airway and an almost immediate increase in the O_2 saturation levels in most patients (a 10- to 20-second delay in response may be noted depending on patient size and location of the pulse oximeter probe).
- *Breathing:* The dentist or assistant performing the previous step places his or her ear 1 inch from the patient's mouth and nose, looking at the patient's chest while listening and feeling for air exiting the patient's mouth and nose and watching the patient's chest for signs of spontaneous ventilatory efforts (Fig. 27.8). In the likely event that the patient is breathing spontaneously but the rate and depth are depressed, the rescuer should assist or control the patient's breathing. Using a positive-pressure O_2 device (Fig. 27.9) or a self-inflating bag–valve–mask device (Fig. 27.10), the rescuer inflates the patient's lungs every time he or she

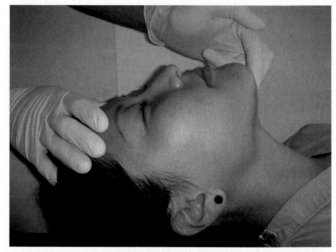

Figure 27.7 Airway maintenance employing head tilt–chin lift maneuver.

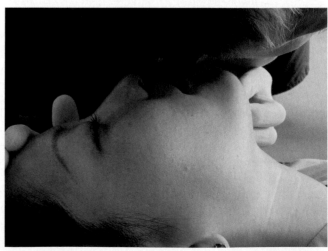

Figure 27.8 Look, listen, and feel while checking for respiration and airway patency.

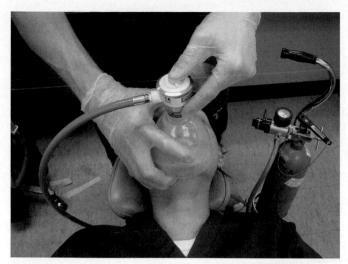

Figure 27.9 Assisted or controlled ventilation using a positive-pressure demand device.

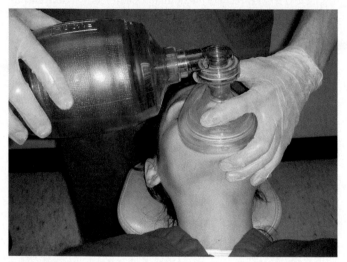

Figure 27.10 Assisted or controlled ventilation using a self-inflating bag–valve–mask device.

initiates a spontaneous respiration. If the patient's respiratory rate is less than 8 breaths/min, the rescuer will increase the rate of breathing by interposing a controlled ventilation between each of the spontaneous attempts by the patient. The self-inflating bag–valve–mask device is not recommended for use in larger adults unless a reservoir bag is added. It is, however, recommended for use in children.

• *Definitive care:* If respiratory depression occurs following opioid administration (either as a sole drug or as one of a combination), an opioid antagonist may be administered. **Naloxone** is the drug of choice for reversing opioid-induced respiratory depression. Naloxone should be diluted from its original 0.4 mg/mL concentration by adding 3 mL of diluent (5% dextrose and water, normal saline), producing a 0.1 mg/mL concentration for injection. The patient is continually observed for signs of increased respiration while 0.1 mg (1 mL) is slowly administered every minute.[22] In most cases, less than

0.4 mg naloxone will be required to reverse opioid-induced respiratory depression. When initially introduced, naloxone was administered in 0.4-mg increments. It was found, however, that larger doses of naloxone also antagonize the analgesic properties of the opioid. If the patient had undergone a painful procedure (e.g., abdominal surgery), the reversal by naloxone of the analgesic actions of the opioid led to an acute onset of pain, which is a significant stimulus to the heart and cardiovascular system. This led to life-threatening emergencies in patients with prior histories of cardiovascular disease.[23] Careful titration of 0.1 mg/min minimizes this reaction. During the time between the administration of naloxone and its onset of action, the required steps of basic life support must be continued.

With the return of deeper and more rapid respiration, the patient begins to look and feel considerably better. O_2 saturation levels will increase. The patient may be unaware of what has transpired because he or she has been deeply sedated during this time. Depending on the status of the patient and clinical experience of the dentist, dental treatment may be continued or halted. If it is elected to terminate the treatment, the patient should not be discharged from the office at this time. Naloxone is a rapid-acting opioid-antagonist; however, its duration of action following IV administration is fairly short. It is therefore possible for respiratory depression to recur approximately 30 minutes after the initial IV dose of naloxone was given. With the use of the shorter-acting opioids, fentanyl, alfentanil, sufentanil, and remifentanil, this is less likely to occur. When meperidine, morphine, hydromorphone, and butorphanol are administered, the likelihood increases. The patient should remain in the office, in a monitored (pulse oximeter) recovery area with O_2 available, for at least 1 hour after the administration of naloxone.

Following the initial IV dose of naloxone and recovery of the patient, it is suggested that 0.4 mg naloxone be administered intramuscularly. The duration of clinical action of IM naloxone is considerably longer than that of an IV dose, further decreasing the risk of recurrence of respiratory depression.

Non–opioid-induced respiratory depression is not reversible with naloxone. The barbiturates are the other drug group most likely to produce respiratory depression. Management of non–opioid-induced respiratory depression is based on the steps of basic life support—circulation, airway, and breathing—until the cerebral blood level of the offending drug has been lowered, through redistribution, to the point at which it no longer depresses respiration. There are no effective antidotal drugs for barbiturates.

Respiratory depression produced by benzodiazepines is significantly less common within the dosage ranges presented previously. That respiratory depression can occur with these drugs was brought to the attention of dentists in the United States by a letter from the manufacturer of midazolam that reemphasized this possibility and recommended appropriate measures to minimize or prevent its development.[24] Management is based on the basic life support techniques described above. The IV administration of the benzodiazepine antagonist flumazenil, in an initial dose of 0.2 mg (2 mL) with subsequent doses administered every minute as needed (to a maximum dose of 1.0 mg), will reverse the respiratory depression (and other clinical actions of benzodiazepines) more rapidly.[25]

Naloxone[22]

Proprietary name:	Narcan
Classification:	Opioid antagonist
Availability:	0 0.4 mg/mL
Average reversal dose (IV):	0.4 mg (adult)
Maximum single dose:	0.4 mg (adult)
Maximum total dose:	1.2 mg (adult)*
	*Lack of improvement after two or three doses usually indicates that respiratory depression is not produced by opioids.

Flumazenil[25]

Proprietary name:	Romazicon
Classification:	Benzodiazepine antagonist
Availability:	0.1 mg/mL
Average reversal dose (IV):	0.2 mg
Maximum single dose:	0.2 mg every 45 seconds
Maximum total dose:	1.0 mg

Emergence Delirium

A complication known as *emergence delirium* has been reported following administration of many CNS depressants and with some adjunctive drugs commonly given intravenously in IV moderate sedation procedures. The patient's response is one of transient delirium, hallucination, anxiety, or rage that develops at some time during or immediately after the sedative procedure. Very often, the response is associated with recall of an upsetting event in the patient's life. Minichetti and Milles[26] reported a case of a 27-year-old patient receiving 7.5 mg IV diazepam in addition to meperidine, atropine, nitrous oxide-oxygen (N_2O-O_2), and local anesthesia for extraction of several teeth. The patient felt quite comfortable and sedated. Following the administration of an additional 2.5 mg diazepam later in the procedure, the patient became progressively more excited. His eyes closed, he began crying, and he would not respond to verbal commands. Attempts made to communicate with the patient were ineffective. He became hyperexcitable and began thrashing about in the dental chair. Removal of the N_2O and administration of 100% O_2 did not resolve the situation, nor did administration of 0.4 mg naloxone. He continued to hallucinate for about 20 minutes, exhibiting rage and anxiety. He

recovered gradually, calmed down, stopped crying, and began responding to his name. When questioned later about the incident, he said that he thought he had merely been dreaming about an unpleasant experience he had had in the Vietnam War.

The drugs most likely to produce emergence delirium are scopolamine, diazepam, and midazolam. Other benzodiazepines, such as lorazepam, have also been reported to produce emergence delirium. Scopolamine, however, is far and away the drug most likely to produce emergence delirium.[27]

The reactions associated with emergence delirium are thought to be manifestations of the central anticholinergic syndrome (CAS).[28,29] CAS includes such paradoxical reactions as acute hyperactivity, anxiety, delirium, hallucinations, and recent memory impairment. In its most severe form, CAS produces apnea, medullary paralysis, coma, and death, although these reactions are extremely rare. The dose of scopolamine or benzodiazepine required to produce CAS is extremely small. CAS is not a dose-related phenomenon. The dentist administering IV anticholinergics or benzodiazepines must be aware of the CAS, its prevention, and its management.

Prevention

The incidence of CAS and emergence delirium is considerably lower in patients between the ages of 6 and 65 years.[30] For this reason, the use of scopolamine is not recommended in patients younger than 6 or older than 65 years. Other anticholinergics, such as atropine and glycopyrrolate, which are less likely to produce CAS, are recommended in these patients. Fortunately the indication for IV moderate sedation in patients younger than 6 or older than 65 years is not great. Slow injection of drugs, titration, and use of minimal doses may aid in minimizing these reactions.

Management

Management of the usual form of emergence delirium, in which the patient may exhibit dreaming and appears uncomfortable but does not respond to verbal questioning, takes two forms.

Symptomatic Management

Positioning, monitoring, ensuring a patent airway and adequate blood supply to the brain (PCAB), and prevention of injury to the patient are the goals of treatment. Given an appropriate time span (which is quite variable), the reaction will end, and the patient will open his or her eyes and be able to respond to commands and questions normally. In one case of emergence delirium witnessed by this author (before the availability of physostigmine and flumazenil), the patient had received scopolamine as a part of the Jorgensen technique and for almost 5 hours continued to dream and make uncoordinated movements in the chair. She was unresponsive to questioning, but had a very adequate airway with her vital signs slightly elevated over baseline. Approximately 5 hours after the administration of the scopolamine, the patient opened her eyes and responded appropriately.

Physostigmine Administration

The second means of managing emergence delirium is the administration of physostigmine, a reversible anticholinesterase. IV administration of physostigmine rapidly reverses emergence delirium and the CAS.

The dose of physostigmine for reversal of emergence delirium is 1.0 mg for the 70-kg adult and 0.5 mg for the child (up to 30 kg), administered intravenously. One milligram of physostigmine may be administered per minute until the reaction is terminated or a maximum dose of 4 mg is reached.[31] Because physostigmine is metabolized within 30 minutes, the patient must be monitored closely to be certain that signs and symptoms do not recur. Rapid administration of physostigmine is associated with the possible development of bradycardia, hypersalivation, emesis, and defecation.[31]

Physostigmine[31]	
Proprietary name:	Antilirium
Classification:	Reversible anticholinesterase
Availability:	1 mg/mL
Average therapeutic dose (IV):	0.5–2.0 mg
Maximum single dose:	2 mg
Maximum total dose:	4 mg

Laryngospasm

Laryngospasm represents a protective reflex of the body. In a fully conscious patient (i.e., no CNS depression), foreign objects are prevented from entering into the airway (trachea) by the swallowing reflex, the epiglottis, and the cough reflex. As a patient becomes more and more CNS depressed through the administration of drugs, these protective reflexes become increasingly depressed. In minimal and moderate sedation, as observed with N_2O-O_2, IV midazolam, and/or diazepam, there is little impairment of these reflexes. Foreign material, such as water, blood, and scraps of dental material, will be easily removed by the patient as he or she spits or swallows. Aspiration of foreign objects into the airway is quite uncommon during moderate sedation. However, as the level of CNS depression deepens with increased doses or the addition of other drugs, protective reflexes are depressed to a greater degree.[32]

In deep sedation, but more so in "ultralight" general anesthesia, foreign material present in the area of the larynx may provoke a protective reflex in which the vocal cords adduct in an attempt to seal off the trachea from entry of foreign material. Though truly a protective reflex, laryngospasm also prevents the passage of air into and out of the trachea and lungs (Fig. 27.11).

Laryngospasm will not occur during minimal or moderate sedation because the other protective reflexes (coughing, swallowing) are still intact. It is only when the patient enters

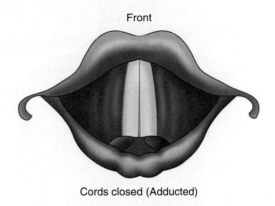

Front

Cords closed (Adducted)

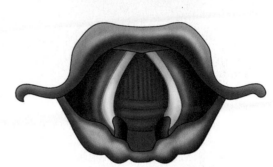

Cords open (Abducted)

Figure 27.11 View of vocal cords. *Top,* Cords are adducted (closed), thus preventing foreign material (this is good) and air (this is bad) from entering trachea. *Bottom,* Cords abducted (open).

into deeper levels of sedation or light general anesthesia that laryngospasm may be observed.

Recognition

Recognition of laryngospasm is based on the presence or absence of sound. Partial laryngospasm is identified by the presence of stridor, defined as an abnormal high-pitched, musical respiratory sound produced as air is forced out through partially adducted vocal folds. Total (complete) laryngospasm is identified by the absence of sound in the presence of spontaneous respiratory efforts, an ominous "sound" indeed.

The patient attempts to breathe against this partially or completely closed airway. Respiratory efforts are exaggerated: Expansion of the chest is greater than usual, and accessory muscles of respiration are used. Substernal, supraclavicular, and intercostal soft tissue retraction may be observed (Fig. 27.12). This occurs as the soft tissues overlying the intercostal spaces between the ribs and sternum are sucked inward as the chest expands and intrathoracic pressure becomes more negative. Soft tissue retraction is a sign of a partially or totally obstructed airway.

Management

1. The first step in management of laryngospasm is to remove any offending material from the patient's airway. A

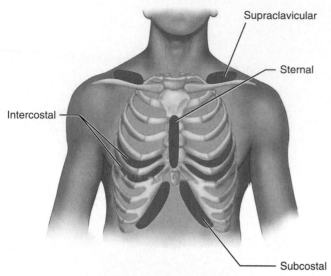

Figure 27.12 Retractions associated with respiratory distress: intercostal, supraclavicular, subcostal, and sternal.

large-diameter suction tip or tonsillar suction is placed into the pharynx to remove any material it finds. This step alone will break laryngospasm in many cases.

2. Following suctioning of the airway, positive-pressure O_2 is administered, either via the self-inflating bag–valve–mask device or positive-pressure demand valve. Often, it is possible to break the spasm by forcing O_2 past the vocal cords.

   Positive-pressure O_2 *should not* be delivered to a patient in partial or complete laryngospasm *before suctioning* of the airway since the material provoking the spasm may be forced through the vocal cords into the trachea or bronchi.

3. **The administration of drugs to terminate laryngospasm is never recommended unless the dentist is well trained in anesthesiology and in management of the apneic patient.** The drug of choice is succinylcholine, a short-acting depolarizing muscle relaxant. Administered in a concentration of 20 mg/mL, an IV dose of 20 to 40 mg is usually adequate to break laryngospasm by paralyzing the muscles of respiration producing apnea. At this point, however, the patient is no longer breathing, and the dentist becomes responsible for instituting controlled ventilation for the 3 to 4 minutes until the typical patient resumes spontaneous ventilation.[33]

4. If no drugs are administered during laryngospasm, the level of carbon dioxide (CO_2) in the patient's blood will increase, their level of consciousness would decrease, and laryngospasm would break spontaneously. Although this technique of managing laryngospasm is acceptable, it is not recommended for the untrained dentist.

Laryngospasm should not develop when lighter levels of sedation (minimal, moderate) are maintained and the airway is kept free of debris, water, blood, and saliva.

SPECIFIC DRUG COMPLICATIONS

Benzodiazepines

The most commonly seen complications associated with midazolam and diazepam administration are as follows:
1. Local venous complications (diazepam)
2. Emergence delirium
3. Recurrences of amnesia
4. Oversedation

Local venous complications and emergence delirium have been discussed previously. The recurrence of amnesia following diazepam administration has occurred in my experience with patients only twice over 40 years; however, it was this phenomenon that caused me to decrease the recommended dose of diazepam used for sedation.

Two patients received diazepam, one a dose of 45 mg and the other a dose of 38 mg, and achieved clinically ideal sedation lasting for the usual 45 minutes. Recovery was normal, with the patients appearing unsedated after 1 hour. It was later reported that for the first 24 hours after they left the clinic (these cases were done at different times and on different dates), their recovery was normal. However, in both cases, approximately 24 hours later, the patients experienced a relapse of amnesia. One patient had driven to work, parked his car, and entered his office building when suddenly he did not remember where he was, how he had gotten there, or what day it was. Within a few minutes, the patient's memory returned. No further relapses occurred. The same type of response occurred in the second patient. I am unaware of similar responses developing in patients who have received less than 30 mg of diazepam at a single treatment; thus the recommendation that this dose not be exceeded as a total for one treatment session.

Oversedation is unlikely to develop with midazolam or diazepam if the drug is titrated at the recommended rate of 1 mL/min. However, if a patient does become oversedated, management is to ensure a patent airway and ventilation (P→ C→A→B). Within a few minutes, redistribution of the drug leads to a lessening of the level of sedation and increased responsiveness. The IV administration of flumazenil will speed recovery (D).[25,34,35]

Promethazine

Promethazine-related complications include oversedation and extrapyramidal reactions. Oversedation is managed through basic life support (P→ C→A→B). There is no effective antidote for promethazine-induced oversedation or respiratory depression. Extrapyramidal reactions, although quite rare, do develop after promethazine administration. Four types of reactions are identified: akathisia (motor restlessness), acute dystonias, parkinsonism, and tardive dyskinesias. These are described in Chapter 7. Management requires administration of IV diphenhydramine, 50 mg for the adult and 25 mg for the child up to 30 kg.

Table 27.2	Percentage of Dentists Who Have Witnessed IV Complications*			
	Malamed (n = 114)		Trieger (n = 117)	
	NO.	%	NO.	%
Hematoma	39	34.2	32	27.0
Infiltration	38	33.3	41	35.0
Pain on injection	29	25.4	50	42.0
Hyperexcitement	29	25.4	11	9.0
Thrombophlebitis	28	24.5	24	20.0
Prolonged sedation	19	16.6	12	10.0
Vomiting	16	14.0	8	6.0
Hypotension	12	10.5	11	9.0
Apnea	1	0.8	0	0.0
Arterial injection	0	0.0	3	2.5

From Malamed SF: Continuing education in intravenous sedation. Part 2: complications and non-use, *Anesth Prog* 28:158, 1981.

*The statistics illustrate the number of dentists who have seen the complication listed, not the number of times they have seen it occur. Therefore a dentist may have seen one case of vomiting in 5000 IV procedures, but because 16 of the 114 reporting dentists reported at least one case of vomiting, it is listed as a 14% incidence.

Opioids

Major adverse side effects of opioid administration are nausea and vomiting, respiratory depression, and rigid chest. The first two complications were discussed earlier in this chapter.

Rigid chest is an uncommon phenomenon that has been observed primarily after administration of fentanyl, but can develop with any opioid.[36-39] It is most commonly seen when N_2O-O_2 has been administered concomitantly.[39] In this situation, the skeletal muscles of the thorax appear to be paralyzed, and inflation of the chest is difficult if not impossible. The cause of rigid chest is unknown. The patient will be unable to breathe. Efforts to force air into the patient will prove futile because the chest does not expand. The chest has a firm boardlike feel during this reaction. Management of rigid chest involves the following:

1. The airway is supported, and an attempt is made to force O_2 into the lungs.
2. IV succinylcholine, 20 to 40 mg, is administered (recommended only for those trained in anesthesiology).
3. Following the release of the rigid chest (caused by the actions of succinylcholine), the patient will be apneic for approximately 3 to 5 minutes, during which time controlled ventilation is absolutely necessary.

Rigid chest has been observed in conjunction with the fentanyl and N_2O combination. The use of combinations of techniques is discussed in Chapter 28.

Scopolamine

The major problem associated with scopolamine administration is emergence delirium, which was discussed earlier.

SUMMARY

Complications can and do occur during IV moderate sedation. Trieger[40] and Malamed[41] conducted independent surveys of dentists having completed basic IV moderate sedation programs to determine which complications did develop most often. Table 27.2 presents their findings.

REFERENCES

1. Mirski MA, Lele AV, Fitzsimmons L, Toung TJ: Diagnosis and treatment of vascular air embolism. *Anesthesiology* 106(1):164–177, 2007.
2. Infusionnurse. IV administration sets: priming volume vs. residual volume. http://infusionnurse.org/2015/02/11/iv-administration-sets-priming-volume-vs-residual-volume. (Accessed 24 March 2016).
3. Philip JH: Intravenous access and delivery principles. In Rogers MC, Tinker JH, Covino BG, et al, editors: *Principles and practice of anesthesiology*, St Louis, 1993, Mosby.
4. Khan ZH, Noorbaksh S: An accidental intra-arterial injection of thiopental on the dorsum of the foot—a case report. *Acta Anaesthesiol Taiwan* 42(1):55–58, 2004.
5. Shenoi AN, Fortenberry JD, Kamat P: Accidental intra-arterial injection of propofol. *Pediatr Emerg Care* 30(2):136, 2014.
6. Joist A, Tibesku CO, Neuber M, et al: Gangrene of the fingers caused by accidental intra-arterial injection of diazepam. *Dtsch Med Wochenschr* 124(24):755–758, 1999.
7. Lopez MA, Delas F, Ledesma M, et al: Accidental intraarterial diazepam injection. *Rev Esp Anestesiol Reanim* 45(1):32, 1998.
8. Hering J, Angelkort B: Acute ischemia of the hand after intra-arterial injection of flunitrazepam. Local combined fibrinolysis therapy in three cases. *Dtsch Med Wochenschr* 131(24):1377–1380, 2006.
9. Myers RA, Schnitzer BM: Hyperbaric oxygen use, update 1984. *Postgrad Med* 76(5):83–86, 89–91, 94–95, 1984.
10. Bittner Ch, Zuber M, Eisner L: Acute ischemia of the hand in a drug addict after accidental intra-arterial injection. *Swiss Surg* 8(6):281–284, 2002.
11. Gelfman SS, Dionne RA, Driscoll EJ: Prospective study of venous complications following intravenous diazepam and in dental outpatients. *Anesth Prog* 28(5):126–128, 1981.
12. Gelfman SS, Driscoll EJ: Thrombophlebitis following intravenous anesthesia and sedation: an annotated literature review. *Anesth Prog* 24(6):194–197, 1977.
13. Driscoll EJ, Gelfman SS, Sweet JB, et al: Thrombophlebitis after intravenous use of anesthesia and sedation: its incidence and natural history. *J Oral Surg* 37(11):809–815, 1979.
14. Margary JJ, Rosenbaum NL, Partridge M, Shankar S: Local complications following intravenous benzodiazepines in the dorsum of the hand. A comparison between midazolam and Diazemuls in sedation in dentistry. *Anaesthesia* 41(2):205–207, 1986.
15. Nordell K, Mogensen L, Nyquist O, Ornius E: Thrombophlebitis following intravenous lidocaine infusion. *Acta Med Scand* 192(4):263–265, 1972.
16. Chambiras PG: Sedation in dentistry, intravenous diazepam. *Aust Dent J* 17(1):17023, 1972.
17. Watcha MF, White PF: Postoperative nausea and vomiting: its etiology, treatment, and prevention. *Anesthesiology* 77(1):162–184, 1992.

18. ClinicalKey. Ondansetron drug monograph. March 17, 2016. www.clinicalkey.com. (Accessed 27 March 2016).

19. Eltaki K, Abdulla H, Sinatra RS: A severe inflammatory cutaneous reaction after continuous epidural analgesia. *Anesth Analg* 106(2):517–519, 2008.

20. ClinicalKey. Epinephrine drug monograph. March 1, 2016. www.clinicalkey.com. (Accessed 27 March 2016).

21. ClinicalKey. Diphenhydramine drug monograph. March 3, 2016. www.clinicalkey.com. (Accessed 27 March 2016).

22. ClinicalKey. Naloxone drug monograph. December 4, 2015. www.clinicalkey.com. (Accessed 28 March 2016).

23. Pallasch TJ, Gill CJ: Naloxone-associated morbidity and mortality. *Oral Surg Oral Med Oral Pathol* 52(6):602–603, 1981.

24. Dosing and titration of midazolam (Versed), Letter to doctors, Nutley, NJ, 1987, Roche Laboratories.

25. ClinicalKey. Flumazenil drug monograph. February 5, 2016. www.clinicalkey.com. (Accessed 28 March 2016).

26. Minichetti J, Milles M: Hallucination and delirium reaction to intravenous diazepam administration: case report. *Anesth Prog* 29(5):144–146, 1982.

27. Olympio MA: Postanesthetic emergence delirium: historical perspective. *J Clin Anesth* 3(1):60–63, 1991.

28. Schneck HJ, Rupreht J: Central anticholinergic syndrome (CAS) in anesthesia and intensive care. *Acta Anaesthesiol Belg* 40(3):219–228, 1989.

29. Rupreht J: The central muscarinic transmission during anaesthesia and recovery: the central anticholinergic syndrome. *Anaesthesiol Reanim* 16(4):250–258, 1991.

30. Voepel-Lewis T: A prospective cohort study of emergence agitation in the pediatric postanesthesia care unit. *Anesth Analg* 96(6):1625–1630, 2003.

31. ClinicalKey. Physostigmine drug monograph. July 2, 2014. www.clinicalkey.com. (Accessed 28 March 2016).

32. Odom JL: Airway emergencies in the post anesthesia care unit. *Nurs Clin North Am* 28(3):483–491, 1993.

33. Roy WL, Lerman J: Laryngospasm in paediatric anaesthesia. *Can J Anaesth* 35(1):93–98, 1988.

34. Longmire AW, Seger DL: Topics in clinical pharmacology: flumazenil, a benzodiazepine antagonist. *Am J Med Sci* 306(1):49–52, 1993.

35. Kulka PJ, Lauven PM: Benzodiazepine antagonists: an update of their role in the emergency care of overdose patients. *Drug Saf* 7(5):381–386, 1992.

36. Klausner JM, Caspi J, Lelcuk S, et al: Delayed muscular rigidity and respiratory depression following fentanyl anesthesia. *Arch Surg* 123(1):66–67, 1988.

37. Vacanti CA, Silbert BS, Vacanti FX: The effects of thiopental on fentanyl-induced muscle rigidity in a human model. *J Clin Anesth* 3(5):395–398, 1991.

38. Ackerman WE, Phero JC, Theodore GT: Ineffective ventilation during conscious sedation due to chest wall rigidity after intravenous midazolam and fentanyl. *Anesth Prog* 37(1):46–48, 1990.

39. Neidhart P, Burgener MC, Schwieger I, Suter PM: Chest wall rigidity during fentanyl and midazolam-fentanyl induction: ventilatory and haemodynamic effects. *Acta Anaesthesiol Scand* 33(1):1–5, 1989.

40. Trieger NT: Teaching intravenous sedation: follow-up of 200 dentists. *Anesth Prog* 25(5):154–156, 1978.

41. Malamed SF: Continuing education in intravenous sedation. Part 2: complications and non-use. *Anesth Prog* 28(6):158–160, 1981.

chapter 28

Practical Considerations

The following are frequently asked questions that relate to intravenous (IV) moderate sedation.

Who can perform venipuncture and administer IV drugs?

Some dentists wish to delegate the duties of venipuncture and drug administration to auxiliary personnel (i.e., the dental assistant, registered dental assistant, dental hygienist, or registered nurse). Although the dental practice act in each state or province must be consulted for specific regulations, it is the law in most states that only the dentist (DDS, DMD or equivalent, or MD) or a certified registered nurse anesthetist (CRNA) may perform venipuncture and administer IV drugs. In some states, registered nurses (RNs) and phlebotomists may perform venipuncture. As mentioned in Chapter 24, an auxiliary may perform virtually all of the duties relating to the IV moderate sedation procedure except for venipuncture and drug administration.

What if the patient does not respond to the maximum dose of the drug?

The response of patients to drugs exhibits great variation, as evidenced by the normal distribution curve. The fact that titration is possible for essentially all intravenously administered drugs (lorazepam is a notable exception) allows us to determine exactly where on this curve each patient lies. Some patients are hyporesponders, in whom the clinically observed effect of a drug at its maximum recommended dose will be suboptimal or may be nonexistent. The most reasonable approach to take when the maximum recommended dose of a drug has failed to produce clinically adequate sedation is to cease further administration of the drug and make an attempt at the planned dental treatment. As mentioned in previous chapters, I have been pleasantly surprised on occasion at the ease with which treatment proceeds on an apparently nonsedated patient. If sedation is truly inadequate to permit the planned procedure to continue, the patient should be allowed to recover (despite the apparent lack of symptoms), discharged (in the custody of a responsible adult), and rescheduled at a later date for a different IV drug technique. For patients in whom midazolam has failed to produce adequate sedation, diazepam has frequently been successful at subsequent visits and vice versa.

Doses of drugs beyond those recommended should not be administered unless the dentist has completed a residency in anesthesiology. In many cases, persons with this training will not administer additional drugs because the administration of other drugs can only prolong and complicate recovery in the ambulatory outpatient setting.

The drug doses and techniques recommended in this section have withstood the test of time. When used as recommended, the success rate of IV moderate sedation approaches, but will never reach, 100%. The occasional failure (either from unresponsiveness to the administered IV drug[s] or inability to successfully gain venous access) will occur and must be accepted by the dentist. Inability to accept failure requires the dentist to inject larger and larger doses of more and more drugs, a situation potentially fraught with problems.

Who should escort the patient from the dental office?

On occasion, usually once in a dentist's career, a patient's escort (ride home) will disappear or never show up. If the IV moderate sedation procedure has yet to begin, I strongly urge that the procedure be canceled unless another suitable escort can be arranged before the start of the sedation/dental procedure. It is tempting and natural for the dentist to want to go ahead with the IV procedure because of the time that has been allotted for it in the day's schedule. This temptation must be resisted.

Patients receiving midazolam or diazepam usually appear clinically recovered 1 hour after administration of one titrating dose. Absent an escort, the patient may opine that he or she is recovered enough to be allowed to leave the office unescorted. This must never be permitted to happen. Explain to the patient that although he or she feels recovered, this is not the case. The feeling is similar to that which occurs when one has had some alcohol and feels normal but is unable to function at normal capacity (e.g., safely operate a motor vehicle).

Alternative escorts that may occur to the patient or the dentist include taking a taxicab, car service (e.g., Uber, Lyft), a bus, or train; walking home; or being accompanied by a member of the office staff. All of these proposed alternatives are unacceptable. The only person who should be permitted to escort the patient home is a relative or close friend of the patient, a person who can remain with the patient until he or she has recovered. I have come to describe the acceptable escort as "a responsible adult, a person who has a vested interest in the health and safety of the patient." This definition precludes use of a taxi, bus, or other form of public transportation in which the escort is a stranger to the patient. The dangers involved in the alternatives are unacceptable. It is good practice for a member of the office staff to contact the patient the day before the scheduled IV procedure to review preoperative instructions, reemphasizing the need for an escort.

What do you recommend when I first introduce IV moderate sedation into my office?

First, members of the office staff, especially chairside assistants, should attend the IV moderate sedation training course with their dentist so that they can learn the procedures firsthand. Very often, remarks made in a lecture are misconstrued, and an important concept may be improperly understood. Having several office personnel attending the course will minimize the chance of this occurring.

Second, the introduction of IV moderate sedation into a dental office will disrupt the normal routine of the office, at least initially. It is a new technique and must be used many times in that environment before it becomes integrated into the practice routine. One must anticipate that extra time may be required during the first 50 or so cases. This can best be accomplished by scheduling IV cases immediately before lunchtime or as the last appointment of the day so that if they do "run over," the dentist will not have to worry about a reception room filled with waiting patients. As the procedure gains the acceptance of the office staff, IV patients can be scheduled earlier in the day, when most apprehensive patients are more ideally treated.

I have more trouble with venipuncture than anything else. How can I become more proficient?

Welcome to the club!

The most difficult part of the technique of IV moderate sedation is becoming adept at venipuncture. Administering drugs intravenously is easy and safe (if basic rules are followed regarding titration). However, without a needle placed within a vein, IV drug administration is impossible.

Venipuncture is a learned technique. Practice makes (almost) perfect. Unfortunately, most dentists do not wish to "practice" venipuncture on their patients. There are several possible places where one might improve his or her technique of venipuncture. A local hospital or blood bank might welcome volunteers to help draw blood. Volunteering 1 hour a week will greatly improve venipuncture technique.

What about the use of combinations of techniques?

Unless the dentist is experienced in general anesthesia or has extensive experience with IV moderate sedation, the use of some combinations of techniques is contraindicated. These include the combination of intramuscular (IM) and IV moderate sedation (absolute contraindication, as per this author) and the combination of inhalation and IV moderate sedation (relatively contraindicated, as per this author).

When nitrous oxide-oxygen (N_2O-O_2) is added to IV moderate sedation, the degree of patient monitoring must increase

significantly because this patient may drift in and out of deeper levels of sedation as the stimulation resulting from the dental treatment changes. Without the suggested training or experience, I do not believe that this combination of techniques should be used.

There are but few indications for the conjoint use of the IM and IV routes of drug administration. One is the use of an IM injection for the induction of sedation in a disruptive child or disruptive adult patient who has a mental or physical disability, after which an IV line is established and used for the administration of any additional drugs that might be needed (see Chapters 35 and 38).

Oral sedation can be used effectively with IV moderate sedation, provided that the level of sedation achieved by the oral route remains light (e.g., minimal sedation) (see Chapter 7).

Oral drugs are administered the night before the appointment and/or immediately (60 minutes) before treatment to "take the edge off" the last few minutes prior to the IV procedure. Oral drugs should not be used for deep sedation because of the lack of titratability of this route of drug administration. Once the IV line is established, as long as the IV drug is titrated, there should be no problem associated with this combination of techniques. Failure to titrate (i.e., administration of a fixed doses of drugs) increases the risk of oversedation and respiratory depression or arrest.

Do I have to titrate IV drugs?

Only if you want to avoid problems. Fixed drug combinations are frequently mentioned in legal depositions where morbidity or mortality has occurred. An oft-heard statement is, "But I gave this same dose of drugs to 10,000 other patients without ever having a problem." Unfortunately, patient number 10,001 was on the extreme hyperresponding side of the bell-shaped curve, and this "usual" dose was too much for this patient. Titration is a safety feature that must always be used. A rule for (almost) all IV moderate sedation drugs is to administer the drug(s) at a rate of 1.0 mL per minute.

Is IV moderate sedation safe?

This is a very interesting and provocative question. Newspapers publish lurid accounts of deaths occurring in dental offices.[1-3] Often these patients have received IV drugs; whether they received IV moderate sedation, deep sedation, or general anesthesia is not often mentioned. If we were to solely consider the newspaper account, we would have to say that intravenously administered drugs are dangerous. The fact of the matter is quite the opposite. When IV moderate sedation is used as taught, it is the safest technique of parenteral drug administration, with the exception of inhalation sedation with N_2O-O_2. The degree of control maintained by the administrator over intravenously administered drugs is second only to that available with inhalation sedation.

If the techniques described in this book are followed and the dentist does not experiment with increased dosages or administer drugs with which he or she is unfamiliar or unprepared to use, serious problems will not occur. In a review of deaths in dental offices related to anesthesia (a very general term implying the use of drugs of any type), The Dentists Insurance Company of California (TDIC) stated that three factors were present in most instances where death or serious morbidity occurred[4]:

1. Inadequate preoperative evaluation of the patient
2. Lack of knowledge of the pharmacology of the drugs administered
3. Inadequate monitoring during the procedure

Though that paper was published in 1983, sadly, these same three factors are still implicated as causations in many recent dental office morbidities and mortalities.[5–8]

Education of the dentist and staff can eliminate these sources of problems. Although no long-term studies have been published regarding morbidity and mortality associated with IV moderate sedation, several papers have been published from which numbers can be extrapolated. Although not scientifically valid, these numbers do illustrate the safety of the basic techniques discussed in this section. More than 15,000 IV moderate sedation cases (diazepam, midazolam, and Jorgensen techniques) were completed without any significant complications occurring during the 38 years of the Basic Intravenous Sedation Course at the University of Southern California School of Dentistry—this by dentists who were neophytes at both venipuncture and IV drug administration. In a 1981 survey of 188 dentists who completed this course, it was found that they had completed more than 53,664 cases in private practice without any serious complications.[9] A very similar basic IV moderate sedation program continues to be presented through the Oregon Academy of General Dentistry and the Oregon Health Sciences University School of Dentistry for 17 years.[10] Approximately 10,000 cases have been completed with no serious complications.[11]

After 6 years of presenting a similar course at the University of Oregon, Foreman et al[12] reported that no complications of a serious nature had been encountered during any of their courses. Extrapolation from the data presented by Foreman et al suggests that IV moderate sedation has been successfully used more than 37,960 times by dentists completing their course.

Rodgers reported on the efficacy and safety of IV moderate sedation in an oral and maxillofacial surgery (OMS) practice over a 7-year period following completion of an OMS residency.[13] During this period, 2889 patients received IV sedation; 60.33% were American Society of Anesthesiologists (ASA) class 1, 39.43% ASA class 2, and 0.24% ASA class 3. Seventy patients experienced 77 adverse events (2.6%). There were no deaths, and no patients required transport to a hospital. Rodgers states that during this period, a number of previously undiagnosed medical problems were discovered.

In a randomized controlled study comparing various IV sedation protocols in 997 patients having third molars extracted, Dionne et al concluded that these data provide evidence that the drugs and doses evaluated resulted in therapeutic benefit to dental outpatients, with minimal incidence of potentially serious adverse effects.[14]

IV sedation is as safe as the person who is administering the drug(s).

REFERENCES

1. Maxwell E: Third patient of dentist being probed dies. Los Angeles Times Feb 20, 1983, p 1.
2. Newcomer K: Dentist waited outside while patient died. Rocky Mountain News Aug 4, 1992.
3. Marks P: Boy lapses into coma after dental surgery. New York Times May 14, 1993, p B5(L).
4. DeJulien LF: Causes of severe morbidity/mortality cases. CDA J 11(2):45–48, 1983.
5. Frazier M: Teen dies after 4 teeth pulled. New York Newsday Dec 22, 2005.
6. Hutton S: Man dies after wisdom tooth operation. Fox 4 News Kansas City, Feb 5, 2007.
7. Owen M, Shelton DL, Gorner J: Patient dies during root canal. Principal's energy in life, work recalled. Chicago Tribune Dec 18, 2007.
8. Leise C: Teen's death while sedated for dental work ruled accidental. Chronicle-Telegram, Elyria, Ohio. April 8, 2011.
9. Malamed SF: Continuing education in intravenous sedation: part 2, complications and non-use. Anesth Prog 28(6):158–160, 1981.
10. Oregon Academy of General Dentistry, Oregon Health Sciences University School of Dentistry. www.learnivsedation.com. (Accessed 9 January 2017).
11. Reed KL: Personal communication. January 8, 2017.
12. Foreman PA, Donaldson D, Jastak JT, Reveal DR: Continuing education in intravenous sedation. Anesth Prog 29(6):163–167, 1982.
13. Rodgers SF: Safety of intravenous sedation administered by the operating oral surgeon: the first 7 years of office practice. J Oral Maxillofac Surg 63(10):1478–1483, 2005.
14. Dionne RA, Yagiela JA, Moore PA, et al: Comparing efficacy and safety of four intravenous sedation regimens in dental outpatients. J Am Dent Assoc 132(6):740–751, 2001.

chapter 29

Guidelines for Teaching

 $\mathcal{E}$ ducation and experience are the critical elements that make intravenous (IV) moderate sedation a safe technique. New drugs, equipment, and monitoring devices become available almost every year, and it is only through continuing education that it is possible for the dentist to evaluate these items properly, some of which are initially touted by their developers as panaceas.

In 1977 the American Dental Association (ADA), the American Dental Society of Anesthesiology (ADSA), and the American Association of Dental Schools (AADS) convened a conference at which Guidelines for Teaching the Comprehensive Control of Pain and Anxiety in Dentistry, part III, were developed for a continuing education program.[1,2] These guidelines have undergone periodic revision, most recently in 2016.[3,4] Sections of part III of the guidelines ("Teaching the Comprehensive Control of Pain and Anxiety in a Continuing Education Program") relating to inhalation sedation were presented in Chapter 19. Material pertaining to continuing education in moderate sedation, which includes the IV route, is presented next.

These guidelines present a basic overview of the requirements for a competency course in moderate sedation. These include courses in enteral moderate sedation and parenteral moderate sedation. The teaching guidelines contained in this section on moderate sedation differ slightly from documents in medicine to reflect the differences in delivery methodologies and the practice environment in dentistry. For this reason, separate teaching guidelines have been developed for moderate enteral and moderate parenteral sedation.

Moderate sedation: a drug-induced depression of consciousness during which patients respond purposefully to verbal commands, either alone or accompanied by light tactile stimulation. No interventions are required to maintain a patent airway, and spontaneous ventilation is adequate. Cardiovascular function is usually maintained.[5]

Note: In accord with this particular definition, the drugs and/or techniques used should carry a margin of safety wide enough to render unintended loss of consciousness unlikely. Repeated dosing of an agent before the effects of previous dosing can be fully appreciated may result in a greater alteration of the state of consciousness than is the intent of the dentist.

Further, a patient whose only response is reflex withdrawal from a painful stimulus is not considered to be in a state of moderate sedation.

The following definition applies to administration of moderate and deeper levels of sedation:

Titration: administration of incremental doses of an intravenous or inhalation drug until a desired effect is reached. Knowledge of each drug's time of onset, peak response, and duration of action is essential to avoid oversedation. Although the concept of titration of a drug to effect is critical for patient safety, when the intent is moderate sedation, one must know whether the previous dose has taken full effect before administering an additional drug increment.

V. Teaching Administration of Moderate Sedation

These guidelines present a basic overview of the requirements for a competency course in moderate sedation. These include courses in enteral and parenteral moderate sedation. The teaching guidelines on moderate sedation contained in this section differ slightly from documents in medicine to reflect the differences in delivery methodologies and practice environment in dentistry.

Completion of a prerequisite nitrous oxide-oxygen competency course is required for participants combining moderate sedation with nitrous oxide-oxygen.

A. *Course Objectives: Upon completion of a course in moderate sedation, the dentist must be able to:*
   1. List and discuss the advantages and disadvantages of moderate sedation.
   2. Discuss the prevention, recognition, and management of complications associated with moderate sedation.
   3. Administer moderate sedation to patients in a clinical setting in a safe and effective manner.
   4. Discuss the abuse potential, occupational hazards, and other untoward effects of the agents utilized to achieve moderate sedation.
   5. Describe and demonstrate the technique of intravenous access, intramuscular injection, and other parenteral techniques.
   6. Discuss the pharmacology of the drug(s) selected for administration.

7. Discuss the precautions, indications, contraindications, and adverse reactions associated with the drug(s) selected.

8. Administer the selected drug(s) to dental patients in a clinical setting in a safe and effective manner.

9. List the complications associated with techniques of moderate sedation.

10. Describe a protocol for management of emergencies in the dental office and list and discuss the emergency drugs and equipment required for the prevention and management of emergency situations.

11. Discuss principles of advanced cardiac life support or an appropriate dental sedation/anesthesia emergency course equivalent.

12. Demonstrate the ability to manage emergency situations.

13. Demonstrate the ability to diagnose and treat emergencies related to the next deeper level of anesthesia than intended.

B. Moderate Sedation Course Content:

1. Historical, philosophical, and psychological aspects of anxiety and pain control.

2. Patient evaluation and selection through review of medical history taking, physical diagnosis, and psychological considerations.

3. Use of patient history and examination for ASA classification, risk assessment, and preprocedure fasting instructions.

4. Definitions and descriptions of physiological and psychological aspects of anxiety and pain.

5. Description of the sedation anesthesia continuum, with special emphasis on the distinction between the conscious and the unconscious state.

6. Review of adult respiratory and circulatory physiology and related anatomy.

7. Pharmacology of local anesthetics and agents used in moderate sedation, including drug interactions and contraindications.

8. Indications and contraindications for use of moderate sedation.

9. Review of dental procedures possible under moderate sedation.

10. Patient monitoring using observation and monitoring equipment, with particular attention to vital signs, ventilation/breathing, and reflexes related to consciousness.

11. Maintaining proper records with accurate chart entries recording medical history, physical examination, informed consent, time-oriented anesthesia record, including the names of all drugs administered including local anesthetics, doses, and monitored physiological parameters.

12. Prevention, recognition, and management of complications and emergencies.

13. Description, maintenance, and use of moderate sedation monitors and equipment.

14. Discussion of abuse potential.

15. Intravenous access: anatomy, equipment, and technique.

16. Prevention, recognition, and management of complications of venipuncture and other parenteral techniques.

17. Description and rationale for the technique to be employed.

18. Prevention, recognition, and management of systemic complications of moderate sedation, with particular attention to airway maintenance and support of the respiratory and cardiovascular systems.

C. Moderate Sedation Course Duration and Documentation: The Course must include:

- A minimum of 60 hours of instruction plus administration of sedation for at least 20 individually managed patients.
- Certification of competence in moderate sedation technique(s).
- Certification of competence in rescuing patients from a deeper level of sedation than intended, including managing the airway, intravascular or intraosseous access, and reversal medications.
- Provision by course director or faculty of additional clinical experience if participant competency has not been achieved in time allotted.
- Records of instruction and clinical experiences (i.e., number of patients managed by each participant in each modality/route) that are maintained and available for participant review.

D. Documentation of Instruction: The course director must certify the competency of participants upon satisfactory completion of training in each moderate sedation technique, including instruction, clinical experience, managing the airway, intravascular/intraosseous access, and reversal medications.

E. Faculty: The course should be directed by a dentist or physician qualified by experience and training. This individual should possess a current permit or license to administer moderate or deep sedation and general anesthesia in at least one state, have had at least 3 years of experience, including formal postdoctoral training in anxiety and pain control. Dental faculty with broad clinical experience in the particular aspect of the subject under consideration should participate. In addition, the participation of highly qualified individuals in related fields, such as anesthesiologists, pharmacologists, internists, cardiologists, and psychologists, should be encouraged.

A participant-faculty ratio of not more than four-to-one when moderate sedation is being taught allows for adequate supervision during the clinical phase of instruction. A one-to-one ratio is recommended during the early stage of participation.

The faculty should provide a mechanism whereby the participant can evaluate the performance of those individuals who present the course material.

F. **Facilities**: Competency courses in moderate sedation must be presented where adequate facilities are available for proper patient care, including drugs and equipment for the management of emergencies. These facilities may include dental and medical schools/offices, hospitals, and surgical centers.

Several specialty groups within dentistry have developed guidelines for their members presenting standards for the use of minimum moderate and deep sedation. These groups include oral and maxillofacial surgery[6,7] and pediatric dentistry.[8,9] The American Academy of Periodontology had published sedation guidelines,[10] although they were rescinded in 2013.[11]

Until the early 1980s, this author presented a continuing education program in basic IV moderate sedation that was 5 days in length (35 hours). The success of this course was apparent because more than 75% of dentists participating in the program continued to use IV moderate sedation in their practices 1 year after the program.[12,13] In a survey of these dentists, it was determined that in no instance did any dentist encounter a serious emergency situation related to the administration of IV medications.[12]

However, because of a number of well-publicized unfortunate occurrences (usually involving dentists who had received little or, more commonly, no formal training in parenteral sedation or general anesthesia), it became evident that the length and depth of training in these valuable techniques had to be increased so as to enhance patient safety. As of December 2008, all 50 states had adopted legislation or regulations that govern the administration of parenteral sedation.[14] In addition, at least three provinces (British Columbia, Alberta, and Ontario in Canada, which has 10 provinces and 3 territories) have enacted similar regulations.[15]

In some extreme instances, a dentist must complete a dental residency in anesthesiology to be eligible to administer IV moderate sedation. Other, more realistic states and provinces have established less restrictive requirements based on the educational and clinical background of the dentist.

The 1- to 2-day short course in IV moderate sedation is a relic of the past. They served only to scare the dentist away from this technique or to create a potentially very dangerous person: a dentist who thought he or she knew how to properly administer IV drugs. Training programs at all levels of education—doctoral (dental school), postdoctoral (residency programs), and continuing education—have been expanded to meet the growing needs of the dental profession and the dental patient.[3,4]

The basic intravenous sedation program offered through the Oregon Academy of General Dentistry and the Oregon Health Sciences University School of Dentistry serves as an example of an outstanding program.[16] The course meets or exceeds the ADA's Guidelines for the Use of Sedation and General Anesthesia by Dentists. It is a 103-hour course and includes a total of 60 hours of didactic education and 43 hours of clinical education. Doctors are required to be accompanied by two dental assistants, so that the IV "team" is trained together. In excess of 10,000 cases have been completed to date (January 2017) with no serious complications.

REFERENCES

1. American Dental Association, Council on Dental Education: Guidelines for teaching the comprehensive control of pain and anxiety in dentistry. *J Dent Educ* 36:62, 1972.
2. American Dental Society of Anesthesiology: Guidelines for the teaching of pain and anxiety control and management of related complications in a continuing education program, part III. *Anesth Prog* 26:51, 1979.
3. American Dental Association, Council on Dental Education: *Guidelines for the Use of Sedation and General Anesthesia by Dentists*, Oct. 2016 ADA House of Delegates. Chicago, 2016, The Association.
4. American Dental Association, Council on Dental Education: *Guidelines for teaching pain control and sedation in dentists and dental students*, Oct. 2016 ADA House of Delegates. Chicago, 2016, The Association.
5. American Society of Anesthesiologists Task Force on Sedation and Analgesia by Non-Anesthesiologists: Practice guidelines for sedation and analgesia by non-anesthesiologists. *Anesthesiology* 96:1004–1017, 2002.
6. American Association of Oral and Maxillofacial Surgeons, Committee on Anesthesia: *Office anesthesia evaluation manual*, ed 8, Rosemont, IL, 2012, The Association.
7. Sims PG, Kates CH, Moyer DJ, et al: Parameters of care: clinical practice guidelines for oral and maxillofacial surgery (AAOMS ParCare 2012). Anesthesia in outpatient facilities. *J Oral Maxillofac Surg* 70(11):e31–e49, 2012.
8. American Academy of Pediatrics and American Academy of Pediatric Dentistry, Cote CJ, Wilson S, Work Group on Sedation: Guidelines for monitoring and management of pediatric patients during and after sedation for diagnostic and therapeutic procedures. *Pediatrics* 118(6):2587–2602, 2008.
9. American Academy of Pediatrics and American Academy of Pediatric Dentistry: Guideline for monitoring and management of pediatric patients during and after sedation for diagnostic and therapeutic procedures. *Pediatr Dent* 30(7 Suppl):143–159, 2008.
10. Committee on Research, Science and Therapy, the American Academy of Periodontology: Guidelines: In-office use of conscious sedation in periodontics. *J Periodontol* 72(7):968–975, 2001.
11. Clarification/Erratum: Guidelines: in-office use of conscious sedation in periodontics. *J Periodontol* 84(4):566, 2013.
12. Malamed SF: Continuing education in intravenous sedation: part 2, complications and non-use. *Anesth Prog* 28(6):158–160, 1981.
13. Malamed SF: Continuing education in intravenous sedation: survey of 188 dentists. *Anesth Prog* 28(2):33–36, 1981.
14. American Dental Association: Department of State and Government Affairs, 30b. Conscious sedation permit requirement. September 2, 2009, The Association. Chicago, IL. http://www.ada.org/~/media/ADA/Advocacy/Files/anesthesia_sedation_permit.ashx. (Accessed 30 March 2016).
15. Dr Mel Hawkins, personal communication, April 2016.
16. Oregon Academy of General Dentistry, Oregon Health Sciences University School of Dentistry. www.learnivsedation.com. (Accessed 9 January 2017).

Section VI

GENERAL ANESTHESIA

Chapter 30: Fundamentals of General Anesthesia

Chapter 31: Armamentarium, Drugs, and Techniques

General anesthesia has been an important aspect of dentistry since 1844, when Horace Wells first administered nitrous oxide (N_2O) to induce the loss of consciousness. (In fact, Dr. Wells was the recipient [the patient], not the administrator of the N_2O.) General anesthesia was, for many years, an integral part of the pain-control armamentarium of dentists, primarily because other techniques of pain control did not exist or were less well developed. With the introduction of local anesthetics (cocaine) in the 1880s and their steady improvement in the 1900s with the introduction of procaine and tetracaine and later of the amides (e.g., lidocaine, mepivacaine) in the 1940s, the need for general anesthesia as a primary means of achieving pain control during dental treatment diminished. A second need for general anesthesia was in the management of dental fears and anxieties. For well more than 100 years, general anesthesia was the primary technique used for this purpose. However, with the development of newer drugs capable of relieving anxiety without inducing the loss of consciousness, our ability to manage dental fears through minimal or moderate sedation techniques increased dramatically, further diminishing the role of general anesthesia in the practice of dentistry.

Despite the decreased reliance placed on general anesthesia in contemporary dentistry, several significant indications for its use remain. These are discussed in Chapter 30. The dental profession has been a leader in the development of general anesthesia, from the early days of Horace Wells and William T.G. Morton, to the more recent advances in the field of outpatient general anesthesia.

I have taken the liberty of categorizing general anesthesia into the following three groups:

1. Outpatient general anesthesia using intravenous (IV) agents
2. Outpatient general anesthesia using conventional general anesthetic agents
3. Inpatient general anesthesia

As becomes clear later in this section, the techniques of general anesthesia are not amenable to teaching in a short course. Extensive training must be obtained by the dentist who contemplates using general anesthesia in his or her practice. The ability to render patients unconscious, safely maintain them in that state during dental treatment, and then return them to their preanesthetic state of functioning requires at least 3 years of full-time training in an anesthesiology residency or its equivalent during an oral and maxillofacial surgery residency program. In addition to the 3 years of training, it is increasingly commonplace for individual state boards of dental examiners to require the dentist to obtain a special license or permit before he or she is allowed to use general anesthesia. As of April 2016, the American Dental Association was aware of 50 states requiring licensure or permits to administer general anesthesia.[1]

Many excellent textbooks are available on the subject of general anesthesia. These books should be consulted by the dentist who is interested in this technique. In the two chapters comprising this section,

Dr. Jason Brady, a dentist anesthesiologist, discusses the indications for general anesthesia in dentistry and some of the drugs and techniques that are currently in use. General anesthesia does indeed form a very valuable technique for the spectrum of pain and anxiety control in both dentistry and medicine.

The primary goals of general anesthesia are to maintain the health and safety of the patient while providing amnesia, hypnosis (lack of awareness), analgesia, and optimal surgical conditions (e.g., immobility).[2]

REFERENCES

1. Department of State Government Affairs: #30a, Statutory requirements for general anesthesia and deep sedation. American Dental Association, Chicago, http://www.ada.org/en/~/media/ADA/Advocacy/Files/anesthesia_general_permit. (Accessed 1 February 2017).
2. Forman SA, Yang RPH: Administration of general anesthesia. In Dunn PF, editor, *Clinical anesthesia procedures of the Massachusetts General Hospital*, ed 7, 2007, Lippincott Williams & Wilkins.

chapter 30

Fundamentals of General Anesthesia

CHAPTER OUTLINE

General anesthesia has been defined as a reversible depression of the higher centers of the central nervous system (CNS) that makes the patient unconscious and insensible to pain.[1] Ideally, general anesthesia represents the simultaneous presence of analgesia (loss of pain), amnesia (loss of memory), and hypnosis, along with reflex inhibition and loss of skeletal muscle tone, which allows for safe surgical procedures.[2]

The techniques of minimal, moderate, and deep sedation have helped patients tremendously; however, there are patients for whom these techniques do not provide adequate sedation for the required treatment. General anesthesia proves to be a much more effective means of successfully completing the planned treatment.

TYPES OF GENERAL ANESTHESIA USED IN DENTISTRY

There are several recognized forms of general anesthesia in dentistry. The most frequent use of general anesthesia is within the specialty of oral and maxillofacial surgery (OMFS). This technique usually falls on the spectrum between deep sedation

and general anesthesia; in many cases the provider can elicit a purposeful response following repeated or painful stimulation. It has many of the same effects as full general anesthesia, as airway intervention may be required and the patient's spontaneous ventilation may be inadequate.[3] The oral maxillofacial surgery patient is usually maintained in the Guedel stage I or stage III of anesthesia (Box 30.1). The oral and maxillofacial surgeon has been responsible, in large part, for the development of outpatient and ambulatory general anesthesia.

The most rapidly growing form of general anesthesia in dentistry involves utilization of a *dentist anesthesiologist in the dental office*. A dentist anesthesiologist is a dentist trained in anesthesia who performs office-based anesthesia for all types of dental specialties and patients. The dentist must have completed clinical anesthesia training in a residency program and hold a valid general anesthesia permit from the state or province in which he or she works. In this form of dental anesthesia, the patient undergoes similar general anesthetic preparation and procedure as does the hospitalized inpatient. Because of the nature of the office-based dental or surgical procedure to be completed, this form of general anesthesia is usually limited to American Society of Anesthesiologists (ASA) 1, ASA 2, and select ASA 3 patients. In addition to an anesthesia residency–trained dentist anesthesiologist, the person administering the anesthesia may be a physician anesthesiologist or, in some states, a certified registered nurse anesthetist (CRNA). Similar procedures may also be executed in an outpatient surgical center. The dentist performing the dental treatment should be familiar with the level of anesthesia being provided but does not need to be trained in anesthesia, as the anesthesiologist is responsible for the administration of the anesthetic for the planned procedure. The corollary for this in the hospital setting is that the surgeon is in charge of the surgery and is not trained in the provision of anesthesia.

A third type of general anesthesia available to the dental patient is the more traditional *inpatient general anesthesia,* in which the patient is admitted into the hospital, anesthesia is induced by an anesthesiologist, and the dental procedure is completed by the dentist. The patient remains in the hospital for monitoring after the procedure in the postoperative anesthesia care unit. Due to rising hospital costs and other factors, this form of anesthesia is waning in popularity and is usually reserved for the more severely medically compromised patient, or in areas where office-based or surgery center anesthesia is not available.

Each of these types of general anesthesia is described in Chapter 31.

ADVANTAGES

There are many advantages to treating dental patients under general anesthesia as opposed to other forms of sedation:

- *The patient is unconscious.* For many patients, dental care may be impossible to tolerate, or the quality of care significantly compromised, if attempted while conscious. An unconscious patient allows the dentist to perform all necessary treatment without concern for movement, cooperation, or anxiety. Many dentists also find that they can complete treatment much more efficiently on an unconscious patient without these concerns being present and without the need for direct dentist–patient communication or patient-requested breaks.

Box 30.1	Guedel Classification

Four stages of anesthesia are described.

Guedel based his observations on the following parameters:
1. Character of the respirations
2. Eyeball activity
3. Pupillary changes
4. Eyelid reflex (presence or absence)
5. Swallowing or vomiting

I. Stage of Analgesia
The first stage of anesthesia starts with the initial administration of a CNS-depressant drug and continues to the loss of consciousness.
1. Respiration is normal.
2. Eye movements are normal, with voluntary movement possible.
3. Protective reflexes are intact.
4. Amnesia (the lack of recall) may or may not be present.

II. Stage of Delirium
Stage II begins with the loss of consciousness and progresses until entry into the stage of surgical anesthesia (stage III).
1. Respirations are irregular early in stage II, but become more regular as stage II deepens.
2. Eyeballs oscillate involuntarily, a movement termed *lateral nystagmus.*
3. Pupils react to light normally.
4. Skeletal muscle tonus is increased, with muscular rigidity present in some patients early in stage II. Muscle tonus decreases as stage II deepens.
5. The laryngeal and pharyngeal reflexes (swallowing and laryngeal closure) are still quite active early in stage II, but become progressively more obtunded as stage II progresses.

III. Stage of Surgical Anesthesia
Entry into stage III is marked by several signs:
1. The respiratory irregularity observed in stage II disappears. Respiration is automatic and involuntary, responding to the level of CO_2 within the blood.
2. Muscular tonus is lost, unlike the increased muscular tonus seen in stage II. The patient's head may now be moved from side to side, and the mouth may be opened with ease.
3. Swallowing and reflex respiratory arrest will not occur if the anesthesiologist suddenly increases the concentration of an inhalational anesthetic. Both of these responses will occur in stage II.

Most surgical procedures are performed at this level of CNS depression when the intercostal muscles weaken and thoracic respiration becomes decreased.

IV. Stage of Respiratory Paralysis
Stage IV begins with the onset of respiratory arrest and ends with the cessation of effective circulation (cardiac arrest).

Box 30.1   Guedel Classification—cont'd

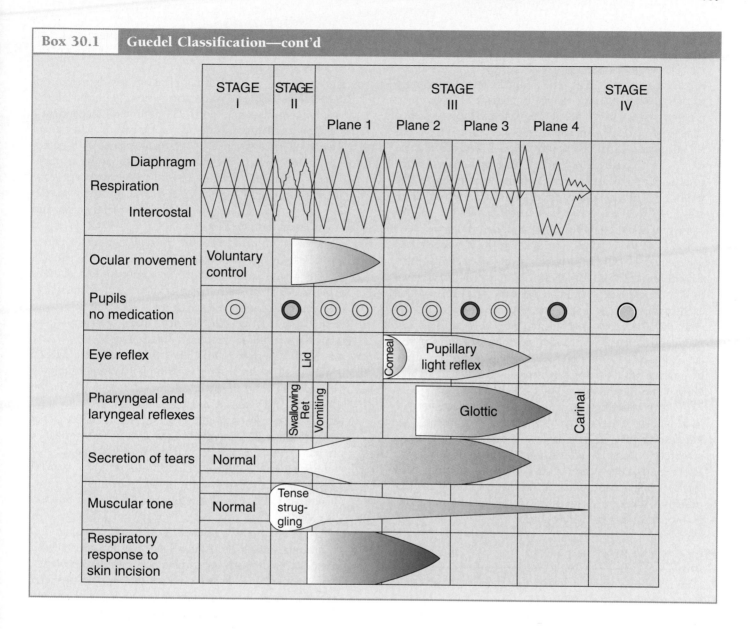

- *General anesthesia, in many cases, is the only technique that will prove successful for certain patients.* Patients who are unable to understand what is occurring, including young children and patients with special needs such as autism or Down syndrome, are often unable to receive treatment without the use of general anesthesia. Likewise, particular manifestations of physical disabilities such as seizure disorders, tremors from Parkinson disease, or involuntary clenching from cerebral palsy can render a patient incapable of receiving dental treatment without general anesthesia.

- *The patient does not respond to pain the same way as the conscious patient.* Although most general anesthetics possess either minimal or no analgesic properties, the level of depression of the patient's CNS in general anesthesia prevents visible response (e.g., movement, phonation) by the patient to the nociceptive stimuli reaching the brain. There will be variation in this response depending on the level of CNS depression.

Technically, there is no need for the administration of local anesthetics during some surgical procedures, including dentistry, performed under general anesthesia. However, it is strongly recommended that local anesthetics be administered during general anesthesia to prevent painful stimuli from ever reaching the brain. In this way, the concentrations or volumes of general anesthetic drugs required to maintain a smooth, even level of general anesthesia will be decreased, thereby minimizing the occurrence of dose-related complications from the anesthetic drugs. Through the administration of local anesthesia, response to painful procedures is prevented, both during the operative procedure and, equally important, into the postoperative period.

- *Patients experience amnesia.* With loss of consciousness, a total loss of memory of the procedure occurs. For extremely dental-phobic patients this can be a major indication for the use of general anesthesia. Recall during general anesthesia procedures is extremely rare and is estimated to occur at a rate of 1 in 1000 patients.[4]

- *Patient cooperation is not absolutely necessary for the success of general anesthesia.* One of the disadvantages of all sedative techniques is that some degree of patient cooperation is necessary for the administered drug(s) to produce the desired clinical effect; uncooperative patients can refuse intravenous (IV) drug administration with excessive movement, avoid inhalational anesthetic via mouth breathing or nasal hood placement refusal, and refuse to swallow oral sedatives. The use of physical restraint is not required with general anesthesia. When loss of consciousness is the goal, patient cooperation, although desirable, is not essential.

- *General anesthesia has a success rate of 100% when the end point of titration of a CNS depressant is the loss of consciousness.* General anesthesia is the highest level of patient management technique obtainable. Minimal, moderate, and deep sedation each require a balancing of the patient's needs versus the risks of either undermedicating (i.e., undersedation) or overmedicating (i.e., oversedation). Loss of consciousness is the desired titration point with general anesthesia. CNS-depressant drug(s) will be administered until the desired clinical effect, loss of consciousness, is achieved.

- *The onset of action of general anesthesia is usually quite rapid.* In general anesthesia, drugs are administered by the IV or inhalation routes, the two routes with the most rapid onset of action. In most situations, loss of consciousness can be achieved in under a minute. In contrast, titration in other levels of sedation depends on the patient's response. The process is longer and can take up to 10 minutes or more, and sometimes is not achievable at all.

DISADVANTAGES

General anesthesia has the following limitations and disadvantages as well:

- *The patient is unconscious.* Mentioned earlier in the list of advantages, unconsciousness must also be listed as a disadvantage because of the many physiologic changes that may occur. When the CNS is depressed to the extent that consciousness is lost, changes take place in the physiology of the patient that would be life threatening in the absence of a "guardian" trained in the management of the unconscious patient. An unconscious patient is completely reliant on the anesthetist's ability to ensure his safety and survival.[5]

- *Protective reflexes are depressed or absent.* Loss of consciousness is accompanied by a progressive depression of the CNS and protective reflexes. General anesthesia has been described as a hypnosis accompanied by the loss of protective laryngeal reflexes (i.e., coughing).[2] Because the dentist is operating in the oral cavity, the potential for debris, water, saliva, or blood to enter the airway and produce airway obstruction or laryngospasm is greater in dental cases than with most other surgical procedures. The potential is high for partial or complete airway obstruction, with the patient unable to

clear the tracheobronchial tree. One of the most important tasks of the anesthesiologist is to ensure the integrity of the patient's airway.

- *Vital signs are depressed.* It is normal to see depression of the cardiovascular and respiratory systems with the administration of general anesthesia. The ability to independently maintain ventilatory function is often impaired. The patient often requires assistance in the maintenance of a patent airway, and positive-pressure ventilation may be required because of respiratory depression or drug-induced depression of neuromuscular function. CNS depression can also lead to hypoxia, hypercapnia, blood gas and pH changes, and cardiovascular depression

- *Intraoperative complications are more likely to occur during general anesthesia than during sedation.* Because the patient's physiology has been altered by the administration of CNS-depressant drugs to a greater degree during general anesthesia than during sedation, complications such as hypotension, tachycardia, bradycardia, dysrhythmias, and respiratory depression are more frequently encountered.[6]

- *Advanced training is required.* In no other technique discussed in this book is the requirement for postgraduate training as important (or as difficult to obtain) as it is for general anesthesia. The physician or dentist who wishes to administer general anesthesia must complete a minimum of 3 years of clinical anesthesia training in a formal anesthesia residency program.[7] Some state requirements mandate that all staff members participating in the administration of general anesthesia must also have received thorough training, including current training in Advanced Cardiac Life Support (ACLS).

- *An "anesthesia team" is required.* For the administration of general anesthesia in a dental office, there must be an anesthesia team, consisting minimally of the anesthesiologist, an assistant, and the dentist. In addition to the dentist and anesthesiologist, it is important to have other staff present: a surgical assistant, anesthesia assistant, and circulating assistant are often utilized in an anesthesia team. The anesthesia team needs to be capable of responding to an emergency. The anesthesia team should have ACLS training, and each team member must know the locations of emergency drugs and equipment and be capable of assisting in emergencies. Teams must be well versed in emergency management and should practice emergency scenarios routinely.

- *Special equipment is required whenever general anesthesia is administered.* Continuous monitoring of the unconscious anesthetized patient is of far greater importance than it is for those who are sedated because of the profound physiological effects caused by the anesthetic drugs. The absence of the ability to communicate with the patient also presents a greater need for patient monitoring. In addition to monitoring equipment, other equipment and drugs are required for the administration of general anesthesia. Examples of additional equipment include a laryngoscope, endotracheal tubes, anesthetic gas circuits, and oropharyngeal and nasopharyngeal airways. It is also necessary to have readily available emergency equipment such as a defibrillator, emergency (ACLS) medications, and equipment needed to rescue and resuscitate a patient.

- *A recovery area must be available for the patient.* Following general anesthesia of any duration or depth, an area must be available in which the patient may remain until he or she exhibits respiratory and cardiovascular stability and appropriate discharge criteria have been met. This area must be equipped with oxygen (O_2) and a suction apparatus. The patient must be monitored continually by a staff member experienced in recovery care while the anesthesiologist is present.[8]

- *A more detailed preoperative patient examination is necessary before performing general anesthesia.* An adequate medical history and thorough physical examination of the patient are absolutely necessary. In some cases, a medical consult with their primary physician or specialist is needed before proceeding with treatment. Complete records showing electrocardiograph reports, blood pressure reports, and pulse oximeter readings must be maintained.

- *The patient receiving general anesthesia must be nil per os (NPO) for 8 hours before the procedure,* meaning nothing to eat or drink. There are variations to specific food and beverage items on the ASA guidelines.[9] These guidelines are important, as food or liquid in the stomach can lead to the extremely dangerous occurrence of regurgitation during anesthesia induction, during the procedure, or upon emergence with the possibility of airway obstruction or aspiration of the vomitus leading to tracheal burning and/or infection of the lung.[10] This risk is negligible during most light sedation procedures.

INDICATIONS

The use of general anesthesia is commonly indicated for several different patient populations:

- *Patients with extreme anxiety and fear.* Many fearful patients can effectively receive treatment under sedation; however, in approximately 3% of such patients, general anesthesia is the only technique that will be successful.[10] In less extreme cases of anxiety and fear, many dentists first opt to try lesser levels of sedation and resort to general anesthesia as an option only if other levels of sedation are ineffective.

- *Adults or children with mental disabilities, dementia, or disoriented patients.* The use of sedation in special needs patients may not be effective, in which case general anesthesia is indicated. This patient population often requires many forms of dental treatment due to dental hygiene issues and lack of prior dental care. This frequently necessitates an extended appointment, for which general anesthesia can prove to be extremely beneficial. This patient demographic is also often unable to understand the necessary treatment and unable to cooperate with routine dental treatment. Patients with

mental disabilities such as Alzheimer disease, dementia, autism, mental retardation, attention deficit hyperactivity disorder (ADHD), and sensory processing disorders can be easily upset by unfamiliar dental treatment. Dentists find that they can complete treatment much more successfully through the use of general anesthesia.

- *Adults or children with physical disabilities.* The patient who is physically compromised, such as with neuromuscular disorders in which the patient makes involuntary movements such as Parkinson disease, cerebral palsy, and certain seizure disorders, can make delivery of dental care difficult and potentially dangerous. General anesthesia arrests these involuntary movements, allowing the dentist to complete treatment more easily. General anesthesia can also be helpful in patients who suffer from a severe gag reflex and are unable to receive adequate dental care as a result.

- *Infants and children.* General anesthesia is indicated in healthy children who are unable to cooperate for office procedures after the standard management armamentarium has been exhausted.[11] The techniques of minimal and moderate sedation may be of little utility in the very young patient primarily because of the patient's inability to cooperate (the 'precooperative' patient). Without anesthesia, extensive treatment plans for children with rampant decay typically take 2 to 4 appointments, with behavioral challenges predictably increasing with each appointment. Failed appointments due to behavior management leave the child with an incomplete treatment plan. When the patient is very young, general anesthesia will be of benefit to both the patient and the dental staff. Many treatment plans can be completed in a single appointment. The trauma involved in dental care is minimized with a properly performed general anesthetic. Dental care may be carried out in a calmer and more controlled environment, more expeditiously, and with the patient's safety ensured by the anesthesiologist. Treatment under general anesthesia has better outcomes, and the need for retreatment is lower than for sedation patients.[12] A positive dental experience ensures that the child will willingly return for regular checkups and examinations, leading to better overall oral health.[12]

- *Traumatic procedures.* Many patients who are not normally fearful of dental procedures elect to undergo general anesthesia when the procedure is traumatic in nature. Third molar extractions and full mouth extractions for dentures are often relatively short procedures, but the amount of pain experienced (either real or imagined) by the patient necessitates general anesthesia.[13] Endodontic procedures are often perceived to be painful, and thus many patients elect general anesthesia to lessen trauma.

- *Prolonged procedures.* General anesthesia is often a viable option for procedures of one or more hours. Many dentists prefer this method to the alternative of breaking the procedure up into multiple appointments, as it is more efficient for both dentist and patient to complete the entire treatment plan in a single appointment. However, the maximum duration that most anesthesiologists will allow a patient to remain under general anesthesia is about 4 to 5 hours, as longer procedures under general anesthesia can negatively affect renal function and blood pressure.[14] The rate of anesthesia-related complications directly increases as the length of procedure under general anesthesia increases.[15–18] Longer procedures are usually broken up into multiple appointments, or general anesthesia is used only for the traumatic portion of the treatment and the patient is awakened for less distressing procedures such as laboratory work following implants.

CONTRAINDICATIONS

The anesthesia provider should perform a risk analysis for each patient before performing general anesthesia. Every medical disability needs to be evaluated on a case-by-case basis for the physiologic effects of undergoing general anesthesia. General anesthesia should never be performed in conditions of uncertainty or beyond the provider's comfort level. The following are contraindications to the administration of general anesthesia for dental treatment in an outpatient facility:

- *ASA 4 and many ASA 3 patients.* Office-based general anesthesia performed in the dental office is generally contraindicated in ASA 4 and many ASA 3 medically compromised patients. It is recommended that these patients be admitted to the hospital to receive dental treatment under general anesthesia. The depression of vital signs caused by general anesthesia can be especially harmful to this patient population. The severely medically compromised patient will benefit from a more thorough preoperative evaluation when hospitalized before the start of treatment and from the more immediate availability of medical consultation and emergency care should the occasion arise. This patient can remain in the hospital following the procedure for more intensive postanesthetic care. Medically compromised patients should be readily identified during the routine medical history and physical examination performed in the dental office.
- *Patients with a history of poliomyelitis in whom the chest muscles have been involved.* Many postpolio patients are at increased risk of complications, especially dysphagia and respiratory muscle weakness.
- *Patients with a history of myasthenia gravis.* It is common for myasthenic patients to develop weakness in both their respiratory muscles and their muscles controlling swallowing, increasing their risk of aspiration.
- *Patients with significantly decreased cardiac and/or pulmonary reserve.* General anesthesia is commonly contraindicated in this patient population, as they are more sensitive to the depressant effects caused by the anesthetic.
- *Morbidly obese patients.* Many obese patients are able to undergo anesthesia without complication. However, certain obese patients, especially those with short, thick necks, will provide difficulty with airway maintenance. Obese patients are also at increased risk of hypoxemia.

- *Patients with a history of malignant hyperthermia (hyperpyrexia).* The onset of anesthetic-induced malignant hyperthermia is life threatening if not treated immediately, so further elective general anesthesia is not generally indicated for this patient demographic.

BENEFITS OF OUTPATIENT VS. INPATIENT GENERAL ANESTHESIA

The use of office-based general anesthesia has grown rapidly in the past few decades, largely in part due to the following benefits.

Quality

The quality and level of care of general anesthesia in an office setting are on par with a hospital operating room or surgery center. Standardized equipment, drugs, and emergency kits are utilized. Providers use their own personalized anesthesia setup and are familiar with the equipment, providing the patient with a practice similar to what they would experience in a hospital. The complication rates of office-based general anesthesia are low and rarely result in serious complications, as patients are typically healthy and receiving routine anesthetic care.

Cost

The cost of outpatient anesthesia is significantly lower than an identical procedure performed in a hospital.[10] A time and cost analysis of office-based general anesthesia compared with in-hospital general anesthesia found that the hospital procedure cost 13.2 times more than the same procedure performed in the office. After adjusting for confounders, the savings to the office-based patient was $5471.[19] A second study found that children with special needs saved an average of $4849 by receiving their general anesthesia in the dental office.[20]

Psychological Benefits

The major psychological benefit of outpatient vs. inpatient treatment is in the field of pediatric and special needs dentistry, in which much of the anxiety associated with the treatment can be greatly reduced by avoiding the hospital. In most cases, the patient is already familiar with the dental office setting and is more comfortable with the familiar location and staff. Inpatient procedures often require separation from parents, whereas in many outpatient general anesthesia procedures the parent is able to remain in the presence of the child until they are under anesthesia.

Reduced Exposure to Nosocomial Infections

A patient in a hospital has a significantly increased risk of developing secondary medical problems, such as infection with methicillin-resistant *Staphylococcus aureus* (MRSA).[21] It has been stated that outpatient general anesthesia in pediatrics results in a decreased incidence of infection because the patient has reduced exposure to health professionals, hospital wards, and their associated pathogens.[15] In most dental office situations, a healthy patient is exposed to a healthy environment with no cross-exposure to superbugs.

Time

The amount of time spent on each step of the procedure was found to be shorter in the office-based procedure than the identical hospital procedure in a time and cost analysis. The mean preop time in the hospital was four times longer than preop in the office-based procedure, with the mean recovery time being up to ten times longer.

Availability

Hospital slots for dental procedures are not always readily available, and many have long wait times, while the patient's dental needs may be urgent. Most dentists are able to schedule the office-based anesthesia procedure during their regular office hours. Many dental offices schedule their anesthesiologist ahead of time and fill patients into those days as needed.

Parental Preference

In surveys of the parents of pediatric patients, the overwhelming majority indicate their preference for outpatient general anesthetic procedures over inpatient procedures.[10]

Dentist Preference

Most dentists prefer having their patients undergo general anesthesia in their own dental office as opposed to in a hospital. In their own office they are able to provide treatment in the location and environment that they are accustomed to, with all their own equipment, materials, and supplies readily available. Many hospitals are not adequately equipped for dental care.

SAFETY

In order for general anesthesia to be administered safely, it is absolutely necessary for certain conditions to be met. First, and arguably the most important, the dentist anesthesiologist must be adequately educated and trained with a 3-year residency in anesthesia and hold a valid state or provincial anesthesia permit. The office staff must also be trained in cardiopulmonary resuscitation (CPR) and emergency preparedness. The procedure must be performed using adequate facilities and using adequate equipment. Under absolutely no circumstances should general anesthesia be administered in the absence of any one of these four vital ingredients.

The mortality rate associated with the operating room type of general anesthesia in ASA 1 and ASA 2 outpatients, administered by qualified persons, is equal to that for hospital inpatients.[10] In healthy ASA 1 patients, the mortality rate has been shown to be 1 death in 593,000 cases,[22] where the general anesthetic was judged to be solely responsible for the death. In cases with ASA 2, 3, and 4 patients in which there was both an anesthesia complication and an underlying disease,

mortality rate was 1 in 148,000 cases. The incidence of hospital admissions as a complication of outpatient general anesthesia is less than 5%[15,23] The rate of complication increases with the duration of general anesthesia; thus the recommendation that the duration of outpatient general anesthesia not exceed 4 hours.[15]

The U.S. Food and Drug Administration (FDA) issued a warning in December 2016 that exposure to general anesthetic and sedation in children younger than 3 years of age or in pregnant women may affect children's brain development. Studies conducted on the use of general anesthetic and sedation in pregnant and young animals show loss of nerve cells resulting in long-term effects on behavior and learning. Some studies on children support these findings; however, all the children in the studies had limitations, and it is unclear whether the negative effects were due to the prolonged exposure to anesthesia or the underlying medical condition that necessitated the surgery. Further research is needed to determine if anesthetic exposure effects children's brain development.[24]

SPECIAL CONSIDERATIONS FOR DENTISTRY

Although widely considered "minor" compared with other forms of surgery such as cardiac and neurosurgery, the administration of general anesthesia for dental procedures is actually more difficult in many ways. The oral cavity is the treatment zone used by the dental provider; thus the potential for airway complications is increased. Familiarity with the peculiar requirements of this combination of surgery and anesthesia serves to increase patient safety.[25]

EDUCATION IN DENTAL ANESTHESIA

In no other area of patient management is thorough educational and clinical experience as important as in the administration of general anesthesia. Unlike most techniques of sedation, it is impossible to teach general anesthesia in short courses. Education in general anesthesia requires no fewer than 3 years of full-time training of the dentist in an accredited anesthesiology residency or its equivalent during OMFS residencies (Box 30.2).[6] General anesthesia must never be taken lightly. The dentist who is considering the use of this valuable but potentially dangerous technique should explore the means of achieving at least 3 full years of residency training in general anesthesia.

Guidelines Relative to the Establishment of a Dental Residency in Anesthesiology

In 1979 the American Dental Society of Anesthesiology (ADSA) established and approved training guidelines.[26] Modern dental anesthesiology residency programs follow the Accreditation Standards for Advanced General Dentistry Education Programs in Dental Anesthesiology from the Commission on Dental Accreditation (CODA).[6]

| Box 30.2 | Accredited Dental Anesthesiology Residency Programs |

University of Pittsburgh Medical Center
School of Dental Medicine
Department of Dental Anesthesiology
G-89 Salk Hall
Pittsburgh, PA 15261
Three Year Program
Michael Cuddy, DMD
Residency Program Director

The Ohio State University Medical Center
Section of Dental Anesthesiology
305 West 12th Avenue
Columbus, OH 43210–1267
Three Year Program
Simon Prior, BDS, PhD, MS
Residency Program Director

University of California, Los Angeles
School of Dentistry
Section of Dental Anesthesiology
Center for Health Sciences
Los Angeles, CA 90095
Three Year Program
Christine L. Quinn, DDS, MS
Residency Program Director

University of Toronto
Faculty of Dentistry
Department of Anesthesia
124 Edward Street
Toronto, Ontario, Canada M5G 1G6
Three Year Master's Degree Program
Carilynne Yarascavich, DDS, MSc
Residency Program Director

Loma Linda University
School of Dentistry
Department of Dental Anesthesiology
Loma Linda, CA 92350
Three Year Program
Dezireh Sevanesian, DDS
Residency Program Director

Stony Brook University Medical Center
Department of Anesthesiology
Division of Dental Anesthesiology
Stony Brook School of Dental Medicine
1104 Sullivan Hall
Stony Brook, NY 11994–8700
Three Year Program
Ralph Epstein, DDS
Residency Program Director

NYC Lutheran Medical Center
Department of Dental Medicine
5800 3rd Avenue
Brooklyn, NY 11220
Three Year Program
Charles Azzaretti, DDS
Residency Program Director

Jacobi Medical Center
Department of Dentistry/OMFS
1400 Pelham Parkway South
Bldg 5, Room 3C15
Bronx, NY 10461
Three Year Program
Barry Langsam, DDS
Residency Program Director

St. Barnabas Hospital
Department of Dentistry
Third Avenue & 183rd Street
Bronx, New York 10457
Three Year Program
Berry Stahl, DMD
Residency Program Director

Wyckoff Heights Medical Center
Department of Dentistry
Division of Dental Anesthesiology
374 Stockholm St.
Brooklyn, NY 11237
Three Year Program
Robert Peskin, DDS
Residency Program Director

All programs listed are CODA credited.
From American Society of Dentist Anesthesiologists. July 2016, http://asdahq.org/schools. Accessed October 24, 2016.

STATE REGULATIONS

Although general anesthesia regulations vary by state or province, many states have proposed regulations limiting the administration of general anesthesia to dentists who meet one or both of the following criteria: (1) a licensed dentist who has completed a residency program in anesthesiology of no fewer than three calendar years that is approved by the CODA or (2) a licensed dentist who has completed a graduate program in OMFS that has been approved by the CODA.

Regulations were passed in 2016 mandating that all dental anesthesia residency programs be a minimum of 3 years. Before this, there were several programs of a minimum of 2 years in length, and in earlier years it was only necessary to have 1 year of training. From this point forward any dentist except OMFS who wishes to perform general anesthesia must complete 3 full years of clinical anesthesia residency training.

Before administering general anesthesia, a dentist must possess a valid anesthesia permit issued by the appropriate state or provincial dental board. In order to obtain a general anesthesia permit, the dentist must hold a valid license to practice dentistry in the state and a current permit to prescribe and administer controlled substances in the state, issued by the U.S. Drug Enforcement Administration. Most states also require that the dentist have a valid (completed within the 2 years before submitting the application) ACLS and/or Pediatric Advanced Life Support (PALS) certificate.

Most states require that the applicant provide proof that they hold all necessary equipment and drugs for administering anesthesia, performing adequate monitoring, and managing emergency situations. The dentist must also provide the credentials of their auxiliary staff, as some states require that anyone involved in the administration of general anesthesia be trained in Basic Life Support and/or ACLS.

Many states require an onsite evaluation of the applicant and an inspection of a single office where general anesthesia will be performed, with some states requiring the inspection take place at every individual office location.

ASSOCIATIONS

The American Society of Dentist Anesthesiologists (ASDA) is composed of dentists who have completed residency training in anesthesiology. The ADSA is a group of dentists, oral maxillofacial surgeons, and dentist anesthesiologists dedicated to pain and anxiety control in dentistry. The American Dental Board of Anesthesiology (ADBA) has established a diplomate status recognizing expertise in the safe and effective administration of general anesthesia.

The history of these organizations can be found in Chapter 41.

More information can be found at the following websites:

- The American Society of Dentist Anesthesiologists: www.asdahq.org
- The American Dental Board of Anesthesiology: www.adba.org
- The American Dental Society of Anesthesiology: www.adsahome.org

REFERENCES

1. *Mosby's dental dictionary*, ed 2, St Louis, 2008, Mosby Elsevier.
2. Pallasch TJ: *Pharmacology for dental students and practitioners*, Philadelphia, 1980, Lea & Febiger.
3. Guidelines for the Use of Sedation and General Anesthesia by Dentists. https://www.ada.org/~/media/ADA/About%20the%20ADA/Files/anesthesia_use_guidelines.ashx. (Accessed 21 October 2016).
4. Geisz-Everson M, Wren KR: Awareness under anesthesia. *J Perianesth Nurs* 22(2):85–90, 2007.
5. Trieger NT: *Pain control*, ed 2, St Louis, 1994, Mosby.
6. Becker DE, Haas DA: Management of complications during moderate and deep sedation: respiratory and cardiovascular considerations. *Anesth Prog* 54(2):59–69, 2007.
7. American Dental Association, Council on Dental Education: Accreditation Standards for Advanced General Dentistry Education Programs in Dental Anesthesiology, as adopted by the Oct 2015 ADA House of Delegates, Chicago, 2015, The Association.
8. Cote CJ, Wilson S: Guideline for monitoring and management of pediatric patients before, during, and after sedation for diagnostic and therapeutic procedures. *Pediatrics* 138(1):1–33, 2016.
9. Practice guidelines for preoperative fasting and the use of pharmacologic agents to reduce the risk of pulmonary aspiration: application to healthy patients undergoing elective procedures: an updated report by the American Society of Anesthesiologists Committee on Standards and Practice Parameters. *Anesthesiology* 3:495–511, 2011.
10. Smith F, Deputy BS, Berry FA, Jr: Outpatient anesthesia for children undergoing extensive dental treatment. *J Dent Child* 45(2):142–145, 1978.
11. Trapp LD: Sedation of children for dental treatment. *Pediatr Dent* 4:164, 1982.
12. Eidelman E, Faibis S, Peretz B: A comparison of restorations for children with early childhood caries treated under general anesthesia or conscious sedation. *Pediatr Dent* 22(1):33–37, 2000.
13. Rosenberg M, Weaver J: General anesthesia. *Anesth Prog* 38(4-5):172–186, 1991.
14. Mercatello A: Changes in renal function induced by anesthesia. *Ann Fr Anesth Reanim* 9(6):507–524, 1990.
15. Steward D: Outpatient pediatric anesthesia. *Anesthesiology* 43:268, 1975.
16. Fahy A, Marshall M: Postanaesthetic morbidity in outpatients. *Br J Anaesth* 41:433, 1969.
17. Steward D: Experiences with an outpatient anesthesia service for children. *Anesth Analg* 52:877, 1973.
18. Schmidt KF: Evaluation of candidates for outpatient anesthesia and surgery. *Int Anesthesiol Clin* 14(2):9–13, 1976.
19. Rashewsky S, Parameswaran A, Sloane C, et al: Time and cost analysis: pediatric dental rehabilitation with general anesthesia in the office and the hospital settings. *Anesth Prog* 4:147–153, 2012.
20. Lalwani K, Kitchin J, Lax P: Office-based dental rehabilitation in children with special healthcare needs using a pediatric sedation service model. *J Oral Maxillofac Surg* 65(3):427–433, 2007.
21. Rehm SJ: *Staphylococcus aureus*: the new adventures of a legendary pathogen. *Cleve Clin J Med* 75(3):177–180, 183-186, 190-192, 2008.
22. Coplans MP, Curson I: Deaths associated with dentistry. *Br Dent J* 153:357, 1982.
23. Smith F, Deputy BS, Berry FA, Jr: Outpatient anesthesia for children undergoing extensive dental treatment. *J Dent Child* 45:38, 1978.
24. U.S. Food and Drug Administration. FDA Drug Safety Communication: FDA review results in new warnings about using general anesthetics and sedation drugs in young children and pregnant women. http://www.fda.gov/Drugs/DrugSafety/ucm532356.htm. (Accessed 17 January 2017).
25. Reed KL, Okundaye AJ: Management of emergencies associated with pediatric dental sedation. In Wright GZ, Kupietzky A, editors: *Behavior management in dentistry for children*, ed 2, Oxford, 2014, Wiley-Blackwell, pp 197–210.
26. American Dental Society of Anesthesiology: Guidelines relative to the establishment of a dental residency in anesthesiology. *Anesth Prog* 26:177, 1979.

chapter 31

Armamentarium, Drugs, and Techniques

CHAPTER OUTLINE

ARMAMENTARIUM
    Anesthesia Machine
    Intravenous Equipment
    Ancillary Anesthesia Equipment
    Monitoring Equipment
    Emergency Equipment and Drugs
DRUGS
    Intravenous Induction Agents
    Opioids
    Neuroleptanalgesia-Neuroleptanesthesia
    Dissociative Anesthesia

    Muscle Relaxants (Neuromuscular
      Blocking Drugs)
    Inhalation Anesthetics
TECHNIQUES
    Ideal Techniques
    Preoperative Procedure
    Preinduction
    Induction
    Airway Management
    Anesthesia Maintenance
    Ending the Case

This chapter presents an overview of the equipment, drugs, and techniques that are important to the success of general anesthesia. Many of the drugs discussed have been reviewed in depth elsewhere in this book and receive only brief mention in this chapter. Other drugs are mentioned for the first time; however, their pharmacology is also reviewed briefly. The scope of this chapter is for brief discussion on the utilities of general anesthesia. As discussed in Chapter 30, this section is meant as an introduction to the vast subject of general anesthesia, not as a complete text in this field.

Following a review of the armamentarium and drugs, each of the major techniques of general anesthesia is discussed.

ARMAMENTARIUM

The equipment required for the administration of general anesthesia may vary according to the technique of anesthesia delivered. In general, the equipment for total intravenous anesthesia (TIVA) varies somewhat from that required for other anesthesia techniques.

The armamentarium for general anesthesia may be divided into the following five groups:
1. Anesthesia machine
2. Intravenous (IV) equipment

3. Ancillary anesthesia equipment
4. Monitoring equipment
5. Emergency equipment and drugs

Anesthesia Machine

The anesthesia machine is able to deliver oxygen (O_2) and inhalation anesthetics to the patient. The inhalation sedation unit used in dentistry to deliver nitrous oxide-oxygen (N_2O-O_2) is a variation of a basic anesthesia machine. The primary difference between the two is the dental nitrous oxide unit delivers only oxygen and nitrous oxide. An anesthesia machine allows a number of halogenated anesthetics. As seen in Fig. 31.1, the anesthesia machine can deliver many gases: N_2O, O_2, sevoflurane, desflurane, and isoflurane. Flowmeters and devices called *vaporizers* that contain the various volatile anesthetics and permit their concentrations to be controlled are integral parts of the anesthesia machine. The flowmeter controls the rate (measured in liters per minute) and type of airflow that will then flow through the vaporizers to collect a percentage of volatile agent. Then, the mixture of anesthetic gases will exit at the common gas outlet to be delivered to the patient through an anesthesia circuit.

Some anesthesia machines are capable of operating with O_2 and N_2O supplied from either a central cylinder system

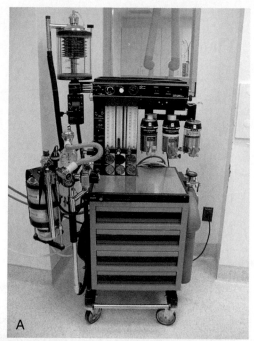

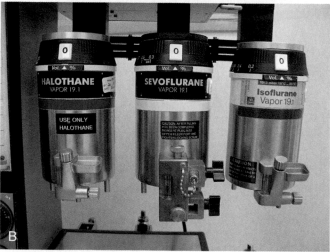

Figure 31.1 A, A general anesthesia machine can deliver a **(B)** variety of volatile anesthetics.

and/or portable cylinders mounted on the unit. Most modern anesthesia machines and nitrous oxide systems have a fail-safe and hypoxic guard system. In addition, most anesthesia machines have O_2 monitors that activate an alarm if the unit fails to provide a preset minimum percentage of O_2 (i.e., 25%).

The modern anesthesia machine also integrates a number of important devices for monitoring patients receiving these agents. Many different monitors can link directly to the modern anesthesia machine, including a blood pressure monitor, electrocardiograph (ECG), pulse oximeter, capnograph (end-tidal carbon dioxide [$ETCO_2$] monitor), and a bispectral (BIS) electroencephalograph (EEG) monitor. Many modern anesthesia machines will also have a ventilator, a device used to control or assist the ventilation of a patient during anesthesia.

Intravenous Equipment

A supply of equipment for venipuncture and IV drug administration is routinely available during general anesthetic procedures. Winged needles are rarely used during general anesthesia, and indwelling catheters are much preferred by the anesthesiologist. Most peripheral IV catheters range from 18 gauge to 24 gauge for common adult and pediatric anesthetic procedures. Larger needles (such as a 16-gauge) are used when a blood transfusion may be required. IV catheters are evolving with primary flash, secondary flash, safety preventative needle-stick, and blood control valves, features that help improve venipuncture success and safety.

IV administration sets and fluids are routinely used during general anesthesia. IV fluids come in different types and sizes. Smaller 100-mL bags may be adequate for short pediatric procedures; larger volume (500 mL or 1000 mL) bags are used for adults and longer procedures. Adults are more susceptible to becoming hypovolemic as a result of a combination of having been NPO (nothing by mouth) before surgery, blood loss during surgery, and evaporation of fluids during surgery (especially where the abdominal or thoracic cavity is exposed). Intravenous fluids help in most circumstances to prevent periinduction hypotension. A variety of *disposable syringes* and *needles* should also be available in addition to various *adhesive tapes* (e.g., paper, hypoallergenic).

Ancillary Anesthesia Equipment

The following items must also be available whenever general anesthesia is administered:
- Full-face masks in an assortment of sizes and appropriate connectors
- Laryngoscope, complete with adequate selection of blades and spare batteries, bulbs, and handles
- Adequate selection of endotracheal tubes and appropriate connectors
- Laryngeal mask airway (LMA)
- Adequate selection of oropharyngeal and nasopharyngeal airways (NPAs)
- Tonsillar suction tips
- Magill intubation forceps
- Child- and adult-size sphygmomanometers and stethoscopes

Anesthesia Face Masks

Anesthesia face masks are rubber or silicone masks that cover both the mouth and nose of the patient. Face masks are used to deliver O_2, N_2O-O_2, and/or other inhalation anesthetics before, during, and after the anesthetic procedure. Because of the variations in the size and shape of faces, several different sizes of face masks should always be available.

Typically, face masks are made from a clear plastic or rubber that allows the patient's mouth and nose to be seen so that foreign material (e.g., vomitus, blood) and condensation may be observed. Many different connectors of various materials,

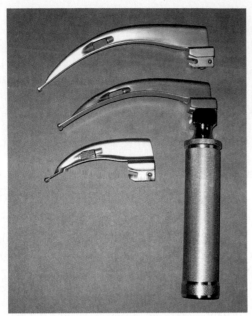

Figure 31.2 Laryngoscope handle and several sizes of curved blades.

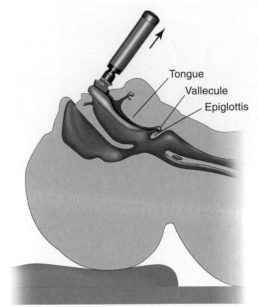

Figure 31.3 Curved blade is placed between the base of the tongue and the epiglottis. The laryngoscope is then lifted, elevating the tongue and exposing the larynx.

shapes, and with or without sample ports attach the face mask to the anesthesia circuit, continuing to connect to the anesthesia machine.

Laryngoscopes

The traditional laryngoscope (Fig. 31.2) is a device designed to assist in the visualization of the trachea during intubation. It consists of two parts: a handle with battery holder and a blade. The handle is usually made of metal (although some are made of plastic) and contains batteries that are used to operate the light bulb found in the blade. Traditional laryngoscopes have progressed to include fiber-optic technology to make them brighter and lighter, and have become much more affordable in recent years.

The blade of the laryngoscope is also usually made of metal, although plastic is also used today as disposable products are becoming increasingly popular in modern medical devices. The laryngoscope blade is designed to be placed into the patient's mouth to aid in visualization of the larynx. A small light that illuminates the laryngeal area is attached to the end of the blade. There are various types of laryngoscope blades: the curved (Macintosh) and the straight (Miller) blades are the most common types. Blades are available in a variety of sizes. The technique for using these blades differs for each style.

The Macintosh blade is more commonly used. The tip of the curved blade is inserted into the vallecula, the cul-de-sac between the base of the tongue and the epiglottis (Fig. 31.3). The handle of the laryngoscope is then lifted straight up and slightly forward, a movement that visualizes the vocal cords. When a straight blade is used, its tip is placed underneath the laryngeal surface of the epiglottis (Fig. 31.4), and the larynx is exposed by an upward and forward lift of the blade. Most

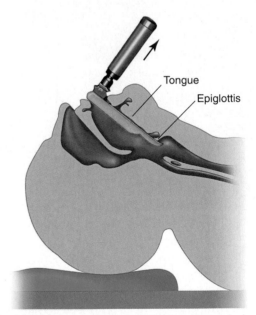

Figure 31.4 Straight laryngoscope blade is placed beneath the epiglottis and lifted, thereby exposing the larynx.

laryngoscopes and blades are designed to be held in the operator's left hand, with the endotracheal tube held in the right. Special laryngoscope blades are available for left-handed operators.

Endotracheal Tubes and Connectors

Endotracheal tubes and connectors (Fig. 31.5) are rubber tubes designed to be placed from the mouth (oroendotracheal) or nose (nasoendotracheal) into the patient's trachea. Reusable

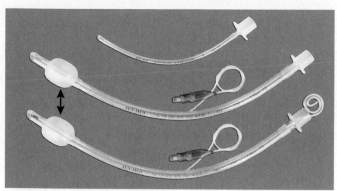

Figure 31.5 Laryngoscope and endotracheal tube. Distal end of tube has inflatable cuff *(arrow)* designed to provide an airtight seal, preventing entry of substances into the trachea. (From Malamed SF: *Medical emergencies in the dental office*, ed 6, St Louis, 2007, Mosby.)

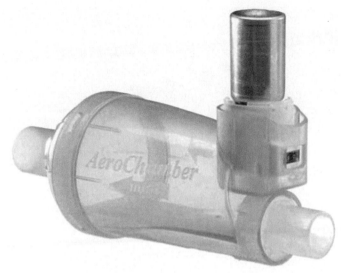

Figure 31.6 AeroChamber Mini. (Used with permission of Monaghan Medical Corporation.)

and disposable endotracheal tubes are available, with disposables more popular today. Because the diameter of the laryngeal opening and the trachea vary from patient to patient, endotracheal tubes are manufactured in a variety of diameters. Endotracheal tubes are commonly referred to by their internal diameter size (e.g., a 7.0 endotracheal tube has an inner diameter of 7 mm). Manufacturers vary in thickness for the outside diameter. The French gauge (Fr.) is represented as three times the size in mm. For example, a 5-mm outside diameter endotracheal tube would be considered a 15 Fr. endotracheal tube. Smaller and larger tubes are available to accommodate the child or larger patient.

Endotracheal tubes can have an inflatable cuff (see Fig. 31.5) located near their distal ends. When a patient is intubated, the endotracheal tube is inserted into the trachea so that the uninflated cuff disappears just beyond the level of the larynx. Air is then injected into a tube that connects with the cuff to inflate it. Enough air is injected into the cuff to seal the trachea off from the pharynx, thereby preventing foreign material, such as blood, saliva, or vomitus, from entering the trachea and bronchi.

Connectors for endotracheal tubes are the same as those used for anesthesia face masks. The dimensions have been standardized for all manufacturers to prevent a potentially hazardous situation. Connectors are used to connect the endotracheal tube to the anesthesia circuit. The design allows for circuits to be connected directly to the endotracheal tube or for various connectors in between for other uses. Connectors may be straight, curved, with a sample port, or with an air chamber for additional aerosol medications to be delivered, as well as others. AeroChamber Mini (Fig. 31.6) is a connector accessory that can connect the endotracheal tube and anesthesia circuit. This device can deliver metered-dose inhaler (MDI) aerosols to the patient while maintaining positive end expiratory pressure.

Laryngeal Mask Airway

Introduced in 1988, the LMA is a supraglottic device designed to provide and maintain airway integrity and to permit spontaneous, assisted, or controlled ventilation in clinical situations in which intubation is either not possible or not practicable. In cases of general anesthesia involving dentistry, the LMA is used as an alternative to orotracheal or nasotracheal intubation. Orotracheal intubation is not indicated for most dental procedures because the tube will compete for space in the oral cavity with both the dental team and dental instruments used. Nasotracheal intubation offers the dental team greater access to the surgical site, but the presence of a tube within the trachea is a potent stimulus (e.g., coughing, gagging, bronchospasm) to the patient and may require a more profound level of central nervous system (CNS) depression for the tube to be tolerated. The flexible LMA is commonly used in dental procedures because it is wire reinforced, permitting it to be repositioned from side to side during surgical procedures without loss of seal of the cuff against the larynx. Additionally the wire-reinforced flexible LMA resists kinking when it is flexed or compressed against a rigid mouth prop. However, the reinforced airway tube does not offer resistance to occlusion by biting.

LMAs are available in multiple sizes to fit the neonate to large adult (Fig. 31.7). The LMA is inserted with the tip of the cuff pressed upward against the hard palate by the index finger while the middle finger opens the mouth (Fig. 31.8, *A*). The LMA is pressed backward in a smooth movement (using the opposite hand to extend the airway) (Fig. 31.8, *B*). The LMA is advanced until definite resistance is felt (Fig. 31.8, *C*), and before the index finger is removed, the opposite hand presses down on the LMA to prevent dislodgment during removal of the index finger (Fig. 31.8, *D*). Following removal of the finger, the cuff is inflated with air.

Oropharyngeal and Nasopharyngeal Airways

Oropharyngeal (Fig. 31.9) and nasopharyngeal airways (Fig. 31.10) are used to assist in maintaining a patent airway at any

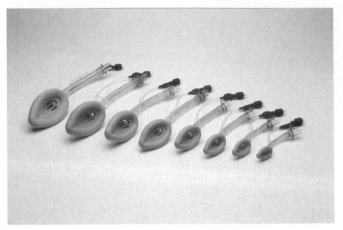

Figure 31.7 LMA (various sizes). (Courtesy LMA North America, Inc., San Diego, CA.)

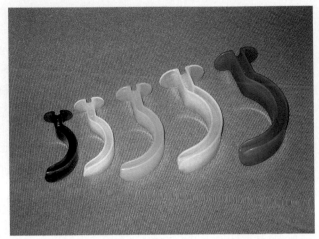

Figure 31.9 Oropharyngeal airways are available in a variety of sizes. (Courtesy Sedation Resource, One Oak, TX.)

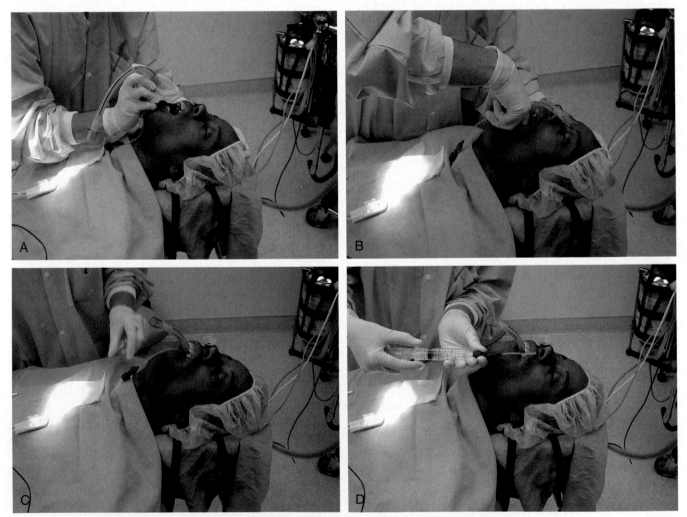

Figure 31.8 A, LMA is inserted by pressing the tip of the cuff upward against the hard palate. **B,** The LMA is advanced backward in smooth movement until definite resistance is felt. **C,** Seated LMA. **D,** LMA cuff is inflated with air to prevent dislodgement. (Courtesy Drs. H. William Gottschalk and Kenneth Lee.)

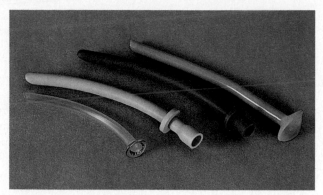

Figure 31.10 Nasopharyngeal airways. (From McSwain N: *The basic EMT: comprehensive prehospital care*, ed 2, St Louis, 2003, Mosby.)

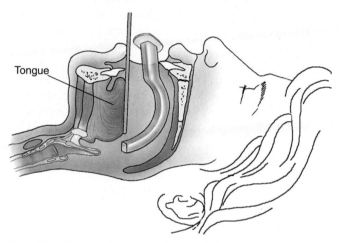

Tongue

Figure 31.11 The oropharyngeal airway is designed to lift the tongue off the posterior wall of the pharynx. (From McSwain N: *The basic EMT: comprehensive prehospital care*, ed 2, St Louis, 2003, Mosby.)

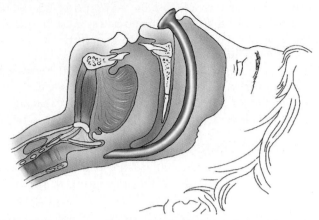

Figure 31.12 The nasopharyngeal airway is designed to rest between the base of the tongue and pharyngeal wall, thus permitting air to pass between the lungs and the nose. (From McSwain N: *The basic EMT: comprehensive prehospital care*, ed 2, St Louis, 2003, Mosby.)

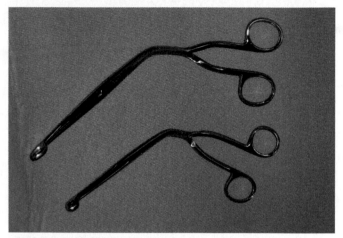

Figure 31.13 Magill intubation forceps are designed to assist in passage of an endotracheal tube, especially during nasal intubation.

point during anesthetic procedure. Oropharyngeal airways are plastic, rubber, or metallic devices designed to lie between the base of the tongue and the posterior pharyngeal wall (Fig. 31.11). The NPA (also known as a *nasal trumpet*) is a thin, flexible rubber tube designed to be inserted through the nares and to rest between the base of the tongue and posterior pharynx (Fig. 31.12). The purpose of both of these devices is to displace the tongue from the pharynx and thereby permit the patient to exchange air either around or through the airway. The NPA is better tolerated than an oropharyngeal airway by the conscious or sedated patient, thereby minimizing the occurrence of gagging and vomiting.

Tonsillar Suction Tips

The immediate availability of suction devices is absolutely essential before general anesthesia is started. Suction is considered an essential emergency device and should be checked before each anesthetic procedure. Excessive salivation, bleeding in the mouth or pharynx, or vomiting can produce airway obstruction, laryngospasm, or possible infection of the trachea or bronchi. Tonsillar suction tips are recommended because

they can be inserted blindly into the posterior pharynx of the patient with minimal risk of producing bleeding. The end of the tonsillar suction tip is rounded, making this device preferable to others that have sharper edges. Several tonsillar suction tips should be available in the event that one becomes clogged.

Magill Intubation Forceps

A Magill intubation forceps (Fig. 31.13) is designed to assist in placing the endotracheal tube. It is most frequently used during nasoendotracheal intubation and is therefore a very important item in the armamentarium for dental general anesthesia procedures.

Sphygmomanometers and Stethoscopes

Sphygmomanometers and stethoscopes are used during general anesthetic procedures. They are used for the monitoring of vital signs, specifically blood pressure, heart rate and rhythm, heart sounds, and breath sounds. Appropriate-size blood pressure cuffs for the sphygmomanometers must be utilized for accurate blood pressure values. An improperly sized blood pressure cuff that is too small will give an incorrectly high reading; inversely, a blood pressure cuff that is too large will give an artificially low reading. The blood pressure cuff should span a minimum of 80% of the patient's upper arm circumference to provide an accurate reading.

Monitoring Equipment

Monitoring of the patient during sedation or general anesthesia is essential to the overall safety of the procedure. During sedation procedures, monitoring of the CNS via direct communication with the patient is of primary importance. Because the patient is able to respond appropriately to verbal commands, other, more complex monitoring devices need not be used routinely.[1] However, once consciousness is lost (increased CNS depression), patients are unable to respond to commands, and other means of determining their status during anesthesia must be used. For this reason, the level of monitoring during general anesthesia is greater than that required for sedative procedures. A monitor is a device that reminds and warns. The Department of Anesthesiology at the Harvard University School of Medicine has designed monitoring guidelines for use during general anesthesia.[2] The recommendations in these guidelines have been well received and widely implemented. The following are some of the methods and devices used to monitor patients during general anesthesia:

1. The stethoscope is used with auscultation to monitor the heart rate, heart rhythm, and/or breath sounds. Taped to the chest in the precordial region, the *precordial stethoscope* provides continuous monitoring of heart sounds, but when placed on the neck directly over the trachea, the *pretracheal stethoscope* (Fig. 31.14) permits monitoring of respiration. The pretracheal stethoscope is recommended for use during all forms of IV sedation and general anesthesia. An

alternative to the precordial stethoscope during general anesthesia is the *esophageal stethoscope* (Fig. 31.15), a rubber tube inserted into the patient's esophagus after intubation. This device provides continuous monitoring similar to that provided by the precordial stethoscope, but is more effective because of its closer proximity to the heart and lungs. Breath and heart sounds can usually be heard more distinctly. Esophageal stethoscopes are not used during sedation procedures and brief outpatient general anesthetics.

2. The *pulse oximeter* (Fig. 31.16) provides a noninvasive means of monitoring the degree of O_2 saturation of hemoglobin in peripheral blood vessels. Pulse oximeters provide continuous monitoring of oxygenation and of the heart rate, permitting a more rapid detection of potential airway problems (there is a time lag of about 20 seconds). The use of pulse oximetry is considered to be standard of care during general anesthesia.

3. *End-tidal carbon dioxide ($ETCO_2$) monitors* also represent standard of care in monitoring during general anesthesia. They evaluate the effectiveness of ventilation. Because the $ETCO_2$ monitor evaluates every breath, airway problems may be detected promptly, permitting correction before they become significant.

4. The *sphygmomanometer,* or *blood pressure cuff,* is used to monitor blood pressure by indirect determination. During general anesthesia, blood pressure, heart rate and rhythm, and respiratory rate are monitored continuously and

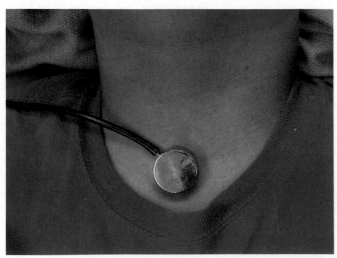

Figure 31.14 Pretracheal stethoscope.

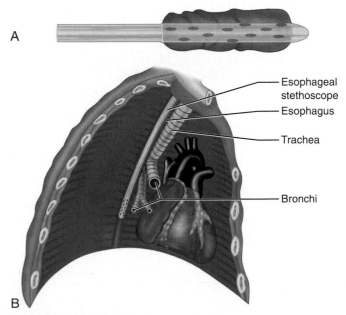

Esophageal stethoscope
Esophagus

Trachea

Bronchi

Figure 31.15 Esophageal stethoscope aids in monitoring both heart and lung sounds. **A,** Distal end of esophageal stethoscope has multiple perforations that aid in picking up sounds in the thorax. **B,** Esophageal stethoscope is inserted into esophagus to the level of the heart, thereby maximizing sound amplification.

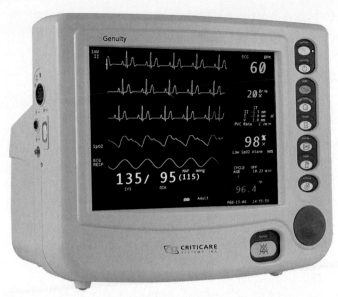

Figure 31.16 Oximeter provides continuous monitoring of arterial O$_2$ saturation, heart rate, respiratory rate, blood pressure, and ECG. (Courtesy Criticare Systems, Inc.)

recorded every 5 minutes. If events warrant, more frequent determinations are obtained.

5. The *electrocardiograph (ECG)* provides a means of monitoring the electrical activity and rhythm of the heart. The ECG permits continuous observation of the rate and rhythm of the heart during general anesthesia. Use of the ECG is considered a standard of care during all forms of general anesthesia.

6. *Continuous temperature monitoring* has become increasingly common since the 1980s with the recognition of malignant hyperthermia. Although not used for all patients undergoing general anesthesia, temperature monitoring is considered a standard of care in children, young adults, patients with fever, and patients undergoing procedures involving induced hypothermia.[2]

7. *Bispectral electroencephalographic monitoring* (BIS monitoring) is described more completely in Chapter 5. The BIS index is a continuous EEG parameter that ranges from an awake, no-drug effect value of 95 to 100 to zero with no detectable EEG activity.[3] The BIS index appears to be a valuable adjunct during the administration of general anesthesia. It primarily measures the effects of hypnotics on the EEG. It is most accurate when used with anesthetic techniques consisting of a low or moderate dose of opioid analgesic and a hypnotic drug titrated to the BIS response. Low opioid doses enable the BIS index to accurately reflect the pharmacodynamics of the hypnotic drugs on the CNS. BIS monitoring provides an important new dimension to the ability to adjust the components of a general anesthetic in a logical manner.

8. Although not used routinely, *direct measurement of arterial blood pressure* is of value in the critically ill patient and during cardiopulmonary bypass, major traumatic surgery, and hypotensive or hypothermic anesthesia. Its major advantage over indirect blood pressure methods is that it provides accurate values of intraarterial or intracardiac blood pressure on a continuous basis.

9. *Collection and measurement of urine output* are easily obtained in the anesthetized patient whose bladder has been catheterized. Urine output is a simple method of determining the degree of hydration of the body. During general anesthesia, the patient should produce urine at a rate approaching the normal rate of 40 to 60 mL/hr. Volumes below this may signify dehydration or poor kidney perfusion and indicate the need for intervention. For routine general anesthetic procedures, the monitoring of urine output is not required.

10. *Central venous pressure (CVP)* measures the pressure exerted by blood returning to the right side of the heart and the ability of the right heart to manage it effectively. Monitoring CVP enables the doctor to distinguish between hemorrhage and congestive heart failure. With extensive blood loss, the CVP will fall, whereas in congestive heart failure or hypervolemia, CVP is elevated. For the typical American Society of Anesthesiologists (ASA) 1 or 2 ambulatory dental patient undergoing general anesthesia, routine use of CVP is not warranted.

Emergency Equipment and Drugs

Many different complications can occur during the administration of general anesthesia. Many of the more frequently observed complications are pulmonary or cardiovascular in nature. These events can lead to hypoxemia, hypotension, and cardiac dysrhythmias. Monitoring of the anesthetized patient enables the entire anesthesia team to be aware of the presence of these and other potentially lethal problems and to initiate appropriate corrective treatment. The anesthesiologist will have available a supply of emergency drugs and equipment for use in these circumstances. The emergency drugs required by the board of dental examiners in the state of California[4] for dentists using general anesthesia are listed here. Suggested emergency drugs and equipment from the American Association of Oral and Maxillofacial Surgeons may be found in Box 31.1.[5] A more thorough discussion of emergency drugs recommended for outpatient facilities is presented in Chapter 33.

Several of the drugs recommended for the emergency tray are also commonly used during the routine administration of general anesthesia. These include succinylcholine, IV replacement fluid, and opioid antagonists.

DRUGS

An array of drugs may be used during the administration of general anesthesia. Many of these drugs have been discussed in other sections of this book and are listed here with minimal discussion. Other drugs make their first appearance at this

---

Box 31.1   Emergency Drugs and Equipment Required for General Anesthesia—California

Drugs
Vasopressor
Corticosteroid
Bronchodilator
Muscle relaxant
IV medication for treatment of cardiopulmonary arrest
Appropriate drug antagonist(s)
Antihistaminic
Anticholinergic
Antiarrhythmic
Coronary artery vasodilator
Antihypertensive
Anticonvulsant
O_2
50% dextrose or other antihypoglycemic

Equipment
Backup lighting system that is battery powered and of
    sufficient intensity to permit completion of any
    operation underway at the time of general power
    failure

Backup suction device that can operate at a time of
    general power failure
O_2 delivery system with adequate full-face masks and
    appropriate connectors that are capable of delivering
    O_2 to the patient under positive pressure together
    with an adequate backup system that can operate at
    the time of a general power failure.
Laryngoscope with complete selection of blades and
    spare batteries and bulb
Endotracheal tubes and appropriate connectors
Oral airways
Tonsillar or pharyngeal type suction tip
Endotracheal tube forceps (Magill intubation forceps)
Sphygmomanometer and stethoscope
Electrocardioscope and defibrillator
Adequate equipment for the establishment of an IV
    infusion
Precordial or pretracheal stethoscope
Pulse oximeter

---

time; however, they, too, will receive only a brief review because it is not the goal of this textbook to provide the reader with an in-depth knowledge of general anesthesia.

The most commonly used drugs in general anesthesia may be divided into the following categories:
- IV induction agents
- Opioids (agonists and agonist-antagonists)
- Neuroleptic agents
- Dissociative agents
- Muscle relaxants
- Inhalation anesthetics

Intravenous Induction Agents

In the adult patient receiving general anesthesia, it is the desire of the anesthesiologist to achieve surgical-depth anesthesia as safely and efficiently as possible.

Barbiturates

Barbiturates used to be the most commonly used IV induction agents, with methohexital, thiopental, and thiamylal most frequently administered. Propofol has since replaced the short-acting barbiturates as an IV induction agent for general anesthesia in most circumstances. Other nonbarbiturate drugs used intravenously during induction of anesthesia include diazepam, midazolam, lorazepam, etomidate, ketamine, and propofol.

Methohexital is a rapid-onset, short-acting barbiturate. It is most often used as the sole agent to provide general anesthesia for short procedures (less than 30 minutes).[6] Methohexital is

less frequently used as an induction agent for general anesthesia. The dosage of methohexital for induction of general anesthesia is 1 mg/kg. It is 2.5 times as potent as the thiobarbiturates (thiopental and thiamylal) and has a more rapid recovery.[7] Proprietary names of methohexital are Brevital (United States) and Brietal (Great Britain). The uses of methohexital in anesthesia are for short-duration outpatient procedures, electroconvulsive therapy,[8] and minor gynecologic or orthopedic procedures.

Thiopental (Pentothal) and *thiamylal* (Surital) are called thiobarbiturates because they possess a sulfa molecule and are quite similar pharmacologically. Following IV administration, the onset of action of these drugs is rapid (within 30 to 40 seconds) and of short duration. Duration of action of thiopental and thiamylal is, however, longer than that of methohexital.[9]

The induction of general anesthesia with a thiobarbiturate is usually produced by IV injection of 150 to 300 mg over a 15- to 30-second interval. Thiopental and thiamylal are used as 2.5% solutions. After induction of general anesthesia, other longer-acting anesthetics are administered for the maintenance of anesthesia.

Absolute contraindications to the administration of barbiturates include status asthmaticus and latent or manifest porphyria.

Benzodiazepines

Several benzodiazepines are also used as induction agents for general anesthesia. These include diazepam, midazolam, and lorazepam.

Diazepam and midazolam are benzodiazepines that are used on occasion to induce general anesthesia.[10] Benzodiazepines provide a slower, more gradual loss of consciousness than do the barbiturates. The patient initially enters into a comfortable level of sedation, at which point additional diazepam, midazolam, or other IV (e.g., opioids) or inhalation agents (e.g., halothane) may be administered to produce the desired level of unconsciousness. Diazepam and midazolam are also used during short IV barbiturate general anesthetic procedures to potentiate the actions of the barbiturate and balance out the anesthesia.

Lorazepam (Ativan) is a benzodiazepine that was not recommended earlier for use in outpatients because of its long duration of action and the inability of the administrator to titrate the drug to clinical effect as a result of its very slow onset of action. Because the need for rapid and "complete" recovery after inpatient procedures is not as urgent, lorazepam may be used like diazepam or midazolam in these patients.

Other Agents

Etomidate was introduced in the United States in 1983 as a nonbarbiturate IV induction agent. Administered in a dose of 0.3 to 0.4 mg/kg, etomidate demonstrates a rapid onset of action combined with less respiratory depression than is seen with the barbiturates.[11] Cardiovascular stability is another positive feature of etomidate. Etomidate is highly lipid soluble, has a half-life of 60 minutes, and is short acting. Recovery of cognitive and psychomotor function is intermediate between thiopental[12] and methohexital.[13] Negative factors associated with etomidate include a burning sensation as the drug is injected in some patients, the occurrence of myoclonic jerks, the inhibition of steroid synthesis, and the occurrence of excitatory effects in approximately 30% of patients receiving it. Etomidate is used for IV induction in children where hemodynamic stability is desirable (hypovolemia) and the hypertension and tachycardia caused by ketamine are unacceptable.

Ketamine, used as either an IV or intramuscular (IM) induction agent, primarily in children, is discussed more fully in Chapter 25. Ketamine is most suitable in children who are hemodynamically unstable or hypovolemic.[14] In addition, ketamine is used in asthmatic children because of its bronchodilating properties.[15] When administered, ketamine is sometimes preceded or accompanied by the administration of atropine or glycopyrrolate to attenuate the increase in airway secretions associated with its administration.[11] In addition, concurrent benzodiazepine administration is recommended to lessen the dysphoric emergence from anesthesia that may be associated with ketamine.[16]

Propofol (diisopropylphenol) is a nonbarbiturate IV anesthetic agent that is used when rapid-onset and short-duration general anesthesia is desired.[17] Propofol has become, in most instances, the preferred IV induction agent for general anesthesia. It is most often compared with methohexital.[18] Pecaro and Houting demonstrated that at usual dosages, propofol has insignificant

cardiovascular and respiratory effects.[19] Moreover, it lacks excitatory or emetic actions. The primary side effect noted with propofol administration was pain on injection (37.5% on dorsum of hand).[20]

The anesthesia induction dose of propofol is 2.5 mg/kg, which makes the drug equipotent with 4 mg/kg of thiopental.[21] McCulloch and Lees[20] suggest an induction dose of 2.25 mg/kg in "younger patients" and a dose of 1.5 mg/kg in "older patients." Pharmacokinetically the terminal half-life of propofol is between 250 and 312 minutes, with clearance ranging from 1678 to 1928 minutes.[22]

Cundy and Arunasalam,[23] comparing propofol with methohexital, found that propofol provided a statistically significant superior quality of anesthesia. No difference was noted in recovery time, and postoperatively, methohexital patients were significantly drowsier. Coughing and laryngospasm did not occur with propofol (0/30) as they did with methohexital (5/30). The proprietary name of propofol is Diprivan.

Opioids

The term *opioid* is used in a broad sense to include both the opioid agonists and opioid agonist-antagonists. The pharmacology of these drugs is discussed in some detail in Chapter 25.

Opioids are frequently used for maintenance of pain control during general anesthesia. General anesthesia is induced with one of the short-acting IV agents previously discussed and maintained with periodic doses of an appropriate opioid. N_2O-O_2 can be administered to minimize the dosage of opioid required. The most commonly used opioids in general anesthesia are morphine, meperidine, fentanyl, and its analogs sufentanil, alfentanil, and remifentanil.

Morphine is the standard opioid analgesic drug against which all others are compared. Morphine has strong analgesic and sedative properties. It is used primarily for longer-duration procedures. Morphine is usually injected as a 1-mg/mL solution.

Meperidine (Demerol) is usually administered in a concentration of 10 mg/mL. Meperidine's duration of action is intermediate between that of morphine and fentanyl.

Fentanyl (Sublimaze) provides a shorter duration than either morphine or meperidine and is commonly used in shorter surgical procedures. It is usually administered in a concentration of 0.01 mg/mL. Fentanyl is the most used opioid in general anesthesia and IV sedation in oral and maxillofacial surgery, where most procedures are of short duration, as well as in outpatient ambulatory general anesthesia primarily because of its short duration of action.[24]

Alfentanil (Alfenta) and *sufentanil* (Sufenta) are rapid-onset, short-duration analogs of fentanyl that have been recently introduced and have gained significant popularity.[25,26] *Remifentanil* (Ultiva) is as rapid acting as alfentanil, but is even shorter acting, requiring its administration via constant infusion (infusion pump) to maintain a therapeutic blood level.[27,28]

Opioid agonist-antagonists, such as *nalbuphine* and *butorphanol,* are also used during general anesthesia. Their primary benefit appears to be the ceiling effect on respiratory depression that is noted with their administration.[29] This contrasts to the dose-related respiratory depression observed with opioid agonists.

The opioid antagonist *naloxone* is used when opioids have been administered and need to be reversed. Titration of naloxone may be necessary to reverse opioid-induced respiratory depression. Careful monitoring of the patient following reversal with naloxone is required because several of the opioids, such as morphine and meperidine, can have a longer duration of action than naloxone and a return of respiratory depression at a later time is possible. To minimize this potential risk, the administration of an IM dose of naloxone can be considered after its IV administration.[30] The slower onset and longer duration of the IM dose of naloxone helps mitigate the risk of a recurrence of significant respiratory depression.

Neuroleptanalgesia-Neuroleptanesthesia

In 1959, Fukuda cited De Castro and Mundeleer, who derived the concept of neuroleptanalgesia, which involved the combination of a major tranquilizer (usually the butyrophenone droperidol) and a potent opioid analgesic (fentanyl) to produce a detached, pain-free state of immobilization and insensitivity to pain.[31] Neuroleptanalgesia is characterized by analgesia, suppression of motor activity, suppression of autonomic reflexes, maintenance of cardiovascular stability, and amnesia in most patients. The addition of an inhaled agent, usually N_2O, improves amnesia and has been called *neuroleptanesthesia*. Neuroleptanesthesia and neuroleptanalgesia are discussed in Chapter 25. The neuroleptic state is produced when a neuroleptic drug (another name for a tranquilizer) and an opioid analgesic are administered together to produce a state characterized by the following[32]:

- Sleepiness without total unconsciousness
- Psychological indifference to the environment
- No voluntary movements
- Analgesia
- Satisfactory amnesia

In clinical practice, neuroleptanesthesia is produced through the administration of the following drug combinations:

- Neuroleptic drug (usually droperidol)
- Opioid (usually fentanyl)
- N_2O-O_2
- Muscle relaxant

The pharmacologic properties of droperidol and fentanyl are discussed in Chapter 25. A brief review follows.

Droperidol, a tranquilizer, produces clinical actions within 5 to 10 minutes after IV administration. Long acting, its actions may be observed for 6 to 12 hours after a single injection. Additional properties of droperidol include its antiemetic and its slight α-adrenergic receptor-blocking effects. Disadvantages of droperidol include its long duration of action (a disadvantage in [short] outpatient procedures); its peripheral vasodilating effects, which may produce hypotension; no pharmacologic antagonist; and large doses produce muscle movements similar

to extrapyramidal effects: dystonia, akathisia, and oculogyric crisis (see Chapter 7).

Fentanyl, a powerful opioid analgesic, acts rapidly after IV administration, with a duration of action between 30 and 60 minutes. The analgesic potency of 0.1 mg of fentanyl is equal to that of 10 mg of morphine. Fentanyl does not release histamine (unlike meperidine), can be reversed by opioid antagonists, produces euphoria, and has negligible effects on the cardiovascular system. Negative features of fentanyl include the fact that it is an emetic and that it produces respiratory depression, miosis, possibly bradycardia and bronchoconstriction, and, with large doses, possibly muscular rigidity (see Chapters 25 and 27).

Neuroleptanesthesia produced by droperidol, fentanyl, N_2O-O_2, and a muscle relaxant is used as an anesthetic technique, especially in the more severely medically compromised patient (ASA 3 and 4). Snow lists the following advantages of neuroleptanesthesia[33]:

- No secretions
- No venous or tissue irritation
- Stable cardiovascular system
- No sensitization of myocardial conduction system to actions of catecholamines
- No toxic effects on liver or kidney function
- Reduced cerebrospinal fluid (CSF) pressure and intraocular pressure
- Nonemetic
- Nonexplosive
- Prompt recovery
- Long periods of analgesia and amnesia
- In recovery room, longer tolerance of endotracheal tube

The following are disadvantages of neuroleptanesthesia[31]:

- Respiratory depression and apnea can be caused by fentanyl and muscle relaxants.
- Assisted or controlled ventilation is required.
- Action of muscle relaxants must be reversed.

Dissociative Anesthesia

Dissociative anesthesia and analgesia, as produced by ketamine, are described in Chapter 25. After IV administration, ketamine produces analgesia and unconsciousness within 30 seconds. The usual general anesthesia–induction dose of ketamine is 1 to 2 mg/kg, injected at a rate of 0.5 mg/kg/min.[34] Ketamine-anesthetized patients have profound analgesia, but keep their eyes open and maintain many reflexes. Corneal, cough, and swallow reflexes may all be present, but should not be assumed to be protective.[35] Patients have no recall of surgery or anesthesia, but amnesia is not as prominent with ketamine as with the benzodiazepines.

Ketamine can be used as an induction agent for general anesthesia and as the sole agent for short diagnostic and surgical procedures that do not require skeletal muscle relaxation. Ketamine is used in children and the special-needs population as a preinduction technique to have enough cooperation for IV placement. It is used especially in surgical procedures in which control of the airway is difficult to maintain, especially for correction of scars and burns of the face and neck—procedures that make intubation and extension of the neck very difficult, if not impossible. The administration of dissociative anesthesia is contraindicated in intraocular surgery and in patients with a history of increased CSF pressure, cerebrovascular accident (CVA), psychiatric problems, and high blood pressure.

Ketamine is nonirritating to blood vessels and tissues. It produces profound analgesia, muscle tone is preserved, and the laryngeal and pharyngeal reflexes are not depressed; therefore a patent airway can usually be maintained without the need for intubation.

Disadvantages of ketamine include increased heart rate, blood pressure, and intraocular pressure; in addition, diplopia, eye movements, and nystagmus can occur during anesthesia—thus the recommendation that ketamine not be used in intraocular procedures. There is no antagonist for ketamine. Probably the most significant disadvantage of ketamine is its ability to produce a confused state, associated with unpleasant dreams and frightening or upsetting hallucinations, which occur most commonly in adults during the recovery period.[36,37] These appear much less frequently in children.

Muscle Relaxants (Neuromuscular Blocking Drugs)

Muscle-relaxant drugs are also known as *neuromuscular blocking drugs*. They provide skeletal muscle relaxation to facilitate intubation of the trachea and controlled mechanical ventilation, and they provide optimal operating conditions. These drugs interfere with the transmission of impulses from motor nerves to muscle at the skeletal neuromuscular junction. Before the introduction of muscle relaxants into anesthesia, skeletal muscle relaxation was obtained during surgery by inducing deeper levels of anesthesia. Along with muscle relaxation, a greatly increased incidence of complications, morbidity, and mortality was seen. With the introduction of muscle relaxant drugs, deep anesthesia can now be avoided, and the concept and technique of balanced anesthesia has developed. Muscle relaxants are a commonly used adjuvant in anesthesia practice.

During short-duration outpatient general anesthesia (e.g., with propofol or methohexital), there is seldom administration of muscle relaxants. For longer-duration procedures, procedures involving the incision of muscles, and where aid is needed in intubation, the use of a paralytic agent is indicated. The short-acting muscle relaxant *succinylcholine* is used frequently in the operating room to aid in intubation. Patients undergoing inpatient dental procedures performed under general anesthesia may receive succinylcholine for intubation and may, if necessary, receive other longer-acting muscle relaxants.

There are four mechanisms by which the physiology of neuromuscular transmission may be interfered with to interrupt nerve impulses arriving at the end plate:

1. In *deficiency block,* the synthesis and/or transmission of acetylcholine is interfered with. Examples of drugs that act in this manner include local anesthetics; neomycin, kanamycin, and streptomycin; *Clostridium botulinum* toxin; calcium deficiency; and magnesium excess.

2. *Nondepolarizing block* is also known as a *competitive* block. The drug attaches to cholinergic receptors, preventing acetylcholine from attaching to the receptor, a form of competitive inhibition. Most commonly used muscle relaxants act in this manner. Examples of nondepolarizing muscle relaxants include d-tubocurarine (Curare), pancuronium, metocurine, vecuronium, atracurium, mivacurium, and gallamine. The actions of nondepolarizing muscle relaxants may be reversed by increasing the concentration of acetylcholine, which is accomplished clinically by administering anticholinesterases, such as neostigmine. Nondepolarizing muscle relaxants do not produce fasciculations (skeletal muscle contractions) when administered intravenously.

3. In *depolarizing block* (also known as *phase I* block), the drug acts in a manner similar to acetylcholine, but for a prolonged time. The drug acts to produce muscle contractions, called *fasciculations* (the equivalent of acetylcholine action), followed by prolonged muscle flaccidity. Two drugs that produce this effect are succinylcholine and decamethonium.

4. *Dual block* is also called *desensitization* block. In dual block, the membrane is depolarized (phase I) and is then slowly repolarized. The drug enters into the nerve fiber and acts as a nondepolarizing agent (phase II), even though the membrane potential is restored.

All neuromuscular blockers impair respiration and can produce apnea; therefore, these drugs must never be administered by persons untrained in endotracheal intubation and who are unable to provide controlled ventilation to the apneic patient. Nondepolarizing muscle relaxants are used more frequently during surgery than depolarizing agents because their duration is somewhat longer (20 to 45 minutes). Depolarizing agents are used for endotracheal intubation, laryngoscopy, bronchoscopy, esophagoscopy, and other short procedures.

Patients with myasthenia gravis should receive nondepolarizing muscle relaxants with great caution because they are extremely sensitive to the actions of these drugs. Such patients usually require as little as one tenth of the usual dose for clinical effect.

Tubocurarine (Tubarine) is the classical nondepolarizing muscle relaxant. After IV administration, the drug produces its actions within 3 minutes and with a duration of more than 50 minutes. The average initial dose in adults is 15 to 20 mg. Supplemental doses may be required for prolonged surgical procedures. Muscle fasciculation and postoperative muscle pain do not develop with tubocurarine. Administration of tubocurarine is contraindicated in patients with myasthenia gravis, renal disease, and bronchial asthma (because it releases histamine).

Pancuronium was introduced in the United States in the early 1970s. It is approximately five times as potent as tubocurarine and has an onset of action within 3 to 5 minutes and

Table 31.1	Classification of Nondepolarizing Neuromuscular Blocking Agents According to Duration of Action		
Clinical Duration			
LONG ACTING (> 50 MIN)	INTERMEDIATE ACTING (20–50 MIN)	SHORT ACTING (10–20 MIN)	
Pancuronium	Vecuronium	Rapacuronium	
Pipecuronium	Rocuronium	Mivacurium	
d-Tubocurarine	Atracurium		
Metocurine	Cisatracurium		
Doxacurium			
Gallamine			
Alcuronium			

a duration of action of more than 50 minutes. Pancuronium does not produce muscle fasciculations, nor does it produce postanesthetic muscle pain. Unlike tubocurarine, pancuronium does not release histamine. The initial IV dose range is 0.04 to 0.1 mg/kg, with supplemental doses required for prolonged procedures. Small doses of pancuronium in patients with myasthenia gravis will produce profound effects.

Other nondepolarizing muscle relaxants include *metocurine, vecuronium, mivacurium, rocuronium,* and *atracurium.* The major advantage of these drugs is an elimination half-life shorter than the 2 hours possessed by pancuronium and d-tubocurarine. Vecuronium has an elimination half-life of 70 minutes, atracurium about 20 minutes.

Commonly used nondepolarizing muscle relaxants are listed by their duration of action in Table 31.1.

Succinylcholine (Anectine) is a synthetic, short-acting depolarizing muscle relaxant. After an IV dose of 60 to 80 mg (for a 70-kg patient), relaxation develops within 1 minute. Recovery of muscle tone is rapid and complete within 5 to 15 minutes. For children the usual dose for intubation is 20 mg. Succinylcholine is used routinely for skeletal muscle relaxation before tracheal intubation. It may also be used by continuous IV drip for relaxation during abdominal operations. Succinylcholine is used during electroconvulsive therapy (ECT) and as an emergency drug during the treatment of laryngospasm (see Chapter 27). Succinylcholine is contraindicated for use in patients with penetrating injuries of the eye and patients with myotonia.

Strong skeletal muscle contractions (fasciculations) are seen after the administration of succinylcholine. Patients receiving this drug may complain of severe muscle pain for several days after its administration. Fasciculations develop first in the eyebrow and eyelids, then in the shoulder girdle and abdominal muscles, and finally in the muscles of the hands and feet. The severity of fasciculations may be diminished by slow administration of the drug or by the prior administration of tubocurarine (3 to 6 mg) or pancuronium (0.5 to 1 mg).

Succinylcholine may produce hyperkalemia (succinylcholine-induced hyperkalemia), which in certain patients may lead to

cardiovascular collapse or cardiac arrest. At-risk patients include those with the following:
- Severe burns
- Massive trauma
- Tetanus
- Spinal cord injury
- Brain injury
- Uremia with increased serum potassium

Succinylcholine has been implicated as a trigger agent in malignant hyperthermia (MH). In MH-susceptible patients, succinylcholine administration is followed by exaggerated fasciculations, rigidity, and difficulty in intubation. Body temperature then increases at an alarming rate. Succinylcholine must not be administered to patients with a history of MH.

Metabolized in the serum by plasma pseudocholinesterase, succinylcholine is usually rapidly inactivated (muscle tonus returns to normal within 5 to 15 minutes). However, 1 in 3000 persons has atypical pseudocholinesterase and will exhibit a prolonged response to succinylcholine.[38] The presence of atypical pseudocholinesterase should be suspected in any patient in whom spontaneous respiration has not returned within 15 minutes after the administration of succinylcholine. Management of prolonged apnea requires continued controlled ventilation until spontaneous ventilation returns or until fresh-frozen plasma or blood is administered to restore the pseudocholinesterase level of the plasma.

Muscle relaxants are important adjuvants to general anesthesia. Their presence has permitted abdominal operations to be completed with much more ease and comfort for the patient, surgeon, and anesthesiologist alike. Their use, especially that of the longer-acting nondepolarizing muscle relaxants, is not recommended in outpatient procedures. Succinylcholine is used in outpatient procedures for intubation and in the emergency management of laryngospasm.

Inhalation Anesthetics

Inhalation anesthetics are very frequently used for producing general anesthesia. They are popular because of their controllability, which is based on the fact that their uptake and elimination are largely affected by pulmonary ventilation. The advantages of inhalation anesthetics are reviewed in Chapters 12 and 13.

The "ideal" inhalation anesthetic has not been found; however, volatile agents that approach the ideal are currently available. The following characteristics are desirable in an inhalation anesthetic:
1. The inhalation anesthetic should be either a gas or a liquid. If it is a gas, it should be easily liquefied at moderate pressures.
2. The blood–gas solubility coefficient (ratio) should be low (in the range of 0.3 to 2) so that a high partial pressure is obtained quickly in the alveoli. This will provide a rapid induction of anesthetic effect and an equally rapid elimination of the agent.

3. The oil–water solubility should also be low so that the drug is not stored in fat, thus avoiding prolonged recovery.
4. The inhalation anesthetic should be neither flammable nor explosive.
5. The inhalation anesthetic should be stable, not decomposing on exposure to moisture, light, or air. It should not corrode or react with rubber, plastic, metal, or carbon dioxide (CO_2) absorbers.
6. The inhalation anesthetic should have a pleasant odor, be nonirritating, and have minimal postanesthetic sequelae.
7. The inhalation anesthetic should be nontoxic to the organs and nonallergenic.
8. The inhalation anesthetic should be potent enough so that it provides good analgesia and anesthesia and so that at least 50% O_2 may be administered with it.
9. The inhalation anesthetic should be completely inert and excreted entirely unchanged through the lungs.

The physical and chemical characteristics of inhalation anesthetics currently used in general anesthesia are presented in Table 31.2. More commonly used inhalation anesthetics include N_2O, enflurane, isoflurane, desflurane, and sevoflurane. Other inhalation anesthetics, such as halothane, cyclopropane, chloroform, diethyl ether, divinyl ether, ethyl vinyl ether, fluroxene, methoxyflurane, and trichloroethylene, are no longer commonly used in general anesthesia.

Among the inhalation anesthetics that are in use today, N_2O is the most common. The pharmacology of this very important inhalation sedative and general anesthetic is presented in Chapter 13. The primary function of N_2O administration during general anesthesia is to potentiate the actions of other, more potent drugs (IV or inhalation) administered to produce a controlled state of unconsciousness. Its administration (along with O_2) permits a smaller dose or lesser concentration of the primary drug to be administered to produce the desired level of general anesthesia. For example, sevoflurane administered with O_2 alone may require a 2% concentration to produce surgical-depth anesthesia; however, with the administration of 60% N_2O, sevoflurane can effectively provide the same

depth of anesthesia at lower concentrations. With IV drug administration, the same is true.

Halothane was introduced into anesthesia practice in 1956 and had profound effects on the practice of anesthesia and surgery in that it was not flammable. This permitted the use of electrocautery by the surgeon and the introduction of extensive electronic monitoring by the anesthesiologist. Unlike ether, which preceded halothane, it permitted a rapid induction and emergence from anesthesia and also allowed rapid changes of anesthetic depth during surgery. With the introduction of newer inhalation anesthetics, halothane is used very rarely today. Minimum alveolar concentration (MAC), the concentration at which 50% of patients do not respond to surgical incision, is 0.75% for halothane.

Disadvantages of halothane include inducing myocardial depression; producing cardiac dysrhythmias (at higher concentrations), resulting in sensitization of the myocardium to the actions of catecholamines; acting as a potent uterine relaxant; and possibly producing shivering or tremor during recovery in patients whose body temperature is low. Probably the most serious disadvantage of halothane is possible hepatotoxicity. Reports also indicate that halothane may produce postanesthetic jaundice or disturbed liver function and even necrosis. The National Halothane Study concluded that if indeed halothane-induced hepatic necrosis occurs, it is rare.[39] Although most inhaled halothane is removed through the lungs, metabolites are slowly removed from the body over 2 to 3 weeks.

Enflurane (Ethrane) was synthesized in 1963 and has clinical and pharmacologic properties similar to those of halothane. Enflurane, however, has the advantage of compatibility with epinephrine, up to 10 mL of a 1:100,000 concentration, with a decreased risk of dysrhythmias developing.[40]

Advantages of enflurane include the following: it has a pleasant odor, there is rapid induction and recovery, it is nonirritating (produces no secretions), it is a bronchodilator and a good muscle relaxant, it keeps the cardiovascular system fairly stable (dysrhythmias are uncommon), it is not an emetic, it

	Partition Coefficient at 37°C		Minimum Alveolar	Inspired Concentrations (%)	
Agent	Fat-Blood*	Blood-Gas†	Concentration (MAC)‡ (%)	Induction	Maintenance
N_2O	2.3	0.47	105.0	75	50–70
Halothane	60	2.3	0.75	1–4	0.5–2.0
Enflurane	36	1.8	1.58	2–5	1.5–3.0
Isoflurane	45	1.4	1.28	1–4	0.8–2.0
Desflurane	27	0.42	4.6–6.0	—	—
Sevoflurane	48	0.59	1.71	—	—

Table 31.2   Characteristics of Inhalation Anesthetics

*Fat–blood partition coefficient—lower value, decreased lipid storage, and more rapid recovery.
†Blood–gas partition coefficient—lower value, rapid onset, and rapid recovery.
‡Minimum anesthetic concentration—gas concentration in alveoli, which, when in equilibrium with the CNS, causes 50% of individuals to move in response to painful cutaneous stimulation (in O_2).

is nonexplosive and nonflammable, and it is compatible with epinephrine. The MAC for enflurane is 1.58%, and anesthesia is induced at concentrations of 2% to 5% and maintained at concentrations of 1.5% to 3%.

Disadvantages of enflurane include the following: myocardial depression, progressive hypotension develops with increase in anesthetic depth, shivering may develop on emergence, the possibility of liver damage, and the production of CNS irritation at higher concentrations (especially if the patient is hypocarbic). In addition, enflurane should be avoided in patients with severely compromised renal function. Clinically, muscle twitching is noted in the jaw, neck, or extremities, and increased spike activity is noted on the EEG. Enflurane undergoes metabolism only to the extent of 2.5%, with the remainder excreted unchanged through the lungs. Enflurane is rarely used in the United States today.

Isoflurane (Forane), synthesized in 1970, is a chemical isomer of enflurane. No abnormal motor activity, such as muscle twitching or convulsions, is noted with isoflurane.

Advantages of isoflurane include a pleasant odor, rapid induction and recovery, is nonirritating (produces no secretions), is a bronchodilator, provides excellent muscle relaxation, keeps the cardiac rhythm stable, is compatible with epinephrine, is not an emetic, and is nonexplosive and nonflammable. The MAC for isoflurane is 1.28%; anesthesia is induced at concentrations of 1% to 4% and maintained at concentrations of 0.8% to 2%.

Disadvantages of isoflurane include production of myocardial depression, depressed blood pressure as the level of anesthesia is increased, postanesthetic shivering, the possibility for hepatotoxicity, and the inadvisability of administering isoflurane to patients with severely compromised renal function.

Sevoflurane (Sojourn, Ultane) is noted for its low solubility and rapid induction of and emergence from anesthesia. It is less irritating to the airway than many other inhalation anesthetics. The MAC for sevoflurane is 1.71%, and the concentration at which amnesia and loss of awareness occur (MAC awake) is 0.6%.

Sevoflurane is a commonly used inhalation anesthetic in ambulatory dental anesthesia cases.

Desflurane (Suprane) also possesses a low blood–gas partition coefficient, thereby producing a rapid onset of anesthesia and equally rapid recovery. Desflurane does not undergo biotransformation in the body. It is not recommended for the induction of anesthesia because of its unpleasant odor and airway irritant properties. Its principal advantage seems to be rapid patient emergence from anesthesia.[41] This may be a valuable property in busy surgical suites where a rapid turnover of patients is required and in surgical outpatients who would especially benefit from the rapid recovery of mental faculties.[42]

TECHNIQUES

Ideal Techniques

General anesthesia as administered to the hospitalized patient represents the fundamental technique from which the other forms of general anesthesia have developed. As a rule, this mode of anesthesia delivery is used in dentistry for the more severely medically compromised patient (ASA 3 or 4) and for patients undergoing extensive and possibly traumatic dental procedures.

A rapidly growing form of general anesthesia in dentistry is a hospital style of general anesthesia performed in the dental office on an outpatient basis. While numerous techniques for delivering general anesthesia exist, there is no "one size fits all" technique for its use. Many factors must go into the determination of which technique to utilize, including the length and invasiveness of the procedure, the patient's medical history, the preference of the dentist, and, importantly, the preference and expertise of the anesthesiologist.

The "ideal" anesthetic technique for an individual case is one that provides the 3 "A's"—anxiolysis, amnesia, and analgesia—meanwhile ensuring cardiovascular and respiratory stability. The anesthesiologist ideally should also have the ability to titrate the anesthetic and quickly and accurately alter the depth of anesthesia, providing a rapid and comfortable induction as well as a rapid, clean emergence. The patient will preferably have postoperative analgesia and no postoperative nausea and vomiting. The anesthesia provider's goal should be to maximize the benefit while minimizing the risk of each drug.

Preoperative Procedure

Before administering general anesthesia, the patient should be evaluated by the anesthesiologist. Additional consults, history and physical, laboratory tests, and test results may also be required. The decision to proceed will be determined by the anesthesiologist once he or she has sufficient information to make a sound clinical judgment.

Preceding the day of service, written preoperative instructions (including NPO instructions) must be provided to and well understood by the patient or parent/guardian. Once the treatment provider has all the necessary information, including information from pretreatment evaluations and information from consulted physicians and specialists, the patient must be involved in the informed consent process and should be educated on the potential risks and benefits.

Some patients benefit from premedication administered at home before arriving at the appointment. In this case, which is frequently experienced in young or uncooperative children or cases of extreme anxiety, the patient will be given a prescription for a benzodiazepine and instructed to take it one hour before arriving at the dental office.

Just before the procedure, the anesthesiologist must confirm NPO status and review medical records and consent forms. The patient should be free of makeup, jewelry, contact lenses, and removable dental prostheses. The anesthesiologist places monitoring devices: an ECG, pretracheal stethoscope, blood pressure cuff, capnograph, and pulse oximeter to acquire preoperative vitals. Baseline vital signs represent the starting point to monitor changing physiology throughout the anesthetic procedure. Vital signs are recorded on the anesthesia record.

Preinduction

In cases involving young, uncooperative children and special-needs patients, the anesthesiologist may opt for one of several preinduction methods before inducing general anesthesia. There are several methods of preinduction, with the end goal of each being to get the patient to a relaxed state in which an IV may be started without complication so that the administration of the anesthetic can proceed.

Intramuscular Ketamine

This preinduction technique requires the provider to administer IM ketamine into the upper arm or other large muscle (e.g., vastus lateralis). The injection is usually performed with the help of the parents and is about as invasive as a standard vaccination. It produces patient sedation and immobility, which can help facilitate separation from parents in pediatric patients to assist in IV placement.

Intramuscular Ketamine + Midazolam

The addition of midazolam to IM ketamine is commonplace in IM preinduction, as it provides amnesia, voiding memory of negative side effects produced by ketamine, such as confusion and agitation.

Intramuscular Ketamine + Midazolam + Anticholinergic

Supplementing the sedatives with an anticholinergic such as glycopyrrolate reduces excessive salivation and secretions, reducing the risk of laryngospasm. Anesthesiologists will sometimes withhold the anticholinergic in the IM injection and utilize it intravenously if needed.

Mask Induction of Sevoflurane

Inhalation induction is achieved via the patient breathing in sevoflurane through a face mask. A vaporizer is required, and additional costs and maintenance are associated with this technique, but many providers find that this method is preferable to their patients in terms of both pain avoidance and postoperative recovery time. Inhalation induction has a rapid onset and is effective in all patients. Anesthesiologists should be aware of the risks of malignant hypothermia associated with sevoflurane.

Premedication

Benzodiazepines such as midazolam can be utilized as a premedication to help aid in preinduction. These oral medications can be mixed with flavored syrup and given to pediatric patients in the waiting room before the appointment.

Induction

The induction phase of general anesthesia brings the pre-induced patient from a state of sedation to a general anesthesia state, either by switching to IV anesthesia or deepening their sedation with inhalation anesthetic. The specific techniques are discussed after the overview of airway management.

Airway Management

After general anesthesia is induced, the anesthesiologist must secure the airway before dental treatment begins. Several techniques are available depending on the patient's medical condition, length of case, preference of dentist, and comfort and expertise of the anesthesiologist. The anesthesiologist must exercise extreme diligence to ensure the airway remains patent and clear of foreign objects. With any airway technique, a partition must be in place to block any foreign object or fluid from getting into the lungs.

Nasopharyngeal Airway

An NPA is a tube that is designed to provide an airway passage from the nose to the posterior pharynx. NPAs can create a patent pathway and help avoid airway obstruction due to hypertrophic tissue. The NPA creates a patent airway throughout the distance of the tube. NPAs can be compromised if the nasal passage is narrow and collapses the inner diameter of the NPA and can also be occluded on the distal end. Patency is the primary goal of an NPA. Oxygenation can be improved by utilizing a nasal hood over an NPA. Oxygen can also be delivered by running a nasal cannula inside the NPA.

Intubation

When a patient is intubated, a tube is placed past the vocal cords. These tubes come in a variety of configurations.

Oral endotracheal tubes are designed to enter through the mouth and end just past the vocal cords in the trachea.

Nasal endotracheal tubes are designed to enter through the nose and end in the trachea. The lubricated nasotracheal tube is placed into a nostril and gently advanced into the nasopharynx (Fig. 31.17). The anesthesiologist visualizes the larynx and the tip of the tube using a laryngoscope. Sometimes Magill intubation forceps are used and the endotracheal tube is gently advanced and inserted into the trachea. Once inserted, the endotracheal tube is attached to the anesthesia machine, and the patient can be ventilated.

Both the oral and nasal endotracheal tubes come with the option of having a cuff at the end to seal off the trachea. A proper intubation will be free of any body fluids, tissue, or foreign material inside the tube. This will allow for the best possible patency for air to travel to the trachea.

Oxygen is delivered through the endotracheal tube typically by an anesthesia circuit that is connected to an anesthesia machine. Other forms of oxygen delivery can be accomplished through an endotracheal tube as they are with NPAs.

Laryngeal Mask Airway

LMAs are a type of supraglottic airway device. LMAs come in many different variations and have many different indications. They are well accepted as a means of establishing an emergency airway. Traditional LMAs occupy space in the oral cavity and

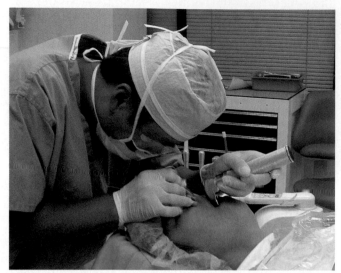

Figure 31.17 Nasoendotracheal tube is passed through the nostril and into nasopharynx. Magill intubation forceps assist in its passage into the trachea.

are not typically used for dental applications. Flexible LMAs provide a means of adjusting the tube and can be positioned out of the way of the working field for the dentist. Flexible LMAs can be utilized for many different types of dental procedures.

Anesthesia Maintenance

The maintenance phase of the anesthesia treatment begins once the patient is induced and the airway is secure. This is the phase of the treatment when the dentist can perform the required dental procedure. The goal in this phase is to achieve "balanced anesthesia" in which the drugs are titrated to the appropriate levels to ensure that the patient is not reactive to the stimuli of the procedure, but their vital signs remain stable. This is also known as the *therapeutic window*. The methods of anesthesia maintenance are primarily IV and inhalation, or a combination of the two.

TIVA is anesthesia delivered completely through the patient's IV. The drugs can either be infused or delivered manually. Infusion of drugs typically requires an infusion pump, lines, and ports to deliver the anesthetic at a constant, steady rate (Fig. 31.18). Manual delivery can be done with a bolus method and entails the anesthesiologist delivering a dose of the anesthetic at regular intervals into the patient's IV.

Inhalation anesthetic is delivered through a vaporizer. Different halogenated anesthetics are picked up through airflow and are adjustable by the percentage of halogenated gas that is desired. These anesthetic gases are then delivered to the patient.

Ending the Case

When the dentist has finished the treatment, the anesthesiologist can begin to conclude the anesthesia treatment. The anesthesiologist stops the administration of drugs and begins

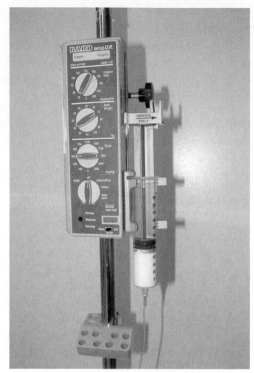

Figure 31.18 Infusion pump with propofol (or remifentanil or alfentanil).

to wean the patient. Return of consciousness is usually quite rapid. The anesthesiologist will determine when to discontinue utilizing the airway management technique that has been in place and will also determine when the patient is stable enough to transition to the recovery process. The patient should continue to be monitored for stability, and vital signs should be recorded. Once the patient has met the discharge criteria, he or she can be placed in the care of a responsible adult.

SUMMARY

The use of general anesthesia in dentistry dates to the origins of anesthesia itself. Dentists were intimately involved in the discovery of this valuable technique of pain and anxiety control and in many of its subsequent advances. Indeed, dentistry has been at the forefront in the recent evolution of outpatient general anesthesia.

General anesthesia is a technique that requires significantly greater training on the part of the dentist and staff for it to be used safely. Under no circumstances should a person without a minimum of 3 years of full-time training in anesthesiology or its equivalent in an oral and maxillofacial surgery training program ever consider the administration of general anesthesia.

The indications for general anesthesia in dentistry have diminished over the years as techniques of sedation have evolved. Yet many indications for its use remain. The selection of the most appropriate type of general anesthesia for use in a given patient must be made after a thorough evaluation of the patient's physical condition, the planned dental treatment, the training and background of the dentist and staff, and the preparedness of the facility.

REFERENCES

1. Rosenberg MB, Campbell RL: Guidelines for intraoperative monitoring of dental patients undergoing conscious sedation, deep sedation, and general anesthesia. *Oral Surg* 71:2, 1991.
2. Eichhorn JH, Cooper JB, Cullen DJ, et al: Anesthesia practice standards at Harvard: a review. *J Clin Anesth* 1(1):55–65, 1988.
3. Stanski DR, Shafer SL: Measuring depth of anesthesia. In Miller RD, Fleisher LA, Johns RA, et al, editors: *Miller's anesthesia*, ed 6, London, 2005, Churchill Livingstone.
4. California State Board of Dental Examiners: General anesthesia and conscious sedation, 2003, Extract from California Code of Regulations.
5. American Association of Oral and Maxillofacial Surgeons, Committee on Anesthesia: *Office anesthesia evaluation manual*, Rosemont, IL, 2006, The Association.
6. Bahn EL, Holt KR: Procedural sedation and analgesia: a review and new concepts. *Emerg Med Clin North Am* 23(2):503–517, 2005.
7. Gilman AG, Brunton LL, Lazo JS, et al: *Goodman and Gilman's the pharmacological basis of therapeutics*, ed 11, New York, 2008, McGraw-Hill.
8. Gaines GY, III, Rees DI: Anesthetic considerations for electroconvulsive therapy. *South Med J* 85:469, 1992.
9. Van Hemelrijck J, Gonzales JM, White PF: Pharmacology of intravenous anesthetic agents. In Rogers MC, Tinker JH, Covino BG, editors: *Principles and practice of anesthesiology*, St Louis, 1993, Mosby.
10. Eldor J: High-dose flunitrazepam anesthesia. *Med Hypotheses* 38:352, 1992.
11. Zelicof-Paul A, Smith-Lockridge A, Schnadower D, et al: Controversies in rapid sequence intubation in children. *Curr Opin Pediatr* 17(3):355–362, 2005.
12. Horrigan RW, Moyers JR, Johnson BH, et al: Etomidate vs thiopental with and without fentanyl, a comparative study of awakening in man. *Anesthesiology* 52(4):362–364, 1980.
13. Miller BM, Hendry JGB, Lees NW: Etomidate and methohexital, a comparative clinical study in outpatient anesthesia. *Anaesthesia* 33:450, 1978.
14. Waxman K, Shoemaker WC, Lipmann M: Cardiovascular effects of anesthetic induction with ketamine. *Anesth Analg* 59:355, 1980.
15. Tobias JD, Martin LD, Wetzel RC: Ketamine by continuous infusion for sedation in the pediatric intensive care unit. *Crit Care Med* 18:819, 1990.
16. Reich DL, Silvay G: Ketamine: an update on the first twenty-five years of clinical experience. *Can J Anaesth* 36:186, 1989.
17. Vanlersberghe C, Camu F: Propofol. *Handb Exp Pharmacol* 182:227–252, 2008.
18. Rutter DV, Morgan M, Lumley J, et al: ICI 35868 (Diprivan): a new intravenous induction agent. *Anaesthesia* 35(12):1188–1192, 1980.
19. Pecaro BC, Houting T: Diprivan (ICI 35868, 2,6-di-isopropylphenol), a new intravenous anesthetic. *Oral Surg* 60:586, 1985.
20. McCulloch MJ, Lees NW: Assessment and modification of pain on induction with propofol (Diprivan). *Anaesthesia* 40:1117, 1985.
21. Grounds RM, Twigley AJ, Carli F, et al: The haemodynamic effects of intravenous induction. Comparison of the effects of thiopentone and propofol. *Anaesthesia* 40(8):735–740, 1985.
22. McCollum JS, Dundee JW, Halliday NJ, Clarke RS: Dose response studies with propofol ('Diprivan') in unpremedicated patients. *Postgrad Med J* 61(Suppl 3):85–87, 1985.
23. Cundy JM, Arunasalam K: Use of an emulsion formulation of propofol (Diprivan) in intravenous anaesthesia for termination of pregnancy. A comparison with methohexitone. *Postgrad Med J* 61(Suppl 3):129, 1985.
24. Webb MD, Moore PA: Sedation for pediatric dental patients. *Dent Clin North Am* 46(4):803–814, xi, 2002.
25. Lysakowski C, Dumont L, Pellegrini M, et al: Effects of fentanyl, alfentanil, remifentanil and sufentanil on loss of consciousness and bispectral index during propofol induction of anaesthesia. *Br J Anaesth* 86(4):523–527, 2001.
26. Scholz J, Steinfath M, Schulz M: Clinical pharmacokinetics of alfentanil, fentanyl and sufentanil. An update. *Clin Pharmacokinet* 31(4):275–292, 1996.
27. Servin FS, Billard V: Remifentanil and other opioids. *Handb Exp Pharmacol* 182:283–311, 2008.
28. Richardson SP, Egan TD: The safety of remifentanil by bolus injection. *Expert Opin Drug Saf* 4(4):643–651, 2005.
29. Lefevre B, Freysz M, Lepine J, et al: Comparison of nalbuphine and fentanyl as intravenous analgesics for medically compromised patients undergoing oral surgery. *Anesth Prog* 39(1-2):13–18, 1992.
30. Elleby DH, Greenberg PM, Barry LD: Postoperative narcotic and nonnarcotic analgesics. *Clin Podiatr Med Surg* 9:365, 1992.
31. Fukuda K: Intravenous opioid anesthetics. In Miller RD, Fleisher LA, Johns RA, et al, editors: *Miller's anesthesia*, ed 6, Philadelphia, 2005, Churchill Livingstone.
32. Bremang JA: Neuroleptic analgesia in ambulatory (nasal) endoscopies. *J Otolaryngol* 20:435, 1991.
33. Snow JC: Intravenous anesthesia. In *Manual of anesthesia*, ed 2, Boston, 1982, Little, Brown.
34. Sinner B, Graf BM: Ketamine. *Handb Exp Pharmacol* 182:313–333, 2008.
35. Taylor PA, Towey RM: Depression of laryngeal reflexes during ketamine anaesthesia. *BMJ* 2:688–689, 1971.
36. Elia N, Tramer MR: Ketamine and postoperative pain—a quantitative systematic review of randomised trials. *Pain* 113(1-2):61–70, 2005.
37. Weerasekera DS, Gunawardene KK: Ketamine as an anaesthetic agent for tubal sterilisation. *Ceylon Med J* 41(3):102–103, 1996.
38. Schweinefus R, Schick L: Succinylcholine: "good guy, bad guy,". *J Post Anesth Nurs* 6:410, 1991.
39. Bunker JP, the National Research Council, Subcommittee on the National Halothane Study: The national halothane study: a study of the possible association between halothane anesthesia and postoperative hepatic necrosis: report, Bethesda, MD, 1969, National Institute of General Medical Science.
40. Ogawa A, Oi K: Use of N_2O/O_2 enflurane anesthesia for dental treatment of the handicapped. *J Oral Maxillofac Surg* 49:343, 1991.
41. Smiley RM, Ornstein E, Matteo RS, et al: Desflurane and isoflurane in surgical patients: comparison of emergence time. *Anesthesiology* 74(3):425–428, 1991.
42. Fletcher JE, Sebel PS, Murphy MR, et al: Psychomotor performance after desflurane anesthesia: a comparison with isoflurane. *Anesth Analg* 73(3):260–265, 1991.

Section VII

EMERGENCY PREPARATION AND MANAGEMENT

Chapter 32: Preparation for Emergencies

Chapter 33: Emergency Drugs and Equipment

Chapter 34: Management of Emergencies

Whenever drugs are administered or prescribed, adverse reactions may occur. Fortunately, with the vast majority of drugs currently used in the management of pain and anxiety, the incidence of adverse drug reactions (ADRs) is low. Indeed, those drugs that, although therapeutically useful, have a greater incidence of ADRs are rapidly replaced in the physician's and dentist's armamentarium by newer, equally useful drugs possessing a decreased risk of ADRs. The barbiturates are an example of such a group.

Indiscriminate drug usage is one of the major causes of the increase in the number of serious incidents of drug-related life-threatening emergencies that are reported in the medical and dental literature.[1,2] It is hoped that whenever a drug is administered or prescribed, a rational purpose exists for its administration. Most drug-related emergency situations are classified as one aspect of iatrogenic disease, a category encompassing a spectrum of adverse effects produced unintentionally by health care providers in the course of patient management.

The frequency of occurrence of ADRs as reported in the medical and dental literature has ranged from 3% to 20% of all hospital admissions.[1-5] Of patients hospitalized for other reasons, 5% to 40% will experience an ADR during their hospitalization. Furthermore, another 10% to 18% of those patients hospitalized because of an ADR will have yet another ADR while in the hospital, which results in increased length of hospitalization.[4] Additionally, more than 100,000 patients die each year as a result of ADRs while hospitalized (in U.S. hospitals).[6]

Because the overwhelming majority of drugs discussed in this text are central nervous system (CNS) depressants administered to patients for the purpose of managing their treatment-related fears and anxieties, it is likely that ADRs will be noted at some time. For this reason, the dentist and the entire office staff must be able to recognize and be prepared to manage these situations rapidly and effectively.

This section is divided into three chapters. The first two chapters discuss the subject of preparation: of the office, office personnel, and the requirement for emergency drugs and equipment. The third chapter reviews the management of systemic emergencies that might arise during sedation procedures. Localized complications have been reviewed with each of the major techniques of sedation (see Chapter 10 for intramuscular sedation, Chapter 16 for inhalation sedation, and Chapter 27 for intravenous sedation).

The need for emergency preparedness exists in a dental or medical practice, regardless of whether sedative techniques are used. Indeed, as discussed in Chapter 4, the medically compromised patient who is fearful or experiences unexpected pain during treatment is more likely to suffer an acute exacerbation of his or her medical problem at this time than is the relaxed, pain-free patient with the same medical problem. In one report, 77% of systemic emergencies associated with dental care occurred either during or immediately after the administration of local anesthetic (54.9%) or during the ensuing dental treatment (22.9%), arguably the most psychologically and physiologically stressful portions of the entire dental experience.[7] The types of dental treatment most frequently taking place at the time the systemic emergency occurred were tooth extraction and pulpal extirpation, procedures in which complete pain control may prove elusive.[7]

Occurrence of Systemic Complications	
Just before treatment	1.5%
During or after local anesthesia	54.9%
During treatment*	22.9%
After treatment	15.2%
After leaving office	5.5%
*See next box for specific treatment during emergency.	

Basic preparation of the dental or medical office and office staff is the same whether or not sedative techniques are used. There are, however, a number of drugs and items of emergency equipment that the dentist using sedation techniques will have available that are unnecessary in the offices of dentists not using sedation. Emergency equipment is reviewed along with the components of the basic emergency kit.

Type of Dental Treatment During Occurrence of Systemic Complication	
Tooth extraction	38.9%
Pulpal extirpation	26.9%
Unknown	12.3%
Other treatment	9.0%
Preparation	7.3%
Filling	2.3%
Incision	1.7%
Apicoectomy	0.7%
Removal of fillings	0.7%
Alveolar plastics	0.3%

Most, but not all, drug-related emergencies can be prevented. The dentist administering or prescribing drugs for a patient must always keep the following three principles of toxicology in mind[8]:
1. No drug ever exerts a single action.
2. No clinically useful drug is entirely devoid of toxicity.
3. Potential toxicity of a drug rests in the hands of the user.

Ideally the right drug in the right dose will be administered by the right route to the right patient at the right time for the right reason and will not produce any unwanted effects.[8] Unfortunately, this clinical situation rarely, if ever, exists because no drug is so specific that it produces only desirable effects in all patients. It must also be remembered that ADRs may occur when the wrong drug is administered to the wrong patient in the wrong dose by the wrong route at the wrong time and for the wrong reason. The most important safety factors in drug administration are the knowledge and ability of the person administering the drug. Before administering any drug, the dentist should be fully prepared to manage any ADR that might develop.

REFERENCES

1. Gomes ER, Demoly P: Epidemiology of hypersensitivity drug reactions. *Curr Opin Allergy Clin Immunol* 5(4):309–316, 2005.
2. Demoly P, Bousquet J: Epidemiology of drug allergy. *Curr Opin Allergy Clin Immunol* 1(4):305–310, 2001.
3. Lundkvist J, Jonsson B: Pharmacoeconomics of adverse drug reactions. *Fundam Clin Pharmacol* 18(3):275–280, 2004.
4. Bates DW, Leape LL, Petrycki S: Incidence and preventability of adverse drug events in hospitalized adults. *J Gen Intern Med* 8(6):289–294, 1993.
5. Boeker EB, Ram K, Klopotowska JE, et al: An individual patient data meta-analysis on factors associated with adverse drug events in surgical and non-surgical inpatients. *Br J Clin Pharmacol* 79(4):548–557, 2015.
6. Bond CA, Raehl CL: Adverse drug reactions in United States hospitals. *Pharmacotherapy* 26(5):601–608, 2006.
7. Matsuura H: Analysis of systemic complications and death during dental treatment in Japan. *Anesth Prog* 36(4-5):223–225, 1989.
8. Pallasch TJ: *Pharmacology for dental students and practitioners*, Philadelphia, 1980, Lea & Febiger.

chapter 32

Preparation for Emergencies

CHAPTER OUTLINE

OFFICE
OFFICE PERSONNEL
  Basic Life Support
  Advanced Cardiovascular Life Support
  Pediatric Advanced Life Support

Team Approach to Emergency
  Management
EMERGENCY PRACTICE DRILLS
OUTSIDE MEDICAL ASSISTANCE

Although the prevention of life-threatening emergencies is always our primary goal, potentially catastrophic situations will develop in spite of our best efforts. With proper patient evaluation before the start of any treatment, appropriate treatment modification if necessary, selection of appropriate techniques and drugs for pain and anxiety control, adherence to proper technique of drug administration, and adequate monitoring throughout the procedure, it is unlikely that serious emergency situations will arise. However, in the event that an emergency does occur, it becomes extremely important for the dental office to be properly prepared and for all office personnel to be trained to recognize and manage such situations in a prompt and effective manner. Box 32.1 summarizes the suggested preparation of the medical or dental office and staff for emergency situations.

OFFICE

With all office personnel trained to recognize and manage life-threatening situations, it should be possible for each one of them to maintain the life of a victim alone or as a member of a trained dental office emergency team. Although management of most emergencies is possible with but a single rescuer, the concerted efforts of a team of trained persons are more efficient. Because most dental and medical offices have numerous staff persons present during working hours, organization of a team approach to emergency management is possible.

OFFICE PERSONNEL

An important factor in preparation of the medical or dental office for management of emergency situations will be the training of *all* office personnel, including non-chairside personnel, in their recognition and management. Training should include an annual refresher course in all aspects of emergency medicine—a course reviewing situations such as seizures, chest pain, unconsciousness, altered consciousness, drug-related emergencies, and respiratory difficulty, not simply basic life support (BLS). Continuing education programs on emergency medicine are available through local, state, and national dental organizations. In a dental office in which sedation is used, refresher courses in these techniques, including their complications, are also recommended. In some states and provinces, dental regulatory bodies make continuing dental education refresher courses in sedation mandatory for permit holders.

Basic Life Support

Of even greater importance than the overall emergency review program is the requirement for the clinical ability to perform BLS, commonly known as *cardiopulmonary resuscitation* (CPR). It is my opinion that no other preparatory step is as important as this one because training in BLS enables a rescuer to recognize an acute life-threatening situation and to know what to do. The steps of BLS require no additional equipment*: the mouth, hands, and knowledge of the rescuer are quite adequate in most cases to maintain a life. In the presence of a drug-related emergency, BLS usually proves to be the first and most important step in management. The acronym PCABD, where P is position, C is circulation, A is airway, B is breathing, and D is definitive

---

*Though no equipment is required for the provision of BLS, health care providers, especially dentists, should be trained to provide rescue breathing (ventilation) using a mask or other barrier device.

care (D also means: Diagnosis, Drugs, Defibrillation), forms the basis of life support and management of all medical emergency situations. The Australian Resuscitation Council (ARC)'s acronym for health care providers is DRSABCD, where D is danger, R is response, and D is defibrillation[1] (Box 32.2).

The dentist should mandate that *all* office personnel remain proficient in BLS techniques after receiving their initial course. There is a rapid decline in CPR skills following an initial BLS training program. Within 6 months of completing a provider-level training program, the average person loses approximately 60% of his or her ability to perform adequate BLS.[2] In a clinical experiment, only 4 of 30 postdoctoral dentists (graduate students), who had been retrained in BLS within the previous 4 months, were able to perform adequate one-person CPR on a mannequin for 1 minute.[3] Maintaining proficiency is important because even when BLS is performed perfectly (a rarely achieved goal), the delivery of oxygenated blood to the victim's brain is only 25% to 33% of normal.[4] Faulty CPR technique leads to diminished cerebral blood flow and to a decreased likelihood of survival, with or without permanent neurologic damage.

If a dentist, assistant, or hygienist was in a dental office with only one other person present and was the victim of cardiac arrest, this second person would be the only one available to provide BLS. *Making certain that **all** personnel are proficient in BLS thus becomes the single most important step in ensuring that medical emergencies are managed efficiently and effectively.*

Advanced Cardiovascular Life Support

Advanced cardiovascular life support (ACLS) involves the use of adjunctive equipment and drugs to further stabilize and manage a victim of cardiac arrest or other serious cardiac rhythm disturbance. The ACLS course includes training and evaluation in techniques of venipuncture and endotracheal intubation, interpretation of electrocardiograph (ECG) rhythms, and management of cardiac dysrhythmias through drug therapy and defibrillation.[5]

Dentists using intravenous (IV) sedation might consider training in ACLS. Many jurisdictions are now mandating ACLS as a requirement for issuing a permit for parenteral sedation (IV, intramuscular [IM], intranasal [IN]).[6] With availability of the IV route of drug administration, an ACLS-trained dentist becomes better able to manage such situations. It is my strongly held conviction that dentists trained in deep sedation or general anesthesia should be experienced in ACLS. Provider-level programs in ACLS are available in most areas to eligible persons. These include the physician, nurse, pharmacist, and dentist who have previously been trained in BLS. In some jurisdictions, paramedical personnel are ACLS trained. ACLS programs are usually presented within a hospital under the auspices of the American Heart Association (AHA). Contact your local AHA affiliate for more information about these courses. The American Dental Society of Anesthesiology has developed a course in airway management for the dental profession.[7]

Pediatric Advanced Life Support

The dentist called on to manage the dental needs of younger children (up to 30 kg) should give serious consideration to becoming trained in pediatric advanced life support (PALS). PALS training includes the following components: BLS (infant and child); use of adjunctive equipment and special techniques to establish and maintain effective oxygenation, ventilation, and perfusion; clinical and ECG monitoring and dysrhythmia detection; establishment and maintenance of vascular access; identification and treatment of reversible causes of cardiopulmonary arrest; therapies for emergency treatment of patients with cardiac and respiratory arrest; and treatment of patients with trauma, shock, respiratory failure, or other prearrest conditions.[8]

Team Approach to Emergency Management

A dental office emergency team consists of two or three members, each of whom has a well-defined role in the management of an emergency situation. The dentist normally directs the team and is the person responsible for monitoring the activities of its other members (unless it is the dentist who is the victim of the emergency). In most situations, the dentist will be responsible for implementing the steps of BLS (P → C → A → B) and will administer emergency drugs (D) to the victim, where indicated.

Member 1 of the team is the first person at the scene of the emergency. Functions of member 1 include (1) staying with the victim (do not leave a person alone during a medical emergency [unless it is absolutely necessary]); (2) "call" for help (activate the dental office emergency team); and (3) provide BLS, as required.

Member 2 of the team is responsible for the maintenance of emergency drugs and equipment. The emergency drug kit and equipment should be checked regularly to ensure that they will be available and fully stocked when needed (see Chapter 33). When an emergency situation does arise, member 2 gathers the emergency kit and equipment (e.g., portable O_2 cylinder and automated external defibrillator [AED]) and immediately brings them to the site of the emergency. Should emergency drugs be required, this team member readies the drugs for administration by the dentist. Other possible roles for member 2 include assisting with BLS, monitoring vital signs, and summoning of medical assistance. In BLS, this team member will be an integral part of the emergency management and will ventilate the victim and/or perform chest compression.

Member 3. A third team member may be used when available. This member reports immediately to the site of the emergency and remains available as a circulating member, assisting as required. Roles for this member include monitoring vital signs, summoning medical assistance (e.g., 911), administering BLS, and keeping records. Member 3 remains available to assist other team members as needed.

If the dental office is located in a large, high-rise multioffice building, a team member is directed to the lobby to ensure that an elevator is readily available for the emergency medical services (EMS) team (emergency medical technicians [EMTs] or paramedics) and to expeditiously lead the EMS team to the proper location.

It is important that all office personnel be capable of participating in the emergency team. In addition, all team members should be able to carry out any of the functions of the entire team. Practice thus becomes vitally important. Box 32.3 summarizes preparation of the dental office, as well as the role of each member of the dental office emergency team.[9]

EMERGENCY PRACTICE DRILLS

If life-threatening situations occurred with more frequency in medical and dental offices, there would be little need for

---

Box 32.3	**Preparation of the Dental Office and Staff for Medical Emergencies**

Basic Life Support
Annually
BLS for health care providers
All dental office employees
In the dental office
Ventilate mouth to mask, *not* mouth to mouth

Dental Office Emergency Team
Member #1
First on scene of emergency
Stay with victim; yell for "help"; administer BLS, as needed
Member #2, on hearing call for "help" …
Obtains (1) emergency drug kit, (2) portable O_2 cylinder, and (3) AED and brings to site of emergency
Member #3, #4, and on …
Assigned ancillary tasks such as:
- Monitoring vital signs (BP, heart rate and rhythm)
- Assisting with BLS
- Activating EMS (911)
- Keeping elevator available in lobby while awaiting arrival of EMS
- Preparing emergency drugs for administration
- Keeping written timeline record during emergency

Doctor remains the "responsible" party during management of medical emergencies.
Tasks can be delegated.
Office personnel should be interchangeable during emergency management.

Activation of EMS
When: As soon as you, the doctor, think it is necessary: for example (1) unable to make a diagnosis, (2) know the diagnosis but are uncomfortable with it (e.g., cardiac arrest), and (3) whenever you think EMS is warranted.
DO NOT HESITATE TO ACTIVATE EMS, if you feel it is needed.
Whom to call: 911 or a nearby physician or dentist *if* you know beforehand that they are well trained in the management of emergency situations.

From Malamed SF. Medical emergencies: preparation and management. MetLife Quality Resource Guide, ed 4. October 2016. www.metdental.com. Accessed January 19, 2017.

emergency practice sessions. Team members would receive their training under actual emergency conditions. Fortunately, life-threatening situations do not occur with any degree of frequency. Because of this, skills in emergency management are quickly lost as a result of the lack of opportunity to use this newly acquired knowledge.[3] Annual refresher courses in emergency medicine are invaluable in maintaining the level of overall knowledge of the emergency team members.

Of greater importance, however, is the team's ability to perform well in the dental office setting. In-office emergency drills are a means of maintaining an efficient emergency team in the absence of true emergency situations. On an irregular basis, the dentist may stage a simulated life-threatening emergency. All team members should be able to respond exactly as they must under emergency conditions. Many dentists have purchased mannequins (CPR "dummies") for practicing BLS and hold frequent practice sessions for their staff.

Oral and maxillofacial surgeons have devised a system of in-office evaluation for general anesthetic technique and emergency preparedness. A group of examiners (other oral surgeons) assesses the preparedness of the oral surgery office by staging mock emergencies (e.g., laryngospasm, cardiac arrest, bronchospasm) and viewing the office staff's response.[10] Created by the Southern California Society of Oral and Maxillofacial Surgeons, the in-office evaluation has become a requirement for membership in the American Association of Oral and Maxillofacial Surgeons. Similar programs have been instituted by dental boards of most of the states that require a dentist to obtain a permit to use general anesthesia or parenteral sedation.[11]

OUTSIDE MEDICAL ASSISTANCE

Although most emergency situations are transient in nature and easily managed by the dental office emergency team (e.g., syncope, bronchospasm, angina), occasions may arise in which outside medical assistance is desired. In situations involving adverse drug reactions following the administration of CNS depressants, follow-up evaluation by well-trained medical professionals may be desired. For these reasons, telephone numbers of emergency services personnel should be readily available and conspicuously posted by each telephone in the office. It is strongly suggested that the following telephone numbers be programmed into a telephone's speed-dial system:
- Local EMS (i.e., 911)
- A *well-trained* (in emergency management) dental or medical colleague
- Emergency ambulance service with BLS-trained or BLS- and ACLS-trained personnel
- An AHA-approved hospital emergency room

Most communities in the United States have instituted the universal (in many, but not all countries [Table 32.1]) emergency telephone number, 911, to expedite activation of their EMS. This number immediately connects the caller to the rescue service (usually fire, police, and medical). When emergency

Table 32.1	Samples of Emergency Medical Services
REGION	**EMS ACCESS NUMBER**
Africa	
Egypt	123
Ghana	999
Kenya	112 or 999
South Africa	10 177
Asia	
Bahrain, Hong Kong, Malaysia	999
People's Republic of China	120
India, Kuwait, United Arab Emirates	112
Indonesia	118
Iran, Vietnam	115
Israel	101
Japan, Republic of Korea, Republic of China (Taiwan)	119
Philippines	117
Saudi Arabia	112 or 911
Singapore	995
Thailand	1669
Europe	
Common number	112
Ireland, United Kingdom	112 or 999
Norway	113
Oceania	
Australia	000
Guam	911
New Zealand	111
North America	
Common number	911
Cuba	104
Mexico	066
Guatemala	128
El Salvador	132
Haiti	116
Jamaica	110
Panama	911
Puerto Rico	911
South America	
Argentina, Bolivia, Ecuador, Paraguay, Peru, Uruguay, Venezuela	911
Brazil	192
Chile	131
Columbia	123

medical assistance is required in the dental office, the community EMS is normally the preferred source of immediate assistance. In an unlikely situation where 911 is unavailable in a community, the seven-digit telephone number should be conspicuously posted and programmed into the telephone.

A *well-trained* (in emergency care) dental or medical colleague can also serve as a source of emergency medical assistance. It is important, however, to discuss this arrangement before its actual need. The dentist seeking assistance must be absolutely certain that the person called is well versed in emergency management and is likely to be available during usual office hours. In dental offices where more than one well-trained dentist is usually present, such a system is easily adopted. It has been my experience that those individuals with the best training in emergency medicine are emergency medicine physicians, anesthesiologists, surgeons (physicians), and oral and maxillofacial surgeons (dentists). Unfortunately for the dentist or physician working in a private dental practice, the first two groups are normally hospital based and thus are not readily available to the non–hospital-based dental practitioner. A surgeon (MD) or an oral and maxillofacial surgeon (DDS, DMD) may be more readily available in this nonhospital setting. Prior arrangement with these persons will prevent potential misunderstandings and increase their effectiveness in emergency situations.

Most emergency ambulance services require their personnel to be trained as EMTs who are capable of providing BLS. This may serve as an alternative source of basic assistance should other rescuers be unavailable. Ambulances staffed with paramedics are capable of providing both BLS and ACLS.

The location of a hospital close to your office that maintains a 24-hour emergency room staffed with fully trained emergency personnel should be determined in the unlikely event that a victim requires transport to that facility for evaluation or management. The AHA evaluates and certifies those emergency rooms that meet their rigid criteria.

SUMMARY

Adequate training of all members of the dental office staff is essential if potentially life-threatening situations are to be adequately managed. Preparation of the staff must occur before emergencies occur. The recommended steps in preparing both the office staff and the office for such situations have been discussed. In the following two chapters, the components of the emergency drug kit and emergency equipment are reviewed, as is the management of specific emergency situations related to drug administration.

REFERENCES

1. Australian Resuscitation Council: Section 8, Cardiopulmonary resuscitation, Melbourne, Australia, January, 2016, Royal Australasian College of Surgeons. http://resus.org.au/guidelines/. (Accessed 19 January 2017).
2. Bhanji F, Donoghue AJ, Wolff MS, et al: Part 14: education: 2015 American Heart Association Guidelines Update for Cardiopulmonary Resuscitation and Emergency Cardiovascular Care. *Circulation* 132(Suppl 2):S561–S573, 2015.
3. Malamed SF: Unpublished data, Dec 2000.
4. Paradis NA, Martin GB, Goetting MG, et al: Simultaneous aortic, jugular bulb, and right atrial pressures during cardiopulmonary resuscitation in humans: insight into mechanisms. *Circulation* 80:361–368, 1989.
5. Link MS, Berkow LC, Kudenchuk PJ, et al: Part 7: adult advanced cardiovascular life support: 2015 American Heart Association Guidelines Update for Cardiopulmonary Resuscitation and Emergency Cardiovascular Care. *Circulation* 132(Suppl 2):S444–S464, 2015.
6. Boynes SG: *Dental anesthesiology: a guide to the rules and regulations of the United States of America*, ed 4, Chicago, 2011, No-No Orchard Publishing.
7. American Dental Society of Anesthesiology: Sim-Man high fidelity human simulation. www.adsahome.org. (Accessed 16 April 2016).
8. de Caen AR, Berg MD, Chameides L, et al: Part 12: pediatric advanced life support: 2015 American Heart Association Guidelines Update for Cardiopulmonary Resuscitation and Emergency Cardiovascular Care. *Circulation* 132(Suppl 2):S526–S542, 2015.
9. Malamed SF: *Medical emergencies: preparation and management. MetLife Quality Resource Guide*, ed 4, October 2016. www.metdental.com. (Accessed 19 January 2017).
10. American Association of Oral and Maxillofacial Surgeons, Committee on Anesthesia: *Office anesthesia evaluation manual*, ed 8, Rosemont, IL, 2012, The Association.
11. American Dental Association: Department of State and Government Affairs, 30b. Conscious sedation permit requirement. September 2, 2009, The Association. Chicago, IL. http://www.ada.org/~/media/ADA/Advocacy/Files/anesthesia_sedation_permit.ashx. (Accessed 19 January 2017).

chapter 33

Emergency Drugs and Equipment

CHAPTER OUTLINE

LEVEL 1: BASIC EMERGENCY KIT
    Injectable Drugs
    Noninjectable Drugs
    Primary (Basic) Emergency Equipment
LEVEL 2: SECONDARY (NONCRITICAL) DRUGS AND EQUIPMENT
    Injectable Drugs

    Noninjectable Drugs
    Secondary (Advanced) Emergency
      Equipment
LEVEL 3: ADVANCED CARDIAC LIFE SUPPORT
LEVEL 4: ANTIDOTAL DRUGS

Emergency drugs and equipment must be available in every medical and dental office regardless of whether or not sedation and/or general anesthetic techniques are used. Although successful resolution of most emergency situations does not require drug administration, on occasion drug administration may prove to be lifesaving. In the anaphylactic reaction, for example, prompt administration of epinephrine is crucial. In most other emergencies, however, drug administration is consigned to a secondary role in overall management. In situations in which adverse drug reactions (ADRs) develop following administration of drugs for sedation or pain control, it may be possible in some cases to significantly improve the clinical picture through the administration of an antidotal drug.

The emergency drug kit is designed in four levels (modules). Module 1, the "bare bones" basic emergency kit, contains drugs and equipment that this author believes should be available in the offices of all practicing dentists and physicians regardless of whether sedative techniques are used. Module 2 consists of drugs that are "nice to have" but are not as essential as those in level 1. Module 3 drugs are recommended for dentists who have received advanced cardiovascular life support (ACLS) training, and module 4 contains drugs required for the management of ADRs associated with parenteral drug administration.[1]

The emergency kit need not and, indeed, should not be overly complex. As Pallasch[2] has stated, "Complexity in a time of adversity breeds chaos."

Because the level of training in emergency management of health care providers can vary significantly, it is impossible to recommend any one list of emergency drugs or any one proprietary emergency drug kit that meets the needs and abilities of all dentists. For this reason, dentists should develop their own emergency drug and equipment kits based on their level of expertise in managing medical emergencies.[3]

The emergency drug kit maintained by the dentist using sedation or general anesthesia will, of necessity, include drugs and equipment not recommended for emergency kits of dentists who are not well trained in anesthesia (used in its broadest sense). The Council on Dental Therapeutics of the American Dental Association, most state dental boards, and specialty organizations have developed and published either recommendations or requirements for the inclusion of specific emergency drugs and equipment for offices in which sedation or general anesthesia is to be administered[4–6] (Box 33.1). In 2010 Massachusetts became the first state to mandate that all dental offices maintain certain emergency drugs and equipment (Box 33.2).[7] West Virginia followed in 2015.[8]

A plastic container or fishing tackle box may be used to store drugs. A more inclusive emergency kit might be developed from a mobile tool chest. Labels are applied to each container with both the generic and proprietary name of the drug and its dosage (e.g., midazolam, 5 mg/mL). The emergency kit must be maintained in an area where it is readily accessible. All emergency drugs and equipment should be checked weekly and replenished before their expiration dates; the oxygen (O_2)

Box 33.1   Suggested Emergency Equipment and Drugs

Suggested Equipment

A. Source of O_2 and equipment to deliver positive-pressure ventilation

B. Respiratory support equipment
- Oral airways and nasal airways
- Endotracheal tubes with stylets (provision for children's airway management)
- Laryngoscope and suitable blades (plus extra bulbs and batteries)
- McGill forceps or other suitable instruments
- Cricothyrotomy set with connector
- Laryngeal mask airway

C. Stethoscope or precordial stethoscope

D. Blood pressure cuff or automatic blood pressure monitor

E. ECG, defibrillator, and automated external defibrillator

F. Pulse oximeter and end-tidal carbon dioxide monitor (if intubated anesthesia is used)

G. Equipment to establish IV infusion
- Angiocaths, needles, syringes, IV sets, and connectors
- Tourniquets for venipuncture
- Tape

Suggested Drugs

The following are examples of drugs that will be helpful in the treatment of anesthetic emergencies. The list should not be considered mandatory or all-inclusive.

A. IV fluids
- Sterile water for injection and/or mixing or dilution of drugs
- Appropriate IV fluids

B. Cardiotonic drugs
- O_2
- Epinephrine 1 mg (10 mL of a 1:10,000 solution)
- Atropine 0.4 mg/mL
- Nitroglycerin (0.4 mg: $\frac{1}{150}$ grain)

C. Vasopressors
- Dopamine 200 mg/5 mL
- Epinephrine 1:1000 or 1:10,000 (1 mg = 1:1000)
- Dobutamine 1, 2, or 4 mg/mL
- Ephedrine 50 mg/mL
- Phenylephrine (Neo-Synephrine) 10 mg/mL

D. Antiarrhythmic agents
- Atropine sulfate 0.4 mg/mL
- Lidocaine 2% (Xylocaine) 20 mg/mL
- Propranolol (Inderal) 1 mg/mL
- Procainamide (Procanbid) 100 mg/mL
- Verapamil (Calan) 5 mg/mL
- Amiodarone (Cordarone et al) 50 mg/mL
- Adenosine 3 mg/mL

E. Antihypertensive agents (immediate)
- Diazoxide (Hyperstat) 15 mg/mL
- Hydralazine (Apresoline) 20 mg/mL
- Esmolol (Brevibloc) 10 mg/mL
- Labetalol (Trandate) 5 mg/mL (20 mL single-dose vial)

F. Diuretics
- Furosemide (Lasix) 10 mg/mL

G. Antiemetics
- Prochlorperazine (Compazine) 5 mg/mL
- Ondansetron (Zofran) 2 mg/mL

H. Reversing agents
- Naloxone (Narcan) 0.4 mg/mL
- Flumazenil (Romazicon) 0.1 mg/mL

I. Additional drugs
- Dextrose 50%
- Hydrocortisone sodium succinate or methylprednisolone sodium succinate (Solu-Medrol) 125 mg
- Dexamethasone (Decadron) 4 mg/mL
- Glycopyrrolate (Robinul) 0.2 mg/mL
- Diazepam (Valium) 5 mg/mL
- Diphenhydramine (Benadryl) 50 mg/mL
- Albuterol (Ventolin) inhaler
- Midazolam (Versed) 5 mg/mL
- Succinylcholine (Anectine) 20 mg/mL
- Morphine sulfate 5 mg/mL
- Dantrolene (Dantrium) 20-mg vials, readily available (36 vials)
- Procaine 10 mg/mL
- Nonenteric aspirin 160 to 325 mg

From American Association of Oral and Maxillofacial Surgeons, Committee on Anesthesia: Office anesthesia evaluation manual, *ed 8, Rosemont, IL, 2012, The Association.*

cylinder should be checked daily. A written record should be kept of these inspections.

The following are guidelines for the development of an office emergency kit. Categories of drugs are listed with a suggestion for specific drug(s) within each grouping. Space precludes lengthy descriptions of the rationale for selecting each drug. Readers desiring more in-depth information are referred to appropriate textbooks.[1,3]

Each of the drug categories presented should be considered for inclusion in the emergency kit; however, dentists should

Box 33.2	Mandatory Emergency Drugs and Equipment – Massachusetts (Effective – 2010)

234 CMR

6.15: Administration of Local Anesthesia Only

(1) Scope of Practice.
  (a) A dentist licensed to practice dentistry may administer local anesthesia under the authority of his or her dental license. The administering dentist shall be currently certified in Basic Life Support (BLS).
  (b) The Board may issue qualified dental hygienists, licensed pursuant to M.G.L. c. 112, § 51, a Permit L which authorizes the holder to administer local anesthesia under the direct supervision of a licensed dentist.
(2) Equipment and Supplies Required. The following equipment and drugs are required where local anesthesia is administered:
  (a) Alternative light source for use during power failure;
  (b) Automated External Defibrillator (AED);
  (c) Disposable CPR masks (pediatric and adult);
  (d) Disposable syringes, assorted sizes;
  (e) Disposable pediatric and adult face masks or positive pressure ventilation with supplemental oxygen;
  (f) Oxygen (portable Cylinder E tank) pediatric and adult masks capable of giving positive pressure ventilation (including bag-valve-mask system);
  (g) Sphygmomanometer and stethoscope for pediatric and adult patients;
  (h) Suction; and
  (i) And any other equipment as may be required by the Board.
(3) Drugs Required. The following drugs and/or categories of drugs shall be provided and maintained in accordance with the AHA/ACLS Guidelines (234 CMR 6.02) or as determined by the Board for emergency use. All drugs shall be current and not expired
  (a) Acetylsalicylic acid (readily absorbable form);
  (b) Ammonia inhalants;
  (c) Antihistamine;
  (d) Antihypoglycemic agent;
  (e) Bronchodilator;
  (f) Epinephrine preloaded syringes (pediatric and adult);
  (g) Two epinephrine ampules;
  (h) Oxygen;
  (i) Vasodilator; and
  (j) Any other drugs or categories of drugs as may be required by the Board.

From Board of Registration in Dentistry. 234 CMR 6.00: Administration of anesthesia and sedation. Section 6.15: Administration of Local Anesthesia Only. Massachusetts Court System. http://www.mass.gov/courts/docs/lawlib/230-249cmr/234cmr6.pdf. Accessed April 18, 2016.

select only those drugs with which they are familiar because they are responsible for having the ability to use each and every one of them. The dentist must carefully evaluate everything that goes into their emergency kit. All drugs come with a "drug package insert" (DPI). The DPI should be saved and read, with important information concerning each drug noted, such as usual dose, contraindications, adverse reactions, and its expiration date. Two categories of drugs, injectables and noninjectables, are included in the emergency kit. Items of emergency equipment also have a very definite place in the management of life-threatening situations. As with drugs, however, it is important for a dentist to know his or her limitations when it comes to using this equipment. Improper use of emergency equipment may further complicate an already tenuous situation. There are two categories of emergency equipment: primary, or basic, equipment, which I believe should be available in every medical and dental office; and secondary, or advanced, equipment, for those persons who have received training and are experienced in its use.

Merely having items of emergency equipment available does not in and of itself make the office better equipped or the staff more prepared to manage emergency situations. Personnel expected to use emergency equipment must be trained in emergency management and in the proper use of these items. Unfortunately, many emergency devices commonly found in dental and medical offices can prove to be useless or, more significantly, hazardous if used improperly or in the wrong situation. Training in the use of some items, such as the laryngoscope and oropharyngeal airway, may best be obtained only by caring for patients under general anesthesia, a situation usually not readily available. Many items of emergency equipment listed in this section are therefore recommended for use only by trained personnel. All secondary equipment falls into this category; unfortunately, several items listed as primary are also included (e.g., O_2 delivery system). Although all dentists and physicians should be trained in the use of O_2 delivery systems, courses in which these techniques are taught to clinical proficiency are particularly difficult to locate.

In the summer of 2008, the Anesthesia Research Foundation of the American Dental Society of Anesthesiology (ADSA) introduced its advanced airway training course.[9] This program consists of an online didactic training session followed by a

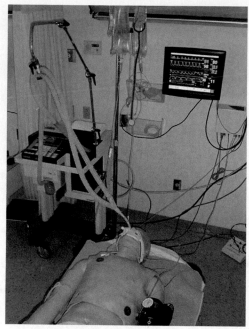

Figure 33.1 SimMan.

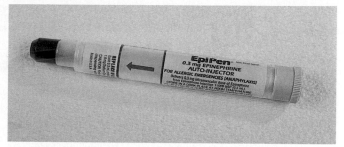

Figure 33.2 Preloaded autoinjector epinephrine syringe. (From Bonewit-West K: *Clinical procedures for medical assistants*, ed 8, St Louis, 2008, Saunders.)

live didactic session and a hands-on component using the SimMan high-fidelity human simulator (Fig. 33.1). SimMan not only allows the user to replicate all of the commonly encountered airway-related medical emergencies seen during sedation and anesthesia but also permits their treatment without the potential for patient harm. All emergency airway devices and procedures may be demonstrated and placed in this valuable educational environment. It is anticipated that most states will eventually accept completion of this course instead of the less ideal ACLS courses currently mandated for sedation and general anesthesia permits.

The types of drugs and equipment included in the emergency kit must be appropriate for the level of training of the office personnel who will be called on to use it. Table 33.1 lists drugs and equipment recommended for inclusion in a basic emergency kit.

LEVEL 1: BASIC EMERGENCY KIT

Injectable Drugs
The following two injectable drugs are considered primary critical drugs and should be included in *all* emergency kits:
1. Epinephrine (for management of life-threatening allergic reactions [e.g., anaphylaxis])
2. Histamine blocker (antihistamine)

Epinephrine (adrenaline), one of the most important drugs in emergency medicine, is the drug of choice in the management of life-threatening allergic reactions (e.g., anaphylaxis) involving the respiratory or cardiovascular system. Additionally, epinephrine administration is indicated for bronchospasm (e.g., asthma) and cardiac arrest. The minimum suggested for the emergency kit is one preloaded syringe (1:1000) (Fig. 33.2).

Preloaded epinephrine syringes are available in a pediatric dosage (1:2000) of 0.15 mg for administration to patients between 15 and 30 kg and of 0.3 mg for patients >30 kg. For the dentist proficient in parenteral drug administration, the use of a 1-mL ampule of 1:1000 epinephrine might be considered.[10,11]

Several *histamine blockers* are available for parenteral administration. Most commonly used in emergency situations are diphenhydramine (Benadryl) and chlorpheniramine (Chlor-Trimeton). Indications for the administration of histamine blockers include management of the delayed allergic response, definitive management of acute allergy, and, potentially, as a local anesthetic when an unconfirmed history of allergy is present.[12] Suggested for the emergency kit are several 1-mL ampules of either 50 mg/mL of diphenhydramine or 10 mg/mL of chlorpheniramine. Though both drugs are equally effective histamine blockers, chlorpheniramine is associated with less sedation than is diphenhydramine, thus its selection as the preferred histamine blocker.

Noninjectable Drugs
Five noninjectable drugs are recommended for inclusion in all emergency kits. *Oxygen* (O_2), the second most important drug in emergency medicine, will also be the drug used most often. Although available in a variety of cylinder sizes (see Chapter 14), the very portable "E" cylinder is recommended for emergency availability. Therapeutic indications for the administration of O_2 include any situation in which respiratory distress is evident. The minimum suggested for the emergency kit is one "E" cylinder (a means of delivering O_2 must also be available and is discussed later).

A *vasodilator* is administered in the immediate management of chest pain. The drug of choice is nitroglycerin. It is available in both a translingual spray and tablets, which are placed sublingually. Though the translingual spray is preferred, as its shelf-life is considerably longer than the sublingual tablets, the cost of the translingual nitroglycerin is substantially greater than the tablets, thus the preference for inclusion of a bottle of sublingual tablets in the emergency kit.

Bronchodilators are required for the definitive management of bronchospasm, seen as the acute asthmatic attack or as a component of anaphylaxis. Epinephrine, the most effective

Table 33.1   Module 1: Critical (Essential) Emergency Drugs

CATEGORY	GENERIC DRUG	PROPRIETARY DRUG	ALTERNATIVE	QUANTITY	AVAILABILITY
Injectable					
Allergy-anaphylaxis	Epinephrine	Adrenalin	None	1 or 2 preloaded auto-inject syringes (e.g., Epi-Pen, Adrenaclick)	1:1000 (mg/mL)
Allergy-histamine blocker	Chlorpheniramine	Chlor-Trimeton	Diphenhydramine (Benadryl)	3 × 1-mL ampules	10 mg/mL
Noninjectable					
O_2	O_2	O_2		1 "E" cylinder	
Vasodilator	Nitroglycerin	Nitrostat sublingual tablets	Nitrolingual Spray	1 bottle (25 tablets)	0.4 mg/metered dose
Bronchodilator	Albuterol (USA) Salbutamol (Canada, Australia, New Zealand, UK)	ProAir, Proventil, Ventolin	Metaproterenol	1 metered-dose inhaler	Metered-aerosol inhaler
Antihypoglycemic	Sugar	Insta-Glucose gel	Orange juice, Nondiet soft drink	1–2 tubes	
Inhibitor of platelet aggregation	Aspirin - powdered	Many	None	2 packets	325-mg packet

EQUIPMENT	RECOMMENDED	ALTERNATIVE	QUANTITY
O_2 delivery system	Positive-pressure demand valve	O_2 delivery system with bag-valve-mask device	Minimum: 1 large adult, 1 child
Face mask	Pocket mask		1 per employee
Automated electronic defibrillator (AED)	Many		1 AED
Syringes for drug administration	Plastic disposable syringes with needles		3 × 2-mL syringes with needles for parenteral drug administration
Suction and suction tips	High-volume suction Large-diameter, round-ended suction tips	Nonelectrical suction system	Office suction system Minimum 2
Tourniquets	Rubber or Velcro tourniquet; rubber tubing	Sphygmomanometer	3 tourniquets and 1 sphygmomanometer
Magill intubation forceps	Magill intubation forceps		1 pediatric Magill intubation forceps

bronchodilator, has previously been discussed as an injectable drug. Other drugs that are effective bronchodilators (β_2 actions) but with fewer cardiovascular (β_1) side effects than epinephrine are available and can be administered by aerosol inhalation directly into the tracheobronchial tree (as can epinephrine, though this is not recommended). Recommended for use in the medical or dental office is albuterol, a drug with excellent β_2 effects but minimal β_1 actions. Salbutamol—albuterol's generic name in many other countries—is used preferentially in Canada, Australia, New Zealand, and the United Kingdom. Therapeutic indications for administration of bronchodilators include respiratory distress as seen in asthma or allergic reactions with a significant respiratory component. Suggested for the emergency kit is one albuterol inhaler.

Hypoglycemia is not an uncommon occurrence. Most hypoglycemic patients, be they diabetic or not, remain conscious but demonstrate bizarre behavior (altered consciousness). Management involves the administration of an *antihypoglycemic* either intravenously, intramuscularly, or orally. Several commercial oral antihypoglycemic products are available, such as Glucola, GlucoStat, and Insta-Glucose. In addition, nondiet soft drinks, fruit juices, and simple sugar are available. Suggested for the emergency kit for management of the conscious hypoglycemic is some form of oral glucose.

Aspirin, an antithrombotic, is recommended for use in the prehospital phase of suspected acute myocardial infarction (AMI). Evidence strongly indicates that aspirin reduces mortality in patients with AMI by 23% when used alone and by 42%

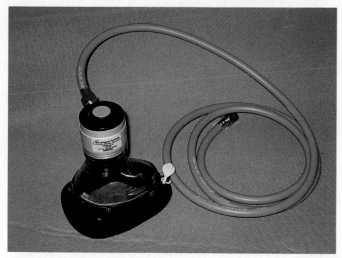

Figure 33.3 Positive-pressure O_2 system. (Courtesy Sedation Resource, Lone Oak, TX. www.sedationresource.com.)

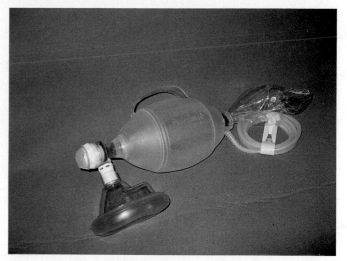

Figure 33.4 Self-inflating bag-valve mask permits delivery of atmospheric air (21% O_2) or O_2-enriched air. Clear face mask is preferred to opaque. (Courtesy Sedation Resource, Lone Oak, TX. www.sedationresource.com.)

when used in combination with thrombolytic therapy.[13] Aspirin, 325 mg, in a powdered form, mixed with water and swallowed, is an integral part of the MONA (morphine, O_2, nitroglycerin, aspirin) acronym for the prehospital management of suspected "heart attack" victims. Suggested for the emergency kit are two packets of powdered aspirin (325 mg).[14]

Primary (Basic) Emergency Equipment

Basic emergency equipment includes the following items:
1. O_2 delivery system
2. Automated external defibrillator (AED)
3. Suction and suction tips
4. Syringes for drug administration
5. Tourniquets
6. Magill intubation forceps

An *O_2 delivery system* adaptable to an "E" cylinder of O_2 must permit the delivery of positive-pressure O_2. Examples of this type of device include the positive-pressure demand valve and the reservoir bag on all inhalation sedation units. The Elder valve (Fig. 33.3) is an example of this device. When positioned properly, these devices provide O_2 on demand whenever the patient breathes spontaneously. Negative pressure created under the mask triggers the device to provide O_2 under positive pressure. In this regard, the positive-pressure demand valve operates similarly to a SCUBA (**S**elf-**C**ontained **U**nderwater **B**reathing **A**pparatus) mask and is readily usable by almost all rescuers. It is in the use of this device for controlled ventilation (positive-pressure ventilation) that potential difficulties arise. To properly ventilate an apneic patient using the positive-pressure mask, the rescuer *must* be able to maintain both a patent airway and an airtight seal with the mask on the patient's face using one or two hands. The second hand (or that of a second rescuer) is used to activate the valve that supplies O_2 to the patient. The positive-pressure demand valve is one means of providing 100% O_2. For this device to be used, a source of 100% O_2 must be available. The positive-pressure demand

valve ceases to function once the O_2 cylinder is depleted. Another potential complication associated with use of the positive-pressure demand valve is overinflation of the lungs (see self-inflating bag–valve–mask [BVM] next).

A self-inflating BVM device is a self-contained unit that is portable and easily transported to any site within the dental or medical office (Fig. 33.4). It does not require a compressed gas cylinder of O_2 to function and therefore has a wider area of potential use than the positive-pressure device. Additionally, overinflation of the lungs is less likely to occur with a BVM device, as the bag contains a fixed volume of "air." As with the positive-pressure device, the rescuer must be able to maintain both a patent airway and an airtight seal of the mask on the patient's face with but one hand; the other is used to squeeze the bellows bag and inflate the victim's lungs (Fig. 33.5). This device has many proprietary names, including the Ambu Bag and CPR Prompt.

The self-inflating BVM device may be used to deliver 21% O_2 (ambient or atmospheric air) or enriched O_2 (greater than 21% but less than 100% O_2) by attaching a delivery tube to the end of the bellows bag.

The self-inflating BVM device is recommended for use in pediatric and smaller adult patients (because of their smaller lung capacity); however, the same device is not recommended for use in the larger than average sized adult. Tests have demonstrated that even in the hands of well-trained ventilators, these devices do not deliver an adequate volume of air to a large adult victim's lungs.[15] Addition of a reservoir bag that provides additional volume can make this device adequate for use in the larger adult.

Face masks must be available if either the positive-pressure mask or BVM is to be used. A face mask should be constructed of a clear plastic or of rubber, which permits the efficient delivery of O_2 or air to the patient while permitting the rescuer

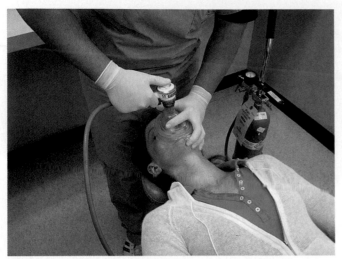

Figure 33.5 Hand position with bag-valve-mask device. (From Malamed SF: *Medical emergencies in the dental office*, ed 7, St Louis, 2015, Mosby.)

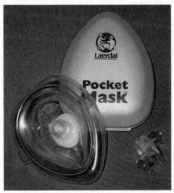

Figure 33.6 Pocket mask. (Courtesy Sedation Resource, Lone Oak, TX. www.sedationresource.com.)

to visually inspect the mouth for the presence of foreign matter (e.g., vomitus, blood) (Fig. 33.6). Several sizes of face masks should be available. Suggested for the emergency kit is one portable O_2 cylinder ("E" cylinder) with a positive-pressure demand valve and/or one portable self-inflating BVM device.

> **COMMENT:** Training is required for the safe and effective use of these devices.

Automated external defibrillator (AED). Though rare in the dental environment, sudden cardiac arrest can occur. Successful resuscitation from out-of-hospital sudden cardiac arrest (OOH-SCA) depends on many factors, most important of which are (1) early initiation of basic life support (BLS) and (2) prompt defibrillation.[16] The most important factor in survival from OOH-SCA is the elapsed time between collapse and defibrillation.[17-19] The shorter this time span, the greater the chance of successful resuscitation. The likelihood

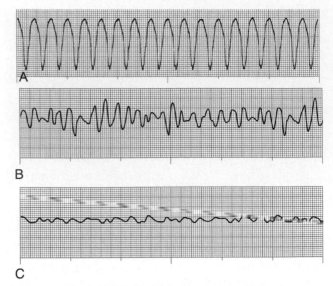

Figure 33.7 "Shockable" dysrhythmias on electrocardiography. **A,** Ventricular tachycardia. **B,** Coarse ventricular fibrillation. **C,** Fine ventricular fibrillation. (A From Aehlert B: *ECGs made easy*, ed 2, St Louis, 2002, Mosby; B and C from McSwain N: *The basic EMT: comprehensive prehospital care*, ed 2, St Louis, 2003, Mosby).

of successful resuscitation from OOH-SCA decreases at a rate of approximately 7% to 10% per minute when BLS is not administered before arrival of EMS, whereas the rate decreases by 3% to 4% per minute when BLS is being administered.[20] Early defibrillation (shock delivered within 5 minutes of receipt of the emergency medical services [EMS] call) is a high-priority goal of EMS care.[21] Unfortunately, this goal is but rarely achieved. Large U.S. cities, such as New York and Los Angeles, have EMS response times of 11.4 minutes and 16 minutes, respectively, with correspondingly low survival rates (to hospital discharge) from OOH-SCA (New York 2%, Los Angeles 1.4%, Chicago 1%).[22] Where rapid response from EMS and early defibrillation are available, survival rates to hospital discharge are significantly higher. Seattle, Washington,[23] reports a 46% survival rate, and Boston, Massachusetts, a 40% rate.[24]

The AED is a sophisticated yet simple battery-operated computerized device that has been shown to be reliable and easy to operate. Simply stated, AEDs are computers that recognize the two "shockable" cardiac dysrhythmias, ventricular fibrillation (VF) and pulseless ventricular tachycardia (VT), which may be effectively treated through defibrillation (Fig. 33.7).

Basic life support (cardiopulmonary resuscitation [CPR]) training is mandated for dental licensure in most states (44 states in the United States [March 2017]) and provinces. "BLS for Healthcare Providers," as defined by the American Heart Association (AHA), includes defibrillation (**P→C→A→B→D**).[25] On February 28, 2006, the Florida Board of Dentistry became the first to mandate the availability of an AED on-site in every dental office location.[26] As of February 2017, three states required on-site availability of AEDs in all dental practices. Forty-six states have requirements for the availability of an AED or defibrillator on-site based on the level of sedation or general

| Box 33.3 | States Mandating Presence of AED in Dental Office as of February 2017 |

Alabama – Minimal and above
Alaska – Parenteral and above
Arizona – Oral and above
Arkansas – Minimal and above
California – General Anesthesia
Colorado – Minimal Sedation and above
Connecticut – Conscious Sedation and above
Delaware – Does not state specifically, but wants
    bradycardia drugs starting at N_2O sedation
Florida – Any and all dentists
Georgia – Starting at Minimal for Pediatrics, Moderate
    for Adults
Hawaii – Moderate and above
Idaho – Moderate and above
Illinois – Moderate and above
Indiana – Light Parenteral and above
Iowa – Minimal and above
Kansas – Parenteral and above
Kentucky – Oral Moderate and above
Louisiana – Deep sedation and above
Maine – Moderate level I and above
Maryland – Enteral Moderate and above
Massachusetts – N_2O and above
Michigan – IV conscious and above
Minnesota – Enteral Moderate and above
Mississippi – Any and all dentists
Missouri – Enteral Moderate and above
Montana – Moderate sedation and above

Nebraska – General Anesthesia
Nevada – Conscious sedation and above
New Hampshire – Moderate sedation and above
New Jersey – Enteral sedation and above
New Mexico – Conscious II and above
New York – Any and all dentists
North Carolina – Minimal and above
North Dakota – Moderate I and above
Ohio – Conscious and above
Oklahoma – Parenteral conscious and above
Oregon – Moderate and above
Pennsylvania – Moderate and above
Rhode Island – Moderate and above
South Carolina – Moderate and above
South Dakota – Minimal and above
Tennessee – Conscious and above
Texas – Moderate and above
Utah – Deep sedation and above
Vermont – Conscious and above
Virginia – Deep and above
Washington – Minimal and above
West Virginia – Minimal and above
Wisconsin – Enteral conscious and above
Wyoming – Conscious and above

Doctors employing any form of sedation should check with their state or provincial dental regulatory agency for more up-to-date requirements.

Source: Healthfirst Corporation, January 20, 2017.

anesthesia the practitioner is performing (Box 33.3). The American Dental Association recommends "that dentists consider purchasing an AED for dental offices in which emergency medical services personnel with defibrillation skills and equipment are not available within a reasonable time frame."

It is essential that effective *suction* and *suction tips* be available in the office. The disposable saliva ejector is entirely inadequate in situations in which anything other than tiny objects must be evacuated from the mouth of a patient. Suction tips should be of large diameter and rounded so that there is little hazard of inducing bleeding should it become necessary to suction the hypopharynx. Plastic evacuators and tonsil suction tips are quite adequate for this purpose (Fig. 33.8). The minimum suggested for the emergency kit is two plastic evacuators or tonsil suction tips. In dental offices where general anesthesia and/or parenteral moderate sedation are employed, most jurisdictions mandate the availability of a nonelectric suction system.

Plastic disposable syringes with an 18- to 21-gauge needle are required for parenteral drug administration. Many syringe sizes are available, but a 2-mL syringe is quite adequate. Suggested for the emergency kit are two to three 2-mL disposable syringes with 18- to 21-gauge needles.

A *tourniquet* is required if IV drug administration is contemplated (see Fig. 22.15). In addition, three tourniquets will be required for management of acute pulmonary edema. A sphygmomanometer (blood pressure cuff) may be used as a tourniquet by inflating the cuff to a pressure that falls between the diastolic and systolic measurements. Suggested for the emergency kit are two to three tourniquets and a sphygmomanometer.

A *Magill intubation forceps* aids in the recovery of small objects that have fallen into the distal part of the oral cavity or pharynx (Fig. 33.9). Table 33.1 summarizes the basic drugs and equipment recommended for the emergency kit.

LEVEL 2: SECONDARY (NONCRITICAL) DRUGS AND EQUIPMENT

Injectable Drugs

A number of injectable drugs—anticonvulsant, analgesic, vasopressor, corticosteroid, antihypoglycemic, antihypertensive, and anticholinergic drugs—are recommended or required for

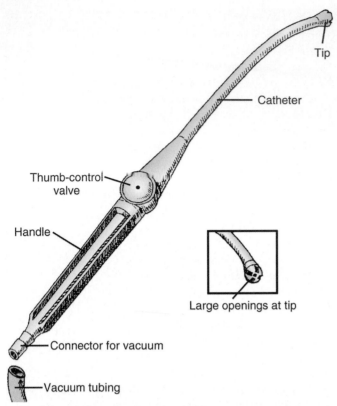

Figure 33.8 Tonsillar suction tip. (From Pilbeam S, Cairo J: *Mechanical ventilation*, ed 4, St Louis, 2007, Mosby.)

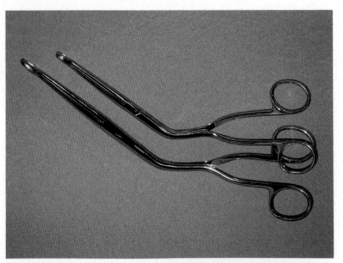

Figure 33.9 Magill intubation forceps, adult *(bottom)* and pediatric *(top)*. (Courtesy Sedation Resource, Lone Oak, TX. www. sedationresource.com.)

inclusion in the emergency kit of dentists with advanced training in emergency medicine and/or anesthesia (Table 33.2). Included are oral and maxillofacial surgeons; dentist anesthesiologists; pediatric dentists, periodontists, endodontists, and other dental specialists who have completed a hospital-based residency program; and general practitioners who have completed a general practice residency, as well as any dentist who has received a permit from their state or province for parenteral sedation.

The *anticonvulsant* of choice is a benzodiazepine, either midazolam or diazepam. Anticonvulsants are administered either intravenously or intranasally to terminate a tonic-clonic seizure, whether in a patient with a history of prior seizure disorders or in management of local anesthetic overdose. Other therapeutic indications for the emergency administration of a benzodiazepine include termination of febrile convulsions, hyperventilation (for sedation), and thyroid storm (for sedation). Suggested for the emergency kit is midazolam 5 mg/mL in a 5- or 10-mL multidose vial. If administered intranasally, the 5-mg/mL concentration is recommended.

An *analgesic* drug will be valuable during situations in which acute pain or anxiety is present. Management of "pain" during AMI represents an important indication for administration of analgesics. Other therapeutic indications include intense, prolonged pain or anxiety and as a sedative in the management of heart failure (HF). Opioid analgesics are the drugs of choice, with morphine sulfate recommended. The administration of nitrous oxide-oxygen (N_2O-O_2) for the management of pain during myocardial infarction has been in use since the 1970s.[27] N_2O-O_2 is administered in a concentration of 50% N_2O and 50% O_2.[27-30] If N_2O is not available, IV morphine sulfate, 10 mg/ mL (two to three 1-mL ampules), is recommended.

Vasopressors are administered to manage hypotension. One vasopressor, epinephrine, has already been included in the basic emergency kit; however, its administration in the management of mild hypotension is not recommended. A vasopressor with less intense actions is usually desirable. Within this category, many drugs are available; ephedrine is selected because of its ability to increase blood pressure with little secondary effect on the workload of the myocardium. Indications for vasopressor administration include management of hypotension, as seen in syncopal reactions, drug overdose reactions, postseizure states, acute adrenal insufficiency, and allergy. Recommended for the emergency kit is 50 mg/ mL of ephedrine (two to three 1-mL ampules).

Parenteral *antihypoglycemics* are administered in the definitive management of hypoglycemia and in the differential diagnosis of unexplained unconsciousness or seizures of unknown origin. A 50% dextrose (D_{50}) solution is recommended, which because of its volume and viscosity must be administered intravenously. One vial (50 mL) of 50% dextrose is recommended for the emergency kit. An alternative is glucagon, available as 1 mg/ mL in a 2-mL ampule. Glucagon may be administered either intravenously or intramuscularly. For patients weighing up to 30 kg, D_{25} is recommended.

Corticosteroids are administered in the management of the acute allergic reaction, but only after epinephrine and the histamine blockers have proven effective. Another indication for their administration is management of acute adrenal insufficiency. Recommended for the emergency kit is 50 mg/mL of hydrocortisone sodium succinate (one 2-mL vial).

The need to administer *antihypertensive* drugs to manage a hypertensive crisis (excessive elevations in blood pressure) is extremely rare. First, the incidence of extreme acute blood pressure elevations is quite uncommon, and second, other

Table 33.2 Module 2: Secondary (Noncritical) Drugs and Equipment

CATEGORY	GENERIC DRUG	PROPRIETARY DRUG	ALTERNATIVE	QUANTITY	AVAILABILITY
Injectable					
Anticonvulsant	Midazolam	Generic	Diazepam	1 × 5-mL vial	5 mg/mL
Analgesic	Morphine sulfate	Generic	N₂O-O₂	3 × 1-mL ampoules	10 mg/mL
Vasopressor	Ephedrine	Generic		3 × 1-mL ampoules	50 mg/mL
Antihypoglycemic	50% dextrose		Glucagon	1 vial	50-mL ampule
Corticosteroid	Hydrocortisone sodium succinate	Solu-Cortef	Dexamethasone	2 × 2-mL mix-o-vial	50 mg/mL
Antihypertensive	Esmolol	Brevibloc	Labetalol	2 × 100-mg/mL vial	100 mg/mL
Anticholinergic	Atropine	Generic	Scopolamine	3 × 1-mL ampules	0.5 mg/mL
Noninjectable					
Respiratory stimulant	Aromatic ammonia	Generic	—	2 boxes	0.3 mL/Vaporole
Antihypertensive	Hydralazine		Nitroglycerin	1 bottle	25 mg/tablet

Equipment*	RECOMMENDED	ALTERNATIVE	QUANTITY
Scalpel or cricothyrotomy needle	Cricothyrotomy set (if trained)	Scalpel	1 set or scalpel
Artificial airways	Nasopharyngeal airways	Oropharyngeal airways	Various sizes (adult, child)
Airway adjuncts	Laryngoscope and endotracheal tubes		1 laryngoscope and various sizes of endotracheal tubes

*All items of equipment require specific training in order to be utilized safely and effectively.

methods may be used to lower blood pressure without the need for parenteral antihypertensive drug administration. Oral drugs, such as nifedipine or nitroglycerin, may be administered in most situations to provide a modest depression of blood pressure. The inclusion of an antihypertensive drug is in response to state and provincial dental board requirements for general anesthesia permits (and in a few states and provinces also for parenteral sedation).

Esmolol (Brevibloc) is a β₁-selective adrenergic receptor–blocking agent with a very short duration of action and is the recommended parenteral drug for acute hypertensive episodes. It is available as a 10-mg/mL formulation, and two ampules of 100 mg/mL (with diluent) are recommended.

Atropine, a parasympathetic *anticholinergic* blocking agent, is recommended for the management of symptomatic bradycardia (adult heart rate of <60 beats per minute). Atropine is also considered an essential drug in ACLS, in which it is employed in the management of hemodynamically significant bradysrhythmias (significant heart block and asystole). It is available as 0.5 mg/mL in 1-mL vials and 1 mg in a 10-mL syringe, and two or three ampules of 0.5 mg/mL (for IM administration) and/or two 10-mL syringes of 1 mg per syringe (for IV administration) are recommended.

Noninjectable Drugs

Two noninjectable drugs, a respiratory stimulant and an antihypertensive (see Table 33.2), are recommended for dentists with some advanced training in emergency medicine. *Aromatic ammonia* is the recommended respiratory stimulant. Its use is not limited to persons with advanced training in emergency medicine. It is included as a secondary emergency drug because it does not represent a "critical" drug in emergency management. Available in a silver-gray vaporole, it is crushed between the rescuer's fingers and held beneath the victim's nose. Indications for aromatic ammonia (aka "smelling salts") include respiratory depression not induced by opioid analgesics and vasodepressor syncope. Recommended for the emergency kit is one box of aromatic ammonia vaporoles.

COMMENT: Aromatic ammonia will be one of the most frequently used drugs in the emergency kit. It is suggested that one or two vaporoles be placed close to every treatment area so that excessive time will not be spent waiting for the emergency kit to arrive. Several vaporoles should remain in the emergency kit for use in other areas of the office (Fig. 33.10).

Secondary (Advanced) Emergency Equipment

Several other items of equipment are available for use in emergency situations. *Training is required for the safe and effective use of these devices.* It is therefore recommended that the

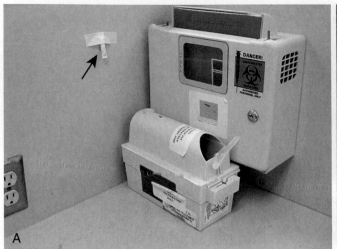

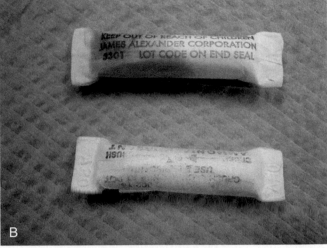

Figure 33.10 A, Aromatic ammonia Vaporole on wall near dental chair *(arrow)*. **B,** Aromatic ammonia Vaporole darkens (bottom) when used. (From Malamed SF: *Medical emergencies in the dental office,* ed 7, St Louis, 2015, Mosby.)

following equipment *not* be included unless adequate training and experience have been obtained:

• Scalpel or cricothyrotomy needle
• Artificial airways
• Airway adjuncts

As a final step in attempting to manage the obstructed airway, cricothyrotomy may be indicated. Although this procedure is highly unlikely to ever be required in the dental environment, there are occasions in which the recommended procedures involving abdominal or chest thrusts may prove to be ineffective in opening an airway that has become obstructed by a foreign object.[31] One clinical situation in which the latter procedures will prove fruitless is laryngeal edema, a form of allergic response in which the soft tissues of the larynx swell, restricting the flow of air into and out of the trachea. The usual airway maneuvers (i.e., head-tilt/chin-lift) fail to provide a patent airway because soft tissue, not a foreign object, is producing the problem. Cricothyrotomy is necessary to provide O_2 to the victim. It is recommended that in the office of a dentist who has been trained in the technique of cricothyrotomy, the emergency kit should contain a *scalpel* or a *cricothyrotomy needle*. The technique of cricothyrotomy is reviewed in Chapter 34. Suggested for the emergency kit is one scalpel with disposable blade and/or one 13-gauge cricothyrotomy needle.

Plastic or rubber *oropharyngeal* and rubber *nasopharyngeal airways* assist in airway management. They are used routinely during and after general anesthesia to assist in airway maintenance in unconscious or semiconscious patients. The oropharyngeal airway is designed to lie between the base of the tongue and the posterior wall of the pharynx, lifting the tongue away from the pharyngeal wall, thus aiding airway maintenance (Fig. 33.11). Use of the oropharyngeal airway (Fig. 33.12) must be restricted to persons trained in its insertion because improper placement can force the base of the tongue back still farther into the pharynx, thereby adding to

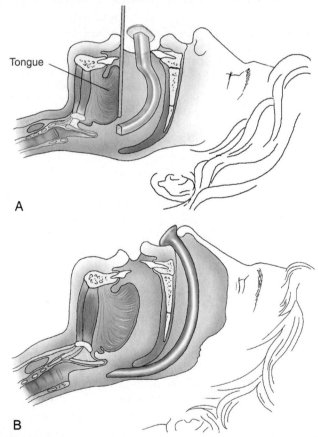

Figure 33.11 Plastic or rubber oropharyngeal **(A)** or nasopharyngeal **(B)** airways are used to help maintain a patent airway in the unconscious patient. (From McSwain N: *The basic EMT: comprehensive prehospital care,* ed 2, St Louis, 2003, Mosby.)

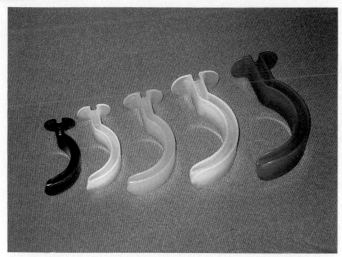

Figure 33.12 Oropharyngeal airways are available in a variety of sizes. (Courtesy Sedation Resource, Lone Oak, TX. www.sedationresource.com.)

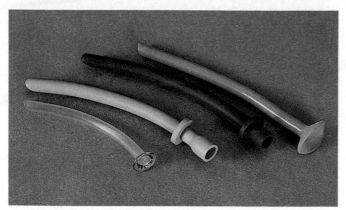

Figure 33.13 Nasopharyngeal airways. (From McSwain N: *The basic EMT: comprehensive prehospital care,* ed 2, St Louis, 2003, Mosby.)

the degree of obstruction. If the oropharyngeal airway is placed into the pharynx of a patient who is not deeply unconscious, the patient will react to the presence of the airway by gagging (not too bad), vomiting or regurgitating (worse), or having a laryngospasm (worse yet). Placing an oropharyngeal airway in a still reactive patient is the equivalent of placing your finger deep down in your throat to the point at which gagging and vomiting occur. In proper insertion of an oropharyngeal airway, the tip of the patient's tongue is held with a piece of gauze and pulled anteriorly while the airway is inserted.

The nasopharyngeal airway (Fig. 33.13) is better tolerated by most patients. It is lubricated (K-Y Jelly or Xylocaine viscous) before insertion into one nostril (usually the right) and then gently advanced into position. Because it is situated in the nasopharynx, not the oropharynx, gagging, vomiting, regurgitation, and laryngospasm rarely develop, even in a conscious patient (see Fig. 33.11, *B*).

Use of these airway adjuncts is recommended only when manual methods of airway maintenance have been ineffective. Training and experience in the use of oral and nasal airways is mandatory if they are to be used effectively and safely.

Suggested for the emergency kit is a set of adult- and child-sized airways (either oropharyngeal or nasopharyngeal).

Endotracheal intubation using a *laryngoscope* and *endotracheal tube* provides the ultimate in airway management. The use of endotracheal intubation must be strictly limited to persons who are well trained in the technique. Quite realistically, this limits its usefulness to physician and dentist anesthesiologists, nurse anesthetists, trained paramedical personnel, and dentists and physicians who have received training in anesthesiology. The most common mistakes noted during intubation are accidental intubation of the esophagus and taking too long to intubate (it should take no longer than 15 seconds to intubate a patient). Table 33.2 summarizes the secondary emergency drugs and equipment.

LEVEL 3: ADVANCED CARDIAC LIFE SUPPORT

Drugs recommended by the AHA for use in ACLS[32] are based on an extensive evidence review initiated by the International Liaison Committee on Resuscitation (ILCOR) after the publication of the ILCOR 2015 *International Consensus on Cardiopulmonary Resuscitation and Emergency Cardiovascular Care Science With Treatment Recommendations.*[33] This review was competed in February 2015.[34]

These drugs should be included in the emergency drug kit or in a separate drug kit in those offices in which the dentist has received training in ACLS. The ACLS-trained dentist is referred directly to the most recent guidelines for more in-depth discussions of the efficacy of these drugs.[32] ACLS drugs include adenosine; amiodarone; calcium channel blockers, including verapamil and diltiazem; β-adrenergic blockers, including atenolol, metoprolol, propranolol, and esmolol; ibutilide; lidocaine; procainamide; and sotalol.[32]

LEVEL 4: ANTIDOTAL DRUGS

Antidotal drugs (Table 33.3) reverse some or all of the actions of drugs that have been previously administered. Specific reversal agents should be available in the emergency drug kit where any technique of parenteral sedation is employed in patient management (IM, submucosal, IN, IV, or general anesthesia). Only a brief description of each drug is given because the pharmacology of the antidotal drugs has been presented in Chapter 25. Antidotal drugs include an opioid antagonist, benzodiazepine antagonist, a drug for reversal of emergence delirium, and a vasodilator.

Opioid antagonists reverse the actions of opioid agonists (i.e., meperidine, morphine, and the fentanyl family [alfentanil, sufentanil, remifentanil]). In clinical practice, opioid antagonists are administered primarily to reverse unwanted respiratory depression produced by opioids. Naloxone (Narcan) is available as a 0.4-mg/mL dosage form (for adults). It is administered at a rate of 0.1 mg every 2 to 3 minutes to the adult up to 2.0 mg, with the patient's response monitored constantly.[35] In children,

Table 33.3	Module 4: Antidotal Drugs				
CATEGORY	GENERIC DRUG	PROPRIETARY DRUG	ALTERNATIVE	QUANTITY	AVAILABILITY
Injectable					
Opioid antagonist	Naloxone	Narcan	Nalbuphine	2 × 1-mL ampules	0.4 mg/mL
Benzodiazepine antagonist	Flumazenil	Romazicon	–	1 × 10-mL vial	0.1 mg/mL
Anticholinergic toxicity Antiemergence delirium	Physostigmine	Antilirium	–	3 × 2-mL ampules	1 mg/mL
Vasodilator	Phentolamine mesylate	generic	Procaine HCl	5 mg/mL powder for injection	1 bottle

an initial IV dose of 0.01 mg/kg is suggested.[35] One must never forget that in addition to reversing the respiratory-depressant actions of opioid analgesics, naloxone reverses its analgesic effects. Therefore patients who receive opioid analgesics for anesthesia and undergo the surgical procedure without the benefit of local anesthesia and then receive naloxone may experience severe postsurgical pain.[36] Nalbuphine, an opioid agonist-antagonist, has also been shown to be effective in reversing opioid-induced respiratory depression. A major advantage of nalbuphine over naloxone is that the analgesic properties of the opioid remain.[37]

Recommended for the emergency kit is 0.4 mg/mL of naloxone (two to three 1-mL ampules) for use in adults. For pediatric use (<30 kg weight) naloxone is available as a 0.02-mg/mL concentration. Naloxone is also available as an INspray.[38]

The *benzodiazepine antagonist* flumazenil (Romazicon) reverses the clinical actions of midazolam and diazepam (and other benzodiazepines). Recovery from sedation is hastened, and the length of amnesia is decreased when flumazenil is administered.[39] It is recommended for IV use only; the initial dose of flumazenil is 0.2 mg administered intravenously over 15 seconds. Additional doses of 0.2 mg may be administered and repeated at 60-second intervals where necessary to a maximum dose of 1.0 mg. Most patients respond to 0.6 to 1.0 mg.[40] Suggested for the drug emergency kit is one 10-mL multidose vial of 0.1 mg/mL flumazenil.

Emergence delirium (central anticholinergic syndrome) is an uncommon ADR developing after administration of anticholinergics (primarily scopolamine) or benzodiazepines. Emergence delirium may be terminated through the administration of *physostigmine* (Antilirium). Dosage is 0.5 to 1.0 mg IM or IV. No more than 1 mg should be administered per minute. Additional doses may be administered every 10 to 30 minutes if the desired patient response is not obtained.[41] Recommended for the emergency kit is 1.0 mg/mL of physostigmine (two to three 2-mL ampules).

A *vasodilator* is recommended for the emergency kit in the event that an extravascular injection of a tissue-irritating drug (e.g., diazepam, pentobarbital) occurs or in the extremely unlikely event of an intraarterial injection of a drug. Phentolamine is the preferred drug. Phentolamine is an alpha-adrenergic receptor antagonist that is administered parenterally and has

a short duration of action. Approved uses of phentolamine include diagnosis of pheochromocytoma and treatment of hypertension in pheochromocytoma, prevention of tissue necrosis after norepinephrine extravasation, and reversal of soft tissue anesthesia.[42] In the treatment of accidental extravasation of drugs with adverse effects on vasculature, 5 to 10 mg of phentolamine is injected into the affected area.[43]

An alternative to phentolamine is procaine (Novocain). Procaine is a potent vasodilator with local anesthetic actions.[44] Procaine is no longer manufactured in the United States.

Recommended for the emergency kit is one vial of phentolamine.

SUMMARY

The selection of emergency drugs and equipment for the dental or medical office must be based on the training and background of the dentist or physician who is responsible for its use. Because of the diversity in emergency preparedness training among both dentists and physicians, no stereotyped emergency kit is appropriate for all practitioners. I have attempted to describe several levels of drugs and equipment that I believe would be appropriate with different degrees of expertise in emergency medicine. In addition, most states and provinces have credentialing bodies that regulate the use of sedation and general anesthesia. Specific mandatory drug lists are included in most of these regulations. Regardless of the nature of drugs and equipment selected for the emergency kit, it is vital for the dentist to become familiar with the indications, contraindications, dosages, and method of administration of each of these drugs and to be able to correctly operate any available equipment.

REFERENCES

1. Malamed SF: Preparation. In *Medical emergencies in the dental office*, ed 7, St Louis, 2015, Mosby., pp 70–102.
2. Pallasch TJ: This emergency kit belongs in your office. *Dent Manage* 16:43, 1976.
3. Hall RE, Malamed SF: Drugs for medical emergencies in the dental office. In *ADA/PDR guide to dental therapeutics*, ed 4, Chicago, 2006, ADA Publishing.
4. American Dental Association, Council on Dental Education: *Guidelines for teaching pain control and sedation to dentists and*

dental students, adopted by the 2016 ADA House of Delegates, Chicago, 2016, The Association. www.ada.org/~/media/ADA/About%20the%20ADA/Files/teaching_paincontrol_guidelines.pdf?la=en. Accessed 30 March 2016.

5. Dental Board of California: Application for conscious sedation permit. Form CS-1, revised 7/08. (Sections 1647 – 1647.9, 1682 Business and Professions Code; Title 16 California Code of Regulations Sections 1043 – 1043.8). www.dbc.ca.gov. Accessed 19 January 2017.

6. American Association of Oral and Maxillofacial Surgeons, Committee on Anesthesia: *Office anesthesia evaluation manual*, ed 8, Rosemont, IL, 2012, The Association.

7. Board of Registration in Dentistry: 234 CMR 6.00: Administration of anesthesia and sedation. Section 6.15: Administration of Local Anesthesia Only. Massachusetts Court System. http://www.mass.gov/courts/docs/lawlib/230-249cmr/234cmr6.pdf. Accessed 18 April 2016.

8. West Virginia Board of Dentistry: Anesthesia emergency drug requirements and equipment list. http://www.wvdentalboard.org. Accessed 31 January 2017.

9. American Dental Society of Anesthesiology: Sim-Man high fidelity human simulation. www.adsahome.org. Accessed 16 April 2016.

10. Sangrik LJ: My Viewpoint: Epipens: dental necessity or extravagance? ADA News 3 October 2016, page 2.

11. Malamed SF: Viewpoint: Epipens: dental necessity or extravagance? ADA News 7 November 2016, page 2.

12. Malamed SF: The use of diphenhydramine HCl as a local anesthetic in dentistry. *Anesth Prog* 20:76–82, 1973.

13. ISIS-2 (Second International Study of Infarct Survival Collaborative Group): Randomized trial of intravenous streptokinase, oral aspirin, both, or neither among 17,187 cases of suspected acute myocardial infarction. ISIS-2. *J Am Coll Cardiol* 12(6 Suppl A):3A–13A, 1988.

14. Haro LH: Initial approach to the patient who has chest pain. *Cardiol Clin* 24:1–17, 2006.

15. Carden E, Hughes T: An evaluation of manually operated self-inflating resuscitation bags. *Anesth Analg* 54(1):133–138, 1975.

16. Becker LB, Pepe PE: Ensuring the effectiveness of community-wide emergency cardiac care. *Ann Emerg Med* 22(2 Pt 2):354–365, 1993.

17. Baker PW, Conway J, Cotton C, et al; Clinical Investigators: Defibrillation or cardiopulmonary resuscitation first for patients with out-of-hospital cardiac arrests found by paramedics to be in ventricular fibrillation? A randomised control trial. *Resuscitation* 79(3):424–431, 2008.

18. Chan PS, Krumholz HM, Nichol G, et al: Delayed time to defibrillation after in-hospital cardiac arrest. *N Engl J Med* 358(1):9–17, 2008.

19. Link MS, Berkow LC, Kudenchuk PJ, et al: Part 7: adult advanced cardiovascular life support: 2015 American Heart Association Guidelines Update for Cardiopulmonary Resuscitation and Emergency Cardiovascular Care. *Circulation* 132(Suppl 2):S444–S464, 2015.

20. Larsen MP, Eisenberg MS, Cummins RO, Hallstrom AP: Predicting survival from out-of-hospital cardiac arrest: a graphic model. *Ann Emerg Med* 22(11):1652–1658, 1993.

21. Wik L, Hansen TB, Fylling F, et al: Delaying defibrillation to give basic cardiopulmonary resuscitation to patients with out-of-hospital ventricular fibrillation: a randomized trial. *JAMA* 289(11):1389–1395, 2003.

22. Eckstein M, Stratton SJ, Chan LS: Cardiac arrest resuscitation in Los Angeles: CARE-LA. *Ann Emerg Med* 45(5):504–509, 2005.

23. Payne P: Seattle's survival rate for cardiac arrest rises. *Puget Sound Business Journal* January 8, 2013.

24. England H, Hoffman C, Hodgman T, et al: Effectiveness of automated external defibrillators in high schools in greater Boston. *Am J Cardiol* 95(12):1484–1486, 2005.

25. Kleinman ME, Brennan EE, Goldberger ZD, et al: Part 5: adult basic life support and cardiopulmonary resuscitation quality: 2015 American Heart Association Guidelines Update for Cardiopulmonary Resuscitation and Emergency Cardiovascular Care. *Circulation* 132(Suppl 2):S414–S435, 2015.

26. Florida Board of Dentistry: Vol. 29, 42, October 17, 2003. 64B5-17.015 Office Safety Requirement. http://floridasdentistry.gov/. Accessed 21 April 2016.

27. Kerr F, Brown MG, Irving JB, et al: A double-blind trial of patient-controlled nitrous-oxide/oxygen analgesia in myocardial infarction. *Lancet* 1(7922):1397–1400, 1975.

28. Castle N: Effective relief of acute coronary syndrome. *Emerg Nurse* 10(9):15–19, 2003.

29. O'Sullivan I, Benger J: Nitrous oxide in emergency medicine. *BMJ* 20(3):214–217, 2003.

30. Siriwardena AN, Shaw D, Bouliotis G: Exploratory cross-sectional study of factors associated with pre-hospital management of pain. *J Eval Clin Pract* 16(6):1269–1275, 2010.

31. Heimlich HJ: A life-saving maneuver to prevent food choking. *JAMA* 234(4):398–401, 1975.

32. Link MS, Berkow LC, Kudenchuk PJ, et al: Part 7: adult advanced cardiovascular life support: 2015 American Heart Association Guidelines Update for Cardiopulmonary Resuscitation and Emergency Cardiovascular Care. *Circulation* 132(Suppl 2):S444–S464, 2015.

33. Morrison LJ, Deakin CD, Morley PT, et al; Advanced Life Support Chapter Collaborators: Part 8: advanced life support: 2010 International Consensus on Cardiopulmonary Resuscitation and Emergency Cardiovascular Care Science With Treatment Recommendations. *Circulation* 122(Suppl 2):S345–S421, 2010.

34. Callaway CW, Soar J, Aibiki M, et al; on behalf of the Advanced Life Support Chapter Collaborators: Part 4: advanced life support: 2015 International Consensus on Cardiopulmonary Resuscitation and Emergency Cardiovascular Care Science With Treatment Recommendations. *Circulation* 132(Suppl 1):S84–S145, 2015.

35. ClinicalKey: Naloxone drug monograph. December 4, 2015. www.clinicalkey.com. Accessed 9 March 2016.

36. Pallasch TJ, Gill CJ: Naloxone-associated morbidity and mortality. *Oral Surg Oral Med Oral Pathol* 52(6):602–603, 1981.

37. Hu C, Flecknell PA, Liles JH: Fentanyl and medetomidine anaesthesia in the rat and its reversal using atipamezole and either nalbuphine or butorphanol. *Lab Anim* 26(1):15–22, 1992.

38. Walley AY, Xuan Z, Hackman HH, et al: Opioid overdose rates and implementation of overdose education and nasal naloxone distribution in Massachusetts: interrupted time series analysis. *BMJ* 346:f174, 2013.

39. Longmire AW, Seger DL: Topics in clinical pharmacology: flumazenil, a benzodiazepine antagonist. *Am J Med Sci* 306(1):49–52, 1993.

40. ClinicalKey: Romazicon drug monograph. February 5, 2016. www.clinicalkey.com. Accessed 21 April 2016.

41. ClinicalKey: Physostigmine drug monograph. July 2, 2014. www.clinicalkey.com. Accessed 9 March 2016.

42. Epocrates.com: Phentolamine drug description. www.epocrates.com. Accessed 21 April 2016.

43. ClinicalKey: Phentolamine mesylate drug monograph. December 4, 2015. www.clinicalkey.com. Accessed 21 April 2016.

44. ClinicalKey: Procaine HCl drug monograph. March 11, 2016. www.clinicalkey.com. Accessed 21 April 2016.

chapter 34

Management of Emergencies

CHAPTER OUTLINE

Despite efforts at prevention, complications and adverse drug reactions (ADRs) will arise during and after the administration of drugs for the management of pain or anxiety. In the office that has prepared for these situations, there is a greater likelihood of a successful outcome than in an unprepared or ill-prepared office. Many states, provinces, and specialty groups require that the dental office team be capable of correctly identifying and managing specific ADRs associated with parenteral sedation and general anesthesia.[1-3] These emergencies are reviewed in this chapter.

Pallasch[4] proposed the following classification of ADRs:

I. Toxicity related to direct extension of pharmacologic effects
   A. Side effects
   B. Abnormal dosage (overdosage)
   C. Local toxic effects

II. Toxicity related to altered recipient
   A. Presence of pathology
   B. Emotional disturbances
   C. Genetic aberrations (idiosyncrasy)
   D. Teratogenicity
   E. Drug–drug interactions
III. Toxicity related to drug allergy

According to Pallasch's system, there are three major methods by which drugs may produce adverse reactions:

1. A direct extension of the pharmacologic actions of the drug
2. A deleterious effect on a chemically, genetically, metabolically, or morphologically altered recipient
3. Initiation of an immune (allergic) response

Most ADRs are not life threatening. There are, however, potential responses that are life threatening, requiring immediate and effective management if the patient is to fully recover. These include the overdose reaction and the allergic response. A third, the idiosyncratic reaction, is also reviewed.

Overdose reaction (also known as *toxic reaction*) refers to those signs and symptoms manifested as a result of an absolute or relative overadministration of a drug producing elevated blood or plasma levels of that drug in specific organs (termed *target organs*) of the body. For central nervous system (CNS)–depressant drugs, an overdose occurs when the blood level of the drug becomes overly high in the cerebral circulation.[5] Clinical manifestations of an overdose are related directly to the normal pharmacologic actions of the drug. For example, in therapeutic doses, opioids produce a mild depression of the CNS, which results in sedation or hypnosis (desirable effects). Opioid overdosage produces a more profound depression of the CNS, with respiratory or cardiovascular depression and a possible loss of consciousness.

Allergy is a hypersensitive state acquired through exposure to a particular allergen, reexposure to which brings about a heightened capacity to react.[6] Clinically, there are a variety of manifestations through which allergy expresses itself. These include drug fever, angioedema, urticaria, dermatitis, depression of blood-forming organs, photosensitivity, and anaphylaxis. Certain drugs are more likely than others to elicit allergic reactions, and allergy is theoretically a possible reaction to any substance.

In contrast to overdose, in which clinical manifestations are related directly to the pharmacology of the causative agent, the clinical response observed in an allergic reaction is mediated by an exaggerated response of the immune system. The degree of this response determines the severity of the allergic reaction. Allergic responses to a benzodiazepine, a local anesthetic, an antibiotic, a bee sting, peanuts, latex, and shellfish are produced by the same mechanism and may appear clinically similar. Management of all allergic reactions is basically the same, whereas overdose reactions to the first three agents listed are quite dissimilar clinically and require different management.

Idiosyncrasy or *idiosyncratic reactions* are those ADRs that cannot be explained by any known pharmacologic or biochemical mechanism. Another definition is that an idiosyncratic reaction is any ADR that is neither an overdose nor an allergic reaction. An example of an idiosyncratic reaction is CNS stimulation (excitation or agitation) produced after the administration of a known CNS depressant such as diphenhydramine.

Idiosyncratic reactions span an extremely wide range of clinical expression. For example, depression after administration of a stimulant, stimulation after administration of a depressant, and hyperpyrexia after administration of a muscle relaxant are all idiosyncratic reactions. It is usually impossible to predict in whom such reactions will develop or, indeed, the nature of the resulting idiosyncratic reaction.

Because of the unpredictability of the nature and occurrence of idiosyncratic reactions, their management is of necessity symptomatic. Of primary importance in the management of idiosyncrasy is basic life support ($P \rightarrow C \rightarrow A \rightarrow B$): ensuring the adequacy of circulation, airway, and breathing, followed by "D" (definitive care). For example, if seizures develop, management is based on airway maintenance and prevention of injury during the seizure.

It is thought today that virtually all instances of idiosyncrasy have an underlying genetic mechanism.[7] These genetic aberrations remain undetected until the individual receives a specific drug, such as succinylcholine, which then produces its bizarre (nonpharmacologic) clinical expression (e.g., hyperpyrexia [malignant hyperthermia]).

Two major forms of ADR, overdose and allergy, are reviewed in this chapter; in addition, other emergency situations are discussed. Successful demonstration of the ability to manage these situations is frequently a requirement of the permitting process for parenteral sedation and general anesthesia. These complications are listed in Box 34.1.

OVERDOSE

Whenever CNS-depressant drugs are administered, the possibility may exist that an exaggerated level of CNS depression might develop. This might be noted clinically as a slightly oversedated patient, or it might result in an unconscious, apneic patient.

The group of drugs most likely to produce an overdose is the barbiturates. Barbiturates represented the first major breakthrough in the pharmacologic management of anxiety, and because of this, adverse reactions, such as allergy, addiction, and overdose, were tolerated. In the 1960s, with the introduction of the benzodiazepines (drugs that do not possess the same potential for abuse and overdose), barbiturate use declined. Description of their use in dentistry was eliminated in the fifth edition of this textbook. Previous editions of *Sedation, a Guide to Patient Management* contain a complete description of their use.[8]

Although the barbiturates present the greatest potential for adverse reaction, it is the opioid analgesics that are involved with the greatest number of clinically significant episodes of

| Box 34.1 | **Emergency Situations Identified for Parenteral Sedation and General Anesthesia** |

1. Airway obstruction
2. Laryngospasm
3. Bronchospasm
4. Emesis and aspiration of foreign material under anesthesia
5. Angina pectoris
6. Myocardial infarction
7. Cardiac dysrhythmias
   a. Bradycardia
   b. Ventricular tachycardia
   c. Ventricular fibrillation
   d. Asystole
   e. Electromechanical dissociation (EMD)
8. Hypotension
9. Hypertensive crisis
10. Acute allergic reaction
11. Seizures
12. Hypoglycemia
13. Syncope
14. Hyperventilation
15. Respiratory depression

Data from California State Board of Dental Examiners: Conscious sedation evaluation protocol, revised July 2008, Sacramento; and American Association of Oral & Maxillofacial Surgeons: Office anesthesia evaluation manual, ed 8, Rosemont, IL, 2012, The Association.

overdose and respiratory depression. As discussed elsewhere (see Chapters 7, 10, and 35), the use of opioids continues to be popular in pediatric sedation. Opioids are often administered intravenously in conjunction with antianxiety drugs to aid in sedation and pain control in the adult patient. Goodson and Moore reported on 14 pediatric dentistry cases in which the administration of opioids (and other drugs) led to seven deaths and three instances of brain damage.[9] Several opioids were implicated in these reactions: alphaprodine (7 cases), meperidine (6 cases), and pentazocine (1 case).

Benzodiazepines are significantly less likely to produce overdose than barbiturates and opioids, a major reason they are the most commonly administered drugs for the management of fear and anxiety.

Predisposing Factors and Prevention

The clinical efficacy of a drug depends, in large part, on its absorption into the cardiovascular system and on subsequent blood levels of the drug in its target organ(s). Only the inhalation and intravenous (IV) routes of drug administration permit titration. With oral, intranasal (IN), and intramuscular (IM) administration, drug absorption is more erratic, as demonstrated by the wide range of variability in clinical effectiveness. The

normal distribution curve becomes important when drugs are administered via those nontitratable routes. "Average" drug doses are based on this curve; therefore diazepam 5 mg orally provides a desired effect (anxiolysis [minimal sedation]) in the majority (~70%) of patients receiving it. For some patients (about 15% of the population), however, the 5-mg dose is ineffective; these patients require a larger dose to attain the same clinical effect. These patients—*hyporesponders*—are not at risk for potential overdose when given an "average" dose because a lack of adequate sedation is the clinical result.

The potential danger in the use of drugs lies with patients for whom an average 5-mg dose of diazepam is too great. These are persons who are quite sensitive (not allergic) to this drug and require smaller-than-usual doses to obtain clinically effective sedation, so-called *hyperresponders*. It is normally not possible to predict the 15% of the population that will react in this manner. A history of a prior ADR may provide a clue to this occurrence. The medical history questionnaire should be examined carefully in relation to all prior drug reactions. When a history of drug sensitivity is obtained, great care should be exercised if opioid analgesics are to be used. Lower-than-average doses should be administered or different drug categories substituted. Nonbarbiturate sedative-hypnotic drugs, such as the benzodiazepines and the opioid agonist/antagonists, may be used in place of these drugs, though also in lower than average doses.

Although the clinical nature of the overdose cannot always be predicted, there is another way in which these drugs can produce this reaction—a way that is preventable. It relates entirely to the goal being sought by the dentist when these drugs are administered. Some clinicians administer CNS depressants seeking to achieve deeper levels of sedation in more fearful patients. When these drugs are used for this purpose via the oral, IN, or IM routes of drug administration, potential for overdose increases. Dentists who administered barbiturates in their practices encountered patients who became uncooperative (less inhibited) after receiving these drugs. The planned procedure could not be completed because of the difficulty in managing a patient who is slightly overdosed on barbiturates. Larger doses of the barbiturate given to a fearful patient in an attempt to produce deeper levels of sedation may produce greater degrees of CNS depression, with possible loss of consciousness and significant respiratory depression. As mentioned multiple times throughout this book, this propensity of the barbiturates is but one reason their continued used cannot be recommended.

Administering any CNS depressant seeking to obtain deeper levels of sedation via routes of administration in which titration is not possible is foolhardy and an invitation to overdose and potential disaster. It can be neither recommended nor condoned. Only those techniques allowing titration should be used when deeper levels of sedation are sought, and then only when the dentist and entire sedation team are thoroughly familiar with both the technique and the drugs to be administered and are able to manage all possible complications associated with the procedure. The concept of "rescue" has been discussed in Chapter 2 (Box 34.2).

The inhalation and IV routes are the only routes that permit titration. A factor to be remembered regarding inhalation and IV sedation is that absorption of the drugs into the systemic circulation occurs rapidly, so drug responses (both therapeutic and adverse) develop quickly. Titration remains the greatest safety feature these techniques possess and should always be used when possible. Table 34.1 summarizes the recommendations made throughout this book for the various routes of drug administration.

Clinical Manifestations
Sedative-Hypnotics, Benzodiazepines, and Barbiturates

Benzodiazepines, but more so barbiturates, produce depression of a number of physiologic properties, including nerve tissue; respiration; and skeletal, smooth, and cardiac muscle. The

Box 34.2	"Rescue"

"Because sedation and general anesthesia are a continuum, it is not always possible to predict how an individual will respond. Hence, practitioners intending to produce a given level of sedation should be able to diagnose and manage the physiologic consequences (rescue) for patients whose level of sedation becomes deeper than initially intended.

For all levels of sedation, the practitioner must have the training, skills, drugs and equipment to identify and manage such an occurrence until either assistance arrives (emergency medical service) or the patient returns to the intended level of sedation without airway or cardiovascular complications."

From *American Society of Anesthesiologists Task Force on Sedation and Analgesia by Non-Anesthesiologists: Practice guidelines for sedation and analgesia by non-anesthesiologists,* Anesthesiology 96:1004–1017, 2002.

mechanism of action (sedation and hypnosis) is depression at the level of the hypothalamus and the ascending reticular activating system (RAS), which produces a decrease in the transmission of impulses to the cerebral cortex. Further increases in drug blood levels produce depression at other levels of the CNS, such as profound cortical depression, depression of motor function, and finally depression of the medulla. This is represented diagrammatically as follows:

Minimal-to-moderate sedation (calming) → *Moderate-to-deep sedation (hypnosis, sleep)* → *General anesthesia (unconsciousness with progressive respiratory and cardiovascular depression)* → *Respiratory arrest*

Minimal Sedation, Moderate Sedation, and Deep Sedation

At low (therapeutic) blood levels the patient appears calm and cooperative (minimal-to-moderate sedation). As the CNS-depressant drug level in the cerebral circulation increases, the patient falls into a rousable sleep (moderate-to-deep sedation). The dentist will notice the patient's inability to keep his or her mouth open despite reminders to do so.

In addition, when barbiturates or (less commonly) propofol are administered, patients at this level of CNS depression tend to overreact to stimulation, especially noxious stimulation. This is rarely observed when benzodiazepines are administered. An unsedated adult patient may grimace in response to a painful stimulus; an adult moderately to deeply sedated with barbiturates will commonly demonstrate an exaggerated response, perhaps yelling or jumping. This reflects a loss of self-control over emotion that is associated with the CNS-depressant action of the barbiturate. This reaction to noxious stimuli is extremely uncommon when benzodiazepines are administered for sedation.

With continued elevation of the barbiturate or propofol blood level, hypnosis (sleep) ensues, with a minor degree of respiratory depression (decreased depth and increased rate of ventilation). At this level of CNS depression, there is usually no adverse action on the cardiovascular system, only a slight decrease in blood pressure and heart rate, similar to that

Table 34.1	Summary of Routes of Drug Administration Control Over Technique		
RECOMMENDED SAFE ROUTE OF ADMINISTRATION	**TITRATE**	**RAPID REVERSAL**	**SEDATION LEVELS**
Oral	No	No	Minimal
Rectal	No	No	Minimal
Intranasal	No	No	Minimal to moderate
Intramuscular	No	No	Adults: minimal to moderate Children: minimal to moderate
Intravenous	Yes	Yes (opioids, benzodiazepines) No (other drugs)	Adults and children*: light, moderate, deep
Inhalation	Yes	Yes	Minimal to moderate

*There is usually little need for intravenous moderate sedation in normal, healthy children. Most children who will permit venipuncture will also permit intraoral local anesthetic administration. The intravenous route is of great benefit in managing children and adults with disabilities and those who are disruptive.

occurring in normal sleep. Dental treatment cannot be continued at this level of CNS depression because the patient is unable to cooperate with the dentist in keeping his or her mouth open and may require assistance in maintaining airway patency (head tilt). The patient still responds to noxious stimulation but in a sluggish manner. If the desired level of sedation was moderate, this patient requires rescue from deep sedation until such time as they return to moderate sedation levels. Though this response is possible following benzodiazepine administration, its occurrence is extremely rare, especially when titration to clinical effect is employed.

General Anesthesia

With further elevation of the barbiturate or propofol blood level, the degree of CNS depression broadens so that the patient is now unconscious (incapable of response to sensory stimulation, loss of protective reflexes with attendant inability to maintain an airway). Spontaneous respiratory efforts may still be present; however, with even further increase in drugs blood level, medullary depression occurs, which is clinically evident as respiratory and cardiovascular depression. Respiratory depression is noted as shallow breathing movements at a slow or rapid rate. Ventilatory excursions of the chest are not an indication that air is entering or leaving the lungs but only that the patient is attempting to bring air into the lungs. Cardiovascular depression is evident as a continued decrease in blood pressure (caused by medullary depression and direct depression of the myocardium and vascular smooth muscle) and an increased heart rate. The patient develops a shocklike appearance and has a weak and rapid pulse and cold, moist skin. Only in an extremely hypersensitive patient, or where the drug is administered for the induction of general anesthesia, would this response be noted with benzodiazepines.

Respiratory Arrest

As the barbiturate or propofol blood level continues to increase, or if the patient is not managed adequately in the previous stage, respiratory arrest will occur. Respiratory arrest is readily managed with controlled ventilation. If ventilation is not adequately provided, cardiac arrest will ensue.

Other nonbarbiturate sedative-hypnotic drugs (i.e., benzodiazepines) also possess a potential to produce overdose, although this is quite a bit less likely to occur as with the barbiturates. The potential for overdose varies greatly from drug to drug, and to varying degrees all sedative-hypnotic drugs have this potential.

Opioid Agonists

Meperidine, morphine, fentanyl, alfentanil, and sufentanil are commonly used parenteral opioids. Fentanyl and meperidine are the most popular.

Meperidine, like most opioid agonists, exerts its chief pharmacologic actions on the CNS. Therapeutic doses of meperidine produce analgesia, sedation, euphoria, and a degree of respiratory depression. Of principal concern, of course, is the respiratory depressant action of the opioid agonists. They are direct depressants of the medullary respiratory center. In humans, respiratory depression from opioid agonists is evident even at doses that do not disturb the level of consciousness. Respiratory depression produced by opioids is dose dependent: The larger the dose, the greater the level of respiratory depression. The opioid agonist/antagonists nalbuphine and butorphanol offer the combination of analgesia and sedation with minimal respiratory depression.

Death from opioid overdose almost always results from respiratory arrest. All phases of respiration are depressed: rate, minute volume, and tidal volume. The respiratory rate may fall below 10 breaths per minute. Rates of 5 to 6 breaths per minute are not uncommon. The cause of this decreased respiratory rate is a reduction in responsiveness of the medullary respiratory centers to increases in carbon dioxide tension ($PaCO_2$) and also a depression of the pontine and medullary centers that are responsible for respiratory rhythm.

The cardiovascular effects of meperidine are not clinically significant when the drug is administered within its usual therapeutic dose range. Following IV administration of meperidine, however, there is normally an increase in the heart rate produced by the atropine-like vagolytic properties of meperidine. Even at overdose levels the blood pressure remains quite stable until late in the course of the reaction, when it falls, primarily as a result of hypoxia. The administration of O_2 at this time will produce an increase in blood pressure despite continued medullary depression. Overly high blood levels of opioid agonists can lead to loss of consciousness.

Overdose reactions to both the sedative-hypnotics (e.g., propofol, benzodiazepines, barbiturates) and opioid agonists are produced by a progressive depression of the CNS that is manifested by alterations in the level of consciousness (leading to airway obstruction) and as respiratory depression that ultimately results in respiratory arrest. The loss of consciousness produced by barbiturates or propofol or opioid agonists is not always the result of unintentional overdose—these drugs are commonly administered as the primary agents in general anesthesia (see Chapter 31). However, when moderate sedation is the goal, unintended loss of consciousness and respiratory depression/arrest must be considered as complications of drug administration.

The duration and the degree of this clinical reaction vary according to the route of administration, the dose administered, and the patient's individual sensitivity to the drug. In most situations oral and rectal administration result in a lesser degree of CNS depression but with a longer duration; IM, IN, and submucosal administration result in a more profound level of depression of relatively long duration, whereas IV administration produces the most profound level of depression, but of shorter duration than that seen with the other techniques. The onset of respiratory depression after IV administration may be quite rapid, whereas that following oral or rectal administration is considerably slower. Onset is intermediate in IM, IN, and subcutaneous administration.

Management
Sedative-Hypnotic Drugs

Management of sedative-hypnotic drug overdose is predicated on correcting the clinical manifestations of CNS depression. Stated another way, according to the definitions of sedation from the American Society of Anesthesiologists[9] and the American Dental Association,[10] the dentist administering sedation must be capable of "rescuing" the patient who inadvertently descends into a level of CNS depression beyond that which is intended.

Of primary importance is recognition and management of respiratory depression through the administration of basic life support (BLS). Benzodiazepines can be reversed through administration of the specific reversal agent, flumazenil. Unfortunately, there is no effective antagonist that reverses the CNS-depressant properties of the barbiturates—another of the many reasons these drugs are no longer recommended for use in sedation.

Diagnostic clues to the presence of an overdose of a sedative-hypnotic drug include the following[11]:

- Recent administration of a sedative-hypnotic drug
- Lack of response, or extremely lethargic response, to sensory stimulation (decreased level of consciousness: sleepy → unconscious)
- Respiratory depression (rapid rate, shallow depth)
- Loss of motor coordination (ataxia)
- Slurred speech

Step 1: **Terminate treatment.** The rate at which clinical signs and symptoms of overdose develop will vary with route of administration. Onset following IV administration will occur within minutes, within 10 to 30 minutes following IM administration, and within 45 minutes to an hour following oral administration.

Step 2: **P**-Position the patient. The conscious patient may be placed in any position that is comfortable for them; however, in the patient who is either semiconscious or unconscious, the supine position with his or her legs elevated slightly is much preferred (Fig. 34.1). The goal in this scenario, regardless of the level of consciousness, is to maintain adequate cerebral blood flow.

Step 3: **C**-Circulation, **A**-Airway, **B**-Breathing (basic life support), as indicated. A patent airway must be ensured and the adequacy of breathing assessed. Head tilt or head tilt–chin lift may be necessary for airway patency at this time (Fig. 34.2). The presence or adequacy of the patient's spontaneous ventilatory efforts is next assessed by the rescuer, who places his or her ear 1 inch from the patient's mouth and nose, listening and feeling for exhaled air while looking at the patient's chest to determine whether spontaneous respiratory efforts are present. **Maintenance of a patent airway is *the* most important step in the management of this patient.** Step 4b (see later discussion), providing adequate oxygenation, is contingent on successfully maintaining a patent airway. The use of capnography and the pretracheal

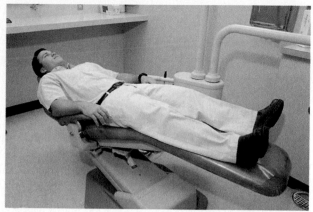

Figure 34.1 The unconscious patient should be placed in the supine position with the legs elevated slightly. (From Malamed SF: *Medical emergencies in the dental office*, ed 7, St Louis, 2015, Mosby.)

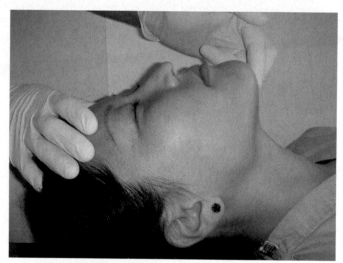

Figure 34.2 The head tilt–chin lift technique.

stethoscope (see Chapter 4) can aid in determining the adequacy of the patients airway and breathing.

Step 4: **D**-Definitive care

Step 4a: **Summon medical assistance,** if needed. In a situation in which the patient loses consciousness following benzodiazepine administration, it might be prudent to consider summoning medical assistance. The requirement for medical assistance will vary depending on the dentist's training in airway management and anesthesiology. If the patient remains conscious but is overly sedated, seeking medical assistance is more of a judgment call by the dentist. When in doubt, it is always wiser to seek assistance sooner rather than later. Inadvertent loss of consciousness is highly unlikely to be noted when benzodiazepines are administered as the sole sedative agent.

Step 4b: **Administer oxygen.** This patient may exhibit different types of breathing. He or she may be conscious but overly sedated, responding, but slowly, to painful stimuli. In this situation the patient will probably be able to maintain his or her own airway and be breathing spontaneously and somewhat effectively (as noted on the pulse oximeter [O_2 saturation readings remain in the very high 90s]). The rescuer need only monitor the patient, assist with airway maintenance (e.g., head tilt–chin lift), and, if desired, administer oxygen through a demand valve or nasal cannula.

The patient might be more deeply sedated and barely responsive to stimulation, with a partially or totally obstructed airway. In this situation assisted ventilation is essential in addition to airway maintenance. With patency of the airway ensured, the patient should receive oxygen via full-face mask or nasal hood. If spontaneous breathing is present but shallow, assisted positive-pressure ventilation is indicated. This is accomplished by activating the positive-pressure mask just as the patient begins each respiratory movement (just as the chest begins to expand). The positive-pressure mask is activated by depressing the button on top of the mask until the patient's chest rises and then releasing the button. With the self-inflating bag–valve–mask device, the bellows bag is squeezed at the start of each inhalation. With both devices, an airtight seal of the mask and head tilt must be maintained at all times. If respiratory arrest occurs (no visible respiratory efforts), controlled artificial ventilation (rescue breathing) must be initiated. The recommended rate for the adult is one breath every 5 seconds (12 per minute) and one breath every 3 seconds for the child aged 1 to 8 years (20 per minute) and the same rate for the infant younger than 1 year old (20 per minute).[12] Expansion of the patient's chest is the only sure sign of successful ventilation. Overinflation should be avoided, as this leads to abdominal distention, resulting in inadequate ventilation and an increased risk of regurgitation. This is more likely to occur with use of the positive pressure mask.

Step 4c: **Monitor vital signs.** The patient's vital signs should be monitored and recorded throughout the episode. Blood pressure, heart rate and rhythm, pulse oximetry, and respiratory rate are monitored constantly and recorded every 5 minutes. A member of the emergency team is assigned to this task. If the blood level of the sedative-hypnotic drug increases significantly, blood pressure may decrease (hypotension) while the heart rate increases (tachycardia). In the absence of blood pressure and pulse (e.g., cardiac arrest), chest compressions must be initiated immediately.

In most cases of nonbarbiturate sedative-hypnotic (e.g., benzodiazepine) overdose, the patient can be managed in this manner until the cerebral blood level of the drug decreases and the patient returns to the desired level of CNS depression (consciousness returns) or until emergency assistance arrives. Recovery occurs as a result of redistribution of the drug within compartments in the body, not biotransformation. The patient becomes increasingly alert and responsive, breathing improves (becomes deeper), and if the blood pressure had been depressed, it returns to near-baseline levels. The length of time for this process to occur depends on the drug administered (short-acting versus long-acting drug) and its route of administration.

Step 4d: **Establish venous access,** if possible. If an IV infusion has not previously been established, it is prudent to obtain one at this time, if training and availability of equipment permit. Although there are no effective antidotal drugs for barbiturate overdose, hypotension may be treated effectively through intravenously administered solutions or drugs. When a benzodiazepine is the cause of the overdose, flumazenil, a benzodiazepine antagonist, can be administered. As blood pressure decreases, however, veins become progressively more difficult to locate and cannulate. Gaining venous access at the earliest possible time may prove invaluable later. Venipuncture should be attempted only if the dentist is trained in this technique, the necessary equipment is available, and the patient continues to receive adequate care (BLS) from other personnel. *A patent airway is more important than a patent vein.*

Step 4e: **Definitive management.** Definitive management of sedative-hypnotic overdose produced by a *barbiturate* is based on maintenance of a patent airway and adequacy of ventilation until the patient recovers. Signs and symptoms of hypotension are evaluated by monitoring vital signs and determining the adequacy of tissue perfusion.*

Benzodiazepine overdosage may be reversed by IV or IM administration of flumazenil, a specific benzodiazepine antagonist. Initially administer 0.2 mg IV. The dose may be repeated after 45 seconds if the desired level of consciousness is not achieved, and subsequently at 1-minute intervals, until a maximum of four doses have been administered (1 mg total over a 5-minute period). If resedation occurs, repeat the regimen at 20-minute intervals, up to a maximum of 3 mg/hour.[13]

Step 5: **Recovery and discharge.** In the event that the overdose is profound, requiring assistance from emergency medical personnel, the patient may need stabilization and transportation to a hospital for observation and full recovery. Should this be necessary, the dentist should always accompany the patient to the hospital. Box 34.3 outlines the steps to follow to manage sedative-hypnotic overdose.

Most cases of sedative-hypnotic overdose involving benzodiazepines are considerably less severe, with diminished responsiveness and slight respiratory depression noted. Management consists of positioning, airway maintenance, and assisted ventilation until recovery. Emergency medical assistance is not usually required. Before discharge in the

---

*Adequacy of tissue perfusion may be determined by pressing on a nail bed or the skin and releasing pressure. Adequate perfusion is present when color returns in not more than 3 seconds. If 4 seconds or more is required for color to return, tissue perfusion is inadequate and consideration must be given to the immediate infusion of IV fluids.

Box 34.3	Management of Sedative-Hypnotic Overdose

Recognize problem
(Recent administration of CNS-depressant drug:
decreased level of consciousness; respiratory
depression; loss of motor coordination;
slurred speech)
↓
Discontinue dental treatment
↓
P—Position patient in supine position with
feet elevated
↓
C→ A→B—Assess circulation, airway, and breathing
↓
D—Provide definitive management as needed
Activate emergency medical service if recovery not
immediate
Administer O$_2$
Monitor vital signs
Establish IV line if possible

Provide Definitive Management:
- Administer intravenous flumazenil for
benzodiazepine overdose
- Continue **P-C-A-B-**for barbiturate overdose
Permit recovery and discharge patient

A, *Airway;* B, *breathing;* C, *circulation;* CNS, *central nervous system;* D, *definitive care;* IV, *intravenous;* P, *position.*

custody of a responsible adult, the patient must be capable of standing and walking without assistance, the same recovery criteria detailed in Chapter 26. In no circumstance should the patient be discharged alone or if not adequately recovered.

Drugs used in management include oxygen and, if benzodiazepines are involved in the overdose, flumazenil. The need for medical assistance with altered consciousness varies with the training and experience of the dentist.

Opioid Analgesics

Oversedation and respiratory depression are the primary clinical manifestations of opioid overdose. Cardiovascular depression typically does not develop until late in the opioid overdose reaction, especially if the patient is positioned supine with their feet elevated slightly. Management of the patient who has received an absolute or relative overdose of an opioid is similar to that described for the sedative-hypnotic drugs with one major addition: A specific antagonist is available to reverse the clinical actions of opioid agonists.

Steps in the management of this situation follow. The clinical picture may vary from minor alterations in consciousness, with minimal respiratory depression, to the unconscious, apneic patient.

Diagnostic clues to the presence of an opioid overdose include the following[11]:
- Altered level of consciousness
- Respiratory depression (slow rate; normal-to-deep depth)
- Miosis (contraction of pupils of the eyes)

Step 1: **Terminate treatment.**

Step 2: **P**-Position the patient. The patient is placed in the supine position with legs elevated slightly.

Step 3: **C**-Circulation, **A**-Airway, **B**-Breathing (basic life support), as indicated. A patent airway is ensured, and breathing is monitored. Opioids produce a decrease in the rate of breathing with little change in tidal volume. Therefore the depth of ventilation is usually increased.

In most cases of opioid overdose the patient remains conscious, although not fully alert or as responsive. Assistance in airway maintenance may be desirable (e.g., head tilt–chin lift). With more profound depression, unconsciousness and respiratory arrest may occur, necessitating reassessment of airway and breathing. Because the cardiovascular system is relatively unaffected by opioid overdose if oxygenation is maintained (airway patency and adequate ventilations are maintained), especially in the supine patient, the blood pressure and heart rate normally remain close to baseline values.

Step 4: **D**-Definitive care.

Step 4a: **Summon medical assistance, if needed.** Depending on the level of consciousness, the degree of respiratory depression, the training of the dentist in emergency care and anesthesiology, and the availability of equipment and drugs, emergency medical assistance might or might not be indicated at this time. As noted in the prior section on sedative/hypnotic overdose, the goal in managing this situation is to "rescue" the patient from this overly deep level of CNS depression, managing them until they either return to the "desired" level or help arrives on the scene to take over management. If unconsciousness and respiratory arrest are present, emergency medical assistance should be summoned immediately if the dentist is not well trained in anesthesiology. In the hands of a dentist well trained in emergency care and anesthesiology (e.g., dentist anesthesiologist), management of the patient may continue to include the administration of antidotal drugs (see Step 4e).

Step 4b: **Administer oxygen.** Oxygen is administered and rescue breathing performed if needed. The administration of oxygen is especially important in the early management of opioid overdose. Minimal cardiovascular depression is normally present and, when present, is usually a result of hypoxia secondary to respiratory depression. The administration of oxygen to a patient with a patent airway prevents or reverses opioid-induced cardiovascular depression, including dysrhythmias that may be evident.

Step 4c: **Monitor and record vital signs.** Vital signs are monitored constantly and recorded every 5 minutes. Should pulse and blood pressure be absent, cardiopulmonary resuscitation (P → C → A → B) is initiated immediately.

Step 4d: **Establish venous access, if possible.** With the cardiovascular system minimally affected by opioid overdose (with the patient in the supine position), it should be possible to establish an IV infusion in most patients. The availability of IV access will expedite definitive therapy.

Step 4e: **Antidotal drug administration.** Definitive management is available when an opioid is the likely cause of the overdose. Even when what could normally be considered a small dose of an opioid has been given (to a hyperresponding patient), an opioid antagonist should be administered to the patient if excessive respiratory depression (or apnea) has developed. No drug will be administered to this patient before the steps of BLS (P → C → A → B) have been assessed and performed, as needed. At this time an opioid antagonist is administered. Naloxone is the drug of choice and should, if possible, be administered intravenously to take advantage of the more rapid onset of action with this route. If the IV route is unavailable, IM administration in the vastus lateralis is acceptable. The onset of action is slower after IM administration, but naloxone will prove to be effective if an opioid is responsible for the respiratory depression. Regardless of the route by which naloxone is administered, the emergency team must continue to provide the necessary steps of BLS from the time of naloxone administration until its onset of action (determined by increased patient responsiveness and more adequate and rapid ventilatory efforts).

Following IV administration, naloxone's actions are noted within 1 to 2 minutes (if not faster) and within 10 minutes following IM administration (in the presence of a near-baseline blood pressure). Naloxone is available in a 1-mL ampule containing 0.4 mg (adult dosage form) or 0.02 mg (pediatric [up to 30 kg] dosage form). Naloxone is initially titrated at 0.1 to 0.2 mg IV at 2- to 3-minute intervals until the desired response is obtained.[13,14] Naloxone is diluted to a concentration of 0.1 mg/mL. This is accomplished by taking 1 mL of the 0.4-mg/mL concentration and adding 3 mL of diluent (e.g., 5% dextrose and water). Every 2 to 3 minutes, 0.1 to 0.2 mg should be injected slowly intravenously while the patient is observed for adequate reversal of respiratory depression: increased ventilatory effort and increased alertness without significant pain or discomfort.

Additional doses of naloxone may be required in some patients, depending on the type and dose of opioid administered and the patient's response to naloxone. If repeated administration of naloxone is necessary, it is recommended that the IM route be given serious consideration because the duration of action of naloxone will be prolonged by this route of administration.

In children 5 years or older or weighing more than 20 kg: initially administer 0.005 to 0.01 mg IV at 2- to 3-minute intervals until the desired degree of reversal is obtained.[15,16] The dose may be administered intramuscularly or subcutaneously if systemic perfusion is adequate. If, for some reason,

naloxone must be administered subcutaneously or intramuscularly, the adult dose is 0.4 mg and the pediatric dose is 0.01 mg/kg. The onset of action is slower; however, the duration of action will be significantly longer than noted after IV administration.

A potential problem when reversing opioid overdose with naloxone is the fact that its duration of clinical activity may be shorter than that of the opioid it is being used to reverse. This is especially true in cases in which a longer-acting opioid agonist such as morphine or hydromorphone is administered; it is less likely to occur with meperidine and even more unlikely with fentanyl and its analogs alfentanil, sufentanil, and remifentanil. When the opioid action is of greater duration than the intravenously administered naloxone, the dentist and staff will notice an initial improvement in the patient's clinical picture as the naloxone begins to act and then see a recurrence of CNS depression approximately 10 minutes or more later (following IV administration of naloxone). Because the opioid producing the overdose continues to undergo redistribution and biotransformation during this time, in the event that such a rebound effect does occur, it would quite likely be less intense than the initial response. In cases in which longer-acting opioids (e.g., morphine) have been administered intramuscularly or submucosally, it is recommended that the initial IV dose of naloxone be followed with an IM dose (0.4 mg [adult] or 0.01 mg/kg [pediatric]). In this way, as the clinical action of the IV naloxone dose is waning, the level of naloxone from the IM dose will be reaching a peak, minimizing the likelihood of a relapse of significant respiratory or CNS depression. The administration of naloxone in opioid overdose is important but not the most critical step in overall patient management (see later discussion).

Step 5: **Permit recovery.** The patient is continuously observed and monitored after the administration of naloxone until clinical recovery becomes evident. The patient may be transported to a recovery area within the dental office but should remain under constant supervision for at least 1 hour. On the other hand, if the dentist considers it prudent, the planned dental treatment may continue. Once again, whether to continue treatment of this patient at this time is a judgment that can be made only by the dentist, and only after taking into consideration the status of the patient and the level of expertise of the dentist and staff in recognizing and managing this situation. A patient demonstrating oversedation with an opioid might be considered an emergency in the office of a less well-trained (in anesthesiology and airway management) dentist, whereas in the office of a more well-trained dentist this same situation could represent nothing more than a minor occurrence, one that is readily managed in a routine manner.

If doubt exists, dental care should be discontinued. Vital signs are monitored constantly and recorded every 5 minutes during the recovery period. Oxygen and suction must be available, and trained personnel must be present.

Step 6: **Discharge.** Patient discharge might require transport to a hospital facility for observation or follow-up care. In most cases, however, hospitalization is unnecessary. Following an adequate period of recovery (minimum 1 hour under observation following naloxone administration) in the dental or medical office, the patient may be discharged in the custody of a responsible adult companion, using the same recovery criteria established for parenteral sedation (see Chapter 26) and general anesthesia.

Box 34.4 outlines the steps to follow in management of opioid overdose.

Drugs used in management include oxygen and naloxone.

The need for medical assistance in the presence of altered consciousness or unconsciousness will depend on the dentist's training and experience.

SUMMARY

The previous discussions dealt with overdose reactions of varying levels of severity that occur after the administration of a single drug. Although single-drug overdose can and does occur, especially after IM, IN, or submucosal administration (because of the inability to titrate to effect), many overdose reactions reported involve the administration of multiple drugs. In many of these cases, drugs such as an antianxiety drug are combined with an opioid to provide a level of sedation and some analgesia. A local anesthetic is then added to manage operative pain. Drugs in all three of these categories are CNS depressants. Added to this, in many cases, will be nitrous oxide (N_2O) and oxygen (O_2), adding yet another degree of CNS depression.

Whenever more than one CNS-depressant drug is administered to a patient, the dosages of all drugs should be reduced from their usual dosage to prevent exaggerated, undesirable clinical responses. As illustrated in Table 34.2, in most of the cases reported by Goodson and Moore, this step was not taken, with catastrophic results often occurring.[9]

Another factor must be considered, one that most health professionals do not, as a rule, give much thought to when using sedative techniques: Local anesthetics themselves are CNS depressants and can produce additive actions when administered in conjunction with drugs commonly used for sedation. The maximal dosage of local anesthetic to be administered to any patient, but especially to patients weighing less than 30 kg (66 lb), should be based on the patient's body weight in kilograms (or pounds). When no other CNS depressants are being administered, this maximal dose could be reached without adverse effects if the patient is an American Society of Anesthesiologists (ASA) 1 and falls within the normal responding range on the bell-shaped curve. Table 34.3 presents the FDA's maximum recommended doses of the most commonly used dental local anesthetics. When a local anesthetic is administered with other CNS depressants, the local anesthetic dosage should be minimized.

| Box 34.4 | **Management of Opioid Overdose** |

Recognize problem
(Altered level of consciousness; respiratory depression; miosis)
↓
Discontinue dental treatment
↓
P—Position patient in supine position with feet elevated
↓
C→A→B—Assess airway, breathing, and circulation
↓
D—Provide definitive management as needed
Activate emergency medical service as needed
Administer O_2
Monitor vital signs
Establish IV line, if possible

Provide Definitive Management:
- Administer IV or IM naloxone
- Continue P→C→A→B as needed
  Permit recovery and discharge patient

A, *Airway*; B, *breathing*; C, *circulation*; D, *definitive care*; IM, *intramuscular*; IV, *intravenous*; P, *position*.

A primary goal of moderate sedation is to produce a cooperative patient who still possesses their protective reflexes (e.g., swallowing, coughing, maintenance of the airway). If possible, this goal should be achieved using the simplest technique available, as well as the fewest drugs possible. Polypharmacy, the combination of several drugs, is necessary in many patients to achieve the desired level of sedation and/or analgesia. The use of drug combinations, however, increases the opportunity for ADRs while making it less obvious which drug might be responsible for any problems that arise, thereby potentially complicating management of the situation.

Within the individual techniques of sedation, it is suggested that single-drug regimens are preferable to combinations of drugs. Rational drug combinations are available for use in certain situations in which they are specifically indicated. With IV drug administration, the problem of severe ADRs should not occur if the technique of titration is strictly adhered to at all times. Titration is not possible with the IM, IN, and oral routes of administration. The dentist must modify individual drug dosages before their administration. Serious ADRs are more likely to occur when the technique used was one in which titration was not possible.

Consideration must also be given to the use of multiple techniques of sedation, as opposed to multiple drugs by one technique of administration. It is not uncommon for patient who is a significant management problem to receive an oral

Table 34.2	Dose Administered Relative to Recommended Maximum Dose			
CASE	NARCOTIC ANALGESICS (%)*	ANTIEMETIC SEDATIVES (%)*	LOCAL ANESTHETICS (%)* N₂O-O₂	RESULT
1	216	36	172	Fatality
2	173	145	237	Fatality
3	336	0	342	Fatality
4	127	27	267	Fatality
5	309	372	230	Brain damage
6	436	?	?	Fatality
7	100	136	107	Fatality
8	167	300	219 +	Brain damage
9	66	0	60 -	Recovery
10	66	92	?+	Recovery
11	183	0	?	Recovery
12	200	558	0 -	Recovery
13	250	136	127 -	Brain damage
14	50	0	370 +	Fatality

*Expressed as a percentage of the maximal recommended dose for that patient.
From Goodson JM, Moore PA: Life-threatening reactions after pedodontic sedation: an assessment of narcotic, local anesthetic, and antiemetic drug interaction, *J Am Dent Assoc* 107(2):239–245, 1983. Copyright by the American Dental Association. Reprinted by permission.

Table 34.3	Maximum Recommended Doses of Local Anesthetics					
	United States			Canada		
	Dose			Dose		
DRUG	MG/KG	MG/LB	MRD*	MG/KG	MG/LB	MRD†
Articaine	7.0	3.2	None listed	7.0 (adults) 5.0 (children)	3.2 (adults) 2.25 (children)	500 mg
Lidocaine	7.0	3.2	500 mg	7.0	3.2	500 mg
Mepivacaine	6.6	3.0	400 mg	6.6	3.0	400 mg
Prilocaine	8.0	3.6	600 mg	8.0	3.6	500 mg
Bupivacaine	None listed	None listed	90 mg	2.0	0.9	200 mg

*United States Food & Drug Administration (FDA).
†Health Canada (Sante Canada).
MRD, Maximum recommended dose.

antianxiety drug before arrival at the office. This is followed by either IM, IN, or IV sedation, and inhalation sedation and local anesthesia during the course of treatment. Whenever oral sedation with CNS depressants is used, the dosages of all subsequent CNS depressants should be evaluated carefully before their administration. This is critical when nontitratable routes of drug administration are used. With inhalation and IV sedation, careful titration of CNS-depressant drugs to the patient who has previously received oral premedication will usually produce the desired level of clinical sedation with minimal risk of adverse response by the patient.

How, then, may overdose reactions best be prevented? Goodson and Moore made the following recommendations concerning the use of sedative techniques involving the administration of opioids[9]:

1. *Be prepared for emergencies.* The cardiovascular and respiratory systems should be monitored continuously. An emergency kit containing drugs such as epinephrine, oxygen, flumazenil, and naloxone should be readily available, in addition to equipment and trained personnel. In their paper, Goodson and Moore state that "because multiple sedative drug techniques can easily induce unconsciousness, respiratory arrest, and convulsions, practitioners should be prepared and trained to recognize and control these occurrences."

2. *Individualize the drug dosage.* When drugs are used in combination, the dosage of each drug must be selected carefully. The toxic effects of drug combinations appear to be additive. Drug selection must be based on the patient's general health history. The presence of significant systemic disease (ASA 3 or 4) usually indicates the need for a

reduction of dosage. Because most sedative drugs are available in quite concentrated form and because children usually require very small dosages, extreme care must be taken when drugs are being prepared for administration.

When possible, fixed-dose administration of drugs based on a range of ages (e.g., 4 to 6 years: 50 mg) should be avoided. Dosages based on body weight or surface area of the patient, or titration, are preferred when possible, keeping in mind that these doses are based on the response of patients lying in the middle of the normal distribution curve.

Should the selected drug dosage administered in a nontitratable technique prove to be inadequate to produce the desired effect in the patient, it is prudent to consider a change in the sedation technique or in the drugs being used (at a subsequent appointment) rather than increasing the drug dosage to a higher and potentially more dangerous level at the same visit.

3. *Recognize and expect adverse drug effects.* When combinations of CNS depressants have been administered, the potential for excessive CNS and respiration depression is increased and should be expected.

The Dentists Insurance Company (TDIC), in a retrospective study of deaths and morbidity in dental practices over a 3-year period, concluded that in most of those incidents related to administration of drugs, there were three common factors.[17] Though published in 1983, sadly these three factors are still relevant.

1. Improper preoperative evaluation of the patient
2. Lack of knowledge of drug pharmacology by the dentist
3. Lack of adequate monitoring during the procedure

These three factors greatly increased the risk of serious ADRs, with a negative outcome being the usual result.

An overdose reaction to the administration of CNS-depressant drugs may not always be a preventable complication; however, with care taken on the part of the dentist, the incidence of these events should be extremely low, with a successful outcome the result virtually every time. With techniques such as IV and inhalation sedation in which titration is possible, overdosage should be rare. With oral, IM, and IN drug administration, in which little control is maintained over the drug's ultimate effect because of the inability to titrate, the dentist must expend greater care in the preoperative evaluation of the patient, in the determination of the appropriate drug dosage, and in monitoring during the procedure so that excessive CNS or respiratory depression may be identified and treated immediately. When the oral, IN, or IM route is used, the onset of adverse reactions may be delayed. An adverse reaction may not develop until after the rubber dam is in place and the dental procedure has been started. For this reason monitoring of the patient throughout the procedure becomes extremely important to the patient's safety. My preferences, as of February 2017, in monitoring during parenteral minimal or moderate sedation are as follows:

1. CNS
   a. Direct verbal contact with the patient

2. Respiratory system
   a. Pulse oximetry
   b. Pretracheal stethoscope
   c. Capnography
3. Cardiovascular system
   a. Continuous monitoring of vital signs
   b. Electrocardiogram (ECG)

ALLERGY

Allergy represents a hypersensitive state acquired through exposure to a particular allergen, reexposure to which produces a heightened capacity to react. Allergic reactions cover a broad range of clinical manifestations, from mild, delayed-onset reactions occurring as long as 48 hours after exposure to immediate and life-threatening reactions developing within seconds of exposure. Although all allergic phenomena are important and require thorough evaluation by the dentist, only one form, the type I, or immediate, reaction is discussed here, for it may present the dentist with a life-threatening emergency situation.

Allergic reactions are mediated through immunologic mechanisms that are similar regardless of the specific antigen responsible for precipitating the response. Therefore an allergic reaction to the venom of a stinging insect may be identical to that seen after aspirin or penicillin administration in a previously sensitized individual. Allergic reactions must be differentiated from the overdose, or toxic, reaction previously discussed, in which the observed signs and symptoms are a direct extension of the normal pharmacologic properties of the drug administered. Overdose reactions are much more commonly encountered than are allergic drug reactions. Of all ADRs, 85% result from the pharmacologic actions of drugs; 15% are immunologic reactions.[18] To the layperson, however, any ADR is frequently labeled "allergic."

Allergy is a frightening word to those health professionals responsible for primary care of patients. Although none of the drugs commonly used for the management of pain and anxiety has a significantly high rate of allergenicity, allergic phenomena may still arise. The only drugs mentioned in this book that, to my knowledge, have never been shown to have produced allergy are N_2O and O_2. Although the concept of prevention has been stressed repeatedly throughout this text, in no other situation is this concept of greater importance than with allergy. Although allergy is not the most common ADR, it is frequently involved with the most serious of these reactions.

Of the many antianxiety drugs used, the barbiturates probably possessed the greatest potential for sensitization of patients. Although not nearly as common as allergy to penicillin or aspirin, barbiturate allergy usually manifests itself in the form of skin lesions, such as hives and urticaria, or less frequently in the form of blood dyscrasias, such as agranulocytosis or thrombocytopenia. Allergy to barbiturates occurs much more frequently in persons with a history of asthma, urticaria, and angioedema.[19] A documented history of allergy to any barbiturate represents an absolute contraindication to their administration.

By contrast, allergy to benzodiazepines, though possible, is extremely rare.[20]

Among the opioids, meperidine can release histamine locally. When meperidine is administered intravenously, this localized histamine release develops along the path of the vein through which the drug travels. This reaction is not an allergy and requires no therapeutic management. The reaction resolves after the drug leaves the area of its administration. Use of meperidine is relatively contraindicated in asthmatic patients because of potential bronchospasm induced by histamine release when the drug enters the pulmonary circulation.

Following IV administration, atropine—an anticholinergic—may produce flushing of a patient's face, neck, and upper chest. Known as *atropine flush*, this is not an allergic reaction and requires no therapeutic intervention because spontaneous resolution occurs within a brief time.[21] Atropine flush is most often seen with overdose of atropine. However, in certain sensitive individuals (those who are hyperresponders on the bell-shaped curve), the usual therapeutic dose may provoke this response.

Prevention of Allergic Reactions

Whenever any drug or combination of drugs is being considered for administration, the dentist must question the patient about any prior exposure to that drug or members of the same drug family. In addition, the patient's medical history questionnaire must be evaluated. All questionnaires include questions concerning current drug use and prior ADRs. These two steps will, in most cases, enable the dentist to assess the possibility of an adverse drug response. Should a positive history be elicited, questioning is undertaken to determine the nature of the previous reaction. Although the questioning may vary, basic questions asked include the following:

1. What drug was used?
2. What happened? (The patient describes the sequence of events that ensued.)
3. What treatment was required? Was epinephrine or a histamine blocker administered? O_2 or aromatic ammonia?
4. Were the services of a physician or emergency paramedical personnel required? Were you hospitalized?
5. What is the name and address of the doctor (physician or dentist) who treated you at that time?

Knowledge of the signs and symptoms of the "reaction" and its management can go far in aiding the dentist in diagnosing the alleged "allergy."

The need for hospitalization or assistance from a second health professional usually indicates that a more serious ADR occurred. If possible, it would be prudent to speak directly to the doctor involved with the patient at that time.

Following a thorough dialog history and review of the medical history questionnaire, it is usually possible to form a general opinion about the true nature of the reaction. If the dentist is convinced that allergy did occur, other drugs that are structurally dissimilar to the offending drug should be selected for administration. In most cases, however, it will become obvious that the "allergy" was in fact a side effect of the drug (e.g., nausea from codeine) or that the response was psychogenic (i.e., tachycardia and/or palpations induced by anxiety). If doubt remains as to the precise nature of the reaction, the patient should be managed, at that time, with drugs unrelated to the one(s) in question, followed by consultation with an allergist (or other appropriate health care professional) so that more definitive testing might be undertaken.

Clinical Manifestations

Most serious (i.e., life-threatening) allergic drug reactions are immediate, in particular the type I, or anaphylactic, reaction. The word *immediate* as it relates to allergic phenomena indicates the development of clinical signs and symptoms within 60 minutes of exposure to the allergen.

A number of organs and tissues are affected during immediate allergic reactions, particularly the skin, respiratory system, cardiovascular system, and gastrointestinal (GI) tract. Generalized, or systemic, anaphylaxis, by definition, affects all the systems mentioned. If hypotension is also a clinical component of the response, the term *anaphylactic shock* is correctly applied.

Immediate allergic reactions also manifest through any number of combinations involving these organs. Reactions involving one system are referred to as *localized anaphylaxis*, for example, asthmatic attack, in which the respiratory system is the sole target, or urticaria, in which the skin is the target organ.

Onset

The time elapsing between exposure of the patient to the antigen and the development of clinical signs and symptoms is of great importance. As a rule, *the more rapidly signs and symptoms evolve after exposure to an allergen, the more intense the ultimate response will be.*[22] Conversely, the greater the length of time between exposure and onset, the less intense the reaction usually is. However, cases of anaphylaxis have been reported to arise many hours after exposure. Of importance, too, is the speed at which signs and symptoms progress once they appear. If they appear and increase in severity rapidly, the reaction is more likely to become life threatening than one that progresses slowly or not at all.

Skin Reaction

Allergic skin reactions are the most common sensitization reaction to drug administration. Many types of allergic skin reaction may occur, the two most important types being localized anaphylaxis and drug eruption. Drug eruption constitutes the most common group of skin manifestations of drug allergy. Included in this category are urticaria, erythema (reddening), and angioedema (localized swelling).

Urticaria is associated with wheals (smooth, slightly elevated patches of skin) and often with intense itching (pruritus).

Angioedema is a process in which localized swelling occurs in response to an allergen. Several forms of angioedema exist, but clinically they appear to be similar. The skin is usually of normal color (unless accompanied by urticaria or erythema) and temperature, and pain and itching are uncommon. The regions most commonly involved are the hands, face, feet, and genitalia. Of special concern is the potential involvement of the lips, tongue, pharynx, and larynx, leading to obstruction of the airway (laryngeal edema).

Allergic skin reactions, if the sole manifestation of allergy, are usually not considered life threatening. However, a skin reaction that develops rapidly after drug administration may be the first indication of the generalized reaction to follow.

Adhesive tape used during IV sedation is a fairly common cause of dermatologic reactions, the adhesive being the allergen. The usual response to this tape is erythema and urticaria developing around the site where the tape has been placed. In adhesive-allergic individuals, hypoallergenic tape is available for use.

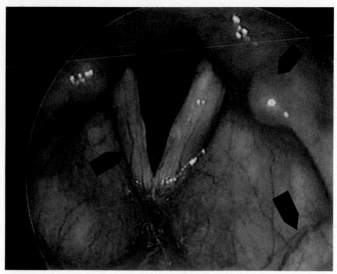

Figure 34.3 Laryngeal edema. (From Dworkin JP: Laryngitis: Types, causes, and treatments, *Otolaryn Clin N Amer* 41(2):419–436, 2008.)

Respiratory Reactions

Clinical signs and symptoms of allergy may be related entirely to the respiratory tract, or signs and symptoms of respiratory tract involvement may develop along with other systemic responses. In a slowly developing generalized allergic reaction, respiratory tract involvement usually follows the skin response but precedes cardiovascular signs and symptoms. Bronchospasm is the classic respiratory manifestation of allergy. It represents the clinical result of constriction of bronchial smooth muscle. Signs and symptoms include respiratory distress, dyspnea, wheezing, flushing, possible cyanosis, perspiration, tachycardia, greatly increased anxiety, and the use of accessory muscles of respiration.

A second respiratory manifestation of acute allergy may be the extension of angioedema to the larynx, producing a swelling of the vocal apparatus with subsequent obstruction of the airway (laryngeal edema) (Fig. 34.3). Clinical manifestations include little or no air exchange from the lungs (chest is not moving, little or no air exchange is felt); wheezing, indicative of partial airway obstruction; or no sound, indicating total obstruction. The occurrence of significant angioedema represents one of the most ominous of clinical signs. Acute airway obstruction leads rapidly to the death of the patient unless immediately corrected.

Generalized Anaphylaxis

Generalized anaphylaxis is the most dramatic and acutely life-threatening form of allergy and may lead to clinical death within a few minutes. It may develop after the administration of an antigen via any route, but is most likely to occur after parenteral administration. The time from antigenic challenge to the onset of reaction varies greatly, but typically the reaction develops rapidly, reaching a maximum within 5 to 30 minutes.[23] Delayed responses of 1 hour or more have been reported. It

is believed that this is the result of the rate at which the antigen enters into the circulatory system.

Signs and symptoms of generalized anaphylaxis are highly variable. Four major clinical syndromes are recognized: skin reactions, smooth muscle spasm (GI and genitourinary tracts and respiratory smooth muscle), respiratory distress, and cardiovascular collapse. In typical generalized anaphylaxis, the symptoms progressively move through these four areas; however, in cases of fatal anaphylaxis, respiratory and cardiovascular disturbances predominate and are evident early in the reaction.[24]

In the typical generalized anaphylactic reaction, the patient may begin to complain of feeling sick with intense itching, flushing, and giant hives developing over their face and upper chest. Nausea, possibly followed by vomiting, may also occur. These early symptoms are primarily related to the skin. Other responses noted early in the reaction include conjunctivitis, vasomotor rhinitis (increased mucus secretion in the nose), and pilomotor erection (the feeling of hair standing on end).

Associated with the development of skin symptoms are various GI and genitourinary disturbances related to spasm of smooth muscle. Severe abdominal cramps, nausea and vomiting, diarrhea, and fecal and urinary incontinence may occur.

Respiratory symptoms normally follow. However, in rapidly developing reactions, all symptoms may occur within a short time with considerable overlap. In particularly severe reactions, respiratory and cardiovascular symptoms may be the only signs present.

Respiratory symptoms begin with a feeling of substernal tightness or pain in the chest. A cough may develop in addition to wheezing and dyspnea. If the respiratory disturbances are severe, cyanosis may develop, noted initially in mucous membranes and nail beds. Laryngeal edema may also develop, producing acute airway obstruction.

Signs and symptoms of cardiovascular disturbance follow and include pallor, lightheadedness, palpitation, tachycardia, hypotension, and cardiac dysrhythmias, followed by loss of consciousness and cardiac arrest. With loss of consciousness, the anaphylactic reaction may more properly be called *anaphylactic shock*.

The duration of the anaphylactic reaction or any part of it may vary from minutes to a day or more. With prompt and appropriate therapy, the entire reaction may be terminated rapidly; however, the two most serious sequelae, hypotension and laryngeal edema, may persist for hours to days despite vigorous therapy. Death may occur at any time, with the usual cause being upper airway obstruction produced by laryngeal edema.

Management
Skin Reactions

Allergic skin reactions may range from localized angioedema to diffuse erythema, urticaria, and pruritus. Management is based on the speed at which they appear after antigenic challenge (drug administration).

Delayed Skin Reactions

Skin reactions appearing more than 60 minutes after antigenic exposure that do not progress are considered non–life threatening. These include a mild skin reaction after IM injection or localized reaction to adhesive tape.

When this occurs during parenteral sedation, the first step in management is the IM or IV administration of a histamine blocker such as diphenhydramine 50 mg for the patient weighing more than 30 kg. The patient is to remain in the dental office for a minimum of 1 hour before considering their discharge (to ensure that the allergic reaction is not progressing). On discharge, the patient is given a prescription for a histamine blocker to be taken orally for 3 to 5 days. Medical consultation should follow with the patient's physician or an allergist to determine the nature of the allergy or allergies.

If the skin reaction is mild but the patient has left the office before it develops, the patient should be requested to return to the office, where the same therapy as described would be employed. Should the reaction be noted at a time when the patient is unable to return to the office for evaluation, the patient is advised to see a physician at a local hospital emergency room. The treating dentist should arrange to meet the patient at the hospital, if possible.

Histamine blockers inhibit the actions of histamine by occupying drug receptor sites on the effector cell (competitive antagonism), thereby preventing the agonist molecules (histamine) from occupying these same sites. The protective responses from histamine blockers include control of edema formation and itch. Other allergic responses, such as hypotension and bronchoconstriction, are influenced little, if at all, by histamine blockers. Histamine blockers are of value only in mild allergic responses in which only small quantities of histamine have been released or to prevent reactions in allergic individuals.

Immediate Skin Reactions

Allergic skin reactions developing in less than 60 minutes should be managed more vigorously. Other allergic symptoms of a relatively mild nature included in this section are conjunctivitis, rhinitis, urticaria, pruritus, and erythema.

Epinephrine is administered intravenously (1 : 10,000), intramuscularly (1 : 1000), or subcutaneously (1 : 1000) in an adult dose of 0.3 mg. A histamine blocker (e.g., diphenhydramine) is then administered. Medical consultation is requested.

Whenever epinephrine administration is required, it is my belief that the patient should be fully evaluated before discharge from the office or hospital. In most cases the patient should be observed for at least 1 hour and, in the absence of a return of signs and symptoms, may be discharged home in the company of a responsible adult. If the reaction is more severe, medical consultation before discharge is indicated.

Respiratory Reactions
Bronchospasm

The most likely situations in dentistry in which an allergic reaction will manifest itself as a respiratory problem (bronchospasm) are (1) in the asthmatic patient who comes into contact with their specific allergens during dental care and (2) the patient who is allergic to aspirin or other NSAIDs.

Diagnostic clues to the presence of an allergy involving bronchospasm include the following:
- Wheezing
- Use of accessory muscles of respiration

Bronchial smooth muscle constriction results in asthma-like reactions. Management of bronchospasm includes the following:

Step 1: **Terminate the treatment.**

Step 2: **P**-Position the patient comfortably. An upright or semierect position is usually preferred by the conscious patient exhibiting difficulty breathing.

Step 3: **C**-Circulation, **A**-Airway, **B**-Breathing (basic life support), as indicated. Assessment of airway and circulation will initially prove adequate. Breathing may demonstrate varying degrees of inadequacy, ranging from mild bronchospasm to almost complete obstruction and cyanosis.

Step 4: **Remove equipment from the patient's mouth.**

Step 5: **Calm the patient.** A conscious person experiencing respiratory distress may become quite fearful. Try to allay any apprehensions.

Step 6: **D**-Definitive care.

Step 6a: **Summon medical assistance.** With clinically evident respiratory distress associated with wheezing and cyanosis, emergency medical care should be sought immediately.

Step 6b: **Administer a bronchodilator.** Albuterol (also known as salbutamol) may be administered by means of an aerosol inhaler (e.g., Ventolin, Proventil, ProAir) or epinephrine by IM or subcutaneous injection (0.3 mL of a 1:1000 dilution for the patient weight of more than 30 kg) or intravenously (0.1 mL of 1:10,000 every 15 to 30 minutes). The potent bronchodilating actions of epinephrine usually terminate bronchospasm within minutes of administration. Epinephrine is the drug of choice as an injected bronchodilator because it effectively reverses the actions of one of the major causes of bronchospasm—histamine; however, like the histamine blockers, epinephrine does not relieve bronchospasm produced by leukotrienes. Inhaled bronchodilators, such as albuterol, also act rapidly in the management of bronchospasm.

Step 6c: **Monitor the patient**. The patient should remain in the dental office for observation because a recurrence of bronchospasm is possible as the epinephrine undergoes rapid biotransformation. Should bronchospasm reappear, epinephrine may be readministered intramuscularly or subcutaneously, or albuterol may be administered by inhalation (aerosol).

Step 6d: **Administer a histamine blocker**. The IM administration of a histamine blocker minimizes the risk of a recurrence of bronchospasm as the histamine blocker occupies the histamine receptor site, preventing a relapse. Diphenhydramine 50 mg intramuscularly (more than 30 kg) or 2 mg/kg intramuscularly or intravenously (up to 30 kg) is suggested.

Step 6e: **Recovery and discharge**. On arrival, emergency medical personnel will stabilize the victim and start any necessary definitive treatment. Additional treatment may involve the administration of one or more of the following: IV bronchodilators, atropine, or steroids (methylprednisolone); intubation and assisted ventilation may be necessary if bronchospasm is persistent and severe. In most cases a patient exhibiting an allergic reaction consisting primarily of respiratory signs and symptoms will require a variable period of hospitalization.

Box 34.5 outlines the steps to take in managing the respiratory allergic reaction.

Drugs used in the management of allergic reactions include oxygen, bronchodilators such as epinephrine (intravenously, intramuscularly, or subcutaneously), albuterol (inhalation), and histamine blockers (intramuscularly).

Medical assistance is required if there is significant respiratory distress.

Laryngeal Edema

The second and usually more life-threatening respiratory allergic manifestation is the development of laryngeal edema. It may be diagnosed when little or no air movement can be heard or felt through the mouth and nose despite exaggerated spontaneous respiratory efforts by the patient or when a patent airway cannot be obtained. A partially obstructed larynx in the presence of spontaneous respiratory movements produces the characteristically high-pitched crowing sound of stridor, in contrast to the wheezing of bronchospasm; total obstruction is

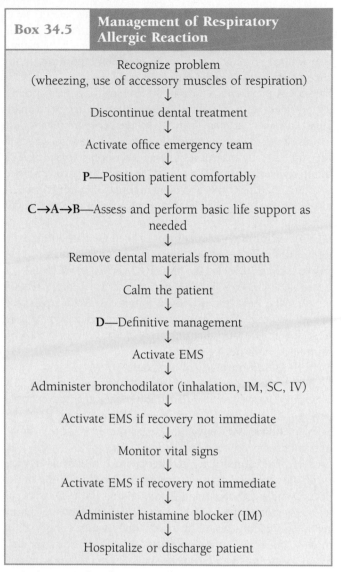

| Box 34.5 | **Management of Respiratory Allergic Reaction** |

Recognize problem
(wheezing, use of accessory muscles of respiration)
↓
Discontinue dental treatment
↓
Activate office emergency team
↓
P—Position patient comfortably
↓
C→A→B—Assess and perform basic life support as needed
↓
Remove dental materials from mouth
↓
Calm the patient
↓
D—Definitive management
↓
Activate EMS
↓
Administer bronchodilator (inhalation, IM, SC, IV)
↓
Activate EMS if recovery not immediate
↓
Monitor vital signs
↓
Activate EMS if recovery not immediate
↓
Administer histamine blocker (IM)
↓
Hospitalize or discharge patient

A, *Airway*; B, *breathing*; C, *circulation*; D, *definitive care*; EMS, *emergency medical services*; IM, *intramuscular*; IV, *intravenous*; P, *position*; SC, *subcutaneous*.

accompanied by silence in the presence of spontaneous chest movement (see Fig. 34.3). The patient loses consciousness from lack of oxygen (e.g., hypoxia, anoxia). Fortunately, laryngeal edema is not common, but it may arise in any acute allergic reaction that involves the airway.

Diagnostic clues to the presence of laryngeal edema include the following:
• Respiratory distress
• Exaggerated chest movements
• High-pitched crowing sound of stridor (partial obstruction) or no sound (total obstruction)
• Cyanosis
• Loss of consciousness

Step 1: **Terminate the treatment**.

Step 2: **P**-Position the patient. An upright or semierect position is usually preferred by the conscious patient exhibiting difficulty breathing. If the degree of edema is severe, the patient's level of consciousness may be significantly altered, and the supine position with the feet elevated is most appropriate. If the patient is unwilling or unable to tolerate the supine position, he or she should be positioned based on comfort.

Step 3: **C**-Circulation, **A**-Airway, **B**-Breathing (basic life support), as indicated. Airway will be the most critical factor in managing laryngeal edema. Initial management should include extension of the neck (head tilt–chin lift or jaw thrust–chin lift), followed by insertion of either a nasopharyngeal tube or oropharyngeal airway. The conscious patient is usually able to tolerate a nasopharyngeal airway, whereas the oropharyngeal airway is likely to elicit a lively gag reflex and, potentially, vomiting.

Step 4a: **Administer epinephrine.** The immediate administration of 0.3 mL of 1:1000 epinephrine intramuscularly in the vastus lateralis muscle (see Figs. 10.3 and 10.4) (0.15 mL for up to 30 kg; 0.075 mL for infant) or 0.1 mL of 1:10,000 epinephrine intravenously over 5 minutes (adult), repeated every 3 to 5 minutes as necessary, is recommended. A maximum dose for 1:10,000 epinephrine of 5.0 mL every 15 to 30 minutes should not be exceeded.

Step 4b: **Summon medical assistance.**

Step 4c: **Maintain airway.** In the presence of a partially obstructed airway, epinephrine administration may halt the progress of, or possibly even reverse, laryngeal edema.

Step 4d: **Administer oxygen.** Oxygen should be administered as soon as it becomes available.

Step 4e: **Additional drug management.** A histamine blocker (diphenhydramine 50 mg [more than 30 kg] or 25 mg [up to 30 kg]) and a corticosteroid (hydrocortisone 100 mg) should be administered intramuscularly or intravenously following clinical recovery, which is noted by airway improvement: normal, or at least improved, breath sounds; absence of cyanosis; and fewer exaggerated chest excursions. Corticosteroids inhibit edema and capillary dilation by stabilizing cell membranes. They are of little immediate value because of their slow onset of action, even when administered intravenously. Corticosteroids have an onset of action approximately 6 hours after their administration. Corticosteroids are used to prevent a relapse, whereas epinephrine, a more rapidly acting drug, is used during the acute phase to halt or reverse the deleterious actions of histamine and other mediators of allergy.

These procedures (steps 1 through 4e) are normally adequate to maintain the patient. Following arrival of emergency medical assistance, the patient will be stabilized and transferred to a hospital for further observation and treatment.

Step 4f: **Cricothyrotomy.** A totally obstructed airway may not be reopened at all, or in adequate time, by the administration of epinephrine and other drugs. In this case an emergency airway must be created to preserve the patient's life. Time is of the essence, and it is not possible to delay action until medical assistance arrives. A cricothyrotomy is the procedure of choice for the establishment of an airway in this situation.[25]

(The reader is referred to Chapter 11 of *Medical Emergencies in the Dental Office*[26] for a complete description of the cricothyrotomy technique.) Once an airway is obtained, oxygen is administered, artificial ventilation initiated (if needed), and vital signs monitored.

Before the arrival of medical assistance, the drugs previously administered may halt the progress of the laryngeal edema and might even reverse it to a degree. The patient will require hospitalization following transfer from the dental office by the paramedics.

Box 34.6 outlines the steps in the management of laryngeal edema.

Drugs used in management of laryngeal edema include oxygen, epinephrine (intravenously or intramuscularly), a histamine blocker (intramuscularly), and a corticosteroid (intravenously or intramuscularly).

Medical assistance is required.

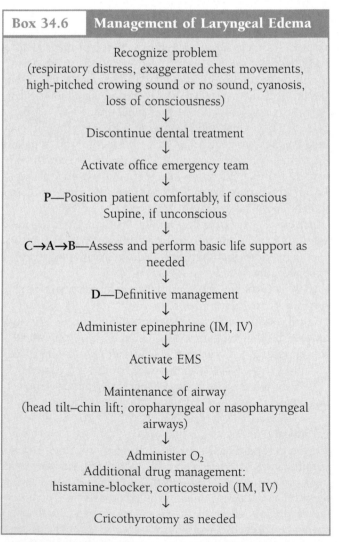

Box 34.6	Management of Laryngeal Edema

Recognize problem
(respiratory distress, exaggerated chest movements, high-pitched crowing sound or no sound, cyanosis, loss of consciousness)
↓
Discontinue dental treatment
↓
Activate office emergency team
↓
P—Position patient comfortably, if conscious
Supine, if unconscious
↓
C→A→B—Assess and perform basic life support as needed
↓
D—Definitive management
↓
Administer epinephrine (IM, IV)
↓
Activate EMS
↓
Maintenance of airway
(head tilt–chin lift; oropharyngeal or nasopharyngeal airways)
↓
Administer O₂
Additional drug management:
histamine-blocker, corticosteroid (IM, IV)
↓
Cricothyrotomy as needed

A, *Airway;* B, *breathing;* C, *circulation;* D, *definitive care;* EMS, *emergency medical services;* IM, *intramuscular;* IV, *intravenous;* P, *position;* SC, *subcutaneous.*

Generalized Anaphylaxis

In generalized anaphylaxis a wide range of clinical manifestations may be noted; however, the cardiovascular system is involved in virtually all systemic allergic reactions. In rapidly progressing anaphylaxis, cardiovascular collapse may occur within minutes of the onset of symptoms. Immediate and aggressive management of this situation is imperative if the victim is to have any chance of survival. In the dental office, this reaction is most likely to occur during or immediately after administration of penicillin or aspirin to a previously sensitized patient. A more remote, although increasingly possible, cause might be latex sensitivity.[27]

Two other life-threatening situations may develop during the injection of a local anesthetic that might on occasion mimic anaphylaxis: vasodepressor syncope and a local anesthetic overdose. In the immediate management of this situation, there must be an attempt to diagnose the actual cause of the problem.

Signs of Allergy Present

Should any clinical signs, such as urticaria, erythema, pruritus, or wheezing, be noted before or after the patient's collapse, the diagnosis is obvious: allergy. Management proceeds accordingly.

Step 1: **P**-Position the patient. The unconscious, or conscious but hypotensive, patient is placed into a supine position with the legs elevated slightly.

Step 2: **C**-Circulation, **A**-Airway, **B**-Breathing (basic life support), as indicated. The airway is opened via head tilt, and steps of BLS are carried out as needed.

Step 3: **D**-Definitive care.

Step 3a: **Administer epinephrine.** The dentist should have previously called for the office emergency team. The immediate administration of 0.3 mL of 1:1000 epinephrine intramuscularly in the vastus lateralis muscle (see Figs. 10.3 and 10.4) (0.15 mL for <30 kg; 0.075 mL for infant) or 0.1 mL of 1:10,000 epinephrine intravenously over 5 minutes (adult), repeated every 3 to 5 minutes as necessary, is recommended. Because of the immediate need for epinephrine in this situation, a preloaded autoinjector of epinephrine should be available in the emergency kit. Epinephrine is the only injectable drug that need be maintained in a preloaded form (to minimize confusion when looking for it in this near-panic situation).

Epinephrine, in one or more doses, usually produces clinical improvement in the patient. Respiratory and cardiovascular signs and symptoms should decrease in severity: breath sounds improve as bronchospasm decreases and blood pressure increases.

Should the clinical picture fail to improve or continue to deteriorate (i.e., increasing severity of symptoms) within 5 minutes of the initial epinephrine dose, a second dose is administered. Subsequent doses may be administered as needed every 5 to 10 minutes if the potential risk of epinephrine administration (e.g., excessive cardiovascular stimulation) is kept in mind and the patient adequately monitored.[22–24]

Step 3b: **Summon medical assistance.** As soon as generalized anaphylaxis is considered a possibility, emergency medical services should be summoned.

Step 3c: **Administer oxygen.** Oxygen, at a flow of 5 to 6 L/min, can be delivered via nasal hood or full-face mask at any time during generalized anaphylaxis.

Step 3d: **Monitor vital signs.** The patient's cardiovascular and respiratory status must be monitored continuously. Blood pressure and heart rate (using the carotid artery) should be recorded at least every 5 minutes and chest compressions begun if cardiac arrest develops. During this acute, life-threatening phase of what is obviously an anaphylactic reaction, management consists of BLS, administration of oxygen and epinephrine, and continual monitoring of vital signs. Until improvement in the patient's status is noted, no additional drug therapy is indicated.

Step 3e: **Additional drug therapy.** Once clinical improvement is noted (e.g., increased blood pressure, decreased bronchospasm, return of consciousness), additional drug therapy is required. This includes the administration of a histamine blocker and a corticosteroid (both drugs intramuscularly or, if possible, intravenously). These drugs function to prevent a recurrence of symptoms and to obviate the need for the continued administration of epinephrine. They are not administered during the acute phase of the reaction because they are too slow in onset and do not do enough immediate good to justify their use while the victim's life remains in danger. Epinephrine and oxygen are the only drugs to administer during the life-threatening phase of the anaphylactic reaction.[26]

In the management of medical emergencies, it is stressed that definitive treatment of emergencies with drugs is of secondary importance to the PCABs of BLS. Drugs need not be administered in all emergency situations. ***Generalized anaphylaxis is one major exception.*** Once a diagnosis of acute, generalized anaphylaxis is made, it is imperative that drug therapy (i.e., epinephrine) be initiated as soon as possible after the start of BLS. Review of clinical reports demonstrates the effectiveness of immediate drug therapy in anaphylaxis. Recovery from anaphylaxis is related to the rapidity with which effective treatment is instituted. Delay in treatment increases the mortality rate. Of those experiencing anaphylaxis provoked by bee stings, 87% survived if treated within the first hour, but only 67% of dying patients were treated in this first hour.[28]

On arrival in the office, emergency personnel will establish IV access, administer appropriate drugs (i.e., histamine blocker and corticosteroid), and stabilize and transport the victim to the hospital emergencyc room for definitive care.

Box 34.7 outlines the steps to take to manage generalized anaphylaxis.

Drugs used in management of generalized anaphylaxis include oxygen, epinephrine (intravenously or intramuscularly), a histamine blocker (intramuscularly), and a corticosteroid (intravenously or intramuscularly).

Medical assistance is required for generalized anaphylaxis.

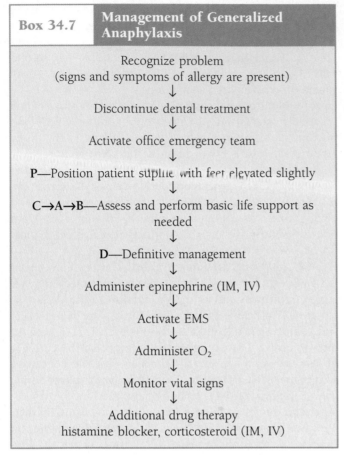

Box 34.7   Management of Generalized Anaphylaxis

Recognize problem
(signs and symptoms of allergy are present)
↓
Discontinue dental treatment
↓
Activate office emergency team
↓
P—Position patient supine with feet elevated slightly
↓
C→A→B—Assess and perform basic life support as needed
↓
D—Definitive management
↓
Administer epinephrine (IM, IV)
↓
Activate EMS
↓
Administer O₂
↓
Monitor vital signs
↓
Additional drug therapy
histamine blocker, corticosteroid (IM, IV)

A, Airway; B, breathing; C, circulation; D, definitive care; EMS, emergency medical services; IM, intramuscular; IV, intravenous; P, position.

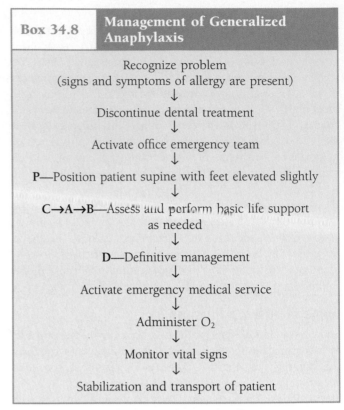

Box 34.8   Management of Generalized Anaphylaxis

Recognize problem
(signs and symptoms of allergy are present)
↓
Discontinue dental treatment
↓
Activate office emergency team
↓
P—Position patient supine with feet elevated slightly
↓
C→A→B—Assess and perform basic life support as needed
↓
D—Definitive management
↓
Activate emergency medical service
↓
Administer O₂
↓
Monitor vital signs
↓
Stabilization and transport of patient

A, Airway; B, breathing; C, circulation; D, definitive care; EMS, emergency medical services; P, position.

No Signs of Allergy Present

A second clinical picture of anaphylaxis might be one in which the patient receiving a potential allergen loses consciousness without any obvious signs of allergy being observed. This picture is disturbing because, in the absence of obvious clinical signs and symptoms of allergy, drug management for anaphylaxis is not indicated.

Step 1: **Terminate dental treatment.**

Step 2: **P-**Position the patient. Management of this situation, which might prove to result from any of a number of causes, requires immediate positioning of the patient in the supine position with the legs elevated slightly.

Step 3: **C-**Circulation, **A-**Airway, **B-**Breathing (basic life support), as indicated. Victims of vasodepressor syncope or postural hypotension rapidly recover consciousness once properly positioned and airway patency is ensured. BLS (breathing and circulation) should be continued in patients who do not recover at this point.

Step 4: **D-**Definitive care.

Step 4a: **Summon medical assistance.** If consciousness does not return rapidly after the steps of BLS have been initiated, emergency medical assistance should be sought immediately.

Step 4b: **Administer oxygen.**

Step 4c: **Monitor vital signs.** Blood pressure, heart rate and rhythm, and respiratory rate should be monitored continuously and recorded at least every 5 minutes, and the elements of BLS should be started at any time they are required.

Step 4d: **Definitive management.** On arrival, emergency medical personnel will seek to diagnose the cause of the loss of consciousness. If this is possible, appropriate drug therapy will be instituted, the patient stabilized, and the patient then transferred to a local hospital emergency room.

In the absence of definitive signs and symptoms of allergy (e.g., edema, urticaria, bronchospasm), epinephrine and other drug therapies are usually not indicated. Any of a number of other situations may be the cause of the unconsciousness, for example, drug overdose, hypoglycemia, cerebrovascular accident (CVA), acute adrenal insufficiency, myocardial infarction (MI), or cardiopulmonary arrest.

Continuing to apply the required steps of BLS until emergency medical assistance arrives represents the most rational management of this situation.

Box 34.8 outlines the steps to take to manage generalized anaphylaxis without obvious signs of allergy being present.

The only drug used in management of this syndrome is oxygen. Medical assistance is always required.

Laryngeal edema is yet another possible development during the generalized anaphylactic reaction. Should ventilation become difficult despite adequate head tilt and a clear pharynx (obtained by suctioning), it may become necessary to perform a cricothyrotomy to obtain an airway. Laryngeal edema is a manifestation of allergy. Once a patent airway has been assured (cricothyrotomy), epinephrine (0.3 mg [more than 30 kg weight]) may be administered, followed by a histamine blocker and corticosteroid as outlined previously. Once stabilized, the patient must be transferred to a hospital for definitive management and observation.

Overdose and allergy represent the most serious complications associated with drug administration for anesthesia and sedation. Other complications may also produce life-threatening situations. These include hypotension, cardiac dysrhythmias, respiratory depression, and laryngospasm. The latter two have been reviewed previously in the discussion of complications of IV sedation (see Chapter 27).

HYPOTENSION

Slight decreases in a patient's blood pressure during general anesthesia or moderate sedation are not unusual. Such decreases in blood pressure are usually minimal, especially during moderate sedation. More significant reductions in arterial blood pressure are clinically important because of the necessity to maintain adequate tissue perfusion. A systolic blood pressure of 90 mm Hg in an ASA 1 adult might not require treatment, whereas the same blood pressure in an elderly hypertensive patient might constitute a life-threatening situation. The need to treat hypotension is based on the ability of the circulation to adequately perfuse the tissues. Clinical signs and symptoms associated with hypotension and inadequate tissue perfusion are found in Box 34.9 and include the presence of chest pain, dyspnea, or a systolic blood pressure (adult) below 90 mm Hg.[29]

Box 34.9	Signs and Symptoms Associated With Significant Hypotension

Chest pain
Dyspnea
Hypotension (systolic blood pressure <90 mm Hg)
Heart failure
Ischemia
Infarction
Restlessness
Anxiety
Disorientation
Pallor
Cold, clammy skin
Dilated pupils
Prolonged capillary refill time (>2 seconds)

In the child, hypotension is characterized by the following[30]:

- Infants from 1 month to 12 months: systolic blood pressure (SBP) <70 mm Hg
- Children older than 1 year to 10 years: SBP <70 mm Hg + (2 × age in years)
- Beyond 10 years: SBP <90 mm Hg

Always consider the difficulty in assessing blood pressure accurately in the smaller child. Use of a blood pressure cuff that is too small (narrow) for the arm produces artificially elevated readings, whereas use of too large a cuff (e.g., an adult cuff on a small child) produces artificially decreased readings. See Chapter 4 for a description of the proper technique of recording blood pressure.

In a conscious hypotensive patient, cerebral ischemia occurs secondarily and is associated with restlessness, anxiety, and disorientation. Circulatory inadequacy is suggested by pallor, cold and clammy skin, and dilated pupils. The rate of capillary refill can be used as a gauge of peripheral perfusion. Normal capillary refill time is <2 seconds. In hypotensive states, capillary refill time is prolonged.

During sedative procedures hypotension can be diagnosed in one or more of several ways:

1. Monitoring of blood pressure throughout the procedure.
2. Observation of, and communication with, the patient.
3. Observation of the operative field during surgical procedures in which bleeding is normal. (The dentist and assistant will notice that the surgical field is considerably "cleaner" than usual. This should lead to an immediate evaluation of the blood pressure.)

If a blood pressure cuff is not immediately available, a quick estimate of SBP may be obtained through palpation of peripheral pulses at the radial, brachial, and/or carotid arteries. For example, if a carotid pulse is palpated but the brachial is absent, the SBP is greater than 60 mm Hg but lower than 70 mm Hg.

Pulse Palpated	Systolic Blood Pressure Is at Least
Radial artery	80 mm Hg
Brachial artery	70 mm Hg
Carotid artery	60 mm Hg

Causes of Hypotension

Possible causes of hypotension include the following:

- Excessive premedication
- The action of therapeutic drugs taken before the sedative/anesthetic procedure by the patient for preexisting disease
- Overdose of sedatives/anesthetics
- Reflex (light anesthesia, pain)
- Vascular absorption of local anesthetics
- Hemorrhage
- Positional changes of patient (postural or orthostatic hypotension)
- Hypoxia and hypercarbia
- Abnormalities of circulatory system
- Adrenocortical insufficiency
- Metabolic derangement (i.e., hypoglycemia or hyperglycemia)

Excessive premedication or the administration of a relative overdose to a "sensitive" patient may provoke hypotension. Following oral CNS-depressant drug administration, this is unlikely to occur; however, hypotension has been documented after IM administration, especially of an opioid agonist. Opioids produce this effect through their depressant actions on the vasomotor center, reducing muscle tone, decreasing ventilation, and dilating peripheral blood vessels.

The influence of other *therapeutic drugs* being taken by the patient to manage preexisting disorders might result in hypotension. Drugs such as corticosteroids, antihypertensives, tranquilizers such as chlorpromazine, and erectile dysfunction drugs (such as vardenafil [Levitra], tadalafil [Cialis], and sildenafil [Viagra]) may produce hypotension.

Overdose of sedatives/anesthetics is unlikely to develop when these drugs are administered carefully via routes in which titration is available and is used. These include the inhalation and IV routes of administration. When these drugs are administered intramuscularly, intranasally, or submucosally, however, there is a greater likelihood of overdose and hypotension because of the lack of control over the drugs' ultimate effect. Conversely, *anesthesia that is too light or the presence of pain* is capable of reflexly inducing hypotension.

Vascular absorption of local anesthetics is another potential cause of hypotension. Many causes for local anesthetic overdose and hypotension exist, including overadministration (relative or absolute), intravascular administration, rapid absorption, slow elimination, or slow biotransformation. The primary means of preventing hypotension and overdose from local anesthetics are aspiration before every injection and slow administration of the smallest volume of solution that will provide adequate pain control. The reader is referred to other texts for a more in-depth description of local anesthetic overdose.[31]

Hemorrhage is unlikely to be severe enough during a dental procedure to produce a drop in blood pressure. However, this is not an uncommon cause of hypotension within the hospital during major surgical procedures.

Positional changes of the patient are more likely to produce postural or orthostatic hypotension, particularly in elderly patients, patients receiving certain drugs (Box 34.10), and those who have received CNS-depressant drugs, particularly opioids.

Positional changes of the dental chair or the patient standing up from the chair should be accomplished gradually to permit the cardiovascular system to adapt to the increased effect of gravity as the patient becomes more upright. It has been mentioned throughout this book that the supine position, with the legs elevated slightly, or a semisupine position is recommended for patients during procedures in which CNS depressants have been administered. The upright (erect) position should be avoided during treatment unless absolutely essential.

Hypoxia and *hypercarbia* are additional possible causes of hypotension. Adequate management of the patient's airway

---

> ### Box 34.10   Drugs and Drug Categories Producing Postural Hypotension
>
> **Category**
> Adrenergic neuron blockers
> α- and β-adrenergic blockers
> Amiodarone
> Angiotensin-converting enzyme inhibitors
> Centrally acting antihypertensives
> Calcium channel blockers
> Diuretics
> Ganglionic blockers
> Levodopa
> Vasodilators

---

during deep sedation or general anesthesia is of critical importance.

Cardiovascular abnormalities are another possible cause of hypotension during sedative or anesthetic procedures. The occurrence of myocardial ischemia or infarction may result in a profound drop in blood pressure. In the conscious, albeit sedated, patient other clinical signs and symptoms would usually be available (e.g., "pain" radiating in a classic pattern, nausea, dusky appearance, cyanosis of mucous membranes) that would aid in diagnosis; however, in the unconscious patient such a diagnosis would be more difficult to establish. Other cardiovascular causes of hypotension, all of which are extremely unlikely to develop in the outpatient setting on ASA 1 or 2 patients, include an embolism in the brain (CVA) or lungs (pulmonary embolism), hypovolemia caused by the patient's poor physical condition before the start of the procedure (unlikely to be observed in the ambulatory outpatient setting), heart failure, and anaphylactic shock.

Adrenocortical insufficiency may produce hypotension and shock. When a patient has received exogenous corticosteroid therapy in the recent past, prophylactic corticosteroid administration may be recommended before the start of any significantly traumatic surgical procedure (see Chapter 4).

Metabolic derangements, such as hyperglycemia (and ketoacidosis) or hypoglycemia, are other possible causes of hypotension that should be considered. A history of diabetes mellitus in a hypotensive patient would provide an indication that this is a possible cause for the hypotension. Hypoglycemia is much more likely to be noted than hyperglycemia in the diabetic patient who is still conscious.

Management of Hypotension

Treatment of hypotension is directed to its cause. However, certain basic steps must be carried out whenever hypotension occurs.

Step 1: **P**-Position the patient. The procedure is terminated, and the patient is placed into the supine position with their

Table 34.4 Vasopressors: Summary of Actions on Receptors

				Usual Dose	
AGENT	α	β_1	β_2	IV	IM
Epinephrine (most potent agent to β-receptor)	+	+	+	0.1 mg	0.2–0.3 mg
Norepinephrine bitartrate	+	+	+	Used as continuous IV drip	Not recommended IM
Isoproterenol	–	+	+	0.025 µg/kg/min IV drip	Not recommended IM
Phenylephrine	+	–	–	0.25–0.5 mg	2–3 mg
Mephentermine	+	+	+	5–15 mg	10–30 mg
Ephedrine	+	+	+	10–25 mg followed by IM dose	25–50 mg
Metaraminol	+	+	–	0.5–2 mg	2–5 mg
Methoxamine	+	–	–	2–5 mg	5–10 mg
Dopamine	–	+	–	Via continuous IV infusion (200 mg in 250 or 500 mL 5% dextrose and water)	
Propranolol		+	+	0.5–1 mg up to maximum of 2 mg IV	

feet elevated to increase blood flow to the brain and aid in return of venous blood from the legs.

Step 2: **C**-Circulation, **A**-Airway, **B**-Breathing (basic life support), as indicated. The patient will likely be attempting to breathe spontaneously, although their airway may or may not be patent. The pulse will be weak and probably rapid (tachycardia usually accompanies hypotension). Blood pressure will be decreased from the patient's baseline values. O_2 may be administered to the patient at any time during management.

Step 3: **D**-Definitive care.

Step 3a. If an inhalation anesthetic such as N_2O (or any other gaseous agent) is being administered, its concentration is decreased. This step alone usually leads to an increase in blood pressure. Although the patient is receiving a concentration of N_2O that is within normal limits, a relative overdose of the drug may be administered if the patient is unusually sensitive to its actions.

If opioids or a benzodiazepine has been administered, the appropriate antagonist (naloxone or flumazenil) may be administered intravenously or intramuscularly. Although the primary effect of naloxone is to improve respiratory depression induced by the opioids, a slight elevation in blood pressure may also be observed because the analgesic actions of the opioid also decrease and the patient begins to respond to painful stimuli if local anesthesia is absent.

If barbiturates have been administered IM or IV, general supportive measures (BLS) must be continued until the patient improves as no effective antagonistic drug for the barbiturates exists.

Step 3b: **Administer fluids.** When hypotension develops during an IV sedation procedure or if an IV infusion can be started, a relatively effective and safe means of managing hypotension is available, especially in the ASA 1 or 2 patient. The rapid IV infusion of solution (5% dextrose and water, physiologic saline, or lactated Ringer's solution) will provide extra fluid volume to the cardiovascular system, thereby increasing the blood pressure. The 250-mL, 500-mL or 1-liter bag of solution should be opened and permitted to flow rapidly until it is observed that the blood pressure has increased. Mild decreases in systemic blood pressure may usually be reversed in this simple manner.

Step 3c: **Administer vasopressors.** The administration of vasopressors is reserved for hypotension that is more severe and that persists after these preceding measures have been undertaken. A number of vasopressors are available. It was recommended in Chapter 33 that ephedrine be available in the emergency drug kit. Ephedrine is selected because of its ability to increase blood pressure with little secondary effect on the workload of the myocardium. In the absence of greater knowledge of the status of the patient's cardiovascular system and heart, the administration of other drugs (Table 34.4) with β-actions or mixed α- and β-actions is not recommended.

Most vasopressors stimulate both α- and β-receptors, but the degree of stimulation by each drug varies. Table 34.4 summarizes clinical actions of the more commonly used vasopressors, and Box 34.11 lists the actions of the various receptors. Other vasopressors may be used in place of ephedrine, provided the dentist is knowledgeable of the pharmacology, indications, contraindications, precautions, adverse reactions, and recommended dosage of the drug. Recommended for the emergency kit is 50 mg/mL of ephedrine (two to three 1-mL ampules). An IM dose of 25 to 50 mg is repeated every 3 to 4 hours as needed[32]; the IV route is reserved for emergency situations in which a more immediate response is required. The onset of activity is 15 minutes after IM administration and 2 to 3 minutes after IV administration. Duration of action is approximately 30 to 60 minutes (with the IV route). Box 34.12 outlines the steps to take to manage hypotension.

Box 34.11	Actions of α- and β-Receptors

α-Receptors
Peripheral vasoconstriction: skin, mucosa, intestine, kidney
Mydriasis
Myometrial contraction

β-Receptors
β-Receptors are subdivided into two groups: β_1- and β_2-receptors.
Stimulation of these receptors produces the following reactions:

β_1-Receptors
Bronchodilation
Tachycardia
Palpitation
Hypertension
Insomnia
Tremor—Increased cardiac contractility

β_2-Receptors
Bronchodilation
Vasodilation

Hypotension in Patients Receiving Corticosteroid Therapy

Patients receiving corticosteroids or those having recently completed a prolonged course of steroid therapy may be more likely to develop hypotensive episodes during significantly traumatic surgery and anesthesia. This is due to their inability to release adequate amounts of endogenous steroids into the circulation in response to the stress of major surgery, leading to acute adrenal insufficiency. Preoperative administration of steroids (in consultation with the patient's physician) may be recommended to minimize this risk. When hypotensive episodes develop during treatment, large IV doses of corticosteroids and vasopressors are required to prevent morbidity or death.

Hypotension in Patients Receiving β-Blockers

Patients receiving long-term β-blocker treatment are unable to respond to exercise with an elevation in their heart rate. When hypotension develops in these patients, management consists of the following[2]:

1. *Isoproterenol* (Isuprel), administered slowly intravenously at a rate of 0.2 mg at 1-minute intervals. The dose is determined by the patient's response. In the presence of a total β-blockade, a large dose of isoproterenol may be required.
2. When the hypotensive episode persists despite isoproterenol administration, IV *glucagon* is administered.

Box 34.12	Management of Hypotension

Terminate the dental procedure
↓
P—Position the patient (supine with the legs elevated)
↓
C→A→B—Assess and perform basic life support, as needed
↓
D—Initiate definitive care
↓
Observe for possible cause of hypotension and manage as necessary

- Decrease concentration of inhalation anesthetics
- Reverse opioid actions with naloxone
- Reverse benzodiazepine actions with flumazenil
- If patient is diabetic, consider hypoglycemia and manage appropriately
- Monitor and seek signs and symptoms of cardiovascular system involvement (e.g., angina, myocardial infarction)
- Determine history of recent corticosteroid therapy, IV administration of corticosteroids
↓
In absence of above, or continued hypotension:
- If IV route is available, administer IV infusate rapidly (up to 500 mL in ASA I, 250 mL in ASA II)
- If IV route is not available, or if hypotension is refractory to preceding steps, administer IM or IV vasopressor
↓
Summon medical assistance as needed
↓
Administer oxygen
↓
Monitor vital signs
↓
Permit recovery and discharge the patient

3. *Atropine* (0.5 to 1.0 mg) is administered intravenously wherever severe bradycardia is present.

HYPERTENSIVE EPISODES

Elevations of blood pressure may be noted during surgical and dental procedures if the level of pain or anxiety control is inadequate. Transient elevations in blood pressure may be prevented through the administration (or readministration) of local anesthesia. Transient minor elevations in blood pressure (hypertensive urgencies) are usually well tolerated and of little danger to the patient. Sustained and/or significant elevations in blood pressure (hypertensive emergencies or crises) require aggressive management. Guidelines for the evaluation of blood pressure in both adult and pediatric patients were presented in Chapter 4.

Causes of episodes of high blood pressure during dental treatment, surgery, and anesthesia (sedation, general anesthesia) include the following[2]:

1. Light anesthesia or sedation
2. Pain
3. Hypercarbia
4. Hypoxia
5. Emergence delirium
6. Fluid overload (overhydration)
7. Hyperthermia

The most common causes of hypertension during dental procedures, surgery, and anesthesia are light anesthesia or sedation and/or the presence of pain. Management is directed at providing adequate sedation, anesthesia, and pain control. Blood pressure returns toward baseline levels as the quality of anesthesia improves.

Hypercarbia and hypoxia are the next most common causes of elevated blood pressure. Catecholamine release is increased with both hypercarbia and hypoxia. Airway management (e.g., head tilt–chin lift) and ventilation reverse this cause of blood pressure elevation.

Postoperatively, pain, hypercarbia, and emergence delirium are common causes of elevated blood pressure. Strict management of the airway and O_2 administration preclude hypoxia and hypercarbia. Physostigmine administration terminates episodes of emergence delirium, and the use of local anesthesia or the administration of nonsteroidal antiinflammatory drugs (NSAIDs) or opioids helps manage posttreatment pain.

Fluid overload is an uncommon cause of high blood pressure in the dental outpatient, especially when the 250- or 500-mL bag of IV infusate is used. ASA 3 and 4 patients with heart failure (HF) may be at risk for acute pulmonary edema when large volumes of IV fluids are received.

Hyperthermia is associated with increased metabolic rates, increased heart rate, and increased blood pressure. Temperature should be recorded before sedation when there is an indication that infection may be present or if the patient appears warm or flushed. Temperature should be recorded preoperatively and intraoperatively whenever general anesthesia is administered.

Management of a Hypertensive Crisis During Sedation or General Anesthesia

Hypertensive crises can be divided into hypertensive emergency or hypertensive urgency according to the presence or lack of acute target organ damage.[33] In general medical practice a hypertensive crisis is said to exist when the SBP is 220 mm Hg or greater and/or the diastolic blood pressure (DBP) is 120 mm Hg or greater.[34]

In the area of sedation and general anesthesia no set blood pressure reading can be used to establish the presence of a hypertensive crisis. An acute rise in blood pressure is more significant than the actual numbers, but a systolic BP of >220 or a diastolic BP of >120 must be treated promptly.[34] Sustained blood pressure elevations of 20% to 30% or greater during dental treatment, whether with or without sedation or general anesthesia, require immediate cessation of the treatment and management. Hypertensive crises are most likely to occur in patients with chronic, stable hypertension. The goal in management is to avoid rapid changes in blood pressure without compromising cerebral perfusion.[35] To this end, antihypertensive therapy is not recommended in any patient unless there is severe hypertension (>220/120 mm Hg).[36] Hypertensive crisis must be distinguished from a modest and transient elevation in blood pressure from causes previously listed. Deepening of the anesthesia or eliminating pain through the readministration of local anesthetics will often bring with it a return of the elevated blood pressure toward baseline values. However, when elevated blood pressure does not return to acceptable levels within a few minutes of onset, or if it continues to increase, the possibility of a hypertensive crisis must be considered and steps initiated to manage it.

Among the possible acute causes of the hypertensive crisis are cardiovascular complications, such as MI and dissecting aortic aneurysm; recreational drug use (e.g., cocaine); monoamine oxidase inhibitor use; pheochromocytoma; and thyroid crisis.[35] It is important when evaluating the hypertensive crisis to distinguish whether the cause is cardiac or noncardiac.[2] When significant elevation is noted in the patient's blood pressure, proceed as follows.

Step 1: **Terminate dental treatment** and **P**-Position the patient. Position the patient in an upright position (45 degrees or more upright).

Step 2: **Assess C**-Circulation, **A**-Airway, **B**-Breathing (basic life support), as indicated. Airway, breathing, and circulation are usually adequate.

Step 3: **D**-Definitive care.

Step 3a: **Monitor blood pressure and heart rate and rhythm** every 5 minutes and administer oxygen.

Step 3b: **Activate EMS.** Emergency medical personnel should be summoned.

Step 3c: **Establish an IV infusion**, if not already present. Where the cause of the hypertensive crisis is cardiac, such as HF, proceed as follows.

Step 3d: **Administer nicardipine (Cardene).** Start at 5 mg/hour and increase by 2.5 mg/hour every 5 to 15 minutes. Maximum dose is 15 mg/hour.

Step 3d: **Titrate nitroprusside** (Nipride) for acute, life-threatening hypertension at an infusion rate of 0.3 mcg/kg/min and increase slowly. The maximum dose is 10 mcg/kg/minute until the blood pressure is lowered to a desired point.

Step 3e: **Administer beta-blockers** (labetalol 5 mg every 2 minutes is preferred because it has both alpha- and beta-blocking properties).

When a noncardiac cause of the hypertensive crisis is present (e.g., anxiety, allergy, CVA), proceed as follows:

Table 34.5	Parenteral Drugs Used in the Treatment of Hypertensive Crisis			
DRUG	**ADMINISTRATION**	**ONSET**	**DOSAGE**	**SIDE EFFECTS**
Sodium nitroprusside	IV fusion	Immediate	0.5–10 µg/kg/min	Hypotension, nausea, vomiting, apprehension
Diazoxide	IV bolus	q5–10 min	6–12 hr 50–100 mg to 600 mg	Hypotension, tachycardia, nausea, vomiting, fluid retention; exacerbates myocardial ischemia, heart failure, or aortic dissection
Nitroglycerin	IV infusion	1–2 min	5–100 µg/min	Headache, nausea, vomiting
Nicardipine	IV infusion	1–2 min	5 mg/hr IV, may increase by 2.5 mg/hr q5–15 min; max 15 mg/hr	Exacerbation of angina; myocardial infarction; ischemic ECG changes; pericarditis; DVT; thrombocytopenia
Labetalol	IV bolus	2 min	20 mg IV over 2 min, then 40 mg to 80 mg IV over 2 minutes in 10-minute intervals.	Maintain patient in supine position to avoid excessive BP drop.
	IV infusion	2 min	2 mg/min IV	Cerebral infarction; optic nerve infarction; angina; ischemic ECG changes

Step 3d: **IV diazoxide** (Hyperstat) should be administered in doses of 1 to 3 mg/kg up to 150 mg. This dose may be repeated every 5 to 10 minutes up to 600 mg.

Step 4: When anxiety is a major component of the hypertensive crisis, midazolam or diazepam, titrated intravenously, may be of some utility in managing the hypertension. Table 34.5 summarizes the drugs employed in management of the hypertensive crisis.

Situations may arise in which an IV infusion cannot be started and/or the appropriate parenteral antihypertensive drugs are not available for administration. In such instances the following regimen is suggested:

Step 1: **Terminate dental treatment** and **P**-Position the patient. Position the patient in an upright position (45 degrees or more upright).

Step 2: **Assess C**-Circulation, **A**-Airway, **B**-Breathing (basic life support), as indicated. Airway, breathing, and circulation are usually adequate.

Step 3: **D**-Definitive care.

Step 3a. **Monitor blood pressure and heart rate and rhythm** every 5 minutes and administer oxygen.

Step 3b. **Oxygen** should be administered.

Step 3c. **Activate EMS.** Emergency medical personnel should be summoned.

Step 3d. **Sublingual nitroglycerin** tablets (2 tablets of 0.4 mg) or two doses of Nitrolingual spray should be administered (spray medication onto the mucous membrane of the tongue). This dose may be repeated every 5 to 10 minutes if necessary.

Step 3e. On arrival of emergency medical assistance, an IV infusion will be established and appropriate antihypertensive drugs administered. The patient usually requires a period of hospitalization to ensure stabilization of blood pressure.

In summary, transient elevations in systolic and diastolic blood pressure can occur during dental procedures utilizing sedation or general anesthesia. These transient spikes in blood pressure are usually secondary to inadequate pain control and/or sedation. Another factor is inadequate maintenance of a patent airway, leading to the development of hypoxia and/or hypercarbia. Transient elevations in blood pressure do not usually require management employing antihypertensive drug administration.

Extremely rare is the situation in which sustained blood pressure elevations are encountered. When such occur following evaluation of the aforementioned etiologies, the administration of antihypertensive drugs may be indicated.

CARDIAC DYSRHYTHMIAS

A dysrhythmia is any deviation from the normal sinus rhythm. It was reported as the most common intraoperative complication, occurring in 112,721 patients studied.[37] The incidence of perioperative dysrhythmias under general anesthesia has been reported by different sources to be from 4% to 60%.[38,39] Driscoll et al have reported the incidence of dysrhythmias during extraction of erupted bicuspids in patients receiving local anesthesia and sedation to be 24.19%.[40]

Fortunately, the majority of dysrhythmias encountered during sedative and general anesthetic procedures rarely require drug intervention. Indeed, if bradycardia (<60 beats per minute) and tachycardia (>100 beats per minute) are discounted, the incidence of dysrhythmias requiring drug treatment is exceedingly low. However, the presence of a dysrhythmia can be a warning that some physiologic or pharmacologic problem exists that does require immediate management. DeRango makes some generalizations about the incidence of cardiac dysrhythmias[41]:

1. The majority of anesthetized patients who are continuously monitored (ECG) will demonstrate some dysrhythmia during the anesthetic period.
2. The incidence of dysrhythmias is higher in patients with a history of heart disease than in those without such a history.
3. The incidence of dysrhythmias is higher in patients whose tracheas are intubated.
4. The incidence of dysrhythmias is more frequent in patients undergoing surgery lasting more than 3 hours than in patients undergoing shorter procedures.
5. Patients receiving digitalis preoperatively have a higher incidence of dysrhythmia than patients not receiving digitalis.

From a review of the preceding information it appears that the incidence of cardiac dysrhythmias during outpatient procedures in ASA 1 or 2 patients should be considerably lower than that for in-hospital procedures. The very nature of the patient (healthier) and the type of procedure (shorter duration, trachea rarely intubated) are reasons for a decreased incidence of clinically significant dysrhythmias during outpatient procedures.

Precipitating Factors

Dysrhythmias may be produced in patients receiving anesthesia and sedation by the following means:

1. Anesthetic agents
2. Elevated levels of carbon dioxide (CO_2)
3. Stimulation under light planes of anesthesia
4. Vagal responses
5. Intubation
6. Anoxia
7. Duration of the procedure

Anesthetic agents may provoke dysrhythmias. Among inhalation anesthetics, halothane (which is rarely used today) is associated with a greater incidence of dysrhythmias than enflurane, isoflurane, desflurane, and sevoflurane.

CO_2 retention (hypercarbia) is a common cause of dysrhythmia during anesthesia and sedation. The mechanism of dysrhythmia generation is the release of catecholamines by the increasing CO_2 tension in the blood. Many anesthetic drugs sensitize the myocardium to the effects of these catecholamines, and dysrhythmia is the result.

Stimulation of the patient during a procedure while the patient is under general anesthesia or sedation is a common cause of dysrhythmias. Stimulation (i.e., pain) leads to vagal and sympathetic responses that are ultimately responsible for most dysrhythmias. Management consists of either deepening the level of general anesthesia or sedation (to decrease patient response to stimulation) or providing more adequate pain control (local anesthesia). In the dental environment the latter is preferred.

Vagal responses produce a slowing of the sinus rate, which can lead to dysrhythmias such as sinus bradycardia, sinus arrest, junctional rhythms, and most frequently, premature ventricular contractions (PVCs). Vagal responses are much more likely to develop during general anesthesia than during sedative procedures. Most often, these responses occur as a result of nondental surgical stimulation, such as traction on intraabdominal structures, traction on extraocular muscles, pressure on the globe, and carotid sinus stimulation.

Tracheal intubation is probably responsible for the greatest incidence of dysrhythmias during general anesthesia, especially when the patient is in a light plane of anesthesia. Most often, the dysrhythmias seen are tachydysrhythmias associated with elevations in blood pressure. These tachydysrhythmias are normally transient and require no drug therapy. Management consists of adequate ventilation and a deepening of the level of anesthesia.

Anoxia or *severe hypoxia* during general anesthesia or sedation is another cause of dysrhythmias. Anoxia is associated with the development of hypercarbia (see previous discussion). Management consists of adequate ventilation.

The *duration of surgery* or of the procedure is related to the incidence of dysrhythmias. The incidence of dysrhythmias occurring during procedures that last less than 3 hours is considerably lower than that during procedures requiring more than 3 hours to complete. The body's ability to handle stress is compromised as the procedure lengthens. Increased levels of catecholamines appear in the blood, resulting in the development of dysrhythmias.

Dysrhythmias are significant because they may indicate dysfunction of the myocardial conduction system, which, if the dysrhythmia results in decreased cardiac output, may lead to cerebral, myocardial, or renal ischemia; HF and pulmonary edema; MI; or ventricular fibrillation.

To reiterate: the overwhelming majority of dysrhythmias seen during general anesthesia and, especially during sedative procedures, are of a transient and relatively benign nature, requiring no formal drug management. Management usually consists of ensuring adequate ventilation, increasing or decreasing (as appropriate) the level of anesthesia or sedation, and providing adequate pain control.

Continuous ECG monitoring of the patient receiving deep sedation or general anesthesia is required; however, the routine use of the ECG during minimal and moderate sedative procedures is not necessary, although if available it should be employed in patients with a history of cardiovascular disease.

Dysrhythmias may be detected through the use of a pulse oximeter or other pulse-monitoring device, or more simply by keeping a finger on the patient's pulse. See Chapter 4 for a review of common dysrhythmias. Advanced cardiovascular life support textbooks should be consulted for in-depth discussion of the significance and management of cardiac dysrhythmias.[42]

ANGINA PECTORIS

Stable angina pectoris is a characteristic thoracic pain, usually substernal, precipitated chiefly by exercise, emotion, or a heavy meal; relieved by vasodilator drugs and a few minutes of rest; and is the result of a mild inadequacy of the coronary circulation.[43] Several anginal syndromes are identified, including stable angina (ASA 3), vasospastic angina (coronary artery spasm, atypical angina, variant angina, Prinzmetal angina: ASA 3), and unstable angina (preinfarction or crescendo angina, intermediate coronary syndrome, and impending MI: ASA 4). Drugs used for the management of acute anginal episodes include nitroglycerin (sublingual tablets, translingual spray, or transdermal patch), which is used for the management of stable and vasospastic angina. Calcium channel blockers (nifedipine, diltiazem, and verapamil) are effective in managing the vasospastic component of angina.

Signs and Symptoms

The "pain" of angina is rarely described as such by the patient. More frequently, an acute anginal episode is described as a "tightness," "constricting feeling," or a "heavy weight" on the chest. The patient usually stops whatever he or she is doing and seeks relief by sitting upright and taking nitroglycerin. A typical anginal episode lasts but minutes with drug therapy but may persist for up to an hour. Chest pain of long duration, however, is more likely to lead to a presumptive diagnosis of MI than angina. Additional signs and symptoms associated with angina include palpitation, faintness, dizziness, dyspnea, and "indigestion."

It is important to note that *the pain of angina is quickly relieved by nitroglycerin administration and that it does not return.* Box 34.13 outlines the steps to take to manage chest pain with history of angina pectoris.

MYOCARDIAL INFARCTION

Prolonged ischemia of the myocardium produced by partial or complete occlusion of blood flow through one or more coronary arteries leads to necrosis of heart muscle. Severe chest pain and dysrhythmias commonly occur during MI. Cessation of effective cardiac function may occur, producing cardiac arrest, necessitating the immediate institution of BLS.

Signs and Symptoms

MI often mimics angina at its onset. One striking difference (in the nondental setting) is that 51% of patients are *at rest* when MI occurs, whereas the onset of anginal pain is associated with an increase in myocardial activity.[44,45]

Patients experience a more severe and more prolonged pain that, although it may seem anginal at onset, progressively increases in severity. The patient is quite apprehensive and may exhibit weakness, diaphoresis, hypotension, and dysrhythmia. Dysrhythmia develops in 95% of MIs and increases the rate of morbidity and mortality associated with MI.[46] Hypotension is noted in 80% of patients with MI.[47]

Management

Management of MI progresses from that described for angina. Box 34.14 outlines the steps to take to manage chest pain.

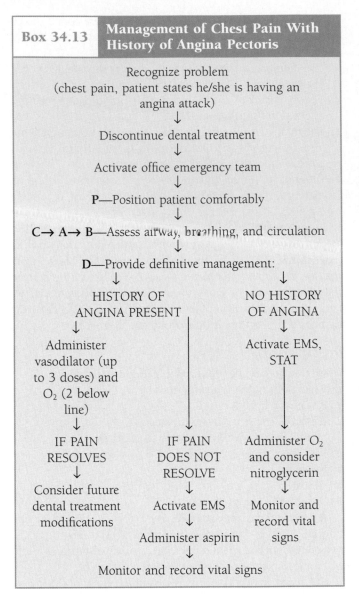

Box 34.13   Management of Chest Pain With History of Angina Pectoris

Recognize problem
(chest pain, patient states he/she is having an angina attack)
↓
Discontinue dental treatment
↓
Activate office emergency team
↓
P—Position patient comfortably
↓
C→ A→ B—Assess airway, breathing, and circulation
↓
D—Provide definitive management:
↓   ↓
HISTORY OF   NO HISTORY
ANGINA PRESENT   OF ANGINA
↓   ↓
Administer   Activate EMS,
vasodilator (up   STAT
to 3 doses) and
O₂ (2 below
line)
↓   ↓   ↓
IF PAIN   IF PAIN   Administer O₂
RESOLVES   DOES NOT   and consider
↓   RESOLVE   nitroglycerin
Consider future   ↓   ↓
dental treatment   Activate EMS   Monitor and
modifications   ↓   record vital
                  Administer aspirin   signs
                       ↓
              Monitor and record vital signs

A, *Airway;* B, *breathing;* C, *circulation;* D, *definitive care;* EMS, *emergency medical service;* P, *position.*
From Malamed SF: Medical emergencies in the dental office, 7e, St Louis, 2015, Mosby.

AIRWAY OBSTRUCTION

The most common cause of airway obstruction during sedation or general anesthesia is posterior displacement of the tongue into the pharynx as muscle tonus is lost as a result of the CNS depression produced by the administered drugs. The presence of a foreign object in the airway, such as a gauze wipe, crown, or tooth that becomes displaced, is a second possible cause of airway obstruction, although the latter commonly do not produce total obstruction but rather a partial airway obstruction.[48,49] Fluids (blood, saliva, water, and vomitus) may also produce airway obstruction.

Partial or complete airway obstruction may occur. Distinctive sounds are associated with airway obstruction produced by

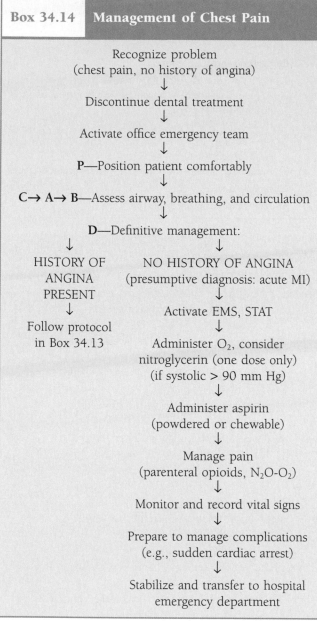

Box 34.14   Management of Chest Pain

Recognize problem
(chest pain, no history of angina)
↓
Discontinue dental treatment
↓
Activate office emergency team
↓
P—Position patient comfortably
↓
C → A → B—Assess airway, breathing, and circulation
↓
D—Definitive management:
↓   ↓
HISTORY OF   NO HISTORY OF ANGINA
ANGINA   (presumptive diagnosis: acute MI)
PRESENT   ↓
↓   Activate EMS, STAT
Follow protocol   ↓
in Box 34.13   Administer O₂, consider
nitroglycerin (one dose only)
(if systolic > 90 mm Hg)
↓
Administer aspirin
(powdered or chewable)
↓
Manage pain
(parenteral opioids, N₂O-O₂)
↓
Monitor and record vital signs
↓
Prepare to manage complications
(e.g., sudden cardiac arrest)
↓
Stabilize and transfer to hospital
emergency department

A, *Airway;* B, *breathing;* C, *circulation;* D, *definitive care;* EMS, *emergency medical service;* P, *position;* M, *myocardial infarction.* From Malamed SF: Medical emergencies in the dental office, 7e, St Louis, 2015, Mosby.

various causes. These sounds must be detected, diagnosed, and managed as expeditiously as possible. Use of the pretracheal stethoscope during parenteral moderate or deep sedation and general anesthesia allows for instantaneous detection of airway problems.

Normal, unobstructed airflow through the mouth and nose has a very distinctive low (barely audible) whooshing sound. Movement of the chest during respiration is minimal and looks "smooth." Soft tissue retraction (intercostal and supraclavicular) is not present. *Complete obstruction* of the airway is associated with the absence of sound. If the patient is attempting

spontaneous ventilation, the observed respiratory movements appear exaggerated, with evident supraclavicular and intercostal soft tissue retraction. The use of abdominal muscles during respiration will also be evident. *Partial airway obstruction resulting from the tongue* being displaced posteriorly is associated with a snoring sound that often can be heard by all persons in the treatment room. The presence of *fluid in the airway* is detected by a gurgling or bubbling sound. One other sound that is heard is wheezing, which results from a partial obstruction of the lower airway caused by *bronchospasm.* Mild bronchospasm is associated with loud wheezing, whereas in more severe bronchospasm, in which little air is being exchanged, wheezing may be absent. Table 34.6 summarizes the sounds associated with breathing and their management.

Management

The dentist should proceed with each of the following steps until a patent airway is obtained, as will be noted by the return of sounds associated with spontaneous breathing. Box 34.15 lists the recommended sequences for removing airway obstruction.

Partial Airway Obstruction Associated With "Snoring"

1. Position patient supine.
2. Perform head tilt–chin lift. If this fails to provide a patent airway, then:
3. Displace the tongue. Physically displace the tongue anteriorly by grabbing it with a hemostat or gauze sponge (Fig. 34.4).

Partial Airway Obstruction Associated With "Gurgling"

1. Position the patient in the supine position.
2. Perform head tilt–chin lift.
3. Suction the airway. Using a tonsillar suction tip, suction the posterior pharynx until all fluids are removed.

Partial Airway Obstruction Associated With "Wheezing"

The management of wheezing is discussed in the earlier section on respiratory allergic reactions. Administration of a bronchodilator is indicated.

Cricothyrotomy

When the preceding steps have failed to reestablish a patent airway, it may be necessary to perform a cricothyrotomy. Cricothyrotomy should be carried out only when the dentist is well trained in the procedure. Cricothyrotomy technique is described in other texts.[25,26]

LARYNGOSPASM

Laryngospasm is a protective reflex that functions to maintain the integrity of the airway by preventing foreign matter from

Table 34.6   **Breathing Sounds and Their Management**

SOUND	PROBABLE CAUSE	MANAGEMENT
Quiet whooshing	Normal, unobstructed airway	None required
None/no chest movement	Apnea	Controlled ventilation efforts
None/exaggerated movement	Complete obstruction	1. Head tilt–chin lift respiratory efforts 2. Anterior displacement of tongue with hemostat or gauze 3. Pharyngeal suctioning 4. Abdominal thrusts 5. Cricothyrotomy
Snoring	Soft tissue (tongue) displaced in pharynx	1. Head tilt–chin lift 2. Anterior displacement of tongue with hemostat or gauze
Gurgling	Fluid in airway	Pharyngeal suction
Wheezing	Bronchospasm	Administration of bronchodilator

Box 34.15   **Recommended Sequences for Removing Airway Obstruction**

A: CONSCIOUS Victim With Obstructed Airway

Identify complete airway obstruction…ask:
"Are you choking?"
↓
Apply abdominal thrusts until foreign body is
expelled or the victim becomes unconscious
↓
Have medical or paramedical personnel evaluate the
patient for complications before dismissal

B: CONSCIOUS Victim With Known Obstructed Airway Who Loses Consciousness

Place victim in supine position with head in
neutral position
Call for help!
↓
Activate emergency medical system (i.e., call 9-1-1) if a
second person is available
↓
Maintain airway (head tilt–chin lift)
↓
Look in mouth for foreign object before ventilation
Attempt to ventilate;
if INEFFECTIVE:
↓
Perform abdominal thrust, repeating until object is
expelled or the victim becomes unresponsive
↓
Check for foreign body
If visible, perform finger sweep to remove
↓
Attempt to ventilate;
if INEFFECTIVE
↓
Repeat abdominal thrusts;
if visible, perform finger sweep to remove and attempt
ventilation until effective
↓
Have medical or paramedical personnel evaluate
patient for complications before dismissal or
hospitalization

C: UNCONSCIOUS Victim, Cause UNKNOWN

Rescuer manages unconscious victim in usual manner:
Assess unresponsiveness
↓
P–Position victim supine with feet elevated slightly
↓
Activate dental office emergency team
↓
A–Open airway (head tilt–chin lift)
↓
B–Assess breathing (look, listen, feel) and
↓
Attempt to ventilate:
if INEFFECTIVE:
↓
Reposition head and attempt to ventilate;
if still INEFFECTIVE:
↓
Activate emergency medical system (i.e., call 9-1-1) and
↓
Look in mouth for foreign object before ventilation
Perform abdominal thrusts:
(5 abdominal thrusts)
↓
Check for foreign body
If visible, perform finger sweep to remove
↓
Attempt to ventilate:
if INEFFECTIVE:
↓
Repeat abdominal thrusts, visualization and finger
sweeps (if visible), and ventilation until successful

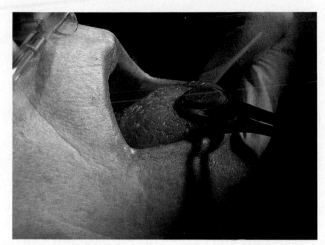

Figure 34.4 Grabbing tongue with forceps. (From Malamed SF: *Medical emergencies in the dental office*, ed 7, St Louis, 2015, Mosby.)

entering into the larynx, trachea, and lungs. In the dental office in which deep sedation and general anesthesia are regularly administered, laryngospasm is considered a complication rather than an emergency.[2]

Laryngospasm is extraordinarily uncommon during minimal and moderate sedation. In moderate sedation, the patient retains his or her protective airway reflexes—coughing, gagging, or swallowing foreign matter—to prevent its entry into the airway. Laryngospasm will also not occur during operating room–depth general anesthesia (see Chapter 2). The degree of CNS depression present at this time is such that the protective reflexes are lost. Material entering into the airway at this level of CNS depression will not provoke a response from the patient. Ensuring the integrity of the airway therefore becomes a prime obligation of the anesthesiologist during general anesthesia.

Laryngospasm may be partial or complete. Partial laryngospasm is associated with a high-pitched crowing sound (stridor) and increased difficulty in ventilation, whereas a complete laryngospasm is associated with an (ominous) absence of sound in the presence of exaggerated respiratory efforts and soft tissue retraction in the supraclavicular and intercostal regions.

Management

On recognition of laryngospasm, the following steps should be taken:

Step 1: **Position** the patient supine.

Step 2: **Administer oxygen.** Administer 100% O_2 via a nasal hood. In most instances the patient will have already been receiving N_2O-O_2 during treatment. The dentist should simply terminate the flow of N_2O and increase the O_2 flow to about 5 to 8 L/min.

Step 3: **Displace the tongue.** The dentist physically displaces the tongue anteriorly by grabbing it with a hemostat or gauze sponge (see Fig. 34.4).

Step 4: **Evaluate the airway.** All materials must be quickly removed from the patient's mouth. If bleeding is noted, the

area should be packed with surgical gauze (4 × 4, **not** 2 × 2) to prevent bleeding into the pharynx at this time.

Step 5: **Suction the airway.** Using a tonsillar suction tip, the dentist completely and rapidly suctions the oral cavity and posterior pharynx to remove any foreign matter.

Step 6: **Reevaluate the airway.** Keeping an ear close to the patient's mouth and nose, the dentist pushes down on the patient's chest. If a rush of air is heard and felt, the spasm has been broken and the airway is patent. If no air is heard or felt, proceed to step 7. Oxygen saturation of the blood will decrease significantly, activating the alarm on the pulse oximeter (which is commonly set at an O_2 saturation of 90).

Step 7: **Positive-pressure oxygen.** Positive-pressure O_2 is administered in an effort to mechanically break the laryngospasm by physically forcing oxygen through the vocal cords. The absolute importance of effective suctioning (see Step 5) before this step is evident, as foreign material may be forced into the trachea by the positive-pressure oxygen flow.

Step 8: **Administer a muscle relaxant.** If the preceding steps are unsuccessful, succinylcholine administration is required. **Succinylcholine should only be administered by dentists who have received prior training in its administration and who are able to manage the apneic patient after its administration.** An initial succinylcholine dose of 10 mg intravenously is recommended for the partial or incomplete laryngospasm, with a dose of 20 to 40 mg recommended for complete spasm or spasm that continues after the initial 10-mg dose is administered.

Step 9: **Assess ventilation and control ventilation,** if necessary. Following succinylcholine administration, apnea may be present for up to 4 minutes. Controlled ventilation is mandatory until spontaneous respiratory efforts return. Succinylcholine administration, especially in larger doses, produces hyperkalemia, which can provoke cardiac dysrhythmias (bradycardia and asystole). Monitoring of the blood pressure, heart rate, and heart rhythm should be continued throughout the recovery period.

EMESIS AND ASPIRATION OF FOREIGN MATERIAL UNDER ANESTHESIA

Emesis (vomiting) and possible aspiration of this material into the airway is one of the most frightening of potential emergencies arising during general anesthesia or deep sedation. Fortunately, it is also one of the least likely situations to develop when recommended patient management techniques are followed. When protective airway reflexes remain intact (minimal or moderate sedation), aspiration of vomitus is unlikely.

Vomiting itself is rarely encountered during sedation and general anesthesia. The act of vomiting requires the forceful contraction of many muscle groups, including the diaphragm, resulting in a projectile expulsion of the vomitus from the patient's GI tract and mouth. Aspiration of vomitus, although possible, is unlikely during minimal-to-moderate sedation.

During deep sedation and general anesthesia, in which protective airway reflexes and muscle tonus are depressed or absent, vomiting does not occur. Regurgitation—a passive reflux of stomach contents into the esophagus and pharynx—can occur and represents a significant danger. Regurgitation is passive (no muscular contraction) and "quiet." In nondental surgical situations, regurgitation may go unnoticed unless someone is actively monitoring the airway. Use of the pretracheal stethoscope enables the gurgling sound associated with vomitus to be detected almost immediately. In dental situations, vomitus will be observed in the posterior of the mouth or pharynx.

Stomach contents have an extremely low pH. Morbidity and death are more likely to occur the lower the pH of the aspirated materials.[50]

When vomitus is aspirated into the trachea, the potential for disaster exists. The makeup of the material aspirated has a profound effect on the resulting clinical situation. The aspiration of solid material may produce acute airway obstruction, progressing to death unless it is managed immediately and aggressively.

When liquid is aspirated, the usual airway response is bronchospasm. Rales, dyspnea, tachycardia, partial airway obstruction, and cyanosis develop within seconds, followed shortly thereafter by hypotension.[2] Pulse oximeter values for oxygen saturation will be depressed (less than 90%) and are likely to remain depressed despite efforts to increase them.

Management

Step 1: **Position the patient.** The patient should immediately be placed into the Trendelenburg position with a head-down tilt of at least 15 degrees. To assist gravity in directing the vomitus into the pharynx (not into the lungs), the patient should be turned onto his or her right side.

Step 2: **Suction.** Using a tonsillar suction, the pharynx should be suctioned, removing any vomitus that may be present.

Step 3: **Secure the airway.** Intubation should be accomplished, if possible. The patient is turned onto his or her back for intubation.

Step 4: **Oxygen.** Oxygen, if not already administered, is administered at this time.

Step 5: **Activate EMS.** The dentist should activate EMS as soon as possible after aspiration has been diagnosed.

Step 6: **Definitive care.**

Step 6a: **Tracheal lavage.** Tracheal lavage should be performed if the patient has been intubated. Following slight elevation of the patient's head, a bolus of 10 to 20 mL of either normal saline or sodium bicarbonate is administered into the endotracheal tube. Larger volumes of solution are contraindicated because this might propel the aspirated material farther into the trachea and lungs. Immediately after lavage, suction and oxygenation are necessary. This procedure can be repeated several times.

Step 6b: **Administer intravenous steroids.** To minimize development of inflammation, edema, and aspiration pneumonitis, steroids should be administered. There is some controversy associated with steroid administration because of its ability to depress the immune response of these patients who may develop aspiration pneumonitis.

Step 7: **Hospitalization.** The patient who aspirated will usually be hospitalized for a variable length of time.

HYPERVENTILATION

In the dental environment, hyperventilation almost always represents an anxiety-induced response to a fear-provoking therapy. Losing control of breathing, the patient breathes both more rapidly (tachypnea) and deeply (hyperpnea) than usual. Large amounts of CO_2 are exhaled, leading to hypocapnia, which is associated with signs and symptoms such as a feeling of coldness and tingling that leads to paresthesia of the fingers, toes, and circumoral region. The patient may become lightheaded or experience a feeling of tightness in their chest (mimicking the discomfort of angina pectoris). This increases the patient's anxieties and intensifies his or her inability to control their breathing. Continued hyperventilation may lead to a spasmodic contraction of the hands and feet, termed *carpopedal tetany* (Fig. 34.5) and then to seizures and the loss of consciousness. Although hyperventilation may occur at any age, it appears that patients between their late teens and late thirties are more likely to hyperventilate.

Management

Management of hyperventilation is predicated on allaying the patient's anxieties and in elevating the CO_2 level of the blood back to normal. This may be accomplished by having the patient rebreathe his or her exhaled air. The preferred method of doing this is to have the patient cup their hands in front of their mouth and nose and simply rebreathe. This has two benefits. First, the warm, moist exhaled air will warm the patient's cold hands—a psychological boost to the frightened patient, and second, the CO_2 level of the patient's blood will increase, relieving the signs and symptoms noted. (Exhaled air contains almost 100 times more CO_2 than inhaled air) It is also possible to have a patient pinch one nostril closed and breathe through the remaining nostril with the mouth shut.

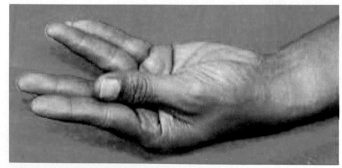

Figure 34.5 Carpopedal tetany. (From Malamed SF: *Medical emergencies in the dental office*, ed 7, St. Louis, Mosby, 2015.)

Box 34.16	Management of Hyperventilation

Recognize problem
(rapid, deep, uncontrolled breathing)
↓
P—Position patient comfortably
(usually upright)
↓
C→A→B—Basic life support as needed
↓
D—Definitive care:
Remove dental material from patient's mouth
Calm patient
Correct respiratory alkalosis
Initiate drug management as needed
↓
Dental care may continue if BOTH doctor and patient
agree
↓
Discharge patient

A, *Airway;* B, *breathing;* C, *circulation;* D, *definitive care;*
P, *position.*
From Malamed SF: Medical emergencies in the dental office,
7e, St Louis, 2015, Mosby.

The older technique of rebreathing exhaled air from a paper bag is no longer recommended.

In the unlikely event that hyperventilation continues, an IV infusion should be started and midazolam or diazepam titrated very slowly until the patient relaxes and his or her breathing becomes normal. Box 34.16 outlines the steps to take to manage hyperventilation.

RESPIRATORY DEPRESSION AND OBSTRUCTION

Respiratory *depression* may develop secondary to the administration of CNS-depressant drugs. It is most likely to be observed during deep sedation and general anesthesia and when certain drug groups, such as the barbiturates and opioids, are used. Respiratory depression is less likely to occur during oral or inhalation sedation and when benzodiazepines are used during minimal and moderate sedation techniques. Benzodiazepines are more likely to produce respiratory *obstruction,* secondary to their muscle relaxant properties.

Respiratory depression may be observed as either a decreased rate of respiration (to apnea) or as decreased ventilatory effort. Monitoring priorities during parenteral sedation and general anesthesia are based primarily on ensuring airway and ventilatory adequacy. The pretracheal stethoscope is the most significant monitor in this regard, permitting evaluation of each and every breath taken by the patient. Respiratory problems may be detected virtually instantaneously with a pretracheal stethoscope, which is suggested for parenteral moderate and deep sedation and general anesthesia cases. Pulse oximetry permits evaluation of the degree of oxygenation of the blood. Although effective, there is a 10- to 20-second time lag between respiratory changes and notification on the oximeter screen. In addition, CO_2 blood levels are not evaluated by the pulse oximeter. Use of the pulse oximeter is recommended for all parenteral moderate sedation, deep sedation, and general anesthesia cases. The capnograph permits virtually instantaneous (2- to 4-second delay) evaluation of the effectiveness of ventilation through monitoring of the end-tidal CO_2 of each breath. Airway obstruction (e.g., tongue "falling back" into pharynx causing obstruction—either partial or total—of the airway, and diminished ventilatory effort (respiratory depression) may be detected immediately, permitting corrective action to be instituted rapidly. Use of the capnograph is currently recommended for operating room general anesthesia and is gaining acceptance in deep sedation and parenteral moderate sedation.

When respiratory depression results from drug administration, it may be possible to administer reversal agents. Naloxone effectively reverses opioid analgesics, and benzodiazepines may be reversed with flumazenil. No specific antagonists exist for either barbiturates or propofol. Propofol, a rapid-acting and short-acting drug, will rarely produce respiratory depression persisting longer than a few seconds.

Respiratory depression or obstruction rarely represents a significant problem where the dentist has received appropriate training in the administration of anesthetic drugs. Outside medical assistance is not usually required, for the period of respiratory depression or obstruction is usually transitory, with no adverse effects to the patient occurring.

Management

Step 1: **Terminate the procedure.**
Step 2: **P**-Position. The patient should be in the supine position.
Step 3: **Assess C**-Circulation, **A**-Airway, **B**-Breathing (basic life support), as indicated. The dentist should provide airway maintenance (e.g., head tilt–chin lift) and evaluate respiratory effectiveness (i.e., look, listen, and feel). In many instances assisted ventilation will be necessary to supplement the patient's inspired air volume. In a few instances in which apnea is present, controlled ventilation is necessary.
Step 4: **D**-Definitive care.
Step 4a. **Blood pressure and heart rate and rhythm should be monitored and recorded every 5 minutes and oxygen administered.**
Step 4b. **Start an IV infusion,** if not already present.
Step 4c. Although their administration is not usually necessary, consider antidotal drug administration:
- When **opioids** have been administered, **slowly titrate naloxone** at 0.1 mg/min until improved ventilation is noted. In children a dose of 0.005 mg/min is administered until improved ventilation is observed.[51]

- Following **benzodiazepine** administration, **flumazenil** should be considered at an IV dose of 0.2 mg/min until respiratory efforts improve. A usual adult dose of flumazenil is 0.5 mg.[52]
- With some drug groups, such as barbiturates, no effective antagonist exists. Continued assisted or controlled ventilation and/or airway management is necessary until spontaneous breathing returns.
- No effective antagonist exists for propofol, but prolonged respiratory depression is unlikely to be observed with this drug because of its short duration of action.

Step 5: **Recovery.** Following return of ventilatory adequacy after a brief period of respiratory depression (rescue of the patient from a deeper level of sedation back to the desired level), it may be possible to continue with the planned dental treatment. If the period of respiratory depression was significant in depth or duration, the dentist may elect to terminate the dental procedure. At the end of the planned dental treatment or after termination of the treatment, the IM administration of an antidotal drug should be considered. In situations in which IM opioids or benzodiazepines have been administered, or in cases in which long-acting drugs such as morphine and lorazepam have been administered intravenously, the potential for a rebound depression exists (although this is highly unlikely to occur). IV antagonists have a rapid onset of clinical action, but their duration after IV administration may be shorter than that of the offending drug. An IM dose of either flumazenil or naloxone should be considered in these situations.

Step 6: **Discharge.** The patient will be discharged from the office in the custody of a responsible adult companion only when the treating dentist believes that the patient's recovery (from sedation or general anesthesia) is adequate to permit his or her safe dismissal from the office and that a rebound sedation is unlikely to occur.

Outside medical assistance is rarely required in respiratory depression.

Box 34.3 outlines the steps to take to manage sedative-hypnotic overdose. Box 34.4 outlines the steps to take to manage opioid overdose.

SEIZURES

Seizures (or convulsions) are not uncommon during dental treatment. Patients with epilepsy are the most likely persons to have seizures in the dental environment because stressful situations may provoke seizures even in epileptics whose seizures are well-controlled. More than 90% of patients with epilepsy have generalized tonic-clonic seizures (GTCS), commonly known as grand mal seizures.[53] Local anesthetic overdose is another possible cause of seizures. The inadvertent intravascular (IV or intraarterial) administration of local anesthetics produces a seizure within seconds of injection, whereas the administration of too large a total dose brings on a more gradual onset of seizure activity (usually within 5 to 10 minutes after local anesthetic administration), with the patient demonstrating increasingly

severe signs and symptoms until frank tonic-clonic convulsions occur. Hyperventilation may also be associated with seizures if the episode goes untreated for an extended period. Seizures are also associated with extreme hypoxia or anoxia and hypercarbia secondary to airway management problems or apnea, as well as with severe hypoglycemia.

Seizures are usually readily managed without resulting injury or mortality. The primary goals in seizure management are preventing injury to the patient during the seizure and ensuring the adequacy of ventilation. Ventilatory adequacy is of particular importance during the local anesthetic-induced seizure because pH changes alter the seizure threshold of the local anesthetic.[54] Acidosis, a result of hypoxia, hypercarbia, and lactic acid production during the seizure, lowers the threshold for local anesthetic-induced seizures, thereby prolonging the seizure and increasing the likelihood of serious postictal morbidity or death. Adequate ventilation will eliminate/prevent CO_2 retention and elevate the seizure threshold of the local anesthetic, thereby decreasing the duration of the seizure.

Anticonvulsants are rarely required to terminate seizures because most seizures are self-limiting, rarely lasting more than 2 to 5 minutes (grand mal epilepsy). However, EMS assistance will, on occasion, be recommended as a part of our management, for two reasons: first, to aid in the definitive management of the patient following the seizure, and second, to administer IV anticonvulsants if the seizure is ongoing on arrival of EMS.

Management

Step 1: **Terminate the procedure.**

Step 2: **P**-Position. The patient should be placed in the supine position.

Step 3: **Assess C**-Circulation, **A**-Airway, **B**-Breathing (basic life support), as indicated. During the clonic phase of a seizure, airway, breathing, and circulation need not be assisted.

Step 4: **D**-Definitive care.

Step 4a: **Prevent injury.** The dentist must protect the patient during the clonic phase of the seizure (alternating generalized muscle contraction and relaxation). Two members of the office emergency team gently hold the patient's arms and legs. Limited movement of the limbs should be permitted so as to prevent injury. Movement should not be completely restricted, as this may cause injury to the patient. Do not attempt to place any object into the mouth of a convulsing victim, as this is a primary cause of injury to persons during seizures (fractured or avulsed teeth and injury to intraoral soft tissues).

Step 4b: **Activate EMS,** if considered necessary by the treating dentist.

Step 4c: **Administer oxygen.** The dentist should ensure airway patency and administer oxygen to minimize hypoxia and hypercarbia.

Most generalized tonic-clonic convulsions cease spontaneously within 2 to 5 minutes. In a few cases a seizure may continue beyond 5 minutes, or a seizure may stop and recur before the patient recovers consciousness. These are the two definitions of status epilepticus, a situation that represents an acutely life-threatening emergency.[55] Seizures secondary to local anesthetic overdose will continue until the cerebral blood level of the local anesthetic falls below the seizure threshold for that drug. With adequate airway maintenance and oxygenation, local anesthetic-induced seizures normally persist for less than a minute. Though unlikely to occur, seizures developing during hyperventilation continue until the CO_2 level of the blood is elevated to close to normal levels. Seizures secondary to airway obstruction or anoxia are associated with extreme morbidity or death. Airway patency and oxygenation must be ensured.

Step 4d: **Establish venous access.** If the seizure persists, an IV infusion should be started, if possible. A catheter is recommended because its flexibility minimizes the risk of its being accidentally dislodged by the seizing patient.

Step 4e: **Anticonvulsant administration.** The administration of IV anticonvulsants should be considered if the seizure is prolonged. To be effective, anticonvulsants should be administered intravenously. Midazolam, the drug of choice, is titrated slowly in a 1.0 mg/mL dilution, at a rate of 1.0 mL per minute—until seizure activity ceases. Anticonvulsant administration should be considered only if the dentist is well trained in management of the unconscious, apneic patient, for this is an entirely possible scenario in the postseizure state when anticonvulsants have been administered. IN midazolam may be administered when venipuncture cannot be established and if the patient is younger and of lighter weight (up to 30 kg). Intranasal dosages of 0.2 to 0.7 mg/kg have been quite effective.[56,57]

Step 5: **Postseizure management.** The epileptic patient who has not received anticonvulsants will normally be sleeping deeply and perhaps snoring in the immediate postseizure (postictal) state. Snoring is indicative of a partial airway obstruction produced by the effect of gravity on the now relaxed muscles of the tongue, forcing the tongue backward into the hypopharynx. Management requires head tilt–chin lift and the administration of oxygen. The postictal patient will also be mentally disoriented. The treating dentist should talk to the patient, explaining where the patient is, what has happened, and that everything is "all right." Complete recovery from a GTCS oftentimes requires several hours. EMS personnel will evaluate the patient to determine whether hospitalization is required or whether the patient may be discharged from the office in the custody of a responsible adult companion.

Patients who have had a local anesthetic-induced seizure normally require hospitalization for an indefinite period so that their neurologic status can be better evaluated. Hospitalization may be suggested after hyperventilation-induced seizures, but the period of observation is usually minimal (several hours).

Seizures secondary to severe anoxia require hospitalization and intensive care for an undetermined period of neurologic

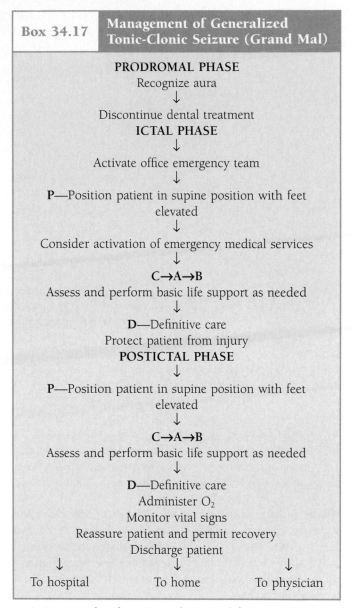

Box 34.17 Management of Generalized Tonic-Clonic Seizure (Grand Mal)

PRODROMAL PHASE
Recognize aura
↓
Discontinue dental treatment
ICTAL PHASE
↓
Activate office emergency team
↓
P—Position patient in supine position with feet elevated
↓
Consider activation of emergency medical services
↓
C→A→B
Assess and perform basic life support as needed
↓
D—Definitive care
Protect patient from injury
POSTICTAL PHASE
↓
P—Position patient in supine position with feet elevated
↓
C→A→B
Assess and perform basic life support as needed
↓
D—Definitive care
Administer O_2
Monitor vital signs
Reassure patient and permit recovery
Discharge patient
↓   ↓   ↓
To hospital   To home   To physician

A, *Airway;* B, *breathing;* C, *circulation;* D, *definitive care;* P, *position.*
From Malamed SF: *Medical emergencies in the dental office, 7e,* St Louis, 2015, Mosby.

assessment. Patients who have received anticonvulsant drugs to terminate their seizures are usually hospitalized.

Box 34.17 outlines the steps to take to manage GTCS. Box 34.18 outlines the steps to take to manage generalized convulsive status epilepticus.

HYPOGLYCEMIA

Hypoglycemia—low blood sugar—is not an uncommon occurrence in patients with type 1, insulin-dependent diabetes mellitus (IDDM). Patients with type 2, noninsulin-dependent diabetes mellitus (NIDDM) are less likely to become acutely hypoglycemic. Changes in recommendations for management

| Box 34.18 | Management of Generalized Convulsive Status Epilepticus |

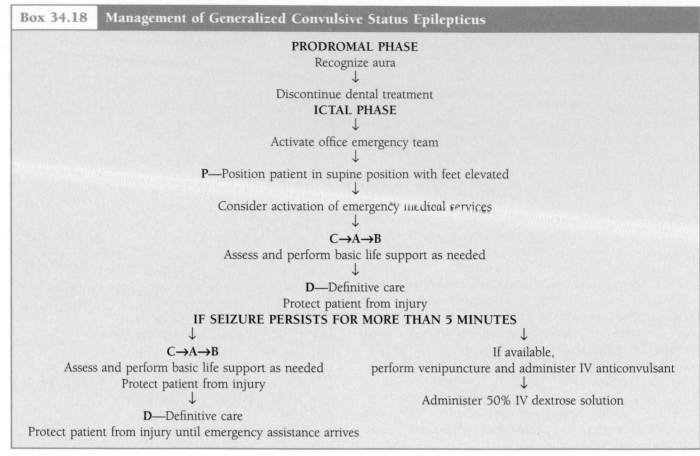

PRODROMAL PHASE
Recognize aura
↓
Discontinue dental treatment
ICTAL PHASE
↓
Activate office emergency team
↓
P—Position patient in supine position with feet elevated
↓
Consider activation of emergency medical services
↓
C→A→B
Assess and perform basic life support as needed
↓
D—Definitive care
Protect patient from injury
IF SEIZURE PERSISTS FOR MORE THAN 5 MINUTES

↓ | | ↓

C→A→B
Assess and perform basic life support as needed
Protect patient from injury
↓
D—Definitive care
Protect patient from injury until emergency assistance arrives

If available,
perform venipuncture and administer IV anticonvulsant
↓
Administer 50% IV dextrose solution

A, Airway; B, breathing; C, circulation; D, definitive care; IV, intravenous; P, position.
From Malamed SF: Medical emergencies in the dental office, 7e, St Louis, 2015, Mosby.

of type 1 diabetes suggest the more frequent administration of insulin (perhaps three to six times per day) as a means of delaying the onset of the chronic complications associated with diabetes. However, increased insulin administration brings with it an estimated threefold increase in the incidence of acute hypoglycemia.[58]

Inadequate cerebral blood glucose levels lead to diminished CNS function. Clinical signs and symptoms associated with mild hypoglycemia include mental confusion, mild muscle tremor, diaphoresis, a feeling of being cold, and tachycardia. This is a likely scenario in a dental practice when the type 1 diabetic patient does not eat before a scheduled appointment. A telephone call the day before the scheduled dental appointment, confirming their appointment and reminding the patient to eat, should minimize this occurrence. If parenteral sedation or general anesthesia is scheduled, a period of fast is mandated. The patient's insulin needs will be decreased and should be so adjusted, either by the patient or after consultation with their primary care physician. The use of 5% dextrose and water as the infusate is not contraindicated in the type 1 diabetic patient. The patient appears in the office slightly hypoglycemic after their fast, and 5% dextrose and water will provide a needed elevation in the blood sugar level. Patients tolerate hyperglycemia much better than they do hypoglycemia.

When blood sugar levels fall too low, consciousness is lost and seizures may occur, although the latter should be unlikely in the dental situation. Mild hypoglycemia is easily managed with a rapid return to normal CNS functioning. The need for EMS and hospitalization is minimal. When hypoglycemia leads to loss of consciousness and/or seizures, EMS assistance is desirable and a period of hospitalization the norm.

Management

Step 1: **Terminate the procedure**.

Step 2: **P**-Position. As soon as signs and symptoms of hypoglycemia are noted, the patient is placed into a comfortable position.

Step 3: **Assess C**-Circulation, **A**-Airway, **B**-Breathing (basic life support), as indicated.

Step 4: **D**-Definitive care. It should be determined whether the patient took an insulin dose and whether he or she has eaten food recently.

Step 4a: **Administer "sugar."** If hypoglycemia is considered a possibility, the dentist should not hesitate to administer sugar to the conscious patient orally. Most type 1 diabetic patients prefer orange juice, feeling that they recover faster than with other liquids ([nondiet] soft drinks). Permit the patient to drink 8 to 12 ounces of orange juice in 4-ounce increments over about 10 minutes. Return to normal CNS status is rapid. Some diabetic patients prefer candy bars. After full recovery the planned dental care may continue if both the dentist and patient are agreeable.

Step 4b: **Activate EMS.** If the episode continues or if consciousness is lost, EMS should be summoned immediately.

Step 4c: **Position.** With the loss of consciousness, the patient is placed into the supine position with their feet elevated slightly and BLS administered as needed. In most instances airway maintenance is all that will be required.

Step 4d: **Venous access.** An IV infusion, if not already present, should be established, if possible.

Step 4e: **Administer an antihypoglycemic.** A dose of 30 mL of 50% dextrose is administered intravenously. The return of consciousness is usually quite rapid. The pediatric dose (patient weight up to 30 kg) is 30 mL of a 25% dextrose solution. If an IV cannot be started or 50% (or 25%) dextrose is unavailable, glucagon may be administered intramuscularly or intravenously.[59] The dose of glucagon is 0.5 to 1.0 mg administered subcutaneously, intramuscularly, or intravenously. Consciousness usually returns within 15 minutes, with the dose repeated every 15 minutes, if necessary. When the patient does not respond to glucagon, IV dextrose 50% must be administered.[59]

Step 5: **Recovery.** Once consciousness returns, the patient should be monitored until EMS personnel arrive. A period of hospitalization is usually necessary when unconsciousness occurs secondary to hypoglycemia. Boxes 34.19 and 34.20 outline the steps to take to manage hypoglycemia.

SYNCOPE

Syncope, a transient loss of consciousness, is not uncommon in the practice of dentistry. In a survey of emergencies in dental practice, 50.3% of 30,608 emergencies were listed as syncope.[60] Produced by a sudden drop in heart rate (bradycardia) leading to a drop in blood pressure (hypotension), which decreases blood and oxygen delivery to the CNS, syncope is also referred to as *vasodepressor syncope, vasovagal syncope, common faint,* and *psychogenic syncope.*

During stressful situations, as might develop in the dental office, such as sudden unexpected pain or the sight of blood or dental instruments (e.g., needles, the drill), blood is directed into the skeletal muscle of the legs and arms to prepare the body for the "fight or flight response." In the absence of movement by the patient (the "macho" patient sits still and "takes it like a man") who is seated upright or semi-upright in the dental chair, the return of venous blood to the heart and the volume of blood flow to the brain decrease (decreased cardiac output). Signs and symptoms of a slight decrease in cerebral blood flow include a feeling of warmth, the loss of color (pale or ashen gray skin tone), diaphoresis, complaints of feeling "bad" or "faint," and nausea, along with the development of a tachycardia. Tachycardia enables the body to compensate for the decrease in cardiac output and to maintain a minimally

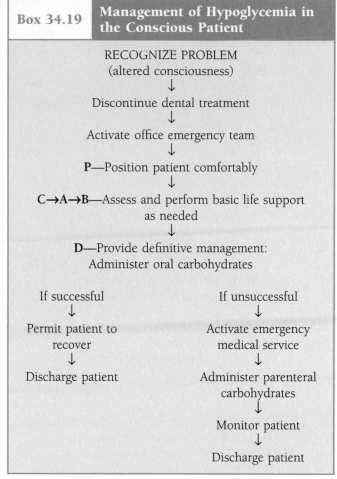

Box 34.19   Management of Hypoglycemia in the Conscious Patient

RECOGNIZE PROBLEM
(altered consciousness)
↓
Discontinue dental treatment
↓
Activate office emergency team
↓
P—Position patient comfortably
↓
C→A→B—Assess and perform basic life support as needed
↓
D—Provide definitive management: Administer oral carbohydrates

If successful
↓
Permit patient to recover
↓
Discharge patient

If unsuccessful
↓
Activate emergency medical service
↓
Administer parenteral carbohydrates
↓
Monitor patient
↓
Discharge patient

A, *Airway;* B, *breathing;* C, *circulation;* D, *definitive care;* P, *position.*
From Malamed SF: Medical emergencies in the dental office, *7e, St Louis, 2015, Mosby.*

adequate blood flow to the brain, which maintains consciousness. In the absence of definitive treatment decompensation occurs, consisting of a significant bradycardia (heart rate <20 beats per minute with periods of asystole frequently observed), which severely decreases cerebral blood flow leading to the loss of consciousness.[61] Placing the patient in the supine position with their legs elevated, significantly increases venous return, and airway maintenance ensures the delivery of oxygen to the blood. Return of consciousness is normally quite rapid, within 10 to 15 seconds following proper positioning and airway management. Rarely is either EMS or hospitalization necessary. Indeed, in a person who "felt faint" but never lost consciousness, the planned dental procedure may continue if both the dentist and patient are comfortable doing so, but only after determining the reason for the faint and taking the steps necessary to prevent its recurrence (e.g., the stress reduction protocol). However, where consciousness was lost for any period of time, however brief, the planned treatment should be rescheduled to a later date. Modifications in subsequent

| Box 34.20 | Management of Hypoglycemia in the Unconscious Patient |

RECOGNIZE PROBLEM
(lack of response to sensory stimulation)
↓
Discontinue dental treatment
↓
Activate office emergency team
↓
P—Position patient in supine position with feet elevated
↓
C→A→B—Assess and perform basic life support as needed
↓
D—Definitive management:
Summon emergency medical service,
Administer carbohydrates:
IV 50% dextrose solution
1 mg glucagon via IV or IM route
Monitor vital signs every 5 minutes
Administer O₂
↓
Allow patient to recover and discharge per medical recommendations

A, *Airway*; B, *breathing*; C, *circulation*; D, *definitive care*; IM, *intramuscular*; IV, *intravenous*; P, *position*.
From Malamed SF: Medical emergencies in the dental office, 7e, St Louis, 2015, Mosby.

dental care should be instituted so as to prevent recurrence of the faint.

Syncope is unlikely to occur in the sedated patient. More likely is the scenario of the fearful, nonmedicated patient collapsing in the reception area or in the dental chair on seeing the needle on the local anesthetic syringe. Pretreatment diagnosis of the patient's dental fears and modifications in dental care should prevent syncope from ever arising. Most incidents of fainting occur with the patient seated in an upright position. With dental patients more commonly placed in a reclined (or supine) position in the dental chair, loss of consciousness from syncope should become less common.

Management

Step 1: **Terminate the procedure.**
Step 2: **P-Position.** The patient is placed into the supine position with the feet elevated.
Step 3: **Assess C-Circulation, A-Airway, B-Breathing** (basic life support), as indicated.
Step 4: **D-Definitive care.**
Step 4a: All dental equipment should be removed from the patient's field of vision.

Step 4b: **Administer oxygen.**
Step 4c: **Administer ammonia.** Ammonia inhalants should be available in every treatment room as well as in the emergency drug kit. Crushed between the rescuer's fingers, the inhalant is held under the patient's nose. Inhalation of ammonia, a noxious odor, provokes muscular movement of the arms and legs, thereby increasing the return of venous blood to the heart and increasing cardiac output and blood flow to the brain (provided the patient has been positioned properly).
Step 5: **Recovery.** The syncopal episode will rapidly resolve, with the patient feeling considerably better once positioned and breathing oxygen. If both the dentist and the patient agree, the planned dental procedure may proceed (if consciousness has not been lost). The dentist should consider modification of dental care to diminish any anxiety that may be present.
Step 6: **Loss of consciousness.** Should loss of consciousness occur, place the patient into the supine position with their feet elevated, and if not already done, head tilt–chin lift performed and the airway assessed. The patient will usually be breathing spontaneously, and the heart rate will be slow (<20 beats per minute).
Step 6a: **Definitive management.** Consciousness should return within 10 to 15 seconds. The postsyncopal period is marked by the patient feeling poorly. The patient is nauseous (and likely to vomit), aches all over, and will require approximately 24 hours to fully return to a normal state of function. Oxygen should be administered to the patient via nasal cannula or nasal hood during this recovery period. Vital signs are monitored and recorded every 5 minutes.
Step 6b: **EMS.** If consciousness does not return within 10 to 15 seconds, EMS should be activated. There are many other potential causes for unconsciousness that do not respond to the treatment described. Whenever unconsciousness persists for longer than 10 to 15 seconds or when the dentist gets a "sense" that the problem is not simply fainting, it is recommended that emergency assistance be sought immediately.
Step 7: **Discharge.** Discharge of the patient from the office should be considered only after a lengthy period of recovery (approximately 1 hour), during which time the patient remains under direct observation. Patients who have lost consciousness should not be permitted to leave the office alone or to drive a car or any other vehicle (e.g., bicycle, skateboard). This patient should be discharged in the company of a responsible adult companion. There is rarely a need for EMS assistance or for hospitalization in the common episode of fainting. Box 34.21 outlines the steps to take to manage vasodepressor syncope.

SUMMARY

Emergency situations can and do arise in the dental and medical office. In this chapter, several potential emergency situations

Box 34.21	Management of Vasodepressor Syncope

Assess consciousness
(lack of response to sensory stimulation)
↓
Activate office emergency system
↓
P—Position patient supine with feet elevated slightly
↓
C→A→B—Assess circulation; assess and open airway; assess airway patency and breathing.
↓
D—Definitive care:
Administer O_2
Monitor vital signs
Perform additional procedures:
Administer aromatic ammonia vaporole; Administer "sugar" (e.g., orange juice, nondiet soft drink)
Administer atropine if bradycardia persists
Do not panic!

(Post syncopal recovery)   (Delayed recovery)
Postpone further dental   Activate emergency
treatment   medical services (911)
                        ↓
            Determine precipitating factors

A, *Airway;* B, *breathing;* C, *circulation;* D, *definitive care;* P, *position.*
From *Malamed SF:* Medical emergencies in the dental office, *7e, St Louis, 2015, Mosby.*

associated with the administration of drugs for anesthesia, sedation, or pain control have been reviewed. The best treatment for these emergencies is their prevention. Adequate preoperative patient evaluation, adherence to recommended technique, intraoperative monitoring, and postoperative management can prevent virtually all of these complications.

Other medical emergencies that occur during medical and dental treatment were described. Patients who are at risk (ASA 2, 3, and 4) are unable to tolerate the stresses normally associated with operative or surgical procedures and are more likely to develop acute exacerbation of their underlying medical problems. The appropriate use of sedation and pain control in these patients will greatly decrease their risk during treatment.

REFERENCES

1. Dental Board of California: Application for conscious sedation permit. Form CS-1, revised 7/08. (Sections 1647 – 1647.9, 1682 Business and Professions Code; Title 16 California Code of Regulations Sections 1043 – 1043.8) www.dbc.ca.gov. Accessed 21 April 2016.

2. American Association of Oral and Maxillofacial Surgeons, Committee on Anesthesia: *Office anesthesia evaluation manual,* ed 8, Rosemont, IL, 2012, The Association.

3. American Academy on Pediatrics; American Academy on Pediatric Dentistry: Guideline for monitoring and management of pediatric patients during and after sedation for diagnostic and therapeutic procedures. *Pediatr Dent* 30(7 Suppl):143–159, 2008-2009.

4. Pallasch TJ: *Pharmacology for dental students and practitioners,* Philadelphia, 1980, Lea & Febiger.

5. Anonymous: Pharmaceutical drug overdose case reports. From the world literature. *Toxicol Rev* 23(1):59–63, 2004.

6. Matzinger P: Tolerance, danger, and the extended family. *Annu Rev Immunol* 12:991–1045, 1994.

7. Uetrecht J: Idiosyncratic drug reactions: past, present, and future. *Chem Res Toxicol* 21(1):84–92, 2008.

8. Malamed SF: *Sedation: a guide to patient management,* ed 4, St Louis, 2000, CV Mosby.

9. Goodson JM, Moore PA: Life-threatening reactions after pedodontic sedation: an assessment of narcotic, local anesthetic, and antiemetic drug interaction. *J Am Dent Assoc* 107(2):239–245, 1983.

10. American Society of Anesthesiologists Task Force on Sedation and Analgesia by Non-Anesthesiologists: Practice guidelines for sedation and analgesia by non-anesthesiologists. *Anesthesiology* 96:1004–1017, 2002.

11. Pollakoff J, Pollakoff K: *EMT's guide to signs and symptoms,* Los Angeles, 1991, Los Angeles Unified School District Vocational Education Program.

12. Kleinman ME, Brennan EE, Goldberger ZD, et al: Part 5: adult basic life support and cardiopulmonary resuscitation quality: 2015 American Heart Association Guidelines Update for Cardiopulmonary Resuscitation and Emergency Cardiovascular Care. *Circulation* 132(Suppl 2):S414–S435, 2015.

13. ClinicalKey. Flumazenil drug monograph. February 5, 2016. www.clinicalkey.com. Accessed 9 March 2016.

14. ClinicalKey. Naloxone drug monograph. December 4, 2015. www.clinicalkey.com. Accessed 9 March 2016.

15. Hospira: Narcan Hydrochloride. Drug package insert, Hospira, Inc., Lake Forest, IL. January 2007.

16. de Caen AR, Berg MD, Chameides L, et al: Part 12: pediatric advanced life support: 2015 American Heart Association Guidelines Update for Cardiopulmonary Resuscitation and Emergency Cardiovascular Care. *Circulation* 132(Suppl 2):S526–S542, 2015.

17. de Julien LF: Causes of severe morbidity/mortality cases. *J Calif Dent Assoc* 11(2):45–48, 1983.

18. Bates DW, Leape LLI, Petrycki S: Incidence and preventability of adverse drug events in hospitalized patients. *J Gen Intern Med* 8(6):289–294, 1993.

19. Dolovich J, Evans S, Rosenbloom D, et al: Anaphylaxis due to thiopental sodium anesthesia. *Can Med Assoc J* 123(4):292–294, 1980.

20. Uchimura A, Yogo H, Kudoh I, Ohmura A: Facial edema and pruritus after intravenous injection of midazolam. *Masui* 55(1):76–78, 2006.

21. Chang KC, Hahn KH: Is alpha-adrenoceptor blockade responsible for atropine flush? *Eur J Pharmacol* 284(3):331–334, 1995.

22. Joint Task Force on Practice Parameters. American Academy of Allergy, Asthma and Immunology. American College of Allergy, Asthma and Immunology. Joint Council of Allergy, Asthma and Immunology: The diagnosis and

management of anaphylaxis: an updated practice parameter. *J Allergy Clin Immunol* 115(3 Suppl 2):S483–S523, 2005.

23. Campbell RL, Hagan JB, Manivannan V, et al: Evaluation of national institute of allergy and infectious diseases/food allergy and anaphylaxis network criteria for the diagnosis of anaphylaxis in emergency department patients. *J Allergy Clin Immunol* 129(3):748–752, 2012.

24. Senna G, Demain JG: Update on the understanding, diagnosis and tailored management of anaphylaxis: making progress. *Curr Opin Allergy Clin Immunol* 14:307–308, 2014.

25. Milner SM, Bennett JD: Emergency cricothyrotomy. *J Laryngol Otol* 105(11).003 885 1991.

26. Malamed SF: Foreign body airway obstruction. In *Medical emergencies in the dental office*, ed 7, St Louis, 2015, Mosby, pp 201–204.

27. American College of Allergy, Asthma, and Immunology. Types of Allergy – Latex Allergy. http://acaai.org/allergies/types/skin-allergies/latex-allergy. Accessed 31 October 2016.

28. Ono SJ: Molecular genetics of allergic diseases. *Annu Rev Immunol* 18:347–366, 2000.

29. National Heart, Lung, and Blood Institute. Types of hypotension. https://www.nhlbi.nih.gov/health/health-topics/topics/hyp/types. November 1, 2010. Accessed 31 October 2016.

30. U.S. Department of Health & Human Services. Chemical Hazards Emergency Medical Management. Definition of hypotension by systolic pressure and age. June 25, 2011. https://chemm.nlm.nih.gov/pals.htm. Accessed 31 October 2016.

31. Malamed SF: Systemic complications. In Malamed SF, editor: *Handbook of local anesthesia*, ed 6, St Louis, 2013, CV Mosby, pp 311–340.

32. ClinicalKey. Ephedrine drug monograph. March 18, 2016. www.clinicalkey.com. Accessed 25 April 2016.

33. Papadopoulos DP, Sanidas EA, Viniou NA, et al: Cardiovascular hypertensive emergencies. *Curr Hypertens Rep* 17(2):5, 2015.

34. Katari A, Kohl BA: Cardiovascular emergencies. In Ruskin KJ, Rosenbaum SH, editors: *Anesthesia emergencies*, Oxford, 2011, Oxford University Press., p 43.

35. Aggarwal M, Khan IA: Hypertensive crisis: hypertensive emergencies and urgencies. *Cardiol Clin* 24(1):135–146, 2006.

36. Patel HP, Mitsnefes M: Advances in the pathogenesis and management of hypertensive crisis. *Curr Opin Pediatr* 17(2):210–214, 2005.

37. Cohen MM, Duncan PG, Pope WDB, Wolkenstein C: A survey of 112,000 anaesthetics at one teaching hospital (1975-1983). *Can J Anaesth* 33(1):22–31, 1986.

38. Atlee JL: *Perioperative cardiac dysrhythmias: mechanisms, recognition, management*, ed 2, Chicago, 1989, Year Book Medical.

39. Wingard DW: What is a normal heart rate prior to surgery? *Anesthesiology* 72(6):1102, 1990.

40. Driscoll EJ, Smilack ZH, Lightbody PM, Fiorucci RD: Sedation with intravenous diazepam. *J Oral Surg* 30(5):332–343, 1972.

41. DeRango FJ: Management of common medical problems. In Lichtiger M, Moya F, editors: *Introduction to the practice of anesthesia*, ed 2, Hagerstown, MD, 1978, Harper & Row.

42. Link MS, Berkow LC, Kudenchuk PJ, et al: Part 7: adult advanced cardiovascular life support: 2015 American Heart Association Guidelines Update for Cardiopulmonary Resuscitation and Emergency Cardiovascular Care. *Circulation* 132(Suppl 2):S444–S464, 2015.

43. Boden WE: Angina pectoris and stable ischemic heart disease. In Goldman L, Shafer AI, editors: *Goldman-Cecil medicine*, ed 25, Philadelphia, 2016, Elsevier Saunders, pp 420–432.

44. Phipps C: Contributory causes of coronary thrombosis. *JAMA* 106:761, 1936.

45. New York Times. Heart Attack Overview. http://www.nytimes.com/health/guides/disease/heart-attack/overview.html#. Accessed 4 May 2016.

46. Ferraris VA, Ferraris SP, Gilliam HS, Berry WR: Predictors of postoperative ventricular dysrhythmias: a multivariate study. *J Cardiovasc Surg* 32(1):17–20, 1991.

47. Liau CS, Hahn LC, Tjung JJ, et al: The clinical characteristics of acute myocardial infarction in aged patients. *J Formosan Med Assoc* 90(2):122–126, 1991.

48. Ospina JC, Ludemann JP: Aspiration of an extracted molar: case report. *J Can Dent Assoc* 71(8):581–583, 2005.

49. Palmer M, Shin T: 24-year old dies after wisdom teeth surgery. April 3, 2013. http://usnews.nbcnews.com/_news/2013/04/03/17580165--24-year-old-dies-after-wisdom-teeth-surgery. Accessed 4 May 2016.

50. Boesch RP, Daines C, Willging JP, et al: Advances in the diagnosis and management of chronic pulmonary aspiration in children. *Eur Respir J* 28(4):847–861, 2006.

51. Barsan WG, Tomassoni AJ, Seger D, et al: Safety assessment of high-dose narcotic analgesia for emergency department procedures. *Ann Emerg Med* 22(9):1444–1449, 1993.

52. Thomson JS, Donald C, Lewin K: Use of flumazenil in benzodiazepine overdose. *Emerg Med J* 23(2):162, 2006.

53. Earnest MP: Seizures. *Neurol Clin* 11(3):563–575, 1993.

54. Covino BG: Toxicity of local anesthetic agents. *Acta Anaesthesiol Belg* 39(3 Suppl 2):159–164, 1988.

55. Fisher RS, van Emde Boas W, Blume W, et al: Epileptic seizures and epilepsy: definitions proposed by the International League Against Epilepsy (ILAE) and the International Bureau for Epilepsy (IBE). *Epilepsia* 46(4):470–472, 2005.

56. Mahmoudian T, Zadeh MM: Comparison of intranasal midazolam with intravenous diazepam for treating acute seizures in children. *Epilepsy Behav* 5(2):253–255, 2004.

57. Kyrkou M, Harbord M, Kyrkou N, et al: Community use of intranasal midazolam for managing prolonged seizures. *J Intellect Dev Disabil* 31(3):131–138, 2006.

58. The Diabetes Control and Complications Trial Research Group: The effect of intensive treatment of diabetes on the development and progression of long-term complications in insulin-dependent diabetes mellitus. *N Engl J Med* 329(14):977–986, 1993.

59. ClinicalKey. Glucagon drug monograph. January 5, 2016. www.clinicalkey.com. Accessed 4 May 2016.

60. Malamed SF: Managing medical emergencies. *JADA* 124(8):40–53, 1993.

61. Dovgalyuk J, Holstege C, Mattu A: The electrocardiogram in the patient with syncope. *Am J Emerg Med* 25(6):688–701, 2007.

Section VIII

SPECIAL CONSIDERATIONS

*I*n this concluding section, several groups of patients for whom the management of pain and anxiety require greater attention are discussed. For these patients the overall risks of unwanted drug effects, acute medical problems, and unsuccessful results are greater than in other groups. For these patients, too, the rewards for successful treatment (in terms of personal satisfaction and accomplishment) are infinitely greater.

The *pediatric patient* represents a group in which the various techniques of sedation and general anesthesia are frequently required, usually for behavioral management. However, pediatric patients cannot be treated as though they were simply small adults. Drug dosages usually must be altered to meet the specific needs of the child patient. Unfortunately, a disproportionate number of the serious problems that have occurred in association with the use of sedative techniques in dental and medical outpatient practices over the past few years have occurred in the pediatric patient.[1-5] In Chapter 35, drugs and techniques that have proved successful in the pediatric patient are reviewed.

The *geriatric patient* (Chapter 36) also represents an increased risk of adverse drug response when central nervous system depressants (and other drugs) are administered. Although the requirement for sedation is not usually as great in this rapidly growing segment of the population as it is in other age groups, there are specific modifications in therapy that are appropriate in managing the geriatric patient.

In Chapters 37 through 39, *medically* and *physically compromised patients* are reviewed. Steadily increasing numbers of these patients are seeking treatment at dental and medical offices. The nature of the patient's underlying medical problem(s) may have a significant impact on the administration of drugs for the management of pain and anxiety. In some cases the patient may prove to be unable to communicate or to cooperate with the dentist, making monitoring during the procedure somewhat more difficult but ever more important. Most of the patients discussed in Chapters 38 and 39 can be successfully treated on an outpatient basis if specific treatment modifications are employed.

In prior chapters of this book, specific contraindications to the administration of drugs were presented as the pharmacology of each drug was discussed. In this section the disease process is introduced and the various techniques of sedation and specific drugs are reviewed as to their appropriateness for these patients.

REFERENCES

1. Goodson JM, Moore PA: Life-threatening reactions after pedodontic sedation: an assessment of narcotic, local anesthetic, and antiemetic drug interaction. *J Am Dent Assoc* 107(2):239–245, 1983.
2. Cote CJ: Round and round we go: sedation—what is it, who does it, and have we made things safer for children? *Paediatr Anaesth* 18(1):3–8, 2008.
3. Cote CJ: Strategies for preventing sedation accidents. *Pediatr Ann* 34(8):625–633, 2005.
4. Lee HH, Milgrom P, Starks H, Burke W. Trends in death associated with pediatric dental sedation and general anesthesia. *Paediatr Anaesth* 23(8):741–746, 2013.
5. Healy M: After child surgery deaths, experts discuss the risks. *USA Today* January 20, 2014.

chapter 35

The Pediatric Patient

CHAPTER OUTLINE

As important as patient management is in the realm of adult dentistry, it is in pediatric dentistry that proper patient management assumes the utmost importance. The young child, approaching a visit to the dentist for the first time, is influenced by a number of sources, some positive, some negative, that will affect his or her attitude and behavior during treatment. Some factors are controllable by the dentist and staff, but others lie beyond their control. Proper patient management, especially in the younger, more impressionable patient, goes far toward producing a patient with positive attitudes about future dental and medical care. Conversely, too many unfavorable influences may cause the patient to look on the prospect of future dental and medical care with increasing fear and trepidation.

In this chapter some of the basic concepts involved in the management of the pediatric patient are discussed briefly. For a more in-depth discussion of this subject, the reader is referred to the following textbooks:

Dean JA: *McDonald and Avery's dentistry for the child and adolescent,* ed 10, St Louis, 2016, Mosby Elsevier.

Casamassimo PS, Fields HW, McTigue DJ, Nowak A: *Pediatric dentistry,* ed 5, Philadelphia, 2012, Saunders Elsevier.

Cameron AC, Widmer RP: *Handbook of pediatric dentistry,* ed 4, St Louis, 2013, Mosby Elsevier.

FACTORS INFLUENCING PATIENT RESPONSE

A number of factors interact to determine whether the pediatric patient will face a scheduled visit to the dentist or physician with eager anticipation or with fearful dread. These include

497

the influences of the parent, of the child's peers, of the dentist, and of the office staff. The child's prior experience with health professionals is yet another factor.

Parental attitudes in general, and toward dentistry in particular, have a profound influence on a child's behavior. Factors thought to be of importance include the age of the parents and their level of maturity. A positive dental attitude in parents creates an environment for the child that is conducive to the acceptance of ideal dentistry. It is frequently heard that the greatest difficulty in patient management occurs when a child is accompanied to the dental office by the grandparent. The grandparents often represent the ultimate authority in the family and will do things as they see fit to do them, not as the dentist may desire. This may be a significant factor when decisions are made regarding the site and route of administration of sedative drugs.

The parents' prior experience with medical and dental health professionals will greatly influence their child's attitudes. Although few, if any, parents will intentionally tell their children of prior traumatic experiences they have had, such attitudes and feelings are transferred to the child nonverbally. Children may overhear their parents discussing their experiences or may see a parent suffering either before or after a dental appointment. Children are surprisingly astute observers and pick up the many clues that parents drop relating to their attitudes toward dental health care.

Parents may make statements to their children that influence the children's behavior or put the children on guard, expecting that something unpleasant might be in the offing. Simply saying to a child, "If you behave yourself at the dentist I will buy you a treat later" may tell the child to anticipate the occurrence of something unpleasant. Children of all ages can be affected by their mothers' anxieties; however, the effect is greatest with those younger than 4 years of age.[1]

The *influence of other children,* either siblings or acquaintances, must never be discounted. Such influence may be either positive or negative. In a family in which several children have undergone dental treatment without difficulty, younger children receive positive reinforcement before their visit. However, if prior appointments have been traumatic, such influence may be extremely negative. The same is true for the friends of the child. I have found that young friends tend to accentuate the more negative aspects of dentistry and medicine.

Another factor influencing the child's behavior during treatment is *his or her own* prior experience with other health care professionals. Traumatic experiences (e.g., a painful vaccination injection) provoke negative behavior in the patient, whereas positive experiences lead to a better-behaved child.

Some children are fearful at their very first visit to the dental office. The collective influence of the parents, siblings, and friends has produced this unwarranted apprehension. Although the goals of the dentist and staff will be somewhat more difficult to accomplish, the attitude of the office staff can dramatically change this child's feelings toward dentistry.

The factors that have been discussed thus far are truly out of the control of the dentist. Fortunately, the dentist is able to control other factors. These include the attitudes of the dentist and staff and the environment (the office) in which the patient will be treated.

The dentist sets the behavior standard in the office. The dress of the dentist is important: White uniforms may provoke negative feelings in younger patients, whereas colorful uniforms (commonly worn today as pastel scrubs or scrubs with designs) evoke a more positive response. With universal precautions (gloves, glasses, and masks being standard of care), explanations and role-playing with the child to make him or her comfortable with our safety garb are suggested.

The same guidelines are important for members of the *office staff.* In the management of the pediatric patient, the auxiliary may have significantly greater contact with the patient than does the dentist; therefore the attitude and attire of the staff are as important, if not more so, than the dentist's.

The time of day at which the appointment is scheduled may have bearing on a child's behavior, especially the younger child. Interference with a child's sleeping or eating habits should, if possible, be avoided. The young child accustomed to a midday nap may be irritable if he or she is in the dental chair instead of napping at that time. Younger patients are most easily managed early in the day. This is also true for the apprehensive adult patient (see Chapter 4). The basic concepts presented in the stress reduction protocols are of great importance in managing the pediatric patient. The length of the appointment should not exceed the child's attention span. Younger patients are less able to tolerate longer appointments than are older, more mature children. Most children are able to tolerate 30- to 45-minute appointments with little difficulty.[2]

The *office environment* is another factor that influences the patient's behavior. An office in which many children are treated should offer an environment that appeals to children. Although most pediatric medical and dental offices are designed with this in mind, even in the office of the busy generalist a separate area in the reception room might be set aside for younger patients. The very fact that this area requires the patient to leave the parent will be more conducive to the separation from the parent that occurs at the time of dental treatment. The color of the office, soundproofing, and odors are important factors to consider in the design of the pediatric office and reception room. Many pediatricians and pediatric dentists offer their patients a gift as they leave the office. These gifts are used as a display of friendship, not as a reward for good behavior.

Klingberg and Broberg, in a review of literature from 1982 to 2006, reported that dental fear/anxiety and dental behavior management problems were relatively common for pediatric dental patients, each affecting 9% of boys and adolescents.[1,3] Girls exhibited more dental anxiety and dental behavior management problems than did boys.

BEHAVIORAL EVALUATION OF THE PEDIATRIC PATIENT

Even though innumerable factors interact to influence a child's behavior in the dental office, the dentist must still be able to evaluate the patient's ability to cope with the planned treatment. A number of systems have been developed to aid in classification of a child's behavior and the potential for successful dental treatment. Two of the most commonly used systems are the Frankl Behavior Rating Scale[4] and the system devised by Wright.[5]

In the Frankl system the observer (dentist) places the child's behavior into one of four categories:

Rating 1. *Definitively negative.* Refusal of treatment, forceful crying, fearfulness, or any other overt evidence of extreme negativism

Rating 2. *Negative.* Reluctance to accept treatment; uncooperativeness; some evidence of negative attitude but not pronounced (sullen, withdrawn)

Rating 3. *Positive.* Acceptance of treatment; cautious behavior at times; willingness to comply with the dentist, at times with reservation, but patient follows dentist's directions cooperatively

Rating 4. *Definitely positive.* Good rapport with the dentist, interest in the dental procedures, laughter and enjoyment

Murphy et al have stated that the Frankl scale appears to be closely related to the attitude of the parent toward dentistry.[6]

The Frankl method of classification has been a popular research tool.[1]

Wright's classification presents three major groups: (1) cooperative, (2) lacking cooperative ability, and (3) potentially uncooperative behavior, with multiple subgroups. Wright has stated that most dentists, either consciously or subconsciously, categorize the behavior of children into one of these groups. These classifications permit the dentist to more readily determine the appropriate means of overcoming the management problems presented by the patient[4]:

1. Cooperative: most children (can be treated by a tell-show-do approach)
2. Lacking cooperative ability (the "precooperative" patient)
   a. Very young children with whom communication cannot be established or comprehension expected
   b. Children with specific debilitating or handicapping conditions
3. Potentially uncooperative behavior
   a. Uncontrolled behavior: tantrums with flailing of arms and legs, suggestive of acute anxiety and fear (usually seen in young children 3 to 6 years old on the occasion of the first dental visit)
   b. Defiant behavior: may use passive resistance (most often seen in older children approaching adolescence)

   c. Timid behavior
      (1) May hide behind the parent, but usually little resistance to separation
      (2) Stalls or hesitates when given directions
      (3) Often withholds tears
      (4) Highly anxious
      (5) Does not always hear or comprehend instructions
   d. Tense cooperative behavior
      (1) Accepts treatment as it is provided
      (2) Voice may have a tremor when speaking
      (3) Body may tremble
      (4) Most often perspires noticeably on the palm of the hand or brow
      (5) Controls emotions
   e. Whining behavior
      (1) Allows dentist to proceed, but whines throughout
      (2) Frequently complains of pain
      (3) Emits sounds constantly

Successful treatment of the patient who lacks the ability to cooperate often requires the use of one of the techniques of sedation (moderate or deep). Should these fail to prove adequate, general anesthesia may be required.

The potentially uncooperative patient may or may not require sedation for successful treatment. The attitudes and technical abilities of the dentist and office staff will be the deciding factors with these patients.

The Functional Inquiry[1]

Before the dentist treats a child, medical, dental, and social histories are essential. However, a functional inquiry from a behavioral viewpoint should also be conducted. Two primary goals are sought: (1) to learn about patient and parental concerns and (2) to gather information to enable a reliable estimate of the cooperative ability of the child. Coupling the findings from the functional inquiry with the clinical experience, the dentist is in a much better position to meet the patient's needs and to apply appropriate behavior guidance strategies to treat individual pediatric patients than by simply proceeding inadequately informed.

Usually, functional inquiries are conducted in two ways: (1) by a paper-and-pencil questionnaire completed by the parent and (2) by direct interview of child and parent. In some offices, one method may predominate, whereas in others both techniques are used. Each method has specific merits.

Written questionnaires can be important tools for gaining information because probing questions can uncover critical facts about child-rearing practices in the home, a child's school experiences, or the patient's developmental status. Four questions with clinical relevance that can be added to medical history forms are listed in Box 35.1. The responses to these questions, originally from behavioral science research, can alert the clinician to a potential behavioral problem. If a parent responds negatively to more than one question, the chance of encountering a behavior problem rises considerably.[1]

Box 35.1	Clinically Relevant Questions That Can Be Added to History Forms

(Circle One)

How do you think your child has reacted to past medical procedures?	Very well Moderately well Moderately poorly Very poorly
How would you rate your own anxiety (fear, nervousness) at this moment?	High Moderately high Moderately low Low
Does your child think there is anything wrong with his or her teeth, such as a chipped tooth, decayed tooth, or gum boil?	Yes No
How do you expect your child to react in the dental chair?	Very well Moderately well Moderately poorly Very poorly

From Stigers JI: Nonpharmacologic management of children's behaviors. In Dean JA, editor, McDonald and Avery's dentistry for the child and adolescent, ed 10, St Louis, 2016, Mosby, pp. 286–302.

DETERMINING THE NEED FOR SEDATION

The decision to use sedation should be made only following consideration of several factors:

1. Assessment of dental need
2. Patient cooperation
3. Parental cooperation and involvement
4. Economic considerations
5. Alternative treatment plans
6. Preoperative health evaluation
7. Preoperative behavioral assessment
8. Training and experience of dentist and staff

When only minimal treatment (e.g., one filling) is necessary, the need for sedation is usually negligible. This is especially true for the parenteral techniques (intramuscular [IM], intranasal [IN], and intravenous [IV]), which involve prolonged durations of drug effects. Inhalation sedation may be the most appropriate technique for this type of procedure. If full-mouth treatment is necessary (e.g., nursing bottle syndrome), the use of IV deep sedation or general anesthesia might be considered.

Patient cooperation is obviously a factor in opting to use a sedation technique. It is the opinion of most pediatric dentists that at least one and preferably two attempts at treatment should be made before considering the use of sedation or general anesthesia. With experience, it may become quite

obvious to the dentist that a patient will require sedation or general anesthesia before the initiation of any treatment. Children who are screaming as they walk or are carried through the parking lot to the dental office are more likely to be candidates for sedation. On the other hand, the patient who sits in the dental chair and cries throughout the treatment may be manageable without the use of adjunctive drug therapy. Crying, in the absence of overt disruptive behavior, may not be an indication for the administration of sedative drugs.

Parental attitudes and desires must be taken into account when considering the use of sedation or nondrug behavior management techniques. Three notable works on parental acceptance are by Murphy and colleagues,[6] Lawrence and associates,[7] and Eaton and coworkers.[8] The three studies are similar in design: Parents are shown videotapes of different behavioral guidance methods and instructed to indicate their acceptability of them on a rating scale. The studies span two decades, provide interesting information, and show how parental attitudes change. In the earliest study (1984),[6] 10 techniques were videotaped. Four of the techniques found to be acceptable were tell-show-do, positive reinforcement, voice control, and use of a mouth prop. Six techniques found to be unacceptable involved restraint methods, sedation, and general anesthesia.

The latter two studies[7,8] used the same videotape and demonstrated eight behavior guidance methods. All studies reported tell-show-do as the most acceptable technique. In the latter two studies, nitrous oxide sedation was found to be the next most acceptable technique. All studies were able to establish a hierarchy of parental acceptance based on the mean ratings of parent responses, allowing for the observation of two interesting changes. Hand-over-mouth became the least accepted technique, whereas general anesthesia became the third most accepted method for behavior guidance.

Unfortunately, the use of sedation in dentistry has periodically received negative publicity,[9] a factor that has conditioned some parents against the use of these techniques in their children. The desires of the parent should always be considered when formulating the patient's treatment plan; however, the dentist must always be the one to make the final decision. A number of pediatric deaths have occurred in part because of the dentist's desires to accommodate the parent's wishes that all the dental treatment be completed at one visit. Though the administration of sedatives to a child patient at home before leaving for the dental office is strongly discouraged,[10] the parent's ability to follow prescribing instructions must be determined when the dentist is considering doing this. When any doubt exists, the child should be scheduled early, with the drug administered by the dentist in the dental office allowing time for the drug(s) to reach maximum effect (usually about 1 hour).

Caleb's Law

On January 1, 2017, Caleb's Law (AB2235)[11] went into effect in the state of California. It was enacted in response to at least five reported deaths of young children receiving deep sedation or general anesthesia in California dental offices. Many of these cases occurred in the offices of oral surgeons who represent the only health care professionals who operate and administer general anesthesia simultaneously without a separate anesthesia provider.[12]

Though designed for providers of deep sedation or general anesthesia, it behooves the dentist providing any form of sedation to minors to become familiar with Caleb's Law.

Economic considerations are also of importance in determining the nature of the sedative procedure to be used. One reason for the increased use of outpatient sedation in dentistry and medicine has been the high cost (in both financial and emotional terms) of hospitalization. Outpatient procedures are usually a fraction of the cost of the same procedure performed in a hospital. (See discussion in Chapter 30.) If the economic status of the family is such that they are unable to afford even the minimal fee for sedation, it might be prudent not to charge the patient for the service. The cooperation of the patient and family is readily obtained, and treatment becomes less traumatic for the entire staff and the patient.

Alternative modes of treatment should be considered. Which technique of sedation is most likely to be effective in this patient? Many dentists develop the disturbing practice of using the same technique (and in some cases the same drugs and dosages) on all patients. Consideration in selection of the technique and drugs involves multiple factors, including the degree of cooperation of the patient and the patient's medical history (i.e., allergies and illnesses). There is no one technique of sedation that will be effective in all patients. Indeed, in pediatric dentistry the failure rate for sedation is considerably greater than that seen in adults. Trapp has stated that a failure rate of 20% to 40% is not unusual unless the dentist is administering general anesthesia.[13] Recent experience with pediatric sedation has demonstrated a 40% to 50% failure rate with oral sedation but a 5% failure rate with IM/IV sedation. As a general rule, the younger the patient, the higher the failure rate of sedation techniques. The greater the number of techniques available to the dentist, the greater the likelihood of a successful outcome.

The preoperative physical evaluation of the child will aid in determining the technique of choice for the patient. Among the items to be determined are the presence of allergies, medications being taken by the patient, and any prior hospitalizations. Behavioral evaluation also aids in a determination of the requirement for sedation or general anesthesia. In addition, training and experience of the dentist and staff are important in determining the appropriate sedative technique. Only those techniques with which the dentist and the staff are well acquainted should be considered for use. The requirements for adequate training in each of the commonly used techniques are discussed earlier in this text.

GOALS AND TECHNIQUES

All techniques of sedation discussed in this book may be used in the pediatric patient. In addition, drug administration by the submucosal (SM) route is occasionally used in pediatric dentistry. Each of these techniques is reviewed with an eye toward its applicability in the pediatric patient.

Kopel has stated that sedation in the pediatric patient should be used to "train" or "retrain" the patient in an understanding of dental procedures and their importance.[14] He continues by listing the following goals of pediatric premedication (sedation):

1. To make the child cooperative and comfortable
2. To decrease anxiety for the patient
3. To decrease strain, apprehension, and excessive fatigue for the dentist and staff
4. To minimize the need for hospitalization and its attendant problems

Listed next are the techniques of patient management involving drug administration that are available in pediatric dentistry. These techniques are presented in the order of their desirability, from the most desirable to the least desirable in the opinion of seven dentist anesthesiologists (DAs)[15]:

1. Inhalation sedation (N_2O-O_2)
2. Oral sedation and inhalation sedation
3. Oral sedation
4. In-office general anesthesia
5. General anesthesia in the hospital

Inhalation sedation (N_2O-O_2) was rated as the most preferred by six of the seven DAs queried. It was listed as second most preferred by the seventh.

The following techniques were considered as **not recommended** for use by a dentist not trained in the management of the unconscious patient and proficient in airway management:

1. IV sedation with or without inhalation sedation
2. IM/IN and IV sedation with or without inhalation sedation
3. Use of the above with body and oral restraints

The goal sought when sedating the pediatric patient is the same as with the adult: to use the most controllable and least profound technique that provides the desired goal.

Once a sedation technique is selected for the pediatric patient, the next task is to determine the appropriate dosage of the drug(s) if the technique selected does not permit titration. Physiologic functions in children may vary considerably from those same functions in the older patient. The metabolic rate is higher in the younger patient. Conversely, enzyme systems responsible for the biotransformation of specific drugs may not yet be fully functional in younger (<4 years of age) patients. This factor and others lead to the increased possibility of higher blood levels developing when pediatric drug dosages are simply calculated from the adult dosage forms commonly supplied with drugs. Instances of morbidity and mortality have been reported in which drug doses within acceptable adult limits were administered to children.

The U.S. Food and Drug Administration (FDA) issued a warning in December 2016 that exposure to general anesthetic and sedation in children younger than 3 years of age or in pregnant women may affect children's brain development. Studies conducted on the use of general anesthetic and sedation in pregnant and young animals show loss of nerve cells resulting in long-term effects on behavior and learning. Some studies on children support these findings; however, all the children in the studies had limitations, and it is unclear whether the negative effects were due to the prolonged exposure to anesthesia or the underlying medical condition that necessitated the surgery. Further research is needed to determine if anesthetic exposure affects children's brain development.[16]

There is no simple answer to the question of proper drug dosage in nontitratable techniques of drug administration. Many factors act to complicate drug selection and drug action in children. In addition, the desired level of drug action varies considerably from patient to patient and from dentist to dentist. The most reliable factor in predicting adequate drug effect is a patient's previous clinical experience with the drug in question. Once a drug has been administered to a patient, subsequent dosages can be modified according to this initial response. This is termed *titration by appointment.*[17] Although previous clinical experience can provide guidelines leading to safer and more effective drug administration, it is still necessary to determine a safe and effective drug dose for a first appointment.

Drug package inserts (DPIs) provide prescribing information concerning pediatric dosages. However, many drugs introduced for the management of pain and anxiety in recent years have not undergone adequate clinical trials in children to permit recommendations concerning pediatric dosage. Conversely, many of these drugs provide only adult dosage forms or indicate that "information [in children] is inadequate to establish dosage." Wilson,[18] in a review of the 1963 *Physicians' Desk Reference,* found that 62% of listed drugs were not indicated for pediatric use, whereas an additional 16% were without recommendation for pediatric dosage. This number has steadily increased in recent years.

In those instances in which pediatric dosages of central nervous system (CNS)–depressant drugs were indicated, the dosages recommended were those used in normal, nonstressful environments. Administration of this dosage form, although adequate to help a child fall asleep at home, often proves to be entirely inadequate for sedation in a stressful environment such as the dental office. Most DPIs and pharmacology textbooks indicate the usual, nondental dosage of a drug. Pediatric dentistry texts should be consulted for appropriate dental treatment doses of these drugs.

Various factors govern the determination of drug dosages for children. These are generalizations, with exceptions to be anticipated:

1. *Age of the child:* In general, the older the child, the larger the dosage required to achieve the desired clinical action. Very young, precooperative children may require larger drug dosages to overcome their extreme level of fear. As we present upper limits of recommended drug dosages, it is to be expected that the failure rate in sedation of younger, precooperative patients will be greater than that for older children.

2. *Weight of the child:* This is very often used as the major factor in determining pediatric drug dosages, especially for parenterally administered drugs. In pediatric drug administration, more and more drugs are being prescribed in terms of body surface area, a factor thought to be a more reliable guide to drug dose than body weight.

3. *Mental attitude of the child:* The greater the degree of anxiety and fear, the larger the dose of drug(s) required.

4. *Level of sedation desired:* The individual dentist will seek to achieve "ideal" sedation in a given patient. However, the definition of ideal sedation will vary considerably. To some dentists, ideal sedation exists only if a patient makes no movement or sound during treatment (i.e., deep sedation); others consider sedation ideal if the planned treatment can be completed in a more relaxed atmosphere (for the staff and patient), even with occasional movement and verbalization from the patient (i.e., moderate sedation). Minimal sedation may prove appropriate for the mildly apprehensive older child, whereas deep sedation or general anesthesia may be required for the precooperative younger patient.

5. *Physical activity of the child:* The hyperactive, overly responsive child commonly requires increased drug dosages.

6. *Contents of the stomach:* Following oral administration, the presence of food in the stomach greatly influences the rate of drug absorption of some drugs into the cardiovascular system.

7. *Time of day:* Larger doses of drugs are required for sedation early in the day, when the patient is fresh and alert; lower doses are in order later in the day, when the patient is more fatigued.[19]

8. *Ability to titrate:* Whenever possible, drugs should be titrated to clinical effect. The ability to titrate eliminates guesswork from determination of the appropriate drug dosage for a patient. The two techniques of drug administration that permit titration, IV and inhalation, are increasingly popular in pediatric dentistry. Oral, IM, IN, and SM administration do not permit titration.

Determination of Drug Dosage for Pediatric Patients

Formulas, such as Young's rule and Clark's rule, have been suggested as aids in determining pediatric drug dosages as a fraction of the adult dose. These methods are used when the manufacturer has not recommended dosages for children. The success of such rules is haphazard at best and cannot be recommended.

Young's rule:

$$\frac{\text{Age of patient}}{\text{Age} + 12} = \text{Fraction of adult dose for children}$$

Clark's rule:

$$\frac{\text{Weight in pounds}}{150} \text{ or } \frac{\text{Weight in kilograms}}{70} =$$

Fraction of adult dose for children

Although age and weight are often used in determining pediatric drug dosage, they present certain problems. Because of significant variation in size among children of the same age, this factor (age) ought not be of primary consideration. Body weight is more commonly used in pediatric dose determination; however, the dose of many drugs is not always a simple linear function of body weight, and to calculate dosages as milligrams per kilogram or per pound leads to inaccuracies, as these values are based on the normoresponding patient (i.e., the 70% of patients in the normal distribution curve ["bell-shaped curve] who respond "normally" to a given drug dosage). Surface area, rather than body weight, has been shown to be a more accurate method of determining drug dosage for a patient. Unfortunately, manufacturers of virtually all drugs marketed today still present dosage recommendations in other units (e.g., mg/kg or mg/lb of body weight).

MONITORING

Monitoring of the sedated patient is discussed in Chapter 5. As important as monitoring is for all sedated patients, in the pediatric patient monitoring is possibly of even greater significance. Because of the relative lack of communication available between the dentist and the very young, precooperative or the handicapped patient, one of the most important means of communication—verbal—is often not present. In addition, because of the inability to titrate drugs administered orally, intramuscularly, or intranasally, the possibility of a relative overdose developing is somewhat enhanced. Constant monitoring of the patient is essential.

In June 2016 the American Academy of Pediatrics (AAP) and the American Academy of Pediatric Dentistry (AAPD) released updated guidelines for monitoring and management of pediatric patients before, during, and after sedation for diagnostic and therapeutic procedures.[10] Anyone considering the use of sedation (minimal, moderate, or deep) in the pediatric patient should become conversant with this document.

Baseline vital signs (blood pressure, heart rate and rhythm, and respiratory rate) should be recorded before treatment if the patient allows it. In the younger, precooperative patient, this often is not possible. Until the child has been sedated, it may be physically impossible to monitor vital signs; however, while the child is screaming, yelling, and moving around, monitoring is actually being done subjectively by simply watching the child's behavior. As soon as the child becomes quiet (sedated), more objective monitoring must be initiated. Vital signs must be recorded and a pretracheal stethoscope placed in position and respirations monitored throughout the procedure.

The pretracheal stethoscope is one of the most valuable pieces of monitoring equipment available (and the least expensive). With it the dentist is able to monitor continuously both breath sounds and, in many cases, heart sounds. The value of the pretracheal stethoscope cannot be overestimated.[20,21]

Monitoring breath sounds in the pediatric patient is of great value because the overwhelming majority of complications seen in sedation of younger patients are associated with respiratory depression or airway management problems. Decreased or altered breath sounds or a slowed rate of breathing should alert the dentist to evaluate the patient's airway and respiratory status. Most cardiac problems in pediatric patients develop secondary to respiratory distress. Recommended monitoring for pediatric sedation includes the following:

1. Preoperative vital signs (if possible [if not possible, the reason should be noted on the patient's anesthesia/sedation record])
2. Vital signs periodically during treatment (recorded every 5 minutes)
   a. Heart rate and rhythm, monitored continuously
   b. Blood pressure, monitored every 5 minutes
3. Pretracheal stethoscope
4. Pulse oximetry – required for moderate and deep sedation
5. End-tidal carbon dioxide (ETCO$_2$) monitoring – recommended for moderate sedation; required for deep sedation
6. Electrocardiograph (ECG) – recommended for moderate sedation; required for deep sedation
   Supplemental O$_2$ or N$_2$O-O$_2$ administration via nasal hood or cannula is recommended for all pediatric sedation cases in which the patient tolerates it.
7. Postsedation vital signs. Initially, vital signs should be documented at least every 5 minutes. Once the child begins to awaken, the recording intervals may be increased to 10 to 15 minutes.[10]

Table 35.1 summarizes pediatric monitoring recommendations as described in the 2016 AAP/AAPD Guidelines.[10]

PHYSICAL RESTRAINT

It occasionally becomes necessary to use physical restraints to treat the pediatric patient properly. Bed sheets may be tied around the patient and then secured with wide adhesive tape to provide restraint. Velcro strips and ties are also available. Parental informed consent *must* be obtained before any form of physical restraint is used in the pediatric patient. Use without prior consent has led to charges of assault and battery being filed against the dentist.[22]

The Papoose Board (Olympic Medical Corporation, Seattle) (Fig. 35.1) is quite effective in restraining the head, torso, and upper limbs. The device should not be wrapped too tightly because the patient may become more agitated; but of greater importance, an overly tight wrap across the patient's chest may

Table 35.1	Recommended Monitoring for Pediatric Patients[10]	
	MODERATE SEDATION	**DEEP SEDATION**
Personnel	An observer who will monitor the patient but who may also assist with interruptible tasks; should be trained in PALS	An independent observer whose only responsibility is to continuously monitor the patient; trained in PALS
Responsible practitioner	Skilled to rescue a child with apnea, laryngospasm, and/or airway obstruction, including the ability to open the airway, suction secretions, provided CPAP, and perform succesfull bag–valve–mask ventilation; recommended that at least one practitioner should be skilled in obtaining vascular access in children; trained in PALS	Skilled to rescue a child with apnea, laryngospasm, and/or airway obstruction, including the ability to open the airway, suction secretions, provided CPAP, and perform succesfull bag–valve–mask ventilation, tracheal intubation, and cardiopulmonary resuscitation; training in PALS is required, at least one practitioner skilled in obtaining vascular access in children immediately available
Monitoring	Pulse oximetry ECG recommended Heart rate Blood pressure Respiration Capnography recommended	Pulse oximetry ECG recommended Heart rate Blood pressure Respiration Capnography recommended
Other equipment	Suction equipment, adequate oxygen source/supply	Suction equipment, adequate oxygen source/supply, defibrillator required
Documentation	Name, route, site, time of administration, and dosage of all drugs administered Continuous oxygen saturation, heart rate, and ventilation (capnography recommended); parameters recorded every 10 minutes	Name, route, site, time of administration, and dosage of all drugs administered Continuous oxygen saturation, heart rate, and ventilation (capnography required); parameters recorded at least every 5 minutes
Emergency checklists	Recommended	Recommended
Rescue cart properly stocked with rescue drugs and age- and size-appropriate equipment	Required	Required
Dedicated recovery area with rescue cart properly stocked with rescue drugs and age- and size-appropriate equipment and dedicated recovery personnel; adequate oxygen supply	Recommended; initial recording of vital signs may be needed at least every 10 minutes until the child begins to awaken, then recording intervals may be increased	Recommended; initial recording of vital signs may be needed for at least 5-minute intervals until the child begins to awaken, then recording intervals may be increased to 10–15 minutes.
Discharge criteria	See Appendix 1	See Appendix 1

Reproduced with permission from Coté CJ, Wilson S: Guidelines for monitoring and management of pediatric patients before, during, and after sedation for diagnostic and therapeutic procedures: Update 2016. *Pediatrics* 138(1), 2016. Copyright © 2016 by the AAP.

restrict respiratory movements that have already been somewhat compromised through the administration of CNS depressants.[23-26]

The use of restraints also makes it more difficult for the dentist and assistant to monitor respiratory movements. The pretracheal stethoscope becomes even more important at these times. AAP and AAPD guidelines recommend that "if a restraint device is used, a hand or foot should be kept exposed, and the child should never be left unattended. The child's head position should be continuously assessed to ensure airway patency."[10]

Allen, Bernat, and Perinpanayagam surveyed 212 pediatric dentists in New York State, receiving 78 replies, regarding their use of sedation.[27] Half of the respondents reported they always used an immobilization device with sedated patients,

whereas 33% used immobilization sometimes, 3% rarely, and 13% never.

MOUTH-STABILIZING DEVICES

Despite the fact that the patient has been restrained, it may still be difficult, if not impossible, for the dentist to examine and treat the patient safely and adequately. Several devices are used as aids to stabilize the mouth during treatment. Rubber bite blocks are available in a variety of sizes; when one is inserted between the teeth of the patient on the side opposite treatment, the patient may bite down onto the block but is unable to close the jaws. A long piece of dental floss should always be tied around the bite block and left outside the patient's

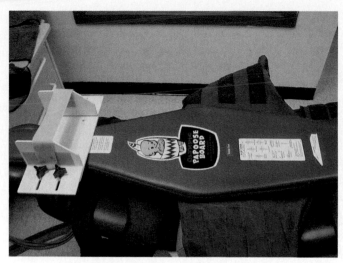

Figure 35.1 Papoose Board restraint device.

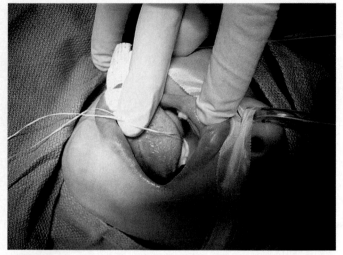

Figure 35.2 Strings of dental floss tied to bite block and gauze pack placed into mouth of sedated patient permits their easy retrieval. (From Malamed SF: *Medical emergencies in the dental office*, ed 7, St Louis, 2015, Mosby.)

mouth to aid in its retrieval, if necessary (Fig. 35.2). A ratchet-type mouth prop (Molt prop) is also available. An advantage to the Molt prop is that the patient need open but a few millimeters for the device to be slipped between the teeth (Fig. 35.3, *A*). Once in the mouth, the device can be ratcheted open to the desired level (Fig. 35.3, *B*). When either device is used, the assistant should remain in contact with it to stabilize it and prevent its accidentally being dislodged.

DRUGS

Before discussing specific routes of drug administration and their use in pediatric dentistry, the sedative drugs and techniques that are in most common use among pediatric dentists in the United States are presented in Table 35.2. This represents the results of a 2002 survey of all 3315 members of the AAPD (1778 responded) concerning their use of sedation in the year 2000 (no more recent surveys have been published).[28]

Regarding inhalation sedation with N_2O-O_2, which was used by the majority of respondents, 47% reported using the technique less than 11% of the time. As to other techniques of sedation, most reported using little, if any, sedation. Eighty-two percent use sedation for less than 11% of their patients. Of the 1778 respondents, 1224 used drugs in addition to N_2O-O_2. In a 3-month period they performed 77,112 sedations. However, of that number, 61,662 (80%) were administered by only 478 pediatric dentists.[28]

An important statistic is the response to the question "What is the typical effect achieved with sedation other than nitrous oxide?" Only 23% (of 1135 answering the question) reported "Excellent" (no or slight crying), 50% "Good" (crying or movement, but no treatment interruption), 25% "Fair" (treatment interrupted but all treatment completed), and 2% "Poor" (treatment interrupted, only partial treatment completed).[28]

Excluding inhalation sedation, almost all sedative drugs were administered orally (95%), with 2% reporting

intravenously, 1% intramuscularly, 1% submucosally, and 1% "other."[28]

Two routes of drug administration predominate: the oral route and inhalation sedation. It also becomes evident that although a variety of drugs are available for the management of anxiety, pediatric dentists seem to rely on a limited number of well-established drugs.

In the Allen et al survey, inhalation sedation was used by 83%, whereas oral sedatives were employed by 38% of pediatric dentists.[23] Of the dentists using the oral route, 66% always used it in combination with inhalation sedation, and 77% of those used N_2O 30% to 50% the majority of the time.

The most commonly used oral sedatives were chloral hydrate (57%), midazolam (33%), hydroxyzine (16%), diazepam (10%), and meperidine (10%). Though the liquid formulation of chloral hydrate is no longer commercially available, some hospitals and pharmacies are compounding their own formulations.*[10,29]

Goals of Sedation in the Pediatric Patient

The goals of sedation in the pediatric patient for diagnostic and therapeutic procedures are as follows[10]:

(1) To guard the patient's safety and welfare; (2) to minimize physical discomfort and pain; (3) to control anxiety, minimize psychological trauma, and maximize the potential for amnesia; (4) to modify behavior and/or movement so as to allow the safe completion of the procedure; and (5) to return the patient to a state in which discharge from medical/dental supervision is safe, as determined by recognized criteria.

---

*Pharmacy compounding is the art and science of preparing personalized medications for patients. Compounded medications are made based on a practitioner's prescription in which individual ingredients are mixed together in the exact strength and dosage form required by the patient.[29]

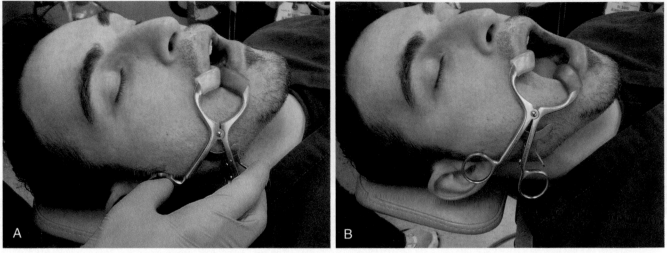

Figure 35.3 A, Molt mouth prop closed. **B,** Molt mouth prop opened.

Table 35.2	Drugs Commonly Used in Pediatric Dentistry	
DRUG		**N =**
Diazepam oral + N₂O-O₂		361
Midazolam (oral) + N₂O-O₂		284
Hydroxyzine + N₂O-O₂		256
Chloral hydrate, hydroxyzine + N₂O-O₂		238
Diazepam alone		195
Meperidine, promethazine + N₂O-O₂		190
Hydroxyzine (Atarax or Vistaril) alone		184
Chloral hydrate + N₂O-O₂		131
Chloral hydrate and hydroxyzine alone		104
Chloral hydrate alone		102
Midazolam (intranasal) + N₂O-O₂		87
Meperidine and promethazine		62
Chloral hydrate, promethazine + N₂O-O₂		54
Meperidine + N₂O-O₂		52
Chloral hydrate and promethazine alone		24
Meperidine alone		16

Adapted from Haupt M: Project USAP 2000—Use of sedative agents by pediatric dentists: a 15-year follow-up survey, *Pediatr Dent* 24:289–294, 2002.

General Rules for Preoperative Medication

The usual preoperative and postoperative instructions given to the parent or guardian of children receiving drugs for the control of their dental fears are listed in Box 35.2. In addition to these instructions, Album lists these general rules regarding the administration of sedatives to pediatric patients[30]:

1. There must be strict supervision of the patient while in the office.
2. Adequate time must be provided for the drug(s) to act.
3. A quiet environment is necessary.
4. Vital signs and reflexes must not be impaired.

Box 35.2	Pediatric Sedation

Preoperative Instructions

It is necessary to use sedative drugs to obtain dental care for your child. Please be aware of the following:

1. It is most important that you tell the dentist of any drug reactions, medical history, or illness and hospitalization your child has had.
2. The child must be accompanied by a parent or guardian for all appointments.
3. The first appointment will be necessary for adjustment of the proper drug dosage; therefore, little dental work may be accomplished.
4. The child may remain sleepy for a time. Do not be alarmed; the drugs are "wearing off." Your child may be irritable as this occurs.
5. Do not allow the child to bite his or her lip, tongue, or cheek if a local anesthetic has been used.
6. After dental care, your child should be under adult supervision and not be allowed to play near streets, stairways, and other areas where he or she may be injured by falling.
7. Cold drinks, such as ginger ale or colas, will help reduce any nausea and help stimulate your child to become more alert.
8. Should any unusual situation arise, please call the dentist and notify him or her as soon as possible.

5. Drugs must not be administered during acute or chronic illness.
6. Parents must be informed of postoperative care.
7. The dentist must be familiar with side effects of medications.
8. Resuscitative equipment must be readily available.

Oral Sedation

Oral sedation is a valuable, although not entirely effective, technique in pediatric dentistry. Failure rates of up to 40% to 50% are to be expected if one is seeking minimal-to-moderate sedation via this route in younger children. One of its major advantages is the fact that there is no need for the use of a needle (in contrast to IM, SM, subcutaneous [SC], and IV techniques) or of a nasal hood (as needed for inhalation sedation) to produce a clinical effect. In the past, it was common to have the parent or guardian of the patient administer the oral drug(s) at home before departing for the office. It is impossible to recommend this practice because of the numerous cases on record in which a parent has inadvertently oversedated the child, thinking perhaps that if 1 teaspoon of the drug is good, 2 or 3 teaspoons (or tablespoons) must be better.[14] Recent pediatric sedation guidelines from the AAP/AAPD strongly recommend against administration of oral sedative drugs outside of the dental/medical office.[10] They emphasize: "Prescription medications intended to accomplish procedural sedation must not be administered without the safety net of direct supervision by trained medical/dental personnel." The admonition continues: "The administration of sedating medications at home poses an unacceptable risk, particularly for infants and preschool-aged children traveling in car safety seats because deaths as a result of this practice have been reported."[31,32]

The oral sedative drug must be administered within the confines of the dental office. The patient is scheduled approximately 1 hour before the start of treatment and the oral drug administered by the dentist. Another consideration, when the drug has been administered in the office, is monitoring of the patient. If the office is busy, it must still be a designated staff member's responsibility to periodically check on the child (who may still be in the reception area with his parent or guardian). In addition, a busy office environment is not conducive to adequate sedation. A more quiet, relaxed environment is desirable during this waiting period. A quiet room, in which the patient and parent may stay, should be used for the administration of oral drugs and during the period of onset of drug action.

Younger children may not tolerate tablets and capsules well, with the parent having to fight with the child to administer the drug. Obviously, if the goal being sought is relaxation of the patient, this type of action is not recommended. Many of the drugs administered orally to children are available as an elixir or syrup, which may prove more palatable to the patient. If the child refuses to accept the liquid medication on a spoon, the drug may be administered through an irrigation syringe, the drug squirted into the buccal vestibule of the patient, not down their throat.

Drugs that have an unpleasant taste or odor may occasionally be mixed with other liquids or food. Orange juice is commonly used; however, the addition of drugs may alter its taste. Acetaminophen (Tylenol) elixir is also commonly used to mask the taste of oral drugs. For smaller children, drugs may be mixed with applesauce, jellies, baby foods, or yogurt, although

these may have an adverse effect on drug absorption from the gastrointestinal (GI) tract. Midazolam syrup for oral administration has become a popular sedative,[33] and fentanyl is available as a lollipop.[34]

The drugs most frequently administered orally in pediatric dentistry are chloral hydrate, hydroxyzine; diazepam; midazolam[28,35]; the combination of chloral hydrate and promethazine; and meperidine in combination with chloral hydrate, hydroxyzine, diazepam, or promethazine. The pharmacology of these drugs was reviewed in Chapter 7. Pediatric use of these agents is discussed here.

Chloral Hydrate

The use of chloral hydrate in pediatric dentistry in the United States has decreased significantly as newer, equieffective, and more effective drugs have been introduced. Both the U.S. Food and Drug Administration (FDA) and the European Medicines Agency (EMA) have withdrawn approval of chloral hydrate.[36-38] The liquid formulation of chloral hydrate is no longer available in the United States, though the drug is still used, prepared by compounding pharmacies.[29] Chloral hydrate is most effective for the very young patient or the patient with a mental or physical disability. It is most effective in the management of mild-to-moderate anxiety. The usual oral dose form of the elixir is 500 mg/5 mL (1 teaspoon).

Initial Dosage

Chloral hydrate is administered 30 to 45 minutes before the planned appointment. The patient should have had nothing to eat or drink for 6 hours.

The dose of chloral hydrate, based on milligrams per kilogram, may range from 500 to 2000 mg, with the usual range between 750 and 1500 mg (Table 35.3). The elixir forms of chloral hydrate usually contain syrups of orange or citric acid to mask its bitter taste. Because of its disagreeable taste and tendency to cause GI upset, chloral hydrate should be diluted still further with water, orange juice, or acetaminophen before being administered. Chloral hydrate must never be diluted in or added to alcohol. The duration of action of chloral hydrate is not more than 1 hour.[38]

Table 35.3	Dose of Chloral Hydrate (to Nearest Half-Teaspoonful)			
WEIGHT (KG)	40 MG/KG	50 MG/KG	60 MG/KG	70 MG/KG
12–14	500	500–750	500–750	750–1000
14–16	500	750	750–1000	1000–1250
16–18	750	750–1000	1000–1250	1250–1500
18–21	750	1000–1250	1000–1250	1500
21–25	750–1000	1000–1250	1250–1500	1500–1750
25–30	1000–1250	1250–1500	1250–1500	1750–2000

> **COMMENT:** In the case of the very young child, it is suggested that a restraint such as a Papoose Board or a Pedi-Wrap be used during treatment.

Inhalation sedation with N_2O-O_2 may also be used as an alternative to increasing doses of the oral drug if moderate to no success has been achieved with the original dose. Because inhalation sedation is titratable, the ideal level of sedation being sought can frequently be achieved by this drug combination. It is my strong belief, however, that when the initial dose of an orally administered sedative drug fails to provide the desired effect, additional oral doses of that same drug should not be administered, nor should different oral drugs be given to the patient at that appointment. Rather, it is more prudent to discharge the patient and reschedule treatment for another day, reevaluating the choice of drugs and their dose. The concept of "titration by appointment" suggests that a different dosage schedule be considered for subsequent appointments based on the response of the patient to the initial dose.

For maximum benefit to be obtained from the use of chloral hydrate, the scheduled appointment should not be longer than 1 hour. The parents of the patient should be advised of the possibility of a postoperative period of irritability or excitation as the effects of chloral hydrate wear off.

Hydroxyzine

Hydroxyzine hydrochloride (Atarax) and hydroxyzine pamoate (Vistaril) are indicated for administration in patients who are older than 3 years, including adolescents. It is most effective in the management of very apprehensive, excited, agitated, and emotionally disturbed children. Additional indications for use of hydroxyzine include hyperactivity, autism, and severe behavioral problems.

Hydroxyzine hydrochloride is available as a syrup in 10 mg/5 mL (1 teaspoon). Hydroxyzine pamoate is available as an oral suspension as 25 mg/5 mL.

Dosage

Hydroxyzine is rapidly absorbed following oral administration. The oral dosages of hydroxyzine pamoate and hydroxyzine hydrochloride are considered equivalent. The onset of effect for hydroxyzine occurs between 15 and 60 minutes, with a usual duration of action of 4 and 6 hours. The recommended dose is 0.6 mg/kg PO.[39]

For the nervous, apprehensive child, 50 mg should be administered 2 hours before the appointment, followed by the same dose 1 hour before the appointment. In the hyperkinetic, agitated patient or patient with a behavioral problem, 25 mg is administered three times the day before treatment, and then 50 mg is administered 2 hours and then again 1 hour before treatment. In the less apprehensive patient, one dose of 50 to 75 mg hydroxyzine may be administered 1 hour before

treatment. Another method of administering hydroxyzine is to give divided doses of the agent; for example, the patient receives 25 mg 1 hour before bedtime the evening preceding treatment, 25 mg on the morning of treatment, and another 25 mg 1 hour before the scheduled appointment (for an appointment between 11 am and 1 pm). Hydroxyzine produces clinical actions within 30 to 60 minutes, with a maximal clinical duration of effective sedation between 1 and 2 hours.[39]

> **COMMENT:** Hydroxyzine is an excellent drug to give for the introduction of N_2O-O_2 to the apprehensive patient. The banana flavored pamoate form of hydroxyzine, Vistaril, is more pleasant tasting to most patients than is the hydrochloride (vanilla flavored). Because of the relatively wide margin of safety observed with hydroxyzine, it may be used effectively with N_2O-O_2 and opioid analgesics, provided that reduced dosages of these drugs are used and that careful monitoring of the patient is maintained.

Promethazine

Promethazine (Phenergan) is most often used in combination with other drugs for preoperative sedation (e.g., chloral hydrate, hydroxyzine, meperidine). As a sole agent for sedation, promethazine is most often used to manage a child with mild anxiety. By itself it is not suitable for management of extreme apprehension or a disruptive, unmanageable child. Promethazine is available for oral administration as a tablet and syrup. Following oral administration onset of action develops within 15 to 60 minutes; sedative effects are sustained for 2 to 8 hours.[40]

Initial Dosage

For children 2 years of age through adolescence, the recommended oral dose of promethazine is 1.1 mg/kg/dose PO.[40] The oral dosage of promethazine, as recommended in pediatric dentistry, is found in Table 35.4.

Midazolam

Along with diazepam, midazolam has become one of the most popular orally administered CNS depressants in pediatric dentistry and medicine. Kain et al studied the effectiveness of oral midazolam in a pediatric population, determining that 14.1% of children receiving a 0.5-mg/kg dose PO exhibited extreme anxiety and distress during the induction of general anesthesia.[41] They further stated that children who are under 4 years of age and highly emotional may not respond well to 0.5 mg/kg oral midazolam. A dose of 0.75 mg/kg should be considered for this group.[41] Similar results were found in a pediatric dental trial using dosages of 0.5 mg/kg and 0.7 mg/kg.[42] Oral midazolam was found to be a useful drug for the management of young children with behavior problems. It was found, however, not to be effective in all cases and for the provision of all types of pediatric dentistry. The results

Table 35.4	Dose of Promethazine
WEIGHT (KG)	**DOSE (MG)**
12–14	12.5
14–16	12.5
16–18	25
18–20	25
20–25	25
25–30	37.5
30–36	37.5
36–45	50

indicate that, when using oral midazolam in children, the treatment should be restricted to simple restorations and extractions over a maximum of two visits.[42] A recent Cochrane Database Review of midazolam concluded that there is some weak evidence that oral midazolam is an effective sedative agent for children.[43] Papineni et al, in reviewing side effects and adverse outcomes associated with oral administration of midazolam in pediatric dentistry, concluded that significant side effects associated with oral midazolam usage for behavior management in children and adolescents requiring dental treatment appear to be rare.[44]

After oral administration, midazolam undergoes extensive first-pass metabolism. Oral midazolam bioavailability is roughly 36% and is independent of age or weight. Onset of anxiolytic and sedative effects usually occur within 10 to 30 minutes of oral administration, with the degree of sedation dependent on the dose administered and the presence or absence of other medications. Food does not appear to affect the extent of absorption, but the indications for oral midazolam often preclude feeding. Recovery times are similar to IV administration of a single dose.[45]

Initial Dosage

For infants and children, 6 months up to 16 years, the recommended dosage of oral midazolam is 0.25 to 0.5 mg/kg (maximum dose 20 mg) as a single dose before treatment.[45] The most commonly reported effective dose was 0.5 mg/kg.[41] Some children may require up to 1 mg/kg PO (maximum 20 mg) for a desired clinical response.

Diazepam

Diazepam is administered orally, in pill form, to the hyperactive, highly anxious, and excitable child more than 4 years old. It is effective in patients with cerebral palsy, especially those with athetoid cerebral palsy, and in patients with mental retardation. Diazepam is available in tablet form (2 mg, 5 mg, 10 mg) and as an oral solution (5 mg/mL, 5 mg/5 mL) in 5 mg/5 mL.[46]

Initial Dosage

Diazepam is the most rapidly absorbed benzodiazepine following an oral dose.[47] The initial dose of diazepam is 0.2 to 0.4 mg/ kg orally 45 to 60 minutes before the procedure. Maximum dose is 20 mg PO.

Oral Combinations

The administration of combinations of oral sedative drugs is not uncommon in pediatric dentistry (see Table 35.2). When two or more sedating drugs are to be administered orally, it must be noted that the potential for an adverse outcome may be increased.[48-52] The lowest dose of drug with the highest therapeutic index should be selected for the procedure. The selection of the fewest number of drugs and matching drug selection to the type and goals of the procedure are essential for safe practice.[10] For example, analgesics, such as opioids, are indicated for painful procedures, although in dentistry local anesthetics are preferred. For nonpainful procedures, sedative/hypnotics are preferred. When both sedation and analgesia are desirable, either single agents with analgesic/ sedative properties (e.g., nitrous oxide-oxygen) or combination regimens are commonly used.[10]

Chloral Hydrate Plus Promethazine

Chloral hydrate is combined with promethazine for administration to the patient younger than 3 years with rampant caries who is too young for the tell-show-do technique to be effective. Other indications for this combination are younger patients with mental or physical disabilities. The combination of chloral hydrate and promethazine is frequently administered in medicine for sedation of children during procedures where patient movement is detrimental.[53] In a study with 90 children undergoing electroencephalography (EEG), they received 40 mg/ kg chloral hydrate and 1 mg/kg promethazine. 96.7% of the children were sufficiently sedated to allow successful completion of the EEG. Mild clinical side effects included vomiting (6.7%), and agitation (3.3%).[53]

Initial Dosage

The dose for the 2- to 3-year-old patient is 1000 mg (2 teaspoons) chloral hydrate combined with 25 mg (1 teaspoon) promethazine. The dose for the 3- to 6-year-old patient is up to 1500 mg (3 teaspoons) chloral hydrate combined with 25 mg (1 teaspoon) promethazine. This combination is mixed together and then added to a fruit drink or soft drink and administered 30 to 45 minutes before the appointment. The patient should take nothing by mouth for 6 hours before its administration. Clinical effectiveness is noted within 45 minutes; maximal clinical benefit occurs at 1 hour.

COMMENT: The availability of a restraint, such as the Pedi-Wrap or Papoose Board, is recommended when managing the very young, apprehensive patient. For greatest benefit to be obtained from this combination of drugs, the maximal length of the appointment ought not to exceed 1 hour. The parents or guardian of the patient must be advised of the possibility of postoperative irritability or excitement as the drug effects wear off.

Promethazine Plus Meperidine

Meperidine (Demerol) and promethazine (Phenergan) are often used in combination for both oral and parenteral administration. The combination is a rational one in that the opioid provides for a sedative and analgesic effect, whereas promethazine potentiates the opioid effect and adds an antiemetic action (to counter any possible nausea produced by meperidine). Indications for the administration of this combination are (1) recalcitrant, defiant, and uncooperative behavior in children over 6 years of age who may require extensive treatment in a prolonged appointment and (2) severe mental retardation in children.

Initial Dosage

For the child weighing approximately 11 kg (25 lb), the initial dose is 25 mg meperidine plus 12.5 mg promethazine. For the child weighing approximately 15 kg (33 lb), the initial dose is 25 mg meperidine plus 25 mg promethazine. For the child weighing approximately 22 kg (50 lb), the initial dose is 50 mg meperidine plus 25 mg promethazine. For ease of administration, the contents of the capsule may be added to a flavored vehicle (liquid or food).

> **COMMENT:** Opioid administration is associated with respiratory depression. The dentist should be experienced in the use of opioids, be able to recognize respiratory depression (monitoring the patient throughout the procedure using pulse oximetry and/or capnography), and have naloxone available whenever this combination is employed.

Benzodiazepines administered orally have become the most commonly used drugs in pediatric sedation, aside from nitrous oxide and oxygen. From a pharmacologic standpoint this is a welcome development, as many of the previously most popular drugs, such as chloral hydrate and meperidine, had significant negatives from a pharmacologic standpoint. The concurrent administration of N_2O-O_2—titrated to effect—can greatly increase the incidence of successful oral sedation procedures.

Parenteral Sedation

Parenteral sedation techniques in pediatric dentistry include the IM, IN, IV, and inhalation routes of drug administration.

In this first section, only IM and IN drug administration are discussed. Use of IM with IV and/or inhalation routes is discussed later in this chapter.

The administration of parenteral sedation (IM/IV/IN) by doctors not well trained in these techniques cannot be recommended.[15]

The IM and IN routes of drug administration are of greater importance in pediatric dentistry than for adult patients, primarily because of the decreased need for patient cooperation in these techniques. To administer a drug via these routes, the patient merely needs to be restrained for a moment during the injection. As discussed in Chapters 3, 9, and 10, there are significant drawbacks to these techniques, the most significant of which is the lack of control over the ultimate drug action maintained by the dentist. Titration is not possible via these routes of drug administration; therefore the risk of oversedation and other adverse events is increased. Because the most commonly used drugs in these techniques have traditionally been the opioids, respiratory depression is an ever-present danger. The introduction and increased usage of IM and IN midazolam has minimized this risk.

Both the IM and IN routes have equivalent onsets of action.[35] IM drug administration is popular because of its ease of administration, rapid onset of action, better absorption (than enteral routes), and greater predictability of the length of the latent period and duration of action. One disadvantage of the IM route is the patient's fear of receiving an injection. A second disadvantage is the potential effect on the parent or guardian of giving their child an IM injection. I have encountered five instances where the parent (usually the father) has fainted while holding his or her child who was receiving an IM injection for sedation. A disadvantage of IN drug administration is the potential for a burning sensation to occur in the nose with some drugs (e.g., midazolam) and a disagreeable taste if the drug should run into the patient's oropharynx. Use of an atomizer on the syringe has been shown to minimize these problems (see Fig. 9.1).[54]

Monitoring of the patient receiving moderate or deep sedation via the IM or IN route is important. The pretracheal stethoscope is an essential piece of equipment. Because parenteral techniques are usually reserved for more difficult management problems, the use of physical restraint is more often required. The possibility of further respiratory embarrassment exists if the physical restraint is too tight around the patient's chest. Supplemental O_2 should always be administered throughout the procedure whenever IM or IN drugs are administered, either as O_2 alone or in combination with nitrous oxide. Monitoring including, but not limited to, pulse oximetry and/or capnography is mandatory.

Meperidine Plus Promethazine

The combination of meperidine and promethazine was discussed previously in the section on oral combinations. It is an effective combination for patients with severe management problems or severe mental retardation. This combination is especially recommended when procedures requiring 2 hours or more are planned.

It is interesting to note that in online pharmacology resources (ClinicalKey, Epocrates), the only indication for administration of the combination of meperidine and promethazine is for the treatment of moderate-to-severe pain.[55]

The premixed combination of these two drugs was available for years as Mepergan (Wyeth) in 10-mL vials and in 2-mL preloaded syringes. Each milliliter contained 25 mg meperidine and 25 mg promethazine. Mepergan is no longer available in the United States (July 2008).

Lytic Cocktail

The combination of meperidine (Demerol), promethazine (Phenergan), and chlorpromazine (Thorazine) is termed the *lytic cocktail,* or DPT.[56] This combination has been in use for many years in both pediatric dentistry and medicine. Its popularity has waned because of erratic patient responses; however, the lytic cocktail is still used within pediatric medicine. *Clinical Practice Guideline: Acute pain management: operative or medical procedures and trauma* raised serious doubt as to the rationale for continued use of this technique.[57] The following is an excerpt from these guidelines:

> Exercise caution when using the mixture of meperidine (Demerol), promethazine (Phenergan), and chlorpromazine (Thorazine), also known as DPT. DPT—given intramuscularly—has been used for painful procedures. The efficacy of this mixture is poor compared with alternative approaches, and it has been associated with a high frequency of adverse effects.[58] It is not recommended for general use and should be used only in exceptional circumstances.

The drugs are combined in one syringe and administered intramuscularly. The patient remains with his or her parent for a few minutes until becoming quiet and is then placed in the treatment environment in a restraint. Monitoring devices are applied, supplemental O_2 and local anesthetic are administered, and the procedure is started.

Extrapyramidal reactions, especially tardive dyskinesia, are not uncommon side effects of the phenothiazines (promethazine and chlorpromazine). Should these develop, management requires the administration of diphenhydramine (see Chapter 7).

Midazolam

The water-soluble benzodiazepine midazolam has received considerable attention as an IM drug for pediatric sedation and has become the IM drug of choice in many institutions, both in dentistry and medicine—primarily pediatric emergency medicine.[59-61] Midazolam has been used successfully intramuscularly as a sole agent for pediatric sedation, and it has been used in conjunction with IV midazolam. This technique is discussed in the section on pediatric IV sedation. The IM dose of midazolam that has been most successfully used is 0.2 mg/kg.[62,63] Following intramuscular administration, the absorption

of midazolam is rapid, with a mean bioavailability greater than 90%. Onset of action following IM is 5 to 15 minutes. Maximum effects are seen in 20 to 60 minutes, with a recovery time of 2 to 6 hours.[45] Patients may usually be placed in the dental chair with minimal difficulty within about 10 to 15 minutes following IM administration. When it is used in conjunction with IV sedation, the duration of dental treatment is indefinite. As with all parenteral sedation techniques, monitoring is essential to patient safety.

The IN route of drug administration has become considerably more popular in recent years[64-69] as a parenteral sedation technique that does not require an injection yet provides a clinical effect equal to that achieved following IM drug administration.[35] Midazolam is one of two drugs (sufentanil is the other) that have received considerable attention via this route of administration. The IN administration of midazolam has proven to provide satisfactory sedation in a majority of cases, enabling child–parent separation to occur with minimal distress.[70] An IN dose of 0.2 or 0.3 mg/kg of midazolam is recommended.[68,70] The drug should be administered slowly into each naris of the patient, preferably with a 1-mL tuberculin syringe with an atomizer attached (see Figs. 9.1 and 9.2).[54,71]

Ketamine

Ketamine, a dissociative anesthetic most commonly used as a general anesthetic, has been administered with success in pediatric dentistry in subanesthetic doses.[70,72,73] When administered intramuscularly, a dose of 3 to 7 mg/kg is administered, with an expected onset of dissociation within about 3 to 4 minutes. The expected duration of anesthesia is between 12 and 25 minutes.[74] The patient can usually be discharged from the office within 90 minutes after the end of the procedure. *It must be stated once again that ketamine should NEVER be administered by anyone who has not completed a residency in general anesthesia and who is not proficient in the management of the unconscious airway.*

Inhalation Sedation

Inhalation sedation with N_2O-O_2 remains the most used technique of sedation, as well as the most nearly ideal sedation technique for pediatric dentistry. In a survey of pediatric dental residents and pediatric dentists in the United Kingdom, Woolley et al found that inhalation sedation was the preferred technique of 98% of practicing pediatric dentists and 97% of pediatric dental residents.[75] Wilson, in 2013, reemphasized the importance of inhalation sedation in pediatric dentistry.[76] The advantages and indications for the administration of inhalation sedation in children are the same as for the adult patient. The major difficulties encountered with this technique in children are twofold: first, the lack of potency of N_2O-O_2 may render the technique ineffective in the management of the more apprehensive patient; and second, some children will object to the placement of the nasal hood. In most cases this second objection can be overcome by altering the usual technique of administration of N_2O-O_2 (see Chapter 15) to meet more realistically the requirements of the pediatric patient. Inhalation sedation was, by a significant margin, the most recommended technique of sedation for pediatric patients when administered by general dentists and pediatric specialists, in a survey of dentist anesthesiologists.[15]

Dosage

The primary advantage of inhalation sedation is the ease with which it may be titrated. Concentrations of N_2O required to provide clinically adequate sedation in the child who readily accepts the nasal hood are virtually identical to those seen in adults. The overwhelming majority of children receiving N_2O-O_2 are adequately sedated at concentrations between 30% and 45% N_2O. Some patients may require less than 30%, and some more than 45% N_2O.

Screaming and crying patients will breathe through their mouths to a much greater degree than is usual and therefore do not receive as great a volume of N_2O being delivered through the nasal hood. A means of overcoming this problem is demonstrated in Fig. 35.4. The dentist removes the nasal hood from the patient's nose and holds it over the mouth so that as the child inhales he or she will receive greater volumes of N_2O. As illustrated in the figure, the patient is rather young and has been placed in a physical restraint. The nasal hood is held over the patient's mouth until he or she quiets down, at which time it is once again placed on the patient's nose and treatment continued. This process may need to be repeated throughout the dental treatment in some patients.

The patient who does not permit the nasal hood to be placed on the nose poses a greater challenge. The following technique will, however, provide the dentist with an increased chance of success. With the child restrained, the nasal hood is placed as close to the child's face as is practical. The concentration of N_2O is maximal (70%), with a high-flow rate (10 to 15 L/min). The patient may be attempting to move his or her face away from the nasal hood and be crying or screaming; however, the patient will be receiving a high concentration of N_2O (not 70% because of significant air dilution) at this time. The nasal hood should be maintained close to, but not on, the face for a few moments until the child quiets. The nasal hood should then be placed onto the nose. At this time, the percentage of N_2O must be lowered to approximately 25% to 30% and then titrated to an appropriate level for the patient.

One of the more unpleasant problems when N_2O-O_2 is used in pediatric patients is vomiting. Though uncommon, the incidence of vomiting in pediatric patients is significantly greater than that seen in adults. Two reasons for this are (1) the lack of ability of the dentist to judge the level of the patient's sedation, which may lead to oversedation, and (2) the greater tendency of children to mouth-breathe. Mouth breathing decreases the volume of N_2O being inhaled and lessens the level of sedation. When the patient returns to nose breathing, the sedation level deepens. Constant fluctuation in N_2O concentration is one cause of vomiting. Two techniques are available that decrease mouth breathing. Simplest, and most effective, is the use of the rubber dam. I highly recommend its application whenever inhalation sedation (or for that matter any sedative technique) is used. It almost entirely prevents mouth breathing. Another method, used in the absence of a rubber dam, is to tell the mouth-breathing patient that some "special water" is being placed into their mouth and that he or she cannot swallow it. A small volume of water from the air–water syringe should be placed into the patient's mouth. To keep the water in the mouth, the patient will have to raise his or her tongue to the roof of the mouth, thereby eliminating mouth breathing.

Several methods of determining a younger patient's level of sedation are available. The first may be used with a patient who is somewhat cooperative and is able and willing to communicate with the dentist. The younger child may be unable to understand the terms usually used to describe the sensations associated with N_2O for the adult patient. The dentist will have to come "down" to the level of the child's understanding. Playing a game with the child is an effective means of determining the level of sedation. The child pretends to be an astronaut, and the nasal hood is the space mask. As the child inhales through this space mask, the "astronaut" will begin to float in space. Questioning the child about his or her feelings can help determine the level of sedation (i.e., floating).

The second technique is used in situations in which the apprehensive child is less communicative. Titration of the N_2O-O_2 continues at the usual rate, with the dentist observing the degree of tension in the patient's body. Watching and touching the patient's hands provides an excellent gauge of the level of sedation. It can be expected that the patient's hands will become more relaxed as sedation increases. The eyelids of the patient begin to close, and the patient may yawn

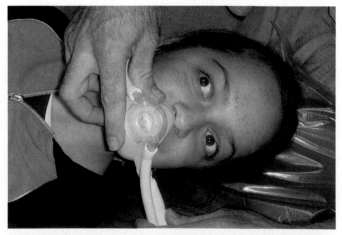

Figure 35.4 In a crying or screaming patient, the nasal hood may be held over the patient's mouth, thereby increasing N_2O delivery.

occasionally. When the dentist believes that the patient is adequately sedated, treatment is attempted. Changes in N_2O-O_2 concentrations are based on the patient's response or lack of response to this treatment.

Nitrous Oxide-Oxygen With Other Techniques

As noted in Table 35.2, N_2O-O_2 is frequently added to other techniques of sedation to enhance effectiveness. As discussed in Chapter 28, I believe that there is potential risk involved in this procedure if used by the inexperienced dentist who is not trained in recognizing unconsciousness and in airway management. When adequate operating room and outpatient moderate and deep sedation experience and training have been received (e.g., pediatric dentistry residency, general practice residency, anesthesiology residency), the combinations of oral plus inhalation sedation, IM or IN plus inhalation sedation, or IM and IV plus inhalation sedation may be used safely. Adequate monitoring of the patient, especially of the respiratory system, is essential. N_2O-O_2 must always be titrated; fixed concentrations should never be administered to all patients because not all patients react in the same manner.

Intravenous Sedation

Traditionally, IV moderate sedation has seldom been used in the management of pediatric dental or medical patients. Although this technique of drug administration is the most reliable and, when used as described, very safe, its use is seldom taught in pediatric dentistry residency programs. It has been my clinical experience that younger patients (under 6 years) who do not respond well (for behavioral reasons primarily) to IM/IN moderate sedation do not respond well to IV moderate sedation either. I emphasize that we are using *moderate,* not *deep,* sedation. Conversely, younger patients who sit quietly allowing an IV line to be established are patients who, in all likelihood, do not require IV sedation for their treatment. Other techniques such as inhalation or oral sedation, either alone or in combination, will likely provide a successful outcome.

Because of the problems that have been associated with the administration of IM/SC/SM opioids in past years,[77] alternative agents and techniques have been vigorously sought. With the introduction of midazolam into clinical use, a new group of drugs, the benzodiazepines, is now being used for IM/IN sedation in pediatrics.

When administered via these routes, the benzodiazepines have a fixed, somewhat short duration of clinical action (<1 hour). It was our thought to combine the administration of IM or IN midazolam (for initial patient management) with IV midazolam or other IV drugs (for continued patient management) in pediatric dental patients.

The technique for IV deep sedation is briefly described.

Following a pretreatment visit at which the patient is thoroughly evaluated (medically, dentally, and psychologically)

Table 35.5	AAP/AAPD Appropriate Intake of Food and Liquids Before Elective Sedation[10,78]	
INGESTED MATERIAL	**MINIMUM FASTING PERIOD (HR)**	
Clear liquids: water, fruit juices without pulp, carbonated beverages, clear tea, black coffee	2	
Human milk	4	
Infant formula	6	
Nonhuman milk: because nonhuman milk is similar to solids in gastric emptying time, the amount ingested must be considered when determining an appropriate fasting period.	6	
Light meal: a light meal consists of toast and clear liquids. Meals that include fried or fatty food or meat may prolong gastric emptying time. Both the amount and type of food ingested must be considered when determining an appropriate fasting period.	6	

for suitability for sedation and after presedation instructions are given to the parent or guardian, the patient returns to the dental office for treatment.

The AAP and the AAPD recommend that guidelines for fasting periods before elective sedation should generally follow those used for elective general anesthesia[10,78] (Table 35.5).

In a quiet room, with the lights turned down, the IM or IN dose of midazolam (0.2 or 0.3 mg/kg) is administered to the patient (if IM, lateral aspect of thigh [vastus lateralis]) while he or she is held by the parent or guardian. A pulse oximeter probe is immediately placed on the patient's toe or finger, and the patient is left with the parent for approximately 10 to 15 minutes. The patient is monitored continuously (via pulse oximetry) during this induction period.

At 10 or 15 minutes the patient is placed into the dental chair, enveloped in a physical restraint, and inhalation sedation added (30% to 50% N_2O). The patient is usually somewhat cooperative but perhaps not relaxed enough to permit the dental treatment to commence. Venous access is obtained in every patient and a continuous IV infusion (D5W with pediatric infusion set) started. Monitors are placed. These include the pretracheal stethoscope, capnograph, ECG, and vital signs monitor in addition to the already placed pulse oximeter.

If possible, dental treatment is started at this time. However, in many situations the patient is not yet cooperative as the stimulation of treatment starts. Small incremental doses (0.5 to 1 mg) of midazolam or other IV drugs are titrated in until the desired level of sedation is reached, at which point local anesthesia is administered and dental treatment commenced. If, at a later time, additional sedation is desired, additional doses of IV drugs or nitrous oxide may be administered.

Fentanyl is occasionally administered to aid in sedation and when a degree of analgesia is desirable at the conclusion of the dental procedure (e.g., multiple extractions).

Propofol has been used during pediatric IV deep sedation when a rapid onset or a short duration of sedation is required. Immediately (20 to 30 seconds) before the administration of a palatal local anesthetic, a dose of 5 to 10 mg of propofol is injected as a bolus. In addition, propofol is administered toward the end of the procedure when the level of CNS depression lightens and the patient begins to make movements that interfere with the completion of the treatment. Increments of 10 mg of propofol enable the procedure to be completed successfully without prolonging the recovery period to any significant degree.

At the completion of treatment, the patient receives 100% O_2, the room lights are turned on (to stimulate the patient), and the dental chair is positioned to make the patient somewhat uncomfortable. The goal at this time is to stimulate the patient to hasten their recovery and discharge. Monitoring is continued throughout the recovery period. When recovery is deemed adequate (see following discussion), the patient is dismissed in the custody of a parent or guardian. A telephone call to the family that evening to inquire as to the patient's status is mandated.

This technique should be used only by persons well trained in deep sedation, general anesthesia, and airway management. During deep sedation there must be one person whose only responsibility is to constantly observe the patient's vital signs, airway patency, and adequacy of ventilation and to either administer drugs or direct their administration. This individual must, at a minimum, be trained in PALS (pediatric advanced life support) and capable of assisting with any emergency event. At least one individual must be present who is trained in and capable of providing PALS and who is skilled to rescue a child with apnea, laryngospasm, and/or airway obstruction.[10]

Using this technique of IM/IV and inhalation sedation, we have been able to manage the dental needs of patients ranging from 18 months to 10 years of age.

DISCHARGE FROM THE OFFICE

From the 2016 AAP/AAPD Guidelines: After the procedure, "the child who has received moderate sedation must be observed in a suitably equipped recovery area, which must have a functioning suction apparatus as well as the capacity to deliver >90% oxygen and positive-pressure ventilation (bag–valve–mask) with an adequate oxygen capacity as well as age- and size-appropriate rescue equipment and devices. The patient's vital signs should be recorded at specific intervals (e.g., every 10 to 15 minutes). If the patient is not fully alert, oxygen saturation and heart rate monitoring shall be used continuously until appropriate discharge criteria are met. Because sedation medications with a long half-life may delay the patient's complete return to baseline or pose the risk of resedation, some patients might benefit from a longer period of less intense observation before discharge from medical/dental supervision.[79,80] A simple evaluation tool may be the ability of the infant or child to remain awake for at least 20 minutes when placed in a quiet environment.[81] Patients who have received reversal agents, such as flumazenil or naloxone, will require a longer period of observation, because the duration of the drugs administered may exceed the duration of the antagonist, resulting in resedation."[10]

Recommended discharge criteria are[82]:

1. Cardiovascular function and airway patency (blood pressure, heart rate and rhythm, respiratory rate, and O_2 saturation) are satisfactory and stable.
2. The patient is easily arousable, and protective reflexes are intact.
3. The patient can talk (if age appropriate).
4. The patient can sit up unaided (if age appropriate).
5. For a very young or handicapped child incapable of the usually expected responses, the presedation level of responsiveness or a level as close as possible to the normal level for that child should be achieved.
6. The state of hydration is adequate.
7. The pediatric patient shall be accompanied to and from the treatment facility by a parent, legal guardian, or other responsible person. It is preferable to have two adults accompany children who are still in car safety seats if transportation to and from a treatment facility is provided by one of the adults.[10,83]
8. In a situation in which the parent or guardian insists on taking the child before the dentist considers the patient adequately recovered, this must be immediately noted in the patient's chart, and it must be countersigned by a second person who is present.

It is the dentist who must be the final arbiter of the patient's ability to be discharged safely from the office. Until such time, the patient should remain in the recovery area of the office. Fig. 35.5 presents a list of objective criteria for discharge of the postsedation patient.

RECORDKEEPING

As with the adult patient, sedation records must be maintained for the pediatric patient. An example of one such form was presented in Chapter 26. The following sedation record is recommended by the AAPD[84] (Fig. 35.6).

GENERAL ANESTHESIA

Approximately 2% to 5% of pediatric patients will require general anesthesia for their dental care to be successfully completed. Dummett[85] lists the following indications for

The following should be completed when considering the discharge of a patient following parenteral sedation. The patient postsedation score must be approximately equal to the baseline (presedation) score.

Physical Signs	(Pretreatment)	Baseline/Discharge Comments
Patient's name: SSN: Date:		
A. MOVEMENT 　2—able to walk (when appropriate) 　1—able to move extremities 　0—unable to move any extremity		
B. RESPIRATIONS 　2—able to breathe deeply and cough 　1—limited respiratory effort 　0—no spontaneous respiratory effort		
C. CIRCULATION 　2—systolic BP ±20% baseline level 　1—systolic BP ±40% baseline level 　0—systolic BP >±40% baseline level		
D. CONSCIOUSNESS 　2—full alertness seen in ability to 　　answer questions qppropriately 　1—aroused when called by name 　0—unresponsive to verbal stimulation		
E. COLOR 　2—normal skin color and appearance 　1—any alteration in skin color 　0—frank cyanosis or extreme pale		
TOTAL SCORE: Dr's signature:		

Figure 35.5 Parenteral sedation discharge criteria.

the administration of general anesthesia to the pediatric patient:

1. Extensive dental needs in uncooperative children who resist all means of conventional management procedures, including premedication and restraints
2. Extensive dental needs in the young, immature, and precommunicative child whose behavior deters dental treatment
3. Multiple pulpally involved teeth in a child with cardiac disease where immediate treatment is indicated for the sake of the child's health
4. Extensive dental needs in patients with severely physical or sensorial disabilities (e.g., deafness and blindness), with whom communication cannot be achieved
5. Extensive dental needs in children with blood dyscrasias who may need transfusions
6. Extensive dental needs in children with mental retardation whose behavior deters dental treatment and impairs dentist–patient communication

As mentioned, before reaching a decision to use general anesthesia, at least two attempts should be made to treat the patient in the office using sedation techniques. Sedation combined with local anesthesia is a highly effective means of managing most patients. When attempts using these procedures have been unsuccessful and signs of progressive improvement in behavior and cooperation have not been demonstrated, general anesthesia should be considered.

Pediatric general anesthesia may be administered in one of three settings: in the dental office, in the hospital or outpatient surgical center as a day admission, or on an inpatient basis in the hospital. For the healthy American Society of Anesthesiologists (ASA) 1 pediatric patient, the potential trauma of separation from the parent in the strange environment of the hospital is a strong indication for the use of either in-office or outpatient day-admission procedures. If the child is ASA 2, 3, or 4, hospitalization and treatment as an inpatient are recommended. General anesthesia is reviewed in Chapter 31.

Sedation Record

Patient Selection Criteria   Date: _____

Patient: _____ ❑ M ❑ F   Age: _____yr____mo   Weight: _____kg   Physician: _____

Indication for sedation: ❑ Fearful/anxious patient for whom basic behavior guidance techniques have not been successful
❑ Patient unable to cooperate due to lack of psychological or emotional maturity and/or mental, physical, or medical disability
❑ To protect patient's developing psyche
❑ To reduce patient's medical risk

Medical history/review of systems (ROS)	NONE	YES*	Describe positive findings: _____	Airway Assessment	NONE	YES*
Allergies &/or previous adverse drug reactions	❑	❑	_____	Obesity	❑	❑
Current medications (including OTC)	❑	❑	_____	Limited neck mobility	❑	❑
Relevant diseases, physical/neurologic impairment	❑	❑	_____	Micro/retrognathia	❑	❑
Previous sedation/general anesthetics	❑	❑	_____	Macroglossia	❑	❑
Snoring, obstructive sleep apnea, mouth breathing	❑	❑	_____	Tonsillar obstruction (___%)	❑	❑
Other significant findings (eg, family history)	❑	❑	_____	Limited oral opening	❑	❑

ASA classification: ❑ I ❑ II ❑ III* ❑ IV* ❑ E   * Medical consultation indicated? ❑ NO ❑ YES   Date requested: _____

Comments: _____
_____
_____
_____

Is this patient a candidate for in-office sedation? ❑ YES ❑ NO   Doctor's signature: _____   Date: _____

Plan   Name/relation to patient   Initials   Date   By

Informed consent obtained from   _____   _____ _____ _____
Pre-op instructions reviewed with   _____   _____ _____ _____
Post-op precautions reviewed with   _____   _____ _____ _____

Assessment on Day of Sedation   Date: _____

Accompanied by: _____   Relationship(s) to patient: _____

Medical Hx & ROS update	NO	YES	NPO status	Airway assessment	NO	YES	Checklist
Change in medical hx/ROS	❑	❑	Clear liquids ____hrs	Upper airway clear	❑	❑	❑ Appropriate transportation home
Change in medications	❑	❑	Milk, other liquids,	Lungs clear	❑	❑	❑ Monitors functioning
Recent respiratory illness	❑	❑	&/or foods ____hrs	Tonsillar obstruction (___%)	❑	❑	❑ Emergency kit, suction, &
Weight: _____kg			Medications ____hrs				O_2 available

Vital signs (If unable to obtain, check ❑ and document reason: _____)

Blood pressure: _____/_____ mmHg   Resp: _____/min   Pulse: _____/min   Temp: _____°F SpO_2:_____%

Comments: _____
_____

Presedation cooperation level: ❑ Unable/unwilling to cooperate   ❑ Rarely follows requests   ❑ Cooperates with prompting   ❑ Cooperates freely
Behavioral interaction: ❑ Definitively shy and withdrawn   ❑ Somewhat shy   ❑ Approachable
Guardian was provided an opportunity to ask questions, appeared to understand, and reaffirmed consent for sedation? ❑ YES ❑ NO

Drug Dosage Calculations

Sedatives
Agent _____ Route _____ _____mg/kg X _____kg = _____mg ÷ _____mg/mL = _____mL
Agent _____ Route _____ _____mg/kg X _____kg = _____mg ÷ _____mg/mL = _____mL
Agent _____ Route _____ _____mg/kg X _____kg = _____mg ÷ _____mg/mL = _____mL

Emergency reversal agents
For narcotic: NALOXONE   IV, IM, or subQ   Dose: 0.1 mg/kg X _____ kg = _____mg (Maximum dose: 2 mg; may repeat)
For benzodiazepine: FLUMAZENIL IV (preferred), IM   Dose: 0.01 mg/kg X _____ kg = _____mg (Maximum dose: 0.2 mg; may repeat up to 4 times)

Local anesthetics (maximum dosage based on weight)

Lidocaine 2%	(34 mg/ 1.7 mL cartridge)	4.4 mg/kg X	_____kg =	_____mg	(not to exceed 300 mg total dose)
Articaine 4%	(68 mg/ 1.7 mL cartridge)	7 mg/kg X	_____kg =	_____mg	(not to exceed 500 mg total dose)
Mepivacaine 3%	(51 mg/ 1.7 mL cartridge)	4.4 mg/kg X	_____kg =	_____mg	(not to exceed 300 mg total dose)
Prilocaine 4%	(68 mg/ 1.7 mL cartridge)	6 mg/kg X	_____kg =	_____mg	(not to exceed 400 mg total dose)
Bupivacaine 0.5%	(8.5 mg/ 1.7 mL cartridge)	1.3 mg/kg X	_____kg =	_____mg	(not to exceed 90 mg total dose)

Figure 35.6 Pediatric sedation records. (From American Academy of Pediatric Dentistry. Sedation Record. 27(6):15-16, 2013.)

Intraoperative Management and Post-Operative Monitoring   EMS telephone number: _____

Monitors: ❑ Observation ❑ Pulse oximeter ❑ Precordial/pretracheal stethoscope ❑ Blood pressure cuff ❑ Capnograph ❑ EKG ❑ Thermometer

Protective stabilization/devices: ❑ Papoose ❑ Head positioner ❑ Manual hold ❑ Neck/shoulder roll ❑ Mouth prop ❑ Rubber dam ❑ _____

TIME	Baseline	:	:	:	:	:	:	:	:	:	:	:	:	:	:	:
Sedatives[1]																
N_2O/O_2 (%)																
Local[2] (mg)																
SpO_2																
Pulse																
BP																
Resp																
CO_2																
Procedure[3]																
Comments[4]																
Sedation level*																
Behavior†																

1. Agent _____ Route _____ Dose _____ Time _____ Administered by _____
   Agent _____ Route _____ Dose _____ Time _____ Administered by _____
   Agent _____ Route _____ Dose _____ Time _____ Administered by _____

2. Local anesthetic agent _____

3. Record dental procedure start and completion times, transfer to recovery area, etc.

4. Enter letter on chart and corresponding comments (eg, complications/side effects, airway intervention, reversal agent, analgesic) below:
   A. _____ B. _____
   C. _____ D. _____

Sedation level*
   None (typical response/ cooperation for this patient)
   Mild (anxiolysis)
   Moderate (purposeful response to verbal commands ± light tactile sensation)
   Deep (purposeful response after repeated verbal or painful stimulation
   General Anesthesia (not arousable)

Behavior/ responsiveness to treatment†
   Excellent: quiet and cooperative
   Good: mild objections &/or whimpering but treatment not interrupted
   Fair: crying with minimal disruption to treatment
   Poor: struggling that interfered with operative procedures
   Prohibitive: active resistance and crying; treatment cannot be rendered

Overall effectiveness: ❑ Ineffective ❑ Effective ❑ Very effective ❑ Overly sedated

Additional comments/treatment accomplished: _____
_____
_____
_____

Discharge

Criteria for discharge
   ❑ Cardiovascular function is satisfactory and stable.
   ❑ Airway patency is satisfactory and stable.
   ❑ Patient is easily arousable.
   ❑ Responsiveness is at or very near presedation level (especially if very young or special needs child incapable of the usually expected responses).
   ❑ Protective reflexes are intact.
   ❑ Patient can talk (return to presedation level).
   ❑ Patient can sit up unaided (return to presedation level).
   ❑ State of hydration is adequate.

Discharge vital signs
   Pulse: _____/ min
   SpO_2: _____%
   BP: _____/_____ mmHg
   Resp: _____/ min
   Temp: _____°F

Discharge process
   ❑ Post-operative instructions reviewed with _____ by _____
      ❑ Transportation ❑ Airway protection/observation ❑ Activity ❑ Diet ❑ Nausea/vomiting ❑ Fever ❑ Rx ❑ Anesthetized tissues
      ❑ Dental treatment rendered ❑ Pain ❑ Bleeding ❑ _____ ❑ Emergency contact
   ❑ Next appointment on: _____ for _____

I have received and understand these discharge instructions. The patient is discharged into my care at _____ ❑ AM ❑ PM

Signature: _____ Relationship: _____ After hours number: _____

Operator
   Signature: _____

Chairside
   Assistant: _____

Monitoring
   Personnel signature: _____

Post-op call

Date: _____ Time: _____ By: _____ Spoke to: _____ Comments: _____

Figure 35.6 cont'd

REFERENCES

1. Stigers JI: Nonpharmacologic management of children's behaviors. In Dean JA, editor: *McDonald and Avery's dentistry for the child and adolescent*, ed 10, St Louis, 2016, Mosby, pp 286–302.
2. Lenchner V: The effect of appointment length on the behavior of the pedodontic patient and his attitude toward dentistry. *J Dent Child* 33(2):61–74, 1966.
3. Klingberg G, Broberg AG: Dental fear/anxiety and dental behaviour management problems in children and adolescents: a review of prevalence and concomitant psychological factors. *Int J Paediatr Dent* 17:391–406, 2007.
4. Frankl SN, Shiere FR, Fogelo HR: Should the parent remain with the child in the dental operatory? *J Dent Child* 29:150, 1962.
5. Wright GZ, editor: *Behavior management in dentistry for children*, Philadelphia, 1975, WB Saunders.
6. Murphy ML, Fields HW, Machen JB: Parental acceptance of pediatric dentistry behavior techniques. *Pediatr Dent* 6:193–198, 1984.
7. Lawrence SM, McTigue DM, Wilson S, et al: Parental attitudes toward behavior management techniques in pediatric dentistry. *Pediatr Dent* 13:151–155, 1991.
8. Eaton JJ, McTigue DJ, Fields HW, Beck M: Attitudes of contemporary parents toward behavior management techniques used in pediatric dentistry. *Pediatr Dent* 27:107–113, 2005.
9. Egerton B: Deadly dentistry: junior's story. The Dallas Morning News. December 9, 2015. www.dallasmorningnews.com.
10. Coté CJ, Wilson S, American ACADEMY of Pediatrics, American Academy of Pediatric Dentistry: Guidelines for Monitoring and Management of Pediatric Patients Before, During, and After Sedation for Diagnostic and Therapeutic Procedures: Update 2016. *Pediatrics* 138(1):e1–e31 :e20161212, 2016.
11. California Legislative Information. Assembly Bill-2235 – Dental Anesthesia and Minors. http://leginfo.legislature.ca.gov/faces/billCompareClient.xhtml?bill_id=201520160AB2235. (Accessed 30 January 2017).
12. Caleb's Law. www.calebslaw.org. (Accessed 30 January 2017).
13. Trapp LD: Special considerations in pedodontic anesthesia. *Dent Clin North Am* 31(1):131–138, 1987.
14. Kopel HM: Lecture notes, AMED 750, August 1983.
15. Malamed SF: Personnel communication with Drs. Jason Brady, Andrea Fonner, H. William Gottschalk, Kenneth Lee, Amanda Okundaye, Kenneth Reed, 27 January 2017.
16. U.S. Food and Drug Administration. FDA Drug Safety Communication: FDA review results in new warnings about using general anesthetics and sedation drugs in young children and pregnant women. http://www.fda.gov/Drugs/DrugSafety/ucm532356.htm. (Accessed 17 January 2017).
17. Johnson R: Lecture notes, AMED 750, August 1983.
18. Wilson JT: Pediatric pharmacology: who will test the drugs? *J Pediatr* 80:855–857, 1972.
19. Chassard D, Bruguerolle B: Chronobiology and anesthesia. *Anesthesiology* 100(2):413–427, 2004.
20. Boriosi JP, Hollman GA: Making a case for use of the pretracheal stethoscope in pediatric procedural sedation. *Paediatr Anaesth* 26:249–255, 2016.
21. Peyton J, Cravero JP: The pretracheal stethoscope useful, but not a necessity. *Paediatr Anaesth* 26:256–258, 2016.
22. American Academy of Pediatrics Committee on Child Abuse and Neglect: Behavior management of pediatric dental patients. *Pediatrics* 90(4):651–652, 1992.
23. American Academy of Pediatrics Committee on Pediatric Emergency Medicine: The use of physical restraint interventions for children and adolescents in the acute care setting. *Pediatrics* 99(3):497–498, 1997.
24. American Academy of Pediatric Dentistry: Guideline on protective stabilization for pediatric dental patients. *Pediatr Dent* 35(5):E169–E173, 2013.
25. Loo CY, Graham RM, Hughes CV: Behaviour guidance in dental treatment of patients with autism spectrum disorder. *Int J Paediatr Dent* 19(6):390–398, 2009.
26. McWhorter AG, Townsend JA, American Academy of Pediatric Dentistry: Behavior symposium workshop A report—current guidelines/revision. *Pediatr Dent* 36(2): 152–153, 2014.
27. Allen SC, Bernat JE, Perinpanayagam MK: Survey of sedation techniques used among pediatric dentists in New York State. *N Y State Dent J* 72(5):53–55, 2006.
28. Haupt M: Project USAP 2000—Use of sedative agents by pediatric dentists: a 15-year follow-up survey. *Pediatr Dent* 24:289–294, 2002.
29. U.S. Department of Health and Human Services: Compounding and the FDA: Questions and answers. http://www.fda.gov/Drugs/GuidanceComplianceRegulatoryInformation/PharmacyCompounding/ucm339764.htm. (Accessed 14 July 2016).
30. Album MM: Meperidine and promethazine hydrochloride for handicapped patients. *J Dent Res* 40:1036, 1961.
31. Coté CJ, Notterman DA, Karl HW, et al: Adverse sedation events in pediatrics: a critical incident analysis of contributing factors. *Pediatrics* 105(4 Pt 1):805–814, 2000.
32. Nordt SP, Rangan C, Hardmaslani M, et al: Pediatric chloral hydrate poisonings and death following outpatient procedural sedation. *J Med Toxicol* 10(2):219–222, 2014.
33. Mittal N, Goyal A, Jain K, Gauba K: Pediatric dental sedation research: where do we stand today? *J Clin Pediatr Dent* 39(3):284–291, 2015.
34. Harrison P: Lollipop successful in providing analgesia to children before painful procedures. *Can Med Assoc J* 145(5):521–524, 1991.
35. de Santos P, Chabas E, Valero R, Nalda MA: Comparison of intramuscular and intranasal premedication with midazolam in children. *Rev Esp Anestesiol Reanim* 38(1): 12–15, 1991.
36. http://www.ashp.org/menu/DrugShortages/DrugsNoLongerAvailable/bulletin.aspx?id=902. (Accessed 24 August 2015).
37. Meadows M: The FDA takes action against unapproved drugs. *FDA Consum* January-February 2007.
38. ClinicalKey. Chloral Hydrate drug monograph, April 18, 2016. www.ClinicalKey.com. (Accessed 11 July 2016).
39. ClinicalKey. Hydroxyzine drug monograph. June 28, 2016. www.ClinicalKey.com. (Accessed 11 July 2016).
40. ClinicalKey. Promethazine drug monograph. June 28, 2016. www.ClinicalKey.com. (Accessed 11 July 2016).
41. Kain ZN, MacLaren J, McClain BC, et al: Effects of age and emotionality on the effectiveness of midazolam administered preoperatively to children. *Anesthesiology* 107(4):545–552, 2007.
42. Day PF, Power AM, Hibbert SA, Paterson SA: Effectiveness of oral midazolam for paediatric dental care: a retrospective study in two specialist centres. *Eur Arch Paediatr Dent* 7(4):228–235, 2006.
43. Lourenco-Matharu L, Ashley PF, Furness S: Sedation of children undergoing dental treatment. *Cochrane Database Syst Rev* (3):CD003877, 2012.

44. Papineni A, Lourenco-Matharu L, Ashley PF: Safety of oral midazolam sedation use in paediatric dentistry: a review. *Int J Paediatr Dent* 24(1):2–13, 2014.
45. ClinicalKey. Midazolam drug monograph. May 11, 2016. www.ClinicalKey.com. (Accessed 11 July 2016).
46. Diazepam drug monograph. www.epocrates.com. (Accessed 11 July 2016).
47. ClinicalKey. Diazepam drug monograph. June 24, 2016. www.ClinicalKey.com. (Accessed 11 July 2016).
48. Coté CJ, Karl HW, Notterman DA, et al: Adverse sedation events in pediatrics: analysis of medications used for sedation. *Pediatrics* 106(4):633–644, 2000.
49. Sanborn PA, Michna E, Zurakowski D, et al: Adverse cardiovascular and respiratory events during sedation of pediatric patients for imaging examinations. *Radiology* 237(1):288–294, 2005.
50. Kamat PP, McCracken CE, Gillespie SE, et al: Pediatric critical care physician-administered procedural sedation using propofol: a report from the Pediatric Sedation Research Consortium Database. *Pediatr Crit Care Med* 16(1):11–20, 2015.
51. Srinivasan M, Turmelle M, Depalma LM, et al: Procedural sedation for diagnostic imaging in children by pediatric hospitalists using propofol: analysis of the nature, frequency, and predictors of adverse events and interventions. *J Pediatr* 160(5):801–806, e1, 2012.
52. Mitchell AA, Louik C, Lacouture P, et al: Risks to children from computed tomographic scan premedication. *JAMA* 247(17):2385–2388, 1982.
53. Fallah R, Alaei A, Akhavan Karbasi S, Shajari A: Chloral hydrate, chloral hydrate—promethazine and chloral hydrate-hydroxyzine efficacy in electroencephalography sedation. *Indian J Pediatr* 81(6):541–546, 2014.
54. Dabir PA, Dummett CO, Musselman RJ, et al: Assessment of intranasal administration of midazolam for conscious sedation, using an atomizer. *J Am Acad Pediatr Dent* 23: 168, 2001.
55. ClinicalKey. Mepergan Fortis drug monograph. March 29, 2016. www.ClinicalKey.com. (Accessed 11 July 2016).
56. Benusis KP, Kapaun D, Furnam LJ: Respiratory depression in a child following meperidine, promethazine and chlorpromazine premedication: report of a case. *J Dent Child* 46(1):50–53, 1979.
57. Acute Pain Management Guideline Panel: Acute pain management: operative or medical procedures and trauma, clinical practice guideline, AHCPR Pub. No. 92-2, Rockville, MD, 1992, Agency for Health Care Policy and Research, Public Health Service, U.S. Department of Health and Human Services.
58. Nahata M, Clotz M, Krogg E: Adverse effects of meperidine, promethazine, and chlorpromazine for sedation in pediatric patients. *Clin Pediatr (Phila)* 24(10):558–560, 1985.
59. Warden CR, Frederick C: Midazolam and diazepam for pediatric seizures in the prehospital setting. *Prehosp Emerg Care* 10(4):463–467, 2006.
60. Corrigan M, Wilson SS, Hampton J: Safety and efficacy of intranasally administered medications in the emergency department and prehospital settings. *Am J Health Syst Pharm* 72(18):1544–1554, 2015.
61. Ghane MR, Javadzadeh HR, Mahmoudi S, et al: Intramuscular compared to intravenous midazolam for paediatric sedation: a study on cardiopulmonary safety and effectiveness. *Afr J Paediatr Surg* 11(3):219–224, 2014.
62. Shashikiran ND, Reddy SV, Yavagal CM: Conscious sedation—an artist's science! An Indian experience with midazolam. *J Indian Soc Pedod Prev Dent* 24(1):7–14, 2006.
63. Malamed SF, Quinn CL, Hatch HG: Pediatric sedation with intramuscular and intravenous midazolam. *Anesth Prog* 36(4-5):155–157, 1989.
64. Chiaretti A, Barone G, Rigante D, et al: Intranasal lidocaine and midazolam for procedural sedation in children. *Arch Dis Child* 96(2):160–163, 2011.
65. Greaves A: The use of midazolam as an intranasal sedative in dentistry. *SAAD Dig* 32:45–49, 2016.
66. Drysdale D: The use of intranasal midazolam in a special care dentistry department: technique and cases. *Prim Dent J* 4(2):42–48, 2015.
67. Wood M: The safety and efficacy of using a concentrated intranasal midazolam formulation for paediatric dental sedation. *SAAD Dig* 27:16–23, 2011.
68. Johnson E, Briskie D, Majewski R, et al: The physiologic and behavioral effects of oral and intranasal midazolam in pediatric dental patients. *Pediatr Dent* 32(3):229–238, 2010.
69. Wood M: The safety and efficacy of intranasal midazolam sedation combined with inhalation sedation with nitrous oxide and oxygen in paediatric dental patients as an alternative to general anaesthesia. *SAAD Dig* 26:12–22, 2010.
70. Lam C, Udin RD, Malamed SF, et al: Midazolam premedication in children: a pilot study comparing intramuscular and intranasal administration. *Anesth Prog* 52(2):56–61, 2005.
71. Primosch RE, Guelmann M: Comparison of drops versus spray administration of intranasal midazolam in two- and three-year old children for dental sedation. *Pediatr Dent* 27(5):401–408, 2005.
72. Shane SM, Carrel R: Ketamine intramuscularly for total dentistry in uncooperative, unmanageable, ambulatory children. *Anesth Prog* 18(1):6–8, 1971.
73. Tarjan I, Mikecz G, Denes J: Ambulatory anesthesia in pediatric dentistry. *Fogorv Sz* 82(2):45–48, 1989.
74. ClinicalKey. Ketamine drug monograph. June 24, 2016. www.ClinicalKey.com. (Accessed 13 July 2016).
75. Woolley SM, Hingston EJ, Shah J, Chadwick BL: Paediatric conscious sedation: views and experience of specialists in paediatric dentistry. *Br Dent J* 207(6):E11, discussion 280-281, 2009.
76. Wilson KE: Overview of paediatric dental sedation: 2. Nitrous oxide/oxygen inhalation sedation. *Dent Update* 40(10):822–824, 826-829, 2013.
77. Moore PA: Local anesthesia and narcotic drug interaction in pediatric dentistry. *Anesth Prog* 35(1):17, 1988.
78. American Society of Anesthesiologists: Practice guidelines for preoperative fasting and the use of pharmacologic agents to reduce the risk of pulmonary aspiration: application to healthy patients undergoing elective procedures. An updated report by the American Society of Anesthesiologists Committee on Standards and Practice Parameters. *Anesthesiology* 114(3):495–511, 2011.
79. Malviya S, Voepel-Lewis T, Prochaska G, Tait AR: Prolonged recovery and delayed side effects of sedation for diagnostic imaging studies in children. *Pediatrics* 105(3):E42, 2000.
80. Terndrup TE, Dire DJ, Madden CM, et al: A prospective analysis of intramuscular meperidine, promethazine, and chlorpromazine in pediatric emergency department patients. *Ann Emerg Med* 20(1):31–35, 1991.
81. Malviya S, Voepel-Lewis T, Ludomirsky A, et al: Can we improve the assessment of discharge readiness? A comparative study of observational and objective measures of depth of sedation in children. *Anesthesiology* 100(2): 218–224, 2004.

82. Coté CJ, Wilson S, American Academy of Pediatrics, American Academy of Pediatric Dentistry: Guidelines for monitoring and management of pediatric patients before, during, and after sedation for diagnostic and therapeutic procedures: update 2016. *Pediatrics* 138(1):e20161212, 2016. Appendix 1.

83. O'Neil J, Yonkman J, Talty J, Bull MJ: Transporting children with special health care needs: comparing recommendations and practice. *Pediatrics* 124(2):596–603, 2009.

84. Coté CJ, Wilson S: Guidelines for monitoring and management of pediatric patients before, during, and after sedation for diagnostic and therapeutic procedures: update 2016. American academy of pediatric dentistry, American academy of pediatrics. *Pediatr Dent* 38(4):E13–E39, 2016.

85. Dummett CO, Jr: Guidelines for hospital admission and discharge of pedodontic patients for restorative dentistry under general anesthesia, New Orleans, 1976, Department of Pedodontics, Louisiana State University School of Dentistry.

chapter 36

The Geriatric Patient

CHAPTER OUTLINE

When the United States was founded, life expectancy was about 35 years. By the mid-1800s it had increased to nearly 42 years. In 1950 life expectancy jumped to 68 years. By 1991 the average life expectancy was 75.5 years. In 2013 the most recent year for which life expectancy statistics were available, the average life expectancy in the United States was 78.8 years (81.2 years for females, 76.4 years for males) (Fig. 36.1).[1] With an estimated life expectancy in 2016 of 79 years, the United States ranks fifty-third worldwide.[2] Monaco (89.47 years) is first, with Japan, Singapore, and Macau all with life expectancies over 84 years.[2] On the basis of mortality experienced in 2013, a person in the United States aged 50 could expect to live an average of 31.6 more years, for a total of 81.6 years. A person aged 65 could expect to live an average of 19.3 more years, for a total of 84.3, and a person aged 85 could expect to live an average of 6.6 more years, for a total of 91.6.[2] Dentists can expect to be treating increasing numbers of elderly patients as life expectancy increases and individuals maintain or prosthetically replace their natural dentition.

Classically, age 65 is considered the beginning of the geriatric period. This is an arbitrary age cut-off that is thought to have originated from two independent sources, the first of which was Imperial Germany.[3] The Bismarck government decided that they had only enough money for those 65 years of age and older. The second source was a group of English physicians who decided to care exclusively for the elderly. They decided, based on population alone, that they would have time for only those older than 65 years.[4]

Adults age 65 and older ("older adults") are the fastest-growing segment of the United States population, and their number is expected to double to 89 million people between 2010 and 2050.[5]

The geriatric population as a group is split into three parts: young-old, ages 65 to 74; old, ages 75 to 84; and oldest-old, age 85 and older. In 1998 12.7% of the general population was 65 and older, and 1.5% was 85 years and older. By July 2015 those percentages had increased to 14.9% and 1.9%, respectively.[6,7] California has the largest population numbers of persons older than 65, but Florida has the distinction of being the state with the largest percentage of residents older than 65 (18.6%).[8,9]

It is important to remember, though, that no matter what age is chosen as the beginning of the geriatric phase, everyone ages in two ways: chronologically and biologically.[4] This makes elderly individuals a physiologically diverse group because there is no correlation of biologic age with chronologic age because of the effects of concomitant diseases.

Almost 75% of young-old persons (in 1992) who were not institutionalized considered their health to be good, very good, or excellent, compared with almost two thirds of individuals older than age 75.[10] It has been found that an individual's *perceived* health is very important. Persons with chronic disease were more likely to die if they considered themselves to be in poor health compared with those who believed themselves to be in good health despite the presence of chronic disease.[10]

Although more people live to advanced age, they do so with increasing illness and disability. Many have diseases, such as arthritis, diabetes, osteoporosis, and senile dementia. These chronic diseases are partially responsible for the functional limitations that some elderly individuals experience. Functional

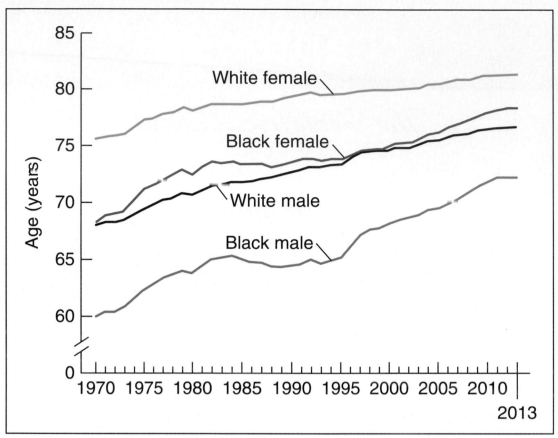

Figure 36.1 Life expectancy by race and sex: United States, 1970–2013. (From CDC/NCHS, National Vital Statistics System, Mortality.)

limitations may include difficulty walking, getting outside, dressing, and other activities of daily living. Individuals with mild impairments usually are living within the community. As individuals acquire more impairments, the likelihood that they will be living in a care facility increases. The active life expectancy becomes an important concept in thinking about elderly individuals. The definition of *active life expectancy* is the expected years of physical, emotional, and functional well-being.[11,12]

The top five causes of death in elderly individuals in 2013 (in the United States) were heart disease, malignant neoplasms, chronic lower respiratory disease, cerebrovascular disease, and Alzheimer disease.[13] As individuals age, heart disease accounts for a larger percentage of the deaths (about 44% of deaths in individuals aged 85 years and older).[13]

The aging process involves both physiologic and pathologic changes that may alter patients' ability to respond to stress and their response to drug administration (Table 36.1). Changes that occur with aging include a decrease in lean body mass, an increase in body fat (more so in women), and a decrease in total body water (more so in men).[14] As a result, the geriatric patient has a smaller central compartment (decreased body water), the rapidly equilibrating compartment is smaller (decreased lean body mass), and the slowly equilibrating compartment is larger (increased body fat).[14] The overall effect

is that when a medication is given intravenously, there will be higher peak concentration because of the smaller central compartment. The volume of distribution should also be increased because of the body fat increases, and there may also be a longer duration of drug effect.[14] The question now is whether geriatric patients really have changes in their pharmacodynamics (what the drug does to the body), or is it that there are changes in the early-phase pharmacokinetics (what the body does to the drug) that make the elderly patient seem more sensitive to medications.[15]

Adverse drug interactions are more common in elderly patients than in younger patients. One reason is that geriatric patients take more medication—medication to control the symptoms of age-related diseases. Approximately half of adults aged 75 years or older take at least two different prescription medications.[16]

Assessing the geriatric patient's physical status can be a challenge. Aging is a process rather than a defined disease. Changes that are seen in all elderly patients are a function of altered tissue and organ system structure and function, whereas changes occurring in tissue and organ system function that are not seen in all members of that population are probably age-related disease.[17] The aging process may alter patients' abilities to respond to stress and their response to drug

Table 36.1	Physiologic and Pathologic Changes in Geriatric Patients	
ORGAN SYSTEM	**ANATOMIC CHANGES**	**FUNCTIONAL CHANGES**
Body composition	Increased lipid fraction Loss of skeletal muscle and other components of lean body mass	Increased half-life for lipid-soluble drugs Decreased O_2 consumption, heat production, and cardiac output
Nervous system	Attrition of neurons Decreased neurotransmitter activity	Deafferentation, neurogenic atrophy, and decreased anesthetic requirement Impaired autonomic homeostasis
Cardiovascular system	Decreased arterial elasticity Ventricular hypertrophy Reduced adrenergic responsiveness	Increased impedance to ejection, widened pulse pressure Decreased maximum cardiac output
Pulmonary system	Loss of lung elastin Increased thoracic stiffness Reduced alveolar surface area	Increased residual volume Loss of vital capacity Impaired efficiency of gas exchange Increased work of breathing
Renal system	Reduced vascularity Tissue atrophy	Decreased plasma flow, glomerular filtration rate, drug clearance, and ability to handle salt and water loads
Hepatic system	Reduced tissue mass	Reduced hepatic blood flow and drug clearance

From Miller R: Effects of aging on body composition and major organ systems. In Miller R, ed: *Anesthesia*, ed 4, New York, 1994, Churchill Livingstone; and Muravchick S: *Geroanesthesia: Principles for management of the elderly patient*, St. Louis, 1997, Mosby.

administration. Geriatric patients therefore are potentially at increased risk during all dental and medical procedures. An organ system approach to preoperative evaluation permits evaluation of the functional status of each major organ system, emphasizing the functional reserve of the systems most greatly affected by anesthetic medications (heart, lungs, central nervous system, and airway). Functional reserve is the difference between basal and maximal organ system function. Each individual organ system's functional reserve should be evaluated by medical history review, laboratory data when appropriate, and physical examination.[17]

Functional reserve is the margin that is needed to meet increased demands for cardiac output, carbon dioxide excretion, and other physiologic parameters. A patient's functional reserve declines with increasing age simply as a result of the aging process.[17] Geriatric patients have a minimal functional reserve; their organs function at or near capacity during ordinary activities. When these individuals are subjected to stress, this minimal reserve contributes to an overall difficulty in responding to a situation or illness. The organ systems most affected by anesthesia and sedation are the central nervous system (CNS), cardiovascular system, respiratory system, hepatic system, and the renal system.

Many physiologic and pathologic changes are encountered in the geriatric patient. A decrease in tissue elasticity is a major physiologic change that significantly affects organs throughout the body. For example, in patients 75 years of age, cerebral blood flow is only 80% of what it was in patients 30 years of age. Cardiac output has declined to roughly two thirds of what it was; renal blood flow has decreased to less than half of its volume at this younger age; and hepatic blood flow has also

decreased.[18] This decrease in renal perfusion is potentially significant with certain drugs, primarily those in which urinary excretion is a principal means of removing the drug and its metabolites from the body. This decrease in renal perfusion is probably the one most responsible for increased plasma drug concentrations. Drugs such as penicillin, tetracycline, and digoxin exhibit greatly increased terminal elimination (β) half-lives.

The effect of aging on the nervous system includes cortical neuron loss and a reduction in neuron density. This does not affect daily function as much as it affects how the patient will respond to sedative and anesthetic agents and stress.[17] Brain atrophy occurs in the elderly; about one third of gross brain mass is involved, mostly evident in the gray matter. There is also a generalized decrease in brain neurotransmitters, but there is no decrease in the affinity for, or density of, CNS benzodiazepine receptors with age,[19] even though elderly patients seem to be more sensitive to the medication.

There is some evidence that older adults may experience some cognitive dysfunction after anesthesia.[20] Delirium is perhaps the most significant age-related postoperative complication of sedation and general anesthesia. It is characterized by an acute decline in cognitive function and attention, with evidence from the patient's history that this is due to physiologic derangement, a medication, or is multifactorial.[21] Importantly, delirium is distinct from chronic cognitive decline and dementia.[22] Depending on the patient population in question, the prevalence of postoperative delirium ranges from 9% to 44%, with the highest rates observed after high-risk procedures, such as cardiac surgery, vascular surgery, and hip fracture surgery.[22] There are three distinct motor subtypes of delirium:

	Diagnosing Delirium: The Confusion Assessment Method – Short Form	
Table 36.2		
FEATURE	**QUESTION**	**ANSWER REQUIRED**
Acute onset and fluctuating course	Is there evidence of an acute change in mental status from baseline, and if so, did it tend to come and go or increase and decrease in intensity?	"Yes" answer
Inattention	Did the patient have difficulty focusing attention?	"Yes" answer
Disorganized thinking	Was the patient's thinking disorganized or incoherent?	"Yes" answer
Altered level of consciousness	What was the patient's level of consciousness (alert, vigilant, lethargic, stupor, or coma)?	Any answer other than alert
SCORING: Suggestion of diagnosis requires the presence of (1) and (2) and either (3) or (4)		

Adapted from Inouye SK, van Dyck CH, Alessi CA, et al: Clarifying confusion: the confusion assessment method. A new method for detection of delirium, *Ann Intern* Med 113(12):941–948, 1990.

hypoactive delirium, which presents with lack of awareness and decreased motor activity; hyperactive delirium, which occurs when a patient is combative or agitated; and a mixed subtype.[23–25]

In order for delirium to be diagnosed, at-risk patients or patients with suspected cognitive impairment should undergo an assessment concerning the following: disturbance of consciousness, a change in cognition, acute onset, and evidence from the history that this is due to physiologic derangement (for example, hypoxia, hypoglycemia, electrolyte abnormality, acid–base abnormality), an intoxicant, medications, or more than one cause.[25] One of the most widely used instruments for assessing postoperative cognitive impairment is the Confusion Assessment Method (CAM)[26] (Table 36.2).

The dental office team should evaluate all postoperative patients who develop delirium for possible precipitating conditions. These include:

a. **Uncontrolled pain**
b. **Hypoxia**
c. Pneumonia
d. Infection (wound, indwelling catheter and bloodstream, urinary tract, sepsis)
e. Electrolyte abnormalities
f. Urinary retention
g. Fecal impaction
h. **Medications**
i. **Hypoglycemia**

Items highlighted in **bold** are more likely etiologies of delirium in the outpatient dental environment.

In the dental office environment, American Society of Anesthesiologists (ASA) 1 and ASA 2 and selected ASA 3 patients are considered candidates for sedation. The risk of a geriatric patient becoming confused following minimal or moderate sedation, though possible, is quite small.

The recommended first-line treatment of delirium following sedation or general anesthesia includes (1) frequent reorientation with voice, calendars, and clocks; (2) a calm environment; (3) avoiding the use of physical restraints; (4) having familiar persons and objects in close proximity to the patient; and (5) ensuring that glasses and hearing aids are readily available.[21,27]

Autonomic functions change with age. Elevations in plasma epinephrine and norepinephrine are seen both at rest and in response to stress. This is to compensate for a reduction in responsiveness of autonomic end organs. In general, the autonomic system is less self-regulated than in the younger adult. As a result, elderly patients are at greater risk for postural hypotension and falls. It is estimated that approximately 30% of people over 65 years of age in the community fall every year.[28,31] Risk factors for falls in the sedated geriatric patient include the following: (1) altered mental status; (2) dehydration (consider NPO status of the geriatric patient); (3) frequent toileting; (4) history of falls; (5) impaired gait or mobility; (6) medications (e.g., sedatives); and (7) visual impairment.[29,30]

Age changes the mechanics of the heart but has little effect on cardiac output.[14] Elderly patients develop some degree of hypertrophy but are able to maintain stroke volume by increasing preload and slightly decreasing the heart rate. The elderly heart compared with a young heart is less tolerant of hypovolemia; it relies on ventricular filling to maintain the length–tension relationship to generate adequate cardiac effort.[31] The elderly heart is more sensitive to the cardiac-depressant effects of anesthetic medications. A decrease in cardiac output is associated with thiopental administration, correlated with a decreased dose requirement in elderly individuals.[32,33]

With aging, elasticity in pulmonary tissues is lost and the intercostal muscles atrophy. The chest wall becomes less compliant as a result of fibrocalcification. In general, there is a decrease in vital capacity and an increase in residual volume.[17,34]

There is an overall decrease in clearance of sedative and anesthetic medications because of decreases in liver volume, blood flow, and intrinsic hepatic capacity. This reflects a loss of tissue mass. Anesthesia also decreases liver blood flow so there is a reduced maintenance dose requirement with drugs that are cleared rapidly by the liver (i.e., propofol).[14]

Albumin concentration decreases with age, and β1-acid glycoprotein increases with age. The influence of age depends on the site of plasma protein binding.[35] If a medication is highly protein bound, a decrease in albumin will result in a greater percentage of the drug available to produce its actions. For example, diazepam is approximately 98.5% bound (1.5% free and available to exert its effect) in younger individuals. In elderly persons, it is only 97% bound. This leaves twice as much diazepam available (3% versus 1.5%) to produce its clinical actions. Given the same drug dosage, the patient with diminished drug binding should exhibit more profound clinical actions.

As age increases, renal blood flow decreases because of tissue atrophy. The net result is an increase in the elimination half-time of anesthetic medications that are cleared by the kidneys, resulting in more elevated blood levels of the drug and potentially an exaggerated clinical or subclinical effect.[14,36]

COMMON HEALTH PROBLEMS

Some of the more commonly seen ailments and diseases of the geriatric population are discussed briefly in the following paragraphs along with possible implications for dental treatment.

Arthritis

The arthritic patient may exhibit difficulty with positioning in the dental chair. Modification of positioning may be necessary for successful and comfortable treatment. The arthritic patient may also have decreased vital capacity because of a decrease in thoracic compliance. Drug management of arthritis commonly includes administration of salicylates and nonsteroidal antiinflammatory drugs (NSAIDs), including COX-2 specific inhibitors.

Hypertension

A desirable level for blood pressure is below 120/80 mm Hg, without the patient experiencing unwanted symptoms. Side effects may be seen with all antihypertensive medications; postural hypotension is the most commonly seen side effect. Antihypertensive agents may accentuate postural hypotension produced by some of the CNS depressants used for sedation. Elderly patients are prone to hypotension even without the presence of antihypertensive medications, because the autonomic system in general and homeostasis specifically is not as tightly regulated. Careful change of patient position and slow titration of sedative medications help minimize the significance of this side effect. Observe extreme caution when permitting the patient to stand following sedation in order to minimize the effect of postural hypotension and the potential for injury secondary to falls.

Heart Disease

Atherosclerotic heart disease (ASHD) is present in differing degrees in all patients older than 65 years. Heart disease is the number-one cause of death in the elderly population. Possible signs and symptoms of ASHD include elevated blood pressure, irregularities in cardiac rhythm, undue fatigue, and "discomfort" in the chest on exertion (e.g., angina pectoris).

The administration of sedative medications may be indicated in these patients to decrease endogenous catecholamine output as a method of minimizing the development of potentially serious complications.

Angina pectoris is a common clinical manifestation of ASHD. Angina may be seen in both the premyocardial and postmyocardial infarction patient. This patient may be at greater risk for a medical emergency during treatment. Inhalation sedation with nitrous oxide-oxygen (N_2O-O_2) is an excellent sedative technique for this patient. Drug therapy for angina includes the administration of nitrates, which are vasodilators. Postural hypotension may develop when these agents are administered in the management of an acute episode. Proper positioning minimizes the development of postural hypotension.

Emphysema

Emphysema is one form of chronic obstructive pulmonary disease (COPD) that may be seen in the geriatric population. Chronic exposure to pollutants (e.g., cigarette smoke, air pollution) is the most common cause. Because the elderly patient's respiratory reserves are already quite diminished, stress reduction becomes important in patient management.

Glaucoma

Glaucoma is an abnormal accumulation of aqueous humor within the eye that leads to an increase in intraocular pressure. Patients with narrow-angle glaucoma may be treated with pilocarpine eyedrops. This medication constricts the pupils so that the aqueous humor may drain. When an anticholinergic medication, such as atropine, is administered, the iris folds back into the angle of the anterior chamber and blocks the outflow of the aqueous humor, increasing intraocular pressure. This effect usually requires larger-than-therapeutic doses of atropine (more than 1 mg). Atropine in the usual therapeutic dose (0.5 mg or less) is not contraindicated in these patients. Timolol, a β-adrenergic blocking agent, is used as an antiglaucoma agent. It is administered alone or in combination with other intraocular pressure–lowering agents.

MANAGEMENT OF PAIN AND ANXIETY

The need for adequate pain control during treatment is as compelling in the 65 years of age and older patient as in any other age group. There are no specific contraindications in the geriatric patient to the administration of any local anesthetic or the use of any anesthetic technique in particular. It is, of course, incumbent on the operator to observe the guidelines for sedation and/or general anesthesia established by the state or province in which they practice. Local anesthetic drug doses should be kept as low as possible in the older age groups because of the unknown degree of hepatic and renal dysfunction that may be present. The elimination half-life of the local anesthetic may, in some instances, be considerably prolonged, and plasma levels may remain elevated for extended periods.

It is also important to be cognizant of all medications that the individual may be taking to prevent possible drug interactions. Block injections are preferred to infiltration because a smaller volume is used to achieve a wider area of anesthesia. The use of vasoconstrictors is not contraindicated in the normotensive patient or the patient with controlled hypertension. Caution should be exercised when using vasoconstrictors in the geriatric patient with uncontrolled hypertension. The benefits should be weighed against the risk of increased heart rate, increased blood pressure, and possible cardiac dysrhythmias.[37]

The geriatric patient may also be dental phobic or noncooperative because of dementia. CNS-depressant drugs may be indicated in these cases. Choosing an anesthetic technique and medication depends on the severity of coexisting disease and age-related disease. The practitioner must also keep in mind that the geriatric patient is more likely to develop adverse drug reactions than is the younger adult patient. The pharmacokinetics and pharmacodynamics of some medications may be profoundly influenced by age. For example, midazolam pharmacokinetics and pharmacodynamics are influenced by age. There is a 75% decrease in effective dose from age 20 to age 90.[38,39]

Since its publication in 1991 the Beers Criteria for Potentially Inappropriate Medication (PIM) Use in Older Adults has been the most consulted source of information about the safety of prescribing medications for older adults.[40] Updates were published in 1997 and 2003.[41,42] The most recent update, in 2012, uses a comprehensive, systematic review and grading of the evidence on drug-related problems and adverse drug events (ADEs) in older adults.[43] The 2012 Beers paper is a valuable resource that should be consulted by any doctor treating an elderly population. Table 36.3, adapted from the Beers Criteria for PIM, lists sedative/anesthetic drugs considered to be deserving of careful scrutiny before being administered to elderly patients.

Inhalation sedation with N_2O-O_2 is the most highly recommended technique of sedation for the geriatric patient. In additional to its titratability, it offers the advantage of providing a light (minimal to moderate) sedative technique with the benefits of supplemental oxygenation.

Oral sedation is indicated in geriatric patients. Age does not seem to affect absorption of oral medications. Because orally administered drugs cannot be precisely titrated, it is recommended that drugs be used in smaller dosages on the initial visit and then titrated by appointment as necessary. Medications such as benzodiazepines and the newer nonbarbiturate sedative-hypnotics, zolpidem and zaleplon, are useful in managing mild anxiety. Benzodiazepines, such as triazolam, are also indicated in the management of anxiety in the elderly patient. The newer nonbarbiturate sedative-hypnotics are chemically unrelated to benzodiazepines but work on a subset of the benzodiazepine receptor. They are both typically prescribed as sleep aids. Both of these medications have an onset of action of about 20 minutes. Barbiturates can no longer be recommended because of their long duration of action and generalized

Table 36.3	Suggested Dose Adjustments for Anesthetic Drugs in Older Patients	
DRUG	**USUAL QUOTED DOSAGE**	**SUGGESTED ADJUSTMENT**
Induction Agents		
Propofol	Bolus 2–2.5 mg/kg Infusion 100–250 µg/kg/min	1.5–1.8 mg/kg or 20% reduction in bolus dose 30% reduction in infusion
Midazolam	0.2–0.3 mg/kg	0.05–0.15 mg/kg in premedicated patients 20% reduction in patients >55 y 75% reduction in patients >90 y
Etomidate	0.3–0.4 mg/kg	0.2 mg/kg
Inhalational Agents		
Isoflurane	1.2%[a]	MAC is decreased by 6% per decade of increasing age
Sevoflurane	1.8%[a]	
Desflurane	6.6%[a]	
Opioids		
Morphine	0.1–0.2 mg/kg intraoperatively 1–2 mg boluses titrated to effect for acute postoperative analgesia	50% reduction in dose No change
Fentanyl	1–2 µg/kg for short-term analgesia	50% reduction in dose
Remifentanil	Bolus 0.5–1 µg/kg Infusion 0.2–0.5 µg/min	50% reduction in bolus dose 33% reduction in infusion

[a]Minimum alveolar concentration (MAC) values show. Adapted from Das et al.[44]

From Sangeeta D, Forrest K, Howell S: General anaesthesia in elderly patients with cardiovascular disorders, *Drugs and Aging* 27(4):265–282, 2010, Springer, with permission.

CNS-depressant effect. They may also occasionally produce delirium in the geriatric patient. Antihistamines may also be used as antianxiety medications.

Intramuscular (IM) sedation is generally not recommended because of the inability to titrate the medication. This technique is usually reserved for the induction of anesthesia in uncooperative patients. When required, midazolam is the medication of choice, keeping in mind the need to decrease the dose of drug in the elderly patient.

Intravenous (IV) moderate sedation is recommended for patients with anxiety. Vascular access in the older patient may be more difficult because of the loss of elasticity and increase in fragility of the veins. Titration is the ultimate safeguard in IV moderate sedation. Titration should occur even more slowly in the geriatric individual because of the pharmacokinetic changes that occur. The patient should be maintained at as light a sedative level as is compatible with comfort. Supplemental O_2 is recommended for all IV moderate sedation procedures in the geriatric patient population.

The use of *outpatient general anesthesia* depends on the overall health of the patient and the absence of significant systemic disease. The elderly patient with dementia is a typical patient requiring outpatient general anesthesia for dental care. This patient may be safely treated in an outpatient setting if he or she does not have significant systemic disease. It is also appropriate to consult the patient's primary care physician about the patient's overall health and presence of coexisting disease, keeping in mind that a "healthy" 80-year-old is not as healthy as a healthy 30-year-old.

Postoperative delirium (see the discussion earlier) is a potential side effect whenever CNS-depressant drugs are administered to an elderly patient.

REFERENCES

1. Xu J, Murphy SL, Kochanek KD, Bastian BA: Deaths: final data for 2013. *Natl Vital Stat Rep* 64(2):1–119, 2016.
2. The world: Life expectancy (2016). www.geoba.se/population. Accessed 15 July 2016.
3. The Editors of Encyclopædia Britannica: Old age, https://www.britannica.com/science/old-age. Accessed 15 July 2016.
4. Gambert SR: Aging: an overview. *Spec Care Dent* 3:147, 1983.
5. Werner C: *The older population: 2010*, Washington DC, November 2011, U.S. Census Bureau.
6. United States Census Bureau: Quick Facts, United States. Persons 65 years and over, percent, July 1, 2015. https://www.census.gov/quickfacts/table/PST045215/00. Accessed 15 July 2016.
7. Administration on Aging: Projected future growth of the older population. http://www.aoa.acl.gov/aging_statistics/future_growth/future_growth.aspx. Accessed 15 July 2016.
8. Colby SL, Ortman JM: Projections of the size and composition of the U.S. population: 2014 to 2060. U.S. Department of Commerce, Economics and Statistics Administration, U.S. Census Bureau, www.census.gov. March 2015. Accessed 15 July 2016.
9. World Atlas: States with the largest elderly population. http://www.worldatlas.com/articles/the-us-states-with-the-oldest-population.html. Accessed 15 July 2016.
10. Rogers RC: Sociodemographic characteristics of long-lived and healthy individuals. *Popul Dev Rev* 21(1):33–58, 1995.
11. Katz S, Branch LG, Branson MH, et al: Active life expectancy. *N Engl J Med* 309(20):1218–1224, 1983.
12. Branch LG, Guralnik JM, Foley DJ, et al: Active life expectancy for 10,000 Caucasian men and women in three communities. *J Gerontol* 46(4):M145–M150, 1991.
13. Centers for Disease Control and Prevention: National Center for Health Statistics. Older Persons' Health. Health United States, 2015. Table 58. http://www.cdc.gov/nchs/fastats/older-american-health.htm. Accessed 15 July 2015.
14. Shafer SL: The pharmacology of anesthetic drugs in elderly patients. *Anesthesiol Clin North Am* 18(1):1–29, 2000.
15. Homer TD, Stanski DR: The effect of increasing age on thiopental disposition and anesthetic requirement. *Anesthesiology* 62(6):714–724, 1985.
16. Schecter BM, Erwin WG, Gerbino PP: The role of the pharmacist. In Abrams WB, Berkow R, editors: *The Merck manual of geriatrics*, Rahway, NJ, 1990, Merck Sharp & Dohme.
17. Muravchick S: Preoperative assessment of the elderly patient: geriatric anesthesia. *Anesthesiol Clin North Am* 18(1):71–89, 2000.
18. Hevesi ZG, Hammel LL: Geriatric disorders. In Hines RL, Marschall KE, editors: *Stoelting's anesthesia and co-existing diseases*, ed 6, Philadelphia, 2012, Elsevier Saunders, pp 642–654.
19. Barnhill JG, Greenblatt DJ, Miller LG, et al: Kinetic and dynamic components of increased benzodiazepine sensitivity in aging animals. *J Pharmacol Exp Ther* 253(3):1153–1161, 1990.
20. Moeller JT, the ISOPCD investigators: Long-term postoperative cognitive dysfunction in the elderly: ISPOCDI-1 study. *Lancet* 351(9106):857–861, 1998.
21. AGS Expert Panel on Postoperative Delirium in Older Adults: American Geriatrics Society Clinical Practice Guideline for Postoperative Delirium in Older Adults. 2014.
22. Mohanty S, Rosenthal RA, Russell MM, et al: Optimal perioperative management of the geriatric surgical patient. American College of Surgeons National Surgical Quality Improvement Program/American Geriatric Society, Best Practices Guideline. 2016, pp. 1-65.
23. Marcantonio E, Ta T, Duthie E, Resnick NM: Delirium severity and psychomotor types: their relationship with outcomes after hip fracture repair. *J Am Geriatr Soc* 50(5):850–857, 2002.
24. Robinson TN, Eiseman B: Postoperative delirium in the elderly: diagnosis and management. *Clin Interv Aging* 3(2):351–355, 2008.
25. American Psychiatric Association: *Diagnostic and statistical manual of mental disorders*, ed 5, Washington, DC, 2013, American Psychiatric Association.
26. Inouye SK, van Dyck CH, Alessi CA, et al: Clarifying confusion: the confusion assessment method. A new method for detection of delirium. *Ann Intern Med* 113(12):941–948, 1990.
27. NICE: Delirium: diagnosis, prevention and management. NICE clinical guideline 103 2010; NICE guideline. Available at: www.nice.org.uk/CG103. Accessed 17 July 2016.
28. Gillespie LD, Robertson MC, Gillespie WJ, et al: Interventions for preventing falls in older people living in the community. *Cochrane Database Syst Rev* (9):CD007146, 2012.
29. Amador LF, Loera JA: Preventing postoperative falls in the older adult. *J Am Coll Surg* 204(3):447–453, 2007.
30. American Geriatrics Society/British Geriatrics Society Panel on Prevention of Falls in Older Persons: Summary of the Updated American Geriatrics Society/British Geriatrics Society clinical practice guideline for prevention of falls in older persons. *J Am Geriatr Soc* 59(1):148–157, 2011.
31. Rooke GA: Autonomic and cardiovascular function in the geriatric patient. *Anesthesiol Clin North Am* 18(1):31–46, 2000.
32. Avram MJ, Sanghvi R, Henthorn TK, et al: Determinants of thiopental induction dose requirements. *Anesth Analg* 76(1):10–17, 1993.
33. Christensen JH, Andreasen F, Jansen JA: Pharmacokinetics and pharmacodynamics of thiopentone: a comparison between young and elderly patients. *Anaesthesia* 37(4):398–404, 1982.
34. Zaugg M, Lucchinetti E: Respiratory function in the elderly. *Anesthesiol Clin North Am* 18(1):47–58, 2000.

35. Macklon AF, Barton M, James O, Rawlins MD: The effect of age on the pharmacokinetics of diazepam. *Clin Sci* 59(6):479–483, 1980.

36. Sieber F, Pauldine R: Geriatric anesthesia. In Miller R, editor: *Miller's anesthesia*, ed 8, Philadelphia, 2015, Elsevier Saunders, pp 2407–2422.

37. Malamed SF: Anxiety and pain control in the older patient. *Spec Care Dent* 7:22, 1987.

38. Bell GD, Spickett GP, Reeve PA, et al: Intravenous midazolam for upper gastrointestinal endoscopy: a study of 800 consecutive cases relating dose to age and sex of patient. *Br J Clin Pharmacol* 23(2):241–243, 1987.

39. Hughes MA, Glass PS, Jacobs JR: Context-sensitive half-time in multicompartment pharmacokinetic models for intravenous anesthetic drugs. *Anesthesiology* 76:334, 1992.

40. Beers MH, Ouslander JG, Rollingher I, et al: Explicit criteria for determining inappropriate medication use in nursing home residents. *Arch Intern Med* 151(9):1825–1832, 1991.

41. Beers MH: Explicit criteria for determining potentially inappropriate medication use by the elderly. An update. *Arch Intern Med* 157(14):1531–1536, 1997.

42. Fick DM, Cooper JW, Wade WE, et al: Updating the Beers Criteria for potentially inappropriate medication use in older adults: results of a US consensus panel of experts. *Arch Intern Med* 163(22):2716–2724, 2003.

43. The American Geriatrics Society 2012 Beers Criteria Update Expert Panel: AGS updated Beers Criteria for potentially inappropriate medication use in older adults. *J Am Geriatr Soc* 60:616–631, 2012.

44. Das S, Forrest K, Howell S: General anaesthesia in elderly patients with cardiovascular disorders: choice of anaesthetic agent. *Drugs Aging* 27(4):265–282, 2010.

chapter 37

The Medically Compromised Patient

CHAPTER OUTLINE

When we previously discussed the management of stress as it is related to medical and dental treatment, it was mentioned that many patients are unable to tolerate the "usual" degree of stress associated with dental therapy and, in some cases, with everyday existence. These persons usually have an underlying medical problem that limits their ability to handle stress in a normal manner. When this patient is faced with a situation in which increased stress is present, there is an increased likelihood of this patient experiencing an acute exacerbation of their underlying disease process. Examples might include the patient with a history of coronary artery disease suffering from chest pain, the epileptic patient having a tonic-clonic seizure, or an asthmatic patient having an acute episode of bronchospasm during periods of increased stress, as might occur during dental treatment.

Advances in medicine and pharmacotherapeutics have made it possible for more medically compromised patients to become increasingly functional to the degree that their existence is no longer confined to their home. Partially or fully ambulatory, they may now be gainfully employed and seek dental and medical care as would any other patient. These persons, however, do represent a greater degree of risk during stressful times. How then can a medically compromised patient be better managed? Reduction of stress associated with treatment is the primary goal in the successful dental management of these patients. Awareness and knowledge of the underlying disease process are essential. In this chapter, disease entities that are more commonly seen in an ambulatory setting are reviewed. Following a brief description of each disease process, we list factors that tend to exacerbate it and review the methods available to successfully minimize perioperative stress in this patient.

CARDIOVASCULAR DISEASE

Cardiovascular disease (CVD) ranks as the number-one cause of death in the United States, United Kingdom, and other industrialized nations. It is estimated that the number of persons in the United States with signs and symptoms of CVD exceeds 83.6 million.[1] In 2014 614,348 persons died from CVD in the United States. Cancer, the second leading cause, was responsible for 591,699 deaths.[2]

Significant advances have occurred in both the surgical and pharmacologic management of many cardiovascular disorders. Patients who once suffered from extremely severe, almost debilitating anginal pains caused by coronary artery disease are today asymptomatic as a result of balloon angioplasty with placement of stents or coronary artery bypass and graft procedures. Newer drugs, such as β-adrenergic blockers (e.g., propranolol), calcium channel blockers (e.g., verapamil, nifedipine), and angiotensin-converting enzyme (ACE) inhibitors (e.g., captopril), have enabled patients to lead more normal lives despite the continued presence of a serious cardiovascular disorder.

In view of the fact that more than 10% of the American population has signs and symptoms of clinically significant CVD, it stands to reason that the dentist will be called on to manage the oral health needs of many cardiovascular-risk patients. Although there are many causes for the various CVDs, there is one factor that, when present, is responsible for dramatically increasing the risk of an acute exacerbation. This is a myocardial oxygen (O_2) requirement that exceeds the supply capability of the coronary arteries. When myocardial O_2 requirements are not satisfactorily met, the patient responds with an acute exacerbation of the underlying disorder. For example, chest pain and/or dysrhythmias may develop in the patient with angina, and dyspnea will occur in the patient with heart failure (HF).

Patients at cardiovascular risk are usually able to tolerate elective and emergency dental care. Modifications in the planned dental treatment are based on the severity (American Society of Anesthesiologists [ASA] 2, 3, or 4) of the disease process as determined through physical evaluation of the patient (see Chapter 4). Sedation and pain control, though important for all patients, are of much greater importance in these patients than in ASA 1 patients. Specific details relating to the management of cardiovascular-risk patients are discussed in the following section.

Angina Pectoris

Angina pectoris is usually a clinical manifestation of arteriosclerotic heart disease, but may occasionally occur in the absence of significant disease through coronary artery spasm, severe aortic stenosis, or aortic insufficiency. The basic mechanism involved in angina pectoris is a discrepancy between myocardial

O_2 demand and O_2 delivery through the coronary arteries. Anginal pain is described as a squeezing or pressurelike pain, retrosternal or slightly to the left of the sternum, that appears suddenly during exertion and may radiate in a set pattern (Fig. 37.1); it typically resolves with rest or the administration of nitrates. Patients with angina may be taking long-acting nitrates, such as isosorbide dinitrate (Isordil, Sorbitrate), to minimize occurrence of acute episodes. Nitroglycerin is available for administration in several forms, including an intravenous (IV) form, translingual spray (Nitrolingual), transmucosal tablet, oral sustained-release form, topical ointment, transdermal patch, and the traditional sublingual tablet.[3]

The patient with stable angina represents an ASA 3 risk. Persons with easily managed and less frequent episodes might be classified as ASA 2 (though stable angina pectoris meets the classical definition of ASA 3), and persons with daily (or more frequent) episodes or episodes that are increasing in frequency or severity (unstable angina) are categorized as ASA 4. An estimated 7.8 million Americans have angina pectoris.[1]

Factors increasing the likelihood of an acute exacerbation of anginal pain include the following:

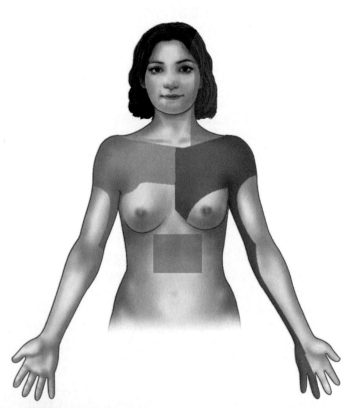

■ Substernal pain projected to left shoulder and arm (ulnar nerve distribution)

■ Less frequent referred sites including right shoulder and arm, left jaw, neck, and epigastrium

Figure 37.1 Radiation patterns of chest pain.

- Physical activity
- Hot, humid environment
- Cold weather
- Large meals
- Emotional stress (e.g., argument, anxiety, sexual excitement)
- Caffeine ingestion
- Fever, anemia, thyrotoxicosis
- Cigarette smoking
- Secondhand smoke (smoke from other persons' cigarettes)
- Smog
- High altitudes

As with all patients, those with a history of anginal pain may exhibit heightened anxiety before dental or surgical treatment. Sedation is especially indicated in these patients because of the effects of anxiety on the cardiovascular system (CVS). Increased blood levels of the catecholamines epinephrine and norepinephrine lead to an increase in the heart rate and an increase in the strength of each contraction. The net result is an increase in the O_2 requirement of the myocardium. In the presence of coronary artery disease, this increased demand may not be met, resulting in an acute anginal episode. Dysrhythmias may also occur at this time. Minimizing stress and maximizing oxygenation of the patient are desired goals in preventing anginal episodes.

Oral sedation is indicated. Minimal-to-moderate levels of sedation minimize the risk of developing possible clinically significant respiratory depression, which could induce myocardial ischemia. Though not essential, the delivery of O_2 through a nasal cannula or nasal hood throughout treatment is recommended, especially in the ASA 3 or 4 patient with a history of angina.

Intramuscular (IM) and intranasal (IN) sedation are not usually indicated. The use of IM or IN sedation in adult patients is rarely indicated in general; these routes are used primarily in pediatric patients (IM, IN) or adults with significant mental or physical disabilities (IM). Should an occasion necessitate the administration of IM sedation to a patient with angina, the level of sedation—though not titratable—should be kept minimal to moderate. O_2 should be delivered via nasal cannula or nasal hood throughout treatment and the recovery period.

Inhalation sedation is most highly recommended. Nitrous oxide-oxygen (N_2O-O_2) inhalation sedation is the preferred technique of sedation for patients with angina. Because anginal episodes are provoked by an unmet myocardial O_2 requirement, the administration of N_2O-O_2 serves the following beneficial purposes: (1) relaxes the patient, (2) increases their pain reaction threshold, and (3) increases oxygenation of the patient, including the myocardium. Not only does N_2O-O_2 minimize any increase in myocardial activity as a result of its sedative and analgesic properties, but also the typical patient will receive more than 50% or, at the very least, approximately 30% O_2. This represents a significant increase in O_2 delivery to the cells

of the patient's body. N_2O-O_2 is the most nearly ideal sedative technique for the management of patients with angina.

IV sedation is recommended for the more fearful patient with a history of angina. Levels of sedation should be kept minimal to moderate (e.g., midazolam or diazepam) to lessen the potential for respiratory depression, hypoxia, or myocardial ischemia. In addition, the patient should receive O_2 via nasal cannula or nasal hood throughout the procedure.

Elective general anesthesia is not recommended for all patients with angina. Outpatient general anesthesia in these patients is generally not indicated because of the increased risk of hypoxia during anesthesia and the inherent increased stress of general anesthesia and of the surgical procedure. Patients with angina who require general anesthesia are usually hospitalized, undergoing treatment as described earlier (Chapter 31) for inpatient procedures.

Unstable Angina

Unstable angina, also known as *intermediate coronary syndrome, preinfarction angina, premature* or *impending myocardial infarction* (MI), or *coronary insufficiency,* is a syndrome intermediate in severity between angina pectoris and acute MI.[4,5]

Because mortality from acute MI is greatest within the first hour, recognition of a syndrome that has an increased likelihood of impending MI mandates immediate hospitalization and monitoring of the patient in an intensive care unit to prevent sudden fatal dysrhythmias and death. Many, if not most, unstable anginal patients are candidates for reperfusion therapy with either thrombolytics or primary balloon angioplasty and cardiac stent.

Unstable angina is recognized by the appearance of pain that is different in character, duration, radiation, and severity from the typical stable anginal episode or pain that, over a period of hours or days, demonstrates progressive ease of induction (decreased exercise tolerance) or that develops at rest or during sleep.

Patients with unstable angina who do not develop signs and symptoms of acute MI are considered to be in precarious balance between coronary artery supply and myocardial demand and should be managed as though they had suffered an MI.

Patients with unstable angina are considered ASA 4 patients and therefore are not candidates for elective dental or surgical care. Immediate medical consultation is recommended. In the event that emergency care is required, hospitalization of the patient should be seriously considered. O_2 delivery via nasal cannula or nasal hood is recommended throughout the procedure, and N_2O-O_2 inhalation sedation is the only sedative technique recommended for this patient. Medical consultation is definitely indicated before any treatment is carried out on this very high-risk patient.

Oral sedation is indicated only if absolutely necessary. Minimal levels of central nervous system (CNS) depression should be sought. The administration of O_2 to this patient throughout the procedure is recommended.

IM sedation is not recommended in patients with unstable angina because of the possibility of hypotension, which further compromises coronary blood flow and respiratory depression. Inhalation sedation is recommended because of the increased O_2 delivery to the patient throughout the procedure. IV sedation is not recommended unless the occasion absolutely demands it. The possibility of hypotension and respiratory depression, although minimal, could further aggravate the precarious balance between coronary O_2 supply and demand. Moderate levels of sedation, such as that seen with benzodiazepines, plus supplemental O_2, would best serve this patient.

Myocardial Infarction

MI is a clinical syndrome resulting from a deficient coronary arterial blood supply to a region of the myocardium, resulting in cellular death and necrosis. Synonyms for MI include *coronary occlusion, coronary thrombosis,* and *heart attack.*

More than 935,000 Americans suffer an acute MI annually (635,000 have a first-time MI; 300,000 have recurrent MIs).[6] In 2011 ischemic heart disease and acute MI were responsible for 787,650 deaths in the United States.[1] CVD accounted for 31.9% of all deaths occurring in the United States in 2011.[1]

Patients who have suffered an acute MI and survived represent a definite risk during dental and surgical treatment. Immediately after an MI, the incidence of reinfarction is high (36% reinfarction rate on surgical patients within 3 months of first MI).[7,8] With time and the formation of a myocardial scar, the incidence of reinfarction declines. Reinfarction rates fall to 16% at 5 months for post-MI patients undergoing surgical procedures and to 5% at 6 months after infarction. Reinfarction rates then level off at 5% and remain at that level indefinitely. By comparison, the risk of infarction during surgical procedures for a patient who has not had an MI is less than 0.1%.

The American College of Cardiology and the American Heart Association published risk stratification guidelines for patients with all types of heart disease who are to undergo noncardiac surgical procedures.[9] Examples include recent MI (defined as having occurred within the past 7 to 30 days) and unstable angina classified as clinical predictors of major risk for perioperative complications.[9,10] A history of past ischemic heart disease—for example, stable angina or a prior history of MI—is considered an intermediate risk factor for perioperative complications, whereas a past history of ischemic heart disease with no other clinical risk factors is unlikely to be associated with significant risk for an adverse event during dental procedures.[9,10]

Patients who have had an MI may be receiving a number of drugs to manage complications, such as HF, angina, and dysrhythmias. Drug categories include nitrates, beta-blockers, calcium channel blockers, ACE inhibitors, lipid-lowering agents, antiplatelet drugs (aspirin is the drug of choice; clopidogrel [Plavix] and ticlopidine may also be used), and various categories of drugs to manage high blood pressure.

The patient who has had an MI is considered an ASA 3 patient if more than 6 months have passed since the initial MI and no further cardiovascular complications have developed. In the event that cardiovascular complications have developed after the MI, medical consultation should be obtained. This patient is classified as either an ASA 3 or 4 patient, depending on the severity of the prior MI and the degree of cardiovascular dysfunction still present. For the 6 months immediately following the MI, the patient should be considered an ASA 4, with all elective care deferred until a full 6 months after the infarction. In the event that emergency care is required, hospitalization should be given serious consideration.

An acute MI may be precipitated when the patient undergoes unusual stress, whether physical (pain) or emotional (anxiety). Unfortunately, the patient need not be undergoing any physical activity at the time of onset of the MI. Scirica and Morrow reported that 51% of patients were at rest and 8% were asleep when the signs and symptoms of MI initially developed.[11] Of the patients, 18% were performing moderate or usual exertion, whereas only 13% were physically exerting themselves. Stewart et al reported on the activity at time of onset of MI by age group (<50, 50 to 60, 60 to 70, and >70 years).[12] Activity was categorized as (1) exercise, (2) in bed, and (3) at rest. Onset of symptoms of MI developed during exercise in 20% to 33.3% of the patients, 27.9% to 40.6% while in bed, and between 38.8% and 40.8% while at rest. There was little age difference in the proportion of patients with symptom onset at rest.

It therefore appears to be more a matter of (bad) timing than a result of dental treatment when an acute MI develops in the dental office. Stress, however, does increase the risk to the patient who has had an MI and must be considered.

Sedation in the patient who has had an MI is extremely valuable because these patients are usually stress intolerant. Any unmet increase in myocardial O_2 demand can lead to serious complications, including anginal pain, increased severity of HF, serious dysrhythmias, and reinfarction.

Oral sedation is recommended for minimal levels (see Chapter 7). More profound (deep) sedation increases the risk of hypotension and respiratory depression with hypoxia. In the event that this does occur, airway management with supplemental O_2 administration is essential. IM sedation is not recommended unless other techniques are unavailable or ineffective, and then only minimal-to-moderate sedation is indicated, with the administration of O_2 via nasal cannula or nasal hood encouraged.

Inhalation sedation is most highly recommended. N_2O-O_2 inhalation sedation provides the myocardium with additional O_2 throughout the procedure. N_2O-O_2 has been used by paramedical and medical personnel for pain management during acute MI and has proven valuable in decreasing or eliminating the associated pain.[13]

IV sedation is recommended in the patient who has experienced an MI when inhalation sedation has proven ineffective. Only minimal-to-moderate levels of sedation are recommended in the ASA 3 patient, with supplemental O_2 administered. Hospitalization is highly recommended for the ASA 4 patient with angina for whom only emergency care is recommended, and then only in a controlled environment.

Both outpatient and inpatient general anesthesia for elective dental or medical procedures are relatively contraindicated in the patient who has had an MI. The risk of reinfarction in this patient during general anesthesia is such that other (conscious) techniques should be attempted before considering the use of general anesthesia.

High Blood Pressure

Approximately 70 million Americans have high blood pressure (HBP) (29% of the U.S. population).[14] About 77% are using antihypertensive medications, but only 54% have their HBP controlled.[6] About 69% of people who have a first MI, 77% of persons having a first cerebrovascular accident (CVA), and 74% who have HF have blood pressure greater than 140/90 mm Hg.[6] Forty-six percent of persons with HBP do not have it under control.[6] Worldwide it was estimated (in 2000) that 972 million adults had hypertension.[15]

Elevations in blood pressure are not uncommonly found in the dental office environment because the stress associated with treatment leads to increased catecholamine release and subsequent elevations in heart rate and blood pressure. In patients who are usually normotensive, this is termed *situational anxiety*.[16,17] In Chapter 4, ASA classifications for blood pressure were presented. The two categories that must be reviewed are ASA 3 and 4. ASA 3 patients have a blood pressure of 160 to 199 mm Hg systolic and/or 95 to 115 mm Hg diastolic. ASA 3 patients may receive elective dental care; however, steps should be taken to prevent any further elevation of blood pressure. Two of the most important steps are the management of pain through the effective use of local anesthesia (vasopressors are not contraindicated in the hypertensive ASA 3 patient) and the management of fear and anxiety. Hypertensive ASA 4 patients have a systolic blood pressure above 200 mm Hg and/or a diastolic blood pressure in excess of 115 mm Hg. Elective dental care should be postponed until the blood pressure is better controlled. Emergency procedures may be performed; however, sedation and effective pain control are absolutely mandatory to prevent any further elevation in blood pressure. Hospitalization of the ASA 4 patient who requires emergency dental care should receive serious consideration.

Further elevation of the hypertensive patient's blood pressure may lead to a number of acute cardiovascular crises, including CVA (stroke, "brain attack"), acute MI, acute renal failure, and acute HF (pulmonary edema). Most patients with HBP are taking antihypertensive drug therapy to lower their blood pressure. Many drugs, each of which has its own side effects, are used to manage high blood pressure. The dentist must be aware of these side effects and any possible drug–drug interactions and take steps to minimize their occurrence, or at least be able to manage them successfully. Table 37.1 lists the major categories of antihypertensive drugs and their more common side effects.

Table 37.1	Side Effects and Drug Interactions of Antihypertensive Medications	
Drug	**Major Side Effects**	**Major Drug Interactions**
ACE inhibitors	Hypotension Reversible renal insufficiency Reversible hyperkalemia	
Clonidine	Drowsiness Orthostatic hypotension Xerostomia	
Guanethidine	Orthostatic hypotension	Alcohol increases orthostatic hypotension
Hydralazine	Tachycardia Palpitation Increased angina Increased CHF	
Loop diuretics	Hypokalemia	
α-Methyldopa	Orthostatic hypotension Drowsiness Depression Xerostomia	
Potassium-sparing diuretics	Hyperkalemia Nausea (triamterene)	
Prazosin	Orthostatic hypotension with syncope Dizziness Weakness Blurred vision Nausea Headache Palpitation	
Propranolol	Bradycardia CHF Increased asthma Weakness Depression	Epinephrine may induce bradycardia
Reserpine	Drowsiness Sedation Weakness Depression Bradycardia	Hypotension with general anesthesia
Thiazide diuretics	GI upset Weakness Hypokalemia Hyperglycemia	

ACE, Angiotensin-converting enzyme; *CHF,* congestive heart failure; *GI,* gastrointestinal.

The primary side effects of antihypertensive drugs of concern during ambulatory patient care are orthostatic (postural) hypotension, CNS depression, and sedation. Prevention of clinically significant orthostatic hypotension requires that alterations in dental chair position occur gradually, allowing the patient to adapt to the increasing effect of gravity as the dental chair becomes more upright. Many CNS-depressant drugs, especially opioids, enhance this effect of antihypertensive drugs. The use of CNS-depressant drugs in patients who may be somewhat CNS depressed from their antihypertensive drugs must be managed with extreme care to prevent excessive sedation from occurring. Titratable techniques are, as always, preferred.

Elevations in a patient's blood pressure can be expected during dental procedures, especially those that are potentially traumatic. The stress-reduction protocols are especially valuable in these patients. Adequate pain control through the use of local anesthetics with vasopressors (if indicated) and anxiety reduction enable these patients to receive dental care with minimal risk.

In the hypertensive patient, increases in stress further elevate blood pressure. Increased blood pressure can precipitate acute medical crises. The use of sedation should minimize or eliminate blood pressure elevations and thereby decrease patient risk during treatment.

Oral sedation, minimal or moderate, is recommended. IM sedation is recommended. Opioid analgesics may enhance orthostatic hypotension associated with some antihypertensive drugs and should therefore be avoided or used with caution.

Inhalation sedation is recommended. Inhalation sedation may be used in patients in whom blood pressure readings are slightly above the ASA 4 level (i.e., 206/112 mm Hg) to determine whether the elevated blood pressure is due to situational anxiety or is truly elevated. N_2O-O_2 is titrated to the point at which the patient is comfortably relaxed. The patient's blood pressure is rechecked at this time. If it has fallen into the ASA 3 range, the planned treatment may proceed; however, when the blood pressure remains in the ASA 4 range (above 200/115 mm Hg), treatment should be postponed and the patient unsedated and dismissed.

IV moderate sedation is recommended. Opioid analgesics may enhance orthostatic hypotension produced by some antihypertensive drugs and should therefore be avoided or used with caution.

General anesthesia is indicated in ASA 2 or 3 hypertensive patients for traumatic procedures in which sedative techniques are not indicated or have proven ineffective. The ASA 2 patient may be managed as an outpatient, whereas the ASA 3 and 4 patients might be better managed as an inpatient.

Dysrhythmias

Myocardial rhythm disturbances are not uncommon. Fortunately, most dysrhythmias are of relatively benign nature in that the myocardium still functions effectively, pumping blood. However, some dysrhythmias are potentially more dangerous, requiring immediate treatment or referral to a physician.

Patients with clinically significant dysrhythmias will be receiving antidysrhythmic drugs. These drugs include quinidine, procainamide, disopyramide, flecainide, propafenone, sotalol, and many others.[18]

In the absence of an electrocardiogram (ECG) and of training in its interpretation, the dentist is frequently unable to determine the precise nature of any dysrhythmia that might develop. Termination of dental treatment, administration of O_2, and consideration for immediate medical consultation are indicated in such cases.

Dysrhythmias may develop in patients with organic heart disease (e.g., in the patient who has had an MI) and in those with a "normal, healthy" heart. Stress, the ingestion (by the patient) of certain drugs (e.g., cocaine) and chemicals or the administration (by the dentist) of certain drugs can precipitate or exacerbate cardiac dysrhythmias. Caffeine (e.g., espresso, Red Bull) and nicotine are examples of substances that may precipitate dysrhythmias; several inhalation anesthetics, including halothane, sensitize the myocardium to catecholamines. Stress causes the release of significant amounts of the catecholamines epinephrine and norepinephrine into the CVS, increasing myocardial work and potentially inducing dysrhythmias.

Sedation is indicated in most patients with rhythm disturbances. Although any technique may be used, it is important that hypoxia and hypotension be prevented because of their dysrhythmogenic characteristics.

Oral sedation is recommended. IM sedation is recommended when other sedative techniques have proven ineffective. The use of supplemental O_2 delivered via nasal cannula or nasal hood is recommended when the IM route is used.

Inhalation sedation is recommended. N_2O-O_2 increases oxygenation, thereby eliminating a common cause of dysrhythmias.

IV moderate sedation is recommended. O_2 supplementation is suggested to minimize the risk of hypoxia.

In patients in whom dysrhythmias are well controlled through the use of drugs and no other CVD is evident, IV outpatient general anesthesia (e.g., propofol, methohexital [uncommonly used today]) is a consideration, although this patient should be considered a candidate for hospitalization. ECG monitoring throughout the procedure is strongly recommended, as is administration of supplemental O_2. The administration of inhalation anesthetics, such as halothane (rarely used today), which sensitize the myocardium to catecholamines, should be avoided, if possible. A commonly used general anesthesia technique for patients with dysrhythmias is N_2O-O_2 and IV opioids.

Local anesthesia is recommended for intraoperative and postoperative pain management. The use of vasopressor-containing local anesthetics is not contraindicated in most ASA 2 and 3 patients.[19] Epinephrine-impregnated gingival retraction cord should be avoided in these patients. Box 37.1 lists contraindications (absolute and relative) to the inclusion of vasopressors in local anesthetic solutions.

Heart Failure

HF is a pathophysiologic state in which an abnormality in cardiac function is responsible for the failure of the heart to pump blood in a volume adequate to meet the requirements of the metabolizing tissues of the body. Left-sided HF is associated with signs and symptoms reflective of pulmonary vascular congestion; right-sided HF commonly exhibits signs and symptoms of systemic venous and capillary engorgement. Left- and right-sided HF can develop independently or they may coexist. The term *CHF (congestive heart failure)* commonly refers to the combination of left- *and* right-sided HF in which there is evidence of both pulmonary and systemic congestion. The terms *HF* and *CHF* are also commonly used interchangeably.

Box 37.1	Contraindications to Use of Vasoconstrictors

Absolute Contraindications:
Unstable angina pectoris (preinfarction angina, crescendo angina)
Recent MI (<6 mo)
Recent coronary artery bypass surgery (<6 mo)
Refractory dysrhythmias
Untreated or uncontrolled severe hypertension (>200 and/or >115 mm Hg)
Untreated or uncontrolled severe HF
Uncontrolled hyperthyroidism
Uncontrolled diabetes
Sulfite sensitivity
Pheochromocytoma
Relative Contraindications:
Patients taking tricyclic antidepressants
Patients taking phenothiazine compounds
Patients taking monoamine oxidase inhibitors (MAOIs)
Patients taking nonselective β-blockers
Cocaine abuser

Modified from Perusse R, Goulet JP, Turcotte JY: Contraindications to vasoconstrictors in dentistry: part I. Cardiovascular diseases, Oral Surg 74:679–686, 1992.

Pulmonary edema is an acute condition marked by excess serous fluid in the alveolar spaces or interstitial tissues of the lungs accompanied by extreme difficulty in breathing.

HF may be produced by a number of causes, including coronary artery disease; myocarditis; hypertension; aortic or pulmonary valve stenosis; hypertrophic cardiomyopathy; aortic, mitral, or tricuspid valve insufficiency; thyrotoxicosis; anemia; pregnancy; and congenital left-to-right shunts. HF is a common sequela of MI.

An estimated 5.8 million Americans have HF,[20,21] with an estimated 550,000 new cases occurring each year.[21] The incidence of HF is equally frequent in men and women, and annual incidence approaches 10 per 1000 population after 65 years of age. Incidence is twice as common in persons with hypertension compared with normotensive persons and five times greater in persons who have had an MI compared with persons who have not. HBP is a common precursor, with more than 75% of patients with CHF having a history of preexisting HBP.[22]

Patients with HF commonly take drugs to control their HBP in addition to preparations of digitalis. Digitalis increases cardiac output, decreases right atrial pressure, decreases venous pressure, and increases the excretion of sodium and water.

There is considerable variation in the severity of HF. A commonly used method of classification of HF is called the *functional reserve category.* Four classes are recognized, based on a patient's ability to climb a normal flight of stairs (Fig. 37.2). The functional reserve classification is defined as follows:
1. Patient is able to climb a normal flight of stairs without pausing and can continue walking without resting.
2. Patient is able to climb a normal flight of stairs without pausing, but must stop at the top of the stairs to catch his or her breath.
3. Patient is able to climb a normal flight of stairs, but must pause before reaching the top of the stairs to catch his or her breath.
4. Patient is unable to climb a normal flight of stairs.

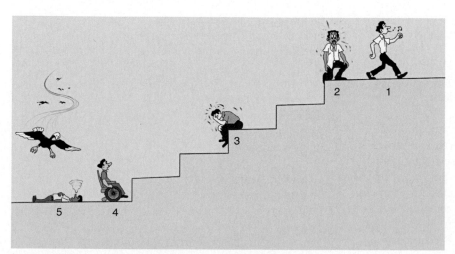

Figure 37.2 ASA classification for HF. (Courtesy Dr. Lawrence Day.)

A.S.A. CLASSIFICATION

These numbers can be considered the ASA physical status classification for HF.

Hypoxia or stress may increase the degree of HF by increasing the workload of the myocardium, thereby increasing its O_2 requirement. The stress reduction protocol is of considerable importance in the management of patients with HF. Scheduling appointments early in the morning, when the patient is well rested and it is generally cooler outdoors; limiting the length of the appointment so as not to exceed the limit of the patient's tolerance; and monitoring vital signs preoperatively are recommended. If the weather becomes extremely warm or humid, or if the patient appears somewhat fatigued before the start of treatment, it may be prudent to postpone the planned treatment to another day. Intraoperatively, the need for effective pain and anxiety control is quite important because increased stress produces an increased myocardial workload and an increase in the degree of HF.

Chair positioning of patients with HF may require modification from that recommended as "ideal" for the sedated patient. Although the supine or semisupine position is strongly recommended for patients during sedative procedures, the patient with HF may exhibit orthopnea that precludes the use of this position. Should this occur, the patient should be placed in the most recumbent position in which he or she can still breathe comfortably.

Local anesthetics containing vasopressors are indicated for pain control in the patient with HF. The recommended concentration of epinephrine is 1:200,000 or 1:100,000.

There are no contraindications to using any of the techniques of sedation in the patient with HF. It is important to remember that the primary problem in this patient is the failure of the heart to deliver an adequate volume of blood (and O_2) to the tissues of the body. Because all sedative drugs are CNS, respiratory, and potentially cardiovascular depressants, it is essential that any additional hypoxia be prevented during the procedure. The ASA 2 patient with coronary heart disease is an excellent candidate for sedation with any technique, whereas the ASA 3 patient with HF should be restricted to minimal-to-moderate levels of sedation by the oral, inhalation, or IV route.

Oral sedation is quite appropriate for the patient with HF (ASA 2 or 3) for preoperative anxiety control. Only light levels of sedation should be sought (minimal to moderate), such as is obtained with the benzodiazepines.

IM sedation should be reserved for the patient in whom other more controllable techniques have proven ineffective. Minimal-to-moderate levels of sedation may be sought, with O_2 supplementation provided throughout the procedure, for the ASA 2 patient only. Potent respiratory-depressant drugs, such as opioids and barbiturates (rarely used today), should be used with extreme care, if at all.

N_2O-O_2 inhalation sedation is an appropriate technique for the ASA 2 or 3 patient with HF because it provides sedation and analgesia and additional O_2 for the patient.

Minimal-to-moderate levels of IV sedation are recommended for the ASA 2 patient with HF. Supplemental O_2 is recommended for all IV sedative procedures. The use of IV sedation is not recommended for use in the ASA 3 patient with HF unless it is considered essential by the dentist, in which case only minimal-to-moderate sedation levels are recommended (with O_2 supplementation).

Outpatient general anesthesia is not usually recommended for the ASA 2, 3, or 4 patient with HF. In-hospital general anesthesia should be considered when other sedative techniques have proven inadequate in patient management.

Congenital Heart Defects

Congenital heart defects affect approximately 1% (about 10,000) of births per year in the United States.[23,24] Some defects develop as a result of genetic abnormalities; however, most congenital heart lesions occur in the absence of any detectable chromosomal abnormality. Although there are a large number of congenital lesions, those listed in Box 37.2 account for more than 80% of those seen in children with congenital heart disease. *Ventricular septal defects* account for approximately one third of all lesions, and *atrial septal defects* and *patent ductus arteriosus* account for 10% each; other relatively common defects include pulmonary stenosis and coarctation of the aorta. Less common are tetralogy of Fallot, aortic stenosis, and transposition of the great arteries.

Box 37.2   Congenital Heart Defects

Acyanotic Heart Lesions With Left-to-Right Shunts
Ostium secundum atrial septal defects
Anomalous pulmonary venous return
Endocardial cushion defects
Ostium primum atrial septal defects
Atrioventricular canal
Ventricular septal defects
Patent ductus arteriosus
Aorticopulmonary window and truncus arteriosus

Acyanotic Heart Disease With Obstructive Lesions
Coarctation of the aorta
Aortic stenosis
Pulmonary stenosis

Cyanotic Heart Lesions
Tricuspid atresia
Pulmonary atresia
Tetralogy of Fallot
Ebstein's anomaly of the tricuspid valve
Transposition of the great arteries

Because great variation in clinical signs and symptoms and relevance toward dental care exists with congenital heart lesions, a thorough medical history, dialog history, and clinical evaluation are absolutely essential. When a history of congenital heart disease is obtained, medical consultation with the patient's (child or adult) physician is recommended.

Primary concerns associated with dental management of this patient include the exacerbation of HF and cardiac dysrhythmias secondary to the stresses associated with dental treatment and the possibility of infection producing bacterial endocarditis. Consulting the most recent American Heart Association (AHA), American Medical Association (AMA), and American Dental Association (ADA) guidelines for prophylaxis, along with possible medical consultation with the patient's primary care physician, will aid in determining the need for prophylactic antibiotics.[25] In many patients with surgically repaired defects, the need for antibiotic coverage during dental care exists for life.

As specifically relates to the management of pain and anxiety in patients with congenital heart disease, pain control through the use of local anesthetics is vitally important as a means of minimizing stress. The administration of vasopressor-containing local anesthetics is not contraindicated in these patients.

Sedative techniques are indicated as a means of minimizing intraoperative stress in this patient. The primary goal during the procedure is to provide adequate sedation without inducing hypoxia. The myocardium of the patient with congenital heart disease may be less able to tolerate hypoxic episodes than healthy heart muscle.

The oral route is indicated for minimal-to-moderate levels of sedation. Deep sedation via the oral route cannot be recommended.

IM sedation should be relegated to a last-choice technique for patients in whom other sedative procedures are unavailable or have proven ineffective. Only minimal-to-moderate sedation levels are recommended by the IM route, along with administration of supplemental O_2 throughout the procedure.

Inhalation sedation is an excellent technique for these patients primarily because of the additional levels of O_2 supplied throughout the procedure.

IV sedation is also recommended, provided the level of sedation remains minimal to moderate. Deep sedation is not recommended because of the increased risk of hypoxia and depression of respiratory and cardiovascular function. Supplemental O_2 should be administered when IV sedation is used.

Outpatient general anesthesia is not recommended in patients with congenital heart lesions, repaired or not. General anesthesia should be reserved for patients in whom sedative procedures have been ineffective. Because of the nature of the underlying disease, the patient is admitted to the hospital before the procedure to receive a more in-depth medical evaluation.

Valvular Heart Disease

Valvular heart disease is a possible sequela of rheumatic fever. The incidence of valvular heart disease secondary to rheumatic fever has diminished over the past four decades; however, congenital valvular lesions are diagnosed with increasing regularity. It is estimated that more than 106,000 cardiac valvular replacements are performed annually in the United States.[26]

Life expectancy is prolonged for most patients receiving valvular replacements. Along with this benefit, however, is the ever-present prospect of bacterial endocarditis. The reader is referred to the guidelines for prophylaxis, which present detailed antibiotic regimens for these patients.[25] The patient's primary care physician may be consulted before dental treatment.

The primary concern during the dental management of the patient with valvular heart disease is the prevention of bacterial endocarditis. In addition, stress should be minimized through the effective use of local anesthesia and sedation, as indicated. Hypoxia should be prevented.

The administration of local anesthetics with vasopressors is indicated in patients with valvular replacement.

Oral sedation is indicated in the management of lesser degrees of preoperative anxiety. Minimal levels of sedation only are recommended.

IM sedation is recommended when other sedative techniques are unavailable or have proven ineffective. Intraoperative O_2 administration is recommended for the minimal-to-moderate sedation recommended by the IM route.

Inhalation sedation with N_2O-O_2 is highly recommended for anxiety control in patients with valvular prostheses.

IV sedation is also recommended, with minimal-to-moderate levels only suggested. Intraoperative O_2 administration is suggested.

Outpatient general anesthesia is not recommended for the patient with a valvular prosthesis. Hospitalization and thorough workup are strongly suggested.

RENAL DISEASE

Chronic kidney disease (CKD) is any condition that causes reduced kidney function over a period of time. CKD is present when a patient's glomerular filtration rate (GFR) remains below 60 mm/minute for more than 3 months or when a patient's urine albumin-to-creatinine ratio is over 30 mg of albumin for each gram of creatinine (30 mg/g).

End-stage renal disease (ESRD) represents total and permanent kidney failure. Persons with ESRD require dialysis and/or kidney transplantation.

An estimated 26 million adults in the United States have CKD—about one in nine adults.[27,28] Glomerulonephritis, pyelonephritis, nephrotic syndrome, chronic renal insufficiency, and chronic renal failure are the most common disorders of renal function. Renal dialysis and transplantation are used in the management of chronic renal failure. In 2006 it was estimated that more than 468,000 persons were undergoing dialysis for ESRD.[27] There were more than 99,357 patients awaiting kidney transplant as of July 26, 2016.[29] Fewer than 17,000 persons receive renal transplants in the United States each year. Every day, 13 people die waiting for a kidney.[27,29]

Most renal failure patients may be safely managed in an outpatient setting, representing ASA 2, 3, or 4 risks. Specific questioning and examination can determine the degree of risk.

All patients with altered renal function, especially those undergoing dialysis in the days just preceding their dialysis appointments, must be managed carefully because their blood chemistries may be in disarray. It is recommended that dental appointments be scheduled on the day following dialysis so that the patient's metabolic status is more optimal and the effects of systemic anticoagulation are minimal.

Vital signs should be closely monitored. Because of the potential for bleeding problems, if an invasive dental procedure is planned, the patient should undergo pretreatment screening for bleeding disorders, and a platelet count should be obtained.[30] Few problems are encountered with nonhemorrhagic dental procedures when the hematocrit is above 25%.[30]

Prophylactic antibiotics may be required before dental care in the patient with renal disease, especially the renal transplant patient. Consultation with the patient's physician (nephrologist) is strongly recommended to determine an appropriate antibiotic regimen.

Many patients with chronic renal disease, especially patients having undergone renal transplantation, receive long-term corticosteroid and antirejection (immunosuppressant) drug therapy. Such therapies diminish the patient's capacity to respond appropriately to increased stress. The administration of supplemental corticosteroid may be recommended before particularly traumatic (emotionally or physically) procedures. Medical consultation is recommended.

Patients undergoing renal dialysis and renal transplant are considered at high risk for contracting hepatitis B and should be evaluated before the start of dental care. Patients who are surface-antigen negative and surface-antibody positive may be treated in the usual manner, whereas those who are surface-antigen positive should be treated using current recommendations to minimize transmission of hepatitis B. There is also an increased risk of HIV and AIDS infection. This increased risk should be considered before the use of parenteral techniques of sedation.

Most drugs are excreted through the kidneys, with a percentage of the drug unchanged along with its major metabolites. Drugs, such as cocaine and gallamine, that are excreted entirely unchanged in the urine should not be administered to patients undergoing renal dialysis. Blood levels of these drugs would become overly high, increasing the risk of overdose (toxic reaction). Approximately 10% to 15% of most amide local anesthetics are excreted unchanged in the urine, whereas virtually no ester local anesthetic is found unchanged in the urine, having undergone biotransformation in the blood. Among drugs used for sedation, there is little problem in that only very small amounts of unchanged drug are found in the urine.

Benzodiazepines and the opioids may be administered in the usual manner in both the patient with renal insufficiency and the functionally anephric patient. Nephrotoxic drugs, including aspirin and other NSAIDs, require dosage adjustments. Aspirin must have its dosage regimen changed from the usual every 3 to 5 hours to every 4 to 6 hours in renal insufficiency and to every 8 to 12 hours in the anephric patient. Acetaminophen, also nephrotoxic, may cause renal tubular necrosis at high doses, but is probably safer than aspirin in ESRD patients because it undergoes metabolism in the liver.[31]

Amide local anesthetics may be administered normally. There are no contraindications to the inclusion of vasopressors.

Oral sedation is indicated for minimal-to-moderate levels of sedation.

IM sedation is indicated for minimal-to-moderate levels of sedation. The increased risk of hepatitis B or HIV in the dialysis patient must be considered before IM sedation.

Inhalation sedation is indicated.

IV sedation is indicated. The increased risk of hepatitis B or HIV in the dialysis patient must be considered before IV sedation.

General anesthesia on an outpatient basis is not recommended in the patient with chronic renal disease. Because of the potential presence of metabolic disorders, the patient should be hospitalized and thoroughly evaluated before general anesthesia.

RESPIRATORY DISEASE

The patient with respiratory disease must be evaluated carefully before dental treatment and especially before the administration of any CNS-depressant drug that may further inhibit the patient's respiratory efforts (e.g., opioids). Many patients with chronic respiratory disorders have respiratory centers that are less sensitive to the normal stimulus for breathing: increased arterial carbon dioxide (CO_2) tension. Instead, these patients develop decreased arterial O_2 tension as their primary respiratory stimulus. Such patients may be described as hypercarbic (increased CO_2 tension) and hypoxic (decreased O_2 tension).

It is likely that many of these patients will be able to tolerate the stresses associated with their dental care, with few, if any, modifications necessary in their treatment. However, the addition of stress can greatly increase the risk of an acute exacerbation of their disease process. Sedative drugs, which possess varying degrees of potential for respiratory depression, must be used with great care to minimize any further reduction in the respiratory drive of these patients.

Evaluation of patients with chronic respiratory disease revolves primarily around the patient's ability to exchange O_2 and CO_2 effectively. Inability to do so is demonstrated by the presence of clinical signs and symptoms. The most commonly observed respiratory disorders include asthma, chronic obstructive pulmonary disease (COPD), bronchiectasis, and pneumonia.

Asthma

Asthma is a clinical state of hyperreactivity of the tracheobronchial tree and is characterized by recurrent paroxysms of dyspnea and wheezing, which are the result of bronchospasm, bronchial wall edema, and hypersecretion by mucous glands. Several forms of asthma—extrinsic asthma (allergic asthma), intrinsic asthma (nonallergic asthma), drug-induced asthma, exercise-induced asthma, and occupational asthma—are recognized.

The number of adults (aged 18 years and older) in the United States who have asthma is 17.7 million.[32] This represents 7.4% of the adult population. An additional 6.3 million children (under 18 years of age) have asthma (8.6%).[32] The typical asthmatic patient is asymptomatic between acute episodes, but demonstrates varying degrees of respiratory distress during the acute asthmatic episode. Although the degree of respiratory distress is usually moderate, many persons die each year in the United States from asthma-related disorders (3630 in 2013 in the United States).[33] The goal in the dental management of the asthmatic patient is to prevent the acute exacerbation.

The acute asthmatic episode may be triggered by any of the following, probably the most significant of which in the dental management of this patient is increased stress:

- Psychological stress
- Antigen–antibody reaction (allergy)
- Bronchial infection
- Dust, fumes
- Climate (e.g., smog, cold)
- Drugs

Of primary importance to the dentist is to determine the type of asthma present and its degree of severity before the start of treatment. The typical asthmatic patient is classified as ASA 2, with the ASA 3 asthmatic patient defined as a patient with a frequency of more than one acute episode per week or with episodes at any frequency that are difficult to manage without seeking medical attention.

Because most asthmatic patients appear asymptomatic between episodes, the dentist must be thorough in the dialog history and physical examination. The dentist should determine which drugs the patient uses for management of acute episodes and request that the drugs be brought to all dental appointments. The acute asthmatic attack is in great part an episode of bronchial smooth muscle spasm (bronchospasm). To this are added bronchial wall edema and the secretion of copious volumes of mucus. The drugs used to manage acute asthmatic episodes are termed *bronchodilators*; the most common are listed in Table 37.2, as well as drugs used in the long-term management of asthma.

Table 37.2	Medications Used in Management of Asthma	
DRUG GROUP	**EXAMPLES (GENERIC NAMES)**	**EXAMPLES (PROPRIETARY NAMES)**
Inhaled short-acting beta-2 agonists	Albuterol sulfate (salbutamol outside of USA)	Accuneb, Proventil-HFA, ProAir-HFA, Ventolin
	Isoetharine HCl	Beta-2
	Isoproterenol HCl	Isuprel
	Levalbuterol HCl	Xopenex, Xopenex-HFA
	Pirbuterol	Maxair Autohaler
	Terbutaline	(None)
Inhaled corticosteroids	Beclomethasone dipropionate	QVAR
	Budesonide	Pulmicort Respules, Pulmicort Flexhaler
	Flunisolide	Aerobid, Aerospan HFA
	Fluticasone propionate	Flovent Diskus, Flovent HFA
	Mometasone furoate	Asmanex Twisthaler
	Triamcinolone acetonide	Azmacort
Inhaled long-acting beta-2 agonists	Formoterol fumarate	Foradil Aerolizer
	Salmeterol xinafoate	Serevent Diskus
Combined medication (inhaled steroid plus long-acting beta-2 agonist)	Fluticasone and salmeterol xinafoate	Advair Diskus, Advair HFA
	Budesonide and formoterol fumarate	Symbicort
Anticholinergics – single medication	Ipratropium bromide	Atrovent, Atrovent HFA
Anticholinergics – combined medication	Ipratropium bromide and albuterol sulfate	Combivent, DuoNeb
Leukotriene modifiers	Montelukast sodium	Singulair
	Zafirlukast	Accolate
	Zileuton	Zyflo CR
Cromolyn and Nedocromil	Cromolyn sodium	Intal
	Nedocromil	Tilade
Anti-IgE	Omalizumab	Xolair

The use of sedative techniques in the asthmatic patient may be important in the prevention of acute episodes in clinical situations in which stress or anxiety levels are increased. However, some commonly used sedative drugs have the potential to provoke an acute episode of bronchospasm. Two examples are the barbiturates (no longer recommended for use) and opioids (especially meperidine), which are histamine-releasing drugs. These drugs should be avoided in the asthmatic patient.

Oral sedation is recommended for minimal-to-moderate levels of sedation. Barbiturates and opioids should be avoided because of the potential for acute exacerbation. Chloral hydrate, hydroxyzine, and midazolam are frequently administered in the management of the asthmatic child, usually with good results.

IM and IN sedation are recommended in the pediatric patient for whom other techniques are ineffective. Opioids and barbiturates, two commonly used drug groups, are relatively contraindicated in the asthmatic patient and should be avoided, if possible. Nasal O_2 throughout the procedure is recommended.

Inhalation sedation with N_2O-O_2 is the most recommended sedative technique for both pediatric and adult asthmatic patients. Although N_2O is not a bronchodilator, its sedative actions and the additional O_2 administered along with it effectively minimize the occurrence of acute asthmatic episodes. The occasional misguided medical consultant recommends against use of N_2O-O_2 because some individuals (mistakenly) believe that N_2O may provoke bronchospasm. Inhalation agents that irritate the respiratory mucosa are capable of provoking bronchospasm; however, N_2O is not an irritating vapor and may be administered without increased risk (in fact, with decreased risk).

IV moderate sedation is recommended, with the addition of O_2 by nasal administration. Opioids and barbiturates are contraindicated (e.g., the Jorgensen technique) in the asthmatic patient.

Outpatient general anesthesia should be avoided in the asthmatic patient because of the increased risk of bronchospasm during general anesthesia. Dental and medical care for the patient with asthma who requires general anesthesia should be completed in the more controlled setting of the operating room of a hospital or day-surgery center.

Chronic Obstructive Pulmonary Disease

Chronic obstructive pulmonary (or lung) disease (COPD, COLD) is the most common cause of death and disability resulting from lung disease in the United States. It represents the third leading cause of death (2013) in the United States.[34] In 2009 133,965 people died of COPD, of which 52.3% were women.[34] Two primary disease entities comprise COPD: emphysema and chronic bronchitis. Unlike the asthmatic patient who is essentially asymptomatic in periods between acute episodes, the patient with COPD appears more debilitated and chronically ill, representing a greater risk during treatment.

The typical patient with COPD is classified as an ASA 3 patient.

Emphysema

Emphysema represents a disease entity in which interalveolar septa (including blood vessels) are destroyed, producing a coalescence of airspaces to form abnormally large cystic or bullous areas in the lungs that do not function in gas exchange. The primary symptom presented in emphysema is a variable degree of dyspnea on exertion. The chest is often enlarged in a hyperinflated (barrel-chest) position. A chronic cough with sputum production may be present, although this is not characteristic of the disease.

There is no effective treatment for emphysema. Medical management is symptomatic, attempting to improve the patient's quality and length of life. Patients are cautioned to avoid all toxic inhalants, such as cigarette smoke and toxic fumes. Minor pulmonary infection may readily lead to respiratory failure in these patients; therefore, extraordinary care is maintained and vigorous treatment instituted at the first signs of infectious respiratory processes. Supplemental O_2 administered via a low-flow nasal cannula (2 to 3 L/min) at home using portable O_2 devices is frequently required for these patients.

Chronic Bronchitis

Chronic bronchitis is among the most common debilitating diseases in the United States. A strong relationship exists between chronic bronchitis and inhalation of irritating substances, most commonly cigarette smoke and various pollutants. Pathologic findings in chronic bronchitis include hyperplasia and hypertrophy of the submucosal bronchial mucous glands, hyperplasia of bronchiolar goblet cells, squamous metaplasia of bronchial mucosal cells, chronic and acute inflammatory infiltrates in the bronchial submucosa, profuse inflammatory exudates in the lumina of bronchi and bronchioles, and denudation of bronchial mucosa. Primary clinical symptoms include chronic cough and sputum production. Chronic bronchitis is most often seen in smokers older than 35 years. For a diagnosis of chronic bronchitis to be established, a productive cough must have been present for a minimum of 3 months a year in at least 2 consecutive years. As the disease progresses, it is marked by recurrent episodes of acute respiratory failure resulting from infectious exacerbations in the bronchi. These episodes are marked by increased cough, change in sputum from clear to purulent, fever, dyspnea, and varying degrees of respiratory distress; management consists of antibiotics, bronchodilators, and respiratory therapy.

Medical management of chronic bronchitis also includes cessation of cigarette smoking and exposure to toxic inhalants and the prevention or vigorous management of any respiratory infections. Other measures included in the management in some of these patients are home O_2 administration via nasal cannula and treatment of right-sided HF (with diuretics), which occasionally develops in chronic bronchitis.

The progression and prognosis of chronic bronchitis are quite variable; however, in general, there is a progressive deterioration of pulmonary function, with increasing frequency of episodes of respiratory failure until death. The life expectancy in the typical patient, once severe symptoms develop, is rarely more than 5 to 10 years.

Typically, the patient with chronic bronchitis represents an ASA 3 risk; those with milder symptoms are ASA 2, but those who require supplemental O_2 at all times, have severe orthopnea, and have a severe, productive cough are classified ASA 4. ASA 4 patients should have elective dental care postponed until such time as their health improves. If dental care is urgent, hospitalization is recommended.

Dental management of patients with COPD usually requires alteration in patient positioning from the recommended supine position because of the presence of orthopnea. These patients should be positioned in the most recumbent position in which they are still able to breathe comfortably. Supplemental O_2 at low flows (2 to 3 L/min) may be administered via a nasal cannula or nasal hood throughout the dental appointment, whether or not a sedative procedure is used.

Local anesthesia is indicated for patients with COPD. Vasopressors are not contraindicated.

Oral sedation may be indicated, but only minimal levels of sedation. Opioids and barbiturates specifically are not recommended because of their greater propensity to depress respiration. Anticholinergics (atropine, scopolamine, and glycopyrrolate) and histamine blockers (hydroxyzine) are contraindicated because they increase the viscosity of secretions in the respiratory tract.

IM and IN sedation are rarely considered in patients with COPD primarily because these disease processes are almost always seen in older adults. Because of the ability of many IM-administered CNS-depressant drugs to produce respiratory depression, this technique of sedation is not recommended. If IM sedation is used, opioids and barbiturates are contraindicated, anticholinergics and histamine blockers should be avoided, and O_2 must be administered in a 2- to 3-L/min flow throughout the procedure. Midazolam, a benzodiazepine, is the preferred IM sedative agent.

Inhalation sedation may be the only sedative technique that can be used in patients with COPD, with an expectation of clinical success that does not also increase the risk of acute respiratory failure. Theoretically, it is possible for the higher levels of O_2 administered with N_2O-O_2 to remove the stimulus for breathing in these patients (decreased arterial O_2 tension). In clinical practice, however, this situation is unlikely to develop, and N_2O-O_2 remains the sedative technique of choice in patients with COPD.

IV sedation is not recommended as a primary technique in patients with COPD because of the increased sensitivity of these patients to hypoxia and respiratory depression. Opioids, barbiturates, histamine blockers, and anticholinergics are contraindicated. Should IV sedation be necessary, minimal or moderate levels of sedation only, with drugs that do not produce significant respiratory depression (benzodiazepines), and the administration of 2 to 3 L/min nasal O_2 throughout the procedure are recommended.

Outpatient general anesthesia is usually contraindicated in patients with COPD. General anesthesia should be relegated to inpatient procedures within the operating room, where thorough preoperative evaluation is obtainable and patients can be observed both during and after the procedure before discharge.

NEUROLOGIC DISORDERS

Neurologic disorders, especially seizures, CVAs, and myasthenia gravis (MG), are of concern to the practicing dentist and physician. The patient who has a CNS disorder must be evaluated carefully, especially when the use of CNS-depressant drugs is contemplated.

Seizure Disorders

Seizure disorders are characterized by abrupt transient symptoms of a motor, sensory, psychic, or autonomic nature, often associated with changes in consciousness. These changes are secondary to sudden transient changes in brain function associated with excessive rapid electrical discharges in the gray matter.

Epilepsy is diagnosed after a person has had at least two seizures not caused by a known medical condition (e.g., idiopathic seizures). It is estimated (2014) that 65 million persons worldwide and 3 million people in the United States have epilepsy.[35]

The incidence of newly diagnosed epilepsy (recurrent seizure activity) among the general population in North America is approximately 150,000 per year.[36] The highest incidence is under age 2 years and over age 65 years. By 20 years of age, 1% of the population can be expected to have developed epilepsy. By 75 years of age, 3% of the population can be expected to have been diagnosed with epilepsy, and 10% will have experienced some type of seizure.[36] It is also estimated that 10% of newly diagnosed epileptic patients fail to gain control of seizures despite optimal medical management.[36] Box 37.3 lists various types of seizure activity.

Seizures encountered most frequently and those possessing the greatest potential for morbidity and mortality are those in group two: generalized epilepsies and syndromes. Within this group are the tonic-clonic convulsive episode, represented clinically as grand mal or major epilepsy and petit mal or minor epilepsy (also termed an *absence attack*).

Among epileptic patients, 70% have only one type of seizure, with the remainder having two or more types. Generalized tonic-clonic seizures are present in 90% of all epileptic patients (60% grand mal only; 30% grand mal plus others). Petit mal seizures are seen in 25% of patients with epilepsy (4% alone; 21% with other types). Petit mal is seen most often in children younger than 16 years. Psychomotor seizures are seen in approximately 18% of epileptic patients (6% alone; 12% mixed)

Box 37.3	International Classification of the Epilepsies and Epileptic Syndromes

1. Localization-related (focal, local, partial) epilepsies and syndromes
   1.1 Idiopathic with age-related onset. At present, two syndromes are established, but more may be identified in the future
      Benign childhood epilepsy with centrotemporal spikes (benign rolandic epilepsy)
      Childhood epilepsy with occipital paroxysms
   1.2 Symptomatic
      This category includes syndromes of great individual variability that will mainly be based on anatomic localization, clinical features, seizure types, and etiologic factors (if known)
2. Generalized epilepsies and syndromes
   2.1 Idiopathic, with age-related onset, listed in order of age
      Benign neonatal familial convulsions
      Benign neonatal convulsions
      Benign myoclonic epilepsy in infancy
      Childhood absence epilepsy (pyknolepsy)
      Juvenile absence epilepsy
      Juvenile myoclonic epilepsy (impulsive petit mal)
      Epilepsy with grand mal seizures on awakening
      Other generalized idiopathic epilepsies, if they do not belong to one of the earlier syndromes, can still be classified as generalized idiopathic epilepsies
   2.2 Idiopathic, symptomatic, or both, in order of age of appearance
      West syndrome (infantile spasms, Blitz–Nick–Salaam–Krämpfe)
      Lennox–Gastaut syndrome
      Epilepsy with myoclonic-astatic seizures
      Epilepsy with myoclonic absences
   2.3 Symptomatic
      2.3a Nonspecific etiology
         Early myoclonic encephalopathy
      2.3b Specific syndromes
         Epileptic seizures may complicate many disease states
         Included under this heading are diseases in which seizures are an initial or predominant feature
3. Epilepsies and syndromes undetermined regarding whether they are focal or generalized
   3.1 With both generalized and focal seizures
      Neonatal seizures
      Severe myoclonic epilepsy in infancy
      Epilepsy with continuous spike waves during slow-wave sleep
      Acquired epileptic aphasia (Landau–Kleffner syndrome)
   3.2 Without unequivocal generalized or focal features
      This heading covers all cases in which clinical and electroencephalographic findings do not permit classification as clearly generalized or localization related, such as in many cases of sleep grand mal
4. Special syndromes
   4.1 Situation-related seizures
      Febrile convulsions
      Seizures related to other identifiable situations, such as stress, hormonal changes, drugs, alcohol, or sleep deprivation
   4.2 Isolated, apparently unprovoked epileptic events
   4.3 Epilepsies characterized by specific modes of seizure precipitation
   4.4 Chronic progressive epilepsia partialis continua of childhood

Modified from: Gilliam F: Diagnosis and classification of seizures and epilepsy. In Winn HR, Berger MS, Dacey RG, Jr., editors: Youmans neurological surgery, *ed 6, Philadelphia, 2011, Saunders/Elsevier, pp. 672–677.*

and are minor seizures in which the victim loses contact with the environment for 1 or 2 minutes.[37]

Anticonvulsant drugs (also known as *antiepileptic drugs [AEDs]*) are used to manage epilepsy; the goal is to prevent the occurrence of seizure activity by depressing the neuronal focus in the brain. Current anticonvulsant drug therapy is effective in 70% to 80% of patients, but about 10% continue to have seizures at intervals of 1 month or less, which severely disrupts their life and work.[38] Tables 37.3 and 37.4 list commonly prescribed anticonvulsants. Major dental treatment concerns with these patients are the prevention of seizure activity and patient management if a seizure does occur. Factors exacerbating seizures include psychological

stress and fatigue. In the presence of apprehension over the planned procedure, sedative techniques should be considered. Alcohol is absolutely contraindicated in epileptic patients because it may precipitate seizure activity. No patient with a history of epilepsy should receive dental treatment if it is obvious that alcohol has recently been ingested. Alcohol should not be used as a sedative in epileptic patients. Most patients with well-controlled epilepsy (seizures developing rarely, less than one a month) are considered ASA 2 risks, with those having seizures more frequently considered ASA 3 risks. The degree of control over seizure activity is a primary factor in determining the risk involved in management of these patients.

Table 37.3	Long-Established Drugs Used to Manage Epilepsy[38]		
GENERIC NAME	**PROPRIETARY NAME**	**TYPE OF SEIZURE**	**SIDE EFFECTS**
Benzodiazepines: Clonazepam, clobazam, lorazepam, diazepam, midazolam		Lorazepam used IV to control status epilepticus	Sedation, withdrawal syndrome
Carbamazepine	Carbatrol, Equetro, Tegretol	All types except absence seizures. Most widely used AED.	Sedation, ataxia, blurred vision, water retention, hypersensitivity reactions, leukopenia, liver failure (rare)
Ethosuximide	Zarontin	Petit mal. May exacerbate tonic-clonic seizures	Nausea, anorexia, mood changes, headache
Phenobarbital	Generic only	All types except absence seizures	Sedation, depression
Phenytoin sodium	Dilantin, Phenytek	Safest drug for grand mal and some cases of psychomotor epilepsy; may accentuate petit mal seizures	Ataxia, vertigo, gingival hypertrophy, hirsutism, megaloblastic anemia, fetal malformation, hypersensitivity reactions
Valproate sodium Valproic acid	Depacon Depakene, Stavzor	Most types, including absence seizures	Generally less than with other drugs. Nausea, hair loss, weight gain, fetal malformations

Modified from Rang HP, Ritter JM, Flower RJ, Henderson G: Antiepileptic drugs. In Rang HP, Ritter JM, Flower RJ, Henderson G. editors: *Rang & Dale's Pharmacology*, ed 8, Oxford, 2016, Elsevier Churchill Livingstone, pp. 546–558.

Table 37.4	Newer Antiepileptic Drugs[38]		
GENERIC NAME	**PROPRIETARY NAME**	**TYPE OF SEIZURE**	**SIDE EFFECTS**
Felbamate	Felbatol	Use mainly for severe epilepsy because of risk of adverse reaction	Few acute side effects but can cause aplastic anemia and hepatic damage (rare but serious)
Gabapentin Pregabalin	Gralise, Neurontin Lyrica	Partial seizures	Few side effects, mainly sedation
Lacosamide	Vimpat	Partial seizures	Nausea, vomiting, dizziness, visual disturbances, impaired coordination, mood changes
Lamotrigine	Lamictal	All types	Dizziness, sedation, rashes
Levetiracetam	Keppra, Spritam	Partial and generalized tonic-clonic seizures	Sedation (slight)
Perampanel	Fycompa	Partial seizures	Dizziness, weight gain, sedation, impaired coordination, changes in mood and behavior.
Rufinamide	Banzel	Partial seizures	Headache, dizziness, fatigue
Tiagabine	Gabitril	Partial seizures	Sedation, dizziness, lightheadedness
Topiramate	Qudexy, Topamax, Trokendi	Partial and generalized tonic-clonic seizures	Sedation. Fetal malformation. Fewer pharmacokinetic interactions than phenytoin
Vigabatrin	Sabril	All types. Appears to be effective in patients resistant to other drugs	Sedation, behavioral and mood changes, visual field defects
Zonisamide	Zonegran	Partial seizures	Sedation (slight), appetite suppression, weight loss

Modified from Rang HP, Ritter JM, Flower RJ, Henderson G: Antiepileptic drugs. In Rang HP, Ritter JM, Flower RJ, Henderson G. editors: *Rang & Dale's Pharmacology*, ed 8, Oxford, 2016, Elsevier Churchill Livingstone, pp. 546–558.

Local anesthesia is indicated in the epileptic patient. Although IV administration or administration of overly large doses of local anesthetics may provoke seizure activity (generalized tonic-clonic), it is unlikely that careful administration, following aspiration and slow injection of minimal volumes of the local anesthetic, will produce a problem. Vasopressors may be included in the local anesthetic.

The use of sedation in the epileptic patient is indicated because it decreases the patient's fears of dentistry. It is important, however, that cerebral hypoxia be prevented because its presence seizures may occur. Adequate oxygenation is therefore quite important for the epileptic patient.

Oral sedation is indicated for the preoperative management of anxiety. When it is used to produce minimal levels of CNS depression only, supplemental O_2 is not required.

IM sedation is indicated in patients in whom other techniques of sedation have proven ineffective. Supplemental O_2 is strongly recommended throughout the sedative treatment.

Inhalation sedation is an excellent technique for use in the epileptic patient. Occasional reports indicate that N_2O is capable of inducing seizure activity (it is allegedly epileptogenic) in seizure-prone patients.[39] Clinical experience with N_2O-O_2 over more than 100 years has conclusively proven its safety in the seizure-prone patient.[39,40]

IV moderate sedation is also recommended in the fearful epileptic patient. Techniques that include the administration of benzodiazepines are preferred because these drugs are excellent anticonvulsants. The administration of supplemental O_2 throughout the procedure, to minimize the possibility of hypoxia, is strongly recommended. IV drugs, such as ketamine, which provokes high-frequency electroencephalographic (EEG) activity, are not recommended in epileptic patients.

General anesthesia in the epileptic patient should be limited to in-hospital procedures.

Cerebrovascular Accident

CVA is a focal neurologic disorder caused by destruction of brain substance as a result of intracerebral hemorrhage (13% of all CVAs), thrombosis, embolism, or vascular insufficiency (87% of all CVAs).[41] Synonyms for CVA include *stroke, brain attack,* and *cerebral apoplexy.*

CVAs are not uncommon in the adult population, although their occurrence in persons younger than age 40 is quite rare.[42] In the United States approximately 795,000 new cases of acute CVA are reported annually.[41] Although mortality rates from various types of CVA differ markedly, the overall rate is relatively high. Deaths from CVAs in the United States were 128,798 in 2015, making it the fifth leading cause of death in the United States.[41] The frequency with which CVAs develop is emphasized by the fact that approximately 25% of routine autopsies (death from all causes) demonstrate evidence of a prior CVA. CVAs are the most common form of brain disease. The average age of persons at the time of their first CVA is approximately 64 years. Fortunately, recent evidence demonstrates a declining incidence of CVAs. For every 100 first episodes of CVAs that occurred in a unit of adult population between 1945 and 1949, only 55 first episodes of CVAs occurred between 1970 and 1974.[43] This decline continues today as the age-adjusted stroke mortality rate has decreased 33% since 1996.[44] This decline occurs in both sexes and all age groups, but is most notable in the elderly population.

Between the ages of 20 and 39 years the prevalence of stroke is 0.2% of the population in males and 0.7% for females.[42] It rises to 1.9% and 2.2% between 40 and 59 years, to 6.1%

and 5.2% between 60 and 79 years, and to 15.8% and 14.0% from 80 years and above.[42]

A number of factors that increase the risk of a CVA have been identified. These factors include HBP, diabetes mellitus, cardiac enlargement, hypercholesterolemia, the use of oral contraceptives, and cigarette smoking. Consistently elevated blood pressure has been demonstrated to be *the* major risk factor in the development of both hemorrhagic and atherosclerotic forms of CVAs.[45] Evidence from the Framingham study and elsewhere has demonstrated that high (systolic) blood pressure may be the major risk factor in the development of an acute hemorrhagic CVA.[46,47] About 77% of people having a first stroke have a blood pressure greater than 140/90 mm Hg.[41] It is estimated that the risk of developing an acute CVA increases by 30% for every 10-mm Hg elevation in systolic blood pressure above 160 mm Hg.

The patient who has had a CVA represents a significant risk within the dental or medical office during treatment. Survivors of CVAs have a good chance of recovering some degree of function. Twenty-five percent of stroke survivors recover with minor impairments, 40% experience moderate-to-severe impairments that require special care, 10% require care in a nursing home or other long-term facility, and 15% die shortly after the stroke.[48] Only 10% exhibited no functional deficit.[49] About 14% of stroke survivors experience a second stroke in the first year following a stroke.[48] Fifteen percent die shortly after the stroke.[48] With independent mobility the status post-CVA patient expects to receive dental and surgical care; however, it must be kept in mind that the recurrence rate of CVAs is high and that pain and anxiety only add to the risk presented by these patients.

Patients who have had an acute ischemic CVA receive some or all of the following drugs: anticoagulants, antihypertensives, and aspirin. Anticoagulants are used in the status post-CVA patient primarily to minimize the risk of recurrent strokes. Antihypertensives are important in status post-CVA patients in whom HBP is present. This includes approximately two thirds of all patients who have had a CVA. The treating dentist must be aware of the many side effects of the antihypertensive drugs (see Table 37.1). Low-dose aspirin therapy has been demonstrated to decrease the risk of a CVA in men with transient cerebral ischemia (TCI).[50,51]

The typical status post-CVA patient represents an ASA 2 or 3 patient—ASA 2 if the patient has had a CVA more than 6 months previously and has no evidence of residual neurologic deficit, ASA 3 if the patient has had a CVA more than 6 months earlier but has some degree of neurologic deficit. The status post-CVA patient is classified as ASA 4 if the CVA occurred less than 6 months earlier or if significant residual deficit remains.

Stress reduction is a top priority in the status post-CVA patient. The stress-reduction protocol, especially shorter appointments, effective pain control, and the management of apprehension, is of great importance in these patients.

All CNS depressants are relatively contraindicated in the patient who has had a CVA. Any of these drugs may produce hypoxia, which may provoke increased confusion, aphasia, and other potentially serious complications, such as seizures. It has been my experience that minimal-to-moderate levels of sedation, as seen with inhalation sedation, are quite safe and highly effective in reducing stress in the status post-CVA patient. However, sedative techniques should be reserved for the patient who has had a CVA in whom their use is truly justified.

Local anesthetics with vasopressors are not contraindicated in the status post-CVA patient, provided that negative aspiration precedes the slow administration of the drug and that blood pressure is not overly elevated. Epinephrine concentration should be 1:200,000, but not more than 1:100,000.

Oral sedation is quite valuable in the status post-CVA patient who demonstrates a greater degree of preoperative anxiety. Only minimal-to-moderate levels of sedation are recommended, using drugs such as the benzodiazepines. Medical consultation with the patient's physician is recommended before administration of these drugs.

IM sedation is contraindicated in the patient who has had a CVA because of the lack of control maintained over the actions of the drugs and the increased potential for hypoxia.

Inhalation sedation is the most highly recommended sedation technique for the status post-CVA patient. Medical consultation before its administration is suggested because some physicians may object to the use of this technique because higher concentrations of O_2 may produce constriction of cerebral arteries, leading to decreased cerebral blood flow and possible hypoxia. However, when sedation is needed in the patient who has had a CVA, inhalation sedation with N_2O-O_2 remains the preferred technique.

IV sedation should be reserved for only the most apprehensive status post-CVA patients and then only following medical consultation. Once again an increased possibility of hypoxia after IV drug administration mitigates against use of this technique. When considered essential to the success of therapy, lighter levels of IV sedation, as obtained with benzodiazepines, are recommended. Supplemental O_2 is strongly recommended.

General anesthesia in the status post-CVA patient should be reserved for the hospital operating room environment, if possible, with the patient admitted for a complete workup before the procedure and permitted to remain in the hospital until recovery is complete.

Myasthenia Gravis

MG is a neuromuscular disorder characterized by a notable weakness and easy fatigability of muscles. Although almost any muscle within the body may be affected, muscles innervated by the bulbar nuclei (facial, oculomotor, laryngeal, pharyngeal, and respiratory muscles) are most often involved. MG is an autoimmune disorder.[52] Muscle fatigability is worsened with exertion and improved with rest.

Recent estimates indicate that the U.S. prevalence is approximately 20/100,000, (60,000 patients total).[53] Epidemiologic studies have shown an increasing prevalence over the past 50 years, related to an increase in the frequency of diagnosis in elderly patients, but also likely due to improved ascertainment, reduced mortality rates, and an increased longevity of the population.[54] Gender and age influence the incidence of MG, with women being affected nearly three times more often than are men before age 40, whereas the incidence is higher in males after age 50 and roughly equal during puberty.[52]

Clinical signs and symptoms include pronounced fatigability of muscles with subsequent weakness and paralysis. Weakness of extraocular muscles results in diplopia and strabismus. Ptosis of the eyelids becomes more pronounced later in the day. Difficulty with speech and swallowing may develop after prolonged use of these functions. The patient may have difficulty using the tongue and may have a high-pitched nasal voice. The so-called *myasthenic smile,* a snarling, nasal smile, may be evident. Fluctuations in the severity of the disease (exacerbations and remissions) are common and unpredictable. Muscle weakness is intensified by infection and certain drugs, such as increased dosages of anticholinesterases (e.g., physostigmine, neostigmine, edrophonium), aminoglycoside antibiotics (e.g., neomycin), and membrane stabilizers (e.g., procainamide, phenytoin).

In recent years the prognosis for patients with MG has improved considerably, largely as a result of advances in intensive care medicine and the use of immunomodulating agents.[55] The therapeutic goal is to return the patient to normal function as rapidly as possible while minimizing the side effects of therapy. A number of therapeutic options are available (Table 37.5),[56] but treatment must be individualized according to the extent (ocular versus generalized) and severity (mild to severe) of disease and the presence or absence of concomitant disease (including, but not limited to, other autoimmune diseases and thymoma).[55]

Corticosteroids were the first immunosuppressants to be widely used in MG. They remain the most frequently used immune therapy today. Prednisone produces marked improvement or complete relief of symptoms in more than 75% of MG patients and some improvement in most of the rest. In a recent review of 1000 MG patients who received immunosuppressants for at least 1 year, all forms of MG benefited from immunosuppression: the rate of remission or minimal manifestations ranged from 85% in ocular MG to 47% in thymoma-associated disease.[57] Prednisone was used in the great majority of these patients, and azathioprine (AZA), was the first-choice nonsteroidal immunosuppressant.

In cases in which pharmacologic management is ineffective or where a thymoma is present or suspected, surgical removal of the thymus (thymectomy) is recommended. Following a review of existing studies, the Quality Standards Subcommittee of the American Academy of Neurology concluded that MG patients undergoing thymectomy are twice as likely to attain

Table 37.5	Drugs Used in Myasthenia Gravis	
	DRUG	**COMMENTS**
Symptomatic relief	Pyridostigmine	Causes worsening in some MG patients
Short-term immune	Plasma exchange (PLEX)	Treatment of choice in myasthenic crisis
	IV Ig	Use in exacerbating MG, children
Long-term immune	Prednisone	First-line immune therapy; rapid response; frequent side effects
	Azathioprine	First-line steroid-sparing
	Mycophenolate mofetil (MMF)	First- or second-line steroid-sparing
	Cyclosporin (CyA)	Steroid-sparing in patients intolerant or unresponsive to AZA, MMF
	Tacrolimus	Steroid-sparing in patients intolerant or unresponsive to AZA, MMF, and CyA
	Cyclophosphamide	Use in refractory/severe MG
	Rituximab	Use in refractory MG

Modified from: Meriggioli MN, Sanders DB: Autoimmune myasthenia gravis: emerging clinical and biological heterogeneity, *Lancet Neurol* 8(5):475–490, 2009 and Sanders DB, Guptill JT: Disorders of neuromuscular transmission. In Darboff RB, Jankovic J, Mazziotta JC, Pomeroy SL, editors: *Bradley's Neurology in Clinical Practice*, ed 7, Philadelphia, 2016, Elsevier.

medication-free remission, 1.6 times as likely to become asymptomatic, and 1.7 times as likely to improve.[58]

Exacerbation of myasthenia gravis occurs with infection and stress. A myasthenic crisis may be induced by a dental abscess or heightened anxiety about impending dental or surgical care. The myasthenic patient with a history of repeated crises should receive dental care within the confines of a hospital or other facility where acute airway management, including intubation, is readily available.

The administration of drugs with muscle-relaxant properties should be reserved for only essential situations. Few such occasions will arise in the typical outpatient dental or surgical setting.

Local anesthetics are the preferred drugs for the management of pain in myasthenic patients. Indeed, even in the hospitalized myasthenic patient, the use of regional nerve block anesthesia is preferred to general anesthesia. Vasopressors are not contraindicated.

Sedative techniques may be used, but care must be taken to avoid the administration of skeletal-muscle relaxants, such as diazepam and midazolam. Medical consultation is definitely indicated before the start of treatment in the myasthenic patient.

Oral, IM, inhalation, and IV techniques may be used on an outpatient basis if it is determined that they are absolutely necessary and only following medical consultation. Drugs that produce muscle relaxation, especially nondepolarizing muscle relaxants, are contraindicated in the myasthenic patient.

LIVER DISEASE

Liver disease is of great importance because the liver is responsible, in large part, for the biotransformation of most drugs. Hepatic dysfunction may be responsible for exaggerated effects of many drugs used for pain and anxiety control. A thorough history must be elicited when liver disease is suspected.

Probably the most recognizable sign of liver dysfunction is jaundice, a yellowish appearance of the skin and sclera. Jaundice is evidence of the accumulation of bilirubin in body tissues. Fatigue and nausea are also commonly seen. Another less common and less obvious sign of liver dysfunction is fetor hepaticus, a sweet, musty odor on the breath of the patient. Liver diseases of significance include viral hepatitis (hepatitis A virus [HAV], hepatitis B virus [HBV], and hepatitis C virus [HCV]), chronic hepatitis, alcoholic hepatitis, fatty liver, nodular cirrhosis, and biliary cirrhosis. Hepatitis is defined as an inflammation of the liver that may result from infectious or other causes.

It is extremely unlikely that the dentist will be called on to treat the patient with active acute hepatitis. In the event that such an occasion arises, the primary concern on the part of the dentist and staff is to prevent cross-contamination. Precautions include masking and gloving and sterilization of all equipment. Vaccination of the dentist and staff with hepatitis B vaccine is recommended. The degree of liver dysfunction present during the acute phase of hepatitis should be determined before treatment. Most local anesthetics (especially the commonly used amides) and CNS depressants undergo biotransformation in the liver. These drugs should be administered only if absolutely essential and then only in the smallest effective dose. Articaine HCl, though classified as an amide local anesthetic, undergoes metabolism in both the liver and blood. Its elimination half-life of 27 minutes, compared with approximately 90 minutes for lidocaine, makes it the preferred local anesthetic in these patients.[59] Medical consultation before initiation of dental treatment is suggested. During the acute phase of hepatitis, the patient may be quite debilitated and unable to tolerate additional stress. Treatment of an emergency nature only is recommended at this time.

Chronic hepatitis is a chronic inflammatory reaction of the liver that persists for more than 6 months. Although different forms of chronic hepatitis exist, the dentist must make a determination of the state of liver dysfunction in the patient before administering drugs. Chronic active hepatitis is characterized by progression to cirrhosis, although milder cases may resolve spontaneously. When deterioration of the patient's condition is evident, approximately 66% of patients die within 5 years of the onset of symptoms.

Alcoholic hepatitis is the most common form of chronic hepatitis. A history of heavy drinking over many years is always found. Parenchymal necrosis of the liver occurs as a result of alcohol abuse. Alcoholic hepatitis is the precursor of alcoholic cirrhosis. Alcoholic hepatitis may be reversible, depending on the degree of liver damage. In patients in whom the prothrombin time has been prolonged (to the degree at which liver biopsy cannot be performed), the mortality rate is 42%.

Drug-induced liver disease may result from toxic responses to the administration of various therapeutic agents. Drug-induced liver disease may mimic viral hepatitis or biliary tract obstruction. Examples of drug-induced liver disease include acetaminophen, amiodarone, bromfenac, cocaine, cyclophosphamide, cyclosporine, methotrexate, niacin, oral contraceptives, tetracycline and toxins such as yellow phosphorus, carbon tetrachloride, *Amanita* toxin, and bacterial toxins.[60]

The most common cause of nodular cirrhosis is the chronic abuse of alcohol. This disease involves hepatocellular injury, which leads to both fibrosis and nodular degeneration throughout the liver. Cirrhosis is a serious and irreversible disease that, when advanced, has a very poor prognosis. Response of this patient to most CNS-depressant drugs may be exaggerated.

Primary biliary cirrhosis is a chronic liver disease manifested by cholestasis. Insidious in onset, it is seen most frequently in women between the ages of 40 and 60 years. Its primary symptom is pruritus, with jaundice developing within 2 years of its onset. Secondary biliary cirrhosis follows chronic obstruction to bile flow, which is usually produced by a calculus, neoplasm, stricture, or biliary atresia.

The major concerns facing the dentist asked to manage a patient with liver disease include the possibly debilitated condition of the patient, the degree of hepatic dysfunction, and the possibility of cross-contamination of the office staff. ASA classifications for patients with liver disease range from ASA 2 to ASA 4, based on signs and symptoms and the results of medical consultation.

In cases in which debilitation is obvious, elective dental care should be deferred until such time as the patient is better able to withstand the stresses involved in treatment. Emergency care should be considered only after consultation with the patient's physician and should be managed in the least traumatic manner. Definitive treatment may be instituted after the patient has returned to an improved state of health.

The administration of drugs to the patient with serious liver damage increases the likelihood of adverse drug reactions because it is likely that the drug will undergo biotransformation into inactive metabolites at a considerably slower rate than usual. For example, the β-half-life of lidocaine in the healthy patient is 90 minutes, whereas with cirrhosis, lidocaine's half-life may approach 450 minutes.[61] Elevated blood levels of the drug develop, potentially leading to a prolonged duration of clinical action of CNS-depressant drugs and a greater risk of side effects and overdose reactions. A significant percentage of the biotransformation of most drugs used in the management of pain and anxiety occurs in the liver. Dosages of these drugs must be determined after careful consideration of the effects of diminished liver function. In general, drug dosages should be decreased to approximately 50% of the usual dose in the ASA 3 or 4 patient with liver dysfunction. It is prudent to avoid the administration of such drugs when possible. The problem of cross-contamination has been previously discussed.

Local anesthesia is recommended. Vasopressors are not contraindicated. Because the half-life of amide local anesthetics may be considerably prolonged when significant liver disease is present, minimal volumes of amide local anesthetics should be administered. Articaine HCl, classified as an amide local anesthetic, has a half-life of approximately 27 minutes. Articaine HCl undergoes biotransformation in the liver, like the other amides, as well as in the blood, via the enzyme plasma cholinesterase, as do the ester local anesthetics. Articaine HCl is a recommended local anesthetic in this situation.[59] Nerve block injection is preferred to infiltration over large areas, except in patients in whom prothrombin times have increased because of their liver damage. In these patients, infiltration or nerve blocks that have a minimal risk of positive aspiration of blood are recommended.

Oral sedation is recommended as an excellent means of providing minimal levels of sedation. Drugs such as the benzodiazepines can be used with little increase in risk in the patient with hepatic dysfunction.

IM sedation should be avoided when possible in patients with hepatic dysfunction because the actions of the drugs may be prolonged and exaggerated. Opioids, drugs commonly used in IM sedation, demonstrate an exaggerated clinical action in the presence of liver dysfunction and should be avoided when possible.

Inhalation sedation with N_2O-O_2 is, without doubt, the safest and most effective sedative technique in patients with hepatic dysfunction. Neither gas undergoes biotransformation in the liver, and neither demonstrates exaggerated clinical actions in the presence of even significant liver dysfunction.

IV sedation is also relatively contraindicated in the presence of severe liver disease (ASA 4). Barbiturates and opioids may result in exaggerated and prolonged responses in these patients. The use of benzodiazepines is preferred in cases in which IV sedation is considered necessary.

Outpatient general anesthesia is also contraindicated in the presence of severe liver dysfunction (ASA 4). The patient for whom general anesthesia is contemplated should be hospitalized for a thorough preoperative evaluation, the condition stabilized, and the procedure completed in the operating room under careful monitoring.

ENDOCRINE DISORDERS

Several potentially important disease entities are related to dysfunction of the endocrine glands, including the thyroid, adrenal, pituitary, and parathyroid glands. Especially important to the practicing dentist and physician are disorders of the thyroid and adrenal glands, specifically hyperthyroidism, hypothyroidism, hyperadrenocorticism (Cushing syndrome), and hypoadrenocorticism (Addison disease).

Thyroid Gland Dysfunction

Located in the neck on either side of the trachea, the thyroid gland produces and secretes hormones that perform an important function in regulating the level of biochemical activity in most tissues of the body. Proper functioning of the thyroid gland is essential for normal growth and development.

Thyroid gland dysfunction is a relatively common medical disorder. If diabetes mellitus is excluded, thyroid dysfunction accounts for 80% of all endocrine disorders. Dysfunction of the thyroid gland may occur through overproduction (hyperthyroidism) or underproduction (hypothyroidism) of thyroid hormones. In both instances, clinical manifestations cover a broad spectrum ranging from subclinical dysfunction to acute life-threatening situations. Fortunately, however, most patients with thyroid dysfunction have milder forms of the disease.

Hyperthyroidism

Hyperthyroidism is known by several other names, including *thyrotoxicosis, toxic goiter* (diffuse or nodular), *Basedow disease, Graves disease, Parry disease,* and *Plummer disease.* It may be defined as a state of heightened thyroid gland activity associated with the production of excessive quantities of the thyroid hormones thyroxine (T4) and triiodothyronine (T3). Because thyroid hormones affect the cellular metabolism of virtually all organ systems, the signs and symptoms of hyperthyroidism may be noted in any part of the body. Untreated hyperthyroidism may lead to thyroid storm or crisis, which manifests itself, in part, as a severe hypermetabolic state.

The incidence of thyroid gland hyperfunction is 3 per 10,000 adults per year and has a female/male ratio of 5 : 1. Hyperthyroidism affects 2% of women and 0.2% of men in their lifetimes.[62] Its peak incidence occurs between the ages of 20 and 40 years. Although its cause is unknown, hyperthyroidism is more common in areas of iodine deficiency and has been demonstrated to have familial (genetic) tendencies. It may manifest itself initially during periods of emotional and physical stress.

Patients with thyroid gland hyperfunction undergo treatment aimed at halting the excessive secretion of thyroid hormones. Management may involve surgical removal of all or part of the thyroid gland (total or subtotal thyroidectomy), long-term drug therapy with antithyroid (thioureylenes) drugs to achieve remission of the disease, or radioactive iodine (RAI) therapy, rather than surgical excision. Frequently prescribed antithyroid drugs include propylthiouracil (PTU), methimazole (Tapazole), and carbimazole. PTU is the third most common cause of drug-related hepatic failure, accounting for 10% of all drug-related liver transplants.[63] Other drugs used, although not antithyroid drugs, include propranolol and nadolol (β-adrenergic

blockers) and glucocorticoids such as prednisolone and hydrocortisone.

Common signs and symptoms of hyperthyroidism are presented in Box 37.4.[63] Milder degrees of thyroid hyperfunction may be mistaken for acute anxiety, with little increase in clinical risk to the patient. It must be noted that several cardiovascular disorders, primarily angina pectoris, are exaggerated in hyperthyroidism. Severe hyperfunction is an indication for immediate medical consultation. Dental care should not begin until the underlying metabolic disturbance has been corrected.

Additional considerations in hyperthyroid patients include contraindications to the administration of several drugs:

1. *Atropine and other anticholinergics* because of their vagolytic properties, which produce an increase in heart rate. This may be a factor in precipitating thyroid crisis.
2. *Vasopressors:* drugs, such as epinephrine, that act as cardiac and cardiovascular stimulants. In the presence of a heart and/or cardiovascular system already stimulated by the hyperthyroid state, cardiac dysrhythmias or thyroid storm may be precipitated. Local anesthetics with vasopressors may be used because they possess minimal epinephrine

Box 37.4	Clinical Manifestations of Hyperthyroidism
General	Heat intolerance
	Perspiration
	Flushing
	Tremor
	Sleep disturbance
	Hair loss
Psychological	Nervousness
	Emotional lability
	Anxiety
	Aggressiveness
	Delusions
Cardiovascular	Palpitations
	Tachycardia
	Supraventricular dysrhythmias
Respiratory	Breathlessness
	Hoarseness
Gastrointestinal	Increased appetite
	Weight loss
	Increased frequency of bowel movements
Reproductive	Gynecomastia
	Irregular menses
Bone	Osteoporosis
Other	Ophthalmopathy
	Dermopathy

Modified from: McIntyre RC, Raeburn CD: Hyperthyroidism. In Harken AH, Moore EE, editors: Abernathy's surgical secrets, *ed 6, Philadelphia, 2009 Elsevier, pp. 288–291.*

concentrations (1 : 200,000 and 1 : 100,000). Of greater risk, however, is the racemic epinephrine cord used in gingival retraction. This more concentrated epinephrine formulation is more likely to precipitate undesirable side effects and should not be used.

Mildly hyperthyroid patients might easily be mistaken for apprehensive patients. The use of sedation is not contraindicated; however, because the cause of this patient's "apparent" nervousness is not truly dental in origin but hormonal, the efficacy of sedative drugs may be less than ideal and/or the dosages required to provide a sedative state may be markedly increased.

Hypothyroidism

Hypothyroidism is a clinical state in which the tissues of the body receive inadequate supplies of thyroid hormones. The clinical picture of hypothyroidism relates to the patient's age at the time of onset and to the degree and duration of hormonal deficiency. *Cretinism* is a clinical syndrome encountered in infants and children, resulting from deficiency of thyroid hormones during fetal and early life. Severe hypothyroidism developing in an adult is termed *myxedema.* Myxedema is the appearance of mucinous infiltrates beneath the skin. Severe, unmanaged hypothyroidism may ultimately lead to the loss of consciousness, a state termed *myxedema coma.*

Hypothyroidism in the adult usually develops as a result of idiopathic atrophy of the thyroid gland (primary hypothyroidism), a process currently thought to occur through an autoimmune mechanism. Primary hypothyroidism occurs in about 5% of individuals. Mild hypothyroidism is present in approximately 15% of older adults.[64] Other causes of hypothyroidism (secondary hypothyroidism) include total thyroidectomy, ablation following radioactive iodine therapy (both procedures are frequently used in the management of hyperthyroidism), and chronic thyroiditis. Hypofunction of the thyroid gland is much more common in women, with its incidence peaking about the time of menopause.

Patients with thyroid hypofunction receive thyroxine replacement (Synthroid, Levoxyl). Other drugs used in the management of hypothyroidism include liotrix (Euthyroid, Thyrolar) and dextrothyroxine (Choloxin).

Clinical manifestations of hypothyroidism are listed in Box 37.5.[65] Clinically, hypothyroid patients may represent an increased risk during medical and dental treatment involving administration of CNS depressants. The hypothyroid patient is unusually sensitive to all CNS depressants, including sedatives, opioids, and local anesthetics. Normal therapeutic doses of these drugs may result in overdose reactions in the hypothyroid patient.

Before commencing treatment on a hypothyroid patient, the following are recommended:
1. Medical consultation with the patient's physician
2. Use of CNS depressants with extreme caution
3. Examination for the presence of CVD

Box 37.5	Clinical Manifestations of Hypothyroidism: Symptoms	
Common Symptoms		**Physical Findings**
Lethargy		Goiter
Weight gain		Low blood pressure and slow heart rate
Constipation		Hair thinning or loss
Slowed mentation, forgetfulness		Dry skin
Depression		Confusion
Hair loss		Depressed affect
Dry skin		Nonpitting edema
Neck enlargement or goiter		
Cold skin		

Modified from: Hueston WJ: Endocrine and metabolic disorders. In Bope ET, Kellerman RD, editors, Conn's current therapy 2016. *Philadelphia, 2016, Elsevier.*

Note that hypothyroid patients have an increased incidence of CVD, especially in cases that have persisted for many years.

The patient who is hypothyroid or hyperthyroid, is receiving medical treatment, and is presently asymptomatic represents an ASA 2 risk, whereas the patient with clinical signs and symptoms is considered ASA 3. The following are recommendations for the use of pain- and anxiety-control techniques for both hypothyroid and hyperthyroid individuals.

Local anesthesia is recommended in both conditions. The use of vasopressors is not contraindicated in the hyperthyroid individual; however, minimal volumes of the least concentrated solution should be employed. In the clinically hypothyroid patient, the volume of local anesthetic should be minimized to prevent local anesthetic blood levels from becoming elevated. Overdose thresholds (blood levels) for local anesthetics may be decreased in the hypothyroid patient.

Oral sedation is recommended in both patients. The use of CNS depressants is relatively contraindicated in the clinically hypothyroid patient. When oral sedation is necessary, barbiturates and opioids should be avoided; instead, the benzodiazepines and other nonbarbiturate sedative-hypnotics (e.g., zaleplon, zolpidem) are preferred.

IM sedation is recommended for use only when other techniques have proven inadequate. The use of opioids and barbiturates is not recommended in the hypothyroid individual.

Inhalation sedation is highly recommended because of the degree of control maintained over the drug's action. In the hypothyroid patient, lower-than-usual concentrations of N_2O may prove adequate, whereas the hyperthyroid individual may require greater-than-usual concentrations or the technique may prove to be unsuccessful. Careful titration of N_2O prevents accidental overdose in this technique in the hypothyroid patient.

IV moderate sedation should be administered with extreme care (e.g., by slower-than-usual titration) in the hypothyroid patient because the actions of most commonly used drugs may be exaggerated. This is especially so for the opioids, but is also true, to a lesser degree, with benzodiazepines. Careful, slow titration minimizes the risk of adverse response. The hyperthyroid patient may prove difficult to sedate adequately within the suggested dosage limits presented earlier (see Chapter 26). Failure of the IV technique to provide adequate sedation is preferable to administration of drug dosages in excess of those recommended.

Outpatient general anesthesia is contraindicated in the clinically hyperthyroid or hypothyroid patient. Hospitalization before the procedure, complete medical evaluation, and stabilization of the disease process should be considered before the administration of any general anesthetic in these patients.

Patients with thyroid gland dysfunction, whether hyperfunction or hypofunction, who are receiving or have received treatment, have normal levels of circulating thyroid hormones, and are asymptomatic are considered to be *euthyroid* (ASA 2). Euthyroid patients may receive dental and medical treatment in the usual manner.

Adrenal Disorders

The adrenal gland is a combination of two glands, the cortex and the medulla, that although fused together, remain distinct and identifiable. The adrenal cortex produces and secretes more than 30 steroid hormones. Cortisol, a glucocorticoid, is considered the most important product of the adrenal cortex. It permits the body to adapt to stress and is therefore extremely vital to continued survival.

Adrenal hypersecretion of cortisol leads to increased fat deposition in certain areas (the face [Fig. 37.3, *A*] and a "buffalo hump" [Fig. 37.3, *B*] on the back), increases in blood pressure, and alterations in blood cell distribution (eosinopenia and lymphopenia). Clinically, cortisol hypersecretion, referred to as *Cushing syndrome,* is usually readily corrected through surgical removal of part or all of the adrenal gland. Cushing syndrome remains one of the most difficult diagnoses in endocrinology. It is a multisystem disorder that develops in response to glucocorticoid excess. Iatrogenic Cushing syndrome is common (e.g., use of corticosteroids in management of medical conditions), but endogenous Cushing syndrome is rare.

The patient with Cushing syndrome represents an ASA 2 risk. The dentist should evaluate the patient carefully for the presence of HBP, signs and symptoms of HF, diabetes mellitus, and possible emotional disorders (depression). The use of local anesthetics and other CNS depressants for sedation is not contraindicated in the patient with Cushing syndrome. Medical consultation is recommended before therapy is started.

Inadequate production and secretion of cortisol, on the other hand, may lead to the relatively rapid development of

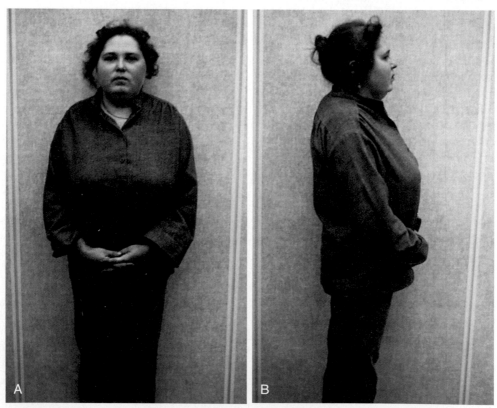

Figure 37.3 Hypersecretion of the adrenal cortex or chronic administration of corticosteroids leads to increased fat deposition in the face **(A)** and back **(B).** (From Zitelli BJ, Davis HW: *Atlas of pediatric physical diagnosis,* ed 5, St Louis, 2007, Mosby.)

signs and symptoms. Primary adrenocortical insufficiency is termed *Addison disease,* an insidious and usually progressive disease. The incidence of Addison disease is estimated at 0.3 to 1.0 per 100,000 persons, occurring equally in both sexes and throughout all age groups. Although all corticosteroids may be deficient in this disease state, it is important to note that the administration of physiologic doses of cortisol corrects most of the pathophysiologic effects. Clinical manifestations of adrenal insufficiency do not develop until at least 90% of the adrenal cortex has been destroyed.

Another form of adrenocortical hypofunction (secondary hypofunction) may occur through the administration of exogenous glucocorticosteroids to a patient with normal adrenal cortices. In the development of acute adrenal crisis, secondary adrenal insufficiency is a much greater potential threat than Addison disease. Glucocorticosteroid drugs are widely prescribed in pharmacologic doses for the symptomatic relief of a variety of disorders. When used in this manner, glucocorticosteroid administration produces a disuse atrophy of the adrenal cortex, decreasing the ability of the adrenal cortex to produce the levels of corticosteroid necessary to cope with stressful situations, in turn leading to the development of signs and symptoms of acute adrenal insufficiency.

Patients with Addison disease require corticosteroid administration in replacement (physiologic) doses for the remainder of their lives. However, patients receiving glucocorticosteroids for symptomatic treatment of their disorders commonly receive larger (pharmacologic or therapeutic) doses. These large doses may produce suppression of the normal adrenal cortex if continued for any length of time.

Recent evidence indicates that the majority of patients with secondary adrenal insufficiency may undergo routine dental treatment without the need for supplemental glucocorticoids.[66-68] At-risk patients for adrenal crisis are those undergoing stressful surgical procedures and have extremely little or no adrenal function.[66]

Because patients in these two categories are unable to adapt to stress in a normal manner, dental treatment must be modified to meet their needs. The stress-reduction protocol is extremely important in the overall management of these patients. Because stress represents a significant factor in increasing the risk involved in treatment of these patients, the requirement for adequate pain and anxiety control is critical.

Local anesthetics, with or without vasopressors, are indicated for use in these patients. All techniques of sedation are indicated. There are no contraindications to any technique or to specific drugs discussed previously.

Outpatient general anesthesia is contraindicated because of the increased stress associated with its administration, even in the best of situations. The patient with adrenal insufficiency, either primary or secondary, should be hospitalized for any general anesthetic procedure.

METABOLIC AND GENETIC DISORDERS

A number of disorders of metabolism and genetics are of potential importance in the management of pain and anxiety. The following disorders—diabetes mellitus, porphyria, malignant hyperthermia (MH), and atypical plasma cholinesterase—are discussed.

Diabetes Mellitus

Diabetes mellitus is a chronic systemic disease characterized by disorders in the production or use of insulin; in the metabolism of carbohydrate, fats, and protein; and in the structure and function of blood vessels. Diabetes is characterized by an inappropriately elevated level of glucose in the blood, termed *hyperglycemia.* Table 37.6 compares blood sugar (glucose) levels.

Diabetes mellitus is present in approximately 9.3% of the population of the United States (2012 statistics).[69] This represents approximately 29.1 million persons. Approximately 1.25 million American children and adults have type 1 diabetes. Of the 29.1 million, 21 million were diagnosed and 8.1 million were undiagnosed.[69] Although diabetes is considered a disease of the elderly (its incidence peaks in the fifth and sixth decades, with 25.9% of persons over age 65 years diagnosed as diabetic), it also occurs in young adults and children as well. Diabetes was the seventh leading cause of death in the United States in 2010.[69]

Two acute complications may develop in the diabetic patient: hyperglycemia (leading to diabetic coma) and, more importantly and much more common, hypoglycemia (leading to "insulin shock"). Whereas these complications must be looked for and managed if they develop, it is other, more chronic complications

Table 37.6	Blood Glucose Results		
	FASTING BLOOD GLUCOSE	RANDOM BLOOD SUGAR (TAKEN ANY TIME OF DAY WITH OR WITHOUT FASTING)	A1C
Preferable result	Less than 100 mg/dL	Less than 140 (even after eating a large meal)	Less than 6%
Prediabetes	100–125 mg/dL	140–200 or greater	6% or more
Diabetes	126 mg/dL and greater	200 or greater	7% or more

that are responsible for the majority of deaths occurring in diabetic persons. Table 37.7 presents the chronic complications associated with diabetes mellitus. Three major categories of chronic complications are large blood vessel disease, small blood vessel disease (termed *microangiopathy*), and increased susceptibility to infection. The dentist treating the diabetic patient should carefully evaluate the patient for clinical signs and symptoms of CVD, which is the most common cause of death in the diabetic patient.[70] Atherosclerotic CVD is the major cause of morbidity and mortality in diabetics. The clinical and pathologic features of CVD in diabetics are generally not distinguishable from those occurring in nondiabetic individuals, but they are manifested at an earlier age, and are more aggressive, and are associated with mortality rates that are two to four times higher in patients with diabetes.[70]

Knowledge on the part of the dentist of the type of diabetes—type 1, or insulin-dependent diabetes mellitus (IDDM), or type 2, non–insulin-dependent diabetes mellitus (NIDDM)—and the degree of control the patient maintains over his or her disease will enable the dentist to establish a risk factor for this patient. In general, the patient with well-controlled type 2 diabetes who demonstrates no associated disease is classified as an ASA 2 risk; patients with type 1 diabetes (patients with no β-cell activity) are ASA 3 or 4 risks, depending on the severity of the disease and their level of control. Table 37.8 compares type 1 and type 2 diabetes.

It is important for the dentist to speak with the diabetic patient before treatment to discuss the possible effect of the dental care on the patient's eating habits. The diabetic patient must attempt to maintain a normal eating pattern so that he or she does not become hypoglycemic after insulin administration. Changes in the management of type 1 diabetes (increasing the frequency of insulin administration) have led to the incidence of hypoglycemic episodes increasing approximately threefold.[71] Modification of insulin dosage may be required in some situations in which alterations in the patient's eating habits are unavoidable. Medical consultation may be indicated before adjustment of insulin dosage.

In the management of pain and anxiety, the diabetic patient does not present any unusual problems. Most techniques of pain and anxiety control are recommended for use in the diabetic patient. Treatment modification is required in ASA 3 and 4 diabetic patients according to the severity of the associated medical comorbidities. The following relates to the diabetic patient who is classified as an ASA 2 risk.

Local anesthesia is recommended for use in the diabetic patient, with no restrictions regarding either the choice of local anesthetic or the vasopressor. If the risk of missing meals is great as a result of prolonged posttreatment soft tissue anesthesia, the use of the local anesthesia reversal agent phentolamine mesylate should be considered.[72]

Oral sedation is recommended for use in the diabetic patient with no restrictions.

Table 37.7	Chronic Complications of Diabetes Mellitus
AFFECTED PART OR CONDITION	**COMPLICATION**
Vascular system	Atherosclerosis Large blood vessel disease Microangiopathy
Kidneys	Diabetic glomerulonephritis Arteriolar nephrosclerosis Pyelonephritis
Nervous system	Motor, sensory, and autonomic neuropathy
Eyes	Retinopathy Cataract formation Glaucoma Extraocular muscle palsies
Skin	Xanthoma diabeticorum Necrobiosis lipoidica diabeticorum Pruritus Furunculosis Mycosis
Mouth	Gingivitis Greater incidence of dental caries and periodontal disease Alveolar bone loss
Pregnancy	Greater incidence of large babies, stillbirths, miscarriages, neonatal deaths, and congenital defects

Table 37.8	Classification of Diabetes	
	TYPE 1	**TYPE 2**
Age at onset	Childhood or early childhood, but may manifest at any age	Middle age or older, but can be manifested in obese children and adolescents
Family history/genetic factors	Genetic risk defined, but most cases are sporadic	Strong genetic component
Environmental triggers	Largely unknown	Obesity, sedentary lifestyle
Requirement for insulin therapy	Universal	Variable
Frequency among diabetics	5%–10%	~90%
Comorbidities	Autoimmunity, especially thyroid, other endocrine disorders	Hypertension, dyslipidemia, metabolic syndrome, polycystic ovary syndrome

Modified from: Crandall J, Shamoon H: Diabetes mellitus. In Goldman L, Schafer AI, editors: *Goldman-Cecil medicine*, ed 25, Philadelphia, 2016, Saunders/Elsevier.

IM sedation is recommended for the diabetic patient when other techniques of sedation have proven ineffective. There are no specific contraindications to the administration of IM drugs.

Inhalation sedation is recommended for use in the diabetic patient with no restrictions.

IV sedation is recommended in the diabetic patient with no restrictions. The use of a 5% dextrose in water infusion will not produce any significant alteration in the patient's blood sugar level, especially when one considers that the patient receiving IV sedation will be NPO (nothing by mouth) for at least 4 hours before the procedure and will be slightly hypoglycemic. As a general rule, diabetics do better if they are a little "sweet" (hyperglycemic) than hypoglycemic.

Outpatient general anesthesia is usually contraindicated in the patient with type 1 diabetes. The patient with NIDDM is a good risk for outpatient general anesthesia. Most insulin-dependent diabetic patients who require general anesthesia should be hospitalized so that their diabetic condition can be stabilized and monitored closely, both during and after the procedure.

Porphyria

Porphyrins are cyclic compounds that are the precursors of heme and other important enzymes and pigments. Heme is the complex of iron and porphyrin that unites with the protein globin to form hemoglobin. The porphyrias are disorders of porphyrin metabolism in which a notable increase in the production and excretion of porphyrins and their precursors is noted. Porphyria may be either hereditary or acquired. Porphyrias are classified in two main categories, hepatic porphyrias and erythropoietic porphyrias, depending on whether the excessive porphyrin production occurs within the liver or in the bone marrow. Most porphyrias are genetic and hertitable.[73]

It is important to be aware of the presence of latent or manifest porphyria because of the potential for some drugs to provoke episodes of acute intermittent porphyria. This rare disorder is exacerbated by the administration of barbiturates, sulfonamides, clonazepam, mephenytoin, phenytoin, and griseofulvin, which cause a marked increase in porphyrin synthesis. Clinically, this is associated with acute episodes of abdominal pain, paresthesia, neuritic pain, convulsions, muscle paralysis, psychiatric disturbances, and the passage of reddish urine. Death, though rare today, results from respiratory paralysis in patients with acute episodes. Such paralysis may not develop for several days after drug administration.

Patients who have porphyria are classified as either ASA 2 or ASA 3 patients, depending on the severity of the disorder and the incidence of acute exacerbations.

Local anesthetics with and without vasopressors are recommended in the patient with porphyria. Oral sedation is recommended; however, *barbiturates are absolutely contraindicated*. IM sedation is recommended, but administration of *any barbiturate is absolutely contraindicated*. Inhalation sedation is recommended in the patient with porphyria. IV sedation is recommended, but the administration of *barbiturates is absolutely contraindicated*.

Fortunately the administration of barbiturates for sedation in dentistry has greatly diminished as newer, more effective, and safer drugs have been introduced into clinical practice.

Outpatient general anesthesia is contraindicated in the patient with porphyria. The patient with porphyria who requires a general anesthetic should be hospitalized before administration of the general anesthetic. *Barbiturates are absolutely contraindicated in the patient with porphyria.*

Malignant Hyperthermia

MH (malignant hyperpyrexia) is a pharmacogenetic disorder in which a genetic variant in the patient alters his or her response to certain drugs. The problem is that before exposure to specific drugs, it may be impossible to recognize an MH-susceptible patient. The genetic defect manifests itself as a flaw in the control of calcium levels in skeletal muscle when the normal intracellular environment is altered by certain drugs.[74] The concentration of calcium in the sarcoplasm is abnormally high. The list of drugs implicated as triggering MH is large and includes many of the most commonly used general anesthetics (Box 37.6). The Malignant Hyperthermia Association of the United States (MHAUS) provides up-to-date information on the safety of anesthetic agents in MH-susceptible patients.[75]

Acute clinical manifestations of MH include the following: *Muscle rigidity,* which occurs in 80% of cases, may appear immediately after the administration of succinylcholine, a muscle relaxant. Because skeletal muscle accounts for approximately 40% of body weight, its increased metabolism has a profound effect on whole-body metabolism.[74] Masseteric rigidity is a common first sign. Rigidity may develop up to 2 hours after the beginning of a procedure when inhalation anesthetics are used. Signs of MH, including tachycardia, increased end-tidal carbon dioxide (CO_2), muscle rigidity, and increased temperature, are related to increased metabolism. *Tachycardia* is almost universally present in MH. *Tachypnea* develops simultaneously with the tachycardia; however, in cases in which muscle relaxants have been administered, this symptom may be masked. *Fever* is the primary feature of MH. It is the rate of rise, not the absolute temperature, that is of importance in MH. In a fulminant MH episode body temperature increases rapidly, by as much as 1° C in 5 minutes.[74] In general anesthetic procedures, the use of a temperature probe is universally recommended. An elevation of temperature of more than 0.5° C should be suspect. Fever is usually a late sign, often noted after tachypnea and tachycardia. Other clinical signs include *dysrhythmias, cyanosis, dark venous blood* in the surgical field, *red urine,* and *hot skin.*

The mortality rate of patients with MH was 63% to 73% before the introduction of dantrolene sodium, an IV agent used to terminate episodes.[76] Dantrolene sodium inhibits the release of calcium from intracellular organelles, such as mitochondria and the sarcoplasmic reticulum. Since its introduction, the mortality rate from MH has decreased to less than 1.4%.[77] Dantrolene sodium is also available in an oral form that has enabled susceptible patients to receive prophylaxis before their exposure to drugs that might induce MH.

Box 37.6	Unsafe and Safe Drugs Used for Sedation, Local and General Anesthesia

Not Safe for Use in MH-Susceptible Patients, the Following Anesthetic Agents Are Known Triggers of MH

Inhaled general anesthetics
Desflurane
Enflurane
Ether
Halothane
Isoflurane
Methoxyflurane
Sevoflurane
Succinylcholine
All other anesthetic agents outside of these two categories of volatile anesthetic agents and depolarizing muscle relaxants are considered safe.

Safe Anesthetic Agents for MH Patients

BARBITURATES/ INTRAVENOUS ANESTHETICS
Diazepam
Etomidate (Amidate)

Hexobarbital
Ketamine (Ketalar)
Methohexital (Brietal, Brevital)
Midazolam
Pentobarbital
Propofol (Diprivan)
Thiopental (Pentothal)

INHALED NON-VOLATILE GENERAL ANESTHETIC
Nitrous oxide

LOCAL ANESTHETICS
Amethocaine
Articaine
Bupivacaine
Dibucaine
Etidocaine
Eucaine
Lidocaine (Xylocaine)
Levobupivacaine
Mepivacaine (Carbocaine)
Procaine (Novocaine)
Prilocaine (Citanest)
Ropivacaine
Stovaine

Proparacaine Hydrochloride
ALCAINE (proparacaine hydrochloride ophthalmic solution)

NARCOTICS (OPIOIDS)
Alfentanil (Alfenta)
Anileridine
Codeine (Methyl Morphine)
Diamorphine
Fentanyl (Sublimaze)
Hydromorphone (Dilaudid)
Meperidine (Demerol)
Methadone
Morphine
Naloxone
Oxycodone
Phenoperidine
Remifentanil
Sufentanil (Sufenta)

SAFE MUSCLE RELAXANTS
Arduan (Pipecuronium)
Curare (The active ingredient is Tubocurraine)
Gallamine
Methocarbamol (Robaxin, Robaxin-750, Carbacot, Skelex)

Metocurine
Mivacron (Mivacurium)
Neromax (Doxacurium)
Nimbex (Cisatracurium)
Norcuron (Vecuronium)
Pavulon (Pancuronium)
Tracrium (Atracurium)
Zemuron (Rocuronium)

ANXIETY-RELIEVING MEDICATIONS
Ativan (Lorazepam)
Centrax
Dalmane (Flurazepam)
Halcion (Triazolam)
Klonopin
Librax
Librium (Chlordiazepoxide)
Midazolam (Versed)
Pail (paroxetine)
Paxipam (Halazepam)
Restoril (Temazepam)
Serax (Oxazepam)
Tranxene (Clorazepate)
Valium (Diazepam)

From Malignant Hyperthermia Association of the United States: Safe and unsafe anesthetics. Hyperthermia Association of the United States. www.mhaus.org/healthcare-professionals/be-prepared/safe-and-unsafe-anesthetics.

The incidence of fulminant MH was reported to be 1 per 62,000 anesthetics administered when known triggering agents were not used. When triggering agents were administered, the incidence rose to 1 case in 4500 anesthetics.[78] The majority of cases occur in children, adolescents, and young adults. Males develop MH more frequently than females. MH is encountered with much greater frequency in certain areas of North America where families with the genetic trait have settled. Three areas of concentration include Toronto, Canada, and Wisconsin and Nebraska in the United States.[79]

Patients with documented MH or those who are possibly susceptible are classified as ASA 3 risks. Definite treatment modification is necessary to minimize risk for these patients during therapy. Medical consultation is recommended, discussing the proposed treatment, including drugs. The MHAUS has an excellent website (www.mhaus.org), which may be accessed for up-to-the-minute information regarding MH.[75]

Local anesthetics of the amide group—articaine, lidocaine, mepivacaine, prilocaine, etidocaine, and bupivacaine—were, at one time, considered absolutely contraindicated in MH

patients. It was believed that these drugs were capable of triggering the MH response. Research has demonstrated conclusively that the *amide local anesthetics are not contraindicated* in the MH-susceptible patient,[80–82] nor is there any contraindication to the administration of the ester local anesthetics. The inclusion of vasopressors in the anesthetic solution is not contraindicated.

Oral sedation is recommended. Opioids and benzodiazepines may be administered with no increased risk in patients with MH.

IM sedation may be administered, although I would probably have serious second thoughts about the administration of any parenteral sedation technique on an outpatient basis to a child with a history of MH. Hospitalization would appear to be a more prudent approach to this patient's management.

Inhalation sedation with N_2O-O_2 is recommended in the patient with MH. Following consultation, the use of inhalation sedation on an outpatient basis might prove to be most favored.

IV sedation is recommended; however, as with IM sedation, I personally believe that it is more prudent to consider hospitalization of the MH-susceptible patient who requires parenteral sedation, unless the patient's condition is well controlled with the administration of dantrolene sodium.

Outpatient general anesthesia is contraindicated in the MH-susceptible patient. Hospital-based care is recommended for the patient with MH who requires general anesthesia. Because of the risk involved in general anesthesia for this patient, the benefits to be gained by using general anesthesia should be carefully weighed against its risk before it is used.

Atypical Plasma Cholinesterase

Atypical plasma cholinesterase is another pharmacogenetic disorder. Two commonly used drugs—succinylcholine, a short-acting, depolarizing muscle relaxant used during intubation in general anesthesia, and the ester local anesthetics, such as procaine, chloroprocaine, tetracaine, and propoxycaine—are metabolized by the enzyme plasma cholinesterase. A form of this enzyme, called *atypical plasma cholinesterase,* is found in 1 in 2820 persons.[83] Patients with atypical plasma cholinesterase are unable to metabolize these drugs at a normal rate and are therefore more likely to exhibit clinical signs and symptoms of (1) prolonged clinical activity and/or (2) drug overdose. When the paralytic agent succinylcholine is administered, the clinical duration of muscular relaxation in these patients is considerably prolonged beyond the usual 5 minutes. In cases in which an ester local anesthetic has been administered, elevated blood levels, which increase the risk of drug overdose, are noted. Clinical duration of action (pain control) is not prolonged when local anesthetics are administered to these patients. Patients with atypical plasma cholinesterase are considered ASA 2 risks.

Amide local anesthetics are recommended in these patients. Vasopressors are not contraindicated. Ester local anesthetics should be avoided in patients with atypical plasma cholinesterase; however, if they must be administered, the smallest effective volume is recommended.

Oral, IM, and inhalation sedation are recommended without specific contraindications. IV sedation is recommended with the warning that succinylcholine not be administered to these patients.

Outpatient general anesthesia may be administered if succinylcholine is not administered to these patients. It is prudent, however, to consider hospitalization of these patients if general anesthesia is required.

HEMATOLOGIC DISORDERS

Several disorders of potential significance to the administration of drugs—anemia, sickle cell anemia, polycythemia vera, and hemophilia—are included in this category.

Anemia

Anemia is defined as a significant reduction in the mass of circulating red blood cells, a result of which is the oxygen-binding capacity of the blood is diminished.[84] Causes of anemia include hemorrhage (either external or internal), diminished manufacture of erythrocytes in the body, and a shortened life span of red blood cells (RBCs). McCarthy has listed the following three categories of anemia[85]:

1. Reduction below the normal number of erythrocytes: megaloblastic anemia, pernicious anemia, folic acid deficiency, aplastic anemia
2. Reduction in the quantity of hemoglobin: iron-deficiency anemia, sickle cell anemia
3. Reduction in the volume of packed red cells: bleeding or destruction (hemolytic anemia)

Signs and symptoms of anemia include ease of fatigability, dyspnea, pallor, palpitation, angina pectoris, and tachycardia. With a normal adult hemoglobin level of 12 to 18 g/100 mL of blood, levels below 9 g/100 mL are considered indicative of anemia. The ASA risk categories for anemic individuals vary according to the severity of clinical signs and symptoms; however, in general, the anemic patient with a hemoglobin level above 9 g/100 mL is classified as ASA 2, whereas the patient with a hemoglobin level below 9 g/100 mL is classified as ASA 3.

Stress reduction is required for the anemic patient. The primary modification is the recommendation that the patient receive O_2 via nasal cannula throughout the treatment.

Local anesthetics are indicated with or without vasopressors. Prilocaine is relatively contraindicated in anemic individuals, especially those with methemoglobinemia.[86] Large volumes of prilocaine may produce cyanosis (managed with the administration of IV methylene blue).[87] Other amide and ester local anesthetics do not produce elevations in methemoglobin.

Oral sedation is recommended with no specific contraindications.

IM sedation is recommended. Supplemental O_2 administered via nasal cannula throughout the procedure is suggested.

Inhalation sedation is recommended. The supplemental O_2 administered along with N_2O is quite beneficial to the patient.

IV sedation is indicated. Supplemental O_2 administered via nasal cannula is suggested.

Outpatient general anesthesia is relatively contraindicated in anemic patients because of the decreased O_2-carrying capacity of the blood. In patients with mild anemia and asymptomatic patients, outpatient general anesthesia may be contemplated. In most cases, however, patients with anemia should be hospitalized for a general anesthetic procedure.

Sickle Cell Anemia

Sickle cell anemia is a hereditary disorder seen almost exclusively in blacks. Abnormal hemoglobin is transmitted as a dominant trait. Heterozygous carriers have mixtures of normal and sickle hemoglobin in all of their RBCs. Sickling of erythrocytes occurs at a low O_2 tension, especially when the pH of blood is also low (acidosis). The S (sickle) hemoglobin (HbS), which is present in this disease, is less soluble in its deoxygenated (reduced) form, leading to an increase in the viscosity of whole blood. Increased viscosity results in stasis and obstruction of blood flow through capillaries, venules, and terminal arterioles, which results in pain and swelling in the involved organs.[88]

It is estimated that 50,000 Americans, primarily blacks, have sickle cell disease, in which HbSS is present in all RBCs. This is approximately 1 per 600 blacks. Sickle cell trait, which another 2 million black Americans may carry, rarely causes signs and symptoms because the RBCs contain both sickle and normal hemoglobin, HbAS.

In African Americans, the incidence of sickle cell anemia at birth is 1 in 600, and the incidence of all genotypes of sickle cell disease is 1 in 300.[89] Sickle cell trait occurs in approximately 300 million persons worldwide, with the highest prevalence of approximately 30% to 40% in sub-Saharan Africa. It is found in nearly 10% of black Americans.[90]

The patient with sickle cell disease represents an increased risk during treatment, particularly treatment that involves the administration of drugs with the potential to produce respiratory depression. A sickle cell crisis might be precipitated by CNS-depressant drugs, infection, or extreme cold. When a sickle cell crisis occurs, the organs most often involved are the brain, kidneys, spleen, liver, and bones. The patient with sickle cell trait, although unlikely to develop crisis, may, in circumstances of extreme stress, such as physical exertion and general anesthesia, suffer a sickle cell crisis.

Most patients with sickle cell disease represent an ASA 3 risk during therapy. Those with sickle cell trait may be categorized as ASA 2 patients. Treatment modifications involve the provision for adequate oxygenation at all times in these patients, the prevention of acidosis, and the management of stress.

Local anesthetics are recommended, either with or without vasopressors. No specific contraindications exist to any drug.

Oral sedation is recommended for minimal levels of preoperative anxiety control. Should moderate levels of sedation be sought by this route, the administration of supplemental O_2 via nasal cannula is recommended.

IM sedation is recommended when other techniques of sedation have been ineffective. O_2 administered via nasal cannula throughout the procedure is recommended.

Inhalation sedation with N_2O-O_2 is ideally suited for the patient with a history of sickle cell disease. Increased levels of O_2 are provided to the patient throughout the procedure.

IV sedation is recommended with no specific contraindications to any drugs. Supplemental O_2 administered via nasal cannula is recommended.

Outpatient general anesthesia is not recommended because the potential risk of hypoxia may be increased. Hospitalization of the patient is strongly recommended for the administration of general anesthesia.

Polycythemia Vera

Polycythemia vera is an overproduction of one or more types of blood cells, such as RBCs, white blood cells, or platelets. Symptoms are produced by an increased viscosity of blood and hypermetabolism. Although polycythemia vera may develop at any age, it is commonly observed after the age of 50. It is more common in men and is seen more often in Jews from Eastern Europe. Polycythemia vera is rarely encountered in blacks and Latin Americans.[91] Clinical signs and symptoms include headache, inability to concentrate, hearing loss, itching, pain in fingers and toes, a decreased feeling of well-being, and a loss of energy.

Complications of polycythemia vera include hemorrhage (gastrointestinal bleeding) and thrombosis, especially in uncontrolled polycythemia vera. Excessive bleeding is common during surgery. Management of polycythemia vera consists of phlebotomy (to keep hematocrit >45% in men and >42% in women. General treatment includes aspirin in patients less than 60 years without history of a prior thromboembolic event.[90] Hydroxyurea and interferon-alpha-2b are also used in management of polycythemia vera patients.[90] Survival without treatment ranges from 6 to 18 months after diagnosis; phlebotomy extends average survival time to 12 years.[90,92] Acute leukemia causes the death of 5% of patients.

The typical patient with polycythemia vera represents an ASA 2 risk during treatment. Excessive bleeding is likely to occur during dental and surgical treatment. The use of supplemental O_2 is recommended during all treatment in these patients.

Local anesthesia is recommended, with no specific contraindications to any local anesthetic drug or vasopressor. Nerve block anesthesia, especially those techniques in which a high percentage of positive aspiration is likely to occur, such as inferior alveolar nerve block, should be avoided because of the potential risk of excessive bleeding. Alternative techniques with lesser risks of positive aspiration of blood, such as the Gow–Gates mandibular block, periodontal ligament injection (PDL), or infiltration, are preferred in these patients.

Oral sedation is recommended without specific contraindications.

Parenteral sedation techniques are relatively contraindicated because of the increased risk of excessive bleeding and venous thrombosis. IM sedation should be reserved for those patients in whom it is absolutely necessary and in whom the benefits of its use outweigh the potential risks. Supplemental O_2 is recommended.

Inhalation sedation is highly recommended.

IV sedation is relatively contraindicated because of the potential for increased bleeding and venous thrombosis. Risks should be carefully weighed against benefits when IV sedation is considered. Supplemental O_2 is recommended.

Outpatient general anesthesia is relatively contraindicated in the patient with polycythemia vera. Hospitalization and treatment as an inpatient should be given careful consideration.

Hemophilia

Hemophilia is an inherited disorder of coagulation characterized by a lifelong history of abnormal bleeding. Hemophilia A and hemophilia B are the most common of the inherited bleeding disorders. Hemophilia A is classic hemophilia resulting from a deficiency of antihemophilic factor (AHF, factor VIII) activity. Because of its absence from plasma, thromboplastin formation is affected. Christmas disease, hemophilia B, is a deficiency in plasma thromboplastin component (factor IX). Patients present with "factor-type bleeding," which results from an inability to form a fibrin clot. These bleeding events include hemarthroses, mucosal bleeding, and intracranial bleeding.[93]

Patients with hemophilia rarely have massive hemorrhages. Bleeding is usually a prolonged oozing that develops after minor surgery or trauma. Of special concern during dental care is the administration of local anesthesia for pain control (see later discussion). Management of patients with hemophilia consists primarily of the prevention of bleeding and the administration of the appropriate factor (VII or IX) to the patient, either prophylactically before surgical procedures or when bleeding does occur, as after dental extractions.

Aspirin-containing analgesics should be avoided in persons with hemophilia because they prolong bleeding for 24 to 48 hours. Acetaminophen, nonsteroidal antiinflammatory drugs (NSAIDs), or other non–aspirin-containing analgesics may be used.

Local anesthesia is recommended, with no specific contraindications to the administration of any local anesthetic drug, with or without a vasopressor. The administration of regional nerve block anesthesia, especially techniques with a greater incidence of positive aspiration (inferior alveolar nerve block, posterior superior alveolar nerve block, and incisive [mental] nerve block), should be avoided in the hemophiliac patient. Alternative techniques, such as the Gow–Gates mandibular block, infiltration, PDL, and intraosseous, are recommended.

Oral sedation is recommended with no specific contraindications.

IM sedation is contraindicated because of the increased potential for prolonged bleeding.

Inhalation sedation is recommended with no specific contraindications.

IV sedation is recommended if the patient has received replacement therapy. Outpatient general anesthesia is contraindicated because of the increased risk of prolonged bleeding. Inpatient general anesthesia is preferred, with the patient well controlled before the procedure. Oral intubation is preferred to nasal intubation because of the reduced chance of bleeding.

REFERENCES

1. Go AS, Mozaffarian D, Roger VL, et al, American Heart Association Statistics Committee and Stroke Statistics Subcommittee: Heart disease and stroke statistics – 2014 update: a report from the American Heart Association. *Circulation* 129(3):e28–e292, 2014.
2. Health, United States: Leading causes of death and numbers of deaths, by sex, race, and Hispanic origin: United States, 1980-2014, Table 19, 2015. www.cdc.gov/nchs/hus/contents2015.htm#$019. (Accessed 31 January 2017).
3. ClinicalKey: Nitroglycerin drug monograph, June 30, 2016. www.clinicalkey.com. (Accessed 20 July 2016).
4. Sami S, Willerson JT: Contemporary treatment of unstable angina and non-ST-segment-elevation myocardial infarction (part 1). *Tex Heart Inst J* 37(2):141–148, 2010.
5. Sami S, Willerson JT: Contemporary treatment of unstable angina and non-ST-segment-elevation myocardial infarction (part 2). *Tex Heart Inst J* 37(3):262–275, 2010.
6. American Heart Association/American Stroke Association: Heart disease and stroke statistics – at-a-glance. www.heart.org/idc/groups/ahamah-public. (Accessed 31 January 2017).
7. Tarhan S, Giuliani ER: General anesthesia and myocardial infarction. *Am Heart J* 87(1):137–138, 1974.
8. Weinblatt E, Shapiro S, Frank CW, Sager RV: Prognosis of men after first myocardial infarction: mortality and first recurrence in relation to selected parameters. *Am J Public Health* 58(8):1329–1347, 1968.
9. Fleisher LA, Beckman JA, Brown KA, et al, American College of Cardiology/American Heart Association Task Force on Practice Guidelines (Writing Committee to Revise the 2002 Guidelines on Perioperative Cardiovascular Evaluation for Noncardiac Surgery); American Society of Echocardiography; American Society of Nuclear Cardiology; Heart Rhythm Society; Society of Cardiovascular Anesthesiologists; Society for Cardiovascular Angiography and Interventions; Society for Vascular Medicine and Biology; Society for Vascular Surgery: ACC/AHA 2007 guidelines on perioperative cardiovascular evaluation and care for noncardiac surgery: a report of the American College of Cardiology/American Heart Association Task Force on Practice Guidelines (Writing Committee to Revise the 2002 Guidelines on Perioperative Cardiovascular Evaluation for Noncardiac Surgery): developed in collaboration with the American Society of Echocardiography, American Society of Nuclear Cardiology, Heart Rhythm Society, Society of Cardiovascular Anesthesiologists, Society for Cardiovascular Angiography and Interventions, Society for Vascular Medicine and Biology, and Society for Vascular Surgery. *Circulation* 116(17):e418–e499, 2007.
10. Little JW, Falace DA, Miller CS, Rhodus NL: Ischemic heart disease. In Little JW, Falace DA, Miller CS, Rhodus NL, editors: *Little and Falace's dental management of the medically compromised patient*, ed 8, St Louis, 2013, Mosby/Elsevier.
11. Scirica BM, Morrow DA: Pathological and clinical manifestations of acute myocardial infarctions. In Mann DL, Zipes DP, Libby P, et al, editors: *Braunwald's heart disease: a textbook of cardiovascular medicine*, 10 ed, Philadelphia, 2015, Saunders/Elsevier, pp 1068–1094.
12. Stewart RAH, Robertson MC, Wilkins GT, et al: Association between activity at onset of symptoms and outcome of acute myocardial infarction. *J Am Coll Cardiol* 29(2):250–253, 1997.
13. Stern MS, Shine KI: Nitrous oxide and oxygen in coronary artery disease. *JAMA* 245(2):129, 1981.
14. Nwankwo T, Yoon SS, Burt V, Gu Q: *Hypertension among adults in the US: National Health and Nutrition Examination Survey, 2011-2012. NCHS Data Brief, No. 133*, Hyattsville, MD, 2013, National Center for Health Statistics, Centers for Disease Control and Prevention, US Department of Health and Human Services.
15. Kearney PM, Whelton M, Reynolds K, et al: Global burden of hypertension: analysis of worldwide data. *Lancet* 365(9455):217–223, 2005.
16. Jeter CR, Bush JP, Porter JH: Situational anxiety and blood pressure lability in the physician's office. *Clin Exp Hypertens A* 10(1):169–185, 1988.
17. Marshall T, Anantharachagan A, Choudhary K, et al: A randomised controlled trial of the effect of anticipation of a

blood test on blood pressure. *J Hum Hypertens* 16(9):621–625, 2002.

18. Olgin JE, Zipes DP: Specific arrhythmias. In Mann DL, Zipes DP, Libby P, et al, editors: *Braunwald's heart disease: a textbook of cardiovascular medicine*, ed 10, Philadelphia, 2015, Saunders Elsevier, pp 748–797.

19. Perusse R, Goulet JP, Turcotte JY: Contraindications to vasoconstrictors in dentistry: part I. Cardiovascular diseases. *Oral Surg* 74(5):679–686, 1992.

20. Mozaffarian D, Benjamin EJ, Go AS, et al, American Heart Association Statistics Committee; Stroke Statistics Subcommittee on behalf of the American Heart Association Statistics Committee and Stroke Statistics Subcommittee: Heart disease and stroke statistics – 2016 update: a report from the American Heart Association. *Circulation* 133:e38–e360, 2016.

21. Roger VL: Heart failure compendium: epidemiology of heart failure. *Circ Res* 113(6):646–659, 2013.

22. National Heart, Lung, Blood Institute: *Congestive heart failure data fact sheet*, Bethesda, MD, 2008, NHLBI.

23. Hoffman JL, Kaplan S: The incidence of congenital heart disease. *J Am Coll Cardiol* 39(12):1890–1900, 2002.

24. Reller MD, Strickland MJ, Riehle-Colarusso T, et al: Prevalence of congenital heart defects in Atlanta, 1998-2005. *J Pediatr* 153(6):807–813, 2008.

25. Wilson W, Taubert KA, Gewitz M, et al, American Heart Association Rheumatic Fever, Endocarditis, and Kawasaki Disease Committee; American Heart Association Council on Cardiovascular Disease in the Young; American Heart Association Council on Clinical Cardiology; American Heart Association Council on Cardiovascular Surgery and Anesthesia; Quality of Care and Outcomes Research Interdisciplinary Working Group: Prevention of infective endocarditis: guidelines from the American Heart Association: a guideline from the American Heart Association Rheumatic Fever, Endocarditis, and Kawasaki Disease Committee, Council on Cardiovascular Disease in the Young, and the Council on Clinical Cardiology, Council on Cardiovascular Surgery and Anesthesia, and the Quality of Care and Outcomes Research Interdisciplinary Working Group. *Circulation* 116(15):1736–1754, 2007.

26. Texas Heart Institute Heart Information Center: Valve repair or replacement. www.texasheart.org/HIC/Topics?vsurg.cfm. (Accessed 31 January 2017).

27. National Kidney Foundation: Fast facts, April 2016. www.kidney.org/news/newsroom/factsheets/FastFacts. (Accessed 31 January 2017).

28. Coresh J, Selvin E, Stevens LA, et al: Prevalence of chronic kidney disease in the United States. *JAMA* 298(17):2038–2047, 2007.

29. U.S. Department of Health and Human Services, Organ Procurement and Transplantation Network, Data, July 26, 2016. https://optn.transplant.hrsa.gov/data. (Accessed 31 January 2017).

30. Little JW, Falace DA, Miller CS, Rhodus NL: Chronic kidney disease and dialysis. In Little JW, Falace DA, Miller CS, Rhodus NL, editors: *Little and Falace's dental management of the medically compromised patient*, ed 8, St Louis, 2013, Mosby Elsevier.

31. Aronoff GR: Dose adjustment in renal impairment: response from drug prescribing in renal failure. *BMJ* 331(7511):293–294, 2005.

32. Centers for Disease Control and Prevention, National Center for Health Statistics: Asthma. www.cdc.gov/nchs/faststats/asthma.htm. (Accessed 26 July 2016).

33. National Vital Statistics Reports, Deaths: Final data for 2013. Volume 64, No. 2, February 16, 2016. www.cdc.gov/nchs/data/nvsr/nvsr64/nvsr64_02.pdf. (Accessed 26 July 2016).

34. American Lung Association, Epidemiology and Statistics Unit, Research and Health Education Division: Trends in COPD (Chronic bronchitis and emphysema): Morbidity and mortality, March 2013. www.lung.org/assets/documents/research/copd-trend-report.pdf. (Accessed 31 January 2017).

35. Shafer PO: About epilepsy: the basics. Epilepsy Foundation, January 2014. www.epilepsy.com/learn/epilepsy-basics. (Accessed 31 January 2017).

36. Epilepsy Statistics, Epilepsy Foundation. www.epilepsy.com/learn/epilepsy-statistics. (Accessed 31 January 2017).

37. Gilliam F: Diagnosis and classification of seizures and epilepsy. In Winn HR, Berger MS, Dacey RG, Jr, editors: *Youmans neurological surgery*, ed 6, Philadelphia, 2011, Saunders/Elsevier, pp 672–677.

38. Rang HP, Ritter JM, Flower RJ, Henderson G: Antiepileptic drugs. In Rang HP, Ritter JM, Flower RJ, Henderson G, editors: *Rang & Dale's pharmacology*, ed 8, Oxford, 2016, Elsevier Churchill Livingstone, pp 546–558.

39. Melon E, Homs JB: Nitrous oxide in neurosurgery: its safety in the seizure-prone patient. *Agressologie* 32:429, 1991.

40. Ito BM, Sato S, Kufta CV, Tran D: Effect of isoflurane and enflurane on the electrocorticogram of epileptic patients. *Neurology* 38(6):924–928, 1988.

41. American Heart Association/American Stroke Association: Heart disease, stroke and research statistics at-a-glance – 2016 update. https://heart.org/dc/groups/ahamah-public/@wcm/@sop/@smd/documents/downloadable/ucm_480086.pdf. (Accessed 28 July 2016).

42. Mozaffarian D, Benjamin EJ, Go AS, et al, American Heart Association Statistics Committee; Stroke Statistics Subcommittee: Heart Disease and Stroke Statistics – 2016 Update: a Report From the American Heart Association. *Circulation* 133(4):e38–e60, 2016.

43. Mackay J, Mensah G, editors: *The atlas of heart disease and stroke*, 2004, World Health Organization. www.who.int/cardiovascular_diseases/resources/atlas/en/. (Accessed January 31, 2017).

44. National Institutes of Health, U.S. Department of Health and Human Services: Research Portfolio Online Reporting Tools (RePORT). Stroke. https://report.nih.gov/nihfactsheets/viewfactsheet.aspx?csid=117. (Accessed 31 January 2017).

45. Ezzati M, Lopez AD, Rodgers A, et al, the Comparative Risk Assessment Collaborating Group: Selected risk factors and global and regional burden of disease. *Lancet* 360(9343):1347–1360, 2002.

46. Fang MC, Coca Perraillon M, Ghosh K, et al: Trends in stroke rates, risk, and outcomes in the United States, 1988 to 2008. *Am J Med* 127(7):608–615, 2014.

47. Brott T, Thalinger K, Hertzberg V: Hypertension as a risk factor for spontaneous intracerebral hemorrhage. *Stroke* 17(6):1078–1083, 1986.

48. National Institute of Neurological Disorders and Stroke: Stroke rehabilitation information. www.ninds.nih.gov/disorders/stroke/stroke_rehabilitation.htm. (Accessed 31 January 2017).

49. Centers for Disease Control and Prevention (CDC): Outpatient rehabilitation among stroke survivors – 21 states and the District of Columbia, 2005. *MMWR Morb Mortal Wkly Rep* 55:204, 2007.

50. Andrews PJ: Critical care management of acute ischemic stroke. *Curr Opin Crit Care* 10(2):110–115, 2004.

51. Lamichhane D: Update on secondary prevention of ischaemic stroke. *J Pak Med Assoc* 64(7):812–819, 2014.

52. Ferri FF: Myasthenia gravis. In *Ferri's clinical advisor 2017*, Philadelphia, 2017, Elsevier, p 835.

53. Phillips LH: The epidemiology of myasthenia gravis. *Semin Neurol* 24(1):17–20, 2004.

54. Carr AS, Cardwell CR, McCarron PO, McConville J: A systematic review of population based epidemiological studies in myasthenia gravis. *BMC Neurol* 10:46, 2010.

55. Sanders DB, Guptill JT: Disorders of neuromuscular transmission. In Darboff RB, Jankovic J, Mazziotta JC, Pomeroy SL, editors: *Bradley's neurology in clinical practice*, ed 7, St Louis, 2016, Elsevier.

56. Meriggioli MN, Sanders DB: Autoimmune myasthenia gravis: emerging clinical and biological heterogeneity. *Lancet Neurol* 8(5):475–490, 2009.

57. Sanders DB, Evoli A: Immunosuppressive therapies in myasthenia gravis. *Autoimmunity* 43(5-6):428–435, 2010.

58. Gronseth GS, Barohn RJ: Practice parameter: thymectomy for autoimmune myasthenia gravis (an evidence-based review). *Neurology* 55(1):5–15, 2000.

59. Malamed SF, Gagnon S, Leblanc D: Efficacy of articaine: a new amide local anesthetic. *J Am Dent Assoc* 131(5):635–642, 2000.

60. Lee WM: Toxin- and drug-induced liver disease. In Goldman L, Schafer AI, editors: *Goldman-Cecil Medicine*, ed 25, Philadelphia, 2016, Saunders/Elsevier, pp 1006–1010.

61. Sawyer DR, Ludden TM, Crawford MH: Continuous infusion of lidocaine in patients with cardiac arrhythmias: unpredictability of plasma concentrations. *Arch Intern Med* 141(1):43–45, 1981.

62. Ferri FF: Hyperthyroidism. In *Ferri's clinical advisor 2017*, Philadelphia, 2017, Elsevier, pp 644–645.

63. Rivkees SA, Mattison DR: Propylthiouracil (PTU) hepatoxicity in children and recommendations for discontinuation of use. *Int J Pediatr Endocrinol* 2009:132041, 2009.

64. Kim M, Ladenson PW: Thyroid. In Goldman L, Schafer AI, editors: *Goldman-Cecil medicine*, ed 25, Philadephia, 2016, Saunders/Elsevier, pp 1500–1514.

65. Hueston WJ: Endocrine and metabolic disorders. In Bope ET, Kellerman RD, editors: *Conn's current therapy 2016*, Philadelphia, 2016, Elsevier.

66. Little JW, Falace DA, Miller CS, Rhodus NL: Adrenal insufficiency. In Little JW, Falace DA, Miller CS, Rhodus NL, editors: *Little and Falace's dental management of the medically compromised patient*, ed 8, St Louis, 2013, Mosby/Elsevier, p 247.

67. Miller CS, Little JW, Falace DA: Supplemental corticosteroids for dental patients with adrenal insufficiency: reconsideration of the problem. *J Am Dent Assoc* 132(11):1570–1579, 2001.

68. Friedman RJ, Schiff CE, Bromberg JS: Use of supplemental steroids in patients having orthopaedic operations. *J Bone Joint Surg Am* 77(12):1801–1806, 1995.

69. American Diabetes Association: Statistics about diabetes. American Diabetes Association. www.diabetes.org/diabetes-basics/statistics. (Accessed 31 January 2017).

70. Crandall J, Shamoon H: Diabetes mellitus. In Goldman L, Schafer AI, editors: *Goldman-Cecil medicine*, ed 25, Philadelphia, 2016, Saunders/Elsevier, pp 1527–1548.

71. The Diabetes Control and Complications Trial Research Group: The effect of intensive treatment of diabetes on the development and progression of long-term complications in insulin-dependent diabetes mellitus. *N Engl J Med* 329(14):977–986, 1993.

72. Hersh EV, Moore PA, Papas AS, et al, Soft Tissue Anesthesia Recovery Group: Reversal of soft tissue local anesthesia with phentolamine mesylate in adolescents and adults. *J Am Dent Assoc* 139(8):1080–1093, 2008.

73. Hift RJ: The porphyrias. In Goldman L, Schafer AI, editors: *Goldman-Cecil medicine*, ed 25, Philadelphia, 2016, Saunders/Elsevier, pp 1408–1416.

74. Zhou J, Bose D, Allen PD, Pessah IN: Malignant hyperthermia and muscle-related disorders. In Miller RD, Cohen NH, Eriksson LI, et al, editors: *Miller's anesthesia*, ed 8, Philadelphia, 2015, Saunders Elsevier, pp 1287–1314.

75. Malignant Hyperthermia Association of the United States: Safe and unsafe anesthetics. Malignant Hyperthermia Association of the United States. www.mhaus.org/healthcare-professionals/be-prepared/safe-and-unsafe-anesthetics. (Accessed 31 January 2017).

76. ClinicalKey: Dantrolene drug monograph, December 21, 2015. www.clinicalkey.com. (Accessed 30 July 2016).

77. Lerman J: Perioperative management of the paediatric patient with coexisting neuromuscular disease. *Br J Anaesth* 107(Suppl 1):i79–i89, 2011.

78. Ording H: Investigation of malignant hyperthermia susceptibility in Denmark. *Dan Med Bull* 43(2):111–125, 1996.

79. Kalow W, Britt BA, Terreau ME, Haist C: Metabolic error of muscle metabolism after recovery from malignant hyperthermia. *Lancet* 296(7679):895–898, 1970.

80. Dershwitz M, Ryan JF, Guralnick W: Safety of amide local anesthetics in patients susceptible to malignant hyperthermia. *J Am Dent Assoc* 118(3):276, 278, 280, 1989.

81. Jelic JS, Moore PA: Malignant hyperthermia and amide local anesthetics. *Pa Dent J (Harrisb)* 55(4):35–36, 1988.

82. Minasian A, Yagiela JA: The use of amide local anesthetics in patients susceptible to malignant hyperthermia. *Oral Surg Oral Med Oral Pathol* 66(4):405–415, 1988.

83. Metrowitz MR, Mauro JV, Aston R, Smith DB: Prolonged succinylcholine-induced apnea caused by atypical cholinesterase: report of a case. *J Oral Surg* 38(5):387–390, 1980.

84. Bunn HF: Approach to the anemias. In Goldman L, Schafer AI, editors: *Goldman-Cecil medicine*, ed 25, Philadelphia, 2016, Saunders/Elsevier, pp 1059–1068.

85. McCarthy FM: Physical evaluation and treatment modification. In McCarthy FM, editor: *Emergencies in dental practice*, ed 3, Philadelphia, 1979, WB Saunders.

86. Bellamy MC, Hopkins PM, Halsall PJ, Ellis FR: A study into the incidence of methaemoglobinaemia after "three-in-one" block with prilocaine. *Anaesthesia* 47(12):1084–1085, 1992.

87. Bhutani A, Bhutani MS, Patel R: Methemoglobinemia in a patient undergoing gastrointestinal endoscopy. *Ann Pharmacother* 26(10):1239–1240, 1992.

88. Sansevere JJ, Milles M: Management of the oral and maxillofacial surgery patient with sickle cell disease and related hemoglobinopathies. *J Oral Maxillofac Surg* 51(8):912–916, 1993.

89. Motulsky AG: Frequency of sickling disorders in U.S. blacks. *N Engl J Med* 288(1):31–33, 1973.

90. Ferri FF: Sickle cell disease. In *Ferri's clinical advisor 2017*, Philadelphia, 2017, Elsevier, pp 1169–1172.

91. Murphy S: Polycythemia vera. *Dis Mon* 38(3):153–212, 1992.

92. Duggan PR, Cerquozzi S: Polycythemia vera. In Boop ET, Kellerman RD, editors: *Conn's current therapy 2016*, Philadelphia, 2016, Elsevier, pp 823–915.

93. Flood E, Pocoski J, Michaels LA, et al: Patient-reported experience of bleeding events in haemophilia. *Eur J Haematol* 93(Suppl 75):19–28, 2014.

chapter 38

The Physically Compromised Patient

CHAPTER OUTLINE

MULTIPLE SCLEROSIS
MUSCULAR DYSTROPHIES
PARKINSON DISEASE

CEREBROVASCULAR ACCIDENT (CVA, STROKE, CEREBRAL ACCIDENT, "BRAIN ATTACK")

*D*ental treatment of the physically compromised patient is in most cases not significantly different from treatment of any other dental patient. Although the level of knowledge of a physician specialist in internal medicine is not necessary for the proper dental treatment of these patients, the more information the dental professional has about these conditions, the more prepared and comfortable they will be when treating them.

MULTIPLE SCLEROSIS

Multiple sclerosis (MS) is a chronic, predominantly autoimmune demyelinating disease of the central nervous system (CNS) characterized by subacute neurologic deficits correlating with CNS lesions separated in time and space, excluding other possible disease.[1] MS, the most common autoimmune disease of the CNS,[2] is second only to head trauma as the leading cause of neurologic disability in young adults.[3]

MS is characterized by a chronic and progressive demyelination of neurons within the CNS frequently manifesting in young adults with episodes of neurologic dysfunction. Eighty-five percent of patients present with relapsing and remitting symptoms.[3] Demyelination is limited to white matter of the CNS, with the peripheral nervous system unaffected.[2,3]

It is estimated that approximately 400,000 persons in the United States have MS,[2-4] and more than 2 million are affected worldwide. The incidence of MS is rising.[4] Clinical manifestations of MS typically occur between the ages of 15 and 50 years, most commonly between 20 and 40 years.[1,4] Females are affected twice as frequently as males.[1,3,4] MS is more common in people raised in northern latitudes and in certain genetic clusters. Prevalence per 10,000 varies from 20 in southern Europe to 150 to 180 in Canada, northern United States, and northern Europe, and <10 in Asia, Central America, and most of Africa.[1,5]

The cause of MS is presently unknown, although it is theorized that it is triggered by an infectious agent.[6,7] Demyelination occurs in the white matter of the CNS producing "plaques" (areas of demyelinated neurons) demonstrating impairment of axonal conduction. Commonly affected areas include the optic nerve, periventricular cerebral white matter, and cervical spinal fluid.[2,3,8,9]

Clinical findings depend on the location of the CNS lesion(s) and may include the following: nonspecific complaints such as fatigue, blurred vision, diplopia, vertigo, falls, hemiparesis, paraparesis, monoparesis, numbness, paresthesias, ataxia, cognitive deficits, depression, sexual dysfunction, and urinary dysfunction.[1] Optic nerve involvement leads to visual disturbances (diplopia, nystagmus) or blindness and represent the most common presenting manifestations.[3]

Subtypes of MS include[1]:

- Relapsing-remitting MS (RRMS): is found in 82%. Relapses followed by complete or near-complete recovery, 50% to 85% of which later become SPMS
- Secondary progressive MS (SPMS): presents with progressive disability with few or no relapses
- Primary progressive MS (PPMS): found in 18%; progressive deterioration from the onset, and relapses are rare
- Progressive relapsing or relapsing progressive courses can be incorporated into PPMS or SPMS, respectively
- Relapses are defined as a subacute onset of neurologic dysfunction that lasts at least 24 hours due to inflammatory demyelination

Treatment of the acute relapse includes high-dose intravenous corticosteroid (methylprednisolone, 3 to 5 days of 15 mg/kg/day) frequently followed by a 7- to 10-day course of tapered prednisone or methylprednisolone.[1,10] High-dose corticosteroids do not alter the long-term course of MS.

Chronic drug management is only approved by the Food and Drug Administration (FDA) for relapsing MS. No therapies are approved for progressive MS.[1]

Disease-modifying injection therapy includes interferon beta-1a (IM Avonex, IM Plegridy, SC Rebif), interferon beta-1b (SC Betaseron, SC Extavia), and glatiramer acetate (SC Copaxone).[11] Disease-modifying oral therapy includes fingolimod (Gilenya), Teriflunomide (Aubagio), and dimethyl fumarate (Tecfidera).[12]

Most MS patients have complete or near-complete recovery within weeks to months after a relapse. The typical RRMS patient will have two relapses per year (75% have more than one relapse).[1] The rate of disease progression is highly variable; however, there is a higher risk of long-term disability associated with higher relapse rates during the first 2 to 5 years and poor recovery from initial relapses, older age at onset, multiple system involvement, male sex, African American, and primary progressive MS.[1,13,14]

Even though local anesthetics exert their clinical actions on nerves and nerve transmission, there are no special considerations associated with the administration of local anesthetics in MS patients. Likewise, inhalation sedation with nitrous oxide and oxygen, enteral (oral) minimal or moderate sedation, parenteral moderate sedation, and general anesthesia are all acceptable in the outpatient dental office. Stress may negatively influence this disease, so all efforts to minimize or ideally eliminate stress are encouraged; of course, this includes all properly performed sedative and anesthetic procedures.

MUSCULAR DYSTROPHIES

Muscular dystrophy is not one disease, but a family of genetically transmitted diseases, each of which encompasses degeneration of musculature but with no definable nerve disturbances. There are nine types of muscular dystrophy[15] (Box 38.1).

Duchenne muscular dystrophy (DMD), also known as *pseudohypertrophic muscular dystrophy,* is the most common. It was first described by the French neurologist Guillaume Benjamin Amand Duchenne in the 1860s. Until the 1980s, however, little was known about the cause of any of the muscular dystrophies. DMD occurs when a specific gene on the X chromosome does not manufacture a protein called *dystrophin;* therefore the disease affects only male subjects. Women may be carriers of the disease. The course of DMD is fairly predictable. Signs of muscle weakness may be seen as early as age 3, with the muscles of the hips, pelvic area, thighs, and shoulders being primarily affected[16] (Fig. 38.1). Within the next 10 years, the heart and muscles of respiration can also be affected. Nearly all children with DMD lose the ability to walk sometime between ages 7 and 12. Muscle deterioration in DMD is not painful, but muscle cramping may occur, normally relieved by over-the-counter analgesics (e.g., ibuprofen). Because muscular dystrophy does not affect the nerves themselves, touch and other senses remain intact, as does control over involuntary muscles of the bladder and bowel, as well as sexual functions.[15] Persons with Duchenne MD usually die in their late teens or early twenties.

Becker muscular dystrophy (BMD) is a milder version of DMD, appearing in the late teens to early adulthood. The course of BMD is slower and less predictable than DMD.[17] Those with BMD can usually walk into their thirties and live further into adulthood.[17]

Myotonic muscular dystrophy (MMD, or Steinert disease) is the most common adult form of muscular dystrophy, affecting more than 30,000 Americans. It is caused by a repeated section of DNA on either chromosome 19 or chromosome 3.[18] This form of muscular dystrophy is quite unusual in that it may trigger many other unrelated symptoms such as hormonal problems, cataracts, heart disease, and myotonia (delayed relaxation of a muscle). Researchers have identified a new genetic form of MMD, a mutation of a gene called *ZNF9*, that may shed light on the nature of mutations causing this and perhaps other diseases.[19]

Other forms muscular dystrophy and neuromuscular disease are summarized in Box 38.1.

There are no particular concerns with local anesthetic administration in patients with muscular dystrophy, nor is inhalation, oral, or parenteral moderate sedation contraindicated. There may be some difficulties with patient positioning, but these are normally minor and of no disruption to the dental office. General anesthesia as normally performed in the dental office (without neuromuscular blocking agents) and is acceptable in select circumstances after appropriate medical consultation, as needed.

PARKINSON DISEASE

Parkinson disease (PD) is a degenerative neurologic disease that primarily affects the specific part of the brain (substantia nigra) that produces the neurotransmitter dopamine (Box 38.2). Symptoms include trembling (tremor), stooped posture, muscular stiffness (rigidity), and slowness of body movements (bradykinesia). The cause of PD is unknown, but some experts believe it may result from toxins, head trauma, or strokes.[20] Others believe PD results from the combination of a genetic predisposition and an as-yet-unidentified environmental trigger.

Approximately 1 million persons in the United States live with PD (this is more than the total number of people diagnosed with MS, MD, and amyotrophic lateral sclerosis [ALS]).[21] In the United States approximately 60,000 persons are diagnosed with PD annually. More than 10 million people worldwide have PD.

PD may appear at any age, but is uncommon in those younger than 30[22]; the risk of developing PD increases with

Box 38.1	Types of Muscular Dystrophy and Other Neuromuscular Diseases

Muscular Dystrophies

Duchenne Muscular Dystrophy (DMD) (also known as pseudohypertrophic)
Onset: 2 to 6 yr of age
Symptoms: generalized weakness and muscle wasting affecting limb and trunk muscles first; the calves are often enlarged

Becker Muscular Dystrophy (BMD)
Onset: adolescence or adulthood
Symptoms: almost identical to DMD, but often much less severe; can be significant heart involvements

Myotonic Dystrophy (MMD) (also known as Steinert disease)
Onset: childhood to middle age
Symptoms: generalized weakness and muscle wasting affecting face, feet, hands, and neck first; delayed relaxation of muscles after contraction

Emery-Dreifuss Muscular Dystrophy (EDMD)
Onset: childhood to early teens
Symptoms: weakness and wasting of shoulder, upper arm, and shin muscles; joint deformities common

Limb-Girdle Muscular Dystrophy (LGMD)
Onset: childhood to middle age
Symptoms: weakness and wasting affecting shoulder and pelvic girdles first

Facioscapulohumeral Muscular Dystrophy (FSH or FSHD) (also known as Landouzy–Dejerine)
Onset: childhood to early adulthood
Symptoms: facial muscle weakness, with weakness and wasting of the shoulders and upper arms

Oculopharyngeal Muscular Dystrophy (OPMD)
Onset: early adulthood to middle age
Symptoms: first affects muscles of eyelid and throat

Distal Muscular Dystrophy (DD)
Onset: 40 to 60 yr of age
Symptoms: weakness and wasting of muscles of the hands, forearms, and lower legs

Congenital Muscular Dystrophy (CMD)
Onset: at birth
Symptoms: generalized muscle weakness with possible joint deformities

Motor Neuron Diseases

Amyotrophic Lateral Sclerosis (ALS) (also known as Lou Gehrig disease in the United States)
Onset: adulthood
Symptoms: generalized weakness and muscle wasting with cramps and muscle twitches common

Adult Spinal Muscular Atrophy (SMA)
Onset: 18 to 50 yr of age
Symptoms: generalized weakness and muscle wasting with muscle twitches common; X-linked form affects men only and involves muscles of mouth and throat and other muscles

Inflammatory Myopathies

Dermatomyositis (PM/DM)
Onset: childhood to late adulthood
Symptoms: weakness of neck and limb muscles; muscle pain and swelling common; skin rash typically affecting cheeks, eyelids, neck, chest, and limbs

Polymyositis (PM/DM)
Onset: childhood to late adulthood
Symptoms: weakness of neck and limb muscles; muscle pain and swelling common; sometimes associated with malignancy

Inclusion Body Myositis (IBM)
Onset: after age 50
Symptoms: weakness of arms, legs, and hands, especially thighs, wrists, and fingers; sometimes involves swallowing muscles

Diseases of the Neuromuscular Junction

Myasthenia Gravis (MG)
Onset: childhood to adulthood
Symptoms: weakness and fatigability of muscles of eyes, face, neck, throat, limbs, and/or trunk

Metabolic Diseases of Muscle

Phosphorylase Deficiency (MPD or PYGM) (also known as McArdle disease)
Onset: childhood to adolescence
Symptoms: muscle cramps usually occurring after exercise; intense exercise can cause muscle destruction and possible kidney damage

Lactate Dehydrogenase Deficiency (LDHA)
Onset: childhood to adolescence
Symptoms: exercise intolerance with muscle damage and urine discoloration possible following strenuous physical activity

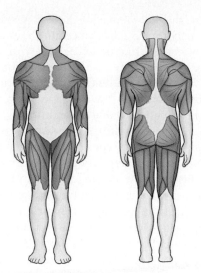

Figure 38.1 Muscles affected in Duchenne muscular dystrophy (DMD). (Used with permission of Muscular Dystrophy Association.)

Box 38.2	Hoehn and Yahr Staging of Parkinson Disease

Stage I
1. Signs and symptoms on one side only
2. Symptoms mild
3. Symptoms inconvenient, but not disabling
4. Usually has tremor of one limb
5. Friends have noticed changes in posture, locomotion, and facial expression

Stage II
1. Symptoms are bilateral
2. Minimal disability
3. Posture and gait affected

Stage III
1. Significant slowing of body movements
2. Early impairment of equilibrium on walking or standing
3. Generalized dysfunction that is moderately severe

Stage IV
1. Severe symptoms
2. Can still walk to a limited extent
3. Rigidity and bradykinesia
4. No longer able to live alone
5. Tremor may be less than earlier stages

Stage V
1. Cachectic stage
2. Invalidism complete
3. Cannot stand or walk
4. Requires constant nursing care

Data from www.parkinson.org/NETCOMMUNITY/Page. aspx?pid=367&srcid=202.

increasing age.[23] Men are affected slightly more often than women. Most patients do not experience the full range of symptoms outlined previously.

Rigidity is always present unless it is temporarily ablated by anti-PD medications. This rigidity may lead to sensations of pain. Bradykinesia is caused by the brain's slowness in the chemical transmission of the instructions to the appropriate parts of the body. Even when the instructions have been received, the body responds slowly in performing them.

Persons with PD may also have a number of secondary symptoms that may include depression, sleep disturbances, dizziness, constipation, and dementia. They may also have difficulty with speech, breathing, swallowing, and sexual function.[24]

Drugs are available to treat the symptoms of PD, but none yet that actually reverse its effects. Levodopa is commonly prescribed for the treatment of PD.[25] Developed in the 1960s, levodopa represented one of the most important breakthroughs in the history of medicine.[26] Structurally, it is a dopamine precursor. Some patients experience unacceptable side effects, including severe nausea and vomiting. Levodopa-carbidopa (Sinemet) represents a significant improvement over previous agents. The addition of carbidopa delays the biotransformation of levodopa and allows more of the levodopa to reach the brain.[27] A smaller dose of levodopa is needed, and side effects are diminished.

Amantadine HCl (Symmetrel) is an indirect-acting dopamine agonist and is widely used as an early single-drug therapy.[28] Sinemet is sometimes added to another regimen involving the drug Symmetrel later in treatment. Anticholinergics act to decrease the activity of the balancing neurotransmitter acetylcholine. Because PD mainly involves a decreased activity of dopamine, one method of treatment has been to decrease the cholinergic system so that it no longer overpowers the dopaminergic system.[29] Selegiline (Eldepryl) has been shown to delay the need for Sinemet when prescribed very early in PD. It is occasionally used in later stages to augment the effects of Sinemet.

COMT (catechol-O-methyl transferase) inhibitors represent a new class of medications used in the treatment of PD. These drugs require levodopa for efficacy; they simply prolong the duration of action of levodopa, requiring lower dosages and therefore diminishing side effects.[30]

There are no particular concerns with local anesthetics in patients with PD, nor is inhalation, oral, or intravenous (IV) moderate sedation contraindicated. Neuroleptics, phenothiazines, and butyrophenones are contraindicated during IV moderate sedation and general anesthesia, but the benzodiazepines, opioids, and alkylphenols are acceptable choices.

Box 38.3	Warning Signs of Stroke*

Sudden onset of the following:
- Numbness or weakness of the face, arm, or leg, especially on one side of the body
- Confusion, trouble speaking or understanding
- Trouble walking, dizziness, loss of balance or coordination
- Trouble seeing in one or both eyes
- Severe headache with no known cause

Every 53 seconds, someone in America has a stroke. Each year, about 600,000 Americans have a stroke, and 160,000 of them will die. Stroke is the number-three cause of death and one of the leading causes of disability in the United States.[31]

Box 38.4	Permanent Neurologic Deficits That Are Commonly Produced by a Stroke

Weakness or paralysis, usually limited to one side of the body

Loss of sensation, usually limited to one side of the body

Problems with vision

Difficulty in talking or in understanding what is said

Difficulty with organization

Clumsiness or lack of balance

Data from www.umassmed.edu/strokestop.

CEREBROVASCULAR ACCIDENT (CVA, STROKE, CEREBRAL ACCIDENT, "BRAIN ATTACK")

Stroke is a sudden loss of brain function caused by occlusion or rupture of a blood vessel within or traveling to the brain, characterized by loss of muscular control, reduction in or loss of sensation or consciousness, dizziness, slurred speech, or other symptoms that vary with the extent and severity of the damage to the brain (Boxes 38.3 and 38.4). It is also called *cerebral accident, cerebrovascular accident,* and *brain attack.* The reader is referred to Chapter 37 for a more in-depth review of CVA.

Local anesthetics themselves are not a problem in patients with a history of stroke, but the vasoconstrictors packaged with them may be a concern. Because acute hypertension is the single most important risk factor for stroke, most patients with a history of stroke also have a history of hypertension. It is very important to obtain baseline vital signs in this patient population before the administration of local anesthetics. A stress reduction protocol should be implemented for each of these patients.

Epinephrine should be limited to the least amount necessary to adequately perform the dental procedure; however, complete elimination of epinephrine is not necessary. In general, up to 40 µg of epinephrine may safely be administered if done slowly and over an adequate time period. Forty micrograms is roughly the amount of epinephrine in two cartridges of any local anesthetic containing 1:100,000 epinephrine (U.S. volume of 1.8 mL of solution per cartridge) or four cartridges of local anesthetics containing 1:200,000 epinephrine (certain bupivacaine, prilocaine, and articaine preparations in the United States).[32] Periodic measurement of vital signs after administration of local anesthetics, with or without vasoconstrictor, is recommended for this group of patients. If vital signs are monitored and recorded on a frequent basis—every 5 minutes—consideration may be given to increasing the total dose of epinephrine beyond the aforementioned 40-µg limit if it may be documented that vital signs are stable and of acceptable values.

Inhalation, enteral minimal and moderate, and IV moderate sedation are generally well tolerated and recommended in many instances because of their anxiolytic and calming effects. Properly sedated patients will be releasing less endogenous catecholamines, with resultant lowered, stable vital signs. The relaxation and slight reduction in blood pressure seen with these techniques are of benefit. Intramuscular sedation is not recommended because most patients with a history of stroke are taking anticoagulant medications of various types and efficacies. If general anesthesia is to be administered, recommended techniques would be those in which opioids are included, with benzodiazepines and alkylphenols administered as indicated.[15]

REFERENCES

1. Ferri FF: Multiple sclerosis. In *Ferri's clinical advisor 2017,* Philadelphia, 2017, Elsevier, pp 825–827.
2. Calabresi PA: Multiple sclerosis and demyelinating conditions of the CNS. In Goldman L, Schafer AI, editors: *Goldman-Cecil medicine,* ed 25, Philadelphia, 2016, Elsevier Saunders, pp 2471–2480.
3. Little JW, Falace DA: Neurologic disorders. In Little JW, Falace DA, Miller CS, Rhodus NL, editors: *Little and Falace's Dental management of the medically compromised patient,* ed 8, St Louis, 2013, Mosby Elsevier, pp 516–519.
4. Multiple Sclerosis Information site: www.msnews.org. (Accessed 31 January 2017).
5. Ramagopalan SV, Sadovnick AD: Epidemiology of MS. *Neurol Clinic* 29(2):207–217, 2010.
6. Bermel RA, Cohen JA: Multiple sclerosis: advances in understanding pathogenesis and emergence of oral treatment options. *Lancet Neurol* 10:4–5, 2011.
7. Sloka S, Silva C, Pryse-Phillips W, et al: A quantitative analysis of suspected environmental causes of MS. *Can J Neurol Sci* 38(1):98–105, 2011.
8. Prat A: Special issue on molecular basis of multiple sclerosis. *Biochim Biophys Acta* 1812(2):131, 2011.
9. Bahr M: Special issue on multiple sclerosis. *Exp Neurol* 225:1, 2010.
10. Jacobs LD, Beck RW, Simon JH, et al: Intramuscular interferon beta-1a therapy, initiated during first demyelinating event in

multiple sclerosis. CHAMPS Study Group. *N Engl J Med* 343(13):898–904, 2000.

11. Kappos L, Wiendl H, Selmaj K, et al: Daclizumab HYP versus interferon beta-1a in relapsing multiple sclerosis. *N Engl J Med* 373(15):1418–1428, 2015.

12. Freedman MS: Present and emerging therapies for multiple sclerosis. *Continuum (NY)* 19(4 Multiple Sclerosis):968–991, 2013.

13. Lublin FD, Baier M, Cutter G: Effect of relapses on development of residual deficit in multiple sclerosis. *Neurology* 61(11):1528–1532, 2003.

14. Scalfari A, Neuhaus A, Degenhardt A, et al: The natural history of MS, study 10: relapses and long-term disability. *Brain* 133(Pt 7):1914–1929, 2010.

15. Duchenne Muscular Dystrophy: www.mda.org/disease/dmd.html. (Accessed 31 January 2017).

16. Yiu EM, Kornberg AJ: Duchenne muscular dystrophy. *J Paediatr Child Health* 51(8):759–764, 2015.

17. Romitti PA, Zhu Y, Puzhankara S, et al: Prevalence of Duchenne and Becker muscular dystrophies in the United States. *Pediatr* 135(3):513–521, 2015.

18. Chau A, Kalsotra A: Developmental insights into the pathology of and therapeutic strategies for DM1: Back to the basics. *Dev Dyn* 244(3):377–390, 2015.

19. Meola G, Cardani R: Myotonic dystrophies: an update on clinical aspects, genetic, pathology, and molecular pathomechanisms. *Biochim Biophys Acta* 1852(4):594–606, 2015.

20. Zigmond MJ, Burke RE: Pathophysiology of Parkinson's disease. In Davis KL, Charney D, Coyle JT, Nemeroff C, editors: *Neuropsychopharmacology: the fifth generation of progress.* American College of Neuropsychopharmacology, Philadelphia, 2002, Lippincott, Williams, & Wilkins, pp 1781–1793.

21. Statistics on Parkinson's. Parkinson's Disease Foundation. www.pdf.org/en/parkinson_statistics. (Accessed 31 January 2017.

22. Mehanna R, Moore S, Hou JG, et al: Comparing clinical features of young onset, middle onset and late onset Parkinson's disease. *Parkinsonism Relat Disord* 20(5):530–534, 2014.

23. Vanitallie TB: Parkinson disease: primacy of age as a risk factor for mitochondrial dysfunction. *Metabolism* 57(Suppl 2):S50–S55, 2008.

24. Gopalakrishna A, Alexander SA: Understanding Parkinson disease: a complex and multifaceted illness. *J Neurosci Nurs* 47(6):320–326, 2015.

25. Kianirad Y, Simuni T: Novel approaches to optimization of levodopa therapy for Parkinson's disease. *Curr Neurol Neurosci Rep* 16(4):34, 2016.

26. LeWitt PA, Fahn S: Levodopa therapy for Parkinson disease: a look backward and forward. *Neurology* 86(14 Suppl 1):S3–S12, 2016.

27. Dhall R, Kreitzman DL: Advances in levodopa therapy for Parkinson disease: review of RYTARY (carbidopa and levodopa) clinical efficacy and safety. *Neurology* 86(14 Suppl 1):S13–S24, 2016.

28. Mazzucchi S, Frosini D, Bonuccelli U, Ceravolo R: Current treatment and future prospects of dopa-induced dyskinesias. *Drugs Today (Barc)* 51(5):315–329, 2015.

29. Mancini M, Fling BW, Gendreau A, et al: Effect of augmenting cholinergic function on gait and balance. *BMC Neurol* 15:264, 2015.

30. Martinez-Martin P, Rodriguez-Blazquez C, Forjaz MJ, Kurtis MM: Impact of pharmacotherapy on quality of life in patients with Parkinson's disease. *CNS Drugs* 29(5):397–413, 2015.

31. American Heart Association/American Stroke Association: Heart disease, stroke and research statistics at-a-glance – 2016 update. https://heart.org/dc/groups/ahamah-public/@wcm/@sop/@smd/documents/downloadable/ucm_480086.pdf. (Accessed 28 July 2016).

32. Malamed SF: Pharmacology of vasoconstrictors. In *Handbook of local anesthesia,* ed 6, St Louis, 2013, Mosby Elsevier, pp 39–51.

chapter 39

Neurologic Illnesses and Other Conditions

CHAPTER OUTLINE

Treatment of patients with various neurologic illnesses is many times more enjoyable than treatment of any other dental patient because patients with these special needs are genuinely a joy to be around. On the other hand, this patient population can present more challenges for the practitioner.

Patients with mental disabilities often suffer more dental disease than other dental patients. Financial considerations may make it difficult to obtain dental treatment, so sometimes treatment is delayed or avoided altogether. Those with neurologic illnesses may be unable to understand the consequences of poor dental hygiene and irregular care, and they may be uncooperative during dental treatment. Many of these disabilities interfere with the ability of the person to perform the fine motor skills needed to properly care for his or her dentition.[1]

DEMENTIA AND ALZHEIMER DISEASE

The Oregonian
Saturday August 18, 2001
HILLSBORO: *"The Oregon Department of Justice reached a settlement Friday with a Hillsboro car dealership it said sold seven vehicles worth $244,708 in one month to an elderly Alzheimer's patient."*[2]

In dentistry, the typical long-term relationships we have with patients allow us to often see the patient's degradation of mental function over time in Alzheimer disease (AD). The informed consent we obtain before performing dentistry may sometimes come from a person other than the patient. Determining the patient's legal guardian may be difficult, but obtaining truly "informed consent" from that person is an absolute necessity.

The term *Alzheimer disease* dates back to a 51-year-old woman admitted to a Frankfurt, Germany hospital in 1901 with signs of dementia. At a meeting held in 1906, Dr. Alois Alzheimer reported on this patient. The title of his lecture was "Über eiene eigenartige Erkrankung der Hirnrinde" (On a peculiar disorder of the cerebral cortex). On her death her brain was examined, and many abnormal clumps—now called *amyloid plaques*—and tangled bundles of fibers—now called *neurofibrillary, or tau, tangles*—were found. A few years later, presenile dementia was designated Alzheimer disease.[3]

AD is a degenerative brain disease and the most common cause of dementia in older people.[4–6] Dementia is characterized by a decline in memory, language, problem-solving, and other cognitive skills that affects a person's ability to perform everyday activities.[6] In AD, the damage and destruction of neurons eventually affect other parts of the brain, including those that enable a person to carry out basic bodily functions such as walking and swallowing. People in the final stages of AD are confined to bed and require around-the-clock care. AD is ultimately fatal.[6]

Common symptoms of AD are listed in Box 39.1.

Occurrence of Alzheimer Disease

Sixty-one percent of AD patients will die before age 80, compared with 30% of those without AD.[6] AD is officially listed as the sixth leading cause of death in the United States and the fifth leading cause of death for persons age 65 and older.[7]

The incidence of dementia increases with aging. In 2016 it was estimated that 5.4 million persons in the United States had AD. Of these, 5.2 million are over 65 years old, with approximately 200,000 persons under age 65 who have younger-onset AD.[8,9]

Eleven percent of people over age 65 have AD.[8,9] Thirty-two percent of people age 85 and older have AD.[8,9] Eighty-one percent of AD patients are age 75 or older.[8,9] Using data from the Framingham Study,[10] the estimated lifetime risk of developing AD, specifically at age 65, was 17% for women and 9% for men.[10]

Box 39.1	Common Symptoms of Alzheimer Disease

- Memory loss that disrupts daily life
- Challenges in planning or solving problems
- Difficulty completing familiar tasks at home, at work, or at leisure
- Confusion with time or place
- Trouble understanding visual images and spatial relationships
- New problems with words when speaking or writing
- Misplacing things and losing the ability to retrace steps
- Decreased or poor judgment
- Withdrawal from work or social activities
- Changes in mood and personality, including apathy and depression
- Increased anxiety, agitation, and sleep disturbances.

Alzheimer's Association: 2016 Alzheimer's disease facts and figures. Alzheimers Dement 12(4):459–504, 2016.

Because AD is underdiagnosed and underreported, a large portion of Americans with AD may not be aware that they have it.[6]

Americans are living longer. Persons over age 85 are called the *oldest-old*. Between 2012 and 2050, the oldest-old are expected to increase from 14% of all people age 65 and older in the United States to 22%, an additional 12 million oldest-old people.[11] These individuals are at greatest risk for developing AD. In 2016 in the United States, approximately 2 million people with AD are age 85 or older, accounting for 37% of all AD patients.[8] In 2031, when the first wave of "baby boomers" (born between 1946 and 1964) reaches age 85, it is projected that more than 3 million people age 85 and older will have AD.[8] By 2050 as many as 7 million people age 85 and older may have AD, accounting for 51% of all people age 65 and older with AD.[8]

Management of Alzheimer Disease

AD is a slowly progressing disease, starting with mild memory problems and ending with severe mental damage. At present there is no one drug or other intervention that will successfully treat AD. Current approaches focus on helping people maintain mental function, manage behavioral symptoms, and slow or delay the symptoms of the disease.[6] The U.S. Food and Drug Administration has approved several drugs to treat mild-to-moderate AD symptoms. These include donepezil (Aricept), rivastigmine (Exelon), and galantamine (Razadyne). Donepezil and memantine (Namenda) are used to treat moderate-to-severe AD. These drugs work by regulating neurotransmitters that transmit messages between

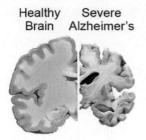

Healthy Severe
Brain Alzheimer's

Figure 39.1 Normal brain (*left*), Alzheimer's brain (*right*).

neurons. They help maintain thinking, memory, and communication skills, but they do not change the underlying disease process.[6] They also are not effective in all AD patients, and the duration for which they are effective is extremely variable.[6]

Brain Changes Associated With Alzheimer Disease

The healthy human brain contains approximately 100 billion neurons, each with long, branching extensions forming connections (synapses) with other neurons.[6] There are approximately 100 trillion synapses in the human brain. The progressive accumulation of the protein fragment beta-amyloid (beta-amyloid plaques) outside neurons in the brain and the accumulation of an abnormal form of the protein tau (tau tangles) inside neurons are two of several changes in the brain believed to contribute to damage and death of neurons resulting in memory loss and other symptoms of AD.[6] Beta-amyloid accumulation is thought to interfere with neuron-to-neuron synaptic transmission and to contribute to neuronal death. Tau tangles block transport of nutrients and other essential molecules inside neurons and are also thought to contribute to neuronal death.[6] Brains of persons with advanced AD demonstrate inflammation, dramatic shrinkage from cell loss (Fig. 39.1), and widespread debris from dead and dying neurons.[6] These changes may begin 20 or more years before the development of symptoms.[12–14]

Considerations for Local Anesthesia, Sedation, and General Anesthesia

Local anesthesia can be used in this patient population without specific concerns. Patients not severely affected with AD may benefit from some sort of sedation for dental therapy. Inhalation sedation is an excellent choice for patients mildly affected with mild-to-moderate AD and others who retain the ability to cooperate for the sedation and dental procedure. Oral sedation is generally not the first choice in this patient population because of its inherent lack of safety related to the inability to slowly and properly titrate the drug. Intravenous (IV) sedation is a good choice precisely because of the ability to slowly and precisely titrate the drugs to a clinical end point. Moderate sedation in moderate-to-severe AD patients may lead to a decrease in cooperativeness as a result of an increase in mental clouding and mental confusion. For these patients, general

Box 39.2	**Common Pervasive Developmental Disorders (PDDs)**

Pervasive developmental disorder—not otherwise specified (commonly referred to as atypical autism): A diagnosis of PDD-NOS may be made when a child does not meet the criteria for a specific diagnosis but there is a severe and pervasive impairment in specified behaviors.

Rett disorder: This is a progressive disorder that, to date, has occurred only in girls. There is a period of normal development and then a loss of previously acquired skills and loss of purposeful use of the hands, replaced with repetitive hand movements, beginning at the age of 1 to 4 years.

Childhood disintegrative disorder: This is characterized by normal development for at least the first 2 years, then significant loss of previously acquired skills.

Data from www.autism-society.org.

anesthesia, possibly office based, may be the most appropriate therapy.

To allow practitioners to keep current with these issues, the *Journal of Alzheimer's Disease* is available online.[15]

AUTISM

Pervasive developmental disorder (PDD) is a general category of disorders that are characterized by severe and persistent impairment in several areas of development.[16] Among others, autism falls under this general category of disorders. Understanding of autism has grown tremendously since Dr. Leo Kanner first described it in 1943.[17] However, there is still no cure for the alterations in the brain that result in what we now call autism. The more common other PDDs are listed in Box 39.2.[18]

Autism is a developmental disability that is typically diagnosed early in life. It is estimated that about 1% of the world population has autism spectrum disorder.[19] Its prevalence in the United States is estimated at 1 in 68 births (1 in 42 boys, 1 in 189 girls).[20] More than 3.5 million people in the United States live with an autism spectrum disorder.[21] The prevalence of autism in U.S. children has increased by 199.4% from 2000 (when it occurred in 1 in 150 births) to 2010 (1 in 68 births).[22] It is four times more prevalent in males than in females and is not related to racial, ethnic, or social groups. Family income, lifestyle, and educational levels do not affect the chance of autism's occurrence. Those with autism typically have difficulties with communication, social interactions, and leisure or play activities. Occasionally, aggressive and self-injurious behavior is seen.[18]

Autism is a disorder with a continuum of presentations, some mildly affected and others severely affected. Two children, both with the same diagnosis, can act very differently from

Box 39.3	Areas That May Be Affected by Autism

Communication: Language develops slowly or not at all; these patients use words without attaching the usual meaning to them; they communicate with gestures instead of words and have a short attention span.

Social interaction: The child spends time alone rather than with others, shows little interest in making friends, and is less responsive to social cues, such as eye contact or smiles.

Sensory impairment: Sensitivities in the areas of sight, hearing, touch, smell, and taste may be noted to a greater or lesser degree.

Play: The child does not participate in spontaneous or imaginative play, does not imitate others' actions, and does not initiate pretend games.

Behaviors: The child may be overactive or very passive; he or she throws tantrums for no apparent reason, perseverates (shows an obsessive interest in a single item, idea, activity, or person), apparently lacks common sense, may show aggression to others or self, and often has difficulty with changes in routine.

Data from www.autism-society.org.

Box 39.4	Effects of Cerebral Palsy[27]

Depending on which areas of the brain have been damaged, one or more of the following may occur:
- Muscle tightness or spasticity
- Involuntary movement
- Disturbance in gait or mobility
- Difficulty in swallowing
- Abnormal sensation and perception
- Impairment of sight, hearing, or speech
- Seizures
- Mental retardation
- Difficulties in feeding
- Bladder and bowel control
- Problems with breathing because of postural difficulties
- Skin disorders because of pressure sores
- Learning disabilities

Box 39.5	Types of Cerebral Palsy

Spastic cerebral palsy
Dyskinetic cerebral palsy
Ataxic cerebral palsy
Mixed types

one another and have varying skill sets. Therefore there is no standard "type" or "typical" person with autism.

Current research links autism to organic alterations in the brain. There might be a genetic basis to the disorder, but to date, no specific gene has been directly linked to autism. If there is a genetic basis to autism, it probably involves interactions among several genes. Some patients with autism may appear to have mental retardation, a behavior disorder, problems with hearing, or even odd and eccentric behavior (Box 39.3).[18]

Autism may coexist with other disorders that have neurologic effects, such as epilepsy, mental retardation, and Down syndrome (DS). It may also coexist with genetic disorders, such as fragile X syndrome, Landau–Kleffner syndrome, Tourette syndrome, or William syndrome.[23–26] It is not unusual for those with autism to test low in IQ. About one in four will develop seizures at some point in their lifetime.[18]

Considerations for Local Anesthesia, Sedation, and General Anesthesia

The more severely affected the individual, the more difficulty he or she will have in cooperating with dental treatment. Autism itself confers no specific contraindications for using common sedative and analgesic or anesthetic drugs. There are no physiologic changes of concern as a result of this specific condition. Patient cooperation may be problematic, however. Local anesthesia, inhalation, enteral, IV moderate sedation, and general anesthesia are all acceptable. As specific disease states are

encountered secondary to autism (i.e., seizures), appropriate alteration to the anesthetic or sedative plan should be made.

CEREBRAL PALSY

The term *cerebral palsy* (*CP*) refers to a group of neurologic disorders that appear in infancy or early childhood and permanently affect body movement, muscle coordination, and balance[27] (Box 39.4). CP affects the part of the brain that controls muscle movements. It is not communicable and is not a disease. CP is the most common motor disability in childhood.[28]

Types of Cerebral Palsy

There are four main types of CP (Box 39.5).[29]

Spastic cerebral palsy. The most common type of CP, accounting for 80% of all cases. People with spastic CP have increased muscle tone. Their muscles are stiff and, as a result, their movements can be awkward. Spastic CP usually is described by what parts of the body are affected:
- Spastic diplegia/diparesis—In this type of CP, muscle stiffness occurs primarily in the legs, with the arms less affected or not affected at all. People with spastic diplegia might have difficulty walking because tight hip and leg muscles cause their legs to pull together, turn inward, and cross at the knees (also known as *scissoring*).

- Spastic hemiplegia/hemiparesis—This type of CP affects only one side of a person's body; usually the arm is more affected than the leg.
- Spastic quadriplegia/quadriparesis—Spastic quadriplegia is the most severe form of spastic CP and affects all four limbs, the trunk, and the face. People with spastic quadriparesis usually cannot walk and often have other developmental disabilities such as intellectual disability; seizures; or problems with vision, hearing, or speech.

Dyskinetic cerebral palsy. People with dyskinetic CP have problems controlling the movement of their hands, arms, feet, and legs, making it difficult to sit and walk. The movements are uncontrollable and can be slow and writhing or rapid and jerky. Sometimes the face and tongue are affected and the person has a hard time sucking, swallowing, and talking. A person with dyskinetic CP has muscle tone that can change (varying from spastic to flaccid) not only from day to day but even during a single day.[29]

Ataxic cerebral palsy. Ataxic CP is the least common type. People with ataxic CP have problems with balance and coordination. They might be unsteady when they walk. They might have a hard time with quick movements or movements that need a lot of control, like writing. They might have a hard time controlling their hands or arms when they reach for something.[29]

Mixed cerebral palsy. Some people have symptoms of more than one type of CP. The most common type of mixed CP is spastic-dyskinetic CP.

Etiology of Cerebral Palsy

CP is caused by abnormal development of the brain or damage to the developing brain that affects a child's ability to control his or her muscles. Between 85% and 90% of CP cases are *congenital,* with the specific cause of the brain damage unknown. The remaining 10% to 15% of CP is caused by brain damage occurring more than 28 days after birth. Called *acquired CP,* common causes include infection, such as meningitis, or head trauma.[29–31]

Population-based studies from around the world report prevalence estimates of CP ranging from 1.5 to more than 4 per 1000 live births of children of a defined age range.[32,33]

About 764,000 persons—adults and children—in the United States have some form of CP.[34,35] Five hundred thousand are children under age 18. Eight thousand to 10,000 infants and 1500 preschool-age children are diagnosed with CP annually.[34,35]

Risk Factors for Congenital Cerebral Palsy[29,36]

- **Low birth weight.** Children weighing less than 2.5 kg (5.5 pounds), and especially those weighing less than 1.5 kg (3 pounds 5 ounces), have an increased risk of CP.
- **Premature birth.** Children born before the thirty-seventh week of pregnancy, especially before the thirty-second week, have a greater chance of having CP.
- **Multiple births.** Twins, triplets, and other multiple births have a greater risk of having CP.

- **Assisted reproductive technology (ART) and infertility treatments.** Most of the increased risk of CP associated with ART is explained by preterm delivery or multiple births, or both.
- **Infections during pregnancy.** Infection can lead to elevated levels of cytokines in the brain and blood of the fetus during pregnancy. Cytokines cause inflammation, which can lead to brain damage.[37] Maternal fever during pregnancy or delivery can also increase cytokine levels. Infections that have been linked with CP include viruses such as chickenpox, rubella, cytomegalovirus (CMV), and bacterial infections of the placenta or fetal membranes, or maternal pelvic infections.
- **Jaundice and kernicterus.** Many newborns have jaundice—an increased level of bilirubin in the blood. When jaundice is untreated, it can cause kernicterus, which can cause CP and other conditions.
- **Medical conditions of the mother,** such as thyroid disorders, intellectual disability, or seizures increase the risk of CP.
- **Birth complications.** Detachment of the placenta, uterine rupture, or umbilical cord problems during delivery can disrupt the flow of oxygen to the newborn, resulting in CP.

Adequate prenatal care may reduce the risk of some rare causes of congenital CP; however, dramatic improvement over the last 15 years in obstetric care at delivery has not reduced the incidence of congenital CP. Some, but not all, cases of acquired CP can be prevented.[38]

Signs and Symptoms of Cerebral Palsy

Early signs of CP usually appear before 3 years of age. Infants with CP are often developmentally delayed, such as in learning to roll over, sit, crawl, smile, or walk (see Box 39.4). Some affected children have hypotonia or hypertonia. The baby may seem flaccid and relaxed, even floppy, or may seem stiff or rigid. In some cases, the baby has an early period of hypotonia that progresses to hypertonia after the first 2 to 3 months of life. Affected children may also have unusual posture or favor one side of their body.[27]

Management of Cerebral Palsy

There is no cure for CP, but management can improve the quality of life for persons with this condition. When discussing long-term goals in CP, *management* is a better word than *treatment.* Management of CP consists of facilitating to the greatest extent possible both growth and development. This requires involvement in the child's movement, learning, speech, hearing, and social and emotional development. Medications, surgical approaches, and braces may be used to improve nerve and muscle coordination and minimize dysfunction.[39]

As children age, they may continue to require more assistance than others, including continuing physical therapy, special education, customized transportation devices, and modified employment opportunities. Depending on their degree of compromise, those affected with CP may attend school, be productive in jobs, raise families, and live independently.[39]

In a 2008 review of 8-year-old children with CP, 58.2% could walk independently, 11.3% walked using a handheld mobility device, and 30.6% had limited or no walking ability.[40] Many of the children had at least one coexisting condition: 41% had epilepsy and 6.9% had coexisting autistic spectrum disorder.

Another study found that 41% of CP children were limited in their ability to crawl, walk, run, or play and that 31% needed to use special equipment, such as walkers or wheelchairs.[41]

Considerations for Local Anesthesia, Sedation, and General Anesthesia

Local anesthesia and inhalation and/or oral minimal-to-moderate sedation can be used in this patient population as in any other dental patient. Sedation is often beneficial in reducing spastic patient movement during dental procedures. In less cooperative patients, intramuscular (IM) or IV moderate sedation may be ideal, allowing patients to cooperate when they really want to but are just physically unable to sit still. If these measures fail, office-based general anesthesia may be safely and effectively performed in the majority of these patients using typical drugs and dosages.

DOWN SYNDROME

Sweatshirt noticed at a DS convention: "The problem is not the way I look but the way you see me."[1]

In 1866 John Langdon Down, an English physician, published an accurate description of a person with what came to be known as Down's syndrome and eventually Down syndrome. Down was superintendent of an asylum for children with mental retardation in Surrey, England, when he made the first distinction between children who were cretins (later to be found to have hypothyroidism) and what he referred to as "mongoloids."[42] In 1959 the French physician Jerome Lejeune identified DS as an abnormality of chromosomes. He found 47 chromosomes in each cell instead of the usual 46.[43] Lejeune's claim that he discovered the extra copy of chromosome 21, however, has been disputed, and in 2014 the Scientific Council of the French Federation of Human Genetics awarded Marthe Gautier the Grand Prize for this discovery.[44]

Types of Down Syndrome

DS is the most commonly occurring chromosomal condition. Approximately 1 in every 691 births (approximately 6000 annually) in the United States results in an extra chromosome of the twenty-first group called *trisomy 21,* or *Down syndrome.*[45,46] DS affects approximately 400,000 persons in the United States.[47] There are three genetic mechanisms for trisomy 21[48]: The first and most common is called *nondisjunction,* in which there is an entire extra chromosome 21 in all cells. This is the case for more than 90% of all patients with trisomy 21. The second

Box 39.6	Genes That May Have Input Into Down Syndrome[49]

Superoxide dismutase *(SOD1):* Overexpression of this gene may cause premature aging and decreased function of the immune system; its role in senile dementia of the Alzheimer type or decreased cognition is still speculative.

COL6A1: Overexpression of this gene may be the cause of heart defects.

ETS2: Overexpression of this gene may be the cause of skeletal abnormalities and/or leukemia.

CAF1A: Overexpression of this gene may be detrimental to DNA synthesis.

Cystathionine β-synthase *(CBS):* Overexpression of this gene may disrupt metabolism and DNA repair.

DYRK: Overexpression of this gene may be the cause of mental retardation.

CRYA1: Overexpression of this gene may be the cause of cataracts.

GART: Overexpression of this gene may disrupt DNA synthesis and repair.

IFNAR: This is the gene for expression of interferon. Overexpression may interfere with the immune system and other organ systems.

is *mosaic DS,* in which trisomy 21 cells are mixed with a second cell line, usually "normal." The third is a *translocation DS,* about 3% to 5% of the total, in which part or all of chromosome 21 is translocated to another chromosome, usually chromosome 14.

Box 39.6 lists genes that may have input into DS.[49] No gene has yet been fully linked to any feature associated with DS

Clinical Manifestations of Down Syndrome

About half of babies with DS have a wide variety of *congenital heart defects,* many of which will require corrective surgery. Other disabilities frequently noted in DS patients include[50]:

- Hearing loss (up to 75% may be affected)
- Obstructive sleep apnea (OSA) (between 50% and 75% affected)
- Ear infections (50% to 70% affected)
- Eye diseases (e.g., cataracts) (up to 60%)
- Eye issues requiring glasses (50%)
- Heart defects present at birth (50%)
- Intestinal blockage at birth requiring surgery (12%)
- Hip dislocation (6%)
- Thyroid disease (4% to 18%)
- Anemia (3%)
- Iron-deficiency anemia (10%)
- Leukemia (1%) in infancy or early childhood
- Hirschsprung disease (<1%)

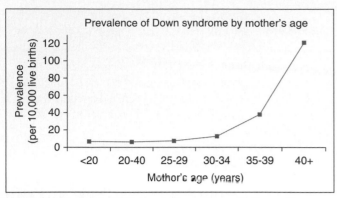

Figure 39.2 Prevalence of Down syndrome by mother's age. (From Centers for Disease Control and Prevention. Down syndrome. Data and statistics. http://www.cdc.gov/ncbddd/birthdefects/downsyndrome/data.html. October 21, 2014. Accessed January 31, 2017.)

- AD (whereas fewer than 10% of the general population will develop AD, about 25% of persons with DS will suffer from this affliction[51])
- DS patients also tend to have many colds in addition to bronchitis and pneumonia

Risk Factors for Down Syndrome

Advancing maternal age is a most significant factor increasing the risk of giving birth to a child with DS[52–55] (Fig. 39.2). It is felt that "older eggs" have an increased risk of improper chromosome division. By age 35, the risk of conceiving a child with DS is about 1 in 350. (The overall risk of conceiving a DS baby is 1 in 691). At age 40 the risk is about 1 in 100, and at age 45 years, the risk is about 1 in 30.[52,53] Due to higher fertility rates in younger women, 80% of children with DS are born to women under 35 years of age.

Previous birth of a DS child increases the risk to about 1 in 100.[53]

Being a carrier of the genetic translocation for DS. Both men and women can pass the genetic translocation for DS on to their children.[53] The vast majority of cases of DS are not inherited. Only in cases of translocation DS, and then in only 1 of 3 cases of this type of DS, is the condition inherited.[53]

Down Syndrome Life Expectancy

Historically, many individuals with DS were killed, abandoned, or ostracized from society. In the twentieth century, it was common for these individuals to be institutionalized, and they did not receive appropriate treatment for the associated medical complications such as heart disorders, vision defects, and intestinal problems. Many children with DS therefore died during infancy or early adulthood.[44]

As the eugenics movement came into being, forced sterilization of individuals with DS was introduced in 33 of the 48 states that then existed in the United States. These sterilization programs reached large proportions until protests from the general public led to their discontinuation. At this point in history, the cause of DS was not understood. It was assumed that several genetic factors, older maternal age, birth injuries, and injury during pregnancy caused the illness.[44]

It was only in the mid-twentieth century (the 1950s) that karyotype techniques were discovered which could be used to help identify the shape and number of chromosomes. This led to the understanding that trisomy 21 was the cause of DS.[44]

Life expectancy for DS patients increased dramatically between 1960 and 2007. Average life expectancy in 1960 was 10 years. In 2007, on average, DS persons lived to about 47 years.[56]

Birth weight has a significant impact on life expectancy with DS. Newborns weighing less than 1.5 kg (3.3 lb—"very-low-birth-weight babies") are 24 times more likely to die within the first 28 days of life compared with DS infants with a normal birth weight (between 2.5 kg and 4.0 kg or 5.5 lb and 8.8 lb).[57]

DS infants with *congenital heart disease* (CHD) are five times more likely to die in the first year of life than DS infants without CHD.[57]

Clinical Signs Associated With DS

The most common clinical signs associated with DS are listed in Box 39.7.[47]

Physiologic changes seen with DS include *mouth breathing*—commonly observed as a result of a small nasal airway; true *macroglossia* is rare; rather, a relative macroglossia is often found in which the tongue is of normal size but the oral cavity is decreased in size as a result of the underdevelopment of the midface.[58]

Box 39.7   Most Common Clinical Signs Associated With Down Syndrome[47]

- Muscle hypotonia (low muscle tone)
- Flat facial profile (depressed nasal bridge and a small nose)
- Oblique palpebral fissures (upward slant to the eyes)
- Dysplastic ears (abnormal shape of the ears)
- Simian crease (a single deep crease across the center of the palm)
- Hyperflexibility (an excessive ability to extend the joints)
- Dysplastic middle phalanx of the fifth finger ("pinky" finger has one flexion furrow instead of two)
- Epicanthal folds (small skin folds on the inner corner of the eyes)
- Relative macroglossia (enlargement of tongue in relation to size of mouth)
- Excessive space between large and second toes

Sleep apnea occurs more often in the DS population than in the general population. One in three children with DS may have an upper airway obstruction.[50,55,59] A 1991 study showed 45% of DS patients with OSA.[60] The decreased airway size and lowered muscle tone predispose these patients to obstructive sleep apnea and airway compromise during general anesthesia and sedation for dentistry.

Considerations for Local Anesthesia, Sedation, and General Anesthesia

Sedative management of the dental patient with DS must consider both the primary disease and other medical problems as a result of or in conjunction with this disease. These patients can usually tolerate dental treatment as well as any other dental patient, with few, if any, modifications. All routes of minimal-to-moderate sedation (inhalation, oral, IM, IV) are acceptable for the patient with DS. However, other coexisting medical problems may be cause for caution (e.g., sleep apnea, bronchitis, pneumonia). The thyroid condition of these patients should be considered. Office-based general anesthesia and deeper levels of sedation are acceptable options, but one must keep in mind the special needs of this patient population related to various airway issues (e.g., relative macroglossia, small nasal airway, mouth breathing) discussed earlier.

INTELLECTUAL AND DEVELOPMENTAL DISABILITIES

Developmental disability is an umbrella term that includes intellectual disability but also includes other disabilities that become apparent during childhood. Developmental disabilities are severe chronic disabilities that can be cognitive or physical or both. The disabilities appear before the age of 18 and are likely to be lifelong. Some developmental disabilities are largely physical issues, such as CP or epilepsy. Some individuals may have a condition that includes a physical and intellectual disability, for example, DS or fetal alcohol syndrome.[61]

Intellectual disability encompasses the "cognitive" part of this definition, that is, a disability that is broadly related to thought processes. Because intellectual and other developmental disabilities often occur together, intellectual disability professionals often work with people who have both types of disabilities.[61]

Incidence and Prevalence of Intellectual Disabilities

Recent estimates in the United States show that about one in six, or about 15%, of children aged 3 through 17 years have one or more developmental disabilities (of all types).[62] Developmental disabilities are a group of conditions due to an impairment in physical, learning, language, or behavior areas. These conditions begin during the developmental period, may affect day-to-day functioning, and usually last throughout a person's lifetime.[63]

Table 39.1	Overall Prevalence of Disabilities for Noninstitutionalized U.S. Children 3 to 17 Years[62]
DISABILITY	**PREVALENCE***
Any developmental disorder	13.9
ADHD	6.7
Autism	0.5
Blind, unable to see	0.1
Cerebral palsy	0.4
Intellectual disability	0.7
Learning disability	7.0
Moderate-to-profound hearing loss	0.5
Seizures	0.7
Stammering/stuttering	1.6
Other developmental delay	3.7

*Prevalence is the proportion of a population who have an event per 1000 population.

The overall prevalence of developmental disabilities in the United States (for noninstitutionalized children ages 3 through 17) is 13.9 per 1000 population (Table 39.1).[62]

Maulik et al published a meta-analysis of studies on intellectual disabilities in all countries from 1980 through 2009.[64] Specifically, the prevalence of *intellectual disability* across all 52 studies included in the meta-analysis was 10.37/1000 population. The estimates varied according to income group of the country of origin, the age group of the study population, and study design. The highest rates of intellectual disability were seen in countries with significant low-to-middle-income populations. Prevalence was higher among studies based on children/adolescents compared with those on adults. Higher prevalence in low- and middle-income-group countries is of concern, given the limitations in available resources in such countries to manage intellectual disability.[64]

The official American Association of Intellectual and Developmental Disabilities (AAIDD) definition of intellectual disability is a disability characterized by significant limitations, both in intellectual functioning and in adaptive behavior, as expressed in conceptual, social, and practical adaptive skills. This disability originates before the age of 18.[61]

Diagnosing Intellectual Disability

The evaluation and classification of intellectual disability is a complex issue. There are three major criteria for intellectual disability: (1) significant limitations in intellectual functioning, (2) significant limitations in adaptive behavior, and (3) onset before the age of 18.[61]

The IQ test is a major tool in measuring *intellectual functioning*, which is the mental capacity for learning, reasoning, problem-solving, etc. A test score below or around 70—or as high as 75—indicates a limitation in intellectual functioning.

Other tests determine limitations in *adaptive behavior,* which covers three types of skills:

- Conceptual skills—language and literacy; money, time, and number concepts; and self-direction
- Social skills—interpersonal skills; social responsibility; self-esteem; gullibility; naïveté (i.e., wariness); social problem-solving; and the ability to follow rules, obey laws, and avoid being victimized
- Practical skills—activities of daily living (personal care), occupational skills, health care, travel/transportation, schedules/routines, safety, use of money, use of the telephone

In defining and assessing intellectual disability, the AAIDD stresses that, in addition to an assessment of intellectual functioning and adaptive behavior, professionals must consider such factors as:

- Community environment typical of the individual's peers and culture
- Linguistic diversity
- Cultural differences in the way people communicate, move, and behave

Causes of Intellectual Disabilities

Chromosomal abnormalities are a more common cause of intellectual and developmental disabilities (IADDs) than are genetic, metabolic, and neurologic abnormalities, although the latter are also causes of IADD. Trisomies involve an additional chromosome (47 chromosomes instead of the normal 46 chromosomes). DS, previously discussed and the most frequently occurring trisomy, results most often from a form of trisomy 21.[47,48]

Mental retardation may result from many other chromosomal abnormalities, including the following:
- Partial deletion of a chromosome (e.g., of chromosome 5 in the *cri du chat* syndrome)[65,66]
- Abnormalities in sex chromosomes (e.g., Klinefelter syndrome [three sex chromosomes, two X and one Y sex chromosome (XXY)])[67]
- Turner syndrome (a single X sex chromosome only)[68]

Those with mild familial IADD may have fragile X syndrome, estimated to affect 1 in 2000 males and 1 in 4000 females. Physical features such as enlarged ears, long face with prominent chin, and macroorchidism are common.[69,70]

Etiologies of Intellectual and Developmental Disabilities

Most developmental disabilities are thought to be caused by a complex mix of factors. These factors include *genetics* (see earlier); *parental health and behaviors* (such as smoking and drinking) *during pregnancy; complications during delivery; infections the mother might have during pregnancy or the baby might have very early in life;* and *exposure of the mother or child to high levels of environmental toxins, such as lead.* For some developmental disabilities, such as fetal alcohol syndrome, caused by drinking alcohol during pregnancy, the specific etiology is known.[71]

Congenital infections are a major cause of IADDs and may occur secondary to exposure to rubella virus, CMV (1 in about 750 live births), *Toxoplasma gondii,* and *Treponema pallidum.*[72]

Considerations for Local Anesthesia, Sedation, and General Anesthesia

Caution should be exercised when contemplating the use of long-acting local anesthetics because of possible lip and cheek biting. Administration of a local anesthesia reversal agent (e.g., phentolamine mesylate [OraVerse]) at the conclusion of a dental procedure in which a vasopressor-containing local anesthetic is used should be considered in these patients. "Plain" local anesthetics do not present any particular concern. Various techniques of minimal-to-moderate sedation (inhalation, oral, or parenteral) as used for other dental patients may be used in the patient with IADD. Intravenous moderate sedation is particularly recommended because of the inherent safety afforded by slow titration. Office-based general anesthesia is typically not necessary for this patient population, but when it is indicated for the more severely affected individuals or its indication is based on degree of difficulty of procedure or other patient management concerns, it may be safely used.

SCHIZOPHRENIA

"People do not cause schizophrenia; they merely blame each other for doing so."
—*E. Fuller Torrey*[73]

Schizophrenia is a severe and debilitating brain and behavioral disorder affecting how one thinks, feels, and acts. Schizophrenics can have trouble distinguishing reality from fantasy, expressing and managing normal emotions, and making decisions. Thought processes may also be disorganized and the motivation to engage in life's activities may be blunted. Those with the condition may hear imaginary voices and believe others are reading their minds, controlling their thoughts, or plotting to harm them.[74,75]

Most people with schizophrenia suffer from symptoms either continuously or intermittently throughout life and are often severely stigmatized by people who do not understand the disease. Contrary to popular perception, schizophrenics do not have "split" or multiple personalities, and most pose no danger to others. However, the symptoms are terrifying to those afflicted and can make them unresponsive, agitated, or withdrawn.

People with schizophrenia attempt suicide more often than people in the general population. The lifetime risk of suicide death is estimated to be 5.6%. The risk is particularly high during the first year of the initial contact with mental health services, being almost twice as high as in the later course of the illness.[76] This is especially noted among young men with schizophrenia.[75,76]

Table 39.2	Age (in Years) at Onset of Schizophrenia[78]	
AGE (YEARS)		PROBABILITY OF DEVELOPING SCHIZOPHRENIA
<16		Rare
16–25		75%
26–40		40%
>40		Rare

Table 39.3	Genetic Associations in Schizophrenia	
GENETIC LINK		PROBABILITY OF DEVELOPING SCHIZOPHRENIA
General population		1%
First cousins		2%
Uncles/aunts		2%
Nephews/nieces		4%
Grandchildren		5%
Half-siblings		6%
Parents		6%
Siblings		9%
Children		13%
Fraternal twins		17%
Identical twins		48%

Incidence and Prevalence of Schizophrenia

The prevalence rate of schizophrenia worldwide is approximately 1.1% of the population over age 18.[77] As many as 51 million worldwide suffer from schizophrenia, including 6 to 12 million in China, 4.3 to 8.7 million in India, 2.2 million in the United States, 285,000 in Australia, >280,000 in Canada, and >250,000 in Britain.[77]

Rates of schizophrenia vary from country to country, but are commonly felt to be between 0.5% and 1% of the population.

In the United States approximately 100,000 persons are diagnosed with schizophrenia annually, more than 1.5 million worldwide.[77]

Schizophrenia affects men and women equally, occurring at similar rates in all ethnic groups around the world. Symptoms such as hallucinations and delusions commonly start between ages 16 and 30 (Table 39.2).[78] Men tend to experience symptoms earlier than women. It is rare for schizophrenia to develop after age 45. Schizophrenia rarely occurs in children, but awareness of childhood-onset schizophrenia (symptoms developing before the age of 13) and early-onset schizophrenia (symptoms developing before the age of 18) is increasing.[79]

It can be difficult to diagnose schizophrenia in teens. This is because the first signs can include a change of friends, a drop in grades, sleep problems, and irritability—behaviors that are common among teens.[79]

Etiology of Schizophrenia

The leading theory of why people get schizophrenia is that it is a result of a *genetic predisposition* combined with *environmental exposures and/or stresses during pregnancy or childhood* that contribute to, or trigger, the disorder (Table 39.3). Researchers have identified several key genes that, when damaged, create an increased risk for schizophrenia. These genes include the *DISC1,* dysbindin, neuregulin, and *G72* genes, but it has been estimated that up to a dozen or more genes could be involved in schizophrenia risk.[80]

Types of Schizophrenia

There are five subtypes of schizophrenia[75]:
- Paranoid schizophrenia — feelings of extreme suspicion, persecution, or grandiosity, or a combination of these

- Disorganized schizophrenia — incoherent thoughts, but not necessarily delusional
- Catatonic schizophrenia — withdrawal, negative affect and isolation, and marked psychomotor disturbances
- Residual schizophrenia — delusions or hallucinations may go away, but motivation or interest in life is gone
- Schizoaffective disorder — symptoms of both schizophrenia and a major mood disorder, such as depression

Signs and Symptoms of Schizophrenia

Schizophrenia can present with very different symptoms from person to person. The manner in which the disease manifests itself and progresses in a person depends on the time of onset, severity, and duration of symptoms, which are categorized as *positive, negative,* and *cognitive.* All three types of symptoms reflect problems in brain function. Relapse and remission cycles often occur; a person may get better, worse, and better again repeatedly over time.[81]

- Positive symptoms, which can be severe or mild, include delusions, hallucinations, and thought disorders. Some psychiatrists also include psychomotor problems that affect movement in this category. Delusions, hallucinations, and inner voices are collectively called *psychosis,* which also can be a hallmark of other serious mental illnesses such as bipolar disorder. Delusions lead people to believe others are monitoring or threatening them or reading their thoughts. Hallucinations cause a patient to hear, see, feel, or smell something that is not there. Thought disorders may involve difficulty putting cohesive thoughts together or making sense of speech. Psychomotor problems may appear as clumsiness, unusual mannerisms, or repetitive actions, and in extreme cases, motionless rigidity held for extended periods of time.[81]
- Negative symptoms reflect a loss of functioning in areas such as emotion or motivation. Negative symptoms include loss or reduction in the ability to initiate plans, speak,

express emotion, or find pleasure in life. They include emotional flatness or lack of expression, diminished ability to begin and sustain a planned activity, social withdrawal, and apathy. These symptoms can be mistaken for laziness or depression.[81]

- Cognitive symptoms involve problems with attention and memory, especially in planning and organizing to achieve a goal. Cognitive deficits are the most disabling for patients trying to lead a normal life.[81]

Treatment of Schizophrenia

Although there is no cure for schizophrenia, the treatment success rate with antipsychotic medications and psychosocial therapies can be high—if medication regimens are fully complied with.[82] Most of those affected by schizophrenia respond to specific drug therapy, and many are able to lead productive and fulfilling lives (Box 39.8).

Antipsychotic medications are proven effective in treating acute psychosis and reducing the risk of future psychotic episodes. The treatment of schizophrenia thus has two main phases: an acute phase, when higher doses might be necessary in order to treat psychotic symptoms, followed by a maintenance phase, which is usually lifelong. During the maintenance phase, drug dosage is often gradually reduced to the minimum required to prevent further episodes and control interepisode symptoms. If symptoms reappear or worsen on a lower dosage, an increase in dosage may be necessary to help prevent further relapse.

Even with continued treatment, patients may experience relapses. The most common cause of a relapse is noncompliance with prescribed medications.[82] The large majority of schizophrenia patients experience improvement when treated with antipsychotic drugs. Some patients, however, do not respond to medications, and a few may seem not to need them.

The first antipsychotic drug, chlorpromazine (Thorazine), was discovered in the mid-1950s. A spate of new drugs followed, including fluphenazine (Prolixin), haloperidol (Haldol), loxapine (Loxapine), perphenazine (Trilafon), thioridazine (Mellaril), thiothixene (Navane), and trifluoperazine (Stelazine).

These drugs, known as *neuroleptics,* though effective in treating the positive symptoms (acute symptoms such as hallucinations, delusions, thought disorder, loose associations, ambivalence, or emotional lability), can cause cognitive dulling and involuntary movements, among other side effects. These first-generation antipsychotics also are not as effective against negative symptoms such as apathy, decreased motivation, and lack of emotional expressiveness.[83] Tardive dyskinesia is the most unpleasant and serious side effect of the antipsychotic drugs. It may cause involuntary facial movements and jerking or twisting movements of other parts of the body. This usually develops in older patients, affecting 20% of those who have taken older antipsychotic drugs for many years. In most, but not all, cases, the tardive dyskinesia slowly goes away when the medication is stopped.[01]

In 1989 a second-generation antipsychotic drug was introduced: clozapine (Clozaril). Clozapine, known as an *atypical antipsychotic,* remains the only drug that has been shown to be effective where other antipsychotics have failed.[85] It is less strongly linked with the side effects mentioned earlier, but it can produce other side effects, including weight gain, changes in blood sugar and cholesterol, and possible decrease in the number of infection-fighting white blood cells.[85,86]

Other second-generation antipsychotics include aripiprazole (Abilify), aripiprazole lauroxil (Aristada), asenapine (Saphris), brexpiprazole (Rexulti), cariprazine (Vraylar), lurasidone (Latuda), paliperidone (Invega Sustenna), paliperidone palmitate (Invega Trinza), quetiapine (Seroquel), risperidone (Risperdal or Risperdal Consta), olanzapine (Zyprexa), and ziprasidone (Geodon) Another atypical antipsychotic, iloperidone (Fanapt), has been approved by the Food and Drug Administration (FDA) for acute (but not long-term) treatment of schizophrenia.[87,88]

The use of all of these medications has allowed successful treatment and release back to their homes and the community for many people suffering from schizophrenia.

Considerations for Local Anesthesia, Sedation, and General Anesthesia

As with all medications patients are taking, reading and understanding the package inserts of these drugs is an absolute requirement. As an example, patients taking trifluoperazine (Stelazine) or haloperidol (Haldol) should have local anesthetics with epinephrine used cautiously because of the possibility of causing paradoxical hypotension.

Sedation for the dental patient with schizophrenia may also be quite complicated. When possible, the avoidance of psychoactive drugs (essentially all sedatives used in dentistry) is highly recommended. If only a very minimal level of sedation is needed, inhalation sedation with nitrous oxide-oxygen is most appropriate, but it must be used with caution. Other routes of minimal-to-moderate sedation (oral, IM, and IV) are generally not indicated. Only after a thorough consultation with the physician managing the patient's antipsychotic medication regimen should these sedative regimens be considered. Office-based general anesthesia with ultrashort-acting medications (e.g., propofol, remifentanil) is generally preferable to moderate sedation because during general anesthesia, the patient's consciousness is removed. This contrasts with an altered state of consciousness seen in minimal-to-moderate sedation (attained through any of the various routes of administration). The fast offset of ultrashort-acting medications is beneficial in the dental patient with schizophrenia in rapidly returning to normal consciousness.

REFERENCES

1. The Resource Foundation for Children with Challenges: www.specialchild.com.
2. The *Oregonian:* www.oregonlive.com/oregonian. August 18, 2001.
3. Eli Lilly and Co: Official prospect of Alzheimer's birthplace: www.marktbreit.de/kultur_bildung/alzheimer_engl.htm.
4. Wilson RS, Segawa E, Boyle PA, et al: The natural history of cognitive decline in Alzheimer's disease. *Psychol Aging* 27(4):1008–1017, 2012.
5. Barker WW, Luis CA, Kashuba A, et al: Relative frequencies of Alzheimer's disease, Lewy body, vascular and frontotemporal dementia, and hippocampal sclerosis in the State of Florida Brain Bank. *Alzheimer Dis Assoc Disord* 16(4):203–212, 2002.
6. Alzheimer's Association: 2016 Alzheimer's disease facts and figures. *Alzheimers Dement* 12(4):1–84, 2016.
7. Xu JQ, Murphy SL, Kochanek KD, Bastian BA: Deaths: final data for 2013. National vital statistics reports; vol. 64, no. 2. Hyattsville MD: National Center for Health Statistics. 2016. http://www.cdc.gov/nchs. (Accessed 31 January 2017).
8. Herbert LA, Weuve J, Scherr PA, Evans DA: Alzheimer disease in the United States (2010-2050) estimated using the 2010 Census. *Neurology* 80(19):1778–1783, 2013.
9. Alzheimer's Association: Early-onset dementia: a national challenge, a future crisis. Washington DC, Alzheimer's Association; 2006.
10. Seshadri S, Beiser A, Kelly-Hayes M, et al: The lifetime risk of stroke: estimates from the Framingham Study. *Stroke* 37(2):345–350, 2006.
11. Ortman JM, Velkoff VA, Hogan H: An aging nation: the older population in the United States. Current population reports. P25-1140. U.S. Census Bureau, Washington DC, 2014. www.census.gov. (Accessed 31 January 2017).
12. Villemagne VL, Burnham S, Bourgeat P, et al; Australian Imaging Biomarkers and Lifestyle (AIBL) Research Group: Amyloid β deposition, neurodegeneration, and cognitive decline in sporadic Alzheimer's disease: a prospective cohort study. *Lancet Neurol* 12(4):357–367, 2013.
13. Jack CR, Lowe VJ, Weigand SD, et al; Alzheimer's Disease Neuroimaging Initiative: Serial PiB and MRI in normal, cognitive impairment and Alzheimer's disease: implications for sequence of pathological events in Alzheimer's disease. *Brain* 132:1355–1365, 2009.
14. Bateman RJ, Xiong C, Benzinger TL, et al; Dominantly Inherited Alzheimer Network: Clinical and biomarker changes in dominantly inherited Alzheimer's disease. *N Engl J Med* 367(9):795–804, 2012.
15. J Alzheimer's Dis: www.j-alz.com.
16. National Institute of Neurological Disorders and Stroke: NINDS Pervasive developmental disorders information page. http://www.ninds.nih.gov/disorders/pdd/pdd.htm, February 1, 2016. (Accessed 31 January 2017).
17. Kanner L: Autistic disturbances of affective contact. *Nervous Child* 2:217–250, 1943.
18. Autism Society of America: www.autism-society.org. (Accessed 31 January 2017).
19. Elsabbagh M, Divan G, Koh YJ, et al: Global prevalence of autism and other pervasive developmental disorders. *Autism Res* 5(3):160–179, 2012.
20. Christensen DL, Baio J, Braun KV, et al; Centers for Disease Control and Prevention (CDC): Prevalence and characteristics of autism spectrum disorder among children aged 8 years – Autism and Developmental Disabilities Monitoring Network, 11 Sites, United States, 2012. *MMWR Surveill Summ* 65(No. SS-3):1–23, 2016.
21. http://www.bloomberg.com/news/articles/2014-06-09/autism-costs-more-than-2-million-over-patient-s-life. (Accessed 31 January 2017).
22. Autism speaks official blog: What is causing the increase in autism prevalence? https://blog.autismspeaks.org/2010/10/22/got-questions-answers-to-your-questions-from-the-autism-speaks%E2%80%99-science-staff-2/ October 22, 2010. (Accessed 4 September 2016).
23. Bailey DB, Jr, Hatton DD, Mesibov G, et al: Early development, temperament, and functional impairment in autism and fragile X syndrome. *J Autism Dev Disord* 30(1):49–59, 2000.
24. Connolly AM, Chez M, Streif EM, et al: Brain-derived neurotrophic factor and autoantibodies to neural antigens in sera of children with autistic spectrum disorders, Landau-Kleffner syndrome, and epilepsy. *Biol Psychiatry* 59(4):354–363, 2006.
25. Verte S, Geurts HM, Roeyers H, et al: Executive functioning in children with autism and Tourette syndrome. *Dev Psychopathol* 17(2):415–445, 2005.
26. Herguner S, Mukaddes NM: Autism and Williams syndrome: a case report. *World J Biol Psychiatry* 7(3):186–188, 2006.
27. National Institute of Neurological Disorders and Stroke: NINDS cerebral palsy information page. http://www.ninds.nih.gov/disorders/cerebral_palsy/cerebral_palsy.htm. March 15, 2016. (Accessed 31 January 2017).
28. Accardo PJ, editor: *Capute and Accardo's neurodevelopmental disabilities in infancy and childhood*, ed 3, Baltimore, 2008, Paul H. Brookes Publishing Co, p 17.
29. Facts about cerebral palsy. Centers for Disease Control and Prevention. https://www.cdc.gov/ncbddd/cp/facts.html. May 2, 2016. (Accessed 31 January 2017).
30. Nelson KB, Grether JK: Causes of cerebral palsy. *Curr Opin Pediatr* 11(6):487–491, 1999.
31. Gibson CS, MacLennan AH, Goldwater PN, Dekker GA: Antenatal causes of cerebral palsy: associations between inherited thrombophilias, viral and bacterial infection, and inherited susceptibility to infection. *Obstet Gynecol Surv* 58(3):209–220, 2003.
32. Paneth N, Hong T, Korzeniewski S: The descriptive epidemiology of cerebral palsy. *Clin Perinatol* 33(2):251–267, 2006.
33. Winter S, Autry A, Boyle C, Yeargin-Allsopp M: Trends in the prevalence of cerebral palsy in a population-based study. *Pediatrics* 110(6):1220–1225, 2002.
34. Prevalence of cerebral palsy. http://www.cerebralpalsy.org/about-cerebral-palsy/prevalence-and-incidence. (Accessed 31 January 2017).
35. Van Naarden Braun K, Doernberg N, et al: Birth prevalence of cerebral palsy: a population-based study. *Pediatrics* 137(1):2016.
36. National Center on Birth Defects and Developmental Disabilities. www.cdc.gov/ncbddd/dd.
37. Dammann O, O'Shea TM: Cytokines and perinatal brain damage. *Clin Perinatol* 35(4):643–663, v, 2008.

38. O'Shea TM: Diagnosis, treatment, and prevention of cerebral palsy. *Clin Obstet Gynecol* 51(4):816–828, 2008.

39. Novak I, McIntyre S, Morgan C, et al: A systematic review of interventions for children with cerebral palsy: state of the evidence. *Dev Med Child Neurol* 55(10):885–910, 2013.

40. Christensen D, Van Naarden Braun K, Doernberg NS, et al: Prevalence of cerebral palsy, co-occurring autism spectrum disorders, and motor functioning—Autism and Developmental Disabilities Monitoring Network, USA, 2008. *Dev Med Child Neurol* 56(1):59–65, 2014.

41. Boulet SL, Boyle CA, Schieve LA: Health care use and health and functional impact of developmental disabilities among US children, 1997–2005. *Arch Pediatr Adolesc Med* 163(1):19–26, 2009.

42. Dunn PM: Dr Langdon Down (1828–1896) and 'mongolism'. *Arch Dis Child* 66(7 Spec No):827–828, 1991.

43. Gautier M, Harper PS: Fiftieth anniversary of trisomy 21: returning to a discovery. *Hum Genet* 126:317–324, 2009.

44. Pain E: After more than 50 years, a dispute over Down syndrome discovery. www.sciencemag.org/news. Science AAAS. February 14, 2014. (Accessed 31 January 2017).

45. Centers for Disease Control and Prevention: Down syndrome. Data and statistics. http://www.cdc.gov/ncbddd/birthdefects/downsyndrome/data.html. October 21, 2014. (Accessed 31 January 2017).

46. Parker SE, Mai CT, Canfield MA, et al; National Birth Defects Prevention Network: Updated national birth prevalence estimates for selected birth defects in the United States, 2004–2006. *Birth Defects Res A Clin Mol Teratol* 88(12):1008–1016, 2010.

47. National Down Syndrome Society: Down syndrome fact sheet. http://www.ndss.org/Down-Syndrome/Down-Syndrome-Facts/. (Accessed 31 January 2017).

48. Canadian Down Syndrome Society: Types of Down syndrome. http://www.cdss.ca/information/general-information/types-of-down-syndrome.html. June 19, 2009. (Accessed 31 January 2017).

49. Hernandez D, Fisher EM: Down syndrome genetics: unraveling a multifactorial disorder. *Hum Mol Genet* 5 Spec No:1411–1416, 1996.

50. Bull MJ; Committee on Genetics: Health supervision for children with Down syndrome. *Pediatrics* 128(2):393–406, 2011.

51. Hill DA, Gridley G, Cnattingius S, et al: Mortality and cancer incidence among individuals with Down syndrome. *Arch Intern Med* 63(6):705–711, 2003.

52. Mai CT, Kucik JE, Isenburg J, et al; National Birth Defects Prevention Network: Selected birth defects data from population-based birth defects surveillance programs in the United States, 2006 to 2010: featuring trisomy conditions. *Birth Defects Res A Clin Mol Teratol* 97(11):709–725, 2013.

53. Alldred SK, Takwoingi Y, Guo B, et al: First trimester serum tests for Down's syndrome screening. *Cochrane Database Syst Rev* (11):CD011975, 2015.

54. Oliver TR, Feingold E, Yu K, et al: New insights into human nondisjunction of chromosome 21 in oocytes. *PLoS Genet* 4(3):e1000033, 2008.

55. Grobman WA, Dooley SL, Welshman EE, et al: Preference assessment of prenatal diagnosis for Down syndrome: is 35 years a rational cutoff? *Prenat Diagn* 22(13):1195–1200, 2002.

56. Presson AP, Partyka G, Jensen KM, et al: Current estimate of Down syndrome population prevalence in the United States. *J Pediatr* 163(4):1163–1168, 2013.

57. Kucik JE, Shin M, Siffel C, et al; Congenital anomaly multistate prevalence and survival collaborative: trends in survival among children with Down syndrome in 10 regions of the United States. *Pediatrics* 131(1):e27–e36, 2013.

58. Chin CJ, Khami MM, Husein M: A general review of the otolaryngologic manifestations of Down syndrome. *Int J Pediatr Otorhinolaryngol* 78(6):899–904, 2014.

59. Baumer N, Davidson EJ: Supporting a happy, healthy adolescence for young people with Down syndrome and other intellectual disabilities: recommendations for clinicians. *Curr Opin Pediatr* 26(4):428–434, 2014.

60. Marcus CL, Keens TG, Bautista DB, et al: Obstructive sleep apnea in children with Down syndrome. *Pediatrics* 88(1):132–139, 1991.

61. American Association on Intellectual and Developmental Disabilities: Frequently asked questions on intellectual disability and the AAIDD definition. https://aaidd.org/intellectual-disability/definition/faqs-on-intellectual-disability#.V9AhhpMrIUE. (Accessed 31 January 2017).

62. Boyle CA, Boulet S, Schieve L, et al: Trends in the prevalence of developmental disabilities in US children, 1997–2008. *Pediatrics* 27:1034–1042, 2011.

63. Rubin IL, Crockere AC, editors: *Developmental disabilities: delivery of medical care for children and adults*, Philadelphia, 1989, Lea & Febiger.

64. Maulik PK, Mascarenhas MN, Mathers CD, et al: Prevalence of intellectual disability: a meta-analysis of population-based studies. *Res Dev Disabil* 32(2):419–436, 2011.

65. Rodriguez-Caballero A, Torres-Lagares D, Rodriguez-Perez A, et al: Cri du chat syndrome: a critical review. *Med Oral Patol Oral Cir Bucal* 15(3):e473–e478, 2010.

66. Hall C, Hallett K, Manton D: The association between Cri du chat syndrome and dental anomalies. *J Dent Child (Chic)* 81(3):171–177, 2014.

67. Groth KA, Skakkebaek A, Host C, et al: Clinical review: Klinefelter syndrome—a clinical update. *J Clin Endocrinol Metab* 98(1):20–30, 2013.

68. Levitsky LL, Luria AH, Hayes FJ, Lin AE: Turner syndrome: update on biology and management across the life span. *Curr Opin Endocrinol Diabetes Obes* 22(1):65–72, 2015.

69. Saldarriaga W, Tassone F, Gonzalez-Teshima LY, et al: Fragile X syndrome. *Colomb Med* 45(4):190–198, 2014.

70. Chen E, Joseph S: Fragile X mental retardation protein: a paradigm for translational control by RNA-binding proteins. *Biochimie* 114:147–154, 2015.

71. Flak AL, Su S, Bertrand J, et al: The association of mild, moderate, and binge prenatal alcohol exposure and child neuropsychological outcomes: a meta-analysis. *Alcohol Clin Exp Res* 38(1):214–226, 2014.

72. Swanson EC, Schleiss MR: Congenital cytomegalovirus infection: new prospects for prevention and therapy. *Pediatr Clin North Am* 60(2):335–349, 2013.

73. www.schizophrenia.com.

74. National Institute of Mental Health: Schizophrenia. www.nimh.nih.gov/healthtopics/schizophrenia/index.shtml. February 2016. (Accessed 31 Januarty 2017).

75. Brain and Behavior Research Foundation: Frequently asked questions about schizophrenia. https://bbrfoundation.org/frequently-asked-questions-about-schizophrenia. 2016. (Accessed 31 January 2017).

76. Nordentoft M, Madsen T, Fedyszyn I: Suicidal behavior and mortality in first-episode psychosis. *J Nerv Ment Dis* 203(5):387–392, 2015.

77. Schizophrenia.com. Schizophrenia facts and figures – 2016. http://schizophrenia.com/szfacts.htm#. (Accessed 31 January 2017).

78. Sham PC, MacLean CJ, Kendler KS: A typological model of schizophrenia based on age at onset, sex and familial morbidity. *Acta Psychiatr Scand* 89(2):135–141, 1994.

79. Lachman A: New developments in diagnosis and treatment update: schizophrenia/first episode psychosis in children and adolescents. *J Child Adolesc Ment Health* 26(2):109–124, 2014.

80. Swerdlow NR, Gur RE, Braff DL: Consortium on the Genetics of Schizophrenia (COGS) assessment of endophenotypes for schizophrenia: an introduction to this special issue of Schizophrenia Research. *Schizophr Res* 163(1-3):9–16, 2015.

81. Lin CY, Tsai GE, Lane HY: Assessing and treating cognitive impairment in schizophrenia: current and future. *Curr Pharm Des* 20(32):5127–5138, 2014.

82. Chang YT, Lee LL: The effectiveness of compliance therapy on drug attitude among schizophrenic patients: a systematic review. *JBI Database System Rev Implement Rep* 13(7):213–240, 2015.

83. Moller HJ, Czobor P: Pharmacological treatment of negative symptoms in schizophrenia. *Eur Arch Psychiatry Clin Neurosci* 265(7):567–578, 2015.

84. Hazari N, Kate N, Grover S: Clozapine and tardive movement disorders: a review. *Asian J Psychiatr* 6(6):439–451, 2013.

85. Hippius H: The history of clozapine. *Psychopharmacology (Berl)* 99(Suppl):S3–S5, 1989.

86. Ayub M, Saeed K, Munshi TA, Naeem F: Clozapine for psychotic disorders in adults with intellectual disabilities. *Cochrane Database Syst Rev* (9):CD010625, 2015.

87. Ventimiglia J, Kalali AH, Citrome L: A review of new atypical antipsychotic launches in the United States. *Psychiatry (Edgmont)* 7(12):13–15, 2010.

88. Vigneault P, Pilote S, Patoine D, et al: Iloperidone (Fanapt), a novel atypical antipsychotic, is a potent HERG blocker and delays cardiac ventricular repolarization at clinically relevant concentration. *Pharmacol Res* 66(1):60–65, 2012.

chapter 40

Medicolegal Considerations

CHAPTER OUTLINE

THE UNIQUE STATUS OF SEDATION IN DENTISTRY

Sedation, particularly parenteral (IV, IM, IN), is generally regulated in states by statute or via dental practice acts.

The reasons for these regulations are multiple, but essentially they are in place because dental students are not routinely trained in advanced forms of sedation. Sedation competency generally requires postgraduate training, beginning with relatively short oral minimal sedation courses. Accredited oral and maxillofacial surgery programs require a minimum of 300 cases involving deep sedation or general anesthesia during a 4- to 7-year residency. Dedicated residency training in anesthesiology lasting 3 or more years produces proficient dentist anesthesiologists. Intravenous sedation courses fall somewhere in the middle temporally. Dr. Malamed's well-recognized intravenous sedation course at The University of Southern California School of Dentistry has been in place since the 1970s.

A second reason that sedation is specifically regulated is that the vast majority of dentists use local anesthesia alone for invasive procedures. It is somewhat ironic that although dentists introduced safe, predictable, and reproducible anesthesia to the world,[1,2] the profession has largely lost that heritage in its gravitation toward local anesthesia. Advanced pain control techniques are not readily available to our patients today despite the overwhelming patient-perceived need and demand. Dentist anesthesiologists and dentists who limit their practices to sedation-only procedures are literally as busy as they desire. It is not uncommon for oral and maxillofacial surgery patients to ask if "all my dental work" can somehow be done with sedation or general anesthesia, as the surgeon has provided.

Anesthesiology is a specialty in medicine, veterinary medicine, and for dentists in Japan and the province of Ontario, Canada. Most of the world recognizes the necessity of formal training to provide anesthesia services; states appropriately are stimulated to ensure that patients are treated by dentists who are competent to provide these services.

For many people, avoiding dental care can be attributed to a deeply ingrained fear.[3] In 2000 the U.S. Surgeon General reported that 4.3% of the population did not avail themselves of dental appointments secondary to fear.[4] Well more than 10% of the population has not seen a dentist professionally for a minimum of 5 years to a maximum time frame of never.[5]

There is no question that dentists who become proficient in the provision of pain control modalities other than local anesthesia will have the opportunity to serve a much larger patient base than colleagues not similarly trained. However, with the additional opportunity to treat patients comes the additional responsibility to be able to safely administer supplemental agents.

LEGAL HISTORY

Health professionals are faced with onerous requirements based on legal issues as we practice in the twenty-first century.

The history of liability for alleged medical errors is long, no doubt dating to times before medical records were even written. It is difficult to find "the good old days" when one considers that health professionals have been under constraint to perform successfully for millennia. Consider Babylon's Code of Hammurabi (1700 BC) that codified the laws of the period and contains the first known written record regulating medical practice.[6]

The code provides, for instance, that "If a doctor treats a man with a metal knife for a severe wound, and has caused the man to die, or has opened the man's tumor with a metal knife and destroyed the man's eye, his hands shall be cut off."[7]

MODERN LIABILITY INSURANCE CRISES

Experienced practitioners today know that we are in the midst of our third modern "liability crisis." Perhaps a more appropriate term would be "liability insurance crisis." As taxing as liability issues are, it appears that most of today's world has accepted the principle of accepting remuneration rather than a literal pound of flesh for medical errors.

Those who were practicing in the 1970s will recall the first modern liability insurance crisis. Physicians in California went on strike for services other than true emergencies. The result of the strike and other types of health professional activism was MICRA, or California's Medical Insurance Compensation Reform Act of 1975.

MICRA provided a multipronged solution to the crisis at that time and included:
1. Limits on noneconomic damages
2. Evidence of collateral sources of payment
3. Limits on attorney's fees
4. Advance notice of a claim
5. Statute of limitations reform
6. Periodic payments for future needs
7. Binding arbitration of disputes

The results of MICRA have been impressive and include findings such as:
1. The time to settlement in California is 3 years, whereas the national average is 4 years.
2. The cost of settlement in California is half of that averaged nationally. Although insurers pay out less, the plaintiffs receive larger average awards during settlement.
3. The cost of liability insurance premiums in California from 1975 to 2000 rose 168%, but nationally, premiums rose 505%.

The second modern liability crisis occurred in the 1980s and resulted in many dentists economically forced to find alternative liability insurance options. One successful experiment involved forming private offshore insurance companies. Despite the significant legal, temporal, and financial logistics involved, this type of planning was successful, as evidenced by the fact that major carrier insurance rates uniformly decreased nationally as the dentist-owned and dentist-operated companies thrived. Rates decreased in part because when the dentists themselves were managers and shareholders, companies quickly settled meritorious claims and aggressively defended frivolous suits. In addition, many health professionals involved in such planning actually profited financially from well-managed concerns. The profits were significant enough that the traditional insurers reentered the marketplace and purchased most of the dentist-owned companies.

Unfortunately, the overall national economic boom of the 1980s did not continue into the 1990s. This, coupled with the loss of personally involved dentist managers and shareholders, resulted in the third crisis, which continues to this day.

Currently, MICRA is still in place in California and appears to continue to be beneficial. Interestingly, there are more than 200,000[8] attorneys in California and approximately 20,000 dentists. Nationally, 1,100,000 attorneys practice, whereas the American Dental Association (ADA) has 170,000 members.

At the time of this writing, tort reform is a major state and national issue. Tort reform involves not only health professionals but all aspects of society where individuals are accused of breaching a duty to another's disadvantage. The trend at this time is logically to revisit California's MICRA-based tort reform. MICRA has stood the test of time and has been shown to be of economic benefit to all interested groups, except that of the trial lawyers (both plaintiff and defense).

The nation has seen a dramatic rise in not only tort-based malpractice lawsuits over the past several years but also the predictable sequelae of such legal action. Trauma centers have closed, dentists are actively and passively (i.e., by limiting their practice or opting for early retirement) leaving lawsuit-friendly communities or states, and patient consumers are now starting to feel directly the loss of health professional availability and other consequences of a litigation system that has never been busier.

As states enact MICRA-based reform, constitutional challenges are predictably foisted in the courts. Recently the Wisconsin Supreme Court invoked the relatively rare rational basis legal theory in a 4–3 decision that eliminated the $350,000 cap on some medical malpractice damages.[9] Time will only tell where the states' machinations lead us, but to many legal commentators, it appears that ultimately a federal resolution is necessary.

LIABILITY INSURANCE COVERAGE

Occasionally, insurance companies will deny coverage for a defendant's claim. For instance, in *Woo v. Fireman's Fund Insurance Co.,*[10] an oral and maxillofacial surgeon was denied coverage for a claim arising from an extraction case done via general anesthesia. Dr. Woo had foisted a "practical joke" on his future former assistant patient. During the procedure, Dr. Woo inserted boar tusk–shaped objects into the plaintiff's mouth and took photographs of the same while the patient was under anesthesia. The patient sued under several theories, in part including outrage, battery, invasion of privacy, false light, public disclosure of private acts, medical negligence, lack of informed consent, and negligent infliction of emotional distress. Fireman's Fund refused to defend Dr. Woo, stating his conduct was outside the scope of his policy.[10]

Dr. Woo sued Fireman's Fund after settling personally with the patient.

The Washington Supreme Court found that Dr. Woo's conduct did fall within the practice of dentistry because the prank occurred within the employer–employee relationship. The court also held that because the practical joke occurred during surgery, the Fireman's professional liability policy applied to the situation. Next the court stated that Fireman's could only be relieved of responsibility if the policy clearly stated that certain conduct was excluded from coverage (similar to the option health insurance policies have of specifically excluding certain conditions or procedures, such as temporomandibular joint [TMJ] pathologic conditions or dental implants). Finally the court warned that the carrier must defer to the insured's interests in ambiguous situations, not the other way around.

THEORIES OF LIABILITY

There are several legal theories by which plaintiffs can seek redress against health professionals.

Statute Violation

Violation of a state or federal statute leads to an assumption of negligence if damage to a patient occurs. In other words, the burden of proof, a significant obligation usually born by the plaintiff, now shifts to the defendant, who must prove that the statute violation was not such that it caused any damage claimed.

Two basic types of statutes exist: *malum in se* and *malum prohibitum*. *Malum in se* (bad in fact) statutes restrict behavior that in and of itself is recognized as harmful, such as driving while inebriated. *Malum prohibitum* (defined as bad) conduct in and of itself may not be criminal, reckless, wanton, etc., but is regulated simply to, for instance, promote social order. Driving at certain speeds is an example of a *malum prohibitum* statute. The difference between legally driving at 15 mph in a school zone and criminally driving at 16 mph in a school zone is not the result of a criminal mind, but a social regulatory decision.

For instance, if one is speeding while driving, several sequelae may result when that statute violation is recognized. The speeder may simply be warned to stop speeding. Second, the speeder may be issued a citation and have to appear in court, argue innocence, pay a fine if found guilty, attend traffic school, etc. Third, if the speeder's conduct causes damage to others, additional civil or criminal sanctions may apply. Fourth, the situation may be compounded civilly or criminally if multiple statute violations are present, such as speeding and driving recklessly or driving while intoxicated.

Occasionally, statute violation is commendable. For instance, a driver may swerve to the "wrong" side of the centerline to avoid a child who suddenly runs into the street from between parked cars. At times, speeding may be considered a heroic act, such as when a driver is transporting a patient to a hospital during an emergency. However, even if the speeder believes that he is somehow contributing to the public welfare, the statute violation is still subject to review.

For health professionals, the administration of drugs without a current state license or Drug Enforcement Administration (DEA) certification is likely a violation of statute. If the type of harm sustained by the patient is the type that would have been prevented by obeying the statute, additional liability may attach to the defendant. As an example, someone without a license may be liable for permanent lingual nerve paresthesia[11,12] after the administration of a local block, but likely would not be liable for temporally related appendicitis.

Occasionally, professional groups, political societies, etc., may publicize opinions that can adversely affect other groups. An example of this is the American Society of Anesthesiologists' (ASA) 1982 policy statement that "anesthesia care is the practice of medicine."[13] Such a policy, if adopted by state boards or other regulatory agencies, could have negative effects on the anesthesia practices within dentistry. Recognizing such, the American Association of Oral and Maxillofacial Surgeons (AAOMS), ADA, and other interested dental professionals entered into negotiations with the ASA soon after the 1982 policy publication. These negotiations resulted in a modified 1987 statement that "[t]he ASA recognizes the right of qualified dentists as defined by the ADA to administer conscious sedation, deep sedation, and general anesthesia to patients having dental procedures only."[14]

Conversely an example of a beneficial regulatory violation and a subsequent positive educational experience for a regulatory agency occurred when a licensee did not fulfill mandatory basic cardiopulmonary resuscitation (CPR) certification, but chose to complete advanced cardiovascular life support (ACLS) certification instead. When admonished by the state board that a violation had occurred, potentially putting the public at greater risk, the licensee pointed out to the regulatory board that ACLS certification is actually more beneficial to the public than CPR. The licensing board then changed the regulation to allow CPR or ACLS certification as a requirement to maintain a license.

Generally, employers are not responsible for statute violations of employees. An exception to this guideline can occur in the health professions. When employees engage in the practice of dentistry or medicine, even without the knowledge or approval of the employer, that employee and the employer may both be held liable for damage. Employer sanctions may be magnified, such as loss of one's professional license, if an employee practices dentistry or medicine with employer knowledge.

Finally, at times, some types of specific conduct are defined statutorily as malpractice per se. For instance, unintentionally leaving a foreign body in a patient after a procedure may be deemed malpractice per se. In these types of cases, theoretically, simply the plaintiff's demonstration of the foreign body, via radiograph, a secondary procedure to remove the foreign body, etc., may be all that is required to establish malpractice.

Contract Law

The relationship between a health professional and a patient is first contractual in that services are provided and payment is received. Any remedies the dentist or patient may have against one another in contract are separate and distinct from tort, or malpractice, claims.

Several contractual relationships are possible. The most common interaction is likely the implied contract. In this instance a patient comes in for treatment, and fees are not discussed in detail. If a controversy arises, the courts will look to see that the fees charged for the procedures provided were reasonable.

Another type of relationship is the express contract, in which the procedures and fees are discussed specifically.

Lastly is a formal written contract regarding services and fees.

A contract is binding whether it is a written agreement, verbal agreement, or implied.

Occasionally, one will read about a case in which a dentist is sued because a contract principle has allegedly been violated. For instance, "guaranteed results" are a particularly worrisome concept and should be avoided.[15]

Criminal Law

Recent history has seen a dramatic increase in the number of suits filed under criminal law theories by government prosecutors. Criminally based suits against health professionals most often fall under three general categories.

The first type of criminal suit is secondary to alleged fraud, particularly involving Medicare or Medicaid.[16]

Second, prosecution for misuse of narcotics is becoming more common. In 2004 John Walters, Chief of the Office of National Drug Control Policy, promised "an unprecedented and comprehensive effort, including increased investigative work by the DEA, to combat the diversion of prescription drugs to the black market."[17]

Third, health professionals are undergoing increased prosecution for plaintiff morbidity or mortality that previously was considered under tort theory only. "A social intolerance of medical mistakes has caused them to be criminalised."[18] Government criminal prosecutors litigating against health providers must in theory be able to prove that a criminal or guilty mind (mens rea)[19] exists in addition to statute violation. In other words, for an act to be criminal, the act must itself be illegal and accompanied by mens rea. Once a criminal act has been shown, mens rea can be documented by proving intentional or knowing commission of a crime. Additionally the government may prove its case by convincing a jury that reckless, wanton, or grossly negligent conduct existed even if specific intent to commit a crime is not seen. If the government does not meet these burdens, acquittal should result.[20]

Finally, occasional criminal conduct is reported in the dental arena that may realistically have only a remote relationship to dentistry. For example, consider the arrest of a correctional center dental auxiliary who allegedly conspired to help a convict escape from prison in Nevada by providing a cellular phone to the inmate.[21]

Tort Law

However, the legal theory covering most health professional activity is that of tort law. A tort is a private civil wrong not dependent on a contract. A tort allegation may be pursued by a plaintiff citizen (civilly) and/or by a plaintiff government (criminally). Classically a viable civil suit in tort requires perfection of four essential elements: duty, a breach of duty, proximate cause, and damage. A health professional may successfully defend a suit in tort by proving no duty existed, no breach of duty occurred, that the health professional's conduct was not the cause of damage, or that no damage exists.

Duty

Briefly the health professional owes a duty to a patient if the health professional's conduct created a foreseeable risk to the patient. Generally a duty is created when a patient and health professional personally interact for health care purposes. Face-to-face interaction at the practitioner's place of practice would most likely fulfill the requirement of a created duty, whereas interaction over the telephone, computer, etc., may not be as clear-cut regarding establishment of a relationship leading to duty.

Breach of Duty

A breach of duty occurs when the health care professional fails to act as a reasonable health care provider. A determination of whether a provider has acted reasonably is contemplated by the jury and involves the battle of the expert witnesses for plaintiff and defendant. A professional has acted reasonably if his conduct has been what a comparable professional in the same or similar circumstances would have done.

Exceptions to the rule requiring experts are cases in which no consent was given or obtained for an elective or urgent procedure. Additional exceptions are cases in which the defendant's conduct is obviously erroneous and speaks for itself (res ipsa loquitur),[22] such as wrong-sided surgery. In addition, as noted previously, some complications are defined as malpractice per se by statute (i.e., statute violation), such as unintentionally leaving a foreign body in a patient after a procedure.

The experts testifying as to the alleged breach of duty are arguing about the standard of care. It is often mistakenly assumed that the standard of the practitioner's community is the one to which he will be judged. Today, the community standard is the national standard. Additionally, if there are specialists reasonably accessible to the patient, the standard may be the national standard for specialists whether the practitioner is a specialist or not.[23–26]

The standard of care may also be illustrated by the professional literature. Health care professionals are expected to be aware of current issues in the literature, such as previously unreported complications to local anesthetics. Often articles will also proffer preventive suggestions and review treatment options.

Simply because an accepted writing recommends conduct other than that which the health care provider used is not necessarily indicative of a breach of duty. For instance, specific drug use other than that which is recommended by the *Physicians' Desk Reference* (PDR) is commonplace and legally acceptable as long as the health care provider can articulate a reasonable purpose for his conduct.[27] Part of this reasoning for off-label drug use may likely include a benefit–risk analysis for various treatment options for a specific patient.

The ordinary standard of care is not necessarily what is statistically most often done by similarly situated health professionals.[28]

Causation

Proximate cause is the summation of the actual cause and legal cause. Actual cause is the cause that exists if a chain of events factually flows from the defendant's conduct to the plaintiff's injury. Legal cause is present if actual cause exists and if the plaintiff attorney can prove that the harm sustained was foreseeable or not highly extraordinary in hindsight.

Damage

Damage, of course, is usually the most obvious of the elements of the tort. Generally the damage must be physical. For instance, plaintiffs who sue for emotional distress must also show a physical manifestation of the emotional distress. The physical damage to one's patient can lead to damages claimed by another individual, such as a patient's spouse's loss of consortium claim.

Reasonableness

An underlying legal principle in all health care–related discussions is the concept of reasonableness. Legal analysis of a controversy usually involves an evaluation of reasonable care (see previous breach of duty: standard of care) and the reasonable man. The reasonable man is a hypothetical person who uses "those qualities of attention, knowledge, intelligence, and judgment which society requires of its members for the protection of their own interest and the interests of others."[29]

Depending on the type of case, the reasonableness of a defendant's conduct can be analyzed by the facts as the defendant perceived them, the facts as the defendant should have known them, or as the facts actually existed as analyzed in hindsight in the courtroom.

Consent

Reasonably the consent process is an essential part of patient treatment for health care professionals. The doctrine of simple consent has been recognized since eighteenth-century English common law. Simple consent can be defined as obtaining permission to perform an act without discussing the ramifications of that act.

The doctrine of consent has historically been well recognized in the United States for over 100 years. In 1914 U.S. Supreme Court Justice Benjamin Cardozo stated, "Every human being of adult years and sound mind has a right to determine what shall be done with his own body; and a surgeon who performs an operation without his patient's consent commits an assault for which he is liable in damages."[30]

Before 1914, obtaining consent was not as predictably accomplished, and this lack of consent was not necessarily secondary to uncaring dentists, but more to the development of the germ theory of disease. For instance, only after the development of penicillin in World War II did the loss of life from combat surpass the loss of life from diseases, such as cholera, dysentery, influenza, smallpox, typhoid, or yellow fever, for deployed combat troops. The same diseases cyclically devastated civilian populations. The physical location of the U.S. government was moved from Philadelphia to Washington, DC, after the friendly city's yellow fever epidemic in 1793.[31]

To combat these epidemics, physicians used human subjects for study. Soldiers would routinely volunteer to be subjects of the experiments, such as is well documented by the yellow fever board in Cuba as "Yellow Jack" was studied in 1900. Yellow fever is a viral disease reminiscent of the more well-known West Nile or Ebola virus today. All these hemorrhagic viral diseases are currently endemic in equatorial jungles and could potentially be devastating to modern human populations. Physicians originally involved in this and other medical studies also routinely tested themselves, occasionally resulting in death or significant morbidity. To the yellow fever board's credit, these experiments were not done without the written and verbal consent of the participating individuals. Personal sacrifices such as William Halsted's self-testing of cocaine and the Curies' self-exposure to X-rays are excellent examples of the scientific era when researchers' very lives were truncated by their desire to solve pressing medical problems.

During these times, occasionally individuals were subjected to medical experiments without knowledge or consent. Almost 10 years before Edward Jenner introduced a safe and successful vaccination for smallpox, he had infected his 10-month-old son with swinepox. Jenner's son remained severely physically and mentally compromised until his death at age 21. Other involuntary and unknowingly heroic individuals in the battles against the devastating plagues of the times came from populations of children, often orphans or the experimenter's own offspring, unknowing patients, prisoners, the mentally impaired, or those already dying.[32] The notorious human experimentation conducted by the Japanese and German Nazis during World War II[33] was sadly postdated by other U.S. events that took place through the mid-1970s, such as the infamous Tuskegee Syphilis study or Holmesburg Prison experiments.[34]

It is now well established legally that an unauthorized (i.e., without consent) touching of another, including a medical touching, is a battery and is subject to civil or criminal remedies.

The specific doctrine of informed consent is a modern concept and was developed in California in 1957.[35]

Essentially, informed consent involves explaining:
1. Nature and purpose of the treatment proposed
2. Risks and consequences of the treatment proposed
3. Alternatives to the treatment proposed, including no treatment
4. Prognosis with or without the proposed treatment

Often treatment planning will result in several viable options that may be recommended by the dentist. The patient makes an informed decision as to which option is most preferable to that patient, and treatment may begin.

Consent is essential because many of the procedures dentists perform would be considered illegal in other settings (i.e., an incision developed by a dentist during surgery versus an equivalent traumatic wound placed in a criminal battery).

Consent may be verbal or written, but when a controversy presents at a later date, a written consent is extremely beneficial. Because many times consent is a standard of care for a procedure, the lack of a written consent may reduce the fact finding to a "he said–she said" scenario. This circumstance may greatly diminish the plaintiff's burden of proving the allegations and may even shift the burden of proof to the defendant.[36]

When treating the mentally challenged or children under the age of majority, consent from a legal guardian is necessary for elective procedures.

Consent obtained before one procedure may not be assumed for the same procedure at a different time or a different procedure at the same time. In addition, consent obtained for one health care provider may not be transferable to another health care provider, such as a partner dentist, an employee dental hygienist, or registered nurse.[37]

It is a recognized legal principle that a patient may not consent to malpractice. The patient who offers to sign a "waiver" to convince a practitioner to provide treatment will not likely be held to that waiver if malpractice is adjudicated to exist.

However, there are several instances when consent may not be required. The first and second, emergencies and good Samaritan rescues, are discussed later.

A third situation when consent may not be required is the extension doctrine. The extension doctrine generally applies during surgery under general anesthesia. An example of a valid use of the extension doctrine would be the removal of an undiagnosed nonfunctional supernumerary tooth found adjacent to and secondary to a molar's removal.

Fourth, revisiting the concept of waiver, a patient may knowingly and voluntarily waive the presentation of a portion of the information that would normally be given during the consent process. However, the patient who wishes to waive some consent information cannot waive all consent information. The practitioner might consider mentioning at least the most significant adverse possibility, such as central nervous system (CNS) compromise or death. The patient who elects to waive routine consent information should sign a document stating that the waiver is known, voluntary, and that the health care provider is ready, willing, and able to provide complete consent.

Finally the doctrine of therapeutic privilege allows dentists to not provide consent if, in the dentist's reasonable and objective opinion, the provision of consent to a patient would be detrimental to that patient; therapeutic privilege allows consent to not be perfected.

The author's (Orr) general consent is included (Fig. 40.1) in this chapter. In addition to the general consent that is essentially used for any and all procedures, verbal consent is obtained and occasionally initialed. Finally, specific written consent for singular procedures is at times obtained.

Statute of Limitations

Statutes of limitations are laws that fix the time in which the litigants, usually plaintiffs, must seek to avail themselves of legal recourse. After the statute of limitations tolls, the parties are barred from seeking legal recourse.

As mentioned previously, modern tort reform, including the MICRA type of laws, usually include statute of limitations clauses. However, statutes of limitations are subject to judicial interpretation and can be predictably extended in situations such as when the plaintiff is a minor or during dental hazardous device recalls years after such devices were placed.[38]

EMERGENCIES DURING SEDATION

The standard of care for emergencies arising as part of sedation treatment is the same as during other situations in that the

ORAL & MAXILLOFACIAL SURGERY CONSENT

The procedures to be performed have been explained to me and I understand what is to be done. This is my consent to the procedures discussed and to any other procedures found to be necessary or advisable in addition to the pre-operative treatment plan. I agree to the use of local, sedation, or general anesthesia depending on the judgment of Dr. Orr.

I have been informed and understand that occasionally there are complications of the surgery, drugs, and anesthesia. The more common complications are pain, infection, swelling, bleeding, bruising and temporary or permanent numbness and/or tingling of the lip, tongue, chin, gums, cheeks or teeth. I understand that pain, numbness, swelling, and inflammation of veins or other structures may occur from injections. I understand death from office procedures has been estimated at 1/400,000. I understand the possibility of injury to the neck and facial muscles, and changes in the bite or jaw joint. I understand the possibility of injury to the adjacent teeth, restorations, and tissues, referred pain to other areas of the head and neck, bone fractures or infections, and delayed healing. I understand the combination of anesthesia and surgery may lead to nausea, vomiting, allergic reactions, and other physical or psychological reactions. I understand sinus complications may include an opening into the sinus from the mouth after the removal of teeth. I understand injury may occur when instruments fail. I understand that many other complications not listed may occur.

I understand medications, drugs, anesthetics and prescriptions may cause drowsiness and a lack of coordination which could be increased by the use of alcohol or other drugs; I have been advised to not operate any vehicle or potentially hazardous devices, or work, while taking medications and/or drugs or until fully recovered from their effects.

I acknowledge the receipt of and understand the postoperative instructions. I understand that there is no guarantee related to treatment. I understand that most complications can be rectified with proper follow up care. I agree to follow up as needed or advised for any concerns or complications. I understand I can receive a review of these and other possible risks by asking.

Signature

Signature

Date

Figure 40.1 Sample of informed consent. (Courtesy Daniel Orr II.)

health care professional must act as a correspondingly qualified health professional would in the same or similar circumstances.

However, by their very nature, emergencies lend themselves to a different analysis of the health professional's conduct. An emergency scenario does not lend itself to typical dentist–patient circumstances. For instance, in an emergency, there is generally not time for leisurely reflection about the problem, consultation with colleagues, the patient, the patient's family, or even proffering of informed consent, let alone bare consent.

Consent During Emergencies

Emergency situations present a different paradigm for consent evaluation. During an emergency, there simply may be no reasonable opportunity to obtain consent.

Defining Emergency

It is important in the law and the health professions to consider how words are defined. Emergency is derived from the Latin *mergere:* to dip, plunge, inundate, engulf, or overwhelm or to bury.[39] *Webster's* defines an emergency as "1. a sudden, urgent, usually unexpected occurrence or occasion requiring immediate action. 2. a state, especially of need for help or relief, created by some unexpected event."[40]

Black's Law Dictionary defines emergency as "a sudden unexpected happening; an unforeseen occurrence or condition; perplexing contingency or complication of circumstances; a sudden or unexpected occasion for action; exigency; pressing necessity."[41] Notice the iteration of "unforeseen" in this definition relative to the comments discussed later.

Thus the patient with chronic odontalgia who "just can't stand it anymore" may define the toothache as an emergency. Clearly a chronic toothache is likely not an emergency because it is, at the least, not sudden or unexpected and likely does not require immediate action. That patients define emergency differently than health professionals is understandable and in part the fault of the health care industry. For instance, patients often avail themselves of an "emergencies welcome" advertisement at the dentist's office. Is the office that advertises "emergencies welcome" soliciting anaphylaxis, massive oral hemorrhage, or something altogether different such as chronic odontalgia? It is well documented that most patients who come to hospital emergency rooms are not actually seen because of an emergency, but secondary to convenience, lack of funds, no previous dentist–patient relationship, etc.[42]

At www.ada.org, the ADA itself lists the following as dental emergencies: "bitten lip or tongue; broken tooth; cracked tooth; jaw-possibly broken; knocked out tooth; objects caught between teeth; toothache."[43]

A chronic toothache, per *Webster's,* may indeed be an "urgent" situation (i.e., "1. compelling or requiring immediate action or attention; imperative; pressing. 2. insistent or earnest in solicitation; importunate. 3. expressed with insistence, as requests or appeals.)"[44]

Urgencies are not emergencies, although at times the definitions may begin to meld together. It is important to not be lulled into a legal confrontation because of a misuse of terms with definitive meanings.

As health professionals, we must be cognizant of how we use the term *emergency,* just as we are with the term *allergy* (as opposed to sensitivity or another physiologic phenomenon). For instance, it has been documented that most patients who give a history of penicillin allergy are not allergic to penicillin.[45]

An important aspect of an emergency situation is the element of unexpectedness. Thus if a certain result is commonly predictable from certain conduct, such as a toothache to chronically neglected decay, it would be difficult to truly categorize such a situation as an emergency.

Per *Black's Law Dictionary,* a complication of circumstances may exist. Emergencies often do seem to be secondary to at least a small series of singular circumstances that would not ordinarily be reasonably expected to occur, particularly sequentially.[46]

Consider the unexpectedness of a chronic toothache progressing to an acute abscess that is in imminent danger of compromising an airway. It is likely an emergency exists. Most toothaches are not expected to progress to life-threatening situations in which immediate action is required.

Notice that pain, a widely variable subjective phenomenon, is not part of the discussion. Further, many health professionals would logically not include pain in any definition of emergency, no matter what the lay public believes.

Two caveats warrant mention in the discussion of the term *emergency.* First, one's state statutes may define emergency differently than authoritative dictionaries or health professionals would. Remember that statutes are generally written by lay legislators with significant input from the legal profession. It is important to know how emergencies are defined in one's own jurisdiction.

The second admonition involves the singular situation of the trial. When one is in the courtroom, the jury itself may be allowed the latitude to define an emergency in the case at hand. The jury's definition may not correspond to *Webster's, Black's,* or statute.

Defining Sedation Emergencies

Not unlike other scenarios in the health professions or in general, one man's emergency will be part and parcel or routine for another. A lifeguard's employment routine involves emergency water rescue. Whereas water rescue and resuscitation would likely be daunting for most individuals, the lifeguard views these acts as "just another day at the office."

Dentists who are trained for and use only local anesthesia might very well define a patient's loss of consciousness and momentary apnea as an emergency. On the other hand, dentists trained in sedation, though unlikely to see loss of consciousness and apnea, should be able to treat these clinical findings seamlessly. Further, dentists who routinely administer general anesthesia actually have as a goal patient unconsciousness and expect to see patient apnea from time to time, so these findings are not emergencies to, for instance, dentist anesthesiologists or oral and maxillofacial surgeons who use general anesthesia.

Importantly, however, dentists should be able to provide successful emergency treatment at a level above what they commonly are comfortable with. For instance, just as dentists who administer local anesthesia only should be able to successfully treat syncope seen secondary to local anesthesia administration, dentists who provide sedation should be prepared to treat complications of sedation (i.e., unconsciousness and apnea). Dentist anesthesiologists who view unconsciousness and apnea as a goal of therapy (for instance, when intentionally paralyzing patients) have been well prepared to treat many more occasional side effects, such as clinical hypertension, hypotension, hypothermia, hyperthermia, fluid retention, fluid loss, electrolyte disturbances, blood gas disturbances, etc., seen when using more potent agents.

EMERGENCY RESCUES—GOOD SAMARITAN STATUTES

Generally, emergencies outside health care settings also do not require consent secondary to Good Samaritan statutes, which apply to rescues. Rescues involve aiding a victim in serious peril that the rescuer's conduct has not created. Interestingly an injured rescuer may have legal recourse against an individual who negligently created the peril, including the victim (rescue doctrine).

It is wise to know what the statute in one's own jurisdiction says. Generally, legislators want to encourage rescues and thus limit potential liability that might be attributed to would-be rescuers.

Under the doctrine of imminent or sudden peril, when a potential rescuer is confronted with an emergent or urgent rescue scenario, he or she is not held to the same degree of duty as one who has time to reflect calmly on the scenario. An individual can lose rescuer status by charging a victim a fee.

Some jobs have required duties of rescue. Whereas law enforcement officers are not required to rescue,[47,48] aquatic lifeguards are. Lifeguards, by the very nature of their employment, are required to rescue, whereas most of society is not. Lifeguards are also held to a higher standard of care, and although a Good Samaritan statute may apply to off-duty professional rescuers, it is less likely that they would receive Good Samaritan protection while on duty.

Statutes in some jurisdictions impose a duty to rescue or perform medical treatment on physicians or other persons employed as professional rescuers.[49]

If a victim is conscious, permission should be sought before aid is rendered. If the victim refuses to allow a rescue, the Good Samaritan has no privilege or duty to attempt a rescue.

Unconscious victims require no consent at all. When treating an emergency victim who is spontaneously or traumatically unconscious, consent is implied.

Consent may be obtained from a legal guardian. The possibility of obtaining consent from a guardian before a rescue is generally time dependent. In an urgent situation, time may be available to discuss the rescue with a guardian. However, during a more emergent situation, taking time to discuss options may actually compromise the patient.

Even though most rescue situations are essentially free from potential legal liability flowing from the victim to the rescuer, a source of liability, even when fully qualified as a "Good Samaritan," is reckless conduct. For instance, reckless conduct in a rescue situation would involve electively and knowingly leaving the victim in a situation that is more desperate than when the rescuer found the victim. An example of such conduct might be when a rescuer offers to transport a victim to a hospital for necessary treatment and then abandons the victim farther from a hospital than where the victim was initially found.

In a recent California case, *Van Horn v. Watson*,[50] the appellate court evaluated the California Health and Safety Code (1799.102) that applies to emergency medical care rendered at the scene of any emergency. Briefly, in this case, an inebriated rescuer stated she removed an inebriated victim from a vehicle after an accident by placing one arm under the victim's legs and one arm behind the victim's back. The rescuer stated that she had seen smoke coming from the top of the vehicle and also saw liquid escaping to the street and was worried about a fire. However, the plaintiff stated that she was removed from the vehicle "like a rag doll" and attributed her subsequent paraplegia to the defendant's extraction.

The court determined that the legislative intent of 1799.102 was to encourage agencies to train people in emergency medical services programs. Further, it determined that the defendant did not provide emergency medical care to the plaintiff and was not entitled to Good Samaritan protection. The case was remanded to the prior court for adjudication under negligence case law.

RELATIONSHIP BETWEEN DENTIST AND EMERGENCY PATIENT

First, already discussed is the Good Samaritan relationship. Generally, any rescuer, including a health professional, is granted wide latitude for conduct as far as reasonableness.

In the second type of emergency situation, based on the dentist–patient relationship, a health provider might find himself or herself called upon to treat a previously unknown patient. An example of this relationship would be when one is called to an emergency room to treat a trauma victim. Often even a basic history or consent of any type is not possible to obtain. Dentists are allowed relatively wide latitude in what is reasonable therapeutic intervention in these scenarios. This latitude may even be legislated at times, for instance, by granting dentists in these situations sovereign immunity, or the same protection the king (state or federal government) enjoys from prosecution in the promulgation of duties.[51]

The third type of association is the one most relevant to the emergencies presented in this text.

Specifically, one needs to consider emergencies that occur during elective procedures for known patients in the private dental office. The standard of care does not change (i.e., one is expected to treat patients in this scenario as another with comparable training would in the same or similar circumstances). However, when the circumstances include an emergency, the guidelines present are less defined because of the unexpected presentation of the problems that need to be immediately addressed.

Foreseeability

Foreseeability is a legal principle that may be used to limit or impose liability for an individual's conduct. A foreseeable result or consequence is one that the reasonable man would expect might occur. Contrarily an unforeseeable result is one that a reasonable man would not expect to occur.

For instance, one might reasonably expect inflammation after a surgical procedure, such as the intraoral administration of local anesthetic. However, one would generally not foresee that a patient would typically lose vision after local anesthetic administration for dentistry, although the phenomenon has been reported.[52-54]

The obvious question at hand is whether or not sedation emergencies in the dental office are foreseeable. If adverse consequences are foreseeable, liability may be imposed. If the adverse consequences are not foreseeable, liability may be avoided.

Sedation emergencies in the dental office do occur and are generally foreseeable. It has been accurately stated that if one practices long enough, a life-threatening event will occur in one's office. This statement is obviously true, but the mere foreseeability of a single life-threatening event sometime during decades of practice does not make that event, when and if it ultimately occurs, expected. Certainly, if dentists routinely expected to be faced with life-threatening events in their offices, the entire nature of the profession would have to change.

LIMITING LIABILITY FOR EMERGENCIES

Just as injudicious practice protocols will lead to an increased incidence of complications and emergencies, careful practice within the standard of care of the profession will minimize adverse sequelae, including emergencies, in an office practice. However, even the most careful practitioner through no fault of his or her own will, given a long enough career, experience emergency situations.

So many factors play a part in the judicious practice that it would be impossible to discuss them in a single text, let alone a chapter. However, several will be briefly discussed.

Prevention and Preparation

Carefully review the prevention and preparation recommendations elsewhere in this text. Following the admonitions therein will do much to maximize the control a practitioner has in reducing the incidence of office emergencies.

Poor Decisions

A poor outcome does not necessarily relate to a poor decision. Examples abound wherein reasonable standard-of-care decisions were made throughout a case in which a bad result occurred. Additionally, patients generally are resilient, and poor clinical decisions do not always lead to adverse outcomes.

However, it has been proposed that three basic types of errors can lead to the development of critical situations that otherwise could be prevented.[55]

The first error is lack of experience. Certainly, most dentists do not routinely treat emergencies. But emergencies may occur secondary to dentists who have extended themselves beyond their routine experiences in medical or surgical therapy. It is never optimal to routinely perform surgical or therapeutic procedures one is not thoroughly familiar with. Ideally, extending oneself to the limits of one's abilities occurs very infrequently and not electively. One legitimate circumstance for such an extension would be when dealing with an emergency. If one desires to expand a practice's scope, appropriate continuing education or specialty training may be considered. Even if one desires to simply maintain status quo licensure, continuing education is usually mandated by most state professional boards. The lesson to be learned is if one is not experienced in providing a certain elective treatment, perhaps that treatment should be deferred.

The second commonly found error is a lack of information for the situation at hand. For instance, an incomplete review of a patient's medical history might result in less-than-optimal treatment for the patient in question.

The third source of poor decisions is due to a lack of aggressiveness when something amiss is noted. As an example, at what blood pressure does one become concerned enough to alter routine treatment protocol?

An example of the third type of poor decision might be demonstrated by alleged conduct reported in March 2008 that led to the closing of multiple southern Nevada endoscopy centers, loss of physician and nursing professional licenses, development of individual and class action civil lawsuits involving more than 40,000 patients, and criminal investigation of those health professionals involved in the situation.

According to a Clark County Health District press release, the centers were initially closed because of unsafe injection practices (using the same syringe on multiple patients). The health district sought to initially alert 40,000 persons who were treated at several clinics to be tested for hepatitis B, hepatitis C, and HIV.[56] It is likely that the pool of potential patients involved will grow significantly as the investigation continues at press time for this text.

Respondeat Superior

Respondeat superior (let the superior reply) is the legal doctrine that assigns liability for employee conduct to the employer. If an employee commits a tort against a patient, in some cases, the employer dentist will have to assume responsibility for the patient's damage.

Even if the dentist is well trained in dealing with various emergencies, if his staff is not trained for their concomitant duties, optimal emergency treatment will be compromised. Any poor performance by one's staff may be attributed to the supervision of the employer dentist.

In addition, peripheral staff, such as answering services, is critical. Perceived or real emergencies may arise after normal office hours, and one must make reasonable arrangements to properly deal with such situations.[57]

Community Standards

Today, automated external defibrillators (AEDs) are commonplace in shopping centers and at sporting events. A dentist would be hard-pressed to explain convincingly why, as a health care provider, his office had no AED when lay providers are so common.

Similarly, if one's own lay patients know CPR better than anyone in the practice, such a discrepancy should be addressed.

Not surprisingly, in the wake of the developing investigation about unsafe injection practices in southern Nevada in March 2008 (see "Poor Decisions" previously), local area hospitals began to distribute guidelines for safe needle and syringe use. Just as it seems health professionals must constantly be reminded about basic concepts, such as hand washing, those using instruments necessary for intravenous sedation or any other treatment must use those instruments in a safe fashion.

Professional Relationships

It would seem judicious to develop relationships with colleagues, including specialist dentists and physicians, for times when consultation would be helpful. Timely consultations can truncate the development of emergency situations.

Similarly a close affiliation with a local hospital can facilitate patient care should admission of one's own patient be necessary.

As mentioned previously, one is responsible for patients after office hours. Patients reasonably expect to have access to their dentist as necessary for perceived or real emergencies. If the primary caregiver is not going to be available, arrangements with another dentist to take calls for the practice are strongly recommended.

Collegiality

Occasionally, patients choose to or are not able to follow up with their original dentist or those designated for follow-up as necessary. This situation results in one's patient seeing a new dentist for evaluation and possible treatment.

A common denominator seen in almost all malpractice litigation is criticism, warranted or not, to the patient from a health care professional seen secondarily about the original treatment. This criticism is usually proffered without consultation with the original dentist.

Unwarranted criticism can often be comfortably eliminated from subsequent treating or consulting dentists by simply contacting the original health professional to compile a more complete history.

Any conduct that promotes frivolous legal action is only in the lawyer's best interests, not in anyone else's, including the patient's. A health professional's highest obligation is to patients, but that duty is part and parcel of other ethical obligations, including those owed to one's colleagues.[58-60]

PHILOSOPHICAL ASPECTS OF TREATING EMERGENCIES

The primary author, Dr. Malamed, occasionally asks a series of relevant questions:

Is a dentist absolutely required to manage a potentially life-threatening emergency?

The "duty to rescue" is an interesting subject for legal analysis. One can easily find eloquent arguments both for and against the societal duty to rescue.

Distilling the question to its elemental issue, does society want to legally mandate rescues, or does society want to preserve individual freedom to accept or reject rescue responsibility and potential liability?

Two well-known tragic incidents seemingly compel mandated rescues. In 1964 a resident of New York City screamed for help from the street outside her apartment when attacked by a knife-wielding criminal. It is well documented that many neighbors witnessed the attack and the wounded woman helpless on the sidewalk. No one responded to the cries for help. After the initial attack, seeing no aid proffered, the criminal returned twice to continue the attack, ultimately leading to the victim's death. The second incident occurred in a Massachusetts tavern in 1983. Patrons watched a rape attack for more than an hour without intervention or a call for help.

A third similar incident occurred in a case the author was involved in as a forensic expert (*NV v. Strohmeyer,* 1997). College student Jeremy Strohmeyer was convicted of the sexual assault and murder of 7-year-old Sherrice Iverson. During the crime, Strohmeyer's friend witnessed a portion of the attack early on as he peered into the bathroom stall Iverson had tried to escape into. A short time later, immediately after Iverson's death, Strohmeyer's friend asked Strohmeyer what happened, and Strohmeyer bragged about the assault and homicide. The two friends subsequently drove home. The public reaction to the lack of any rescue effort by Strohmeyer's friend led to a flurry of legislative proposals to legally require rescues.

Regularly, such cases in which a life could have likely been saved by minimal intervention come into the legal system. Almost uniformly, courts decline to impose any liability on individuals who decline the responsibility and potential liability involved in a rescue.

However, persons with special relationships to the victim may be required to attempt to effect a rescue. Some such persons considered to have special relationships include family members, the individual who is the cause of the victim's duress, an employee duty bound to rescue (i.e., a lifeguard), and a property owner who has invited the victim onto the owner's property.

Occasionally, states will consider requiring its citizens to rescue. Currently, only Minnesota and Vermont have statutes requiring rescue under certain circumstances. However, Good Samaritan statutes are found uniformly in state law because legislatures want to encourage rescues by removing potential liability, although some liability may always attach.

Good Samaritan statutes are aptly named and intended by states to promote moral behavior. Religious and philosophic leaders throughout history have championed selfless service to others.[61,62] Jesus' New Testament story of the Good Samaritan[63] simply builds on a well-known tenet of the Old Testament,[64] thus reasonably representing and uniting the views of at least the world's Jews, Christians, and Muslims, which all recognize Abraham as a patriarchal ancestor.

Briefly the biblical Good Samaritan rescued a victim despite potential physical and/or legal harm to himself, contrary to existing social mores regarding his nation's sworn enemies and only after others who might have been expected to give aid refused. Interestingly the question leading to Jesus Christ's narrative was posed by an adversarial lawyer. The lesson offered is that if the Samaritan can rescue his enemy, we are thus admonished to also serve our neighbor and fellow man.

The ADA's Code of Professional Conduct states an ethical obligation for dentists to: "… make reasonable arrangement for the emergency care of their patients of record. Dentists shall be obliged when consulted in an emergency by patients not of record to make reasonable arrangements for emergency care."[65]

Thus it appears after this brief analysis that dentists are likely obligated morally, ethically, and often legally to treat both established and emergency patients who need care.

Is calling 911 sufficient to fulfill responsibility for the rescue?

Calling 911 is likely the minimal effort that would be required to fulfill rescue obligations in the dental office and requires no professional expertise whatsoever. Depending on the emergency and the dentist's prior conduct, much more responsibility might be mandated by the body that evaluates the case, be it one's regulatory board or a criminal or civil court. For instance, a known epileptic in the waiting room who has a seizure would likely be evaluated differently than a child who seizes secondary to an absolute or relative local anesthetic overdose.

What is the dentist's responsibility when another with more emergency expertise arrives?

The dentist who calls 911 and goes to lunch is in a different position than one who is actively helping treat the emergency by, for instance, maintaining an airway. The dentist who is deciding whether or not to relinquish the emergency care of his patient to another must reasonably weigh the risk and benefit of such conduct. It is possible that emergency medical technicians (EMTs), paramedics, oral and maxillofacial surgeons, and some physicians (i.e., anesthesiologists) will have more expertise in maintaining an airway than a general dental practitioner. Some physicians, such as radiologists, pathologists, or psychiatrists, may have minimal airway training. What reasonably appears to be in the patient's best interests is the correct course of action.

Unfortunately, the one considering relinquishing care can be legally liable for damage no matter which decision is made.

Is a dentist legally required to maintain an emergency drug kit and/or CPR certification?

Many dentists are indeed legally required to have an emergency drug kit. Specifically, those who have special general anesthesia or sedation permits issued by the various state boards are required to have such kits. The states of Massachusetts[66] and West Virginia[67] have enacted laws mandating the presence of emergency drugs and equipment in every dental office in the state.

Dentists who do not have general anesthesia or sedation permits would do well to consider the package inserts from the various local anesthetic solutions, which state that drugs, equipment, and personnel for management of drug-related emergencies must be immediately available.

Such package inserts coupled with the almost universal state board requirement that licensed dentists must be proficient in CPR appear to imply that dentists are likely responsible for reasonable efforts in maintaining airways and cardiovascular function in the event of a local anesthetic reaction requiring this.

What drugs should be contained in an emergency kit?

Depending on the patients treated, modalities used, and personal preference, the recommended contents of an emergency kit are myriad.

Dentist anesthesiologist and educator Dr. Ken Reed offers a reasonable suggestion for the basic emergency kit for dental offices using local anesthesia and nitrous oxide.[68] Dr. Reed's basic kit includes oxygen, epinephrine, diphenhydramine, albuterol, aspirin, nitroglycerin, a form of sugar, and an AED.

Most often, practitioners who administer intravenous sedation will be required by state statute or their dental practice act to have available certain specific emergency drugs, such as those used during ACLS.

What is the dentist's ultimate responsibility during a medical emergency in the office?

For years, Dr. Malamed has iterated the reasonable response that the dentist's responsibility is to "try to keep the victim alive by treating the victim until recovery or until another more qualified individual assumes responsibility for treatment."[69]

REFERENCES

1. Wells H: *A history of the discovery of the application of nitrous oxide gas, ether, and other vapors, to surgical operations*, Hartford, CT, 1847, J Gaylord Wells.
2. Fenster JM: *Ether day*, New York, 2001, Harper Collins.

3. Thibodeau E, Mentasti L: Who stole Nemo? *J Am Dent Assoc* 138(5):656–660, 2007.

4. National Institute of Dental and Craniofacial Research: *Oral health in America: a report of the surgeon general*, Rockville MD, 2000, U.S. Department of Health and Human Services, U.S. Public Health Service.

5. Lethbridge-Cejku M, Vickerie J: Summary health statistics for U.S. adults: national health interview survey. *Vital Health Stat* 10(225):104–2005, 2003.

6. Lyons AS, Petrucelli RJ: *Medicine: an illustrated history*, New York, 1978, Harry N Abrams, p 59.

7. Lyons AS, Petrucelli RJ: *Medicine: an illustrated history*, New York, 1978, Harry N Abrams, p 67.

8. McCarthy N: 200,000 lawyers and counting. *Calif Bar J* 1, Feb 2005.

9. Gibeaut J: Med-Mal ruling has doctors reeling. *ABA J Rep* 1–4, July 29 2005.

10. Woo v Fireman's Fund Ins Co, 164 P.3d 454 (Wash, 2007).

11. Pogrel MA, Thamby S: Permanent nerve involvement resulting from inferior alveolar nerve blocks. *J Am Dent Assoc* 131(7):901–907, 2000.

12. Pogrel MA, Schmidt BL, Sambajon V, et al: Lingual nerve damage due to inferior alveolar nerve blocks: a possible explanation. *J Am Dent Assoc* 134(2):195–199, 2003.

13. American Society of Anesthesiologists: Transactions of the house of delegates, 1982.

14. American Society of Anesthesiologists: Board of directors, 1987.

15. Heffner v. Reynolds, 777 N.E. 2d 312 (Ohio).

16. Florida v. Harden, Fla App Lexis 623, 2004.

17. Associated Press, Mar 2004.

18. Holbrook J: The criminalisation of fatal medical mistakes. *BMJ* 327:1118, 2003.

19. *Barron's law dictionary*, ed 2, New York, 1984, Barron's Educational Services.

20. Associated Press: Jury acquits Pasadena dentist of 60 child endangering charges, Mar 5, 2002.

21. USA Today state news, Nev, Aug 29, 2005.

22. *Barron's law dictionary*, ed 2, New York, 1984, Barron's Educational Services.

23. Pollack BR: *Handbook of dental jurisprudence and risk management*, Littleton, MA, 1980, PSG Publishing.

24. Keeton WP, et al: *Prosser and Keeton on the law of torts*, St Paul, MN, 1984, West Publishing.

25. Sandbar SS, et al: *Legal medicine*, Philadelphia, 2004, CV Mosby.

26. Tierney K: Legal consideration in dentistry. *Dent Clin North Am* 26(2):284–285, 1982.

27. Johnson LJ: Off-label prescribing and the standard of care. *Med Econ* 78(16):97, 2001.

28. Williamson v. Elrod, 72 S.W. 3d 489 (Ark 2002).

29. Restatement of torts 2d, 283(b).

30. Schloendorff v. Society of New York Hospital, 105 N.E. 92, 93 (NY 1914).

31. Wilson G, Girard S: *The life and times of America's first tycoon*, Boston, 1996, DaCapo Press.

32. Crosby MC: *The American plague*, New York, 2006, Berkley Books.

33. Bradley J: *Flyboys*, New York, 2003, Little, Brown.

34. Hornblum A: *Acres of skin*, New York, 1998, Routledge.

35. Salgo v. Leland Stanford, Jr., University Board of Trustees, 317 P. 2d 170, 181 (Calif App Ct, 1957).

36. Orr DL, 2nd, Curtis B: Obtaining written informed consent for the administration of local anesthetic, in dentistry. *J Am Dent Assoc* 136(11):1568–1571, 2005.

37. Starozyntk v. Reich, Superior Ct of NJ, Case #A-4706-03T1, *Leg Med Perspect* pp. 75-76, Sep/Oct 2005.

38. Cox v. Paul, Ind. LEXIS 575, 2005.

39. *The new college Latin & English dictionary*, New York, 1995, Bantam Books.

40. *Webster's encyclopedic unabridged dictionary of the English language*, New York, 1996, Gramercy Books.

41. *Black's law dictionary*, ed 5, St Paul, MN, 1979, West Publishing.

42. Carpenter D: Our overburdened ERs. *Hosp Health Netw* 75(3):44–47, 2001.

43. Dental emergencies & injuries, 2005. Available at www.ada.org/public/manage/emergencies.asp.

44. *Webster's encyclopedic unabridged dictionary of the English language*, New York, 1996, Gramercy Books.

45. Arroliga ME, Wagner W, Bobek MB, et al: A pilot study of penicillin skin testing in patients with a history of penicillin allergy admitted to a medical ICU. *Chest* 118(4):1106–1108, 2000.

46. Gava DM, Fish JK, Howard SK: *Crisis management in anesthesiology*, 1994, Churchill Livingstone.

47. Weiner v. Metropolitan Authority, Shernov v. New York Transit Authority, 55 NY 2d 175. 948 NYS 2d l4l (1982).

48. Warren v. District of Columbia, 444, A. 2d 1 (1981).

49. State v. Perry, 29 Ohio App 2d 33, 278 NE 2d 50, 53.

50. Van Horn v. Watson, 148 Calif App 4th 1013 (4th Dist, 2007).

51. Nevada Revised Statutes, Chapter 41.

52. Goldenberg AS: Transient diplopia as a result of block injections mandibular and posterior superior alveolar. *NY State Dent J* 63(5):29–31, 1997.

53. Penarrocha-Diago M, Sanchis-Bielsa JM: Ophthalmologic complications after intraoral local anesthesia with articaine. *Oral Surg Oral Med Oral Pathol Oral Radiol Endod* 90(1):21–24, 2000.

54. Sawyer RJ, von Schroeder H: Temporary bilateral blindness after acute lidocaine toxicity. *Anesth Analg* 95(1):224–226, 2002.

55. Klein G: *Sources of power how people make decisions*, Cambridge, MA, 2001, MIT Press.

56. Kulin D: County suspends business licenses today, Clark County Nevada Health District press release, Mar 4, 2008.

57. American Dental Association: Principles of ethics and code of professional conduct, sec 4B.

58. American College of Dentists: *Ethics handbook for dentists*, 2004, American College of Dentists.

59. American Association of Oral and Maxillofacial Surgeons: Code of professional conduct, V, A1, 2006.

60. Orr DL: A plea for collegiality. *J Oral Maxillofac Surg* 64(9):1086–1092, 2006.

61. *The teaching of Buddha*, Tokyo, 1989, Kosaido Printing.

62. *The analects of Confucius*, New York, 1992, Harper Collins.

63. King James Bible, Luke 10:25–37, 1979, Intellectual Reserve.

64. King James Bible, Leviticus 19:18.

65. American Dental Association: Principles of ethics and code of professional conduct, sec 4B.

66. 234 CMR: Board of Registration in Dentistry—6.15: Administration of Local Anesthesia Only (3) Drugs Required, August 2010. http://www.mass.gov/eohhs/docs/dph/regs/234cmr006-20100820.pdf.

67. West Virginia Board of Dentistry: Anesthesia emergency drug requirements and equipment list. http://www.wvdentalboard.org. Accessed 31 January 2017.

68. Reed K: personal communication, 2005.

69. Malamed S: personal communication, 2005.

chapter 41

The Controversial Development of Anesthesiology in Dentistry

CHAPTER OUTLINE

The development of advanced pain control modalities in dentistry has never been without controversy, legal and otherwise, from both without and within the profession. Professional society, state regulatory agency, judicial, and individual files are well stocked with attorney-generated missives to cease and desist, allegations of antitrust conduct, accusations of defamation, and defensive replies about First Amendment rights and the truth as an absolute defense to defamation. In addition to the moral and ethical machinations such issues lead to, there is almost always a significant, generally not publicly addressed or argued, economic component affecting all individuals involved in the controversies. Everyone seems to have concerns about his or her piece of the pie when it gets right down to it. Such has been the state of affairs even since the very day dentistry gave safe, reproducible anesthesia to the world, a bequest recently called one of the three greatest advances in modern medical history (i.e., since 1840) by the British Medical Association.[1]

Today, the vast majority of dental procedures are accomplished by means of the administration of local anesthesia, which has been in constant use in dentistry since William Stewart Halstead, a physician who understood perhaps better than most surgeons patients' abhorrence to pain,[2] began performing nerve conduction blocks in 1884.[3,4] Halstead recruited Dr. Nash, a dentist, to care for an upper incisor after injection of cocaine near the infraorbital nerve at the infraorbital foramen. Halstead thereafter performed an inferior alveolar nerve block on a medical student volunteer.[5]

These two injections have evolved to more than 300 million dental local anesthesia administrations performed annually in the United States.[6] Dentists likely administer more local injections per capita than any other health professional. Halstead's introduction of nerve blocks to the profession was secondary to his melding of Alexander Wood's 1855 use of the hollow needle[7] and Carl Koller's demonstration of the effectiveness of cocaine as a local anesthetic.[8]

HORACE WELLS AND WILLIAM T.G. MORTON

However, as popular and effective as local anesthesia is today in dentistry, our dental ancestors might be surprised that dentistry has drifted so far from other pain control techniques. Local anesthesia was indeed preceded by the development of sedation and general anesthesia by dentists. In 1844 Horace Wells (see Fig. 11.4) first publicly demonstrated the use of nitrous oxide for a surgical procedure at Massachusetts General Hospital.[9] In 1846 dentist William T.G. Morton demonstrated the use of ether, also at Massachusetts General Hospital.[10] In a short period of time, a controversy developed between Wells, Morton, and other individuals as to who should be given primary credit for the discovery of anesthesia.

In Morton's case, it is ironic that credit for one of the most beneficent gifts to mankind was claimed by a classic, chronic scoundrel. That notices were published in Rochester, New York,[11] and St Louis, Missouri,[12] warning the populace to "look out for" and "beware" of the "villain" Morton is not surprising. Morton's legal and moral transgressions are numerous and well documented and include, but are not limited to, embezzlement, excommunication from his church for profanity and dishonesty, passing bad checks, the theft of U.S. mail seals, forgery, abandoning fiancées, and even skipping out on medical bills.[13]

As far as Morton's place in the history of anesthesiology, one of the earliest legal rulings concerning medical procedure patents was *Morton v. New York Eye Infirmary*, 17 E. Cas. 879 (C.C.S.D.N.Y. 1862). Dr. Morton sued the infirmary for infringing on his patent for the use of ether for surgical procedures. The court determined that Morton's patent was invalid because the use of diethyl ether during surgery was determined to be a discovery of a new use for a common chemical compound as opposed to an invention.[14] Following this case, medical procedure patents were generally considered inappropriate, which may ultimately be Morton's greatest contribution to patient health.

The issue of whom the honor of the initial development of anesthesia belonged grew to involve even the U.S. Congress[15] and health professionals in Europe. Other authors[16] have pointed out that for millennia mankind has attempted to reproduce the biblical account of Adam's "deep sleep"[17] to reduce pain during surgery. However, until Wells, who had completed fewer than 15 nitrous oxide cases before his appearance at Massachusetts General Hospital, no one had publicly reported a safe and predictably reproducible pain control technique for surgical procedures. Ultimately, it seems that Wells likely has prevailed in the primacy argument, as he is recognized by the lay public and the professions in the United States[18–27] and Europe.[28]

Specifically, in 1864 the American Dental Association (ADA) adopted the resolution that "… to Horace Wells, of Hartford, Connecticut, (now deceased) belongs the credit and honor of the introduction of anesthesia in the United States of America, and we do firmly protest against the injustice done to truth and the memory of Dr. Horace Wells, in the effort made during a series of years and especially at the last session of Congress, to award the credit to other persons or person."[29] This resolution was reaffirmed in 1872.[30] In 1870 the American Medical Association (AMA) resolved that "… the honor of the discovery of practical anesthesia is due to the late Dr. Horace Wells, of Connecticut."[31]

As strange as it may seem, the development of pain control techniques for surgical procedures was in and of itself somewhat controversial. Until Wells' demonstration, the attitude of surgeons worldwide can be summed up by French surgeon Alfred Louis Marie Velpeau's 1839 statement that "[t]o escape pain in surgical operations is a chimera which we are not permitted to look for in our days. A cutting instrument and pain in operative medicine are two ideas which never present themselves separately to the mind of the patient, and it is necessary for us surgeons to admit their association."[32]

Historically, dental procedures were one of the most common examples of a singularly excruciating (Latin "of the cross") surgical pain experience, as exemplified by the patron saint of dentistry, Apollonia (Fig. 41.1), who was immolated in third-century Alexandria only after undergoing torture (Latin "to twist") involving dental and facial fractures. The trend emphasizing the pain of dentistry is continued in the popular culture today, for instance, in movies such as *Little Shop of Horrors, Marathon Man,* and *The Dentist.*

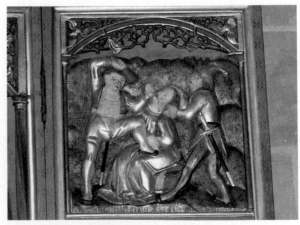

Figure 41.1 St. Apollonia.

EARLY RESISTANCE TO ANESTHESIA

Anesthesia controversy has not been limited to internecine conflicts within the health professions. Once anesthesia was quickly adopted by medicine, it was denounced not only by some surgeons but even from the pulpit. It is understandable that surgeons would decry the use of anesthesia, particularly when it was not readily available to all surgeons, some of whom witnessed their patients gravitating to competitors who could offer the administration of anesthesia. In 1859 a physician at a public meeting opined that "[p]ain is the wise provision of nature, and patients ought to suffer pain while their surgeon is operating; they are all the better for it, and recover better."[33]

In opining that anesthesia was somehow immoral and the diminution of pain an unnecessary truncation of "God's will,"[34] preachers often ignored Adam's "deep sleep" and instead quoted Genesis 3:16: "Unto the woman he said, I will greatly multiply thy sorrow and thy conception; in sorrow thou shalt bring forth children ..."[35] James Simpson, a physician of Edinburgh, Scotland, and an early European advocate of inhalational anesthesia, received a letter from a preacher stating that ether anesthesia was a "decoy of Satan" and that it would "rob God of the deep earnest cries which arise in time of trouble ..."[36] As late as 1929 H.W. Haggard opined that "the very suffering which a woman undergoes in labor is one of the strongest elements in the love she bears for her offspring!"[37] Circumspectly this author's spouse asked if there are any similar quotes regarding the use of anesthesia in childbirth from women.[38]

During these years, religion often entered into public controversies. Organized dentistry was not shy about speaking to, for instance, both sides of the debates about darwinian theories of the origin of species. In 1873 American Dental Convention President I.J. Wetherbee devoted his annual session opening address to the criticism of Darwin's work.[39] *Dental Cosmos* editor J.H. McQuillen had previously published: "Whenever a new and startling fact is brought to light in science, people first say, 'it is not true'; then, that 'it is contrary to religion' and lastly, 'that everybody knew it before.'"[40]

In spite of dental scriptures, such as Psalms 3:7: "... thou hast smitten all mine enemies upon the cheek bone; thou hast broken the teeth of the ungodly,"[41] it is problematic that the use of anesthesia in dentistry was harshly criticized by some in organized dentistry. At the very least, not everyone with a broken tooth is likely ungodly. The American Society of Dental Surgeons (ASDS) stated: "... in all minor operations in surgery, (anesthetic) administration is forbidden; and that (the) demand in the practice of dental surgery is small ..."[42] The ASDS, the first national dental organization, was only in existence from 1840 to 1856. However, the ultimate demise of the ASDS was primarily caused by the amalgam controversy. The ASDS first fought against the use of amalgam and sought to enforce its views primarily by legislative fiat rather than scientific study, but ultimately rescinded its amalgam policy, disgusting many members in addition to historical antagonists.[43]

In addition to criticism of anesthesia from the quarters mentioned, surgical procedures were considered as a last resort, after all else in medicine had failed. Reminiscent of the medical science fiction in television and motion picture versions of *Star Trek*, the Dr. McCoy–like working theory in the first decades of the nineteenth century was that the true triumph of medicine would result in the obsolescence of surgery.[44]

PROFESSIONAL LITERATURE, THE *DENTAL COSMOS*

The *Dental Cosmos*, published from 1839 to 1936, was the precursor of the *Journal of the American Dental Association* and the primary professional publication of dentistry for nearly 100 years, particularly as it was present before the many supplemental specialty and other journals in publication today.

Anesthesiology was a regularly discussed, if not debated, topic in the *Dental Cosmos*. For instance, volume 53, published in 1911, had several articles of interest. Dentist Charles Teter argued for the preeminence of nitrous oxid [sic] as the agent of choice for dental procedures, stating: "I am sure that in the judgment of the thoughtful, experienced man there can be no favorable comparison" (with nitrous oxide with any other agent). Of course, techniques of nitrous oxide administration differed somewhat from those recommended today. Dr. Teter advised that "this gas must be given *at least* 80 per cent pure" (oxygen could be added for longer cases). Dr. Teter also supplemented his nitrous oxide with the "intelligent use of preanesthesia narcotics, such as morphin [sic], atropin [sic], and scopolamin [sic]." Confidently "... the accomplished dentist can keep his patient under the anesthetic as long as may be necessary to complete his work ... I almost consider it an insult to my intelligence and skill when a patient or physician makes the remark, 'Doctor, I would like so many teeth extracted, but if you can't get them all, I wish you would remove certain ones,' etc. I think this is disgraceful and a stigma on the profession. If the dentist is not capable of anesthetizing his patient and keeping him anesthetized to the completion of this work, he should send his patients to one more competent."

Prophetically, Dr. Teter admonished that "[t]here is an increasing demand for general anesthetics in dental surgery" and "[t]he time is soon coming in this country when there will be laws passed to restrict the administration of anesthetics, and it behooves the dental profession to see that the subject is given a prominent place in the curriculum of our colleges ... Unless this is done, the dental profession will be greatly humiliated by having the right to administer anesthetics annulled."[45]

Volume 53 also held an article by Dr. Guido Fischer of the University of Greifswald, Germany, who argued for the use of local anesthesia in dentistry. Dr. Fischer proposed: "The efforts of modern medicine are more and more concentrated upon an endeavor to limit general anesthetics as much as possible, and to have local anesthetics take their place, by the endeavor to develop these to the highest perfection. I need only refer to the introduction of the anesthesia of the medulla by Bier

..." He noted that organic agents "… can produce fatty metamorphosis of the inner organism" and that with ether narcoses, one sees death once in every 3000 or 4000 cases.

Paradoxically, Dr. Fisher opined: "In dentistry local anesthetics should be the only kind used, and one should resort to general anesthetics only in exceptional cases." Although Dr. Fischer never defines "exceptional," he does admit that "obstinate or timid" patients may need to be narcotized with ether or ethyl bromid [sic]. Also: "There is one inconvenience which still attaches to cocain, viz, its often very toxic influence on the living tissues." Toxic effects besides death "often observed" from the "smallest dose" include rapid pulse, difficult respiration, nervous excitement, nausea, vomiting, convulsions, dyspnea, and collapse.[46]

Finally, one last reference from volume 54 is titled "Stimulants in Cases of Heart Failure Due to Cocaine." This clinical tip was offered: "In view of the almost universal use of cocaine and the fact that owing to idiosyncrasies even its use topically sometimes brings about alarming symptoms, we should be especially prepared to meet conditions of heart failure." The author's generally employed prescription for heart failure is a mixture of ether, camphor, and olive oil, but if that or "everything else fails," he recommended the 1911 version of advanced cardiac life support (ACLS) of "artificial respiration, about twenty beats to the minute."[47]

Predictably, patients, whether they studied the arguments in the professional literature or not, when given the option of having anesthesia or not availed themselves of anesthesia for even minor[48] surgical procedures when possible. Patients did so despite the condemnation of anesthesia by professional society spokespersons after controversial dental entrepreneurs, such as Gardner Q. Colton[49,50] and Edgar R.R. "Painless" Parker,[51] popularized techniques other than local anesthesia only. Parker believed that patients avoided dentistry because of pain, ignorance, procrastination, and lack of money, and of these, fear was the strongest deterrent.[52]

Working with a local druggist, Parker developed hydrocaine, an analgesic that contained cocaine. He aggressively advertised his services, reportedly removed 357 teeth in 1 day on a vaudeville stage, and coincidentally developed 30 West Coast dental offices that grossed more than $3 million annually in the early twentieth century. Not surprisingly the profession gradually began to embrace anesthesia not only as a morally acceptable form of therapy but also one that would attract patients.

VARIED ANESTHESIA PROVIDERS

At the turn of the century, anesthesia in the United States was administered by dentists, physician general practitioners, surgeons, interns, medical students, nurses, orderlies, and often whoever was handy. In October 1905 a small group of nine physician-anesthetists met and formed the Long Island Society of Anesthetists, the precursor of the American Society of Anesthetists (1936) and ultimately, in 1945, the American Society of Anesthesiologists (ASA).[53] Today, the ASA limits its membership to licensed physicians and osteopaths.

The International Anesthesia Research Society (IARS), the premier group of anesthesia providers in the world, was formed in 1922 to foster progress and research in all phases of anesthesia and is the publisher of *Anesthesia & Analgesia*. Based in Cleveland, Ohio, the 15,000-member IARS is nonpolitical and accepts as full members all doctorate-level anesthesia providers, including dentists.[54]

Anesthesiology became a specialty of medicine in 1938 and of veterinary medicine in 1975.[55] Anesthesiology has been a specialty in dentistry in Japan since 1973,[56] in Ontario, Canada, and is the nation's oldest nursing specialty, dating back to the Civil War.[57] Medical and veterinary anesthesiologists and dental anesthesiologists in Japan are, of course, recognized as the most knowledgeable experts in their fields of surgical pain control. Local anesthesia is also commonly used by specialists, and most surgical procedures can be performed with local anesthesia only.[58–60] However, not surprisingly, patients not only often believe that they need, but also demand, sedation or unconsciousness from these practitioners.

In the early twentieth century, dental anesthesia services continued to be provided by a cadre of dentists, but the profession as a whole began to gravitate to the administration of local anesthesia for almost all dental procedures.

AMERICAN SOCIETY OF EXODONTISTS

Anesthesiology in dentistry gradually became part and parcel of the practice of the American Society of Exodontists, founded in 1918 in Chicago. It can be argued that what set the exodontists apart from other generalists who also removed teeth was the provision of pain control modalities, other than local anesthesia, administered as single-operator anesthetists. Many members of the American Society of Exodontists became very proficient at removing a great number of teeth in the time it took a patient administered 100% nitrous oxide to regain normal skin color after intentionally induced cyanosis. A case can be made that the provision of general anesthesia by the exodontists is what directly led to the development of the specialty of oral and maxillofacial surgery.

ORAL AND MAXILLOFACIAL SURGERY ANESTHESIA PIONEERS

As an example, consider the pioneering efforts of University of Southern California Dental School graduate Adrian Orr Hubbell. In 1937 Dr. Hubbell started a postdoctoral course of training that would include 2 years of surgery and an additional year of general anesthesia. Hubbell experimented with sodium thiopental and found it to be a wonderfully appropriate drug for oral surgery that had advantages over techniques such as 100% nitrous oxide.[61] At this time, a prevailing attitude in medicine was shared that no general anesthetic should be given to any patient without an overnight admission, a concept Dr. Hubbell and other dentists knew was unnecessary. In addition, at times dentists found that they were unable to gain staff privileges at hospitals because of a prejudicial requirement for medical school training.

Many oral surgeons predictably began providing the anesthesia needed and demanded by their patients in their own offices. Beginning in the 1930s, oral surgeons developed not only the first outpatient surgical centers (a concept not embraced by medicine until the 1970s), but also became the experts at single-operator anesthetist procedures, a technique that is a recognized standard of care today.

AMERICAN DENTAL SOCIETY OF ANESTHESIOLOGY

In 1950 the ASA determined to not continue to allow dentists full membership. Dentists had been part of the ASA from its founding and one, Charles Teeter, had even been its president. In 1952 as the medical specialty in anesthesiology grew, dentistry began to believe that the role of anesthesiology in dentistry might be threatened. The American Dental Society of Anesthesiology (ADSA) was formed in 1953 after dentist anesthesiologist William B. Kinney suggested the development of a society for those interested in all forms of pain control for dental patients. The ADSA was composed of, in part, dentist anesthesiologists, although a significant majority of the membership consisted of oral and maxillofacial surgeons, who were providing most of the nonlocal limited anesthesiology in the profession.[62]

Interestingly the founding purposes of the ADSA were "to encourage the study of anesthesiology; to encourage specialization in anesthesiology; to foster higher standards of education in the dental schools as regards the teaching of anesthesiology; and to raise the standards of practice of anesthesiology by providing more and better training programs at the graduate level and to meet together for the purpose of exchanging information and reporting progress in the field of anesthesiology."[63] The first application for specialty status for anesthesiology in dentistry was submitted in the early 1950s.[64]

HISTORICAL DENTAL ANESTHESIOLOGY TRAINING

After the first formal anesthesiology training programs were established beginning in 1927, dentists routinely were enrolled as anesthesiology residents. For decades, there were dozens of AMA-approved anesthesiology residency programs that accepted dentists as residents. Dentist graduates of these programs were trained equivalently to their physician colleagues and provided anesthesiology services for the full scope of surgical procedures. Many of these dental anesthesiology graduates went on to become dental specialists, educators training dentists and/or physicians in anesthesiology, and chairmen of hospital and professional school departments of anesthesiology. Participating in a more limited fashion in these residency programs were hospital-based oral surgery residents who spent at least 3 months of their residencies training with anesthesia residents. During these years, it was the opinion of the ADA's Council on Judicial Procedures that dentists enrolled in AMA-approved anesthesiology training programs were "in a situation parallel to a residency program accredited by the ADA's Commission on Accreditation."[65]

AMERICAN SOCIETY OF DENTIST ANESTHESIOLOGISTS

In the late 1970s a group of singular dentists felt the need to form an organization that had not yet existed. This group would be composed of dentists who had 2 or more years of full-time training in anesthesiology. Their purpose in part was to establish advanced programs for continuing education in pain and anxiety control for dentistry and pursue the development of a specialty in anesthesiology in dentistry.[66] In February 1980 the American Society of Dentist Anesthesiologists (ASDA) was formed.[67]

Because some individual dentist anesthesiologists had allegedly opined that the operator/anesthetist model may be a less-than-optimal way to provide anesthesia services, contrary to the ASDA's officially published statement supporting that paradigm,[58] organized oral and maxillofacial surgery abruptly accomplished a complete turnaround of their previous support of a specialty of anesthesiology in dentistry.

AMERICAN ASSOCIATION OF ORAL AND MAXILLOFACIAL SURGEONS

Organized oral and maxillofacial surgery, the American Association of Oral and Maxillofacial Surgeons (AAOMS) in particular, now vigorously sought to protect and preserve the single-operator anesthetist concept. In spite of the fact that the ASDA published an official statement supporting "[t]he right of all ADA-approved specialties ... and other dental organizations to set practice guidelines and standards in anesthesia pertaining to their own areas of interest,"[68] AAOMS did not want to gamble with compromising their model of anesthesia service. The Southern California Society of Oral Surgery (SCSOMS) had been particularly progressive in documenting the safety of the oral surgical provision of anesthesia services since the days of Adrian Orr Hubbell and others.

A 1974 study was completed that reported results of a questionnaire sent to SCSOMS members that indicated the safety record for office-based oral surgical anesthesia compared very well with that of inpatient anesthesia services. According to the paper, office-based oral surgery anesthesia had one death per 432,000 anesthetics.[69] This was compared with 1 death per 10,000 inpatient tonsillectomies.[70] A follow-up study from the same author in 1978 reported a death rate of 1 for every 860,000 anesthetics administered from 1968 to 1977.[71] The 1974 SCSOMS statistics are nearly identical to historical and current data reported by the ASA in 2007 for hospitalized patients: "During the past 20 years, anesthesia-related deaths have dropped dramatically from one in 10,000 anesthetics delivered to one in 400,000 for outpatient procedures."[72]

Another finding of the study was that many oral surgeons were providing general anesthesia for well more than 1500 patients annually. Although the surgical duration of these anesthetics was often very brief, the sheer average number of cases provided by individual oral surgeons was significantly more than the vast majority of any other type of anesthesia provider.

As recently as 2000, AAOMS initiated another outpatient anesthesia study. The purpose of the study was to combat those who were perceived as planning to take away traditional oral and maxillofacial surgery office anesthesia. "Those" were specifically identified as dentist anesthesiologists. Such statements were disconcerting to dentist anesthesiologists, who again pointed out that the ASDA not only had members who practiced as single-operator anesthetists and that the ASDA had never called for a discontinuance of the single-operator anesthetist concept, but had in fact endorsed "the right of all ADA-approved specialties, the Academy of General Dentistry, and other dental organizations to set practice guidelines and standards in anesthesia pertaining to their own areas of interest."[73]

OFFICE ANESTHESIA EVALUATIONS

In the 1970s the SCSOMS was also the first anesthesia provider organization to initiate voluntary in-office anesthesia evaluations for its members. That program has evolved to the point that to be a component of AAOMS at the present time, all state oral and maxillofacial surgeon (OMS) societies must follow AAOMS national bylaws mandating in-office examinations for members every 5 years.

Similarly, state dental boards now also require the successful completion of an in-office examination before issuing a permit to dentists desiring to administer sedation or general anesthesia to their patients. Dentists who administer advanced pain control owe a debt of gratitude to the foresight of the SCSOMS, whose in-office examination concept kept the evaluation of dental anesthesia legally and appropriately within the profession.

MEDICAL ANESTHESIA'S STATUS IN OFFICE-BASED ANESTHESIOLOGY

As dentist anesthesia providers led the professions in the development of outpatient anesthesia techniques, which were provided in private oral and maxillofacial surgery offices initially, so dentists are decades ahead of other professions in establishing office-based anesthesia practices. Although the ASA acknowledges that office-based anesthesiology is a rapidly emerging specialty within the field of anesthesiology, current medical anesthesia residents are receiving minimal, if any, exposure to office-based anesthesia during their training.[74]

In addition, whereas all states have dentist-generated statutes in place to regulate the safe practice of office-based anesthesia, organized medicine is just entering the formative stages of the process. As the 2007 ASA *Office-Based Anesthesia and Surgery* brochure states:

> There is one fundamental and very important difference between office-based anesthesia and receiving anesthesia in a hospital or surgical center: The strict, well-defined (Joint Commission) standards and regulations that help keep surgery and anesthesia very safe in hospitals and surgical centers do not uniformly apply to physicians' offices in the United States. Currently, only a few states and the District of Columbia require the same standards and regulations in doctors' offices as they do in hospitals and surgical centers.[75]

Despite the admitted lack of office-based training and nascent status of regulation in office environments, medical anesthesiologists have also recently recognized the potential market in providing services to dentists.[76] The dental literature has published articles expounding the benefits of mobile office anesthesia provided by physicians that not only does not mention dentist anesthesiologists, but also suggests that such historically founded services are innovative.[77]

A growing concern among dentist anesthesiologists is that their professional innovations and services will be subsumed or even eliminated by the rapidly growing cadre of medical mobile anesthesia providers. In addition, it would be surprising if the current cooperation between oral and maxillofacial surgery and anesthesiology was continued as far as anesthesiology's support for the single-operator anesthetist model (as dental anesthesiologists have officially continuously supported)[58] once medical anesthesiologists realize that market's potential availability. There is no question that an alleged advantage medical anesthesiologists will trumpet is the additional safety available from a dedicated anesthesia provider rather than a single-operator anesthetist who provides both anesthesia and surgical services. This is despite the fact that no studies have ever shown such to be true and have shown that single-operator anesthetist office-based oral and maxillofacial procedures are historically safer than comparable hospital-based procedures.[61-64]

Certainly, there would not appear to be any comparative increase in risk between a single-operator anesthetist performing dental surgery versus an anesthesiologist placing additional intravenous, arterial, or central lines; placing urinary catheters; or performing any number of additional ancillary procedures, often far more distant corporally from the airway than the oral cavity, contemporaneously with the anesthesia.

EXTRAPROFESSIONAL CRITICISM OF DENTAL ANESTHESIOLOGY

Nondental groups have historically formally expressed disfavor with the OMS anesthesia and other dental anesthesia models. The Accreditation Council for Graduate Medical Education (ACGME) for Anesthesiology training, consisting of ASA members, in 1993 forwarded a letter to the Council on Dental Education stating that "the anesthesia community in general, will be quite intolerant of what you call 'deep sedation' and general anesthesia being administered by the same individual who is performing the dental work. In the interest of patient safety, this situation must be forbidden... . I hope this will serve to clarify our position ..."[78]

Astonishingly, on another front, in 1993, Certified Registered Nurse Anesthetists (CRNAs) presented a statement to the Illinois State Anesthesia Committee critical of dentists administering nitrous oxide-oxygen analgesia and questioned the competence of dentists to use this anesthetic.[79]

AAOMS RESPONSES

AAOMS has historically responded effectively to challenges to its single-operator anesthetist model, no matter the origination of the challenges. Dentistry is indebted to the AAOMS' defense of dental anesthesia from outside the profession.

However, AAOMS has also aggressively responded to perceived threats from within dentistry. For instance, in 1989 the ADSA had been in contact with ASA President James Arens and found that rumors that the ASA was opposed to specialty status for dental anesthesiology were false. However, the ADSA also advised the ASDA that "oral surgeons primarily seem to be concerned that anesthesia specialists will be pitted against them in legal matters concerning anesthesia and that they will come up short most of the time."[80] ASDA's president wrote back to the ADSA that the concern made no sense and that ASDA's posture was one of strengthening, rather than weakening, relationships between dental anesthesia provider groups.

With regard to such concerns of a potential specialty in anesthesiology, AAOMS leadership, still fearing an attack on the single-operator anesthetist model from dentists, also orchestrated the truncation of anesthesiology residency training opportunities for dentists so that instead of scores of programs accepting dentists for anesthesia training, only a handful remained.

During the ongoing efforts to silence the dentist anesthesiologists, AAOMS nearly had its own anesthesia training compromised. The ASA issued a policy statement opining: "anesthesia care is the practice of medicine."[81] Such statements had been made previously, beginning at least in 1912 and repeated in the 1920s during the ASA-supported litigation against nurse anesthetists. Courts routinely found that anesthesia care is the practice of medicine, but is also the practice of dentistry, nursing, and even veterinary medicine. This time, intense negotiations between AAOMS, the ADA, the AMA, and the ASA produced a nonlitigated statement from the ASA that "[t]he ASA recognizes the right of qualified dentists as defined by the American Dental Association to administer conscious sedation, deep sedation, and general anesthesia to patients having dental procedures only."[82] Although dentists were now recognized as able to provide anesthesia for dental procedures, it became more difficult politically for dentist anesthesiologists to provide care for nondental surgical procedures.

POSWILLO REPORT AND ALASKA

Dentistry's potentially tenuous grasp on the provision of anesthesia services in the face of political onslaught was demonstrated in 1990 with the release of the Poswillo report from Great Britain.[83] In part the report recommended graduate education for dentists in anesthesiology. However, without a specialty in anesthesiology in dentistry in Great Britain, there were no advanced training opportunities for dentists. As a result of the Poswillo report, dentists in Great Britain now have lost the ability to administer general anesthesia.

Whereas the Poswillo report and its adverse sequelae were frightening revelations to dental anesthesia providers in most of the United States, the information was all old news to dentists in Alaska, who had lost their privilege as single-operator anesthetists in the 1970s.[84]

1990S DENTAL ANESTHESIOLOGY SPECIALTY APPLICATIONS

Founding goals of the ADSA, such as more graduate training programs and specialty status for anesthesiology in dentistry, were abandoned secondary to the influence of its oral and maxillofacial surgery members as oral and maxillofacial surgery sought to maintain its single-operator anesthetist niche. The dentist anesthesiologists of the ASDA now were the champions of the goal of specialization. Following the early application championed by the ADSA in the 1950s, applications for specialty status were submitted via the ASDA to the ADA and successfully passed on through the various committees until they were forwarded with strong recommendations for passage to the ADA House of Delegates (HOD) in 1994, 1997, and 1999. Single-digit losses in the house prevented dentistry from having a specialty in anesthesiology. In 1999 five of the six mandatory requirements for specialty recognition were met, but, interestingly, the house did not believe that there was a sufficient "need or demand" for recognized anesthesiology-mediated advanced pain control services in dentistry.

The last anesthesiology specialty application submitted to the ADA occurred in 2012. This application once again handily passed through the comprehensive ADA process until reaching the HOD, when it was again defeated after intense political maneuvering. The ASDA has now determined to no longer pursue specialty recognition through the ADA but instead pursue other options. Negotiation and litigation have resulted in several states now acknowledging other pathways to specialization separate and distinct from the ADA. State recognition of specialty status is not a new concept. Oral and maxillofacial surgery was recognized as a specialty before ADA recognition in states such as Michigan, Oklahoma, Illinois, and Tennessee.[i]

Alternatively, many medical specialties today are overseen by the American Board of Medical Specialties.

---

[i]MacIntosh RB, Kelly JP: *The American Board of Oral and Maxillofacial Surgery, a history,* ed 2, Chicago, 2010, ABOMS.

After the 2012 ADA HOD vote, the American Board of Dental Specialties (ABDS) was incorporated in order to recognize dental specialties according to traditional criteria, not as a political issue. Finally, in 2013 the federal government issued a singular dentist anesthesiologist taxonomy number (1223D0004X). Because of the ADA HOD's historical reluctance to recognize new specialty areas, dentists now have the option of pursuing specialty recognition via states, the ABDS, and the federal government in addition to the ADA.

NEED AND DEMAND

That the ADA's HOD found no need or demand for enhanced anesthesia services is fascinating, even considering the intense political legerdemain involved in defeating the specialty application. Not surprisingly the Centers for Disease Control and Prevention (CDC) has reported that 12% of the population had not seen a dentist in more than 5 years, if ever, and only 46% availed themselves of a dental appointment within the preceding 6 months.[85] That the popular public perception of dentists throughout history nearly always includes significant concepts of pain and fear[86] was confirmed even for our era by a U.S. Surgeon General's report in 2000.[87]

ORAL SEDATION ENTREPRENEURIAL GROUPS

The fallacy of an insufficient need or demand for advanced pain control services in dentistry was bluntly demonstrated beginning in 2000 with the founding of the Dental Organization for Conscious Sedation (DOCS), an entrepreneurial enterprise whose founder also recognized that indeed millions of potential dental patients were not availing themselves of dental treatment secondary to the fact that local anesthesia alone was not, in many patients' minds, adequate for their treatment. The DOCS and other similar regimens are relatively straightforward and essentially involve the administration of an oral sedative before the administration of local anesthesia. Despite the fact that the DOCS protocol has been shown to be safe, as administered well more than a million times by more than 22,500 DOCS-trained dentists, such protocols have been subject to logically inexplicable criticism, as seen surrounding other dental anesthesia entrepreneurs, such as Edgar Randolph Rudolph "Painless" Parker, one of the first to routinely offer local anesthesia to patients.

FROM THE SOCIETIES, STATES, CONGRESS, AND THE U.S. SUPREME COURT

The legal history of anesthesiology in dentistry has been controversial since Horace Wells first demonstrated for the world his safely reproducible technique using nitrous oxide. Debates related to Wells reached the U.S. Congress.[88] Organized dentistry has always been sensitive to issues regarding advertising, although it has not always been circumspect in differentiating between charlatans and effective entrepreneurs, such as Painless Parker. Dr. Harry Semler challenged dental advertising restrictions in Oregon and ultimately lost an appeal against the Oregon State Board of Dental Examiners, the state dental society, and the ADA, heard by the U.S. Supreme Court in 1935. Two interesting footnotes resulted from the Semler case. First, the profession also subsequently successfully opposed an effort to amend the Oregon constitution to allow any person to advertise, providing the advertisement was true.[89] Second the Semler case resulted in U.S. Supreme Court Chief Justice Charles Evans Hughes' famous definition of professional ethics: "what is generally called the 'ethics' of the profession is but the consensus of expert opinion as to the necessity of such standards."[90]

Modern dental anesthesiology is equally as legally impressive. For instance, dentists have had to fight many battles within state legislatures to provide anesthesia and other services,[91] which they are trained to do. Dentist anesthesiologist Gaither Everett was forced to litigate and appeal his right to practice as a dentist anesthesiologist in the state of Washington to the Washington Supreme Court. The court found Dr. Everett's issue moot secondary to the Washington legislature contemporaneously confirming the right of properly trained dentists to administer anesthesia for any surgical procedure.[92] Dr. Russell Paravecchio's dental anesthesia cause was appealed to the doors of the U.S. Supreme Court, a case in which the author acted as amicus curiae[93] (Fig. 41.2). The AAOMS continues to serve dentistry well by aggressively monitoring and reacting to nondental threats to dental anesthesiology that predictably arise. In contrast to the 1993 letter previously mentioned, in 2004 the ASA acknowledged to AAOMS that "… members of AAOMS have a long history of safely using general anesthesia in the care of their patients."[94]

COMPETING DENTAL FACTIONS

The major factions with vested interests in advanced pain control in dentistry today, excluding those who limit themselves to nitrous oxide-oxygen, include dentist anesthesiologists, dentists who provide conscious (minimal or moderate) sedation, DOCS type of oral sedation entrepreneurs, and OMSs.

Those who opine that single-operator anesthetist sedation and general anesthesia models for anesthesia delivery are outdated or less than optimal are ignoring the enviable safety record that OMSs have built over decades since that specialty's anesthesia pioneers first developed the concept of single-operator anesthetist *and* outpatient surgery in the 1930s. Similar to controversies regarding dental amalgam, which would likely never be accepted with the techniques and materials that are available in the twenty-first century, the historical oral and maxillofacial model of anesthesia delivery remains unsurpassed as far as cost effectiveness and relative safety for patients who undergo similar procedures within the hospital environment.

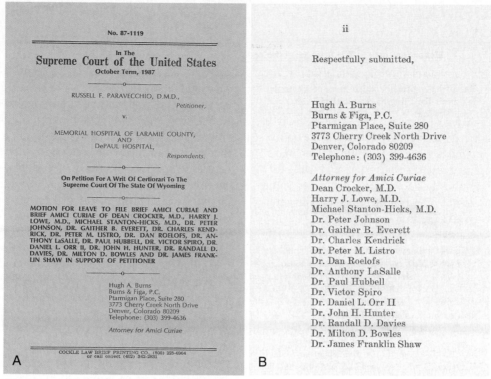

Figure 41.2 A, Petition for a writ of certiorari, The Supreme Court of the United States, Russell F. Paravecchio, DMD, Petitioner. **B,** Amicae for Dr. Paravecchio.

There also exists a group of dentists who provide intravenous sedation during which the practitioners assiduously avoid doses of drugs that would render patients not only unconscious or apneic, but simply nonresponsive to verbal communication or without adequate spontaneous ventilation. This group is composed primarily of generalists and non–oral and maxillofacial surgery specialists who avail themselves of intravenous sedation courses, such as those that have been offered by Stanley Malamed, this text's primary author, during his tenure at the University of Southern California School of Dentistry. Because of a changing emphasis in the training of OMSs, many of this specialty's newer graduates have not received the extensive single-operator anesthetist general anesthesia training of their predecessors and thus limit themselves to intravenous sedation only. Dentists who provide intravenous sedation are the least controversial of the factions with an interest in advanced pain control in dentistry.

Conversely, OMSs who opine that their enviable single-operator anesthetist niche constitutes the apex of anesthesia expertise within dentistry and others who state there is no need or demand for more esoteric anesthesia techniques are ingenuous at best.

Three or 4 months of incidental anesthesia training within a surgical specialty does not equate with 2 or more years of a dedicated residency in anesthesiology. Despite oral and maxillofacial surgery's unsurpassed single-operator anesthetist expertise, outpatient surgery primacy, and outstanding safety record, there is no question that dentist anesthesiologists are overall the most well-trained anesthesia providers of all the factions in dentistry.

Dentistry may owe a significant debt of gratitude to the DOCS type of entrepreneurs. Within a few short years of its organization, more dentists have been trained annually in oral sedation protocols than graduate in all dental anesthesiology, oral and maxillofacial surgery, and intravenous sedation training programs combined. DOCS has effectively demonstrated that dentistry's underserved patient base is huge, but amenable to regular treatment if its simple *need and demand* for services beyond local anesthesia or advanced pain control modalities provided by the present inadequate number of dental anesthesia providers is met, the ADA HOD's denial of need and demand notwithstanding.

Finally, one additional group needs to be mentioned: future dental practitioners. Dental students are like all students in that they are students for a reason (i.e., they do not have the knowledge, expertise, technical skills, political savvy, or historical perspective to effectively proffer their craft until they are graduates). Further, it takes time to develop into efficient dental professionals after graduation. However, despite their student and/or recent graduate status, even such individuals readily recognize that their education is sadly lacking in pain control modalities needed and demanded by their future patients. This is evidenced by the fact that those contemporary recent graduates surveyed would support an increase in tuition and fees to gain more, or even any, advanced pain control knowledge while in school.[95]

FUTURE OF DENTAL ANESTHESIOLOGY

Dentists introduced safe, effective, and reproducible anesthesia to the world. Dentists administer more local anesthetics and general anesthetics per trained provider than any other health profession. Dentists perfected outpatient general anesthesia techniques decades before their medical colleagues even considered outpatient general anesthesia a reasonable option. Dentist anesthesia providers have at least equivalent, if not better, morbidity and mortality statistics compared with other professions providing anesthesia services. Throughout the United States, state dental boards have fully implemented statutes designed to ensure the qualified provision of dental anesthesia, whereas such statutes are currently in place in only a few states for medicine. Yet when one looks at the relatively minimal patient-perceived presence of dentistry in the anesthesia world, it is apparent that dentistry has not handled its gift of pain control to the world with the fiduciary care anesthesiology should have been afforded.

In January 2007, the Council on Dental Accreditation (CODA) published a standards document entitled "Advanced Dental Education Programs in Dental Anesthesiology." As of the date of that publication, standards now exist for dental anesthesia residencies to be accredited. Before this publication, no such accreditation was possible for the many decades that dentists were trained in general anesthesia. These standards are quite stringent. For instance, each resident must do a minimum of 500 deep sedations or general anesthetics, 200 of which must be intubated general anesthetics, and at least 50 must be nasotracheal intubations, and 20 cases must incorporate advanced airway techniques, such as fiber-optic intubation, laryngeal mask airway, etc. A minimum of 100 cases must be for children 6 years old or younger, and 50 cases must be for special-needs patients.[96] In 2008 most of the existing dental anesthesiology programs were successfully accredited, and two new dental anesthesiology residency programs were established, with several more planned.

There are three major benefits to the profession that will be derived from the accreditation of dentist anesthesiologist residency programs[97]:

1. Because there is a huge increased need and demand for dentists to provide advanced sedation and anesthesia services for other dentists, accreditation should provide increased funding opportunities to support more residents and residency programs to meet that need and demand.
2. Accreditation by dentistry helps cement anesthesia at its highest level as within the scope of dental education and within the scope of the clinical practice of dentists.
3. Finally, accreditation keeps the highest level of anesthesia education within the control of dentistry and maintains dentistry's ability to control the quality of anesthesia training that dentist anesthesiologists receive to protect the safety of the public that we serve. State dental boards now have an appropriate measuring stick to judge the adequacy of anesthesia training for dentist anesthesiologists. They should now recognize that future dentist anesthesiologists must be graduates of CODA-accredited training programs to be eligible for anesthesia permits (with, of course, traditional grandfathering for those who completed training before accreditation).

But for the historical and current internecine battles waged within dentistry over dental anesthesiology, the profession would have an ADA recognized specialty in the art, similar to that present in medicine, veterinary medicine, nursing, and dentistry in other parts of the world, to the benefit of the entire profession and its patients. All the current dental models of anesthesia delivery mentioned earlier have been shown to be safe and effective. Mutual respect and collegial cooperation between dental groups, currently struggling against economically competing dental colleagues to maintain their anesthesia status quo from perceived threats within the profession, would lead to synergistic and exponential growth of anesthesiology in dentistry. A specialty would also be the most effective buffer against compromising attacks from nondental anesthesia providers. If dentistry continues its noncooperative and self-destructive conduct, it is the author's opinion that the ability to continue safely administering advanced pain control modalities within the exact profession that gave safely reproducible anesthesia to the world may be severely truncated. Compromise will likely occur from timely opportunistic pressure exerted by significantly more numerous anesthesia provider groups outside of dentistry (Table 41.1) that covet dentistry's patient base, including dental patients currently ignored by the profession who subjectively need and demand advanced pain control for dental procedures.

Of course, legal colleagues will be more than willing to continue to adjudicate the controversies.

Table 41.1	U.S. Organizational Memberships 2007
Dental Organizations	
Dentist Anesthesiologists	250
Oral Sedation Entrepreneurs	>25,000
AAOMS	7,000
ADSA	1,500*
Nursing Organizations	
AANA (CRNAs)	35,000
Medical Organizations	
ASA	35,000

*Many ADSA members have been charted elsewhere as dentist anesthesiologists, oral sedationists, or oral and maxillofacial surgeons (i.e., approximately 60% of the members of the ADSA are oral and maxillofacial surgeons, already accounted for in AAOMS). There are likely approximately 1500 members of the ADSA actively providing advanced anesthesia services separate and distinct from those accounted for in other groups.

REFERENCES

1. BMJ website, January 19, 2007. Available at www.bmj.com.
2. Halstead WS: Available at www.quotegarden.com/medical.html.
3. Halstead WS: Water as a local anesthetic. *NY Med J* 42:327, 1885.
4. Halstead WS: Practical comments on the use and abuse of cocaine; suggested by its invariably successful employment in more than a thousand minor surgical operations. *NY Med J* 42:294, 1885.
5. Fink RB: *Neural blockade in clinical anesthesia and management of pain*, ed 2, Philadelphia, 1988, Lippincott.
6. Malamed SF: *Handbook of local anesthesia*, ed 5, St Louis, 2004, Elsevier.
7. Wood A: New method of treating neuralgia by the direct application opiates to the painful points. *Edinburgh Med Surg J* 82:265, 1855.
8. Koller C: On the use of cocaine for producing anaesthesia on the eye. *Lancet* 2:990, 1884.
9. Wells H: *A history of the discovery of the application of nitrous oxide gas, ether, and other vapors, to surgical operations*, Hartford, CT, 1847, J Gaylord Wells.
10. Fenster JM: *Ether day*, New York, 2001, Harper Collins.
11. Look out for a villain! *Rochester Daily Democrat*, February 11, 1841.
12. Beware a villain, *St Louis Daily Evening Gazette,* September 30, 1840.
13. Ether day, *St Louis Daily Evening Gazette*, 10, 81-94.
14. American College of Legal Medicine. *Leg Med Perspect* 17:2, 3–7, 2008.
15. Fenster JM: *Ether day*, New York, 2001, p 219.
16. Keys TE: *The history of surgical anesthesia*, 1945, Dover Publications.
17. Holy Bible, King James Version, Genesis 2:21.
18. *Boston Med Surg J* 35:397, 1847.
19. *Boston Med Surg J* 36:494–497, 1847.
20. Transactions of the American Medical Association, 1:178, 1848.
21. Proceedings of the Sixty-Seventh Annual Convention of the Conn Medical Society, 10, Hartford, CT, 1859.
22. American Dental Association: Transactions of the fourth annual meeting, Niagara Falls, NY, 1864.
23. American Dental Association: Transactions of the eleventh annual meeting, White Sulphur Springs, NY, 1872.
24. American Medical Association: Transactions of the twenty-first annual meeting, Washington, DC, 1870.
25. *JAMA* 126:779, 1037, 1944.
26. *J Am Dent Assoc* 31:1659–1665, 1944.
27. Vandam LD: The history of anesthesiology, nitrous oxide, 1981, American Society of Anesthesiology Wood Library-Museum of Anesthesiology reprint series.
28. Paris Medical Society, 1848.
29. American Dental Association: Transactions of the fourth annual meeting, Niagara Falls, NY, 1864, p. 17.
30. American Dental Association: Transactions of the eleventh annual meeting, White Sulphur Springs, NY, 1872, p. 18.
31. American Medical Association: Transactions of the twenty-first annual meeting, Washington, DC, 1870, p. 19.
32. Velpeau AALM: *Nouveaux elements de medicine operatoire*, ed 2, Paris, 1839, JB Bailliere.
33. *An appeal to patrons of science*, Boston, 1857.
34. Fenster JM: *Ether day*, New York, 2001, Harper Collins, p 23.
35. Holy Bible, King James version, Genesis 3:16.
36. Welch WH: *A consideration of the introduction of surgical anaesthesia*, Boston, 1908, Barta Press.
37. Haggard HW: *Devils, drugs, and doctors*, New York, 1929, Harper & Brothers.
38. Orr AM: personal communication to the author, 2007.
39. American dental convention. *Dent Cosmos* XV:530, 1873.
40. McQuillen JH: Proceedings of the Odontographic Society of Pennsylvania. *Dent Cosmos* IX:201n, 1867.
41. Holy Bible, King James version, Psalms 3:7.
42. American Society of Dental Surgeons: Resolutions of the eighth annual meeting. *Am J Dent Sci* 9:1, 1848.
43. McCluggage RW: *A history of the American Dental Association, 1859-1959*, Chicago, IL, 1959, Lakeside Press, RR Donnelley & Sons.
44. Fenster JM: *Ether day*, New York, 2001, Harper Collins, p 32.
45. Teter CK: Nitrous oxid and oxygen pre-eminently the anesthetic of choice in dentistry. *Dent Cosmos* 53:37–43, 1911.
46. Fischer G: Local anesthesia in dentistry. *Dent Cosmos* 53:168–177, 1911.
47. Webster GO: Stimulants in cases of heart failure due to cocaine, dental review. *Dent Cosmos* 53:380, 1911.
48. Walton B: *Sports Illustrated* 1980.
49. Colton GQ: *Anesthesia—who made and developed this great discovery?*, New York, 1886, Sherwood & Co.
50. Malamed SF: *Sedation: a guide to patient management*, ed 4, St Louis, 2003, CV Mosby.
51. Christen AG, Pronych PM: *Painless Parker: a dental renegade's fight to make advertising "ethical,"*, Canada, 1998, Dental Tobacco Cessation Consultants.
52. Giangredo E: *The life and times of Painless Parker*, Mesquite, NV, 2007, Pierre Fauchard Academy Museum.
53. American Society of Anesthesiologists: The diamond jubilee, 1980.
54. www.iars.org.
55. www.acva.org.
56. Matsuura H: Modern history of dental anesthesia in Japan. *Anesth Prog* 40(4):109–113, 1993.
57. www.aana.com.
58. Covino BG, et al: *Handbook of spinal anaesthesia and analgesia*, Philadelphia, 1994, WB Saunders.
59. Katz J: *Atlas of regional anesthesia*, Norwalk, CT, 1985, Appleton-Century, Crofts.
60. Cousins MJ, Bridenbaugh PO: *Neural blockade in clinical anesthesia and management of pain*, ed 2, Philadelphia, 1988, Lippincott.
61. Hubbell AO, Adams RC: Intravenous anesthesia for dental surgery with sodium ethyl (1-methylbutyl) thiobarbituric acid. *J Am Dent Assoc* 27:1186, 1940.
62. American Association of Oral and Maxillofacial Surgeons: The building of a specialty: oral and maxillofacial surgery in the United States 1918-1998. *J Oral Max Surg suppl* 56(7,3):22–23, 1998.
63. American Dental Society of Anesthesiology: Constitution, 1959.
64. Allen DL: The future of dental education. *Anesth Prog* 39:1–3, 1992.
65. Dunn WE, ADA Secretary, Council on Judicial Procedures, Constitution and Bylaws: letter, February 19, 1976.
66. American Society of Dentist Anesthesiologists: The American Society of Dentist Anesthesiologists: who we are and what we avow, 2007. Available at www.asdahq.org/about.html.
67. Reed KL: A brief history of anesthesiology in dentistry. *Texas Dent Assn J* 119(3):219–225, 2002.

68. Reed KL: p 51.
69. Lytle JJ: Anesthesia morbidity and mortality survey of the Southern California Society of Oral Surgeons. *Oral Surg* 32(10):739–744, 1974.
70. Alexander DW, Graff TD, Kelley E: Factors in tonsillectomy mortality. *Arch Otolaryngol* 82:409, 1965.
71. Lytle JJ, Yoon C: 1978 anesthesia morbidity and mortality survey: Southern California Society of Oral and Maxillofacial Surgeons. *J Oral Surg* 38(11):814–819, 1978.
72. www.asahq.org/patientEducation/officebased.htm.
73. www.asahq.org/patientEducation/officebased.htm.
74. Hausman LM, Levine AI, Rosenblatt MA: A survey evaluating the training of anesthesiology residents in office based anesthesia. *J Clin Anesth* 18:499–503, 2006.
75. Hausman LM, Levine AI, Rosenblatt MA, p 58.
76. Yee TC: I am the baby-sitter; you are the baby, 2007, promotional dental office anesthesia pamphlet.
77. Hoffman J: Growth plan, mobile anesthesiologists expands well beyond its base areas. *Dent Tribune* 2:28, 2007.
78. Prevoznik S: Findings Association of Anesthesia program directors, November 1993.
79. CRNA targets dentists. *ASDA Newsletter* 13(2):5, 1993.
80. ADSA requests position paper. *ASDA Newsletter* 9:2, 1989.
81. American Society of Anesthesiologists: Transactions of the House of Delegates, 1982.
82. American Society of Anesthesiologists: Board of directors, 1987.
83. Dental Advisory Council: *General anaesthesia, sedation, and resuscitation in dentistry, report of an expert working party*, London, 1990.
84. Alaska 12 AAC 28.020: Operative procedure. A dentist administering a general anesthetic may not perform any operative procedures for the duration of the anesthesia.
85. Lethbridge-Cejku M, Vickerie J: Summary health statistics for U.S. adults: national health interview survey, 2003. *Vital Health Stat* 10(225):104, 2005.
86. Thibodeau E, Mentatsi L: Who stole Nemo? *J Am Dent Assoc* 138(5):656–660, 2007.
87. National Institute of Dental and Craniofacial Research: *Oral health in America: a report of the surgeon general*, Rockville, MD, 2000, U.S. Department of Health and Human Services, U.S. Public Health Service.
88. National Institute of Dental and Craniofacial Research.
89. National Institute of Dental and Craniofacial Research.
90. Rosenthal LA, et al: Semler v. Oregon State Board of Dental Examiners, 294 US 608, 1935.
91. American Association of Oral and Maxillofacial Surgeons: Governor Schwarzenegger approves bill giving California citizens greater access to reconstructive and elective cosmetic surgical care of the head and neck, 2006, press release.
92. The Supreme Court for the State of Washington: Everett and Everett v. The State of Washington, Case #49163-1, 1982.
93. The Supreme Court of the United States: No 87-1119, Paravecchio v. Memorial Hospital of Laramie County and DePaul Hospital, on petition for a writ of certiorari to the Supreme Court of the state of Wyoming, 1987.
94. American Society of Anesthesiologists: Propofol letter to AAOMS, 2004.
95. Boyles SG, Lemak AL, Close JM: General dentists' evaluation of anesthesia sedation education in U.S. dental schools. *J Dent Educ* 70(12):1289–1293, 2006.
96. Reed KL: The history and current status of dental anesthesiology in dentistry. *J Nev Dent Assoc* 11(1):15–18, 2009.
97. Weaver JM: Accreditation of dentist anesthesia residencies is approved by CODA. *Anesth Prog* 54(2):43–44, 2007.

Index